NEW HANDBOOK of
AUDITORY EVOKED
RESPONSES

JAMES W. HALL III

University of Florida

Boston | New York | San Francisco
Mexico City | Montreal | Toronto | London | Madrid | Munich | Paris
Hong Kong | Singapore | Tokyo | Cape Town | Sydney

Executive Editor and Publisher: *Stephen D. Dragin*
Editorial Assistant: *Katie Heimsoth*
Production Managing Editor: *Joe Sweeney*
Editorial–Production Service: *Walsh & Associates, Inc.*
Composition and Prepress Buyer: *Linda Cox*
Manufacturing Buyer: *Linda Morris*
Cover Administrator: *Kristina Mose-Libon*
Electronic Composition: *Omegatype Typography, Inc.*

For related titles and support materials, visit our online catalog at www.ablongman.com

Library of Congress Cataloging-in-Publication Data

Hall, James W. (James Wilbur), 1948–
New handbook of auditory evoked responses / James W. Hall, III.
p.   cm.
Includes bibliographical references (p.).
ISBN 0-205-36104-8
1. Auditory evoked response.   2. Audiometry, Evoked response.   I. Title.

RF294.5.E87H35   2006
617.8'075—dc22

2006051541

Printed in the United States of America

5 6 7 8 9 10   V0CR   13 12

With love and appreciation

to my wife,

Missy

and to my children,

Jason C. Hall, M.S.

Cpl. Austin S. Hall, 3/6 2nd Div. U.S.M.C.

Victoria G. Hall

CONTENTS

10 ABR: Adult Diseases and Disorders and Clinical Applications   366

14 Mismatch Negativity (MMN) Response 548

A NEW WORLD

When the original *Handbook of Auditory Evoked Responses* was published in 1992, there was no easy way to access the literature. Audiologists and other professionals with membership in professional organizations could, of course, sample some literature published in journals received as a benefit of their membership. Professionals with university affiliations also had the resources of health science center, hospital, and department libraries. However, the typical practitioner did not have ready access to a wide variety of scientific journals and, therefore, couldn't thoroughly review the literature, or easily research a specific topic. Within the past decade, development of the World Wide Web has altered remarkably the world we live and work in. Virtually all that is known about a topic is now as close as the computer keyboard. Academics and practitioners alike can at any time conduct a personally directed review of the literature. An efficient starting point is the National Library of Medicine (NLM) in the National Institutes of Health (NIH) in Bethesda, Maryland. The titles of most published papers, and a formal abstract, can now be found by visiting the website www.nlm.nih.gov and entering keywords (for subjects or authors) to research a specific topic.

The original *Handbook of Auditory Evoked Responses* was a comprehensive review of the topic. The 871-page tome included hundreds of figures and tables and well over a thousand references. The scope of the book encompassed five major types of auditory evoked responses (AERs): electrocochleography (ECochG), the auditory brainstem response (ABR), the auditory middle latency response (AMLR), the auditory late response (ALR), and the auditory P300 response. The book included, in addition to detailed discussions of these responses, an overview of two nonauditory evoked responses: electrical AERs and electroneuronography (ENoG). Entire chapters were devoted to specific clinical applications of certain AERs, such as newborn hearing screening with the ABR. One chapter presented an overview of basic audiologic principles and procedures for the non-audiologist reader. Another lengthy chapter summarized various pathologies, especially neuropathologies that might be encountered by clinicians applying AERs in real-world settings. And, the final two chapters were filled with presentations of case reports illustrating AER findings for pediatric and adult patients with diverse disorders. The original *Handbook* was clinically focused, with a distinct emphasis on responses and clinical applications of interest to audiologists. Over a thousand additional articles published since 1992 have described new techniques and strategies for measurement and clinical application of AERs or refinements of existing techniques. Nonetheless, since the reader of the *New Handbook of Auditory Evoked Responses* has direct access via the Internet to most of the literature on auditory evoked responses, fewer references are cited in the book. The *New Handbook of Auditory Evoked Responses,* however, maintains a clear clinical focus with an emphasis on information required by practicing audiologists and others involved in measurement and application of AERs. Indeed, the *Handbook* has been reorganized to better meet the demands of clinicians.

ORGANIZATION OF THE *NEW HANDBOOK OF AUDITORY EVOKED RESPONSES*

The first part of the book covers general information on the topic of auditory evoked responses, including general measurement principles and a review of anatomic and physiologic underpinnings. Most students and also clinicians without formal education on auditory evoked responses should first read Part I of the Book. Subsequent chapters are devoted to separate reviews of major auditory evoked responses that include information important for measurement and analysis, and then clinical applications. The presentation of information on auditory evoked responses is organized anatomically, beginning with chapters on auditory responses arising from the cochlea and progressing to those arising from the cortex.

The *New Handbook of Auditory Evoked Responses* reflects new trends and developments in clinical neurophysiology and new applications of auditory evoked response in patient populations. To cite three examples of such changes, the discussion of electrocochleography (ECochG) includes a section on "auditory neuropathy." A chapter is devoted to techniques used for frequency-specific estimation of auditory sensitivity in infants and young children—that is, the tone-burst-elicited auditory brainstem response (ABR) and the auditory steady-state response (ASSR), and the review of nonauditory evoked responses includes a review of the vestibular evoked myogenic potential (VEMP).

The relative attention given to each auditory evoked response in the *New Handbook of Auditory Evoked Responses* is intended to correspond to the likelihood of application of that response by audiologists in various clinical settings. This guideline for preparation of the book explains the obvious emphasis on the earlier latency auditory evoked responses—ECochG and ABR—and the more modest coverage of cortical auditory evoked responses and the non-auditory electrophysiologic procedures. We may be on the threshold of greater clinical application of cortical evoked responses. For example, there appears to be increased interest in the use of the auditory late response in the assessment of higher level auditory processing of diverse patient populations, such as children with suspected auditory processing disorders (APD) and children and adults with cochlear implants. Another exciting new application of cortical AERs is documentation of treatment for auditory disorders. These applications are highlighted in the chapters devoted to the auditory middle latency response (Chapter 11), the auditory late response (Chapter 12), the P300 response (Chapter 13), and the mismatch negativity (MMN) response (Chapter 14). Those researchers who focus on investigations of cortical evoked responses may be disappointed at the relatively superficial discussions just noted. To be sure, the length of the chapters on cortical responses, such as the P300 response, in no way reflects the amount of research reported on the response. For example, a Medline search will quickly reveal thousands of articles on the P300 response—far more than for ECochG and ABR combined. The majority of these papers are published in journals not regularly read by practitioners who apply auditory evoked responses in the clinical setting. In contrast to this clear imbalance toward the cortical auditory responses in the literature, the earlier latency AERs—ECochG and ABR—are most often applied clinically by audiologists.

Admittedly, this book is not an exhaustive review of the literature on AERs. Experimental AER findings for thousands of articles are not summarized in the book. The literature yields a wealth of basic scientific data recorded from a variety of animal specials on most of the different AERs, from ECochG to the cortical responses. Much of this information has, or someday will have, implications for the clinical application of AERs. For example, animal research offers an obvious approach for the description of anatomic generators for auditory evoked response components. The disadvantage of this experimental approach, however, is equally obvious. One cannot generalize with confidence to humans the conclusions from studies of the neuroanatomy of AERs

that are drawn from studies involving small (subprimate) animals, e.g., gerbils and rats, to humans. Another substantial chunk of the literature not included in the book consists of articles published in languages other than English. With few exceptions, these papers were either not reviewed, or only details of the study cited in the abstract of the paper were included in the book. The policy of including mostly English-language papers does not in any way suggest that the articles published in other languages, and other journals, are in some way inferior or contribute less to our understanding of AERs. Rather, papers not published in English were largely bypassed for two practical reasons. First, length constraints for the book precluded an unlimited review of the literature. Also, lacking proficiency in a variety of languages, the author was unable to review thoroughly and accurately the non-English literature. Indeed, some readers may question the author's mastery of English alone.

A final thought for prospective readers that was included in the Preface of the original *Handbook of Auditory Evoked Responses* will be reiterated herein:

> A little learning is a dangerous thing;
> Drink deep, or taste not the pierian spring:
> There shallow draughts intoxicate the brain,
> and drinking largely sobers us again.
>
> —Alexander Pope (1688–1744) [*An Essay on Criticism*]

ACKNOWLEDGMENTS

During the five years required for preparation of the manuscript for this book ("after hours" on week nights and on weekends), I benefited from the assistance of hard-working persons who were, at the time, students in the Doctor of Audiology program at the University of Florida, including Katie Gray, Katie Curran, Amy Thomas, Colleen Burns, and Andrea Cossetini. My (our) son Austin Hall helped with the conversion of the manuscript of the original *Handbook of Auditory Evoked Responses* created with a now-defunct word processing program and stored on dozens of delicate floppy disks to a current word processing program backed up on a flash drive. I am grateful to reviewers of portions of the manuscript for the book, particularly Albert R. De Chicchis, University of Georgia; Catharine Pettigrew, University College, Cork; and Steve D. Smith, Auburn University. Finally, I thank Steve Dragin, my editor at Allyn and Bacon, for agreeing to publish the book and for patience as it was created.

James W. Hall III
March 23, 2006
Gainesville, Florida

CHAPTER

Overview of Auditory Neurophysiology
Past, Present, and Future

This chapter introduces auditory evoked responses (AERs) to those readers who are unfamiliar with the topic. With the exception of the passages on historical development of AERs, information within the chapter is presented in greater detail elsewhere in the book. Advanced students, and clinicians with experience in recording AERs, may wish to go directly to the next chapter.

INTRODUCTION TO AUDITORY EVOKED RESPONSES

What Are Auditory Evoked Responses?

An auditory evoked response (AER) is activity within the auditory system (the ear, the auditory nerve, or auditory regions of the brain) that is produced or stimulated (evoked) by sounds (auditory or acoustic stimuli). Anatomic origins of the major auditory evoked responses are reviewed in the next chapter. Representative waveforms of major AERs are shown in Figure 1.1. In the simplest of terms, AERs are brain waves (electrical potentials) generated when a person is stimulated with sounds. The sounds that can be used to elicit AERs range from clicks (very brief, sharp sounds) to tones, and even to speech sounds. The intensity or strength of the sounds (corresponding to how loud they are) may be high (loud) to low (faint). As a rule, sounds with greater intensity produce larger auditory brain responses. The sounds are presented to a person with some type of an acoustic transducer, such as an earphone. An acoustic transducer is a device for converting electrical energy into acoustic (sound) energy.

Activity from the ear and brain evoked by the sounds is picked up by electrodes placed usually at specific places on the scalp (e.g., high on the forehead) and near the ears (e.g., on the earlobes). A typical electrode consists of a wire with a disc or adhesive patch at one end that makes contact with the skin, and a pin at the other end, which plugs into an electrode box or preamplifier. The activity evoked by the sounds arises from structures within the ear, nerve, and brain, at some distance from these skin electrodes. Stimulus-evoked sensory and neural activity is conveyed from the auditory structures through body tissue and fluids to the surface electrodes. Then the wires lead this electrical activity to a preamplifier, to filters, to an analog-to-digital converter, and then to a computer.

A logical question at this juncture is, If the electrodes are relatively far removed from the generators of the responses, then how does one know where the response is coming from in the brain? Since the stimulus is a sound, it is clear that the response arises from the auditory system. The specific source of the response within the auditory system is often difficult or impossible to pinpoint. Nonetheless, by analyzing the pattern of the response and by calculating the time period after the stimulus in which the response occurs, it is usually possible to determine the regions in the auditory system generating the response and, sometimes, specific anatomic structures. The time after the stimulus at which AERs occur is invariably less than 1 second. Therefore, the post-stimulus times (latencies) of peaks in the response pattern (waveform) are described in milliseconds. A millisecond is one-thousandth of one second.

Responses with the shortest latencies are generated by the inner ear and the auditory nerve. A few milliseconds later, there are unique response patterns reflecting activity within the auditory brainstem. Recorded still later are response patterns due to activity in higher auditory portions of the brain, such as the cerebral cortex. Extensive experience in recording AERs from normal human subjects and patients with pathologies involving different regions within the brain has produced some useful correlations among response patterns, the periods after the stimulus, and the generators of AERs. In fact, the terms used in referring to different categories of AERs are sometimes related to the auditory structures that give rise to the response. Examples are electrocochleography (from the cochlea or inner ear) and auditory brainstem response (from the brainstem). To a large extent, however, AER terminology is inconsistent and quite confusing.

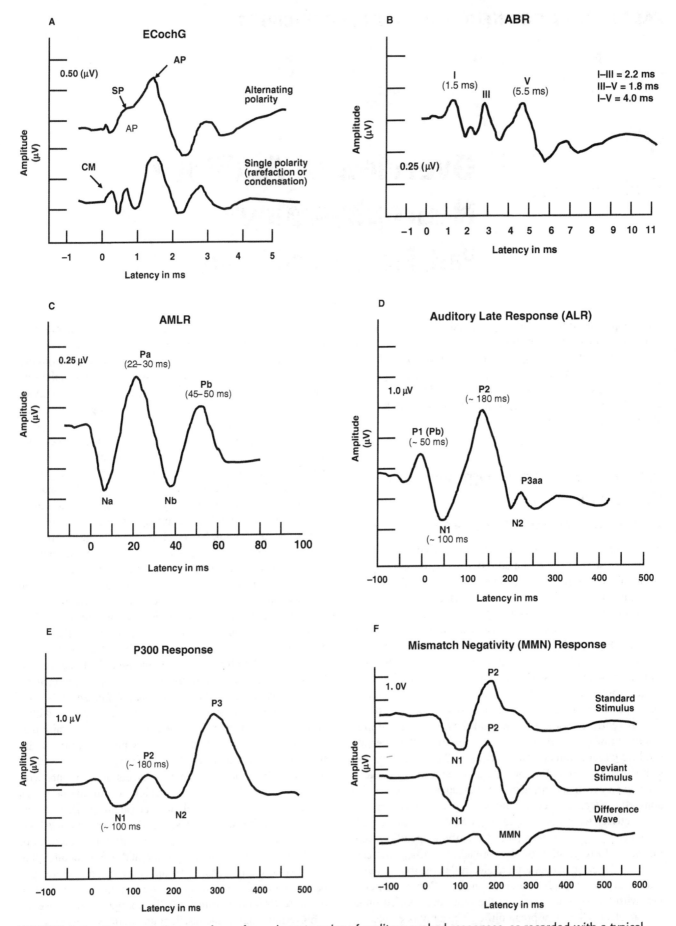

FIGURE 1.1. Representative waveforms for major categories of auditory evoked responses, as recorded with a typical stimulus, including: A. electrocochleography (ECochG), B. auditory brainstem response (ABR), C. auditory middle-latency response (AMLR), D. auditory late response (ALR), E. auditory P300 response, and F. mismatch negativity (MMN) response.

The brain activity underlying AERs is of extremely small voltage (refer again to Figure 1.1) and is measured in microvolts (μvolts). A microvolt is one-millionth of a volt, or one-thousandth of a millivolt (one millivolt is one-thousandth of a volt). Activity arising from the higher regions of the auditory system (the cerebral cortex) involves hundreds of thousands, perhaps millions, of brain cells. The electrodes are also relatively close to the sources of this activity. Therefore, these responses tend to be somewhat larger in size (amplitude), on the order of 5 to 10 μvolts. In contrast, activity generated by the ear, auditory nerve, and brainstem, which involves fewer neural units and may arise at a further distance from the electrodes, may be extremely small, on the order of 0.10 to 0.50 μvolts.

Because auditory evoked brain activity is of very low voltage, two processes are essential for detecting AERs. The brain activity must be increased, or amplified. Smaller voltage activity from the ear, auditory nerve, and brainstem is typically made 100,000 times larger by amplification before any analysis of the response takes place. The second process is signal averaging. The signal (the actual auditory evoked bioelectric signal) is buried within other brain activity (general background brain activity or electroencephalogram, EEG) and even electrical signals from sources outside of the auditory system, such as fluorescent lights in the test room and muscle potentials related to movement of or tension in the jaw or neck. Electrical activity that is not related to the auditory stimulus is referred to as noise. If a sound were presented to a person just once, it would be impossible to distinguish the tiny signal from the ear, auditory nerve, or brain activity (signal) produced by the sound from the much larger ongoing background electrical activity, the noise, which is also detected by the electrodes.

Different techniques are available for increasing the size of the signal (AER) and reducing the size of the noise (other electrical activity)—that is, improving the signal-to-noise ratio (SNR). The most important technique is signal averaging. Every time a stimulus is presented, brain activity detected with the electrodes, including the auditory response if there is one, is stored in computer memory. During the signal averaging process, hundreds, and often thousands, of stimuli are presented, and brain activity is stored. The basic assumption is that the pattern of auditory brain activity produced by each stimulus will almost always be the same. At any specific time after the stimulus, there will a similar voltage in the response. That is, the response is generally time-locked to the stimulus. With each additional presentation of a stimulus, then, the resulting AER will be added to and strengthen previous responses. From time to time, the number of stimulus presentations is divided into the sum of waveforms, that is, an average is calculated. Meanwhile, background electrical activity, also detected by the electrodes, is simultaneously being added up. This activity is considered random, however, and does not have the same pattern after each stimulus presentation. At any specific time after one stimulus is presented, the "noise" may have, for example, a positive voltage (e.g., +1 μvolt), and yet after another stimulus presentation the voltage at this time may be negative (e.g., −1 μvolt). As these subsequent patterns of random background activity are added together, they are eventually cancelled or averaged out, or reduced in size, leaving mostly the AER.

As detailed below, AERs have an interesting and varied history dating back to 1930. The most dramatic growth in AER clinical use, however, has occurred since the 1970s and is directly related to the increased availability of relatively small and inexpensive, yet powerful, computers. Now, there are over a dozen manufacturers of user-friendly computerized instruments for recording AERs. As more devices have been introduced commercially and different types of health care professionals have incorporated AERs into the scope of their practice, the clinical uses for AER have correspondingly expanded. Just a few examples of these clinical uses include estimation of auditory sensitivity in newborn infants who are at risk for hearing impairment as well as older children, diagnosis of inner ear disease (e.g., Ménière's disease), detection of tumors and other pathology of the auditory central nervous system (auditory nerve, brainstem, or cerebrum), monitoring central nervous status during nerve and brain surgery, and even diagnosis of brain death. These and many other clinical applications of AERs are reviewed in this book.

Factors in the Measurement of AERs

Instrumentation for recording auditory evoked responses (AERs) and important factors influencing AER recordings are summarized schematically in Figure 1.2. The information highlighted by this figure is discussed in detail throughout other portions of the book for specific responses. What follows here is a brief review of this topic. Accurate, reliable, and clinically meaningful AER measurement depends on an appreciation and understanding of how the factors in Figure 1.2 affect each type of response.

SUBJECT FACTORS IN AER MEASUREMENT. | Subject characteristics are a logical starting point for a review of factors, since there can be no AER without a living organism. With rare exceptions, the information in this book is limited to human AERs. Among subject variables, the anatomical and physiologic bases of AERs are perhaps the least understood yet most important clinically. For example, application of AERs in frequency-specific assessment of auditory sensitivity requires knowledge of which portions of the cochlear partition (basilar membrane) contribute to the averaged response for given tonal stimulus parameters. Use of AERs in evaluation of central nervous system (CNS) pathophysiology, such as identification and localization of brain lesions, is directly dependent on knowledge of the neural generator(s) of the specific wave components. Other subject characteristics that are known to influence AERs, and which must be considered clinically in the interpretation of findings, are age, gender (male versus

**Instrumentation for Auditory
Evoked Response Measurement**

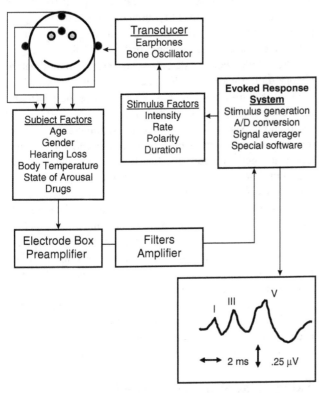

FIGURE 1.2. Schematic diagram of instrumentation used in recording auditory evoked responses (AERs) and selected factors influencing AER measurement. Information in the figure is discussed in the text.

female differences), body temperature, state of arousal, muscular artifact, and the effect of drugs. There may be important variations in the effects of these factors on the different AERs. For example, gender mostly affects ABR, age seriously affects all AERs, and state of arousal and certain drugs influencing the central nervous system are not important factors in interpretation of earlier latency responses (ECochG and ABR) but must be taken into account for valid measurement of later latency responses (ALR and P300). Effects of nonpathologic subject characteristics on ECochG and ABR are reviewed in Chapters 4 and 7, respectively. Finally, one must consider the relation between AERs and pathology of the peripheral auditory system (middle ear, cochlea, and eighth cranial nerve) and central auditory system (brainstem and cerebrum). There are myriad interactions among pathologies.

STIMULUS PARAMETERS. | Major stimulus parameters or factors influencing AERs are also shown in Figure 1.2. The transducer, usually some type of earphone, is an important component of auditory evoked response instrumentation. Selection of the stimulus parameters that are appropriate for a given subject depends largely on the type of AER to be recorded and the objective of the assessment. The consequence

of selecting an inappropriate stimulus parameter may vary greatly. For example, if a low-frequency tone stimulus with excessively long rise-fall times and plateau, e.g., a 500 Hz tone burst with rise-plateau-fall values of 10 ms–30 ms–10 ms, respectively, is chosen for ABR measurement, rather than a more transient (brief) stimulus, e.g., 4 ms–0 ms–4ms, there will be little or no response, even in a normal subject. These same stimulus parameters, however, would be appropriate and effective for generating an auditory middle latency response (AMLR) or an auditory late response (ALR). Rate of stimulus presentation is another example of a parameter that has very different effects on various AERs. Increasing the rate of click stimulation to 21.1/sec will have no serious influence on the auditory brainstem response (ABR), whereas this relatively fast rate would abolish the auditory late response (ALR). Stimulus rates as slow as 1 stimulus very few seconds, or even slower, are required to elicit the ALR. Information from published studies on the effect on AERs of stimulus parameters, including type (e.g., click or tone burst), duration characteristics, intensity level in decibels (dB), rate of presentation, acoustic polarity, mode of presentation (e.g., monaural versus binaural), and type of transducer, are reviewed for subsequent chapters.

ACQUISITION PARAMETERS. | To a large extent, the type of AER recorded (for example, ECochG versus ALR), and the success with which it is recorded, is determined by acquisition factors. Essential acquisition parameters are illustrated in Figure 1.2. The type of electrode used in many clinical AER settings is a either metal-alloy, disk-shaped EEG electrode or a disposable self-adhesive cloth electrode attached to the skin, although other types are often used for special applications, such as intraoperative neurophysiologic monitoring. Electrode placement (the electrode array) is a crucial factor in all AER recordings and varies greatly depending on the type of AER to be recorded and the purpose of the assessment. Also, post-stimulus evoked response analysis time has a fundamental impact on the AER that will be recorded. If the analysis time period does not encompass the latency region of the response, for example, at least 10 ms for the ABR or 500 ms for the later latency response, the desired evoked activity will not be observed, even if all other measurement parameters are appropriate. There is a relation between analysis time, the number of data points sampled in recording an AER, and the time resolution of the recording. This interaction, along with comments about selection of the number of stimuli to be presented, is included in a discussion of an essential element of evoked response measurement—signal averaging. Filtering out the frequency regions of the unwanted activity greatly facilitates the detection of an AER in the presence of ongoing neurogenic, myogenic, and environmental activity (or noise). With inappropriate filtering, however, part or all of the desired evoked response may also be eliminated from analysis.

AER measurement is often referred to as an "objective" method of assessing status of the peripheral and central auditory system. The description of AERs as objective is probably used because, in distinction to traditional auditory measurement, a behavioral subject response is not required. AERs are electrophysiologic responses, not behavioral responses. That is, for most AERs (except the P300 response), the subject will, with the appropriate measurement conditions, produce a response without performing any behavioral task. However, analysis of the AER waveform is often dependent on subjective analysis. Response interpretation is influenced by clinical skill and experience. There are exceptions to this statement. For example, the P300 (P3) response is a "cognitive" evoked response that is recorded with a protocol often requiring subject attention to a listening task. Also, within the past ten to fifteen years, devices have been developed for "automated" response analysis. Automated ABR measurement is especially common in specific clinical applications, e.g., newborn hearing screening. Nonetheless, for many applications of AERs a clinician must identify some feature of the response (such as a wave component), calculate a measure or index of this component (such as latency or amplitude), and form a judgment about response reliability and the accuracy of the calculations. No standardized protocols for AER measurement or universally accepted criteria for definition or analysis of responses exist. Guidelines and clinical conventions are followed, as cited throughout this book. Response parameters other than wave latency or amplitude, such as morphology or frequency composition (spectrum) are not routinely analyzed clinically. There is no single measurement technique or approach that can or should always be used in recording AERs. The best technique or approach is the one that produces the most reliable, well-formed, and accurate response. There are, conversely, many ways that measurement of AERs can run afoul. These two themes are reiterated and illustrated often in this book. Put simply, AER measurement is a far more challenging clinical task than sticking a few electrodes on a head, presenting some sounds to an ear, pressing some buttons, and determining at a glance whether the resulting response is normal or abnormal.

Next, each major AER will be reviewed briefly and placed into a historical perspective. The order of the presentation of each AER is generally related to the latency and anatomic origin of the response, beginning with the ear and progressing to the cerebral cortex.

Electrocochleography (ECochG)

GENERAL DESCRIPTION AND WAVEFORM TERMINOLOGY. | In contrast to the rather confusing and varied terminology used to describe other AERs, there is relative consistency in referring to this response. Aside from very early references to "cochlear potentials" and some confusion of "cochlear action potentials" with "cochlear microphonic" potentials, most authors and clinicians adhere to the conventional term "electrocochleography" or "electrocochleogram," as abbreviated ECochG or ECoG. The former abbreviation is possibly more precise, since ECoG may also refer to "electro-

corticogram," an EEG-type recording. Along the same line, the abbreviation "ECG" is not advised because it is also an abbreviation of a diagnostic measure of heart function, the "electrocardiogram." In this book, therefore, ECochG (electrocochleography) will be used exclusively.

Typical ECochG waveforms were shown in Figure 1.1. The response, arising from the cochlea and eighth (auditory) cranial nerve, occurs within the first 2 or 3 milliseconds after an abrupt stimulus. The first component observed, under certain measurement conditions, is the cochlear microphonic (CM). The CM is an alternating electrical potential generated at the hair cell level in the cochlea. With a single polarity stimulus (rarefaction or condensation), the CM appears as a waveform with a series of repeated upward and then downward peaks (bottom ECochG waveform in Figure 1.1). The CM component can obscure other later components in the ECochG waveform because it continues as long as the stimulus is presented. Use of an alternating polarity stimulus effectively reduces the CM. The upward-going bumps to the positive voltage polarity stimuli are averaged in with the downward-going bumps to the negative voltage polarity stimuli. In this way, the CM is usually cancelled out. This is usually desirable in ECochG measurement.

The next two ECochG components (top ECochG waveform in Figure 1.1) are the summating potential (SP) and the action potential (AP). Other terms for the AP are N1 and ABR wave I. The SP may appear as a separate peak preceding the AP, going in the same direction as the AP or in the opposite direction. It may also appear as a ledge or hump on the beginning slope of the AP. The AP is generally the larger of the two peaks and has a latency (time after the stimulus) of about 1.5 ms. Whether the AP (and sometimes SP) is upward- or downward-going depends on the location of the two (noninverting an inverting) recording electrodes. In this book, however, AP is plotted upward in order to be consistent with other AERs. The term N1 (N referring to negative peak), therefore, is not used. The SP arises from the cochlea, whereas the AP (actually the compound or combined action potentials of many nerve fibers) is generated by fibers in the distal (cochlear) end of the auditory (eighth cranial) nerve. Even with this earliest latency AER there is, therefore, some inconsistency in terminology. That is, electrocochleography (ECochG) includes components that do not arise directly from the cochlea. A second major peak is usually observed following the AP and sometimes described in reference to ECochG. Again, whether this peak is upward- or downward-going depends on the electrode configuration. The label N2 (implying the second negative peak), often used as a label for this peak, is not technically appropriate if the component is positive (upward-going). The N2 also does not arise directly from the cochlea. It is equivalent to the wave II component of the auditory brainstem response (ABR).

HISTORICAL OVERVIEW. | Table 1.1 displays a chronological summary of major AER developments, including those for ECochG. The first paper on ECochG was also the first

TABLE 1.1. Chronological Summary of Major Early Auditory Evoked Response
(AER) Developments

YEAR	AER	INVESTIGATOR(S)	FINDING
1929	ALR	Berger	Human EEG discovered
1930	ECochG	Wever, Bray	Cochlear microphonic (CM) in animal
1933	FFR	Davis, Derbyshire, et al.	Response noted in animal
1935	ECochG	Fromm et al.	CM recorded from round window in human through tympanic membrane (TM) perforation
1935	ECochG	Davis, Derbyshire	Action potential (AP) recorded from round window in animal and analyzed by superposition
1939	ECochG	Andreev et al.	CM recorded from round window in human through TM perforation
1939	ALR	Davis P	Alteration in EEG with auditory stimulation in human
1939	ALR	Davis H, Davis P, Loomis et al.	"K-complex" observed in EEG of human during auditory stimulation
1941	ECochG	Perlman, Case	CM recorded from round window in human through TM perforation and photographed
1942	ALR	Woolsey, Walzl	Auditory evoked responses from animal cortex
1947	ECochG	Lempert et al.	CM recorded from round window in human through TM perforation
1950	ECochG	Davis	Summating potential (SP) in animal
1951	All AERs	Dawson	Averager for evoked responses
1953	ECochG	Tasaki	Action potentials (APs) in single fibers of auditory nerve in animal
1954	ECochG	Goldstein R	SP in animal
1954	ECochG	Tasaki et al.	SP in animal
1958	AMLR, ALR	Rosenblith	Computer averaged evoked responses
1958	AMLR	Geisler	Response first recorded in man (with Rosenblith)
1959	ECochG	Ruben et al.	Round window CM in human with hearing impairment
1960	ECochG	Ruben et al.	Round window AP in human with ear pathology
1961	All AERs	Clark	Description of average response computer (ARC)
1961	ALR	Kiang	Cortical evoked response in animal
1962	ALR	Williams et al.	Response in sleep; components labeled in lowercase (p1, n1, p2, n2)
1963	ECochG	Ruben et al.	Direct eighth nerve AP in human
1963	ALR	Davis, Yoshie	Among first of many studies of stimulus parameters; components labeled in uppercase (P1, N1, P2, N2)
1964	AMLR	Bickford et al.	Response described as myogenic (a muscle response)
1964	P300	Davis	Response first noted in ALR
1965	ECochG	Kiang	Classic monograph on discharge patterns of auditory nerve
1965	AMLR	Mast	Further evidence of a neurogenic origin
1965	P300	Sutton et al.	Response first investigated
1966	ALR	Davis, et al.	Further study of effects of stimulus parameters
1967	ECochG	Yoshie et al.	Promontory CM in human with transtympanic (TT) electrode
1967	ECochG	Yoshie et al.	AP with ear canal electrode
1967	ECochG	Portmann et al.	Promontory AP with TT electrode in human
1967	ECochG	Sohmer, Feinmesser	AP with earlobe electrode

YEAR	AER	INVESTIGATOR(S)	FINDING
1967	ABR	Sohmer, Feinmesser	Response first shown but described nonspecifically in paper on ECochG
1967	AMLR	Goldstein, Rodman	First of numerous studies on response; system for labeling components
1967	ALR	Rapin, Graziani	Response applied in normal, brain-damaged, and hearing impaired infants
1968	ECochG	Aran et al.	Promontory AP recorded in human with TT electrode
1968	ECochG	Yoshie	Promontory AP recorded in human with TT electrode
1968	FFR	Marsh, Worden	Described in human
1968	AMLR	Celesia	Identified in exposed human cortex
1968	ALR	Davis et al.	Further study of effect of stimulus parameters
1969	ECochG	Aran et al.	Promontory AP recorded in children with TT electrode
1969	ALR	Jerger	Findings in temporal lobe pathology
1970	ECochG	Coats	AP recorded in human with external ear canal electrode
1970	ABR	Jewett	Response first described in animal
1970	ABR	Jewett, Romano, Williston	Response first described in human
1970	ALR	Vaughan, Ritter	Scalp topography and generators in human
1971	ECochG	Salomon, Elberling	AP recorded in human with external ear canal electrode
1971	ABR	Jewett, Williston	Systematic study in human
1971	ABR	Moore E	Unpublished Ph.D. study
1971	ALR	Kooi et al.	Scalp topography restudied
1972	ECochG	Cullen et al.	AP recorded in human with tympanic membrane (TM) electrode
1973	FFR	Moushegian et al.	Response described in human
1973	ABR	Terkildsen, Osterhammel, et al.	Series of studies on stimulus and acquisition parameters
1973	P300	Hillyard	Systematic study of measurement factors
1974	ECochG	Coats	CM, SP, & AP recorded in human with ear canal electrode
1974	ECochG	Eggermont	Diagnosis of Ménière's disease
1974	ECochG	Eggermont	Frequency specific response with masking
1974	ECochG	Berlin et al.	Recorded from TM in human
1974	ABR	Hecox, Galambos	Description in infants and children
1975	ABR	Schulman-Galambos, Galambos	Response in premature infants
1975	ABR	Starr	Response described in patients with varied CNS pathology
1975	ALR	Barnet et al.	Age effect described in infants and young children
1976	ABR	Salamy	Development of the response in neonates
1976	ABR	Robinson, Rudge	Response described in multiple sclerosis
1976	SN10	Davis	Response described in human
1976	ABR ALR	Greenberg R	Application in acute head injury
1977	ECochG	Gibson et al.	Diagnosis of Ménière's disease
1977	ECochG	Gibson et al.	Application in diagnosis of Ménière's disease
1977	ABR	Selters, Brackmann	Response applied in acoustic tumor detection
1977	ABR	Clemis	Response applied in acoustic tumor detection

(continued)

TABLE 1.1. (continued)

YEAR	AER	INVESTIGATOR(S)	FINDING
1977	ABR	Terkildsen et al.	Response applied in acoustic tumor detection
1977	ABR	Stockard, Rossiter	Findings in patients with varied CNS pathology
1977	ECochG, ABR	Arlinger	Responses recorded with bone stimulation
1977	ABR, AMLR	Robinson, Rudge	Findings in multiple sclerosis
1977	P300	Squires	Effect of stimulus parameters
1978	ABR	Stockard, Stockard, Sharbrough	Monograph on measurement techniques
1978	ABR	Don, Eggermont	High pass masking for frequency specific response
1978	P300	Goodin, Squires	Effects of aging; findings in dementia
1978	MMN	Näätänen	Discovery of MMN response
1979	ECochG	Eggermont	Diagnosis of Ménière's disease
1979	ABR	Jerger, Mauldin	Response described for bone conduction stimulation
1979	ABR	Yamada	Effects of cochlear hearing impairment described
1979	ABR	Chiappa	Normal variations in waveforms
1979	ABR	Dobie, Berlin	Binaural response investigated
1979	ABR	Don	Frequency specific response with masking paradigms
1979	P300	Ford, Pfefferbaum	Effects of aging, dementia, alcohol
1980	ABR	Jerger, Hall	Effect of age and gender on response
1980	ALR	Knight, Hillyard	Application in cortical pathology
1980	P300	Halgren et al.	Neural generators in human
1980	P300	Roth et al.	Findings in schizophrenia
1981	ECochG	Coats	Diagnosis of Ménière's disease
1981	40 Hz	Galambos	Response described in human
1981	ABR	Møller	Neural generators studied with depth electrodes from human eighth nerve and brain
1981	ABR	Hashimoto	Neural generators studied with depth electrodes from human eighth nerve and brain
1981	ABR	Borg	Effects of recording parameters, cochlear hearing impairment, bone conduction stimulation
1981	ABR	Grundy	Application in intraoperative monitoring
1981	ABR	Rosenhamer et al.	Systematic study in peripheral auditory pathology
1982	ECochG	Goin et al.	Diagnosis of Ménière's disease
1982	ABR	Hall et al.	Systematic application in intensive care unit monitoring
1982	AMLR	Kraus et al.	Hemisphere recordings in cortical pathology in human
1982	ALR	Wood, Wolpaw	Scalp topography and neural generators in human
1984	ABR	Pratt et al.	Lissajous geometric analysis
1984	ABR	Burkhard	Effect of stimulus parameters and ipsilateral noise
1984	ABR	Elberling	Computerized analysis of response
1984	AMLR	Lee, Leuders, et al.	Neural generators studied with electrodes on surface of exposed human brain

TABLE 1.1. (continued)

YEAR	AER	INVESTIGATOR (S)	FINDING
1984	ASSR	Rickards, Graeme, Rance, et al.	Discovery by Australian research group
1984	ASSR	Picton, Stapells, et al.	Discovery by Canadian research group
1985	ECochG	Ferraro et al.	Applied in management of Ménière's disease
1985	ECochG	Mori et al.	Management of Ménière's disease
1985	ECochG	Yanz, Dodds	Improved ear canal electrode in human
1985	ABR	Hall et al.	Determination of brain death
1985	ABR, AMLR	Scherg	Dipole localization in human
1987	ECochG	Stuplkowski, Staller	TM electrode in human
1987	ABR	Gorga, et al.	Comprehensive neonatal and pediatric normative data
1987	ABR	Martin W	3-channel Lissajous trajectory analysis
1987	AMLR	Kileny et al.	Neural generators and findings in human cortical pathology
1987	AMLR, ALR	Woods, Knight, Clayworth, et al.	Generators of responses in patients with CNS pathology
1988	ECochG	Ruth et al.	Ear canal vs. TM electrodes in human
1988	AMLR	Kraus et al.	Computed topography in normal humans
1988	ABR, AMLR	Kileny et al.	Electrically elicited response in human
1989	ECochG	Schwaber, Hall	Simple TT electrode technique
1989	ALR	Pool, Finitzo	Computed topography in patients with CNS pathology
1997	ABR	Don et al.	Discovery of stacked ABR technique
2003	ALR, MMN	Kraus et al.	Neural representation of speech processing

publication on AERs in general. In 1930, Ernest Glen Wever and Charles W. Bray, both of Princeton University, published a two-paragraph summary of observations on auditory physiology investigations in cats.

In their article, entitled "Auditory Nerve Impulses," Wever and Bray cautiously described the ECochG. The passage, a true classic, is reproduced in its entirety as follows:

> By placing an electrode on the cat's auditory nerve near the medulla, with a grounded electrode elsewhere on the body, and leading the action currents through an amplifier to a telephone receiver, the writers have found that sound stimuli applied to the ear of the animal are reproduced in the receiver with great fidelity. Speech is easily understandable. Simple tones, as from tuning forks, are received at frequencies which, so far as the observer can determine by ear, are identical with the original. Frequencies as high as 3000 cycles per second are audible.
>
> Numerous checks have been used to guard against the possibility of artifact. No response was obtained when the active electrode was placed on any other tissue. After destruction by pithing of the cochlea on the electrode side, the intensity of the response was diminished; after destruction of the cochlea on the other side as well, the response ceased. However, the possibility is still conceivable that these results are due to purely mechanical action of the nerve, which is brought about by mechanical vibrations transmitted from the cochlear structure acting as a special receptor and transmitter. Further experiments are in progress. (Wever & Bray, 1930, p. 215)

Investigators within the next few years (e.g., Saul & Davis, 1932) confirmed these general observations in animals and attributed the response to cochlear activity. Then, in 1935, Fromm, Nylen, and Zotterman of Stockholm successfully recorded the CM from two patients with tympanic membranes perforated secondary to chronic otitis media and replicated the findings in a cat, a guinea pig, and a rabbit. Russian investigators also reportedly detected cochlear potentials from human subjects during this period with the aid of a cathode ray oscilloscope. Perlman and Case (1941) published the first figure showing a human ECochG. The remarkable feature of these early studies and, in fact, evoked response investigations through the late 1950s, was that the electrical activity was recorded without the benefit of computer averaging. However, it is possible with a electrode placed on the cochlea and with proper amplification to detect an AP component evoked by a single high-intensity stimulus.

The major ECochG developments within the next ten years were additional studies of the CM in human subjects. Almost all studies were conducted with patients either having perforated tympanic membranes or undergoing ear surgery (myringotomy), with the middle ear exposed. Either case permitted electrode placement on the promontory or near the round window. However, within this period the first attempts at recording ECochG with transtympanic (TT) placement of electrodes on the promontory were also reported. As early as 1947 and 1950, Julius Lempert and colleagues, Dr. Weber and another prominent auditory physiologist from Princeton (Merle Lawrence), recognized the optimal site for ECochG recordings and wisely predicted the clinical value of ECochG, stating:

> Our observations thus confirm those previously reported that the round window membrane is the only suitable location for the electrode (Lempert, Wever, & Lawrence, 1947, p. 67). . . . Here we envisage their being used both for general diagnosis and for surgical guidance. (Lempert et al., 1947, p. 65)

These investigators clearly established the feasibility of the TT electrode approach, commenting:

> It is possible, as we have found, to pass a needle electrode through the tympanic membrane and to make contact with the bony promontory beyond. The needle electrode then may be maintained safely in position for the time necessary for a series of cochlear response tests. After the needle is withdrawn, the drum membrane heals perfectly in a short time. (Lempert et al., 1947, p. 310)

Lempert and colleagues, however, questioned the technique's clinical utility, noting:

> We have concluded, after these considerable efforts, that the recording of the cochlear potentials is not a practical clinical procedure. . . . a clinical method ought to be routinely applicable and reliable in results, and we have not been able to adapt the procedure to meet these conditions. (Lempert et al., 1947, p. 311)

Also during the 1950s, the SP and AP components of ECochG were described in animal models (e.g., Tasaki, 1954; Tasaki & Eldredge, 1954).

By the late 1950s and early 1960s, Robert Ruben (then at Johns Hopkins University Medical School) and colleagues were regularly reporting the results of CM and AP recordings intraoperatively in patients with conductive and sensorineural hearing impairment. Quality of these recordings was often very good (e.g., see Ruben, Bordley, & Lieberman, 1961), although electrode placement still followed surgical exposure of the middle ear space for access to the promontory. Amplitude of the "cochlear response," which was actually the AP (N1) component, for tonal stimuli (250 to 8000 Hz) was calculated before and after surgical correction of middle ear pathology (e.g., otosclerosis). The effectiveness of surgery was demonstrated by a postoperative increase in the size of the response. Ruben and colleagues also similarly applied ECochG in the operating room setting to estimate sensorineural hearing status in a series of seven children, most with suspected concomitant middle ear dysfunction. The Hopkins group by 1961 reported that ECochG recording was attempted in thirty-four patients, and was successfully obtained in twenty-eight. Within the next few years, ECochG data were reported for an additional series of adult patients with middle ear pathology and children with communicative disorders. These studies collectively constitute the earliest consistent diagnostic application of ECochG.

Four subsequent events profoundly influenced the clinical application of ECochG. The event with the most far-reaching implications, which had an unprecedented effect on all AER measurement, was the development of an averaging computer in this same time period (late 1950s to early 1960s). This will be reviewed below in a discussion of the AMLR. Two other developments were reported in 1967. One was the finding that the CM component of the ECochG (Yoshie, Ohashia, & Suzuki, 1967) and the AP component (Aran & LeBert, 1968; Aran et al., 1969) could be consistently recorded by placing a needle electrode through the tympanic membrane and onto the promontory after local anesthesia of the tympanic membrane. The obvious advantage of TT placement of a needle electrode was that high-quality ECochG waveforms could be recorded from persons with intact tympanic membranes; i.e., tympanic membrane perforation was no longer a prerequisite for clinical ECochG. The tympanic membrane typically heals within hours of the removal of the TT needle. With the advent at this time of averaging computers, the TT ECochG technique met the necessary criteria for clinical feasibility and reliability noted previously by Lempert and colleagues.

The other advance in 1968 was an ear canal electrode designed for noninvasive measurement of the ECochG (Yoshi, 1968). This was soon followed by another, improved ear canal electrode design by Coats (1974). Related to these advances in electrode types was the report by a former student of Ruben's at Johns Hopkins University, Chuck Berlin and colleague Jack Cullen of Louisiana Medical Center Kresge Hearing Laboratory of the South, of ECochG recorded noninvasively from the tympanic membrane (Berlin et al, 1974; Cullen, Ellis, Berlin, & Lousteau, 1972). As noted in Chapter 3, there are now a wide variety of types of electrodes for ECochG and, many years later, renewed clinical application of the TM electrode approach for recording ECochG.

The final factor dramatically affecting clinical interest in and, consequently, application of ECochG was the discovery in the late 1970s by an international array of investigators of a correlation between alterations of the SP/AP ratio and Ménière's disease. These researchers included Gibson and colleagues in England, Eggermont in the Netherlands, Coats in Texas, Mori and colleagues in Japan, and Dauman and colleagues in France. The role of ECochG in Ménière's disease is discussed in greater detail in Chapter 5, as is the latest clinical application of ECochG in children, diagnosis of auditory neuropathy.

Essential information on ECochG is summarized in the form of a "fact sheet" in Table 1.2.

Auditory Brainstem Response (ABR)

GENERAL DESCRIPTION AND WAVEFORM TERMINOLOGY. | Essential information on ABR is summarized in the form of a fact sheet in Table 1.3. From the first descriptions of the human ABR, independently by Jewett and Williston (1971) and Lev and Sohmer (1972), the response has been described with a variety of terms and acronyms, and different schema have been used to denote wave components. To begin with, numerous terms have been, and still are, used in referring to the response. This was implied in the legend of Table 1.3. Inconsistencies in terminology abound in the literature. Even now, when more than one department within a medical facility offers auditory evoked response services, the inconsistency in terms contributes to mistakes by physicians, nurses, and ward clerks when auditory evoked response services are ordered for a patient in a hospital. As noted by Goldstein (1984), all AERs can be described along various different dimensions, such as time (early versus middle versus late responses), speed (fast versus slow), anatomy (electrocochleography versus auditory brainstem response), a general property of response generation (exogenous or endogenous), or some more specific generator property (stimulus-related versus event-related). Unfortunately, although our current system of terminology involves a mixture of these dimensions, primarily combining anatomic and time (latency) terms, it will be followed in this text for the sake of consistency with common usage.

In 1979, Hallowell Davis formally introduced the term "ABR" in a report of a United States–Japan seminar on "auditory responses from the brain stem." A review of the references for this book by the reader will clearly indicate that the ABR is described with a variety of terms. The most common two alternate terms for the ABR are brainstem auditory evoked response (BAER), used consistently in neurology, and brainstem auditory evoked potential (BAEP). The term brainstem evoked response (BSER), popular in the late 1970s, is improper because it does not specifically refer to the auditory system. Responses from other sensory systems, such as the somatosensory system, also have brainstem components. The same limitation applies to the popular term "middle latency response (MLR)," as noted below. Arguments for use of the specific term "potential" instead of "response," and apparent

distinctions in the neurophysiologic meanings of these terms, have been presented in the past. While it is possible that the term "response" might imply to some readers an overt, voluntary, behavioral reaction to a sensory stimulus, no difference in meaning will be argued here. In the interest of consistency, the term "response" will typically be used in this book, and it will be considered interchangeable with the term "potential." Furthermore, the term auditory brainstem response, abbreviated ABR, will be used exclusively.

Commonly used nomenclature for ABR waveform description is shown in Table 1.3. As noted throughout this chapter, auditory evoked response wave components are denoted with a variety of labels including Roman numerals (e.g., wave III), by positive (P) and negative (N) voltage indicators plus Arabic numerals (e.g., N1, P3), and with just Arabic numbers (1) . There are inconsistencies, as noted above, in the polarity of the response for the vertex electrode (negative versus positive). With the Roman numeral labeling system as introduced by Jewett and Williston (1971), vertex positive waves are plotted upward (shown in Figure 1.1). That is, the electrode at the vertex (or high forehead) is plugged into the positive voltage input of the amplifier while the earlobe (or mastoid) electrode is plugged into the negative voltage input. This produces the typical ABR waveform. However, some investigators, usually Japanese (e.g., Hashimoto) or European (e.g., Terkildsen), reverse this electrode arrangement (negative voltage input is at the vertex or high forehead), and major peaks in the resulting waveform are plotted downward. Not all well-known European electrophysiologists adhere to this arrangement. On the other hand, several prominent auditory neurophysiologists in the United States (Aage Møller) and Canada (Terence "Terry" Picton) also continue to follow the convention of showing positive peaks downward and negative peaks upward.

There is inconsistency even in the sequence of labeled ABR wave components. Some investigators (Lev & Sohmer, 1972; Thornton, 1975) labeled the wave IV–V complex with the number 4 and used number 5 (or P5 or N5) as the label for what is conventionally shown as wave VI. This labeling practice may have evolved because the ABR often lacks a distinct wave IV versus V, as typically recorded with a vertex-to-ipsilateral ear (earlobe or mastoid) electrode array. Traditionally, little attention has been given to the troughs following ABR peaks, even though the troughs may correspond to different anatomical regions than the peaks and, therefore, have clinical value. In this text, nomenclature prevailing in the United States and recommended by many well-respected auditory neurophysiologists (Davis, 1979) will be used in description of ABR waveforms. Namely, Roman numerals are used as labels for waves I through VII, with positivity plotted upward.

At relatively high stimulus intensity levels (70 dB HL and above) and with click stimuli, the wave I component normally appears at approximately 1.5 ms after the stimulus, and then each subsequent wave occurs at approximately

TABLE 1.2. Essential Information on Electrocochleography (ECochG)

Electrocochleography is also referred to as electrocochleogram, cochlear potentials, cochlear receptor potentials, and cochlear action potentials, and the early response.

History

- Earliest of AERs discovered (cochlear microphonic described in animal in 1930 by Wever & Bray).
- Clinical application (intraoperatively) by Ruben and colleagues in early 1960s.
- Routine clinical use with transtympanic and ear canal electrodes demonstrated by numerous groups in late 1960s and early 1970s.
- ECochG is currently the topic of renewed interest in diagnosis of Ménière's disease (summating versus action potential relation).
- Combined ECochG/ABR technique is valuable for enhancing eighth nerve action potential during intraoperative monitoring of auditory status.

Components

- ECochG consists of three major components: cochlear microphonic (CM), summating potential (SP), and action potential (AP or N1) occurring in sequence within the first 1.5 to 2.0 ms after an acoustic stimulus.

Anatomy

- CM is alternating current cochlear activity arising from outer hair cells.
- SP is direct current cochlear activity probably reflecting distortion products mainly in inner hair cell function.
- AP (equivalent to ABR wave I) is the compound action potential reflecting activity within eighth (auditory) nerve afferent fibers as they leave the cochlea (the distal portion of the nerve).

Stimulation

- The optimal stimulus is an abrupt, brief duration sound (e.g., a click) that produces synchronous activation of many hair cells and firing of neurons in the eighth nerve.
- The AP is most robust for click stimuli presented at a slow rate and at high stimulus intensity.
- Single polarity stimulus (rarefaction or condensation) required for recording the CM, whereas an alternating polarity stimulus is optimal for detection of the SP (with cancellation of CM).

Acquisition

- The site of the recording electrode is very important since ECochG is a near-field AER. Optimal responses are recorded with electrodes as close as possible to the cochlea.
- Amplitude of ECochG components is largest with promontory (transtympanic) electrode placement and decreases by approximately 90% for tympanic membrane (noninvasive) electrode and then by approximately 50% for ear canal electrode. Earlobe and mastoid electrode sites are inadequate for measurement of the ECochG.
- Conventionally recorded with a horizontal electrode array (noninverting and inverting electrodes at the level of the ears).
- Optimal response (including SP) recorded with extended a high-pass filter setting, i.e., less than 30 Hz.

Important Factors

- The click-evoked ECochG is dependent on high-frequency hearing sensitivity (mostly in the 1000 to 4000 Hz region).
- The ECochG is resistant to effects of drugs and subject state of arousal.

Clinical Applications

- Simultaneous ECochG/ABR enhances eighth nerve activity (ABR wave I). Wave I is important in calculation of ABR interwave latency values.
- Contributes to diagnosis of Ménière's disease.
- ECochG measurement (e.g., of CM) is clinically useful in the diagnosis of auditory neuropathy.
- A form of ECochG, referred to as the electrical compound action potential (ECAP) contributes to electrophysiological documentation of cochlear implant performance.
- Intraoperative monitoring of cochlear and eighth nerve activity is performed with ECochG techniques during surgery putting auditory system at risk (e.g., in the posterior fossa).

Clinical Limitations

- Does not provide information on auditory system beyond the eighth nerve.
- The ECochG is not a test of hearing, as only status of the auditory periphery is assessed.
- Variability (inter- and intrasubject) in conventional SP/AP analysis can lead to false-positive and false-negative findings in Ménière's disease.
- Click evoked ECochG does not provide frequency specific information on auditory sensitivity but, instead, is dependent only on high-frequency audiometric region.

TABLE 1.3. Summary of Practical Information about the Auditory Brainstem Response, or ABR

The ABR has also been referred to as brainstem auditory evoked response (BAER), brain stem evoked response (BSER), brainstem auditory evoked potential (BAEP), and the early or fast response.

History

- The first thorough and published description was by Jewett and Williston in 1971.
- Over 1,000 published clinical studies on myriad applications for auditory assessment and neurodiagnosis have appeared in the literature since the early 1970s.
- In recent years, with the advent of universal newborn hearing screening, ABR has assumed an essential role as an electrophysiologic technique for estimating auditory threshold in infants at risk for hearing loss.

Components

- Major peaks in the ABR waveform are labeled by Roman numerals, i.e., waves I through wave V.
- The response occurs within a 5 to 6 ms period following the presentation of a high-intensity transient (e.g., click) acoustic signal.

Anatomy

- Evidence from human investigations by Møller, Hashimoto, and others indicates that the generator for wave I is the distal eighth nerve and, probably, for wave II the proximal (brainstem portion) of the eighth nerve. Later waves each have multiple generators within the auditory brainstem.
- The response presumably reflects synchronous activation primarily of onset-type neurons in axons within the auditory system.
- ABR waves I, II, and III arise from auditory pathways ipsilateral to the side of stimulation, whereas wave V reflects activity in midbrain auditory structures contralateral to the stimulus.
- ABR waves reflect compound action potentials along auditory pathways, although latencies for later components are also dependent on synaptic activity in major brainstem auditory centers.
- For persons with normal hearing, the click-generated ABR is mostly dependent on activation of the higher frequency (i.e., 3000 Hz) region of the cochlea.

Stimulation

- The optimal stimulus is a brief duration (e.g., 0.1 ms) click that enhances synchronous neural activity of many neurons.
- Tone burst stimuli also are effective in eliciting the ABR.
- The ABR is detected within background electrical activity (i.e., EEG) and other bioelectric and extraneous signals by means of a process called "signal averaging." The main objective is to achieve an adequate signal-to-noise ratio. The ABR is the signal, and all other activity detected by the electrodes is the noise.
- A stimulus rate of 20/second or even faster is effective in evoking the ABR.
- As stimulus intensity increases, response latency values decrease and response amplitude increases. Above approximately 70 dB nHL, latency remains stable while amplitude continues to increase.
- Another property of the stimulus that must be taken into account in ABR measurement is polarity.

Acquisition

- The ABR is recorded minimally with one electrode located either at the top of the head (vertex) or high in the midline on the forehead and with another electrode located near the ear (e.g., earlobe) on the stimulated side. A ground (common) electrode can be located anywhere (e.g., low forehead).
- The ABR is detected within a post-stimulus analysis time of 15 seconds, although shorter or longer analysis times may be appropriate under certain test conditions.
- Band-pass filter settings of 30 or 100 to 1500 or 3000 Hz are appropriate to encompass spectrum of response while reducing undesirable electrical activity (e.g., electrical noise, muscle artifact).

Important Factors

- The ABR is influenced by subject age (under age 18 months and over the age of 60 years), gender, and body temperature.
- Even though the ABR is generated by the eighth cranial nerve and auditory brainstem, the response is influenced by, and useful in detecting, conductive (middle ear) and sensory (cochlear) hearing impairment.
- The response is not seriously affected by subject state of arousal (including sleep) or most drugs, including sedatives and anesthetic agents.

Selected Clinical Applications

- Newborn infant auditory screening.
- The estimation of auditory sensitivity in infants and difficult-to-test children, including frequency specific information at audiometric frequencies.
- Neurodiagnosis of eighth nerve or auditory brainstem dysfunction.
- Monitoring eighth nerve and auditory brainstem status intraoperatively during surgery potentially affecting the auditory system.
- Diagnosis of auditory neuropathy.

Clinical Limitations

- With click stimuli, the ABR only estimates hearing sensitivity in the 1000-to-4000 Hz region and not for lower frequencies. The ABR, however, can also be evoked with frequency specific (tone burst) signals.
- The ABR is *not* a test of hearing. It is evoked with simple acoustic signals and is generated mostly by onset neurons. Also, the ABR provides no information on auditory function above the level of the brainstem (e.g., the auditory cortex).

1.0 ms intervals (wave II at 2.5 ms, wave III at 3.5 ms and so forth). An approximation of normal absolute latencies of each of the ABR waves can be recalled, therefore, by counting the number of waves beyond wave I, and adding this number to 1.5 ms. For example, wave III is two waves after wave I, and 2 ms + 1.5 ms equals 3.5 ms. Estimation of average interwave intervals is also rather simple since there is usually about 1.0 ms between each wave. The wave I–V latency interval (an important response parameter in neurodiagnosis with ABR) is estimated by subtracting 1 (or I) from 5 (or V), or by adding up the intervals (1.0 ms) between each of the intervening waves (for wave I–II, wave II–III, wave III–IV, and wave IV–V). Either way, the result is an average normal wave I–V latency interval of 4.0 ms. Another handy mnemonic for remembering vital ABR normative data for high-intensity level stimulation is to keep in mind that the wave V occurs at about *5.5* ms and has an amplitude of about *0.5* μvolts (here 5 is the magic number). In a further extension of this theme, the upper cutoff for a normal wave I–V interval in adults (actually persons over 1.5 years of age) is in the region of 4.5 ms, whereas a newborn infant typically has a wave I–V latency interval of no greater than 5.0 ms. Additionally, the cutoff for a normal wave V/I amplitude ratio (the lowest amplitude still considered normal) is 0.5 μvolt. As stimulus intensity levels are decreased below 70 dB HL, absolute latency values for all components systematically increase and the guidelines just offered no longer apply. Also, latency values are increased considerably with young children (less than 18 months) and for tone (versus click) stimulation.

The relation between these ABR wave components and underlying neural generators—that is, the anatomic structures in the auditory system whose activity gives rise to the response—has been the source of confusion and even some controversy. Information on generators is summarized in Table 1.3 and reviewed in detail in Chapter 2.

HISTORICAL OVERVIEW. | A chronological summary of major ABR developments is included in Table 1.3. There are two sources of debate, and perhaps even controversy, regarding the initial discovery of the ABR. As early as 1967, Harvey (Haim) Sohmer and Moshe Feinmesser, of Israel, in a paper entitled "Cochlear Action Potentials Recorded from the External Ear in Man" showed waveforms resembling what we now would recognize as the ABR. Although these investigators were interested in recording the ECochG only, their electrode array (noninverting electrode on the earlobe and inverting electrode on the bony bridge of the nose) was actually quite similar to that employed in ABR measurement (see Chapter 6 for a detailed description of electrodes). Not surprisingly, distinct waves following the ECochG N1 (AP), including N2 (or ABR wave II) and, perhaps, waves III, IV, and V were apparent in their published waveforms. Keep in mind that with the electrode convention employed in this study, so-called "vertex positive" waves are plotted down-

ward (see discussion above), rather than the more familiar upward orientation. At the end of their paper, Sohmer and Feinmesser rather casually note that:

> The recorded responses were usually made up of four negative peaks. The first two of these may be interpreted as the N1 and N2 components of the cochlear action potential. The succeeding negative peaks, which are also observed in recordings in animals, may be due to repetitive firing of auditory nerve fibers . . . or may be due to the discharge of neurons in brain stem auditory nuclei (which, like the N1 and N2 components, reach the recording site by volume conduction). (Sohmer and Feinmesser, 1967, p. 434)

Within two or three years of this article, other investigators were independently discovering similar fast, early latency auditory evoked responses by scrutinizing the waveform just after the response of interest (ECochG) or well before the response of interest (auditory middle latency or late response). Ernest J. Moore was one of these investigators who, in the late 1960s, was conducting ECochG research in human subjects. Although his Ph.D. dissertation (at the University of Wisconsin in 1971) was entitled "Human Cochlear Microphonics and Auditory Nerve Action Potentials from Surface Electrodes," Moore, like Sohmer and Feinmesser, attributed components observed immediately after the ECochG to the auditory brainstem. Apparently, Moore's attempts to publish these observations were met with an incredulous response from journal reviewers (see preface to Moore, 1983). Therefore, although Moore soon began to apply the ABR clinically, his work did not generate widespread research interest or clinical excitement.

Credit for discovery of the ABR without doubt appropriately goes to Don Jewett (Figure 1.3). In the late 1960s, Jewett was a fledgling neurophysiologist with a D.Phil. degree from Oxford University who had just left a research position in the laboratory of Robert Galambos at Yale University for his first faculty appointment in the Physiology Department of the University of California–San Francisco.

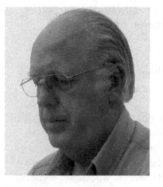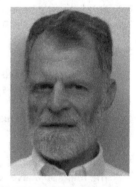

FIGURE 1.3. Dr. Don Jewett (left) who, with colleague John Williston (right), first described the auditory brainstem response (ABR) in humans in 1970, and then in 1971 published a systematic study of the response.

[The reader is referred to Jewett's Introduction to Moore's book *Bases of Auditory Brain-Stem Evoked Responses* (1983) for a fascinating, humorous, and insightful narration of the events that led to discovery of the ABR.] Jewett repeatedly, and even publicly, dismissed his observation of ABR components as "nothing but artifacts," mainly because his primary interest was in higher level CNS functions. However, needing desperately to publish, and assisted by a then graduate student (Michael Romano) and a post-doctoral fellow (John Williston), Jewett began to seriously investigate these early components. Ironically, the studies were carried out mostly with human subjects in order to generate more interest in the overall focus of their research, animal ABR findings. Through a series of personal contacts between Jewett and other highly respected auditory neurophysiologists in California and elsewhere (e.g., R. Galambos, A. Starr, and H. Davis), clinical interest in ABR quickly spread, even before additional papers on the topic were published. The Jewett group also encountered some difficulty in getting their findings published (in *Science*), but they persevered (Jewett, Romano, & Williston, 1970), and, as the saying goes, the rest is history.

The paper on ABR published in 1971 by Jewett and Williston in the journal *Brain* is truly a classic and should be considered mandatory reading for all clinicians who record auditory evoked responses. The authors displayed unprecedented figures of the now familiar ABR waveform (Figure 1.4), identified major features of the ABR, and investigated, at least in a preliminary fashion, many of the factors that influence the response. The following collage of statements from the article on various ABR observations is presented to illustrate this point.

On anatomy:

Under the conditions of skull and scalp boundaries and intracranial inhomogeneities, recordings from a single electrode position offer little indication as to the location of a wave's neural generators. . . . the evidence that wave I is volume-conducted from the eighth nerve is good . . . wave II most likely arises from the cochlear nuclei . . . double firings from the eighth nerve might contribute to wave II . . . later waves are undoubtedly composites from multiple generators, both ascending and descending in algebraic summation. (pp. 681, 692)

On nomenclature:

A remarkably distinct series of waves in the first 9 msec after a click stimulus can be averaged from the human vertex . . . with a likelihood approaching inevitability, we chose to label the waves sequentially with roman numerals. (p. 683)

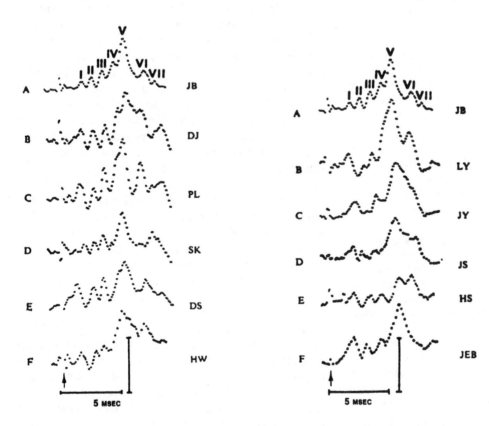

FIGURE 1.4. Auditory brainstem response (ABR) waveforms from the classic paper on the topic by Jewett and Williston (1971). ABR waveforms were recorded from eleven normal subjects. The arrow indicates stimulus presentation.

On subject state:

It was our impression that recordings with the most distinct waves were obtained when the subjects were relaxed and well adapted to the experimental procedure. . . . no differences between awake and asleep records were noted but this was not systematically investigated. The provision of a micro-switch, which allowed the subject to turn off the averager (but not the click) prior to voluntary movements, was important in obtaining sufficient relaxation of the subject. (p. 688)

On stimulus rate:

The distinctiveness and replicability of the earliest waves were markedly affected by the click repetition rate. (p. 688)

On filter settings:

When . . . the average at a bandpass of 1.6 Hz was re-averaged with a bandpass of 1.6 to 100 Hz, the wave shapes showed less detail and an apparent increase in latency . . . the apparent latency of the early waves is markedly influenced by the high frequency cut-off filter . . . 300 Hz low-frequency cut-off filter . . . distorted the low frequency components of the waveform, making interpretation of the waves difficult. (pp. 690, 691)

On electrode sites:

If the vertex-recorded waves reported here are to meet the criteria of far field responses, recordings made short distances apart should be similar . . . similar waveforms [were] obtained simultaneously from three electrode locations (at the vertex, 7 cm anterior to the vertex, and 7 cm lateral to the vertex) . . . If there are significant potentials at the ear lobe, then the use of the ear lobe as a grounding point could, under some circumstances, influence the wave shapes obtained. (pp. 687, 693)

On response reliability:

After careful perusal of the similarities of [waveforms shown in Figure 1.4], we could, with courage of conviction, find all the waves through VI in all of the traces. (pp. 684, 685)

On clinical application:

While the constancy of pattern and amplitude suggests that the early auditory field potentials presented here may have considerable use for empirically based clinical and experimental work, the usefulness of this method will be enhanced if the neural generators of the waves can be identified. The responses from the same individual were remarkably constant [see Figure 1.4]. . . . Wave V will probably be the best basis of comparison across individuals and between different laboratories because its amplitude makes it easiest to record. . . . Certainly this response might be considered when objective audiometry based upon latency of response to one or a few fixed intensities is developed. (pp. 684, 685, 687, 694)

Jewett and Williston clearly appreciated the major clinical advantages of ABR over later latency AERs, namely, reliability and independence from the patient's state of arousal. They also accurately predicted some valuable audiologic and neurologic applications. With this publication, the course of clinical auditory neurophysiology was radically altered. Even though selected research teams continued to investigate AERs earlier in latency than ABR (for example, groups headed by Eggermont, Coats, Aran, and Portmann; Yoshie, Elberling, and Berlin) or later in latency than ABR (for example, groups headed by Goldstein and Hillyard), ABR quickly became the major clinical focus in AER research.

For many years, a long list of clinical investigators had searched for an "objective" auditory test for very young children or those difficult to test by traditional audiometry. Not unexpectedly, therefore, pediatric auditory assessment was high on the list of popular clinical ABR applications during these formative years and, of course, and remains so even now. Notable among the early publications were papers by Robert Galambos and colleagues (Hecox & Galambos, 1974; Schulman-Galambos & Galambos, 1975) and fellow Californian Alan Salamy. Other investigators, especially in neurology (such as Stockard, Sharbrough, Starr, Robinson, and Rudge), began in the mid-1970s to explore the clinical utility and diagnostic value of ABR in detecting and localizing varied CNS pathologies, ranging from multiple sclerosis to brain tumors.

During this era, a series of articles published in the otolaryngologic and audiologic literature by Selters and Brackmann, Clemis, Thomsen, Terkildsen, and others confirmed the remarkable power of ABR in diagnosis of acoustic tumors, and posterior fossa lesions in general, in comparison to behavioral auditory tests and radiologic procedures of the day. Other applications of ABR reported during this period, but not enjoying immediate clinical acceptance, included estimation of outcome in severe traumatic head injury (Greenberg & Becker, 1976) and confirmation of brain death (Starr, 1976). Systematic normative studies and descriptions of the effects of fundamental subject characteristics (e.g., age and gender) and measurement parameters (e.g., stimulus factors, filter settings, electrode locations) appeared somewhat belatedly in the late 1970s, after the initial explosion of clinical ABR research (e.g., Jerger & Hall, 1980; Stockard, Stockard & Sharbrough, 1978). Monographs reporting the proceedings of major conferences on ABR also began to be published shortly thereafter (e.g., *Scandinavian Audiology* Supplement 11 in 1980 and Supplement 13 in 1981). The end of the 1970s saw the introduction of instrumentation for ABR measurement that combined the clinically attractive features of simplicity in operation (lots of knobs arranged in a logical way), mobility (a cart with relatively large wheels), and dependability. One popular first-generation clinical evoked response system—the Nicolet CA-1000—was remarkably user friendly and so durable that beloved vintage units are still in service today a quarter of a century after they were manufactured (see Figure 1.5).

The early 1980s saw a variety of textbooks on clinical measurement of sensory evoked responses, including ABR. Also in the same era, dogma regarding the neural generators of ABR was challenged. Previously, a one-to-one re-

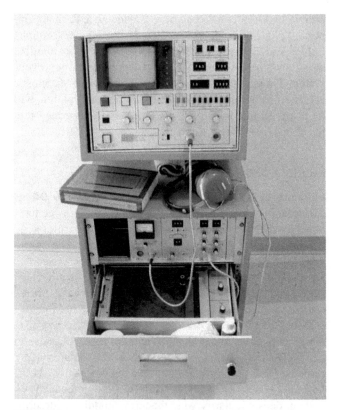

FIGURE 1.5. A Nicolet CA-1000 evoked response system (manufactured in 1980) representing the type of equipment used by hundreds of audiologists during the early years of ABR clinical application. With this device, clinicians were required to select and manipulate stimulus and acquisition parameters manually, rather than relying on existing software programs. In a typical workday, the rather heavy CA-1000 was transported (rolled) from the audiology clinic to various test settings throughout a hospital, e.g., patient rooms, the intensive care nursery, the operating room, and the neuro-intensive care unit.

lationship between successive ABR waves and separate anatomic structures in the ascending auditory system was assumed, largely on the basis of small animal (rat and cat) research and clinical findings in CNS pathology. As foreshadowed by Jewett and Williston's insightful comments above, this anatomic schema, while clinically appealing, was highly simplistic and inaccurate. The outcome of depth electrode recordings of ABR activity from the surface of the eighth nerve and brainstem in human subjects prompted a reassessment of the original anatomical schema for ABR.

In the more than three decades since Jewett and Williston discovered the ABR, effects of virtually every possible measurement parameter on the response have been investigated and described in the literature. Nonetheless, some of these research findings are conflicting, and, in addition,

many clinically important questions remain unanswered. Early studies of pediatric ABR application laid the foundation for the later emphasis on newborn hearing screening and, more recently, electrophysiologic estimation of the audiogram with frequency-specific (tone burst) ABR measures and the auditory steady-state response (ASSR). Finally, exploitation of the neurodiagnostic value of ABR continued unabated until the advent of magnetic resonance imaging (MRI) technology. The routine clinical application of MRI for localizing even small retrocochlear lesions contributed to a dramatic reduction in the demand for neurodiagnostic ABRs, at least in adults. The ABR, however, is still a powerful diagnostic tool in clinical audiology today as evidenced, for example, by its use in the identification and evaluation of auditory neuropathy (see Chapters 5 and 9 for information on auditory neuropathy).

Auditory Steady-State Response (ASSR)

Although not really an ABR or an auditory middle latency response (AMLR), the auditory steady-state response (ASSR) will be mentioned at this juncture. The ASSR was first described independently in the 1980s. Multiple investigators from around the world were involved in this research effort, including groups in Australia (e.g., Rickards & Clark, 1984), the United States (e.g., Kuwada, Batra, & Maher, 1986). England (e.g., Rees, Green, & Kay, 1986), Finland (e.g., Mäkelä & Hari, 1987), and Canada (e.g., Stapells, Linden, Suffield, Hamel, & Picton, 1984; Picton et al., 1987). Since its discovery, the ASSR has been referred to by different terms and abbreviations, such as the envelope following response, or EFR (e.g., Dolphin & Mountain, 1992), the amplitude modulated frequency response, or AMFR (e.g., Kuwada et al., 1986), and the steady-state evoked response (SSER) or steady-state evoked potential, or SSEP (e.g., Rickards et al., 1994). A problem with these latter acronyms (SSER and SSEP) was soon recognized—namely, they were already used for another sensory evoked response, the somatosensory evoked response or potential. As the technique began to be applied clinically, the phrase "auditory steady-state response" was coined, with the abbreviation ASSR, to minimize confusion in terminology. A team of researchers from the Royal Victorian Eye and Ear Hospital and the University of Melbourne in Australia, including Field Rickards, Gary Rance, Graeme Clark, and colleagues, developed instrumentation for automatic detection of an auditory response to rapid modulations in the frequency and/or amplitude of a sinusoidal (steady-state) tone. The group soon applied the new technique in the electrophysiological estimation of auditory thresholds of infants and young children suspected of hearing loss, including auditory neuropathy, as reported in a series of publications. During the same time period, Terrence Picton (Figure 1.6) and a group of Canadian colleagues also constructed instrumentation for measuring a steady-state evoked response to amplitude and frequency modulated pure tone stimuli. For

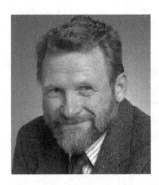

FIGURE 1.6. Dr. Terrence (Terry) Picton, a Canadian auditory neurophysiologist who, with students and colleagues, has published extensively on auditory evoked responses including the auditory steady-state response (ASSR).

about twenty years, the technique was refined and further developed in the laboratory setting. More recently, the technique, described as **m**ultiple **a**uditory **s**teady-**s**tate **e**voked **r**esponse (MASTER) has been applied clinically in different patient populations. Both of the research groups, Australian and Canadian, have made numerous contributions to auditory electrophysiology, in addition to their work on the ASSR.

The ASSR has emerged as a clinically valuable electrophysiological measure of auditory sensitivity, especially for infants and young children with severe-to-profound hearing loss. Clinical application of the ASSR was accelerated as instrumentation and algorithms from the Australian and Canadian research groups were acquired and adapted for clinical use by several major manufacturers of audiologic equipment and, following FDA approval, marketed in the United States. Other manufacturers soon followed with devices, or software updates for existing evoked response systems, permitting the measurement and automated analysis of the ASSR. The impetus for the rapid emergence of the ASSR as a clinical procedure was universal newborn hearing screening (UNHS) and the subsequent need to diagnose and define hearing loss one or two months after birth, well before it's possible to obtain ear-specific and frequency-specific estimations of hearing sensitivity with behavioral audiometry. Evidence is quickly mounting that the ASSR plays an important role in the pediatric audiologic test battery. Due to intensity constraints of transient acoustic signals, the maximum effective hearing loss that can be estimated with the ABR, for either click or tone burst stimuli, is about 80 to 85 dB HL. Accurate hearing fitting requires an estimation of auditory thresholds, even for children with severe-to-profound hearing loss. Prescriptive hearing aid fitting algorithms require specific values for hearing thresholds at, minimally, three or four frequencies over the range of 500 to 4000 Hz. When electrophysiologic estimation of hearing threshold levels above 80 to 85 dB HL is lacking, appropriate hearing fitting is impossible for children who cannot be evaluated adequately with behavioral audiometry, e.g., infants and young or difficult-to-test children. As reviewed in Chapter 9, the ASSR permits estimation of hearing thresholds at audiometric test frequencies across the intensity range of 0 to as high as 120 dB HL. Despite the clear clinical value of the ASSR in defining hearing thresh-

olds in children before audiologic management, many important clinical questions remain unanswered. For example, little is known about the effects on the ASSR of maturation, aging, sedation and anesthesia, and central auditory nervous system dysfunction. Indeed, it's likely that other diagnostic applications of the ASSR, in adults as well as children, will be demonstrated as the technique becomes integrated into the clinical audiologic test battery.

Auditory Middle-Latency Response (AMLR)

GENERAL DESCRIPTION AND WAVEFORM TERMINOLOGY. |

Essential information on AMLR is summarized in the form of a fact sheet in Table 1.4. As with the ABR, terminology is confusing for AMLR. Other terms used in referring to this response are listed at the beginning of the table. The most common two, "middle-latency response" (abbreviated MLR) and "auditory middle response" (abbreviated AMR), are not applied in this book in the interest of both clarity and consistency. MLR, without the descriptor "auditory," is rather ambiguous, for it might as appropriately refer also to components of other responses, such as the somatosensory response, that occur within the same latency region. Auditory middle response (AMR), while specifying the auditory system, does not clarify what the term "middle" is describing. Since other AERs have been labeled on the basis of the optimal recording site (e.g., auditory "vertex" response), the term AMR could imply that the response is best recorded from the middle of the head. As noted below, this is not the case.

The AMLR is observed in a time period between about 12 ms and 50 ms, a time frame that is after the ABR and before the auditory late response (ALR), thus the term "middle latency." Admittedly, such a definition for the AMLR is both arbitrary and artificial, since with the appropriate measurement conditions almost all of the so-called "exogenous" or stimulus-dependent (versus attention-dependent) AERs really form a continuum of electrical activity arising from peripheral and, later, central regions of the auditory system (refer back to Figure 1.1). Indeed, the term "middle latency" was only coined following discovery of the ABR. Prior to this, the current middle-latency components were viewed as "early" or "fast" responses, in comparison to still later components (the ALR).

The AMLR is typically recorded with a noninverting electrode on the scalp of the head, either in the midline at the vertex or high forehead location (for some clinical applications), or on the side of the head approximately midway between the ear and vertex (for neurodiagnostic applications), and with another (inverting) electrode near the ear(s). With this electrode array, AMLR waves appear with positive voltage plotted upward (Figure 1.1). Following nomenclature introduced by Goldstein, each positive voltage wave is labeled with an uppercase "P," and each negative voltage wave is labeled with an uppercase "N." The sequence of waves is

TABLE 1.4. Summary of Information on the Auditory Middle-Latency Response (AMLR)
It is also referred to middle latency response (MLR), middle response, or early component of averaged evoked response or potential.

History

- Initially described by Dan Geisler in 1958.
- Extensive studies by Robert Goldstein and colleagues at the University of Wisconsin in late 1960s and during the 1970s.
- Recent renewed interest in measurement of response with multiple electrode arrays.

Components

- Major sequential peaks are labeled N (negative voltage waves) and P (positive voltage waves) with typical electrode arrangement. They are Na, Pa, Nb, and Pb. The Pb wave is also referred to as the P50 (it occurs in the latency region of 45 to 50 ms).
- The response occurs within the interval of 15 to 50 ms after presentation of an acoustic stimulus at a moderate intensity level.

Anatomy

- Evidence in humans suggests that generators in the auditory thalamus and primary auditory cortex contribute to the Pa component of the response, and the Pb component is dependent on activity in the secondary auditory regions.
- Anatomy of the response may differ when recorded with an electrode located on the midline (subcortical) versus electrodes over the temporal-parietal hemispheres (cortical).
- Anatomy probably includes reticular formation, in addition to lemniscal auditory pathways.

Stimulation

- The AMLR can be recorded with click or tone burst stimulation, but tonal stimuli with relatively long duration are more effective than highly transient click stimuli.
- A stimulus rate of less than 11/second is optimal, with rates as slow as 1/second or less for generating the AMLR in infants or the AMLR Pb component in patients of all ages.
- High stimulus intensity may produce post-auricular muscle (PAM) artifact.
- A response can be elicited by electrical as well as auditory stimulation.

Acquisition

- AMLR recording with electrodes located over left and right hemispheres is indicated for neurodiagnostic application.
- A high-pass filter setting of 10 Hz or lower is necessary to encompass response spectrum and minimize filter artifact components in waveform.

Important Factors

- The response is often not adult-like until age 8 to 10 years.
- There is an interaction between age (under 10 years) and stimulus rate (slower rates are necessary for younger children).
- Amplitude of the Pa wave may be influenced by sleep and sedation.
- Anesthetic agents and other CNS suppressants seriously alter or abolish response.

Clinical Applications

- Electrophysiologic documentation of auditory CNS dysfunction, including auditory processing disorders (APD) above the level of the brainstem.
- Frequency specific estimation of auditory sensitivity in older children and adults (e.g., malingerers).
- Electrophysiologic evaluation of cochlear implant performance.
- The Pb component (P50) is applied in the measurement of "sensory gating" in various neuropsychiatric disorders.
- The AMLR has been investigated clinically as a measure of depth of anesthesia during surgical procedures.

Clinical Limitations

- The response often cannot be reliably recorded from younger children under sedation or in some sleep stages.
- Identification of the major components is confounded by muscle artifact and movement interference.

---

denoted alphabetically in lowercase (e.g., Na, Pa, Nb, and Pb). Some AMLR waveforms will show a small positive wave before Pa. Usually labeled "P_0," this component is not an invariant feature of AMLR waveforms, and its origin has been debated. It is likely that P_0 is actually not a true component in the AMLR, that is, not a neurogenic component

(arising from the nervous system) but, rather, a reflection of postauricular muscle activity.

As with the ABR, there are some general consistencies in the latency and amplitude of AMLR components that facilitate their recall. At a high intensity level for most types of stimuli (clicks or brief duration pure tone stimuli), the prominent peak (Pa) normally occurs with a latency of about 25 ms. The next positive peak (Pb), highly variable and often not present even in normal subjects, occurs another 25 ms later. Amplitude of the Pa component is, on the average, about 1.0 μvolt in normal adult subjects. It is important to note at this point that there are complex interactions among AMLR latency and amplitude values and subject age (below about 10 years), subject state of arousal (awake, different sleep states, sedated, anesthetized), stimulus rate, filter settings and electrode sites, and other factors. Consequently, latency and amplitude values cited in studies of AMLR may vary widely due to differences in methodology.

HISTORICAL OVERVIEW. | A chronological summary of major AMLR developments is listed in Table 1.4. Although auditory components in the EEG were discovered earlier (as summarized below) using rather simple superimposition methods, the AMLR was the first AER to be recorded with computer-averaging techniques (Geisler, Frishkopf, & Rosenblith, 1958). At this point, therefore, major technical advances leading to computer averaging of AERs will be reviewed. During the 1930s and up to 1950, AER waveforms (for ECochG and ALR) to successive individual stimuli were superimposed, either on a piece of paper or on an oscilloscope, in an attempt to determine the presence of repeatable responses appearing often in the midst of considerable larger background activity. G. D. Dawson, a neurophysiologist at the National Hospital on Queen Square in London, had been studying cortical somatosensory evoked responses in human subjects for several years by superimposing many individual recordings. He, and others who relied on the technique (e.g., Derbyshire & Davis, 1935), remained dissatisfied with the results, mainly because for all but a few subjects the responses were obscured by large spontaneous brain activity. Dawson recognized the detection of the responses "would be greatly increased if the records in some way [could] be added instead of superimposed" (Dawson, 1951, p. 65). In a lengthy paper entitled "A Summation Technique for the Detection of Small Evoked Potentials," published in 1954, Dawson presented a detailed description of a technique, first introduced three years earlier (Dawson, 1951). In his words:

> The method uses a rotating switch to sample the signal voltages at regular intervals examined continuously on a cathode ray tube and photographic records may be made of the average they represent.

Dr. Dawson noted that the concept of averaging dated back at least to eighteenth-century scientists—for example, the French mathematician and astronomer Pierre Simon (Marquis de) LaPlace—who were interested in other phenomena as far afield as lunar tides. Dawson generously credited earlier investigators in the 1930s and 1940s who had attempted to develop devices to perform this task and, modestly, stated with foresight that his device may become outdated but had the advantage of simplicity.

For the serious student of evoked responses, the Dawson article would be well worth reading. It is filled with numerous statements that have stood the test of time, such as:

> . . . it may be noted that any gain in signal-to-noise ratio brought about by a change in the recording method must be paid for . . .

and

> . . . any attempt to improve the signal-to-noise ratio by reducing the bandwidth below certain limits, which are set by the time course of the signal, must result in the distortion and loss of information.

Also,

> The gain in accuracy to be expected from averaging a series of observations which are disturbed by random errors is proportional to the square root of the number of observations added. (all Dawson, 1951, p. 66)

Dawson even went so far as to discuss the advantages and disadvantages of autocorrelation and cross-correlation in evoked response analysis, techniques that are even today undergoing study.

The time was ripe for routine application of signal averaging techniques in evoked response measurement. Hallowell Davis at Central Institute for the Deaf (CID) was, naturally, on the forefront of this effort in the 1950s with a device referred to with the acronym HAVOC, for histogram, average, and ogive computer. Studies of human cortical auditory evoked responses were also underway at MIT by Rosenblith and colleagues with a digital device designed by Clark, the ARC (average response computer). Dr. Daniel Geisler (Figure 1.7), then a student in this laboratory, conducted doctoral research on the topic that led to the first published account of the human AMLR in 1958 (Geisler, Frishkopf, & Rosenblith, 1958). The following passage is taken from this pioneering work:

> We have observed responses to acoustic clicks from ordinary scalp electrodes in man. These average responses [see Figure 1.8] are characterized by onset latencies of approximately 30 ms and peak latencies of approximately 30 ms and by response amplitudes and latencies that depend upon the intensity and the rate of presentation of the stimulus. The threshold for

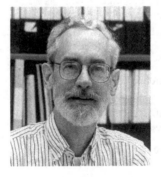

FIGURE 1.7. Dr. Daniel Geisler who, as a Ph.D. student at MIT, described a cortical response evoked from humans that is now known as the auditory middle-latency response.

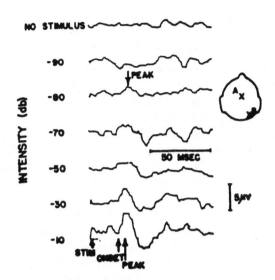

FIGURE 1.8. The earliest published auditory middle-latency response (AMLR) waveforms, reported by Geisler, Frishkopf, and Rosenblith in 1958. AMLR waveforms recorded from a normal subject are shown for different intensity levels. Electrode locations (vertex and mastoid) for the recordings are also depicted. A peak (the Pa component) is present in the 30 ms region.

Reprinted with permission from Geisler, C. D., Frishkopf, L. S., & Rosenblith, W. A. (1958). Extracranial responses to acoustic clicks in man. *Science, 128,* 1210–1211. Copyright © 1958 AAAS.

the appearance of a detectable average response agrees closely with the minimum intensity at which the subject reports that he hears clicks. . . . The response to monaural clicks is bilateral: electrodes placed symmetrically about the midline record virtually the same response. . . . These data, and the latency of the surface-negative component of evoked responses to clicks, in cats and monkeys, suggest that the responses which we obtain are cortical in origin. (Geisler, Frishkopf, Rosenblith, 1958)

Among AERs, history of the AMLR is in many respects the most interesting, mainly because of the tendency of even well-respected investigators to occasionally reach what were, in retrospect, inaccurate conclusions on the basis of incomplete facts. To quote Oliver Wendell Holmes, Jr.: "Upon this point a page of history is worth a volume of logic." This unfortunate tendency of early AMLR investigators spawned at least two major controversies. The AMLR debate that was cited most often over the years was generated by a claim in 1964 that the response was nothing more than muscle artifact. Bickford, Jacobson, and Cody, well-known neurologists from the Mayo Clinic, were involved at the time in comprehensive investigations of motor systems in human subjects. In an interesting study, they recorded electrical activity in the middle latency region during click stimulation from 30 normal subjects and 4 patients with known pathology of the auditory system. Each subject's head was put in a traction arrangement so that pressure could be applied in a forward or backward direction. With forward traction, a very large

response (many μvolt) was reliably recorded in the 12 to 50 ms latency region. The response disappeared with backward traction, subject relaxation, and also after administration of a muscle paralyzer (curare). Their conclusions were unequivocal:

> A human "sonomotor" response system has been described in which click stimuli produce widespread activation of the muscular system with latencies ranging from 6 msec (inion, cervical) to 50 msec (leg). These responses can be detected throughout the cranial musculature and are believed to be the basis of the so-called cortical responses to auditory stimulation reported by Geisler, Frishkopf & Rosenblith. (Bickford, Jacobson, & Cody, 1964, p. 217)

and furthermore,

> There seems little doubt that Geisler's results relate to myogenic components. . . . (Bickford et al., 1964, p. 216)

The Bickford paper was initially presented at a conference on "Sensory Evoked Response in Man" held in 1963 by the New York Academy of Sciences. Dr. Geisler, who had since relocated from MIT to the University of Wisconsin (where he remained on the faculty until his retirement in 1996), took the opportunity to respond to these contradictory findings. His remarks are published in the proceedings, immediately after the Bickford article. After clarifying that he and his coauthors never really said the response was definitely from the cortex and then providing some details of the methodology of the original investigation, Geisler noted:

> . . . for even though muscle activity can be recorded from the scalp, brain potentials can also be recorded there. (Geisler, 1964, p. 218)

and

> . . . on the basis of our first set of experiments, therefore, we feel that the muscular origin of the responses to clicks recorded on the scalp has not been proven. On the basis of our second set of experiments, we feel that further experimentation is necessary before the mechanism by which these responses are generated are [sic] clear. (Geisler, 1964, p. 219)

Since the mid-1960s accumulated evidence has clearly vindicated Geisler and confirmed that the AMLR is indeed "neurogenic," although post-auricular muscle (PAM) contamination of the response remains a troublesome clinical problem. One lesson suggested by this sequence of events is that researchers often seem to find what they are looking for, sometimes against formidable odds.

During the late 1960s and early 1970s, before ABR assumed a major clinical role, AMLR challenged ALR as the major research focus for auditory neurophysiologists. The late Robert Goldstein of the University of Wisconsin and his students (D. MacFarland, J. Madell, C. McRandle, M. Mendel, M. Vivion, K. Wolf, and others) published the majority of papers on AMLR during this period. Hallowell

Davis had, in turn, directly influenced Dr. Goldstein in previous years. Goldstein spent the years from 1952 to 1958 in the auditory research laboratories as Central Institute for the Deaf in St. Louis, and then at The Jewish Hospital of St. Louis, before moving on to Wisconsin. From 1966 through 1980, Dr. Goldstein was the author of at least 30 publications on myriad variations of the AMLR theme, including investigations of the effect of stimulus parameters (among them AERs to synthetic sentence stimuli) and other factors (all-night sleep, alcohol), and measurement of AMLR in neonates. Goldstein's prolific AMLR research is further confirmation that Davis is, as Robert Galambos (1976) stated, the "father of the AER." The AER "children" and "grandchildren" of Davis, among them Goldstein and his former students, have contributed to our understanding of the AMLR.

The second source of AMLR controversy was sparked by Dr. Goldstein and colleagues in the 1960s and 1970s when they reported normal-appearing AMLR recordings in newborn infants. The controversy, in fact, highlights many important and timely principles about AMLR measurement. Beginning in 1967, the Goldstein group conducted dozens of studies in normal-hearing adult subjects and clearly demonstrated well-formed, reasonably reliable AMLR waveforms when certain measurement parameters were used. Namely, these measurement parameters were electrodes located at the vertex and ear (often the earlobe contralateral to the stimulus), a stimulus (click) rate of 10/sec, and filter cutoff settings on the order of 30 Hz to 100 Hz, even though the settings originally employed (e.g., Goldstein & Rodman, 1967) were 1 Hz to 50 Hz. Goldstein and colleagues were obviously excited about the potential clinical value of AMLR, yet prudently commented:

> Review of our data suggests that the early components of responses to rapidly repeated stimuli can be of value in determining threshold sensitivity, at least to a broad range click stimulus such as we used. . . . further investigations are planned in which the patterns of responses to short bursts of pure tones will be studied. (Goldstein & Rodman, 1967, pp. 703, 704)

Similar measurement parameters were therefore applied in investigations of AMLR in young children, including neonates. For example, as late as 1978 Wolf and Goldstein described AMLR findings recorded from 5 newborn infants (24 to 96 hours after birth). Stimuli were 1000 Hz tone bursts presented at a rate of 5.4 stimuli per second. The response was detected with electrodes located at the vertex and ears, and filtered at 25 to 75 Hz (48 dB/octave rejection slope). The objective of these studies was to validate AMLR as a technique for auditory threshold estimation in this population. Their findings prompted the following conclusion:

> Although the present results are not interpreted as threshold measures, they demonstrate that middle components can be obtained at levels approaching voluntary adult behavioral thresholds with these stimuli. Thus, an abecedarian step has

been taken toward the long-range goal of defining an objective response and quantifying hearing sensitivity in individual neonates. (Wolf & Goldstein, 1978, p. 513)

The word "quantifying" referred to the precocious application in this study of a technique for computerized scoring of the AMLR. Actually, the possible use of an "automatic peak detector" for AMLR analysis was first proposed by Goldstein as early as 1967 (Goldstein & Rodman, 1967) and then used in several investigations before the 1978 paper. On the topic of vocabulary, the term "abecedarian" is defined in the context above as "elementary, rudimentary."

Unfortunately, it would appear that assumptions regarding test strategy were based on the outcome of AMLR measurement in normal subjects under ideal conditions, that is, robust and smooth-looking waveforms, rather than fundamental principles of measurement. For example, one of the first questions to ask in selecting filter settings for any evoked response is "What is the spectrum (frequency composition) of the response?" and a logical second question might be "What effect will filtering have on the response?" The question "How smooth is the resulting waveform?" should be far down on the list. We now know that AMLR energy is in the region of 20 to 40 Hz and that restrictive filtering, especially with high-pass filters (the low-frequency cutoff) with relatively steep slopes, may substantially distort a response. A filter setting of 25 to 75 Hz is, consequently, not appropriate on two counts. In fact, with highly restricted filter settings, especially with steep skirts or slopes, a waveform component that resembles the Pa component may be produced entirely by filter ringing (distortion), even if there is no real AMLR present.

Another question apparently not asked in pioneering investigations is "What is the optimal rate of stimulation for AMLR, that is, the rate that produces quality responses with minimal test time?" Also, does this optimal rate vary as a function of other factors, such as subject age, sleep state, central nervous system pathology, and perhaps additional factors? The presence of a reliable AMLR at rates of 10 stimuli per second in healthy, alert, normal-hearing adult subjects in a laboratory setting does not necessarily imply that equivalent response patterns will occur when recorded in varied clinical settings from patients who do not meet these rather strict criteria. And yet, some early investigators of the AMLR speculated that an even faster rate might offer a clinical advantage, as suggested by the following statement:

> We felt no constraint in presenting stimuli at the rate of 10 per second because no evidence could be adduced from our records of adaptation or habituation of the early components of the evoked responses. Pilot studies have already been initiated with the goal of shortening the test time at each level through a reduction in the number of stimuli and through an increase in the repetition rate. (Goldstein & Rodman, 1967, p. 704)

We now realize that, with appropriate filter settings (e.g., 10 to 250 or 1500 Hz), an AMLR is not typically present in young children, at least with a relatively rapid stimulus rate of 10/sec. Rates as slow as 1/sec may be necessary before a response is obtained in young children.

Finally, early investigators soon demonstrated that a large and reliable AMLR is usually detected with a midline electrode at the vertex or high forehead and that response amplitude diminished for recording electrodes over each hemisphere, particularly for lower sites (over the temporal lobe regions and near the ears).

Whether the AMLR detected at these different electrode locations arose from the same or different generators, however, was apparently not considered. Electrode site is an important factor in AMLR measurement. There is evidence that responses recorded with a midline electrode versus electrodes located over each cerebral hemisphere may reflect activity in different parts of the brain. These multiple and still poorly understood interactions among subject characteristics and measurement parameters on the AMLR are more fully reviewed elsewhere in the book. In any event, such methodological concerns of the early AMLR studies limit the validity of their conclusions. Our understanding of AMLR in various patient populations, including children, is to a large extent based on studies conducted only since the early 1980s, when the above noted measurement principles began to be appreciated.

The AMLR continues to be the topic of ongoing clinical investigation, as reviewed in Chapter 11. Musiek and colleagues (1999) have explored AMLR test performance in patients with confirmed and localized brain pathologies. These authors described the sensitivity of various measurement approaches (e.g., scalp electrodes located at midline versus over the left and right cerebral hemispheres) and the diagnostic value of different analysis approaches (e.g., latency versus amplitude). The Pb component, largely ignored during the first forty years of AMLR research, has attracted the attention of researchers from diverse disciplines, e.g., audiology, psychiatry, neurology, and cognitive psychology. Nelson, Hall, and Jacobson (1997) reported a clinically feasible test protocol for consistently recording the Pb component in children and adults. The P50 component (another term for the Pb wave), evoked by stimulus pairs (the so-called double-click paradigm), is now applied as an index of "sensory gating" in investigations of habituation and the brain's ability to rapidly differentiate relevant versus nonrelevant stimuli (e.g., Adler et al., 1998; Boutros & Belger, 1999). This research has led to detailed descriptions of the influence of nonpathologic subject factors on the AMLR, such as such as age and sleep (it is present during awake and REM sleep states), and to the dependence of the AMLR on the reticular activating system and cholinergic neuron groups within the mesopontine region of the brainstem (Buchwald, Rubenstein, Schwafel, & Strandburg, 1991). The P50 (Pb) component of the AMLR has been studied in a wide range of patient populations, among them posttraumatic stress disorder (PTSD), schizophrenia, Parkinson's disease, Alzheimer's disease, and autism. Another fascinating and nonaudiologic line of research for the AMLR has to do with monitoring depth of anesthesia. Related directly to the dependence of the AMLR on cortical and subcortical regions controlling state of arousal and consciousness, this intraoperative clinical application has potential implications for improving the effectiveness and efficiency of anesthesia and, possibly, the short- and long-term neurologic and cognitive outcome of millions of patients undergoing surgery each year.

40 Hz Response

GENERAL DESCRIPTION AND WAVEFORM TERMINOLOGY. | The 40 Hz event-related potential (ERP) is recorded similarly to the AMLR, with the exception that stimulus rate is faster, approximating a rate of 40/sec versus a rate of 11.1/sec or less. In fact, the 40 Hz ERP is in many respects just a variant of conventional middle-latency responses that can be elicited with somatosensory as well as auditory stimulation. The 40 Hz ERP is referred to as a steady-state potential versus a transient response (the distinction was discussed above). Briefly, with a steady-state response the waveform of the response approximates the pattern of periodic stimulation (the stimulus is repeated rapidly again and again). Terminology used in referring to the 40 Hz ERP is rather confusing and not always accurate. To begin with, any term that includes reference to "40 Hz" is technically incorrect, since this AER often is recorded for stimulus rates slightly higher or lower. In children, the response may actually be best recorded for stimuli presented at a rate of 20/sec or less.

The phrase "event-related potential" traditionally has been applied in description of late latency responses, such as the P3 response, that usually involve subject attention to a specific sensory "event." Another term commonly used is auditory "steady-state evoked potential" or SSEP, or now known as the auditory steady-state response (ASSR). This should not be mistaken for the acronym for short-latency somatosensory evoked potential. The term SSEP implies a distinction between a response that occurs repeatedly and overlaps during stimulus presentation and a transient response, as the other AERs might be called, which terminate after a single stimulus presentation and before the next stimulus is presented. The 40 Hz ERP has also been called a "high rate response," a "high rate driven" response, and "composite response" (Stach, 1986). The term 40 Hz ERP, although admittedly not perfect, will be used in this book. The characteristic waveform of a transient response (e.g., the ABR), in contrast, is produced by a single presentation of the stimulus, although averaging the response to many stimulus repetitions may be necessary to detect it.

A stimulus rate of about 40 per second produces an evoked response waveform with a peak every 25 ms, or

40 peaks per second, i.e., at 40 Hz. That is, a time interval of 1 second (1000 ms) divided by 25 yields a quotient of 40. Major components of the AMLR occur at intervals or with a period of about 25 ms. With a stimulus rate of about 40/sec, and adequately long analysis time (at least 25 ms), the ABR that will occur at a frequency of about 40 times per second (one for each stimulus) and the AMLR components recorded for a typical rate of 10/sec (e.g., Na, Nb, Pa, and Pb) will be in phase (occur at the same time relative to the stimulus) and will become superimposed. With a stimulus time of 100 ms, it is possible to view about four cycles of this waveform (e.g., a sequence of four complete waveforms from beginning to end).

At least three characteristics of the 40 Hz ERP suggested to early investigators that it would be useful for estimation of auditory threshold in children. Due to the large amplitude (usually well over 1.0 μvolt), it could be quickly detected and observed for intensity levels very close to actual hearing threshold level in children. Moreover, tone burst stimuli were equally, or even more, effective in eliciting the auditory 40 Hz response, permitting frequency specific estimation of audiometric thresholds. Along with early excitement about these audiometric applications of the 40 Hz response was interest in its possible neurodiagnostic value for evaluating the status of the CNS above the level of the brainstem, perhaps specifically in the thalamic region. Some features of the 40 Hz ERP seriously limit its clinical value, among them the pronounced effects of age, sleep, and sedation.

HISTORICAL OVERVIEW. | A chronological summary of major 40 Hz ERP developments was displayed in Table 1.1. Beginning in 1972, Basar and his German colleagues conducted a series of studies of a 40 Hz resonance or enhancement phenomenon elicited by auditory stimulation, with the first data from human subjects reported in 1976 (Basar, Gonder, & Ungan, 1976a, 1976b). A major objective of this work was to define the relationship of the response to other CNS-mediated activity (e.g., EEG, memory, and learning) and to determine the neural generators. Schimmel, Rapin, and Cohen (1975) also noted the possibilities for relatively simple automated analysis or "machine scoring" of a response produced by stimulus rates in the 40 to 45/sec region. Over the years, anonymous clinicians no doubt also noted, perhaps quite by accident, a 40 Hz phenomenon upon AMLR measurement with stimulus rate of about 40 Hz. The author happened upon this observation in 1980 when attempting to record a conventional AMLR after someone had tampered with equipment settings of his trusty Nicolet CA-1000 evoked response equipment, including the stimulus rate knob. Nonetheless, the term 40 Hz ERP was coined by Galambos, Makeig, and Talmachoff in their description of this AER in 1981, as demonstrated in the following passage (a photograph of Dr. Galambos is shown in Figure 1.9).

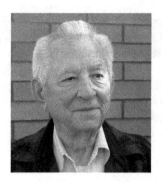

FIGURE 1.9. Dr. Robert Galambos, who in 1981 described the 40 Hz response and who, in the mid-1970s, was among the first clinical investigators to apply the ABR in hearing screening and audiologic assessment of infants.

This phenomenon, the 40-Hz event related potential (ERP), displays several properties of theoretical and practical interest. First, it reportedly disappears with surgical anesthesia, and it resembles similar phenomena in the visual and olfactory system, facts which suggest that adequate processing of sensory information may require cyclical brain events in the 30- to 50-Hz range. Second, latency and amplitude measurements on the 40-Hz ERP indicate it may contain useful information on the number and basilar membrane location of the auditory nerve fibers a given tone excites. Third, the response is present at sound intensities very close to normal adult thresholds for the audiometric frequencies, a fact that could have application in clinical hearing testing. (Galambos, Makeig, & Talmachoff, 1981, p. 2643)

This publication generated excitement in the audiology community and prompted considerable research on potential clinical application of the 40 Hz ERP.

Auditory Late Response (ALR)

GENERAL DESCRIPTION AND WAVEFORM TERMINOLOGY. | Essential information on the auditory late response (ALR) is summarized in the form of a fact sheet in Table 1.5. Characteristics of the waveform are apparent in Figure 1.1. There are, in fact, a variety of auditory evoked response components in the latency region of 50 to about 500 ms, such as the N100 complex (N1a, N1b, N1c), the processing negativity, and the N400. Within the past fifty years since the ALR was first discovered, it has been referred to by many, and often confusing, terms. One of the earliest and most descriptive terms for the ALR was "on-effects in the waking human brain" to acoustic stimuli. There is, in addition, a rather lengthy list of terms for the ALR, including "evoked response audiometry (ERA)," which was one of the more popular terms apparently coined by Hallowell Davis, "averaged evoked EEG audiometry (AEA)," "averaged electroencephalic response (AER)," "electroencephalic audiometry," "evoked auditory response (EAR)," "cortical audiometry," "human vertex (or V) potential," "sound evoked cerebral response," "cerebral evoked response," "auditory cortical response (ACR)," "auditory evoked cortical response," "averaged evoked potentials," "acoustic evoked response," and simply "auditory evoked response (AER)."

TABLE 1.5.   Essential Information on Auditory Late Response (ALR)

Also referred to as vertex (V) response; vertex (V) potential; auditory cortical response (ACR); auditory evoked potential (AEP); averaged electroencephalic response (AER); and slow averaged evoked potential or response, cortical evoked response audiometry (ERA), electroencephalic response (EER), or audiometry (ERA).

___

History

- Noted in 1939 by Pauline Davis as an auditory component in the EEG.
- Hallowell Davis and colleagues conducted systematic investigations of effect of measurement parameters on the response from the mid-1960s into the 1970s.
- Topographic mapping of the response by Vaughan and Ritter in 1970.
- Recent resurgence of interest in clinical application of the response with computed evoked potential topography techniques and sophistical stimulation (e.g., speech stimuli).

Components

- Sequential peaks labeled by N (negative voltage) or P (positive voltage), including P1, N1, P2, N2, as recorded with a vertex electrode.
- Major components occur within 75 to 200 ms after a moderate stimulus intensity level (e.g., N1 in the range of 75 to 150 ms and P2 in the range of 150 to 200 ms).

Anatomy

- The N1 and P2 components arise from auditory cortex.
- Response reflects dentritic neural activity (versus action potentials).

Stimulation

- Optimally evoked by tone burst stimuli of relatively long duration (greater than 10 ms).
- The ALR can also be elicited by speech or electrical stimuli.
- Stimulus rates of 1/second or less are appropriate.
- The maximum response is typically obtained for moderate- (50 to 60 dB) versus high-intensity stimuli.

Acquisition

- The typical recording electrode sites are on the midline (e.g., Fz, Cz, or Pz).
- High-pass filter settings as low as 0.1 Hz are required to record this low-frequency response.

Important Factors

- The response is highly susceptible to alterations in state of arousal (sleep stages) and to the effects of drugs, such as sedatives.

Clinical Applications

- Electrophysiologic assessment of higher level auditory CNS functioning and auditory processing.
- Assessment of cognitive functioning in persons with neuropsychiatric disorders.
- Documentation electrophysiologically of benefits of auditory training.
- Frequency-specific estimation of hearing sensitivity in cooperative children and adults.

Clinical Limitations

- Considerable intra- and intersubject variability.
- Susceptibility of the response to subject state and to drugs.

___

Auditory late response (ALR) components are recorded in a time period from about 50 to 400 ms after acoustic stimulation at a relatively slow rate (one stimulus every 1 or 2 seconds, or even slower rates). In comparison to earlier responses, amplitude for the ALR is large, usually within the 3 to 10 µvolt range, and occasionally larger. The main components, and their characteristic latency values, as shown in Figure 1.1, are P1 (50 to 80 ms), N1 (100 to 150 ms),

P2 (150 to 200 ms), and N2 (180 to 250 ms). The labels for these peaks refer to the expected voltage polarity of the response as recorded from the vertex ("P" for positive and "N" for negative). Note that with accepted nomenclature both ECochG and ALR share an N1 component.

HISTORICAL OVERVIEW. | Table 1.2 displayed a chronological summary of major AER developments, including those for ALR. The ALR was actually the first auditory electrical response to be recorded from the CNS (Figure 1.10). In 1939, Pauline Davis and colleagues discovered an "on-response" to sound in the EEG and coined the term K complex to describe it (Davis, 1939; Davis, Davis, Loomis, Harvey, & Hobart, 1939). The term "K complex" was selected because it had not been previously used to describe any other EEG phenomenon. As seen from these literature citations, one of Pauline Davis's colleagues in these pioneering investigations was Hallowell Davis, her husband at that time. Dr. Davis (Figure 1.11), whose first publications in neurophysiology appeared in 1925, was by 1939 already a respected auditory scientist conducting research in essentially all areas of auditory physiology. During the 1950s, a handful of other investigators

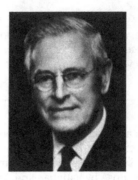

FIGURE 1.11. Dr. Hallowell Davis, who deserves the reputation as the "father of auditory evoked responses." For over fifty years, Dr. Davis has published seminal papers covering the gamut of AERs, from the cochlear microphonic (CM) and the summating potential (SP) in the ECochG to the P300 response.

from around the world independently described this auditory complex in the EEG using, by today's computer world standards, primitive instrumentation and techniques (e.g., Abe, 1954; Bancaud, Bloch, & Paillard, 1953; Roth, Shaw, & Green, 1956; Suzuki & Asawa, 1957). As electronic computers and signal averaging became in some of the premier auditory research laboratories in the early 1960s, a proliferation of studies of ALR as "an accurate, objective method of evaluating auditory acuity in man" (Cody & Klass, 1968, p. 76) were reported (e.g., Barnet & Goodwin, 1965; Bickford, Jacobson, & Cody, 1964; Borsanyi & Blanchard, 1964; Davis, 1964, 1965; Goodman, Appleby, Scott, & Ireland, 1964; Gross, Begleiter, Tobin, & Kissin, 1965; Keidel & Spreng, 1965; McCandless & Best, 1964; Rapin, 1964; Suzuki & Taguchi, 1965; Teas, 1965; Weitzman, Fishbein, & Graziani, 1965; Williams, Tepas, & Morlock, 1962).

Virtually no potential clinical application was overlooked during this intensive period of research in the 1960s. Patient populations ranged from normal and brain-damaged newborn infants (e.g., Rapin & Graziani, 1967) to adults with well-defined cerebral pathology (e.g., Jerger, Weikers, Sharbrough, & Jerger, 1969). Interestingly, many prominent names in the fields of audiology, otolaryngology, and neurology were in the thick of the ALR action during this period, even though some of them did not continue to conduct evoked response research. Among these names are H. A. Beagley, R. G. Bickford, C. L. Blanchard, L. Doerfler, E. Donchin, M. Engebretson, R. Goldstein, J. Jerger, W. D. Keidel, L. Lamb, F. Lassman, G. A. McCandless, E. J. Moore, D. Nielsen, R. Nodar, P. A. Osterhammel, R. Roeser, D. E. Rose, W. T. Roth, H. Shimizu, P. Skinner, T. Suzuki, D. Teas, H. G. Vaughan, B. A. Weber, N. Yoshie, S. Zerlin, and, of course, H. Davis.

Investigation of ALR continued unabated throughout the decade (see Reneau & Hnatiow, 1975, for a comprehensive historical review) and, by the second half of the 1960s, development of instrumentation specifically for clinical measurement of late auditory evoked responses was reported in the scientific literature (Davis, Mast, Yoshie, & Zerlin, 1966). This device, designed by Hallowell Davis, was referred to as HAVOC (**h**istogram, **av**erage, and **o**give **c**omputer) and resembled the CAT (**c**omputer of **a**verage **t**ransients) developed earlier at MIT. HAVOC was coupled to GATES (**g**enerator of

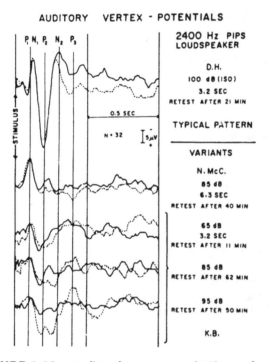

AUDITORY VERTEX - POTENTIALS

P₁ N₁ P₂ N₂ P₃

2400 Hz PIPS
LOUDSPEAKER

D.H.
100 dB (ISO)
3.2 SEC
RETEST AFTER 21 MIN

0.5 SEC

TYPICAL PATTERN

N = 32   5 μV

VARIANTS

N. McC.
85 dB
6.3 SEC
RETEST AFTER 40 MIN

65 dB
3.2 SEC
RETEST AFTER 11 MIN

85 dB
RETEST AFTER 62 MIN

95 dB
RETEST AFTER 50 MIN

K.B.

FIGURE 1.10. Auditory late response (ALR) waveform as reported in one of the earliest papers on the topic by Hallowell Davis and colleagues (Davis et al., 1966). Positive voltage peaks are plotted downward. The typical ALR waveform is illustrated in the top portion of the figure. Stimulus conditions are also indicated in this portion.

Reprinted with permission from Davis, H., Mast, T., Yoshie, N., & Zerlin, S. (1966). The slow response of the human cortex to auditory stimuli. *Electroencephalography and Clinical Neurophysiology, 21*, pp. 105–113. Copyright © 1966 Elsevier.

acoustic transients) and a system for amplifying and filtering the incoming EEG (Davis et al., 1966). ALR waveforms of high quality were recorded group with this early computer by Hallowell Davis and his colleagues.

Papers on ALR appeared after this time, but interest in the ALR as a clinical procedure for auditory assessment declined sharply following the first volley of clinical reports on ABR around the mid-1970s. ALR recordings are at best highly variable between and among healthy, adult subjects. ALRs are very much influenced by subject state of arousal and cannot be obtained reliably from a sedated patient. ABR, in short, offered a distinct clinical advantage over ALR in these respects. Although many of the studies of ALR were conducted over thirty years ago, and despite the above noted clinical limitations, the ALR must not be thought of simply in a historical context. Time spent learning about past clinical experiences with ALR is likely to contribute to a better understanding of the renewed interest in clinical application of cortical evoked responses today (reviewed in Chapter 12).

Auditory P300 Response

GENERAL DESCRIPTION AND WAVEFORM TERMINOLOGY. | Essential information on the auditory P300 response is summarized in the form of a fact sheet in Table 1.6. The P300 was among the collection of event-related or endogenous evoked responses described first in the mid-1960s (Davis, 1964; Sutton, Braren, Zubin, & John, 1965). The P300 response even today is the topic of many publications. The term "endogenous" means originating from within, whereas "exogenous" means originating from outside. This terminology is ambiguous and not entirely adequate, to be sure, since all evoked responses actually arise from within the subject and, conversely, all these responses are evoked by externally produced auditory stimuli.

Exogenous responses are dependent directly on stimulus characteristics and independent on the subject processing or attending to the stimuli. For example, whether a subject listens closely to click stimuli or, at the other extreme, is comatose or anesthetized has no effect on the outcome of measurement of the ECochG or ABR. Furthermore, well-formed waveforms for the AMLR, the 40 Hz ERP, and even the conventional ALR can be recorded from an awake subject who is totally oblivious to the sounds presented. The important point is that no active participation in the testing or attention to the stimulus is required to obtain an optimal exogenous response. In contrast, even a minor alteration in certain stimulus characteristics (e.g., a reduction in stimulus intensity) can dramatically affect the exogenous response, and may even abolish it. The perceptive reader has by now probably recognized, from the waveforms shown in Figure 1.1 and the preceding discussion, a fundamental problem in classifying AERs according to latency. Namely, more than one type of AER may occur within the ALR time frame (approximately 50 ms through about 400 ms). Yet all are, by a time-based definition, "late" or "slow" auditory responses. Despite the inadequacy of the terms, all of these responses will be designated here as "endogenous" or as "event-related potentials (ERPs)," consistent with the literature and existing convention.

Evoked responses classified as exogenous (e.g., ECochG, ABR, AMLR, ALR) are described throughout the book. There are a variety of other types of responses within the general category of endogenous or event-related responses and in the latency period from 50 ms and beyond, such as the P50, N100, P100, N130, N400, P600, and, of course, the P300. Clearly, these various endogenous components are not observed together in every waveform. Rather, each component, or possibly several in combination, is recorded with rather unique test paradigms, including in some cases a particular type of stimulus (e.g., words vs. tones, constant vs. shifting acoustic features) and/or a particular task (e.g., attending or ignoring stimuli). Exogenous responses are relied on by most audiologists for audiometric and neurodiagnostic assessment of the auditory system, whereas exogenous responses are used by neurophysiology or psychophysiology investigators as electrophysiologic probes of higher level function in diverse CNS disorders, such as dementia, schizophrenia, chronic alcoholism, and Alzheimer's disease. The P300 response, and all other endogenous responses, are primarily distinguished by their dependence on stimulus context, rather than stimulus factors, and on subject attention characteristics, rather than subject characteristics.

One test approach or "paradigm" commonly used in recording the P300 response involves the presentation of an "oddball" or target stimulus. The stimulus used in the frequent condition is presented most of the time, but occasionally a different stimulus is presented instead. That is, there is a series of maybe five or six identical stimuli (e.g., 1000 Hz tone bursts) and then, unpredictably, a different or oddball stimulus (e.g., 2000 Hz) is presented. The oddball stimulus may differ in its frequency, as in this example, or some other parameter, such as intensity or duration or, for speech signals, in a more subtle characteristic, such as voice onset time or an articulation difference. The oddball stimulus may even be, in fact, the absence of an expected stimulus. The term "high probability" is sometimes used to describe the frequent stimulus, whereas the oddball stimulus is also referred to as the "infrequent," "rare," "task significant," "probe," or "target" stimulus. By definition, a target stimulus cannot occur predictably (with high probability) or very often (frequently). Using the example just noted, if the 2000 Hz tone burst was presented 50 percent of the time (and the 1000 Hz tone burst the other 50 percent of the time), then the 2000 Hz stimulus would be considered neither odd, infrequent, nor rare. Usually, the target stimulus occurs only about 10 to 20 percent of the time. If the target (rare) stimulus always occurred regularly after the same number of frequent stimuli (e.g., a series of nine frequent stimuli was always followed by a rare stimulus; every tenth stimulus was rare),

TABLE 1.6. Summary of Information on the Auditory P300 Response

Also referred to as the P3 response, endogenous auditory evoked potential, cognitive auditory evoked response, event-related potential (ERP), late potential complex, and late or very late auditory evoked potential.

History

- Described first, independently, by Hallowell Davis in 1964 and Samuel Sutton and colleagues in 1965.
- Extensive investigation of test paradigm influences on P300 and other endogenous responses began during late 1960s and continues today.
- There is ongoing research on clinical value of P300 in electrophysiologic assessment of higher level auditory processing.
- Application of evoked-response topography with multiple scalp electrodes includes study of the P300 response.
- Two relatively new oddball paradigms for measurement of the P300 response are the single stimulus (only rare stimulus) and passive (versus attention demanding) P300 techniques.

Components

- The major peak is a large positive voltage wave (5 μvolts or greater) occurring at approximately 300 ms after a rare (oddball) auditory stimulus.
- P3 label is often used for major component because it is the third positive going wave in late response time frame.
- The term "endogenous" is often used to describe the P300 response and other auditory evoked-response components that are highly dependent on subject attention to certain auditory stimuli (versus exogenous responses).
- A P3a component, with shorter latency and smaller amplitude than conventional attention-dependent P3 (i.e., P3b), is elicited in the passive measurement paradigm.

Anatomy

- Human depth electrode studies provide evidence of contributions to the P300 response from auditory cortex and also the medial temporal lobe (hippocampus) region.
- Reflects dendritic neuronal brain activity.

Stimulation

- The P300 response is optimally evoked by unpredictable, infrequent acoustic stimuli presented randomly with a probability of 15 to 20% in an "oddball" test paradigm.
- Sophisticated stimuli, including speech sounds, are effective in elicitation of the P300 response.
- The P300 can also be elicited by a single stimulus (only the rare stimulus).
- A relatively slow rate of stimulation (2/sec or less) is appropriate.

Acquisition

- Acquisition factors are generally equivalent to those for ALR.

Important Factors

- Subject attention to the "oddball," but not the frequent, stimuli is an important (though not essential) feature in P300 measurement.
- A "passive P3" response can be recorded without subject attention to the rare stimulus.
- The response is profoundly affected by alterations in subject state of arousal, by sleep stage, and by drugs.
- Instructions to the subject regarding the listening task produce marked effects on the type of response recorded.
- Response latency decreases and amplitude increases during childhood and then the process reverses in aging during adulthood.

Clinical Applications

- Electrophysiologic assessment of higher level auditory processing.
- Documentation of the effectiveness of medical and nonmedical management for different disorders, e.g., ADHD and auditory processing disorders (APD).

Clinical Limitation

- Minor, perhaps unappreciated, alterations in attention or the listening task produce marked effects on the response.

then it would cease to have low probability or predictability. The target stimulus, then, must be infrequent, unpredictable (occurring at random), and, in some way, different to meet criteria for the oddball paradigm. The question of how different the stimulus must be to produce a P300 response cannot be easily answered. This aspect of P300 measurement,

in fact, offers a potentially valuable approach for evaluating a subject's level of performance on a cognitive task. Importantly, frequent versus infrequent stimuli used in P300 measurement need not be simple, pure tones. There is considerable theoretical and clinical interest in P300 responses for speech stimuli differing along an acoustic dimension. For example, the frequent stimulus may be /ta/ and the infrequent or oddball stimulus /da/.

The main distinctions between ALR versus P300 waveforms were evident in Figure 1.1. The waveform in the upper left portion of the figure was recorded to repetitive (frequent) stimuli that the subject was instructed to ignore. This is the typical test condition for ALR recordings. That is, the response is obtained by presenting a series of hundreds of signals, usually tone burst, to an awake but inattentive subject. However, even when a subject is instructed to attend to a series of repetitive and identical stimuli, the response does not change. The stimuli are all the same, very predictable, carry no new information, and require no processing or decision making on the part of the subject.

According to the conventional view of the oddball paradigm, the rare signal does not produce a P300 response if the subject is instructed to ignore all stimuli. A P300 response, however, can be elicited when an oddball stimulus is presented and when the subject is not attending to either set of signals—that is, during passive listening (e.g., Polich, 1989). The passive listener is making no active attempt to discriminate or identify the oddball stimuli and is not required to perform a task to assure attention, such as counting rare stimuli. However, the P300 response is typically larger in amplitude when the subject listens for (attends to) the oddball (rare) stimulus. The P300 response appears as a large (5 to 20 μvolt) wave, usually the third positive component (P3) in region of 300 ms. As noted below, latency and amplitude of the P300 component can vary tremendously depending on measurement conditions. A P300 response can even, in fact, be produced by the absence of a stimulus (Sutton, Tueting, Zubin, & John, 1967).

HISTORICAL OVERVIEW. | Table 1.2 displayed a chronological summary of major AER developments, including those for the P300 response. The P300 response, and endogenous responses in general, have a long and varied history, dating back at least to the mid-1960s. Hallowell Davis summarized findings of a 1964 paper entitled "Enhancement of Evoked Cortical Potentials in Humans Related to a Task Requiring a Decision" as follows:

> The averaged, slow response evoked by auditory stimuli and recorded from the vertex of the human skull can usually be enhanced by requiring the listener to make a rather difficult auditory discrimination. An easy routine reaction is not effective. (Davis, 1964, p. 182)

In their often-cited early paper on the P300 in 1965, Samuel Sutton, along with colleagues Braren, Zubin, and John, noted that within the previous two to three years no less that six studies had been published on the topic, including the paper by Davis. These papers described the relation among human evoked responses and "such variables as fluctuations of vigilance, direction of attention, distraction, habituation, conditioning, meaningfulness, type of task, and

difficulty of discrimination" (p. 1187). One of the illustrations of responses obtained by Sutton et al. (1965) is reproduced in Figure 1.12. These investigators noted that:

> There are differences between the waveforms evoked by certain and uncertain stimuli in each of the five components which were measured. However, the most dramatic difference is in the large positive deflection whose latency at peak amplitude is about 300 msec. The amplitude of this late positive component was larger for the uncertain stimulus in 36 out of 36 experiments with eight subjects. (Sutton et al., 1965, p. 1187)

They conclude:

> These data and the studies cited indicate that the evoked-potential waveform recorded from scalp of human subjects may reflect two kinds of influences. One of these is largely exogenous and related to the character of the stimulus. The other is largely endogenous and related to the reaction, or attitude, of the subject to the stimulus. The reaction of the subject is at least in part amenable to quantitative experimental manipulation. (Sutton et al., 1965, 1188)

During the mid- to late-1970s, a collection of neurophysiology research groups intensely studied the effects of various measurement conditions on the P300 response and, in addition, explored other endogenous response types (noted above and in Table 1.2). Prominent among the investigators in these groups were J. Desmedt, E. Donchin, J. Ford, D. Goodin, S. Hillyard, A. Pfefferbaum, T. Picton, W. Roth, S. Sutton, and K. Squires. Since then many hundreds of published papers have described P300 measurement with simple and complex stimuli (e.g., tone versus speech), with different stimulus conditions (e.g., one-, two-, or three-stimulus oddball paradigms), and in varying subject attention states (e.g., active versus passive). There is also a substantial literature on the application of the P300 response in evaluating information processing, memory, and attention in diverse patient populations (e.g., those with alcoholism, Alzheimer's disease, and schizophrenia).

The heavy weighting in this book toward exogenous responses, and the P300, was determined by clinical practice and not motivated by philosophic bias, as noted above. The reader interested in more than a cursory awareness of endogenous responses is strongly encouraged to consult the texts listed at the end of this chapter and to survey relevant literature cited in the reference section of this book or obtained by an internet search. Along this line, most articles on endogenous responses are published not in clinical audiology or medical journals but, rather, in journals devoted to neurophysiology, psychology, neuropsychology, and neuroscience. Examples of journals often containing articles on the P300 response include *Cortex, Brain, Psychophysiology, Physiological Psychology, Psychiatric Research, Neuropsychobiology, Progress in Brain Research, Progress in Clinical Neurophysiology, Electroencephalography and Clinical Neurophysiology,* and the highly prestigious journal *Science.*

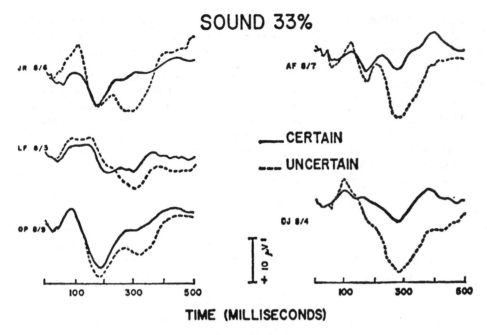

FIGURE 1.12. One of the earliest figures showing P300 waveforms for frequent (certain) versus rare (uncertain) stimuli from five normal subjects, as reported in 1965 by Sutton and colleagues. Positive voltage peaks are plotted downward. For each subject, a large positive peak can be seen in the 300 msec region in the rare, uncertain, but not the certain, condition.

Reprinted from Sutton, S., Braren, M., Zubin, J., & John, E. R. (1965). Evoked potential correlates of stimulus uncertainty. *Science, 150,* 1187–1188. Copyright © 1965 AAAS.

Mismatch Negativity (MMN) Response

In the mid-1970s, Risto Näätänen and colleagues, while investigating aspects of the P300 response with a variation of the conventional oddball stimulus paradigm, described a response to the rare stimulus that was not related to subject attention (Näätänen, Gaillard, & Mäntysalo, 1978). The discovery of the MMN response occurred during experiments conducted during the summer of 1975 at the Institute for Perception TNO in Soesterburg, The Netherlands. Using a dichotic stimulus presentation protocol, subjects in the experiment were instructed to ignore certain tones presented to both ears, and to listen for an oddball or "deviant" stimulus (a tone of a slightly higher frequency or intensity level) in one ear. The researchers observed that both of the deviant sounds, including the unattended sound, produced a negative wave within the 100 to 200 ms region (see Figure 1.13 from Näätänen, Gaillard, & Mäntysalo, 1978). The negativity was most evident when the waveform for the standard stimuli was subtracted from the waveform for the deviant stimulus, referred to as the "difference wave."

As noted by Dr. Näätänen in the original paper on the MMN response (Näätänen et al., 1978),

> . . . it may well be that a physiological mismatch process caused by a sensory input deviating from the memory trace ("template") formed by a frequent "background" stimulus is

such an automatic basic process that it takes place irrespective of the intentions of the experimenter and the subject, perhaps even unmodified by the latter. This view is supported by the fact that the mismatch negativity was similarly observed for both the attended and unattended sides. Hence, we may

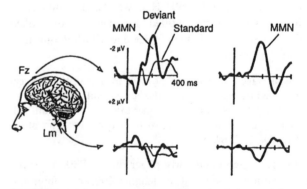

FIGURE 1.13. One of the earliest depictions of the mismatch negativity response (MMN) reported in 1978 by Risto Näätänen and colleagues.

Reprinted from Näätänen, R., Gaillard, A. W. K., & Mäntysalo, S. (1978). Early selective-attention effect on evoked potential reinterpretation. *Acta Psychologica, 42,* 313–329. Copyright © 1978 with permission from Elsevier.

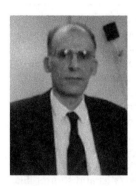

FIGURE 1.14. Dr. Risto Näätänen, who, with Finnish colleagues, first described in 1978 the mismatch negativity response (MMN).

here be dealing with a deviation effect rather than relevance effect, whereas the much larger P300 in the EPs to the attended signals than to the unattended signals certainly represents a relevance effect (pp. 324–325). . . . the mismatch negativity reflects specific auditory stimulus discrimination processes taking place in the auditory primary and association areas. . . . The latter processes are suggested to be largely automatic, beyond the control of will, instructions, etc. . . ." (pp. 326–328).

And, more recently, Dr. Näätänen (see Figure 1.14) adds, "the irrelevant stimulus sequence included deviant stimuli that were physically equivalent to the deviant stimuli (targets) of the attended input sequence" (Näätänen, 1995, p. 6). Information on the MMN response is summarized in Table 1.7. Hundreds of published investigations of the MMN response have subsequently been conducted under Dr. Näätänen's direction in the Cognitive Brain Research Laboratory at the University of Helsinki in Finland. In the thirty plus years since the report of the discovery of the response—appropriately called the mismatch negativity—extensive laboratory and clinical investigations have produced evidence in support of generators in the auditory cortex of the temporal lobe and the frontal lobe, and also contributions from subcortical regions. The MMN is perhaps the most accurate objective measure of auditory processing within the central nervous system. Many hundreds of published studies, perhaps more than a thousand, by various research groups and individual investigators around the world have confirmed that the MMN response can be elicited with a wide range of distinctions among stimulus characteristics and categories including tones, speech and music, and even acoustic cues in speech signals that are not reflected by behavioral measurements (see Schröger, 2005, for a review). The MMN has also been studied in subjects representing the extremes of the age spectrum—newborn infants to aging adults—and in diverse clinical populations, such as patients with auditory processing disorders, learning disabilities, neuropsychiatric diseases, alcoholism, and HIV. Dr. Näätänen's review of the MMN is an excellent source of information on the response, including its research potential and application in multiple clinical populations (Näätänen, 2000).

CLINICAL CONCERNS ABOUT AERs

Around the time that Dawson began his study of averaging techniques for sensory evoked response measurement in human subjects, Geoffrey Tooth, a British colleague, opened an article with the statement:

> Where knowledge of a medical condition is incomplete, there is a danger that the results of ancillary aids, especially when expressed in numerical terms, may acquire an unwarranted appearance of infallibility. (Tooth, 1947)

Such a concern may apply to AERs. There are myriad measurement factors that may conspire to invalidate AER findings. In the measurement process, there is also ample opportunity for technical errors. Even if AERs are recorded optimally and without technical mistakes or mishaps, they must, in most cases, be analyzed and interpreted manually (versus automatically or by computer). This final step in the process introduces the possibility of human error or misjudgment. The simplest and most clear-cut examples of such errors would be normal AERs interpreted as abnormal AERs and vice versa. Unfortunately, AER latency and amplitude data reported numerically and in milliseconds and microvolts can lead to a false sense of security and precision. The problem with reliance on AERs in clinical settings is further confounded by the complex and often poorly understood relation among AER patterns and a multitude of peripheral and central auditory system pathologies and dysfunctions.

Another important issue to consider, and in fact debated in the literature (e.g., Bodis-Wollner, 1985; Chiappa & Young, 1985; Cracco, 1985; Kimura, 1985) is the possibility of "overuse, underuse, or misuse" of AERs clinically. There is a natural tendency, when new technology becomes commercially available, for these misapplications to occur. A sample of quotations offers illustration of such concerns. Cracco, after reviewing various valuable clinical applications of sensory evoked responses in neurodiagnosis of CNS disorders, comments that

> The value and cost-effectiveness of evoked potential monitoring in these procedures [surgical operations of the brain and spinal cord] have not yet been conclusively demonstrated. Despite their usefulness in some situations, there is some controversy concerning the indications for and limitations and possible overuse of evoked potentials in clinical diagnosis. (Cracco, 1985, p. 3490)

In a positive light, Chiappa and Young (1985) comment that:

> Although some of the information these tests [evoked responses] provide is similar to that elicited at the bedside by an experienced clinician, EPs are essential to the modern practice of medicine because they also provide data unobtainable without the use of amplifiers and oscilloscopes, EPs quantify and objectify data that the clinician may sense, EPs can localize lesions within a long sensory pathway, and EPs may be more

TABLE 1.7 Summary of Information on the Mismatch Negativity (MMN) Response

History

- Näätänen, Gaillard, and Mäntysalo discovered the MMN response in 1978.
- Dr. Risto Näätänen and colleagues at the Cognitive Brain Research Unit at the University of Helsinki in Finland have since published the findings of hundreds of investigations of the MMN response in normal subjects and a wide range of patient populations.
- Dozens of Dr. Näätänen's former students and research fellows have gone on to conduct MMN studies around the world.
- Many other research centers in Europe, North America, Asia, and Australia are actively and prolifically producing original data on the MMN response, including findings with various permutations of speech stimuli and studies documenting response the effect of training and intervention electrophysiologically with the MMN.

Components

- The MMN response is a broad negative voltage wave occurring in the latency region of 100 to 300 ms, with amplitude of about 1 μV. It is typically derived as a difference waveform by subtracting the waveform elicited by standard stimuli from the waveform elicited by deviant stimuli.
- In recording the MMN response, it is important to minimize the potential influence (contamination) by other auditory evoked response waves or subcomponents within the same general latency region (e.g., N1, N2, P300).
- The MMN reflects automatic preattentive (preconscious) processing of auditory stimuli and cognitive processes such as sensory memory.
- The MMN is an objective and electrophysiologic index of "stimulus-feature representations in auditory sensory memory" (Näätänen, 1992).

Anatomy

- Generators of the MMN are widespread and include structures in the primary and secondary auditory cortex within the temporal lobe in each cerebral hemisphere.
- Frontal lobe activity also contributes importantly to generation of the MMN response.
- There are age-related (developmental) differences in the anatomic origins and topographic distribution of the MMN response.
- MMN response reflects activity in the cerebral hemispheres evoked by speech and nonspeech stimulation. Speech stimuli tend to generate more activity in the left hemisphere.

Stimulation

- The MMN response is evoked by deviant stimuli—that is, unpredictable—infrequent acoustic stimuli presented randomly, usually with a probability of < 10 percent in an "oddball" test paradigm, after a sensory memory trace is established by standard frequently occurring stimuli.
- A wide variety of stimuli can effectively elicit the MMN response, ranging from simple differences between to pure-tone frequencies, durations, or intensities, to complex tonal patterns, music, and speech sounds (e.g., phonemes, syllables, and words).
- The MMN is best elicited, and differentiated from the P300 response, by the reliance on small or "fine" differences between standard and deviant stimuli.
- The effect of stimulus rate and interstimulus interval (ISI) on the MMN is in contrast the effect of these related variables on other late latency responses. That is, slower rates and longer ISIs are associated with larger amplitudes for most responses (e.g., the ALR), whereas due to immediate memory constraints the MMN response is more robust with faster rates and shorter ISIs.

Acquisition

- Acquisition factors are similar to those for the ALR and the P300 response (see Chapters 12 and 13).
- Recommended electrode locations for recording the MMN generally include two or three on the midline (e.g., Fz, Cz, and Pz), one electrode over each cerebral hemisphere (e.g., F3 and F4), and inverting electrodes ear the ear (e.g., ear lobe or mastoid). These electrode locations are appropriate at the MMN has fronto-central scalp distribution.
- An analysis time of 500 ms or less is adequate since the MMN occurs usually within the first 300 ms after stimulation.
- Filter settings can be rather restrictive and still encompass the MMN, as spectral energy is mostly in the frequency region of 1 to 25 Hz.

Important Factors

- Subject attention to stimuli is not important, in fact undesirable, in MMN measurement.
- Generation of the MMN response is determined by a person's discrimination of small differences between repetitive sounds that are on the same order as behavioral discrimination thresholds.

Clinical Applications

- Electrophysiological assessment of higher level auditory processing, including speech and music perception, and developmental changes in processing.
- Documentation of the effectiveness of medical and nonmedical management for different disorders, e.g., ADHD and auditory processing disorders (APD).
- Electrophysiological documentation of central auditory nervous system plasticity in language, including learning of a second or foreign language.
- Hundreds of publications describe clinical investigations of the MMN for a variety of neuropsychiatric disorders (e.g., schizophrenia, Alzheimer's disease, Parkinson's disease), neurodegenerative diseases, alcoholism, traumatic brain injury, aphasia, and dyslexia.

Clinical Limitations

- Routine clinical application of the MMN response is hampered by problems in identification due to small amplitude of the MMN wave and modest signal-to-noise ratio, imprecise latency calculations, relatively poor reliability, and undefined sensitivity and specificity for major clinical entities.

"efficient" and "cost-effective" because the time consuming testing itself is usually done by paramedical personnel. . . ." (p. 76)

However, there are those who have openly questioned or even condemned the clinical application of evoked responses on the grounds that they contribute little or no nonredundant clinical information, that they are "lucrative" procedures adding unnecessary patient cost, and that indications for use are poorly defined (Eisen & Cracco, 1983). Kimura (1985) adds:

The flaws in current [evoked response] practice are multitude and include such fundamental matters as the lack of technical knowledge, limited expertise in interpretation, and the absence of appropriate control values for comparison. The test is often conducted without due regard to the rigorous criteria required of any diagnostic procedure. Substandard techniques may actually be preferred in a busy practice since nonadherence to rigid rules is a major time-saving maneuver. The most disturbing fact, however, relates to the overuse of EP without a specific clinical indication. (p. 78)

Kimura goes on to note that:

Distinction must be made between the diagnostic and investigative use of EP. One need not resort to EP testing if the disease entity is already clinically known, even though such studies contribute to elucidating the nature of the disease. . . . Even with unequivocal EP abnormalities, clinical localization of lesions based on this test requires extreme care because the neuroanatomic substrates of the various peaks are still unknown. The concepts of EP are not new, but recent evolution of the technique and its popularity, together with its profitability, are forcing many clinicians to perform the test without proper training or experience."(p. 79)

Concluding, Kimura (1985) states:

Abuse and misuse are common with any new diagnostic procedures. The problem, however, is particularly acute in EP studies that have become routine before their time, while the technique is still evolving very rapidly. (p. 79)

These sentiments clearly imply that auditory evoked responses, while unquestionably a major step forward in auditory and neurologic diagnosis, require continued basic and clinical investigation and judicious clinical application. The concerns remain valid more than twenty years later and now may apply also to other auditory evoked responses, such as the ASSR and the MMN response.

TEXTBOOKS AND MONOGRAPHS ON AUDITORY EVOKED RESPONSES

General

Aminoff MJ (ed). (1980). *Electrodiagnosis in clinical neurology.* New York: Churchill-Livington.

Chiappa R (1983). *Evoked potentials in clinical medicine.* New York: Raven Press.

Chiarenza GA, Papakostopoulos D (eds). (1982). *Clinical applications of cerebral evoked potentials in pediatric medicine.* Amsterdam: Excerpta Medica.

Courjon J, Mauguiere F, Revol M (eds). (1982). Clinical applications of evoked potentials in neurology. *Advances in Neurology 32.* New York: Raven Press.

Davis H (1976). Principles of electric response audiometry. *The Annals of Otology, Rhinology & Laryngology 85* (supplement 28).

Goldstein R, Aldrich WM (1998). Evoked potential audiometry: Fundamentals and applications. Boston, MA: Allyn and Bacon.

Halliday AM (ed). (1982). *Evoked potentials in clinical testing.* London: Churchill Livingstone.

Malhotra A (1997). *Auditory evoked responses in clinical practice.* Berlin: Springer-Verlag.

Naunton, RF, & Fernandez C (eds). (1978). *Evoked electrical activity in the auditory nervous system.* New York: Academic Press.

Nuwer MR (1986). *Evoked potential monitoring in the operating room.* New York: Raven Press.

Nodar RH, Barber C (eds). (1984). *Evoked potentials II. The Second International Evoked Potentials Symposium.* Boston: Butterworth Publishers.

Owen JH, Davis H (eds). (1985) *Evoked potential testing: Clinical applications.* Orlando, FL: Grune & Stratton.

Spehlmann R (1985). *Evoked response primer: Visual, auditory, and somatosensory evoked potentials in clinical diagnosis.* Boston: Butterworth Publishers.

Stalberg E, & Young RR (eds). (1981). *Neurology I: Clinical neurophysiology.* London: Butterworth Publishers.

Whipple HE (ed). (1984). Sensory evoked response in man. *Annals of the New York Academy of Sciences 112: 1–546.*

Electrocochleography (ECochG)

Ruben RJ, Elberling C, & Salomon G (eds). (1976). *Electrocochleography.* Baltimore: University Park Press.

Auditory Brainstem Response (ABR)

Hood LJ (1998). *Clinical applications of the auditory brainstem response.* San Diego: Singular.

Hood LJ, Berlin CI (1986). *Auditory evoked potentials.* Austin TX: Pro-Ed.

Jacobson JT (ed). (1985). *The auditory brainstem response.* San Diego: College-Hill Press.

Lundborg T (ed). (1981). Scandinavian Symposium of Brain Stem Response (ABR). *Scandinavian audiology (Supplement 13).*

Moore E (ed). (1984). *Bases of brainstem auditory evoked responses.* New York: Academic Press.

Newman-Ryan J (2000). *Auditory brainstem evoked potentials. Laboratory exercises and clinical manual.* Boston, MA: Allyn and Bacon.

Worthington DW (guest ed.). (1988). Auditory evoked response measurements in children. *Seminars in Hearing 9.*

Cortical and Event-Related Responses

Callaway E, Tueting P, Koslow SH (eds.) (1978). *Brain event-related brain potentials in man.* New York: Academic Press.

Cohen J, Karrer R, Tueting P (eds). (1984). *Proceedings of the 6th international conference on event-related slow potentials of the brain.* New York: New York Academy of Sciences.

Desmedt JE (ed). (1977). *Cerebral ERPs.* Basel: Karger.

Donchin E, Lindsley DB (eds). (1969). *Average evoked potentials: Methods, results and evaluations.* NASA SP-191. Washington, DC: Government Printing Office.

Gazzaniga MS (ed). (1995). *The cognitive neurosciences.* Cambridge MA: MIT Press.

Handy TC (2005). *Event-related potentials: A methods handbook.* Cambridge MA: The MIT Press.

Karrer, R, Cohen J, Tueting P (eds). (1984). Brain and information: Event-related potentials. *New York Academy of Science 425*: 1984.

Kornhuber, HH, Deeke L (eds). (1980). Motivation, motor and sensory processes of the brain: Electrical potentials, behavior and clinical use. *Progress in brain research 54:* 1980.

Lehmann D, Callaway E (eds). (1979). *Event-related potentials in man: Applications and problems.* New York: Plenum Press.

McCallum WC, Knott JR (eds). (1973). Event-related slow potentials of the brain: Their relations to behavior. *Electroencephalography and clinical neurophysiology, supplement 33:* 1973.

McPherson DL (1995). *Late potentials of the auditory system.* San Diego: Singular.

Otto DA (ed). (1978). *Multidisciplinary perspectives in event-related brain potential research.* EPA-600/9-77-043. Washington, DC: U.S. Environmental Protection Agency.

Picton TW (ed). (1988). *Handbook of electroencephalography and clinical neurophysiology.* Volume 3: Amsterdam: Elsevier.

Reneau J, Hnatiow G (1975). *Evoked response audiometry: A topical and historical review.* Baltimore: University Park Press.

Rugg MD, Coles MGH (eds). (1995). *Electrophysiology of mind: Event-related brain potentials and cognition.* New York: Oxford University Press.

Zani A, Proverbio AM (eds). (2003). *The cognitive electrophysiology of mind and brain.* New York: Academic Press.

2 CHAPTER

Anatomy and Physiology Principles of Auditory Evoked Responses

Anatomic and physiologic bases of AERs are reviewed in this chapter. The discussion begins with a summary of neurophysiologic properties important in generation of near-field and far-field evoked responses. Then, anatomy of the auditory system contributing to AERs, from ECochG to the MMN response, is summarized. The chapter does not introduce principles of neuroscience, nor provide a comprehensive review of anatomy and physiology of the auditory system, even though such information is important for successful clinical application of AERs. Within the confines of this book, such a discussion would be superficial and inadequate.

GENERAL CENTRAL NERVOUS SYSTEM (CNS) ANATOMY AND PHYSIOLOGY

Principles of Neurophysiology

The distribution of current flow in the extracellular (extraneuronal) space is a potential field. The transmembrane ionic current flow of the cell, in the case of evoked responses the neuron, is the origin of voltage potentials that underlie AERs. Transmembrane current flow can be associated with an action potential that travels along an axon of a neuron or with synaptic activity between two or more neurons. Current flow into one portion of the cell creates depolarization and is related to a negative charge potential in the nearby extracellular region, often termed the current "sink." This current inflow is balanced by current outflow at another portion of the cell, which is related to a positive voltage potential. The resulting electrical field with a negative polarity at one end and a positive polarity at the other end is called a *dipole*. A positive potential, therefore, forms the leading edge of propagated neuronal activity, that is, neuronal transmission. Following activation of the sensory organ, the cochlea for AERs, such sequential transmembrane current flow evoked by the stimulus occurs in neurons in a peripheral to central direction, i.e., from the ear to the cerebral cortex.

The concept of *volume conduction* is important in understanding the neuroanatomy and neurophysiology underlying AERs and sensory evoked responses in general. Responses arising from anatomic pathways deep within the brain are conducted to rather distant electrodes through a complex media consisting of diverse substances, including fluids, brain tissue, bone, and skin. A number of factors contribute to and affect the surface-recorded, volume-conducted AER. One factor in detecting volume-conducted AERs is the location of recording electrodes relative to the electrical field or dipole. Evoked responses recorded by electrodes close to or within the potential field, as in intracranial depth electrode studies (e.g., Lee et al., 1984; Møller, 1981), are called *near-field* responses. Evoked responses detected at a relatively great distance from the source, such as the scalp-recorded ABR, are *far-field* responses. Increasing the distance between the recording electrodes and the voltage source has two major effects on the volume-conducted evoked response. First, spatial resolution is reduced, as illustrated in Figure 2.1. As depicted in the top portion of the figure, the evoked response waveform from a single electrode on the scalp and distance from a dipole generator yields a broad less distinct waveform, whereas the wave recorded from an electrode closer to the electrical field is sharper. Also, a response recorded at some distance from two intracranial sources (dipoles) appears to consist of a single wave component (lower portion of the figure). The individual contribution of each dipole cannot be distinguished. With an electrode located closer to the two electrical fields, the waveform is resolved into two distinct peaks (one for each dipole).

The second effect of increased distance between recording electrode and voltage source is a dramatic reduction in response amplitude. This is shown diagrammatically in Figure 2.2, highlighting the major distinction between near- versus far-field responses. Amplitude of near-field responses is large, but decreases sharply when the electrode is moved even a small distance (a centimeter or less) from the generator (dipole). In contrast, amplitude of far-field responses is

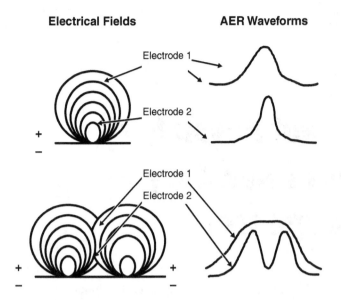

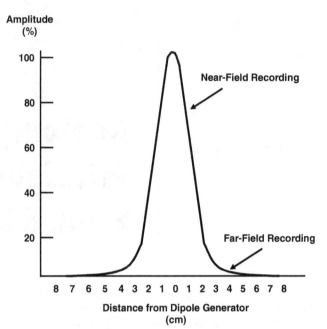

FIGURE 2.1. Reduction in the spatial resolution or precision of evoked responses recorded with far-field techniques in detecting and representing underlying neuronal activity. Electrical fields are illustrated in the left portion of the figure. Hypothetical AER waveforms recorded from two sites in one electric field are shown in the top portion of the figure, and waveforms recorded from two sites within two adjacent electric fields are shown in the bottom portion of the figure.
Adapted from Wood & Allison, 1981.

FIGURE 2.2. Comparison of the effect of electrode distance from the generator for an auditory evoked response amplitude when recorded with near-field versus far-field electrode techniques.
Adapted from Allison, 1968, cited in Wood & Allison, 1981.

very small, but doesn't change appreciably with large alterations in electrode location. The generators (dipoles) of AERs are located within the skull, either within the temporal bone or the cranium. Clinically, however, most AERs are recorded with far-field techniques, that is, with electrodes located outside of the skull (extracranially), and usually at the scalp. Two exceptions this rule are during intraoperative monitoring, when recording electrodes may be placed, for example, directly on the eighth cranial nerve and during transtympanic membrane ECochG, when a recording electrode may be placed on the promontory. The promontory, a landmark on the medial wall of the middle ear consisting of the bone between the middle ear space and cochlea, is only millimeters from the generators of the ECochG.

The geometric orientation of the activated neurons also exerts an important influence on volume conduction. Over fifty years ago, Lorente de No (1947) noted that synchronous depolarization of a group of neurons that are oriented in the same direction produces an enhanced electrical field (dipole) that can be detected a relatively great distance, whereas with cells that are oriented in different directions, there may be cancellation of electrical fields. Figure 2.3 illustrates this arrangement of cell bodies that are in a line and the axons that are parallel. Lorente de No (1947) referred to these as *open* and *closed* potential fields. The orientation of fiber tracts,

and of the dendrites within nuclei, plays an important role in the generation of far-field responses. In fact, with the closed field neuron orientation, it is conceivable that a sensory stimulus could evoke neuronal activity that is not measurable by volume conduction.

The spatial and temporal characteristics of the current flow for individual neurons also play a role in generation of evoked responses. Evoked responses are directly dependent on temporal synchronization of neuronal activity. AERs are optimally generated by action potentials or synaptic potentials arising almost simultaneously from many neurons within a specific anatomic region. When transmembrane current flow occurs in a very restricted part of the neuron, spatial summation of extracellular potential fields from many neurons is less likely. Similarly, when transmembrane current flow produces a rapid transient voltage potential, the likelihood of temporal summation of extracellular potential fields (synchronous activity among neurons) is reduced. Consequently, volume-conducted evoked responses are greatest for neurons with relatively widespread and extended duration changes in voltage. Spatial and temporal characteristics apply to transmembrane neuronal activity in the region of the cell body (i.e., synaptic transmission), but are not important for propagation of action potentials along long axons.

Finally, neurons can be differentiated on the basis of structure and function. In the eighth cranial nerve and pontine auditory brainstem, for example, there are at least five types of neurons, each with its own distinctive appearance

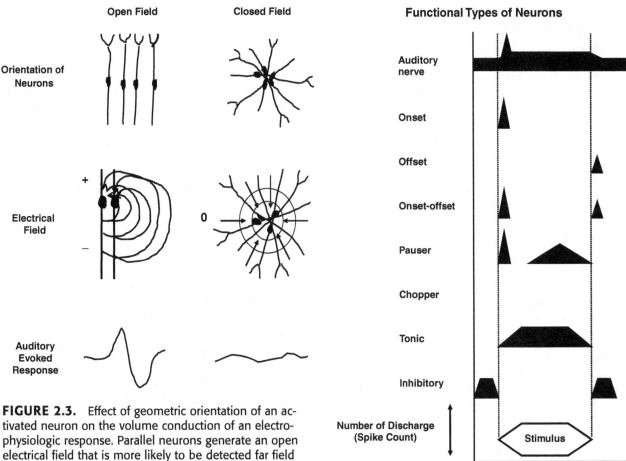

FIGURE 2.3. Effect of geometric orientation of an activated neuron on the volume conduction of an electrophysiologic response. Parallel neurons generate an open electrical field that is more likely to be detected far field as an auditory evoked response (bottom left portion of the figure) than the neuron orientation producing a closed field (bottom right portion of figure).
Adapted from Wood & Allison, 1981.

(e.g., pyramidal, octopus, globular, stellate, and spherical or bushy) and, respectively, its own response pattern (e.g., pauser, onset, primary-like with notch, chopper, primary-like). Types of neurons categorized on the basis of function, i.e., the pattern of response (firing) to acoustic stimuli, are illustrated in Figure 2.4. Whether different AER components are effectively evoked by different subpopulations of neurons is not known. Also, the relationship between structural types (shape) and functional types (response) of neurons is not clear.

In summary, evoked responses actually reflect electrical potential fields that consist of summated transmembrane electrical activity for thousands of neurons, located in nerve fiber tracts or CNS nuclei. In general, the greater the number of neurons contributing to the potential field, the larger the amplitude of the AER, although other factors cited here certainly qualify this statement. Sensory evoked responses have, to a large extent, rapidly been accepted as a routine clinical procedure because they can be successfully recorded noninvasively, that is, without placing a needle or catheter into the body. For AERs to be detected clinically, electrical current

FIGURE 2.4. Different types of neurons in the auditory system according to their response characteristics (i.e., functional types) following acoustic stimulation. The response pattern of neurons in the auditory system following acoustic stimulation, also known as "histograms" in reference to the firing rate of nerve fibers, is indicated by the black shapes.
Adapted from Kiang, 1975; Musiek & Baran, 1986.

must be conducted (must flow) from its intracranial neural voltage source(s), the generator site of the response, through a volume consisting of brain tissue and interstitial fluid, and across a skull and skin barrier to surface electrodes located on the scalp.

ANATOMY AND PHYSIOLOGY OF THE AUDITORY SYSTEM

The following cursory review pertains mainly to the anatomical and physiological bases of human AERs. The auditory system, peripheral and central, is an extremely complex sensory system that remains inadequately understood. At least seven features contribute to this complexity:

1. Cochlear physiology is a complicated interaction between metabolic and biomechanical properties of the cochlea.

2. Major auditory system nuclei, such as the cochlear nuclei, olivary nuclei, and inferior colliculus, are structurally complex, each consisting of numerous subdivisions.

3. There are varied relations between structural and functional neuron types (e.g., stellate and chopper, bushy [spherical] and primary-like, octopus and onset).

4. The number of neurons and potential synapses between neurons increases geometrically from the eighth nerve (approximately 30,000 fibers) to auditory cortex (over 10 million neurons).

5. Multiple decussations, or midline crossings, of fiber tracts connect the right and left sides of the brainstem and cortex.

6. The afferent auditory system has components within the reticular activating system.

7. The efferent (descending) auditory system can influence function of the afferent (ascending) auditory system.

A brief review of auditory system anatomy and physiology would necessarily be superficial and simplistic. However, an understanding of the structure and function of the auditory system is an essential prerequisite for successful clinical and experimental AER measurement and interpretation. At the least, the clinician must appreciate principles of anatomy and physiology for the middle ear; cochlea and eighth nerve (sensorineural apparatus); afferent and efferent brainstem pathways and centers; thalamus, corpus callosum fibers; and primary, secondary, and tertiary auditory cortical regions. For supplemental reading, which is strongly advised, the reader is referred to numerous introductory and advanced texts on general neurophysiology and, specifically, auditory system structure and function. The Internet, of course, also offers ready access to a wealth of information on the neuroscience of auditory function. Information found on websites for universities with hearing research centers is particularly relevant and often includes figures of important anatomic structures and even simulations of essential auditory functions.

ECochG

The ECochG consists of two sound-evoked cochlear potentials and the compound eighth (auditory) cranial nerve action potential. The location of the cochlea and eighth nerve within the temporal bone is illustrated in Figure 2.5. Important structures within the cochlea, including the inner and outer hair cells, are enlarged on the right side of Figure 2.5. ECochG potentials are the cochlear microphonic (CM) and summating potential (SP). The CM was first recorded by Wever and Bray in classic auditory neurophysiology experiments over fifty years ago (Wever & Bray, 1930) and has been studied extensively since then (history of AERs is re-

viewed in Chapter 1). The CM is an alternating current (AC) potential that follows the waveform of the stimulus and the vibrations of the basilar membrane, hence the term *microphonic*. A pure tone stimulus, for example, produces a CM that appears as a sine wave of the same frequency. In fact, in the initial classic Wever and Bray (1930) experiment, speech was presented to the experimental animal while an electrode was placed within the auditory nerve and the resulting electrical activity, when transduced (converted) back to sound and amplified, was transmitted as clear speech. The CM has no latency, since it begins with the stimulus. The CM arises from hair cells and, in the normal cochlea at least, mainly from outer hair cells (Dallos, 1973; Sellick & Russell, 1980). As recorded from outside the cochlea—for example, from the promontory in the middle ear or from an electrode in the external ear canal—the CM reflects outer hair cell activity in the basal portion of the basilar membrane (Aran & Charlet de Sauvage, 1976; Hoke, 1976; Sohmer, Kinarti, & Gafni, 1980). Mechanisms underlying CM production include velocity or acceleration of hair cell movement, displacement of the basilar membrane, and receptor potential activity generated at the apex of outer hair cells secondary to bending of the stereocilia. Single polarity (rarefaction or condensation) stimuli are most effective for eliciting the CM, whereas alternating these stimulus polarities effectively cancel out the CM. Stimulus factors in ECochG measurement are reviewed in more detail in Chapter 4.

The SP is a DC potential that can be recorded following a continuous tone or a transient acoustic stimulus, such as a click or tone burst. It is a reflection of nonlinear properties of the cochlea. As shown previously in Figure 1.1, and elsewhere in Part I of the book, the SP can be viewed as a shift in the baseline of an ECochG recording, usually occuring in the same direction and just prior to the compound action potential (AP) of the eighth nerve. The precise source of the SP within the cochlea has been questioned since its discovery in the early 1950s. The origin of the SP has been attributed to distortion products associated with irregularities in basilar membrane and hair cell displacement, subsequent generation of electrical current (Eldredge, 1974; Whitfield & Ross, 1965), and to both inner and outer hair cell activity (Dallos, 1973). Durrant and colleagues (Durrant, Wang, Ding, & Salvi, 1998) concluded that the inner hair cells primarily generate the SP. These authors showed that carboplatin administered to chinchilla caused severe damage to inner hair cells and eliminated most of the direct current (DC) potential that corresponds to the SP. Outer hair cells, at low intensity levels, contribute to inner hair cell activation and may, therefore, also play a role in the generation of the SP component (Wuyts et al., 2001). The SP, unlike the AP, is clearly observed even with extremely rapid stimulation and is relatively more prominent when recorded with a high-frequency tone burst stimulus than other types of stimuli. Within recent years, there has been increased interest in the application of tone burst signals for generation of ECochG components, es-

ANATOMY OF THE HUMAN EAR

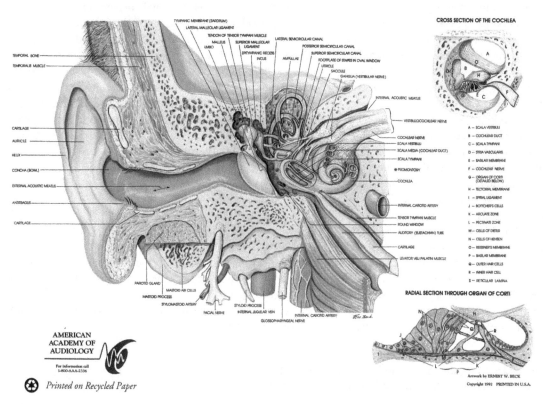

FIGURE 2.5.   A schematic representation of the peripheral auditory system, including outer ear, middle ear, cochlea (inner ear), and distal portion of the eighth cranial nerve. Expanded views of the scala within the cochlea and the organ of Corti are shown in the right portion of the figure.
Courtesy of the American Academy of Audiology.

pecially in certain clinical populations, e.g., endolymphatic hydrops. The literature on ECochG measurement with tone bursts, and the application of this technique in clinical populations, is reviewed in Chapters 4 and 5.

The AP component of the ECochG waveform is the far-field representation of the compound action potential of the eighth (auditory) cranial nerve. The AP component, also referred to as N1, is the same as the ABR wave I. However, with an electrode array sometimes used in ECochG the AP is recorded with negative (N) electrical polarity and is plotted downward-going (see Chapter 4 for more discussion). Since the AP reflects synchronous firing of many eighth nerve fibers, amplitude is largest for transient stimuli with abrupt and rapid rise times, such as clicks. AP amplitude also increases, and latency decreases, with increased stimulus intensity. The intensity-related increase in amplitude is due to an increase in the number of eighth nerve fibers contributing to the response, that is, there is more neuroelectric activity summating at essentially the same time. Other important factors affecting AP latency and amplitude changes as a function of stimulus intensity include synaptic properties of the

hair cells—for example the rate of excitatory post-synaptic potentials, or EPSPs (e.g., Møller, 1983; Pickles, 1988). The intensity-related decrease in AP latency is thought to reflect a more basal origin of cochlear activity as the basilar membrane traveling wave for higher intensities extends in that direction.

A second wave, labeled N2 (or P2 if plotted with positive upward), is sometimes noted in discussions of ECochG. There are two apparently conflicting theories on the origin of N2. Based on study of derived (frequency specific) ECochG, the AP (N1) reflects eighth nerve firing due to activity in the basal (first turn or high-frequency) portion of the cochlea and N2 reflects eighth nerve firing due to activity in more apical (second turn or lower frequency) regions of the cochlea (Eggermont, 1976b; Elberling, 1976). Stimulus intensity is an important factor in these theories on the AP (N1) versus N2 generators. High-intensity stimuli produce mostly basal cochlear activity, whereas low-intensity stimuli may also activate lower frequency (second turn) portions of the cochlea (Yoshie, 1976). It is generally agreed that AP (N1) component amplitude decreases directly with intensity, but according to some authors, N2 component amplitude increases as stimulus intensity decreases, and at very low intensities only the N2 component is present (Gibson, 1978). Latencies for both components increase as intensity decreases. The effect of intensity on ECochG is discussed in greater detail in Chapter 4. For click stimuli at high intensity levels, at least, this N2 component is probably equivalent to ABR wave II, and therefore its anatomy will be discussed in the following section.

The velocity of the traveling wave on the basilar membrane is considerably faster in the basal turn (20 meters/sec for a frequency of 10,000 Hz) than in the apical turn (2 meters/sec at 500 Hz). In the apical region of the cochlea, traveling wave velocity is inadequate to produce synchronous firing of associated eighth nerve afferent fibers. The traveling wave requires approximately 2 ms for transit from the 10,000 Hz region to the 500 Hz region (Békésy, 1960; Borg, 1981a; Elberling, 1976; Ozdamar & Dallos, 1976; Parker & Thornton, 1978; Zwislocki, 1975). Manipulation of a stimulus parameter that results in more basalward cochlear activation, such as increasing the frequency or intensity, will therefore decrease response latency of the AP component. For tone burst stimuli (versus clicks), the decrease in latency

with increased intensity is, based on animal experiments (Møller, 1983), most pronounced for relatively low frequencies (e.g., 2000 Hz) and minimal for very high frequencies (e.g., 20,000 Hz). Anatomical structures and regions contributing to generation of the ECochG, and other AERs, are summarized in Table 2.1. There are other potentials within the cochlea, referred to as standing or resting potentials, that are present continuously in the ear and are not evoked by acoustic stimuli. The major direct current (DC) electrical potential is the endocochlear potential (Békésy, 1960; Dallos, 1973; Møller, 1983; Pickles, 1988), which appears to depend on activity within the stria vascularis.

ABR

Available information on anatomic and physiologic underpinnings of the ABR is based comes from at least five different sources:

1. Associations between surgically induced CNS lesions and ABR findings in experimental animals (most commonly cat and rat).
2. Associations between clinically confirmed brain pathology and ABR findings in man.

TABLE 2.1. Summary of Anatomic Regions Contributing to Auditory Evoked Response (AER) Components and Major Sources of Blood Supply for These Regions

AER	ANATOMY	BLOOD SUPPLY
ECochG		
CM	Outer hair cells	Vertebrobasilar artery, AICA, internal auditory artery
SP	Inner hair cells	[same]
AP	Distal eighth nerve	[same]
ABR		
I	Distal eighth nerve	[same]
III	Cochlear nucleus, trapezoid body, superior olivary complex	Vertebrobasilar artery, complex para-median arteries
V	Lateral lemniscus termination in inferior colliculus	
SN10	Inferior colliculus	Posterior cerebral artery
ASSR		
	Brainstem (fast modulation rate)	
	Cortex (slow modulation rate)	
AMLR		
Na	Thalamus ?	
Pa	Auditory radiation fibers	Internal carotid artery
	Primary auditory cortex	Middle cerebral artery
ALR		
N1	Auditory cortex (posterior superior temporal gyrus)	[same]
P2	?	
P300		
	Hippocampus	Vertebrobasilar artery
	Auditory cortex	Middle cerebral artery
MMN		
	Auditory cortex	Middle cerebral artery

3. Analyses of single neural unit and averaged evoked responses recorded directly from localized auditory structures in experimental animals.
4. Analyses of surface-recorded ABR waveforms with different electrode locations and arrays in humans.
5. Analyses of averaged evoked responses recorded directly with depth electrodes from specified regions of the auditory system in humans during neurosurgical procedures.

Valuable insights as to the anatomic and physiologic bases of the ABR have been gleaned from each of these approaches. Animal findings, in fact, formed the basis for the speculation on anatomy underlying ABR until the early 1980s. Important differences in auditory CNS anatomy in man versus animal models (especially small animals such as guinea pig and even cat) are now well appreciated (Møller, 1985; Moore, 1987a,b). In an excellent review article, Moore (1987a) contrasts auditory brainstem anatomy for humans versus other mammals. Because of these interspecies anatomical differences, information from depth electrode recordings in humans with normal auditory CNS status and, to a lesser extent, correlations among documented brain pathophysiologic processes and ABR findings in humans, are most pertinent for clinical application of ABR.

NORMAL ANATOMY AND PHYSIOLOGY. | Information on the anatomic origins of the ABR is less precise and more conflicting for later components (waves III, IV, V, VI) than for the earlier components (waves I and II). In their classic clinical studies of the ABR, Sohmer and Feinmesser (1967) and Jewett and Williston (1971) confidently attributed wave I to eighth nerve compound action potential activity, but refrained from speculating on the specific neural origins of other ABR components. Rather, with appropriate caution Sohmer and Feinmesser (1967) stated "the succeeding negative peaks, which are also observed in recordings in animals, may be due to repetitive firing of auditory nerve fibers . . . or may be due to the discharge of neurons in brain stem auditory nuclei (which, like N1 and N2 components, reach the recording site by volume conduction)" (p. 434) and Jewett and Williston (1971) noted, "later waves are undoubtedly composites from multiple generators both ascending and descending in algebraic summation" (p. 692).

Despite the caveats expressed by these early investigators, a clinically appealing yet overly simplistic anatomic schema for the ABR soon appeared repeatedly in the literature. The inaccurate schema, often presented in the form of a diagram, associated a single structure or region in the ascending auditory system with each successive major ABR component, as follows: wave I, eighth (auditory) cranial nerve; wave II, cochlear nuclei; wave III, superior olivary complex; wave IV, nucleus of the lateral lemniscus; wave V, inferior colliculus; wave VI, medial geniculate body of thalamus. This incorrect information on the anatomical

generators of the ABR is perpetuated among physicians-in-training by the clever, but wrong, mnemonic ECOLI. In a large measure, this representation of ABR generators was inferred from analyses of ABR abnormalities in small animals with experimental lesions (Buchwald & Huang, 1975; Huang & Buchwald, 1978; Lev & Sohmer, 1972). However, there are, in the human brainstem, numerous examples of auditory cell groups and nuclei that are smaller, or not even observed, when compared to brainstem anatomy of lower animals, such as cat (Moore, 1987a,b). A major auditory brainstem center in an animal, giving rise to a prominent ABR component, may in the human brainstem not be of sufficient size to generate a detectable ABR component. There are important differences in anatomic dimensions between small animals and humans even for the auditory nerve. The length of the auditory nerve, for example, is approximately 2.6 cm (26 mm) in an adult human, but only 8 mm long in cat (Møller et al., 1995). As Møller (1985; Møller, Jhon, Yokota, & Jannetta, 1995) points out, distinct differences in auditory neuroanatomy between man and typical small experimental animals (rat, cat, guinea pig) severely limit any hypotheses regarding ABR component generators that are based on these studies.

There are at least two other factors influencing traditional inferences on the anatomic bases of ABR. Most clinical studies correlating ABR findings to underlying brain pathology have a technical limitation related to electrode placement. The conventional differential recording arrangement, with one electrode on the vertex and the other on the mastoid, may produce results that are not equivalent to those recorded with a true reference electrode located, for example, at a noncephalic (neutral or inactive) site. This latter recording approach is more appropriate for inference of the neural generators of AERs (Møller, 1985). Also, the propensity for reducing a potentially complex relationship among ABR wave components and auditory anatomy to a clinically useful schema is understandable, but the schema is not compatible with the concept of volume conduction of far-field potentials from spatially compact neuroanatomic structures in the human brainstem (refer back to Figure 2.3). In fact, the anatomy of the ABR is rather complex. Multiple anatomic sites may contribute to a single ABR wave and, conversely, a single anatomic site may generate multiple ABR waves. Without doubt, the most accurate information available on the anatomic origins of the ABR in humans derives from intracranial measurements using near-field techniques (electrodes close to the dipole generators of the response). What, then, do we know about the generators of the five major ABR components?

Wave I. The anatomic origin of the first component of the ABR waveform is clearly defined. The ABR wave I component is the far-field representation of the compound action potential in the distal portion of the eighth nerve, that is, afferent activity of eighth nerve fibers as they leave the

Auditory Pathways

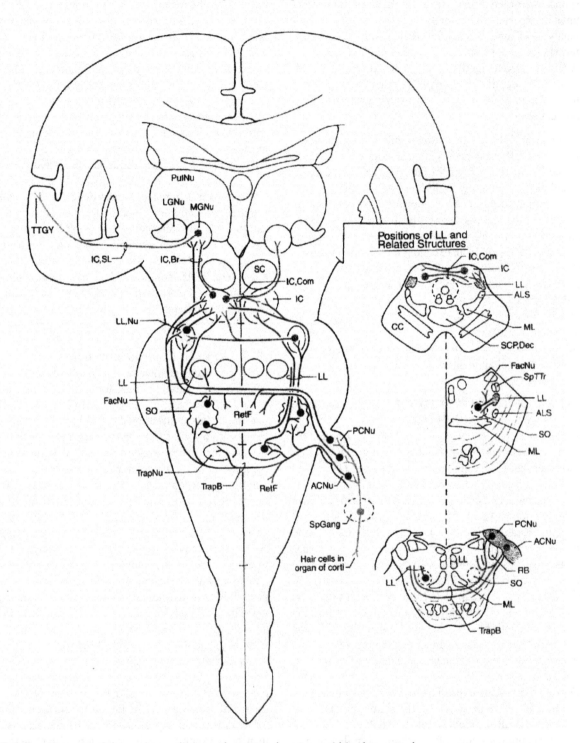

FIGURE 2.6. Diagram of the major auditory pathways and centers within the central nervous system. Abbreviations shown in the figure are defined in Table 2.2.

cochlea and enter the internal auditory canal. The relationship between anatomy and the ABR is shown in a highly schematic fashion in Figures 2.6 and 2.7. The unequivocally accurate statement that ABR wave I arises from the auditory nerve is based on evidence from direct recordings of eighth nerve potentials in man by numerous investigators (Hashimoto, Ishiyama, Hoshimoto, & Nemoto, 1981; Møller & Jannetta, 1981, 1989, 1983a,b; Møller, Jannetta,

TABLE 2.2. Abbreviations of Terms Used in Referring to Auditory System Anatomy (arranged alphabetically), Neurochemistry, and Blood Supply

TERM	DEFINITION	TERM	DEFINITION
Anatomy		PC	paracentral nuclei
		PVCN	posterior ventral cochlear nucleus
AC	auditory cortex	RF	reticular formation (also, RAF = reticular
A I	primary auditory cortex (koniocortex) in		activating system, RAS = reticular activation
	monkey and cat		system, or ARAS = ascending RAS)
A II	secondary auditory cortex in monkey and cat	SG	spiral ganglion
AN	auditory (VIII or eighth) cranial nerve	SH	stria of Held (intermediate acoustic stria)
AR	auditory radiation to cortex	SM	stria of Monakow (dorsal acoustic stria)
AS	acoustic stria	SOC	superior olivary complex
AVCN	anterior ventral cochlear nucleus	STP	superior temporal plane
BIC	brachium of the inferior colliculus	TA	tegmental areas
CANS	central auditory nervous system	TB	trapezoid body
CC	corpus callosum	TBT	trapezoid body tract (also VS = ventral stria)
CIC	commissure of the inferior colliculus	TL	temporal lobe
COCB	crossed olivo-cochlear bundle	UCOCB	uncrossed olivo-cochlear bundle
CN	cochlear nucleus	VCN	ventral cochlear nucleus
CP	commissure of Probst	VMGB	ventral medial geniculate body (of thalamus)
CX	cortex of inferior colliculus		
DAS	dorsal acoustic stria	**Neurochemistry**	
DCLL	dorsal commissure of the lateral lemnisicus		
DCN	dorsal cochlear nucleus	*Excitatory Neurotransmitters*	
DMGB	dorsal medial geniculate body (of thalamus)	ACh	acetylcholine
EP	ectosylvian posterior area	asparate	
GC	Gudden's commissure	glutamate	
HG	Heschl's gyrus	NMDA	N-methyl-D-asparate
IAS	intermediate acoustic stria		
IC	inferior colliculus	*Inhibitory Neurotransmitters*	
INS	insula area	dynorphin	
LL	lateral lemniscus	enkaphalin	
LLD	dorsal nucleus of the lateral lemniscus	GABA	gamma aminobutyric acid
LLV	ventral nucleus of the lateral lemniscus	glycine	
LSO	lateral superior olive		
MCP	middle cerebellar peduncle	**Blood Supply**	
MGB	medial geniculate body (of thalamus)		
MSO	medial superior olive	AICA	anterior inferior cerebellar artery
MTB	medial trapezoid body	IAA	internal auditory artery
MTL	medial temporal lobe	MCA	middle cerebral artery
NLL	nucleus of the lateral lemniscus	PCA	posterior cerebral artery
OCB	olivo-cochlear bundle	PICA	posterior inferior cerebellar artery

& Møller, 1982; Møller, Jho, Yokota, & Jannetta, 1995) and is universally supported by numerous electrocochleographic studies, as noted above in the discussion of the ECochG AP component. A distal eighth nerve generator for ABR wave I is also suggested by 3-channel Lissajous trajectory clinical ABR analysis and by spatio-temporal dipole models (Grandori, 1986; Ino & Mizoi, 1980; Scherg & von Cramon, 1985a,b) and by clinical findings in retrocochlear pathology (Sohmer, Feinmesser, & Szabo, 1974; Starr & Achor, 1975; Starr & Hamilton, 1976; Stockard & Rossiter, 1977). Spatiotemporal dipole modeling of ABR also implies that the negative trough following wave I reflects activity arising from the region of the eighth nerve as it exits the internal

auditory canal at the porus acousticus (Scherg & von Cramon, 1985a,b).

Wave II. According to Møller's intracranial recordings in man, wave II is also generated by the eighth (auditory) nerve (Møller, 1985; Møller & Jannetta, 1982, 1983a,b; Møller, Jannetta, & Møller, 1982; Møller, Jho, Yokota, & Jannetta, 1995). A proximal eighth nerve generator site (the end of the nerve near the brainstem) for wave II is supported by the relationship between the latency of waves I and II and the relatively slow conduction time expected for the auditory nerve (10 to 20 m/sec), which is on the average 25 mm in length (Lang, Happonen, & Salmivalli, 1981)

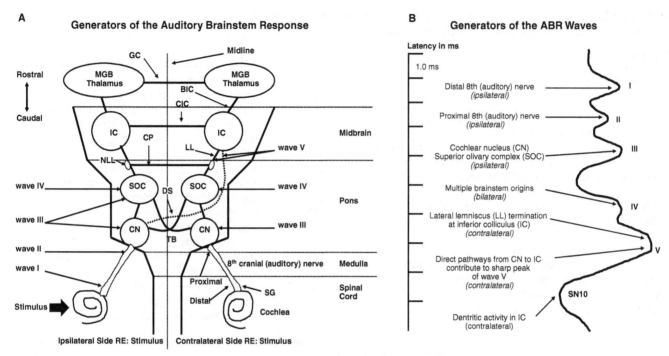

FIGURE 2.7. A. A schematic drawing of the presumed generators of the auditory brainstem response (ABR). Abbreviations are defined in Table 2.2. (Courtesy of the American Academy of Audiology.) B. Auditory brainstem response (ABR) waveform showing presumed anatomic correlations of major peaks. Note that one anatomic structure may give rise to more than one ABR wave, and, conversely, more than one anatomic structure may contribute to a single ABR wave.

with a diameter of approximately 2 to 4 micrometers (μm) in adults (Lazorthes, LaComme, Ganbert, & Planel, 1961). In small children, wave II is not consistently recorded. Møller attributes this observation to shorter eighth nerve length that results in fusion of wave I and wave II. Spatio-temporal dipole studies showed that "wave II appeared to be a result of overlapping activities, predominately from the second peak in the triphasic shape of dipole [for wave] I" (Scherg & Von Cramon, 1985a, p. 295). Based on esti-mations of eighth nerve velocity and synaptic delays, wave II must reflect activity of the first order neuron (i.e., the eighth nerve itself versus the auditory brainstem). A cra-nial nerve origin for wave II in humans is also supported by clinical evidence of the persistence of a reliable wave II in brain death and by intraoperative recordings directly from the eighth nerve at the root entry zone, as it enters the brainstem (e.g., Hall, 1992; Hall, Mackey-Hargadine, & Kim, 1985).

Wave III. On the basis of experimental lesion studies in small animals (Buchwald & Huang, 1975; Lev & Sohmer, 1972), wave III was traditionally associated with neural activity in the superior olivary complex (SOC) within the brainstem contralateral to the side of stimulation. General anatomy of the human auditory brainstem is illustrated in Figure 2.6. Subsequent findings, also based on animal experiments, were

conflicting. For example, Achor and Starr (1980) recorded activity in the wave III latency region mainly from the ip-silateral superior olivary complex in cat. In contrast, Gardi and Bledsoe (1981) concluded from electrophysiologic and histopathologic data in guinea pig that wave III arises largely from the contralateral medial nucleus of the trapezoid body. There is general agreement that wave II in small animals ac-tually corresponds to wave III in humans. In small animals, therefore, an ABR component corresponding to wave II in humans is not recorded.

Information from human intracranial recordings is, again, most useful for clinical application of the ABR in neurodiagnosis. Møller and colleagues (Møller & Jannetta, 1982, 1983; Møller et al., 1995) found an association be-tween the latency of potentials recorded directly from the cochlear nucleus (ipsilateral to the stimulated ear) and the surface-recorded wave III. Spatiotemporal dipole model in-vestigations, conducted by Scherg and colleagues (Scherg & Von Cramon, 1985) and Grandori (1986), also are very help-ful in defining the generator(s) for ABR wave III in normal humans. Wave III arises from second order neuron activity (beyond the eighth nerve) in or near the cochlear nucleus, whereas the negative trough following wave III appears to arise from the trapezoid body. Based on these collective ob-servations from depth electrode recordings in man, we can confidently presume, at the least, that wave III is generated in the caudal portion of the auditory pons, and probably on the same side as the stimulus (refer again to Figures 2.6 and 2.7). The cochlear nucleus consists of approximately 100,000 neurons, most of which are innervated by eighth nerve fibers (Moore, 1987a,b). Dentrites show a parallel arrangement in the dorsal nucleus, although in the ventral nucleus the orientation follows no pattern. In view of the size of the cochlear nuclei, the opportunity for synchronous innervation of neurons by the eighth nerve in response to sound, and the evidence of optimal orientation of dendrites (refer to Figure 2.3) for an evoked response dipole generator, cochlear nuclei would be expected to generate a major ABR component (Moore, 1987a,b), such as wave III.

Wave IV. Wave IV, as recorded clinically in far-field measurements, often appears as a leading shoulder on wave V and for this reason is sometimes referred to only as the wave IV/V complex. (ABR morphology, including details on normal variations in the wave IV and V complex, is described in Chapter 7.) Wave IV has attracted relatively little attention in clinical applications of ABR. On the basis of early animal studies, wave IV was attributed to the nucleus of the lateral lemniscus, but there are no human data to support this claim. Determining the precise generators of wave IV (and V for that matter) is complicated by the likelihood of multiple crossings of midline (decussations) for auditory fibers beyond the cochlear nucleus. Intracranial investigations by Møller and colleagues (e.g., Møller et al., 1995) imply that wave IV arises from pontine third-order neurons mostly located in the superior olivary complex and "a horizontally oriented dipole located through the entire cross section of the brainstem, with a slight preponderance to the ipsilateral side" and "perhaps representing parallel processing" (p. 604) of multiple generators. Neuroanatomic studies support this suggestion. In humans, the medial nucleus of the superior olivary complex is prominent. According to Moore (1987a,b),

> the medial nucleus has a distinctive morphology which should make it an effective dipole generator. . . . the pronounced parallel orientation of the dentrites should enhance efficacy of the medial nucleus as a generator. (p. 37)

Evidence for second-order, as well as third-order, neuron contributions to wave IV was also provided by spatiotemporal dipole model investigations (Scherg & von Cramon, 1985a,b). Anatomic features argue against a major role in ABR generation for nuclei of the lateral lemnisci. The human ventral lemniscal nucleus is extremely small. Although the dorsal lemniscal nucleus is relatively larger and also has dendrites arranged horizontally, the dorsal nucleus is still smaller that other centers (e.g., medial olivary nucleus). In addition, it receives innervation from different pathways, thus reducing the likelihood of simultaneous firing of the majority of neurons. For these reasons, Moore (1987a,b) concludes that the contribution of the nucleus of either lateral lemniscus to human ABR is probably minor.

Wave V. Wave V is the component analyzed most often in clinical application of the ABR. Accurate information on the origin of wave V is, therefore, critical. As noted above, the generator of wave V was traditionally thought to be the inferior colliculus, based on experiments in small animals (Buchwald & Huang, 1975) and clinical correlations of waveform abnormalities with pathology. Depth electrode and spatiotemporal dipole model findings in man reported since 1980 have prompted a major revision of this concept. In these studies, the distinctly peaked and positive voltage wave V is generated at the termination of lateral lemniscus fibers as they enter the inferior colliculus that is *contralateral* to the stimulated ear (e.g., Møller et al., 1995), in contrast to generators of ABR wave III that are on the same side as the stimulus. In other words, the ABR wave V evoked by stimulation of the right ear is generated from the lateral lemniscus on the left side of the brainstem, and vice versa (shown in Figures 2.6 and 2.7). A sizable proportion of auditory fibers (more than one-third) leave the cochlear nuclei and cross to the other side of the brainstem en route directly via the trapezoid body and lateral lemniscus to the inferior colliculus (e.g., Ponton, Moore, & Eggermont, 1996). Other fiber pathways in the ascending auditory system have multiple synapses along the way in the olivary complex and/or nucleus of the lateral lemniscus, still on a contralateral route through the brainstem. The inferior colliculus that is ipsilateral to the ear stimulated, and ipsilateral pathways in general, appear to contribute little to generation of the ABR wave V. The morphology of the ABR waveform also appears to be related to anatomy. For example, according to Møller et al. (1995), "the sharp portion of peak V reflects the activity in the lateral lemniscus that has not been interrupted in the superior olivary complex or the nucleus of the lateral lemniscus" (p. 602).

The large, broad negative voltage trough following wave V is attributed to dendritic potentials within the inferior colliculus. The slow-going (low-frequency) negative wave, recorded only with an appropriately open high-pass (low-frequency) filter setting, corresponds to the SN10 (i.e., slow negative wave at 10 ms) described by Davis and Hirsh (1976) and others. Surface-recorded ABR waveforms most closely resemble the waveforms recorded intracranially by Møller and colleagues when a noncephalic reference electrode is used, rather than the typical placement of the inverting, or voltage negative, electrode on the earlobe (or mastoid) on the side of the stimulus. Electrode terminology and concepts are described in Chapter 3. Hashimoto et al. (1981) also concluded from their intracranial human studies that the inferior colliculus was the primary origin of this slow negative deflection (SN10) following wave V. It is possible, however, that second-order neuron activity may contribute in some way even to wave V.

Why isn't the largest wave in the normal ABR—wave V—generated by the largest nucleus in the auditory brainstem—the inferior colliculus? The inferior colliculus is a major and complex auditory brainstem structure, approximately 6 to 7 mm in diameter. Its location is illustrated in Figures 2.6 and 2.7. The inferior colliculus is composed of an intricate collection of subdivisions with different neuronal types, myriad synapses among neurons, and varied afferent inputs. Organization of inferior colliculus in the cat and rodents has similarities to organization in man (Moore, 1987a,b). According to Moore (1987), the main structural characteristics of the inferior colliculus across these species are a central nucleus with multiple neuron types and dendritic fields that are arranged in layers and oriented parallel to ascending lateral lemniscus axons. Almost all axons (over 99%) from lower auditory brainstem regions course via the lateral lemniscus to the inferior colliculus and then synapse within this complex structure (Goldberg & Moore, 1967). Activation of the inferior colliculus is not highly synchronized but, rather, staggered because the arriving pathways have varying lengths and varying numbers of synapses. The complex organization of the inferior colliculus presumably results in a closed field arrangement for neurons and, specifically dentrites. As noted above and displayed in Figure 2.3, auditory evoked responses are not generated with a closed field but, rather, with an open electrical field. Therefore, we would not expect a sharp and well-defined peak (wave V) to arise from the inferior colliculus.

Waves VI and VII. Generators of subsequent ABR wave components (VI, VII) are likewise open to question. A thalamic (medial geniculate body) origin is suggested on the basis of clinical observations (Stockard & Rossiter, 1977). Evidence for a thalamic generator is also available from depth electrode recordings from humans reported by some investigators (Hashimoto et al., 1981) and from such recordings in subhuman primates (Arezzo, Pickoff, & Vaughan, 1975). Yet Møller and colleagues (1995) attribute these peaks to continued synchronous firing of neurons in inferior colliculus.

Summary of Anatomic Bases of ABR. Moore (1987b) summarizes a likely sequence of neural events in the auditory brainstem after a stimulus is presented to one ear as follows:

> a synchronized somatodendritic depolarization in the cochlear nuclear complex would be followed shortly by a depolarization in both medial olivary nuclei. Somewhat later, a much smaller depolarization would occur in the dorsal lemniscal nuclei and shortly after that a large, but less well synchronized depolarization would occur in the inferior colliculus. During this time, action potentials would be continuously present in both the direct and relayed pathways connecting the cochlear nuclei with the colliculus. (p. 39)

Furthermore, data from human investigations suggest that the positive peaks in the ABR reflect combined or "compound" afferent (and probably efferent) activity from axonal pathways in the auditory brainstem (e.g., trapezoid body, lateral lemniscus) and the negative troughs reflect somatodendritic potentials in major cell groups (e.g., cochlear nuclei, superior olivary complex, nucleus of the lateral nucleus and

the inferior colliculus). According to Moore (1987a,b), the characteristics of the negative ABR waves (e.g., amplitude, morphology, and latencies) are compatible with the size and caudal-rostral location of these major cell groups in the human brainstem. However, as noted by Møller et al. (1995), "No evidence exists that only the peaks of the vertex-positive peaks of the BAEP [sic ABR] that are conventionally labeled by Roman numerals have clinical significance. Also, no evidence exists that only the vertex-positive peaks can be related to specific neural generators" (p. 597).

The generator sites for waves III, IV, and V are not entirely clear. Several principles of auditory brainstem anatomy are important for an understanding of components of the ABR following wave II. The major pathways, such as the lateral lemniscus, consist of thinly myelinated axons of 2 to 4 μm in diameter. There may be as few as two synapses along the most direct route from the caudal extreme (cochlear nucleus) to the rostral end (inferior colliculus), or as many as four synapses if the superior olivary complex and nucleus of the lateral nucleus are involved. Additional synapses contribute to neural conduction time, that is, latency of wave components. Also, as Moore (1987b) states: "human auditory centers, and their evoked responses, are neither totally independent nor totally interdependent" (p. 41).

Therefore, with the exception of wave I and wave II, each ABR component presumably has multiple generators. There is contribution of activity from more than one anatomic structure to a single wave. Conversely, the same anatomic structure (e.g., the cochlear nucleus) can contribute to more than one peak (see Figures 2.6 and 2.7). Auditory information is simply not passed on sequentially from one relay station to another, as implied by the clear but inaccurate anatomic schematics often shown to depict the anatomy of ABR. The complexity of auditory brainstem anatomy and the timing of activity arising from different structures are certainly important factors in the anatomy versus ABR wave component relationship (Scherg & von Cramon, 1985a,b). The cochlear nucleus and inferior colliculus in the caudal and rostral brainstem, respectively, are the only two auditory centers where synapses are always made in the ascending auditory system. There are numerous and varied alternate routes for transmission of auditory information between these two centers. It is reasonable to expect that structures that are located close to one another in the auditory brainstem or that are activated at or about the same time after the stimulus each contribute in varied amounts to the wave. With this spatial and temporal summation of auditory brainstem activity, a wave component could be generated mostly by one structure, even though more than one structure was activated by the stimulus. And, as noted above, only a subset of neural units within any anatomic region may actually contribute to the ABR. For these reasons, the specific anatomic generators contributing to each of the peaks after wave I and wave II are not precisely defined, at least in humans.

PATHOLOGIC ABR ANATOMY. | There are hundreds of clinical ABR reports describing findings in a wide range of brain pathologies. Clinical findings are reviewed in Chapters 9 and 10. A handful of early articles by an even smaller number of investigators, however, described correlations between documented CNS lesions and pattern of ABR abnormalities. Because these classic papers were instrumental in highlighting the potential value of ABR in neurodiagnosis, they will be reviewed briefly here. Within several years after the discovery of the human ABR, Arnold Starr and colleagues first described patterns of ABR findings in patients with carefully defined CNS insults, pathologies, and disorders, among them drug overdose, hypoxia, metabolic abnormalities, trauma, subarachnoid hemorrhage, epilepsy, brainstem infarcts, and various types of mass lesions (tumors) that involve the brainstem (Starr & Achor, 1975; Starr & Hamilton, 1976). In addition to documenting unequivocally the neurodiagnostic value of ABR, Starr and associates were among the first to correlate ABR findings and brainstem anatomy, as indicated by the following summary from their second (1976) paper:

> Far-field auditory brainstem responses were recorded in ten patients in whom the distribution of pathology was defined at autopsy or at operation. . . . Interruption of auditory pathway at the juncture of VIII nerve with brainstem results in loss of response components after Wave I. Interruption of auditory pathway at midbrain results in loss of response components after Wave III. We conclude that Wave I reflects activity of VIII nerve, Waves II and III reflect activity of cochlear nucleus, trapezoid body, and superior olive and Waves IV and V reflect activity of lateral lemniscus and inferior colliculus. The generators of Waves VI and VII were not defined. (Starr & Hamilton, 1976, p. 607)

In this same time period, neurologists James Stockard, Janet Stockard, Frank Sharbrough, and colleagues carried out meticulous studies of ABR in confirmed brain pathology (Stockard & Rossiter, 1977; Stockard, Rossiter, Wiederholt & Kobayashi, 1976; Stockard, Stockard, & Sharbrough, 1978). Reporting findings for over 100 patients, these authors correlated changes in latency and amplitude for each wave component (waves I through VII) with a wide variety of pathologies. Stockard, Sharbrough, and colleagues also examined the accuracy of ABR findings in localizing lesions within the peripheral and brainstem auditory system. Their rather prophetic, and succinctly stated, conclusions also warrant repeating:

> In summary, scalp recording of brain stem auditory responses is a relatively simple, noninvasive neurophysiologic test that has proved clinically useful in 1) detecting and localizing brain stem demyelination not revealed by other ancillary neurologic tests, 2) localizing neoplastic and vascular lesions to peripheral, pontomedullary, pontine, midbrain, and thalamic levels of the auditory pathway, 3) monitoring the evolution and response to therapy of brain stem tumors, contusions, demyelination, and inflammatory processes, and 4) differentiating metabolic from structural etiologies of coma and confirming

brain death in the presence of electrocerebral silence. (Stockard & Rossiter, 1977, p. 325)

Frequency Following Response. Continuous presentation of low-frequency tone stimuli can produce a scalp-recorded evoked response of the same frequency. Moushegian and colleagues (Moushegian, Rupert, Stillman, 1973) adapted the term *frequency following response*, abbreviated FFR, to refer to this type of evoked response. The term *FFR* had been previously used in auditory neurophysiology studies by Worden and Marsh (1968). There is substantial evidence that the anatomic generator for the FFR, at least for humans, is in the rostral brainstem (Marsh, Brown, & Smith, 1974; Smith, Marsh, & Brown, 1975; Sohmer, Pratt, & Kinarti, 1977; Worden & Marsh, 1968;). However, Yamada, Marsh, and Handler (1982) recorded an FFR with scalp electrodes from a 5-year-old severely brain-damaged child with an ABR characterized by an apparent absence of brainstem components (only a wave I and II component were reliably observed). The interval between the tonal stimulus (a 500 Hz tone burst of 30 ms duration and with abrupt rise-fall times presented at a rate of 10/sec), and the measured FFR was reported to be considerably shorter than one would expect for a neural response. These investigators concluded that the cochlear microphonic must contribute to the scalp-recorded FFR. In an earlier study, Sohmer and Pratt (1976) reduced the contribution of the ABR to the FFR with masking techniques. These authors suggested also that the FFR can, in part, be a far-field reflection of the cochlear microphonic. Electrode location during FFR recording is, presumably, an important factor in determining the contribution of the cochlear microphonic. In the studies just noted, the inverting electrode was located on the mastoid ipsilateral to the stimulus and therefore relatively close to the cochlea. It is likely that the use of a noncephalic site for the inverting electrode (e.g., cervical neck), as suggested by Yamada, Marsh, and Handler (1982), would reduce the contribution of the cochlear microphonic to the scalp recorded FFR in man. Nonetheless, the preponderance of independent evidence (cited above) supports neural generators for the FFR within rostral brainstem structures. In addition, studies of the FFR evoked by speech stimuli confirm phase locking of neurons in the brainstem to certain features or presentations of speech stimuli, e.g., formants and dichotically presented vowels (Galbraith & Arroyo, 1993; Krishnan, 1999).

ASSR

The auditory steady-state response (ASSR) is evoked by a pure-tone signal that is modulated in either amplitude and/or frequency. The anatomic generators of the ASSR vary as a function of the rate of pure-tone stimulus modulation. Multiple anatomic generators for other auditory evoked responses, such as the P300 and the MMN response, have also been demonstrated with manipulations of stimulus or acquisition parameters. Clinical investigation of ASSR abnormalities in patients with well-defined lesions within the auditory system or recordings of the ASSR with depth electrodes from persons without auditory system pathology is limited. Knowledge of the anatomic and physiologic bases of the ASSR is, to a large extent, based on animal research and on localizing possible anatomic sites in humans using the brain electric source analysis (BESA) technique. Experimental studies consistently show that the ASSR evoked by fast rates of amplitude modulation arises from brainstem structures (e.g., Batra, Kuwada, & Stanford, 1989; Creutzfeldt, Hellweg, & Schreiner, 1980; Kuwada et al., 2002). Kuwada et al. (2002) conducted a systematic investigation of the anatomic sources of the ASSR using an animal model (rabbit). Information on the anatomic sources of the ASSR was gleaned from evaluation of the effects on the response of manipulations in placement of recording electrodes (near versus away from auditory cortex), stimulus modulation frequency (low versus high rates), both behavioral stimulation (e.g., touching the rabbits) and pharmacological stimulation (e.g., CNS stimulation with cocaine), pharamacological depression (with pentobarbital), and anesthesia (ketamine). Even though this study was conducted in rabbits, each of these factors influencing generation of the ASSR has clinical implications. Kuwada and colleagues (2002) note,

> At every level of the auditory system, neurons can temporally follow the envelopes of modulated signals. However, the upper limit of modulation frequencies that neurons can follow decreases as the information ascends along the auditory pathways. . . . Since neurons in all structures can follow low modulation frequencies, the surface recorded AMFR [aka ASSR] to these frequencies can reflect contributions from all levels of the auditory pathway. In contrast, responses to higher and higher modulation frequencies can only reflect contributions from lower and lower auditory structures. (pp. 199–200)

The modulation transfer function (MTF) of neurons differs for each level or region of the auditory system, e.g, auditory nerve (cut off frequency of about 800 Hz), inferior colliculus (below 100 Hz), and auditory cortex (below about 20 Hz). The reader will recall a brief discussion in the beginning section of this chapter of functional types of neurons. There is some evidence that in the cochlear nuclei one functional type, onset neurons, are more synchronized to changes in modulation frequency than those neurons with a sustained discharge pattern (Rhode & Greenberg, 1994). However, a different relation between stimulus modulation and the functional type of neuron is found in other regions of the auditory brainstem, such as the superior olivary complex (Kuwada & Batra, 1999). And, within one auditory region of the brain, MTF for neurons is dependent on stimulus factors other than modulation frequency (e.g., stimulus intensity).

With manipulation of the various experimental parameters noted above (stimulus modulation rate, behavioral stimulation, and pharmacologic stimulation and depression of the CNS), Kuwada et al. (2002) found evidence that for pure tone stimuli at carrier frequencies of 60 Hz up to 40,000 Hz low modulation frequencies (80 to 100% amplitude modulation at a rate of <80 Hz) were associated with a cortical source for the ASSR. Faster rates of amplitude modulation (>80 Hz) had two sources within the brainstem, one probably in the midbrain, and the other possibly within the superior olivary complex or cochlear nucleus. It is important to keep in mind that the ASSR data were recorded in the rabbit and that there may be differences in ASSR generators among animal species. Findings for the ASSR reported by Kiren et al. (Kiren, Aoyagi, Furuse, & Koike, 1994) in the cat were at variance with the results of the study conducted by Kuwada et al. (2002), although the discrepancies between the two investigations may be due to methodologic variables (e.g., the response parameters analyzed) rather than animal species. Also, one must recall that ABR generators localized in experiments with small animals did not invariably agree with findings in human subjects. However, clinical evidence with ASSR, in combination with findings for the AMLR and 40 Hz response, support the assumption that low stimulation rates evoke activity throughout the auditory system and the largest responses from cortical regions, whereas the responses to fast stimulation rates are exclusively generated in subcortical (e.g., brainstem) regions. In addition, the work of Kuwada et al. (2002) suggests that the ASSR evoked by slow stimulus modulation rates arises from regions of the auditory cortex contralateral to the side of stimulation. Furthermore, the frequency of neural activity for the ASSR is comparable when recorded with a far-field technique and with a microelectrode from single cortical neurons. The interaction of stimulus factors (e.g., rate of amplitude modulation) and subject factors (e.g., behavioral status and drugs) on the ASSR will be revisited when clinical applications of the response are discussed in Chapter 8.

Herdman et al. (2002) recorded from 10 right-handed adult subjects (5 male and 5 female) the ASSR evoked by a 1000 Hz tone that was 100 percent amplitude modulated at three rates (12, 39, and 88 Hz) and presented at 70 dB SPL (about 60 dB nHL). Subjects rested comfortably during a two-hour data collection session while reading (to remain awake and alert). The ASSR was detected simultaneously with 46 scalp electrodes with analysis of frequency (Fast Fourier Transform or FFT) and phase topography and data processing with the BESA technique. Brain activity following presentation of the 1000 Hz tone modulated in amplitude at 12 Hz was relatively small and difficult to differentiate from ongoing EEG noise. Stimuli at the other two amplitude modulation rates (39 and 88 Hz) produced both brainstem and cortical activity, but the slower of the two rates generated more energy within cortical sources. It is likely the ASSR evoked by rapid amplitude modulation of a tonal stimulus (e.g., > 80 Hz) arises from the auditory brainstem with generators including caudal structures (e.g., cochlear nucleus) to more rostral regions (e.g., inferior colliculus). Limitations in the source modeling approach used to localize generators of the ASSR precluded determination of the laterality of the response. In the waking subjects, amplitude of the ASSR was about five times larger for slow (39 Hz) than for fast (88 Hz) rates of stimulus amplitude modulation. The differential anatomic sources of the ASSR for slow versus fast rates of amplitude modulation have clinical implications, as reviewed in Chapter 8.

AMLR

NORMAL AMLR ANATOMY. | Fifty years ago in the first report of scalp-recorded responses recorded in the middle latency region from man, Geisler, Frishkopf, and Rosenblith (1958) cautiously concluded that the generator was cortical and, perhaps a "deep location of the auditory cortex" (p. 1211). Although the generator(s) of the AMLR has since been debated, there is long-standing evidence from exposed cortex recordings and other localizing techniques in humans that the Pa component of AMLR, at least in part, arises from the superior temporal gyrus within the auditory cortex (Celesia, Broughton, Rasmussen, & Branch, 1968; Cohen, 1982; Goff, Matsumiya, Allison, & Goff, 1977; Lee et al., 1984). The Na component of the AMLR, on the other hand, arises mostly from subcortical structures with prominent contribution from the inferior colliculus within the midbrain region (Hashimoto, 1982; Kileny, Paccioretti, & Wilson et al., 1987; McGee, Kraus, Comperatore, & Nicol, 1991). Multiple anatomic regions have been hypothesized for the localization of the Pb component, including the reticular activating formation (e.g., Erwin & Buchwald, 1986), the auditory regions of the temporal lobe, such as the planum temporale, and even the hippocampus (e.g., Goff et al., 1978; Woods et al., 1987). The reticular activating system has been suggested as a generator because detection of the Pb component is very dependent on state of arousal. Techniques, such as the magnetoencephalography (MEG) technique described below have appeared to localize the Pb component to the auditory cortex, although both anterior and posterior sites have been implicated. The information about the anatomic origins of AMLR components derived from intracranial recordings in normal human subjects and in animal models (described below) are in general agreement with numerous clinical reports of findings in patients with radiologically or surgically defined cortical pathology in the auditory regions of the temporal lobe (e.g., Kileny et al., 1987; Kraus, Özdamar, Heir, & Stein, 1982; Parving et al., 1980; Pool et al., 1989; Scherg & von Cramon, 1986; Woods et al., 1987).

The intracranial study by Lee et al. (1984) was a comprehensive attempt to localize the neural origin of the human AMLR. AERs were recorded from five patients with seizure disorders (aged 11 to 29 years) with an array of 16 subdural stainless steel disc electrodes placed 1 cm apart. During temporal craniotomies, the electrodes are placed over the mid and posterior peri-sylvian region. The general approach for

relating AMLR waveform to electrodes located on the dura mater over the cerebral cortex is illustrated in Figure 2.8. Amplitude of the evoked response components in the AMLR latency region (e.g., 24 to 30 ms and especially the Pa component) is usually greatest for electrodes on the banks of the Sylvian fissure. Decreased amplitude of responses recorded from electrodes located away from this region suggest a near-field origin.

Information on the anatomic structures that are involved in the generation of the AMLR is also available from a sophisticated technique referred to as "dipole source analysis" (Scherg & von Cramon, 1986). Studies in normal subjects and patients with defined cerebral pathology once again confirmed the role of the pathways from the thalamus to, and including, the auditory regions of the temporal lobe in the generation of the AMLR Pa component, whereas the Pb component appears to be also generated and/or modulated to some extent by the reticular activating system. Generator sites estimated with the technique were, however, variable among subjects. For example, Nakagawa et al. (1999) reported that there were three variations for generator of the Pa component in normal subjects, including each (right and left) supratemporal cortex in three subjects, the right

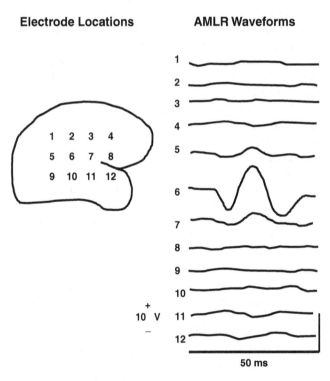

FIGURE 2.8. Auditory middle latency response (AMLR) as recorded intracranially with a grid of electrodes on the brain surface from human subjects with epilepsy undergoing neurophysiologic studies prior to surgical management. Numbers indicate electrode sites corresponding to the AMLR waveforms in the right side of the figure.
Adapted from reports of Lee et al., 1984; Hall, 1992; and others.

temporal cortex for one subject, and in the right midbrain for another subject. For the other thirteen subjects in the group, all equivalent dipoles were in the midbrain. Equivalent dipoles were not localized for the Na component.

Liegeois-Chauvel and colleagues (Liegeois-Chauvel et al., 1994) also described a comprehensive investigation of the generators of the AMLR in 37 adult epileptic patients (aged 20 to 56 years) using a chronic stereotactic, intracerebral recording technique the authors referred to as "stereo-electro-encephalographic exploration (SEEG)." The AMLR was evoked with 1000 Hz tone burst signals with rise/fall times of 0.3 ms and a plateau of 30 ms, presented a rate of 0.7/second and at an intensity level of 70 dB SL (above the behavioral thresholds for the signal). The bandpass filter settings were 5 to 1500 Hz and the analysis time was 100 ms. To summarize the authors' detailed discussion of the topography of the AMLR, the P30 was recorded from the Heschl's gyrus, specifically the medial portion of primary auditory cortex that the authors describe as the dorso-postero-medial region of the gyrus (Liegeois-Chauvel et al., 1994, p. 211). The P50 was localized more laterally in primary auditory cortex (specifically the dorso-postero-lateral region), although there was overlap with the region generating the P30. A component (P16) was recorded at the tip of Heschl's gyrus that might be equivalent to the scalp-recorded Na component. However, the authors do not speculate on the anatomic origin of the Na component. Latency values of these intracerebrally recorded components were in agreement with those previously reported for AMLR components recorded from the scalp. Other responses were recorded from the region of the planum temporale of the superior gyrus of the temporal lobe.

These investigations suggested that another less appreciated peak within the middle latency time frame—referred to as the TP41 or T45 component—is also generated by structures in the same anatomic region of the auditory CNS (e.g., Cacace, Satya-Murti, & Wolpaw, 1990; Kraus, Kileny, & McGee, 1994). The TP41 component, with a latency of about 40 to 45 ms, is recorded with an AMLR test protocol than includes noninverting electrodes located at somewhat lower sites, over the temporal lobe (T3 or T5 and T4 or T6), than the customary electrode sites (C3 and C4). In the initial series of studies of the P41 (P45) reported by Cacace and colleagues (Cacace, Satya-Murti, & Wolpaw, 1990), the inverting electrode was placed at a balanced noncephalic (Stephenson & Gibbs, 1951) site, i.e., a true reference. The authors presented an argument for why other investigators had not previously identified the P41 (P45) component, and why the component was neurogenic, and not myogenic. Based on the analysis of responses mapped for 32 scalp electrodes, these authors described Pa and Pb components of the AMLR at central and fronto-central locations, and the P41 component recorded over the auditory cortex in the temporal lobe.

Magnetoencephalography (MEG) is another technique that has been applied to identify the dipole generators of the AMLR (e.g., Godey et al., 2001). MEG has adequate resolution for localization of brain activity, particularly the dipoles (equivalent current dipoles, or ECDs) from axons in the auditory cortex that are oriented perpendicular to the scalp. The ECDs are described as vectors with three properties . . . an origin (the dipole), a phase angle or direction, and strength, i.e., length (Kaga et al., 2004). Waves identified with MEG are labeled with an "m" (e.g., Pam or P30m and Pbm or P50m.) There are apparently no published MEG investigations MLR of the generator(s) of the Na component (Nam). MEG studies show that the Pa component (P30m) arises from the posterior medial region of Heschl's gyrus within the primary auditory cortex (Kaga, Kurauchin, Yumoto, & Una, 2004). There is disagreement as to the generators of the Pb (P50m) component. Although MEG findings are consistent with a primary auditory cortex generator, the precise site of origin is not clear, with some investigators suggesting that the generator is in the lateral portion of Heschl's gyrus, and anterior to the generator of the Pa (P30m) component (Godey et al., 2001). A planum temporale origin has also been offered for the Pb (P50m) component of the AMLR. These anatomic correlations with AMLR components must be tempered by the possibility that generators of the magnetic components are not identical to AMLR components (Kaga et al., 2004). In addition, generators localized with MEG do not necessarily align directly with superficial recordings of the AMLR from multiple electrode locations (e.g., 28 to 30) on the scalp. For example, Woods et al. (1995) reported a fronto-central scalp distribution for the Na, Pa, and Pb (P1) components, with centro-parietal distribution for the Nb component. The results of these recordings from the scalp, however, are predicted from the orientation of the generators within the superior temporal plane and the Sylvian fissure (e.g., Woods et al., 1995).

In addition to these clinical studies, experimental investigations with various animal models (guinea pig, cat, monkey) have, for many years, produced information on the anatomic structures contributing to the AMLR (Arezzo, Pickoff, & Vaughan, 1975; Brett, Watkins, & Barth, 1994; Kaga, Hink, Shinoda, & Suzuki, 1980; Knight & Brailowsky, 1990; Kraus et al., 1994; Kraus, Smith, & McGee, 1988; Littman, Krauss, McGee, & Nicol, 1992; Pribram, Rosner, & Rosenblith, 1954; Reese, Garcia-Rill, & Skinner, 1995; Shaw, 1991; Uno, Kaga, Tsuzuku, & Kuroki, 1993; Woolsey & Walzl, 1942). Animal research has provided more direct access to cortical and subcortical anatomic structures and the pharmacological manipulation of neurophysiological activity within these structures. These experimental studies yielded evidence indicating that the AMLR components are produced by multiple generator sites depending on measurement factors, such as the location of the noninverting electrode, the rate of signal presentation, the mode of signal presentation (monaural versus bilateral), and different developmental time courses. Contributing to the formation of the AMLR in animal species are subcortical structures (i.e., the medial geniculate body in the thalamus and the reticular formation within the medial brainstem) and cortical structures (i.e., primary auditory cortex [Heschl's gyrus] within the temporal lobe). The AMLR components produced by subcortical regions are usually detected with recording electrodes located on the midline of the scalp (from the forehead back to the parietal area), whereas AMLR components produced by cortical generators are recorded with noninverting electrodes located on the scalp over the temporal lobe of the brain (e.g., Kraus et al., 1988). Furthermore, drugs that selectively suppress cortical activity have a more pronounced effect on temporal lobe versus subcortical generators of the AMLR. There is ample evidence that the reticular formation plays an important role in the generation of the AMLR Pa component based the effect of sleep on the response in humans (reviewed in Chapter 11) and on experimental investigations (e.g., Kraus et al., 1992) and clinical studies (Hall, Huangfu, & Gennarelli, 1982). As noted by Kraus, Kileny, and McGee (1994), accumulated findings on the anatomic generators of the AMLR suggest two fundamentally different sources. The primary, or thalamocortical, sensory pathways are important in processing auditory information and related, therefore, to basic audiologic measurements, such as word recognition and the perception of auditory signals in the presence of background noise. The secondary or "nonprimary" anatomic structures, also referred to as "association" or "extralemniscal" pathways, mediate very different auditory functions, such as auditory attention and the integration of information from auditory and other modalities (e.g., vision) (Kraus, Kileny, & McGee, 1994).

PATHOLOGIC AMLR ANATOMY. | Clinical reports by Kileny and his colleagues (Ho, Kileny, Paccioretti, & McLean, 1987; Kileny, Paccioretti, & Wilson, 1987), Kraus and her colleagues (Kraus et al., 1982; Özdamar & Kraus, 1983), and Scherg (Scherg & Von Cramon, 1986) support the notion that the AMLR Pa component receives contributions from primary temporal lobe. According to these authors (Ho, Kileny, Paccioretti, & McLean, 1987; Kileny, Paccioretti, & Wilson, 1987), the Pa component is characteristically reduced in amplitude or not detectable when recorded by an electrode located over a pathologic primary auditory cortex (e.g., at C5 or C6), but is unaffected by lesions in the main auditory portion of the thalamus (medial geniculate body), known auditory association areas of the cortex, and frontal or parietal operculum areas. The use of hemisphere-specific electrodes (versus a midline electrode at Cz or Fpz for example) appears to be essential for this type of neuroanatomic localization of the AMLR in clinical applications.

Woods, Clayworth, Knight, Simpson, and Naeser (1987), despite the foregoing clinical evidence in support of a primary auditory cortex role in AMLR generation, offer a conflicting viewpoint. These authors present a critical review of the literature, summarizing the findings of twenty-three previous clinical reports on AMLR and/or ALR findings in brain pathology. Woods et al. (1987) also describe results of a clinical investigation of five patients with carefully documented and localized lesions involving both temporal lobes. Normal subjects, young and old, showed slightly larger Na-Pa component amplitude over the hemisphere contralateral to the ear stimulated than over the ipsilateral hemisphere, and they showed greater amplitudes for binaural than monaural stimulation. Notably, all patients with bilateral temporal lobe pathology had reliable Na and Pa components. Woods et al. (1987):

> found no simple relationship between Na-Pa amplitude and the extent of damage to primary auditory cortex or auditory association areas. . . . thus our data provide little support for the hypothesis that Pa is generated exclusively in primary auditory cortex or auditory association areas (p. 143). . . . if cortical lesions affect the Pa generator, they must extend outside of classical auditory areas. . . . another possibility is that extensive lesions are required to assure that the cortical generator of the Pa has been destroyed. (p. 144)

The anatomic generator of the AMLR recorded with a midline noninverting electrode may, as the above studies indicate, be a summation of far-field activity from subcortical (e.g., thalamic) generators with contributions also from primary auditory cortex in each hemisphere. Parving et al. (1980) recorded normal-appearing AMLRs from a patient with bilateral temporal lobe infarcts. The results of this study are sometimes cited as evidence that the AMLR Pa component does not have an auditory cortex origin. In the context of the studies noted above, one could infer from the findings of Parving et al. (1980) that the midline-recorded AMLR does, indeed, reflect activity in subcortical auditory regions.

In a recent study of the MEG technique in patients with radiologically confirmed cortical pathology, Kaga et al. (2004) found that the magnetic Pa component (Pam) was abnormal or absent in patients with pathology involving the left or right auditory cortex or radiation fibers, but the Pa component of the AMLR was preserved in some cases. The authors explain this discrepancy by postulating that the Pam is exclusively generated by primary auditory cortex, whereas the AMLR Pa component receives contributions from thalamic and reticular formation structures, as well as the primary auditory cortex. Conversely, damage to or dysfunction of these subcortical regions (thalamus and reticular formation) may affect the Pa component even with integrity of the primary auditory cortex (Kaga et al., 2004).

Relatively less clinical attention has been given to the possible generator(s) for AMLR components other than Pa (that is, Na, Nb, and Pb). From the data reported by Woods et al. (1987), it is reasonable to consider the possible role of the thalamic medial geniculate body in the generation of the Na component. However, Hashimoto (1982) did not record slow wave activity in the corresponding latency period from electrodes placed on this auditory structure.

AUDITORY 40 HZ EVENT-RELATED RESPONSE. | When they described the auditory 40 Hz event-related response in 1981,

Galambos, Makeig, and Talmachoff speculated on a possible neuroanatomic origin within the polysensory areas of the thalamus. The generator, however, is still open to question. Spydell, Pattee, and Goldie (1985) recorded a midline auditory 40 Hz event-related response from sixteen neurologically normal subjects and ten patients with radiologically confirmed CNS lesions (five in midbrain and/or thalamus and five in temporal lobe). Abnormally low 40 Hz response phase values were consistently calculated for patients with midbrain lesions, while patients with temporal lobe lesions showed normal 40 Hz responses.

ALR

NORMAL ALR ANATOMY. | The neuroanatomic origins of the major ALR components (N1 and P2) occurring in the range of approximately 60 to 250 ms have, for many years, been the subject of study and debate. More than fifty years ago, Davis (1939) showed that the ALR could be recorded from electrodes at numerous locations on the scalp, with maximum amplitude from midline electrodes over frontal regions. Diffuse, nonspecific generators in thalamo-cortical regions were suspected. On the basis of this general scalp distribution, subsequently confirmed by others, Picton, Hillyard, Krausz, and Galambos (1974) postulated a generator site or region in the association cortex of the frontal lobe. On the other hand, the results of a series of investigations of the scalp topography of ALRs in man (Peronnet, Michel, Echallier, & Girod, 1974; Vaughan & Ritter, 1970; Wood & Wolpaw, 1982), as well as intracranial electrode recordings in the monkey (Arezzo, Pickoff, & Vaughan, 1975) and man (Chatrian, Petersen, & Lazarte, 1960; Liegeois-Chauvel, Chauvel, Marquis, Musolino, & Bancaud, 1994), placed the generator or generators in the region of the Sylvian fissure and superior temporal plane in the temporal lobe. Accurate definition of the generators of ALR waves and subcomponents is complicated by a number of subject factors, e.g., age (in young children and advancing age in adults) and attention, and various measurement parameters, e.g., signal type, duration, and presentation rate (or ISI).

By recording ALRs simultaneously with scalp electrodes arranged in a coronal array, Vaughan and Ritter (1970) demonstrated in six normal subjects a clear polarity inversion at the Sylvian fissure level for a component in the 200 ms range. Superior to the Sylvian fissure, this component was of positive voltage and below it was negative voltage. The concept of polarity inversion of the ALR for recording electrodes in the region of the generator sites is illustrated schematically in Figure 2.9. Vaughan and Ritter (1970) suggested, based on their investigation, that the source of the ALR was a dipole within the primary auditory projection cortex on the supratemporal plane. In the Vaughan and Ritter (1970) study, the inverting electrode site (so-called reference electrode) was the tip of the nose (a cephalic location). One year later, Kooi, Tipton, and Marshall (1971) reported an in-

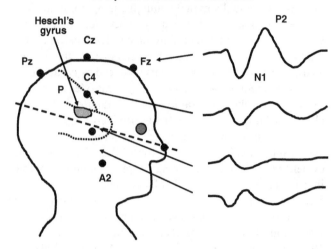

Scalp Distribution of the ALR

FIGURE 2.9. A display of the scalp distribution of the auditory late response. Polarity inversion at the Sylvian fissure for a component in the 200 ms latency region is illustrated by waveforms in the right portion of the figure. The inverting electrode ("reference" electrode) is indicated by the black circle on the nose.

Adapted from a paper by Vaughan & Ritter, 1970.

vestigation of ALRs recorded with a noncephalic reference electrode that failed to confirm this polarity conversion and cast doubt on the theory of a auditory temporal cortex origin. Then, in a two related papers in 1982, Wood and Wolpaw clearly showed that some commonly used cites for inverting ("reference") electrodes, such as the nose, ear, and mastoid, were active with regard to AER measurement. These authors recommended a balanced sterno-vertebral reference for an indifferent electrode that is not seriously contaminated by EKG artifact. Although Wood and Wolpaw did not confirm some of the noncephalic electrode voltage gradient patterns of Vaughan and Ritter (1970), they did support, with a sterno-vertebral (noncephalic) reference electrode, the theory of a dipole source layer generator in the auditory cortex. Data did not differentiate between a generator site located within the superior temporal plane versus the lateral temporal surface.

The auditory evoked response neuromagnetic fields (AEF) can provide information on the origin of the electrophysiologically recorded ALR waves. One of the most stable and easily detected AEF components is the N100m, which is equivalent to the ALR N100 wave. Tonotopic organization within the primary auditory cortex, including variations in generator positions along the anterior-posterior and medial-lateral dimensions for different frequencies, was clearly demonstrated with the N100m component (Huotilainen et al., 1995; Pantev et al., 1995).

Within the N1 wave complex (described in Chapter 12), multiple individual components can be recorded under certain stimulus and subject conditions, among them Nb, Nc and the "processing negativities." The major N1 and P2 components receive contributions from in primary auditory cortex and the supratemporal plane located anterior to this region, and with the downward-sloping plane of the Sylvian fissure, vertically oriented dipoles angle toward frontal (e.g., Fz) electrode sites. It appears that both tonal and speech signals elicit N1 and P2 components generated within the auditory cortex (Tiitinen et al., 1999). Mäkelä, Alku, May, Makinen, and Tiitinen (2004), however, provide evidence that the source (estimated ECD) for N1 activity elicited by vowels is limited to the left auditory cortex, consistent with the specialization of the left hemisphere for speech processing. Subcomponents (e.g., N1b, Nc) may reflect different orientations (vertically or laterally oriented) for the dipoles underlying the N1 (e.g., Scherg & von Cramon, 1986) and temporal lobe regions related to primary auditory cortex, (e.g., association auditory cortex) within the superior temporal gyrus. In addition, with selective attention to specific acoustic features of signals, cerebral regions outside of the temporal lobe (e.g., frontal motor and pre-motor cortex) probably play a role in the generation of early and later components within the N1 wave complex, with influence also from subcortical structures, including the thalamus, hippocampus, and the reticular activating system (Näätänen & Picton, 1987). The later negative waves—N2 and perhaps its variants or subcomponents—are dependent at least to some extent on activity within the limbic system and reticular activating system in the region of the thalamus (Perrault & Picton, 1984).

The generators of the P2 component are not yet well defined. Based on topographic recordings, techniques for estimating equivalent current dipoles (ECDs), and MEG studies, it appears that the P2 wave receives contributions from multiple anatomic sources (e.g., Godey et al., 2001; Perrault & Picton, 1984). The subcortical reticular activating system plays a role in the generation of the P2 wave (Näätänen & Picton, 1987). Auditory cortex structures also probably contribute to the P2 wave, including the planum temporale and the auditory association (area 22) regions. These suspected generator sites are anterior to and different from those noted above for components comprising the N1 wave complex. Additional support for the idea of different anatomical substrates for the N1 versus P2 waves is provided by findings from patients with CNS pathology (e.g, Knight, Hillyard, Woods, & Neville, 1980) and by the very different timetable for maturation of individual ALR waves. The P2 wave is essentially mature by age 2 to 3 years whereas developmental changes of the N1 wave may continue until age 16 years (e.g., Ponton et al., 2000).

Selected ALR components beyond the N1 (e.g., N250 and N450), when elicited with speech sound signals (e.g., vowels), produce larger amplitudes as detected by left versus right hemisphere recording sites (Ceponiene et al., 2001). Given the strong linkage of the N400 response to language (semantic) processing and the complexity of the processes involved in tasks required to evoke the response, multiple structures and pathways in different regions of the brain presumably contribute to the generation of the N400, e.g., auditory cortex, language areas in the temporal and parietal lobes, and even the frontal lobe (Kutas & Hillyard, 1982). Utilizing the MEG technique, Mäkelä et al. (2001) found the the apparent generator site for the N400(m) response differed for short- versus long-duration Finnish words. Short-duration words at the end of improbable sentences produced a very sharp-peaked N400 response that was localized to neuronal sources within the auditory cortex. Longer duration words, in contrast, elicited a broad, less well-defined negative wave that could not be localized using an equivalent current dipole (ECD) estimation technique.

A fundamental concern about the anatomic bases of AERs has to do with laterality. That is, with monaural stimulation, does the response originate from the same (ipsilateral) side of the brain, the opposite (contralateral) side of the brain, or from both sides (bilateral)? Although seemingly straightforward, the laterality of anatomic structures generating auditory evoked responses is a controversial topic for all but one. The exception, of course, is the ECochG that assuredly originates from the cochlea and eighth nerve ipsilateral to the stimulus. In man and certain animal models (e.g., cat), dominance of contralateral auditory pathways and centers has long been appreciated, at least on the basis of gross anatomical studies and for tasks involving processing of speech stimuli (Kimura, 1961). Whether the same contralateral advantage also exists for electrophysiologic responses in man and other animals is less clear (Mononen & Seitz, 1977).

Investigations of ALR laterality in human subjects likewise have yielded conflicting results, including no amplitude difference between hemispheres for verbal stimuli and shorter latency and larger amplitude values for ALRs recorded from the hemisphere contralateral versus ipsilateral to the stimulus (Butler, Keidel & Spreng, 1969; Majkowski et al., 1971). Mononen and Seitz (1977) conducted a comprehensive study. Stimuli were clicks presented monaurally and dichotically and temporally embedded in a sentence. Attention was assured by requiring the subject to indicate the location of the click in relation to the sentence. AERs were detected over the parietal lobes (C3, C4 electrode sites). There was significantly decreased latency for the dichotic click-sentence stimulation recorded from the contralateral side. There was no laterality difference for response amplitude or for the monaural click condition. Clearly, it is impossible to discuss AER anatomy independent of stimulus factors (e.g., monaural vs. binaural presentation) and acquisition factors (e.g., electrode sites).

PATHOLOGIC ALR ANATOMY | In contrast to vast clinical experience with ABR, fewer investigators have recorded ALRs from patients with CNS pathology. (Kileny, 1985; Knight, Hillyard, Woods, & Neville, 1980; Squires & Hecox, 1983; Peronnet & Michel, 1977; Scherg & von Cramon, 1986). Woods et al. (1987) reviewed critically the literature on

ALRs in CNS pathology. The clinical implications of these papers are reviewed in the following section on neurodiagnosis. An early study by Knight, Hillyard, Woods, and Neville (1980) is one of the more comprehensive. These researchers studied ten patients with unilateral frontal lobe lesions and ten patients with unilateral temporal-parietal lesions, all carefully defined by CT scan. The ALR N1 component was not decreased by frontal lobe pathology, yet actually appeared to be larger than expected with contralateral stimulation. Amplitude of this component was very reduced (by 57% on the average) in patients with posterior temporal-parietal pathology, of either hemisphere, whereas anterior and middle temporal lobe lesions did not appear to be a factor. The results of Knight et al., study were in agreement with those reported earlier by Peronnet et al. (1974), although results of other studies are not entirely in agreement. Woods et al. (1987) recorded ALRs, as well as AMLRs, from five patients with precisely localized brain pathology. Based on clinical data and interpretation of findings reported in the literature, these authors conclude that the ALR N1 component is always reduced in amplitude when temporal lobe lesions extend into the parietal lobe, involving angular and supra-marginal gyri. Pathology limited to the superior temporal plane, on the other hand, spares the N1 component.

Attempts to determine the generators of the ALR by multiple electrode, topographic scalp recordings, even utilizing computerized evoked potential topography techniques, are complicated by the factors involved in all far-field measurements, discussed earlier in this chapter. Based on existing evidence from scalp and intracranial recordings in normal subjects and studies of patients with temporal lobe lesions, it seems reasonable to presume overlapping generators of the ALR—that is, the posterior portion of the superior temporal plane, lateral temporal lobe, and especially adjacent parietal lobe regions. Other anatomic structures probably contribute in some combination to components of the ALR in the 60 to 250 ms region. Although there does not appear to be an ALR generator in frontal cortex, portions of this brain region probably do modulate the response in some way.

P300

NORMAL P300 ANATOMY. | The P300 response to auditory or other sensory modality stimulation is typically defined in operational terms, rather than by its neural generators. That is, the P300 is referred to as a cognitive response or a reflection of attention to a stimulus. As with other AERs, neuroanatomy of the scalp-recorded P300 (event-related potential, or ERP) can really only be inferred with confidence by correlating these recordings with depth electrode recording mapping of potential fields from neurologically normal human subjects, although this is rarely possible. Even when this opportunity presents itself, the geometry or orientation of the potential fields of underlying neural tissue must always be kept in mind as noted at the outset of the section on

neuroanatomy and physiology in this chapter. The concept of open versus closed electrical fields was illustrated in Figure 2.3. Open fields are characterized by parallel or columnal organization that is ideal for summing or enhancement of local electrical activity (micro-fields) and transmission of the activity to the scalp via volume conduction. In contrast, activity at the micro-field level near the neuron is minimized or even cancelled out when neurons are in a closed-field arrangement. Although neuronal activity may be strong, it cannot be recorded with scalp electrodes at some distance from the dipoles. Vaughan and Arezzo (1988) succinctly state the problem:

> In the case of the ERP, the distinction between the "open" and "closed" field generator is critical. If current flows within the active region are fully symmetrical, no external currents and thus no differential potential gradients will be generated beyond the immediate vicinity of the active neurons. Thus, surface recorded ERPs are blind to closed field generators. (p. 535)

As a consequence of practical and ethical limitations, functional anatomy of P300 has been more extensively investigated in subhuman primates (Vaughan, 1982; Vaughan & Arezzo, 1988) than in man. Experimental investigations of P300 anatomy in lower animals (e.g., cat) would have limited value in understanding the human P300, since there are marked interspecies differences in the responsiveness of relevant anatomical structures (i.e., hippocampus) to auditory stimulation.

Vaughan and Arezzo (1988) point out that even under the best research circumstances:

> The complexity of these potentials and the variations in morphology and timing of components with respect to the surface recorded ERP dictate caution in implicating particular intracranial structures in the generation of specific ERP components. (p. 536)

The motivation for pursuing such study is strong, however, because of the potential clinical applications of the P300 and other event-related potentials as "direct indices of brain activity underlying human perception, cognition and behavior" (Vaughan & Arezzo, 1986, p. 539).

The P300 response, along with other late-latency responses, reflect electrical activity or currents (i.e., excitatory or inhibitory postsynaptic potentials) originating from neurons (dentrites) and, specifically, from extracellular dipoles that are recorded with a far-field technique (refer back to Figure 2.2). According to Frodl-Bauch, Bottlender, and Hegerl (1999), the neurotransmitter substance glutamate plays a primary role in the generation of the excitatory postsynaptic potentials (EPSPs) that underlie the P300 response and other cortical AERs. Other neurochemicals may influence the role of glutamate in generating the P300 response (Frodl-Bauch et al., 1999; Oranje et al., 2000). For example, acetylcholine is associated with an increase in amplitude and decrease in latency of the P300 response, whereas administration of ketamine and GABA is followed by a reduction in P300 amplitude and increased latency. Other substances, such as serotonin, dopamine, and noradrenaline, may exert a secondary influence on the P300 response by modulating the action of acetylcholine. Multiple anatomic regions within the brain contribute to generation of the auditory P300 response. More recent papers in the literature on neural generators of the P300 make a distinction between those contributing to the P3a versus P3b components.

Over a span of fifteen years, Eric Halgren and colleagues (e.g., Halgren, Baudena, Clarke, Heit, Liegeois, Chauvel, & Musolino, 1995; Halgren, Squires, Wilson, Rohrbaugh, Babb, & Crandall, 1980; Halgren, Stapleton, Smith, & Altafullah, 1986) published comprehensive reports on the origins of the human auditory P300 response as measured with the oddball signal paradigm. The P300 (P3) was defined as a scalp-recorded response with a latency in the 250 to 700 ms range and recorded as voltage positive over much of the head, but of largest amplitude at midline electrode sites (Cz or Pz). The P300 response is most evident when the subject attends to rare stimuli, the auditory "oddball" task. Based on their intracranial electrode recording technique, mostly with patients undergoing careful evaluation for possible surgical management of epilepsy, Halgren and colleagues identified multiple likely cortical and subcortical regions involved in generation of scalp-recorded P300 components (P3a and P3b). The list included medial temporal lobe limbic structures (hippocampus, para-hippocampal gyrus, and amygdala), portions of the frontal lobe, the parietal lobe, and the parietal occipital junction. Other investigators have, likewise, implicated a variety of brain regions in the generation of the P300 response, including the thalamus, auditory cortex (posterior superior temporal plane), temporal-parietal cortical areas, and portions of the frontal lobe (Courchesne, 1978; Knight, Scabini, Woods, & Clayworth, 1989; Tarkka, Stokic, Basile, & Papanicolaou, 1995). The P3a response appears to reflect the brain's detection of novel signals and does not require active attention during the recording. In contrast, active attention is important in recording the P3b component, a reflection of voluntary detection of a signal.

Functional magnetic resonance imaging (fMRI) has more recently been combined with electrophysiologic measurement of the P300 response in studies attempting to localize the anatomical generators of the response (e.g., Horovitz, Skudlarski, & Gore, 2002; Linden, Prvulovic, Formisano, Vollinger, Zanella, Goebel, & Dierks, 1999; Stevens, Skudlarski, Gatenby, & Gore, 2000). Importantly, functional neuroimaging offers an approach for investigating the origins of the P300 response in humans that is not compromised by the well-appreciated limitations of lesion studies. The fMRI documents metabolic and hemodynamic activity during auditory stimulation, including Blood Oxygenation Level Dependent (BOLD) activity. Information from fMRI studies have generally confirmed previously reported findings for P300 generators, including perisylvian regions (e.g., supra-marginal gyrus), the frontal operculum, the insular cortex, thalamic regions, inferior parietal areas, and a region in the right medial frontal gyrus (Linden et al., 1999). Finally, the corpus callosum should not be neglected in a discussion of the anatomical bases of cortical auditory evoked responses, particularly the P300 response. As reviewed in Chapter 13, differences in the size of the corpus callosum for right- versus left-handed persons have been cited in explanations of the effect of handedness on the P300 response. Inter-hemispheric communication of sensory information, including attention processing, appears to play a role in the generation of the P300 response (see Polich & Hoffman, 1998, for brief review). In addition, functional neuroimaging has provided support for the clinical evidence of discrete differences in the multiple generators for the P3a versus P3b components of the P300 response. The P3a component appears to be more dependent on anterior generators, whereas the P3b component receives greater contributions from posterior cortical regions. In summary, the clinical value of the P300, in contrast to other AERs, apparently will not be in localizing lesions (Halgren et al., 1986). CT, magnetic resonance imaging (MRI), and positron emission tomography (PET) techniques are better suited for this neurodiagnostic role.

PATHOLOGIC P300 (P3) ANATOMY. | Explanations of the neural origin of the P300 are complicated by variable clinical findings in CNS pathology. Although P300 amplitude is usually diminished in patients with anatomically small medial temporal lobe regions (Halgren et al., 1986), there are patients with distinct P300 components as recorded directly from the limbic structures yet no apparent surface P300. The reverse pattern was also reported. Unilateral removal of most of the medial temporal lobe, as part of anterior temporal lobe removal in surgical treatment for epilepsy, does not necessarily affect surface-recorded and tone-stimulated P300 latency or amplitude (Wood, Allison, Goff, Williamson, & Spencer, 1980), whereas removal of the left anterior temporal lobe, in right-handed subjects, is associated with abnormalities of a P300 response evoked by repeated words. The P300 response has been recorded from patients representing a diverse collection of pathologies involving the medial temporal lobe, such as hypoxia, infarction, encephalitis, tumors, and even anterior temporal lobe removal or lobectomy (Johnson, 1988; Polich & Squires, 1993). In general, amplitude for the P300 response recorded with scalp electrodes in lateral temporal and frontal locations is reduced by medial temporal lobe pathology. Amplitude is also reduced for patients with lesions in the temporal-parietal region (superior temporal plane and sulcus) when the P300 response is recorded with more posterior scalp electrode sites. It is likely that these clinical findings indicate interactive roles in the generation of the P300 response for structures the medial temporal lobe and the temporal-parietal region that are related to basic cognitive activities (e.g., memory, attention, detection of novel stimuli) that are important in generation of the response. Structures within the prefrontal cortex may also play a part in the modulation of P300 activity originating from posterior regions of the cortex.

Mismatch Negativity (MMN) Response

According to various techniques for localizing evoked responses, including scalp current density (SCD), magneto-encephalography (nMMN), positron emission topography (PET), functional magnetic resonance imaging (fMRI), intracranial recordings, and clinical studies in patients with confirmed pathology (e.g., infarctions of the middle cerebral artery), the MMN response receives neural contributions from a rather broad region extending from the frontal lobes to the auditory portions of the temporal lobe. Neural generators of the MMN response, as well as the mechanisms underlying generation of the MMN, change as a function of maturation over the age range from birth to at least adolescence (e.g., Martin et al., 2003). In adults, the MMN response is maximal when recorded with electrodes over the fronto-central scalp, with major neural generators in primary and secondary cortex (transverse temporal gyrus and superior temporal gyrus), and secondary contributions from centers within the frontal lobe of the cerebrum and from subcortical regions of the auditory system (e.g., Alain, Woods, & Knight, 1998; Deouell, Bentin, & Giard, 1998; Döller et al., 2003; Giard, Perrin, Pernier, & Bouchet, 1990; Javitt et al., 1992; Müller et al., 2002; Opitz, Mecklinger, von Cramon, & Kruggel, 1999; Rinne et al., 2000). As a general rule, major generators for the MMN response are considerably more medial (midline) and anterior than generators for other cortical auditory responses (e.g., the N100 wave). When recorded with the magneto-encephalographic technique, the neuromagnetic MMN dipole typically has an inferior-posterior orientation. However, the dipole locations for the MMN response vary as a function of the nature of the standard versus deviant stimulus difference (e.g., frequency, intensity, or duration), showing a spatial separation or distribution as a function of the processing and analysis acoustic features. For example, the MMN response to frequency deviant stimuli (there is a frequency difference between standard and deviant stimuli) is generated anterior to the MMN response for duration deviant stimuli. Coupling MMN response measurement with simultaneous fMRI (blood-oxygenation-level dependent, or BOLD) studies reveals with a frequency stimulus condition hemodynamic activity in the temporal lobe (right superior gyrus) and in the opercular portion of the right prefrontal region (inferior and middle frontal gyri), with the locus of activity (and the amplitude of the MMN response) varying as a function of the size of the difference between standard and deviant stimuli. There is also strong evidence of hemispheric specialization in processing of acoustic stimuli for the MMN response (Döller et al., 2003; Liebenthal et al., 2003; Schall et al., 2003). That is, perception of pitch (nonverbal information) is processed in the right auditory cortex (superior temporal gyrus, superior temporal plane, and Brodmann area 22), whereas temporal processing of speech sounds takes place within the left auditory cortex. Published findings suggest that the processing of deviant stimuli in the MMN measurement paradigm involves an interaction between anterior and posterior brain regions and, furthermore, can be divided into earlier and later stages, with the former ("automatic change detection") dependent mostly on temporal lobe regions and the latter (attention switch mechanism) on prefrontal regions of the cortex (Döller et al., 2003; Schall et al., 2003). A complex "neural network" involving other brain regions, including the parietal cortex, insular cortices, and perhaps even the cerebellum, may also be involved in processing auditory information during MMN measurement (Schall et al., 2003).

There are, in addition, developmental changes in the MMN response. In contrast to the fronto-central predominance in adults, the MMN response in young children appears to be dependent more on brain activity in lateral (versus midline) regions, reflecting specifically neural events in the supra temporal plane and/or lateral portion of the temporal gyrus (e.g., Halgren, Marinkovic, & Chauvel, 1998) and posterior regions.

BLOOD SUPPLY

There are two major vascular systems serving the nervous system. Each of these—the vertebrobasilar system and the internal carotid system—send blood to anatomical regions generating AER components. When consulting textbooks to review peripheral and central auditory nervous system anatomy and physiology, the reader is advised to also study the vascular systems that supply blood to the ear, the brainstem, and the cerebrum. Beginning from the periphery, the cochlea and eighth cranial nerve receive blood from the vertebrobasilar system. The anterior inferior cerebellar artery (AICA) leads from this system to the internal auditory artery (also referred to as the labyrinthine artery), which travels to the cochlea through the internal auditory canal. Branches of the internal auditory artery then distribute to the vestibular labyrinth and to the cochlea, where the stria vascularis is the major destination and internal source of blood. The two vertebral arteries join on the ventral surface of the brainstem at the pons–medulla boundary and form the basilar artery. The basilar artery continues along the brainstem ventral surface and then divides into the two posterior cerebral arteries. The pontine blood supply is, to a large extent, from paramedian and short circumferential branches of the basilar artery. The cerebellum receives its blood from the superior and anterior inferior cerebellar arteries, also branching off the basilar artery. Vertebrobasilar distribution includes upper spinal cord, medulla, cerebellum, pons, parts of midbrain, and posterior and medial regions in the temporal lobes, along with the occipital lobes.

The vertebrobasilar system supplies regions of the auditory system involved in generation of ECochG and, to some extent, the ABR and ASSR. The vertebral arteries may not be of equal size, and branches from both vertebral and basilar arteries, and their distribution, are variable from one person to another. Consequently, the same site for obstruction of a vessel may produce different signs and symptoms clinically. The effect of impaired posterior cerebral artery blood circulation depends on the status of the circle of Willis. Brainstem, cerebellum, and thalamus infarction and dysfunction may result from stenosis or occlusion of the basilar artery or both vertebral arteries. There is often occlusion of the penetrating branches of the basilar artery, causing brainstem infarction.

The internal carotid artery system supplies, presumably, most regions of the auditory system above the level of the brainstem, which give rise to the 40 Hz ERD, AMLR, ALR, P300 response, and the MMN response. The P300 response, arising in part from hippocampus, is also dependent on vertebrobasilar system blood supply. The anterior cerebral artery sends blood to the anterior three-fourths of the medial portions of the cerebral hemispheres. The middle cerebral artery supplies the lateral three-fourths of the cerebral hemispheres. Anatomic regions thought to be important in generation of AMLR and ALR, including the superior temporal gyrus, Heschl's gyrus, the insula, and inferior parietal regions, are thus served by the middle cerebral artery.

3
CHAPTER

Introduction to Auditory Evoked Response Measurement

Selected principles of electrophysiological measurement, including stimulus and acquisition parameters, test strategies, and patient instructions shared by most auditory evoked responses, are reviewed in this chapter. There is a common perception that AERs are "objective" measures of auditory function, implying that by following a fixed test protocol any tester with minimal technical skills will consistently obtain reliable, valid, and clinically useful data. This is, in fact, a misperception. First of all, it is not possible to follow a fixed and inflexible test protocol and still assess many patients efficiently, effectively, and successfully. Test protocols must often be tailor-made for individual patients. Test protocols are highly dependent on the reason for the assessment. Moreover, because of unpredictable environmental or subject variables, a clinician is frequently required to revise his or her test strategy. To be regularly successful in AER assessment, the clinician must constantly think on his or her feet. The clinician must be prepared to make adjustments in the assessment approach on the basis of clinical judgment and ongoing analysis of data as it is collected during AER recordings. There are myriad interactions among the effects of subject characteristics, stimulus and acquisition parameters, auditory pathology, and other factors on AERs. The complexity of these interactions precludes their prediction or evaluation entirely by computer or the adherence by a clinician to a fixed test sequence. The responsibility for adapting strategy to obtain optimal AER results remains with the clinician. Clinical expertise goes beyond both a superficial "cook book" understanding of AER measurement and extensive "book knowledge" of AER principles. Consequently, interpretation of AERs will probably always be largely dependent on judgment by an experienced clinician. Automated data collection and scoring certainly has assumed an important role in some AER applications, such as newborn auditory screening and neuromonitoring. Automation is even incorporated to some extent into routine AER measurement, for example, with auditory steady-state responses (ASSRs). However, automation is not likely to be routinely relied upon

for diagnostic clinical AER applications. Perhaps the most dangerous consequence of the assumption that AERs are "objective tests" is an oversimplification of the complexity of clinical assessment and a false sense of security about one's ability to carry out the testing. Consistency in test instrumentation and protocol is always desirable, but should not and cannot be maintained at the expense of test feasibility, efficiency, or accuracy. Major components of the AER evaluation will now be reviewed.

AER MEASUREMENT WITH PATIENTS IN THE REAL WORLD

To reiterate a theme stated at the outset of this book, AER measurement is technically and clinically challenging. Ideally, the audiologist or clinical neurophysiologist first develops a firm grasp of the principles underlying AERs, and then begins to develop necessary technical and clinical skill by recording responses from dozens of normal persons under optimal measurement conditions. Ideal subjects are friendly, cooperative, healthy young adults who are known to have normal hearing sensitivity and auditory CNS function. The test setting is a quiet and familiar clinical facility. There is a relaxed atmosphere, with virtually unlimited test time and no demand for an interpretation and a report of findings. Technical mistakes may not be detected until after the test or, blissfully, not at all. In either case, no harm is done.

Contrast this relatively serene description with one of the following, and not atypical, clinical scenarios.

• A restless newborn infant with suspected peripheral and/or central auditory dysfunction undergoes ABR measurement in an intensive care nursery late on a Friday afternoon. The procedure must be repeatedly halted because of excessive electrical interference from the incubator and physiologic monitors or an ambient noise level that forces the testers to literally shout in order to communicate. The infant's parents are waiting anxiously in an adjacent room.

After a two-month hospital stay beginning at birth, the parents are looking forward to the infant's discharge as soon as "hearing testing" is complete. The attending neonatologist has asked to be paged and informed of the findings as soon as possible.

• ABR assessment is requested for a 9-month-old child with bilateral congenital aural atresia and possibly maximum conductive hearing loss in each ear. The surgeon needs to verify sensorineural auditory status for each ear in order to plan otologic management. If the hearing loss is, indeed, conductive bilaterally, surgery is indicated. If either or both ears have sensorineural component, surgery is contraindicated. The assessment is completed in the operating room under general anesthesia immediately before high-resolution temporal bone CT scanning. About 45 minutes are allotted for the ABR assessment. Again, the physician wants a prompt report of findings. The family is from a distant city, and he will discuss the management plan with parents immediately after the ABR and CT scan so that they can leave for the airport and return home. The outcome of the ABR assessment will largely determine the surgical management approach.

• ABR assessment is carried out in the clinic for neurodiagnosis with an adult having an asymmetric sensorineural hearing loss. The patient understands that the procedure is being performed to rule out a tumor involving the auditory nerve and is understandably anxious and tense. Waveform morphology is poor, in part because of muscular artifact. Pure tone audiometry showed bilateral high-frequency sensorineural hearing impairment and, as recording begins, a wave I component cannot be recorded from either ear. There is an interaural wave V latency difference, but could it be consistent with the difference in hearing sensitivity between ears? The patient is scheduled to return to the neurotologist the same day after the testing, with ABR waveforms and a report in hand.

• Repeated attempts to obtain valid behavioral audiometry findings from a 7-year-old mentally retarded child with Down syndrome have failed, and AERs are requested. Not unexpectedly, middle ear dysfunction is suspected. Sedation is required. Chloral hydrate is administered, but the child actually becomes more active and testing is aborted. What next steps will lead toward successful auditory assessment?

• Combined ECochG/ABR intraoperative recordings are requested to monitor eighth nerve and auditory brainstem function during surgical removal of a moderate-sized meningioma from the cerebellopontine (CP) angle. One objective of surgery is hearing preservation. Preoperative ABR assessment failed to show a distinct wave I on the involved side. In the OR on the day of surgery with this case, AER measurement is made more difficult by excessive electrical artifact. The neurotology-neurosurgery team is expecting moment-to-moment information on functional status of the auditory system as well as information that will be useful in predicting postoperative hearing outcome. How can high-quality AER waveforms be quickly and reliably recorded intraoperatively under these hostile conditions?

• AER assessment in the ICU is requested for a comatose young adult within 24 hours after severe head trauma. The patient is unresponsive to any sensory stimulation. Brain death is suspected. The organ transplant team has been consulted and has already initiated the initial contact with the patient's family. CT scanning showed evidence of unilateral temporal bone fracture as well as diffuse cerebral edema. Medications at the time of testing include sedatives, chemical paralyzing agents, and aminoglycoside antibiotics. The patient is hypothermic. The referring physician requires an immediate report of the findings. What possible influences do the temporal bone fracture, medications, and temperature have on ABR and AMLR outcome? When are AER findings compatible with brain death?

• An ABR assessment of a 2-year-old girl with severe language delay is conducted in the OR under light anesthesia and immediately after insertion of ventilation tubes. Previous behavioral audiologic assessment yielded inconsistent responses. OAEs were absent, but that was anticipated as the patient had a history of middle ear disease. There is no ABR to click stimulation at maximum signal intensity levels (95 dB nHL). Likewise, there is no response to tone burst stimulation at equipment limits. The parents ask whether their daughter will benefit from amplification or whether she is a candidate for a cochlear implant. How will you fit a hearing aid without an estimation of auditory threshold, and is the child even likely to benefit from amplification?

These are just a few examples of the numerous types of clinical challenges faced regularly in AER measurement. For consistently successful AER measurement, the clinician must master relatively straightforward technical skills, such as proper electrode placement and operation of the evoked response system. The clinician must also continuously adapt to unexpected difficulties in testing. The clinician must apply whatever techniques and strategies seem to be useful in dealing with measurement problems presented by a given patient and test setting. Finally, the clinician must know what AER information is needed and must be guided by one overall objective: to get this AER information if at all possible, often as quickly as possible. In this chapter, commonly encountered problems in AER measurement are cited and clinically feasible solutions presented. Admittedly, this is an inadequate format for presenting strategies for troubleshooting in AER measurement because problems do not always occur in isolation. In fact, they are often multiple and related. Also, AER interpretation is largely a matter of detecting dynamic patterns in waveforms. Measurement problems usually are detected first as some aberration in a waveform. Therefore, whenever possible, measurement problems are illustrated here with actual AER recordings. Valuable information is available clinically from AER data as it is acquired, rather than after the waveform is averaged. Unfortunately, this measurement process cannot be presented in a book format. The emphasis in this chapter is on general problems and solutions. Measurement difficulties encountered most often in specific responses (e.g., ECochG, ABR, ASSR, and AMLR) or in special AER applications, such as intraoperative and ICU neuromonitoring and newborn auditory screening, or in recording nonauditory evoked responses, are also reviewed in more detail in the chapters devoted to each of these topics. Inevitably, not all of the difficulties that may arise in clinical AER measurement are cited in this chapter. I hope, however, that the principles of AER problem solving reviewed here will also be of value in resolving other unmentioned problems.

AER measurement problems can be divided into two general categories. The first category consists of operator errors. That is, a less than optimal, perhaps totally inadequate, AER is recorded because of a technical mistake. Examples of these types of errors are an improper electrode placement or an incorrect equipment setting. The second type of measurement problem, one related to the subject or the test environment, is often more frustrating and its solution more challenging. This second type of problem may plague AER measurement for the experienced clinician as well as the novice. The author, in recording AERs clinically during the course of the past thirty years, has made each of the operator errors described in this chapter, and then some. He has also faced all of the other problems. As noted in the introduction of the book, clinicians cannot expect to record AERs flawlessly, but should always view their results critically and attempt to detect possible measurement problems during recording. In this way, problems can be solved while there is still an opportunity to obtain valid and adequate AER data, i.e., the patient is still in the clinic and hooked up. Put another way, in clinical AER measurement and in life in general, "all's well that ends well."

PREPARATION AND PRECAUTIONS BEFORE THE TEST

An important ingredient in successful AER assessment is adequate preparation before patient contact. Although the degree of preparation required and its impact on the outcome of AER assessment varies among applications, at least three main concerns should be addressed. First, it is extremely valuable to know what kind of patient is scheduled for assessment and why. There are many questions to be asked. What is the patient's age? Is the patient a newborn (premature or full-term?), a young child or older child, a young adult or older adult? Is the primary objective of testing information on auditory or neurological status? What is the tentative diagnosis or what are the likely etiologies to be ruled out in the differential diagnosis? If a diagnosis is suspected, the reader can refer to other portions of this book and additional reference sources to determine the specific AER findings or pattern of findings that are characteristic of the diagnosis and any special recording problems that might be encountered.

Has an AER assessment been carried out before? What did it show and are the results available? Does the referral source want an immediate report on the results? Will the patient be reasonably alert, lethargic, or comatose? Is he or she currently on medications that might affect AERs? Why can't behavioral auditory evaluation techniques be used? If previous behavioral testing was done, what did it show? Does the patient have normal hearing and, if not, what is the type and degree of hearing impairment? Is it likely that sedation will be needed? Are there any contraindications to sedation? Is an order for sedation and, if necessary, additional sedation, available? Who will administer the sedation, and is this person ready?

Second, before the testing is scheduled to begin, it is important to ensure that the necessary equipment and supplies are in place. This determination is, in part, based on the answers to the questions above. For example, are there enough clean electrodes of the proper type or enough disposable electrodes on hand? Is there an adequate supply of tape, abrasive liquid, and conducting paste for electrode application and unused insert ear cushions? If the instrumentation is programmable, are programs for the planned test protocols prepared and accessible? Is there a sufficient supply of data record sheets and report forms? These concerns are especially important for mobile AER assessments away from the evoked response laboratory or audiology clinic, because retrieving even a minor missing item might be very time consuming or even impossible. Special steps may be necessary in preparation for certain AER applications, such as newborn auditory screening and neuromonitoring.

Patient Instructions

With the exception of recordings made in the operating room or intensive care unit, some explanation of the AER procedure to the patient is required. For adults and older children who will be tested without sedation, the explanation is given directly to the patient. The parents or caregiver of infants and younger children also benefit from some description of the upcoming test. Instructions vary in detail for different types of AERs, as noted next. As a rule, the time taken instructing the patient is time well spent. Patients who understand what will be done during the procedure, and what will be expected from them, are less likely to be anxious about testing and more apt to be cooperative and relaxed during testing. Recording AERs is, in many respects, a high-tech procedure. The relatively sophisticated equipment (computer, electrodes, earphones), often in combination with a clinical environment (e.g., white lab coats, austere test room), tend to make the typical patient rather apprehensive. AER assessment may be a familiar and comfortable daily routine for the clinician, but for a patient on the initial visit, it is likely to be foreign and even frightening. The electrodes alone often conjure up scenes of horror. Patients may even incorrectly assume that the electrodes are used to present a shock to their

> The clinician should never forget that there is a person—a human being—between the stimulus transducer and the recording electrodes. Each and every patient deserves a simple, but complete, description, in everyday language, of the auditory evoked response procedure that is about to be performed.

head, rather than to passively detect brain activity containing the AER.

The clinician should never forget that there is a person—a human being—between the stimulus transducer and the recording electrodes. Each and every patient deserves a simple, but complete, description, in everyday language, of the AER procedure that is about to be performed. Good clinicians are not only technically skilled in recording AER data, but also sensitive and caring in the approach taken with patients and family members before, during, and after test sessions. Not unexpectedly, some patients undergoing neurodiagnostic assessment have communication impairment secondary to pathologies or disorders, for example, patients with receptive language impairment following a cerebrovascular accident (stroke). Care must be taken to be sure that all patients understand the explanation of the nature of the AER assessment and specific instructions.

It is always helpful for clinicians to put themselves in the patient's or family member's shoes before the test. Often these people are already anxious about the possibility of a health problem, ranging from a hearing impairment to a brain tumor. Perhaps they have traveled many miles. Patients from a rural area may have been frightened by urban traffic and may have had difficulty finding a parking space or may have become lost in a medical center maze. Parents of young children may be worried about possible dangers of sedation or that the testing will be painful to their child. Any patient may, of course, have concerns about the cost of procedure and whether insurance will cover this cost. New clinicians will become sensitized to potential patient concerns about evoked response assessment by undergoing AER measurement themselves. Actually, the clinician can learn much about recording techniques by practicing (behind closed doors) AER measurement while serving as both the subject and the tester.

Some guidelines on patient instructions are offered below for each major AER. For patients who, during their first visit to the clinic, are scheduled to return for AER assessment, a brief explanation of the scheduled test procedure may reduce anxiety. Simply written summaries of these instructions may also be given to patients at that time, mailed before the test, and or handed to the family when they arrive on the AER test date. Many clinics and centers now include on their website patient information about test procedures, diseases, and disorders, as well as clinical services offered at the facility.

GENERAL EXPLANATIONS. | Some patient instructions are appropriate for all types of AERs, whereas others are uniquely suited for one type of AER or another. The common features of AER patient instructions are discussed here, while details specific to each AER follows. The detail and vocabulary of instructions will vary depending on the age and educational background of the patient or family member. Two fundamental components of patient instructions are (1) what procedure will be performed and (2) how it will be done. In many cases, some mention of why testing is being done is also in order, although this latter information is optional and dependent on the objectives of testing—for example, hearing threshold estimation versus neurodiagnosis. A rather typical explanation for ABR procedure is as follows:

> In this test, I [or we] will record a response from your ear, a response of the nerve that runs from your ear to your brain, and even brain waves caused by sounds. [The phrases auditory evoked response, auditory brainstem response, and other technical terms are used only with patients having some knowledge of the procedures or medical terms in general.] The response from your ear and the brain waves will be picked up with these wires. The wires will be taped onto your head and ears. You will hear clicking sounds [or beeping tones] through these earphones. They sound like this [click your tongue]. You do not have to listen to these sounds. I just need for you to lie here very quietly. Try to stay relaxed and to keep your jaw loose. We'll recline this chair just before the test begins. It's OK if you fall asleep [for ECochG and ABR; see specific instructions below for AMLR, ALR and P300]. In fact, we'll turn down the lights when the test begins to help you to rest and maybe fall sleep.
>
> First, I will scrub the skin on your forehead and earlobes (or the outer part of your ear canal) with a scratchy liquid. This is the most uncomfortable part of the test. Then, I'll put some paste on these wires [electrodes] and tape them to these locations. I'll clean the paste off your skin when we are done with the test. During the test, you will wear these earphones or [for inserts] I will place these soft foam plugs in each of your ears. This test may give us (or whoever referred the patient) important information on your hearing.

ECochG. | Much information explained to patients is similar for all AERs, as noted above. Instructions specific to ECochG depend mostly on electrode type. If earlobe electrodes are

---

Important points to be clarified for each patient:
- AER recording is a routine clinical procedure, used even with newborn infants.
- The procedure does not pose any risk to the patient.
- The procedure is noninvasive and not painful (ECochG may be an exception).
- There are no side effects for unsedated AER recordings.
- Results may not be immediately available.
- The assessment can be stopped at any time upon patient request.

used, ABR instructions apply as well for ECochG. With ear canal electrodes, the patient is told that the outer portion of the ear canal will be scrubbed lightly with a scratchy liquid. Then, a soft foam plug will be placed within this portion of the ear canal. Note that a patient's hearing will be attenuated by about 20 dB after the foam plugs are inserted in the ear canal, and the tester may need to speak very loudly to be heard. If a tympanic membrane electrode type is used (typically without anesthesia), the patient is told that a soft plastic tube will be inserted into the ear canal. The patient will feel the tube within the ear canal. During insertion of the electrode the patient might experience a tickling feeling, and it may be slightly uncomfortable. The patient will have a sensation of pressure or fullness when the soft flexible end of the tube rests on the eardrum. The patient is encouraged to tell the tester what the electrode feels like, especially if it is too uncomfortable. Transtympanic electrode instructions, of course, are slightly different. Following the general instructions just noted, the patient is told that the doctor (physician) will numb the eardrum with a liquid (e.g., Phenol). This may cause a stinging sensation. It is the most uncomfortable part of the test. Then the doctor will place an electrode into the ear canal and through the eardrum. Finally, a foam plug will be inserted gently into the ear canal. At this point in the instructions, the typical patient will no doubt appreciate an estimate of test time. Generally, after electrode placement, transtympanic ECochG can be completed in less than 10 minutes. The foam plug and needle electrode will be removed as soon as testing is completed. There should not be any discomfort after testing. The author, who has acquired ECochG experience with this electrode type, has not yet encountered a patient who has refused to undergo the procedure or who complained of excessive discomfort during the procedure. Patients, in fact, occasionally fall asleep during testing and often do not realize when the electrode is extracted from the tympanic membrane.

ABR. | The general instructions cited above are sufficient for most patients undergoing ABR assessment. Adults and children are encouraged to sleep during the test. Sleep is facilitated by making the patient comfortable (stretched out with a pillow under the his head) and by lowering lights in the test room. Administration of sedation (usually chloral hydrate) to induce sleep is often indicated with children between the ages of 3 to 6 months and 6 years (see Chapter 8). Sedation is occasionally helpful as well for tense adults, although another drug (e.g., Valium) is typically used. With any AER assessment, patients usually rest in the supine position on a gurney or bed. It may be necessary to ask how the patient can be made more comfortable. For example, readjusting the pillow under the head may serve to relax the neck muscles and promote sleep. The patient may wish to remove his or her eyeglasses and shoes. Also, men may wish to loosen their ties and women may want to remove earrings. If the test

room is cool, a blanket is useful to keep the patient comfortable and to maintain normal body temperature. Low body temperature (hypothermia) may influence ABR findings (see Chapter 7). Finally, patients should be given the opportunity to visit the restroom before electrodes are applied and testing begins (and after to freshen up).

AMLR. | Encouraging a relaxed state is very important for quality AMLR recordings. Post-auricular muscle (PAM) artifact, which can seriously interfere with identification of AMLR components (see Chapter 11 for details), is more likely with tense patients. The challenge in AMLR measurement, however, is to maintain a relaxed patient state without necessarily allowing the patient to fall asleep. Sleep may reduce AMLR amplitude, and changes in sleep status during testing contribute to variability in findings. If the choice facing the tester is a tense versus sleeping patient, quality of waveforms is more likely to be enhanced by sleep. Naturally, in describing electrode placement to the patient, the tester should mention also that an electrode may be placed on the scalp (and in hair) on each side of the head.

ALR. | Either an awakened patient (for adults) or a deep sleep state (for infants and young children) is essential for optimal ALR measurement conditions. Again, the challenge is to keep the patient awake while also encouraging the patient to relax. The patient is asked to rest comfortably, but not to fall asleep. Usually, it is best for the patient to lie still with eyes open. Also, arranging for the patient to view silent video material (e.g., cartoons or movies with subtitles) is helpful in facilitating a quiet yet awake state of arousal. A number of investigators have described in their protocols for recording late latency AERs the use of videos or DVDs to maintain an awakened state for pediatric and adult patients. While AERs are recorded, the patient watches a cartoon or movie, with the audio either at a low volume or muted. The tester still should periodically assure that the patient has not fallen asleep. As noted in the section on test strategy above, the proper patient state for each AER when recorded as part of a test battery may be facilitated by the following sequence: ALR, P300, AMLR, and ABR/ECochG. This is based on the premise that the patient will begin the testing alert, and then will tend to fall asleep as the testing continues.

P300. | Patient instructions are typically an extremely important component in successful P300 measurement. Whenever possible, the patient must clearly understand the attention-related task, if attention is required for the P300 recording. For example, the patient may be told that there will be two kinds of sounds, one with a lower pitch and the other with a higher pitch. He or she will hear the lower pitched sound quite often, but will occasionally hear the higher pitched sound. The task is to listen carefully for the occasional higher pitched sound, and to count how many of these sounds he or she hears during the test. The patient will be asked to report the number of these sounds at the conclusion of the test. Of course, throughout the test the patient should remain alert and not doze or fall asleep. A passive P300 response (P3a) can be recorded without the requirement of subject attention to the stimuli, as reviewed in Chapter 12.

STIMULUS PARAMETERS

Acoustic stimuli are necessary for generation of all AERs. Stimulus properties, such as frequency, duration, intensity, rate, and polarity, exert profound and often interrelated effects on AER measurement. There are, in addition, complex interactions among some stimulus factors and subject characteristics (e.g., age, cochlear hearing impairment). Equally important is the transducer that converts an electrical signal into the acoustic signal that elicits the response. Further, mode of stimulus presentation, such as monaural versus binaural, may also affect the response that is recorded. Finally, the presence of masking sounds affects auditory response. Proper stimulus selection, definition, calibration, and presentation is one of the most challenging, yet essential, aspects of AER measurement. General stimulus factors in AER measurement are reviewed in this chapter. Three simple principles important for all auditory evoked responses are stated in Table 3.1. Terminology used in reference to acoustic stimuli is defined briefly throughout the chapter. However, the reader without background in psychoacoustics and hearing science will require additional information, available from numerous textbooks as well as on the Internet.

Stimulus Type and Frequency

For neurophysiologic reasons, early latency AERs are recorded optimally with very brief (transient) stimuli having an almost instantaneous onset. In fact, the rapid onset of the transient stimulus is important in producing the synchronous firing of numerous auditory neurons that underlies these responses. Therefore, the brief duration (e.g., 0.1 ms or 100 μsec) click, which has an abrupt onset, is by far the most commonly used stimulus for ECochG ABR measurement. The click stimulus may actually be one of several somewhat different acoustic signals, including a rectangular voltage electrical pulse, diphasic square-wave pulses, triangular waves, or a single period of a high-frequency haversine or half-sine wave. Terminology used in describing electrical signals and acoustic stimuli in AER measurement is defined in Table 3.2. Selected types of stimuli (click, tone, burst) that may be used in AERs are illustrated in Figure 3.1. An abrupt signal, such as a rectangular electrical pulse, has a very broad spectrum and, when delivered to a transducer, results in an acoustic signal encompassing a wide range of frequencies. In theory, then, this range of frequencies activates the cochlea and, specifically, the hair cells, over an extensive region of the basilar membrane. The frequency content of the stimulus

TABLE 3.1. Three General Principles of AER Measurement

Stimulus Principle

- The optimal stimulus rate for an AER is directly related to the speed of the response.
- Early AERs (e.g., ECochG and ABR) are fast responses that can be elicited with faster stimulus rates, whereas later AERs (e.g., AMLR or P300) are slower responses that require slower stimulus rates.

Filter Principle

- Elimination of unwanted electrical activity (noise) with preservation of desired electrical activity (response).
- Early AERs (e.g., ECochG and ABR) are fast responses with more high-frequency content, whereas later AERs (e.g., AMLR or P300) are slower responses with more low-frequency content.

Averaging Principle

- The extent of signal averaging (time) needed to record a detectable AER depends on the size of the signal (the AER) and the amount of noise (electrical and myogenic) within the recording (the signal-to-noise ratio, or SNR).
- Early responses have smaller amplitude and require more averaging, whereas later responses have larger amplitude and require less averaging (when noise is constant).

actually generating the AER for a given subject, however, depends on a variety of factors, such as (1) stimulus intensity, (2) the electro-acoustic properties of the transducer, (3) ear canal and middle ear properties affecting sound transmission, and (4) the integrity of the cochlea.

Higher frequencies in the click acoustic spectrum are responsible for generating the ABR in the normal ear. An ABR evoked by a moderately intense (e.g., 60 dB nHL) click stimulus and delivered with insert earphones reflects activation of the high-frequency regions (roughly 1000 through 4000 Hz) of the cochlea. Reported differences in the frequency region most important for generation of the ABR (such as 1000 to 4000 Hz, 4000 to 8000 Hz, 3000 Hz, 4000 Hz, 2000 Hz and above, and so forth) are probably, to a large degree, due to the differences in stimulus intensity and the upper frequency limit of the acoustic transducers used in the studies to present the clicks (Bauch & Olsen, 1986; Coats, 1978; Coats & Martin, 1977; Eggermont & Don, 1980; Gorga, Reiland, & Beauchaine, 1985; Gorga, Worthington, Reiland, Beauchaine, & Goldgar, 1985; Hoke, Lutkenhoner, & Bappert, 1980; Jerger & Mauldin, 1978; Kileny, 1981).

More apical (low-frequency) regions of the cochlea are also activated by the click but, for two reasons, do not

TABLE 3.2. Definition of Terms Used to Describe Auditory Evoked Response (AER) Stimulus Characteristics

TERM	DEFINITION
air conduction	The process by which sound is conducted to the inner ear (cochlea) through the air in the external acoustic meatus (ear canal) as part of the pathway.
alternating	The polarity of the stimulus pressure wavefront is alternated on successive trials (between rarefaction and condensation).
bone conduction	Transmission of sound to the inner ear mediated primarily by mechanical vibration of the cranial bones.
brief tone[a]	A tone pulse with a duration of less than 20 ms.
click	Acoustic signal produced by a rectangular electric pulse of a specified duration, delivered to a transducer.
condensation	A stimulus polarity that initially causes the pressure wavefront of a transducer to move toward the eardrum.
filtered click	Acoustic signal produced by a rectangular electric pulse of a specified duration, passed through a filter, and subsequently delivered to a transducer.
gating function	The time function that modulates the amplitude of a continuous signal in order to determine the turn-on and turn-off characteristics.
hearing level (HL)	For a specified stimulus, for a specified type of transducer, and for a specified manner of application, the HL is the SPL, or the vibration force level, of the signal set up by the transducer with a specified coupler minus the appropriate reference equivalent threshold level for air and bone conduction, as applicable. It is measured in decibels (dB) relative to a standard reference threshold for the specified stimulus.
masking	The process by which the threshold of audibility of a signal is raised by the presence of another sound.
peak sound pressure	The peak sound pressure for any specified time interval is the maximum absolute value of the instantaneous sound pressure in that interval. The reference for 0 dB peak sound pressure is 20 µPa (micropascals).
peak-to-peak equivalent sound pressure level (peSPL)[a]	The peSPL of a short-duration signal is the sound pressure level calculated as (RMS) of a pure tone, which, when fed to the same transducer under the same test conditions, has the same peak-to-peak amplitude as the short-duration signal.
plateau duration	When measurable, this is the time during which the envelope of the burst is at 100% amplitude.
polarity	The initial direction of the pressure wavefront in the stimulus waveform, measured at the face of the transducer.
rarefaction	A stimulus polarity that initially causes the pressure wavefront of a transducer to move away from the eardrum.
repetition rate	The number of stimuli presented per unit time.
rise/fall times	The time interval for a waveform to go from zero amplitude to maximum amplitude (rise time) or from maximum to zero (fall time).
sensation level (SL)	The level of the sound above its threshold of audibility for an individual subject.
sound pressure level (SPL)	Based on a physical reference for the (RMS) sound pressure. For any sound, it is equal to 20 times the logarithm to the base 10 of the ratio of the pressure of the sound to the reference pressure. The typical reference for 0 dB RMS SPL is 20 µPa.
tone burst	Specifiable carrier frequency with a specified envelope function by which the carrier is modified.
total duration	The time between each instance of zero amplitude on the waveform envelope.
white noise	A noise for which the spectrum density is substantially independent of frequency over a specified frequency range. The slope of the pressure spectrum level of white noise is 0 dB per octave.

[a] From Working Group 10 (Specification of Reference Audiometric Test Signals of Short Duration).
Source: The first draft of American National Standard entitled "Stimulus Specifications for Instruments Used to Measure Auditory Evoked Potentials" and proposed by the Acoustical Society of America Accredited Standards Committee, Working Group S3–72, Measurement of Auditory Evoked Potentials. Courtesy of Chair: R. A. Ruth.

Two Stimuli Used to Elicit Auditory Evoked Responses

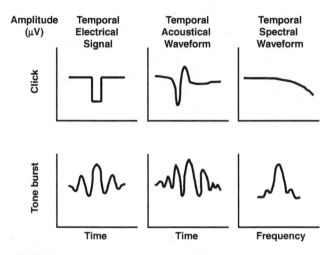

FIGURE 3.1. Two types of stimuli (clicks and tone bursts) used to elicit auditory evoked responses.

contribute much to the ABR, at least in normal hearers. First, the neurophysiologic response elicited by cochlear activation in the higher frequency regions (near the base of the cochlea) has already occurred by the time the traveling wave reaches the apex and has activated hair cells in this region. Second, the leading "front" of the traveling wave is more gradual (less abrupt) when it reaches the apical region and consequently not as effective introducing synchronous firing of many eighth-nerve afferent fibers over a concentrated portion of the basilar membrane. Instead, smaller numbers of afferents sequentially fire over a more dispersed stretch of the basilar membrane. In persons with an impairment of auditory sensitivity for the higher frequency region, generation of the ABR may not necessarily follow this pattern. In addition, the portion of the cochlea contributing to the ABR varies as a function of the components (e.g., wave I vs. wave V) and stimulus intensity. For example, wave I appears to reflect basal activation, whereas wave V may reflect activity from portions of the basilar membrane closer to the apex. Also, at high stimulus intensity levels, there is spread of activation toward the apex, whereas at lower intensity levels, activation is limited more to the basal region.

There are, therefore, two general principles to keep in mind in considering stimuli for evoking auditory responses. First, frequency specificity of a stimulus (i.e., the concentration of energy in a specific frequency region) is indirectly related to duration (Burkard, 1984; Gabor, 1947; Gorga, Reiland, & Beauchaine, 1985; Harris, 1978). With very brief stimuli, energy tends to be distributed over more frequencies, whereas stimuli with longer duration (including rise/fall times and plateau time) are spectrally constrained. Second, there is generally a direct relationship between duration of the response and duration of the stimulus. That is, slower responses (longer latency) are activated best by slower (lower

rate of stimulation, and longer onset and duration) stimuli whereas faster (shorter latency) responses require faster (higher rate of stimulation and shorter onset and duration) stimuli.

Duration

Stimulus duration is the sum of the rise time, plateau time, and fall time. These terms were defined in Table 3.2 and are illustrated in Figure 3.2. This definition is actually oversimplified, primarily for illustrative purposes. Duration for the electric waveform used in generating the stimulus can be determined by means of an oscilloscope. Duration of the acoustic waveform of the stimulus also can be measured with an oscilloscope, along with a standard coupler and a sound level meter. Whether measurements of duration are made electrically or acoustically, a consistent definition must be used. Other examples of definitions for rise/fall times are the time interval from the onset of any amplitude to maximum amplitude, the time interval between the 10 percent and the 90 percent amplitude points, or the number of cycles of a sinusoidal stimulus occurring during the rise or fall portion of the stimulus. Plateau time likewise can be described in different ways, such as the time interval between the 50 percent amplitude points on the rise versus the fall envelopes of the stimulus or simply the time from one end of the plateau to the other for the click. Both rise/fall times and plateau time were incorporated into the concept of "equivalent duration," defined by Dallos and Olsen (1964) as two-thirds of the rise time plus the plateau duration.

There are two common approaches for classifying tonal stimuli based on their duration characteristics. One is to define a constant rise time for all nonclick stimuli. For example, Stapells and Picton (1981) suggest that tonal stimuli at any frequency consistently have a 5 ms rise time. Kodera, Yamane, Yamada, and Suzuki (1977) and by Klein (1983)

Stimulus Duration

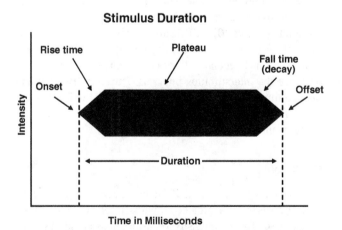

FIGURE 3.2. An illustration of stimulus components that contribute to duration, including rise time, plateau, and fall time.

employed the constant rise-time approach. With a fixed rise/fall time, temporal features of the stimulus are clearly constant, but spectral splatter will be greater for lower versus higher frequencies. The other approach, introduced by Hallowell Davis and colleagues (Davis, Hirsh, Popelka, & Formby, 1984) and recommended also by others (Coats, Martin, & Kidder, 1979; Hall, 1992) is to define tone-burst rise-time duration on the basis of a constant number of cycles. Specifically, Davis suggested using tones with rise and fall times of 2 cycles and a plateau of 1 cycle. This is referred to as the 2-1-2 paradigm for stimulus duration. Because 1 cycle for a 1000 Hz tone (i.e., by definition 1000 cycles per second) lasts 1 ms, the 2-1-2-rule would define a tone burst with rise/fall times of 2 ms and a plateau of 1 ms. A 500 Hz stimulus, with cycles each lasting 2 ms (i.e., 1000 ms/500) would, by the 2-1-2 rule, have rise-plateau-fall values of 4 ms–2 ms–4 ms, and so on. As described in Chapter 8, the most common current duration of tone bursts used now for frequency-specific ABR measurement is 2 cycles for the rise and fall times and no (0 ms) plateau. With this approach, duration features of various stimulus frequencies vary, yet energy is held constant for different frequencies.

Complex interactions among stimulus parameters influence AER recordings. Stimulus duration is particularly closely related to the frequency content of the stimulus and to the rate and interstimulus interval (ISI). Duration inversely affects spectral (frequency) content. For stimuli of extended durations, frequency content may consist of a single pure tone. In critically reviewing studies of stimulus duration and AERs, and also in attempting to define the clinical implications of altering stimulus duration, it is always reasonable to question whether changes in AERs that appear to be due to duration are, in fact, a result of a broader stimulus frequency content. This concern is enhanced for patients with auditory pathology. The connection between stimulus duration, stimulus rate, and interstimulus interval can be understood intuitively. If a certain number of stimuli are presented within a specific amount of time, such as 20/sec, then increasing the duration of each stimulus while keeping the number constant (e.g., at 20) will result in decreased interstimulus intervals. Alternatively, increasing the number of stimuli presented within 1 second will, of course, increase the rate and decrease the interstimulus intervals. Duration (rise/fall and plateau times) is first reviewed as a factor in AER measurement, followed by a discussion of stimulus rate and interstimulus interval.

Intensity

As a general principle, AER latency decreases and amplitude increases with greater stimulus intensity. The physiologic bases for the intensity versus response relations were reviewed in Chapter 2. Effects of intensity on AERs have probably been studied more than those of any other stimulus parameter. Intensity does not necessarily affect all AERs

in the same way and does not produce simple linear effects, even for a single AER (e.g., ABR), or equivalent effects for both latency and amplitude. Also, intensity often interacts in a complex fashion with a variety of subject characteristics and other stimulus parameters. Terms use in describing intensity were defined in Table 3.2. The unit of measure for intensity is the dB (decibel). A full discussion of the dB is beyond the scope of this book. As many as five references may be used to describe stimulus intensity in AER measurement:

1. dB sound pressure level (SPL)
2. dB peak-equivalent SPL (peSPL)
3. dB hearing level (HL) (according to ANSI standards)
4. dB sensation level (SL)
5. dB normal hearing level (nHL).

The most common convention clinically is to define intensity with a biological or behavioral reference, that is, in dB relative to the normal behavioral hearing threshold level for the stimulus, e.g., click or tone burst, usually indicated as "dB nHL." Threshold level for the click stimulus (i.e., the intensity level on the evoked response system at which the click is just audible [detectable]) is determined in a clinical facility (where the AERs will be recorded with patients) for a group of ten to fifteen normal-hearing young adults. The average of these threshold levels, in dB, is referred to as 0 dB nHL and is the reference level for indicating clinical intensity level. For example, if the average dB level for detection of the click by the normal subjects was 5 dB, then a dial or screen setting (equipment setting) of 75 dB would actually correspond to 70 dB nHL (75 minus 5 dB). It is important to keep in mind, as noted in the next section on stimulus rate, that faster click rates will enhance behavioral hearing levels, so at a high rate (e.g., 70 or 80 per second) the click threshold will be about 5 to 6 dB lower (better) than at a slow rate (e.g., 5 to 10 per second).

Another intensity reference sometimes reported in AER studies, and commonly used in hearing science, is dB SPL. The reference for 0 dB SPL is typically 0.0002 dynes/cm^2, or 20 microPascals (μPa). Devices for measuring dB SPL often cannot capture rapid onset, short-duration AER stimuli, such as clicks. A common practice, therefore, is to describe the peak sound pressure of these stimuli in terms of dB SPL for puretone stimulus. The peak of the click voltage waveform on an oscilloscope is compared to the peak for a long-duration pure tone of known intensity in dB SPL and is referred to as peSPL (peak equivalent SPL). The equivalent of 0 dB nHL under typical stimulus conditions (a 0.1 ms click presented at a rate of about 10 to 20 per second with conventional audiometric earphones) is 36.4 dB peak SPL and 29.9 dB peSPL (Burkard, 1984; Klein & Teas, 1978; Stapells, Picton, & Smith, 1982).

Rate

Rate is a stimulus parameter that must be selected by the operator in AER measurement. Therefore, an understanding of the effects of stimulus rate is needed to make rational decisions regarding which rate to use for different types of AERs and for different clinical applications. In the hands of an experienced clinician, stimulus rate can be manipulated to permit the fastest data collection in the least amount of time, thus either saving test time or permitting a thorough AER assessment in the time available (e.g., while a small child sleeps after sedation). There is no single correct rate, one that is appropriate for all patients under all test circumstances. The effects of rate are distinct for each of the AER types, particularly the shorter (ECochG, ABR) versus longer (ALR, P300) responses. For each AER type, rate effects are a product of the interactions among rate, a variety of subject characteristics (such as age, body temperature, and drugs), and various other stimulus parameters (such as intensity and duration). Finally, rate appears to be a factor in the diagnostic power of certain AERs. That is, rate may interact also with neuropathology.

A simple, yet statistically and clinically significant relationship exists between rate for transient stimuli and behavioral auditory threshold. From a stimulus rate of 5/sec to a stimulus rate of 80/sec, threshold is enhanced by 5 dB (measured in peak SPL). Presumably, this is due largely to temporal summation of acoustic energy, similar to the effect of increasing acoustic stimulus duration, although other processes are likely involved and the effect has not been consistently demonstrated (Klein & Teas, 1978; Picton, Oulette, Hamel, & Smith, 1979). The rate-versus-intensity relation itself is in turn influenced by frequency. Significantly less threshold improvement with increasing rate is observed for high- versus low-frequency stimuli. Stimulus rate must be considered in collecting normative AER data.

Interstimulus Interval (ISI) and Rate

For transient (very brief) stimuli, the interval between successive stimuli can be determined by dividing a discrete time period by the number of stimuli presented within that period (i.e., 1 second/rate = ISI). If a transient stimulus, for example, is presented at a rate of 20/sec, the accumulated time of the actual stimulus presentation is negligible. A total of 1000 ms (i.e., 1 second) divided by 20 results in an ISI of 50 s. With a rate of 10/sec, the ISI is 100 ms; for a 100 stimuli/second rate, the ISI is 10 ms, and so forth. For nontransient stimuli, calculation of ISI is not as straightforward because duration times for each individual stimulus accumulate and consume some of the time. If total duration of each stimulus is 5 ms (2 ms rise and fall times plus a 1 ms plateau), then for a rate of 20 stimuli/second, the accumulated stimulus time is 100 ms (20 stimuli at 5 ms each). Within a 1 sec (1000 ms) time frame, therefore, only 900 ms are available for the ISIs. Thus, 900 ms/20 yields an ISI of 45 ms. Analysis time could not be greater than this without including the response from the subsequent stimulus presentation within the same time period. If stimuli are presented at such a rapid rate that they occur within the analysis period, they will not contribute to the response and can actually degrade the averaged response.

Fast responses, such as the ECochG or ABR, occur within a relatively brief time period (5 to 6 ms or less), require relatively brief ISIs, and permit more rapid stimulus rates. Slower responses, such as the ALR or P300, last from 250 to 300 ms, require relatively extended ISIs, and limit effective stimulation rate to no faster than approximately 2 stimuli/second. When refractory times are also considered, optimal rate may be as low as 1 stimulus/2 second, or much lower. The effect of ISI on AERs is related to basic neurophysiologic mechanisms. Following every neural event (an AP or a postsynaptic membrane potential), there is a recovery or refractory period during which the neural unit is either incapable of being activated or has a higher threshold for activation. If the ISI time period exceeds this recovery period, then the neural unit can fully recover and will be responsive to the next stimulus. When ISIs are shorter than the recovery period, however, some stimuli will not contribute fully to the response because they are presented during the recovery period for the neural units generating the response. The result may be alteration of the response, such as increased latency or decreased amplitude. Physiologic processes presumably underlying these alterations are variations in the neural refractory period, changes in neural transmission factors, and adaptation and fatigue of neural receptor elements. Among AERs, there are different recovery times and, therefore, different requirements for ISIs. The neurophysiologic events of longer latency AERs, such as the ALR, require longer recovery periods. For example, amplitude of the auditory late response increases with progressively longer ISIs, up to 8 seconds. Onset neurons underlying the ABR, on the other hand, have relatively rapid recovery times. Therefore, even very brief interstimulus intervals (ISIs < 10 ms) are sufficient in measurement of the ABR.

Polarity

There are three categories of stimulus polarity in AER measurement—condensation, rarefaction, and alternating. With a positive electrical pulse or signal and movement of the transducer diaphragm toward the tympanic membrane, a click signal with a positive pressure wave is generated. Movement in a positive direction, or a positive polarity, is also known as "condensation polarity." A pressure wave in a negative direction (negative polarity), produced by a movement of the transducer diaphragm away from the tympanic membrane, is called "rarefaction polarity." Alternating polarity is a switching between condensation and rarefaction polarities at subsequent stimulus presentations. Polarity is an important feature for a click stimulus. Clinically, polarity is not as critical a feature for tonal stimuli. A tonal stimulus, by definition, oscillates in a sinusoid fashion from one polarity to the other.

The polarity (phase) of the initial portion of a tone stimulus may also play a role in AER measurement.

An understanding of some basic principles of cochlear physiology is required to appreciate the effects of click polarity on AERs, especially ECochG and ABR (see also Chapter 2). According to different investigators (Brugge, Anderson, Hind, & Rose, 1969; Dallos, 1973; Davis, 1976b; Tasaki, 1954; Zwislocki, 1975), the afferent auditory nerves are activated primarily by the portion of a stimulus that moves the basilar membrane upward, in the direction of the scala vestibuli. This cochlear activity occurs when a rarefaction (negative) polarity or phase stimulus is presented, theoretically producing an outward movement of the tympanic membrane and in turn the stapes footplate in the oval window (Figure 3.3). With the resultant basilar membrane deviation upward toward the scala vestibuli in the cochlea, stereocilia on the hair cells in the organ of Corti are bent in the direction of the tallest stereocilia, receptor potentials are produced at the apex of the outer hair cells, and a negative CM is generated in the scala vestibuli while a positive CM is generated in the scala tympani. Bending of the stereocilia on the inner hair cells secondary to the effects of endolymph flow generates a bioelectrical event, synaptic transmission via the neurotransmitter glutamate, and afferent activity in the eighth (auditory) cranial nerve.

The apparently simple relationship between stimulus polarity and cochlear physiology, as just outlined, is complicated by at least four factors:

• Polarity of the stimulus may be reversed by ear-canal acoustics in its course from the transducer diaphragm to the tympanic membrane and/or by middle ear or inner ear mechanics in its transformation from eardrum to hair cell (Borg & Lofqvist, 1982; Dallos, 1975; Gerull, Mrowinski, Janssen, & Anft, 1985). Of course, if stimulus polarity is reversed twice before the afferents are activated (once in the ear canal and again in the middle ear), the original polarity will be maintained.

• The outward (lateral) movement of the oval window (the stapes footplate) with rarefaction clicks may be greater than the inward (medial) displacement due to condensation clicks (Guinan & Peake, 1967), and this polarity difference may be intensity dependent.

• Polarity effects are probably not comparable for conventional rectangular-wave clicks (with almost vertical onset and offset) versus for clicks with rapid onset but gradual offset. Clicks with rapid onset and offset produce basilar membrane movement in first one and then the other direction (in response first to onset and then to offset), even though polarity of a stimulus is designated by the onset direction.

• The initial component of the acoustic click waveform may be followed by an even larger amplitude and opposite-polarity (phase) second component, which is actually effective in generating the response. Some acoustic transducers "ring" when delivering a transient stimulus, resulting in oscillation and alternating polarities.

TRANSDUCERS

A transducer is a device for converting energy from one form to another. For most AER applications, the stimulus

Stimulus Polarity and Activation of the Auditory Brainstem Response (ABR)

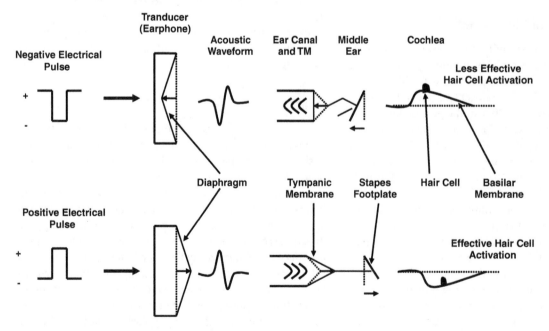

FIGURE 3.3. Schematic illustration of the sequence of events related to activation of the ear with by acoustic stimuli with rarefaction polarity.

is acoustic and the transducer is an earphone. Electrically elicited AERs, recorded most often in cochlear implant patients, are an exception to this rule (see Chapter 15). Transducers for AER measurement receive an electrical signal and produce a sound that is presented as an air-conduction stimulus. An air-conduction acoustic stimulus may also be presented with a loudspeaker. Even though loudspeakers are a common transducer type in behavioral audiologic assessment, they are rarely used in AER measurement. In some instances, AERs are elicited with bone-conduction (versus air-conduction) stimulation. An oscillator or vibrator is placed on the skull. The electrical signal with this type of transducer does not produce a sound; instead, mechanical oscillation is transmitted to the inner ear fluids, largely by vibration at the test frequency of the temporal bone (within which the inner ear is encased). The use of bone-conduction oscillators in eliciting AERs is discussed in a later subsection.

TDH-39 Earphone with MX41/AR Cushion

An array of transducers that are used in presenting stimuli in AER measurement is shown in Figure 3.4. Until the early 1990s, acoustic stimuli were presented via a Telephonics TDH-39 earphone mounted in an MX41/AR cushion. The apparent reasons for selection of the TDH-39 earphone in AER measurement were its availability, the security of knowing that it was routinely used in clinical audiometry, and the existence of pure-tone and speech audiometry standards for this earphone. However, there is really no rationale for continued reliance on the TDH-39 earphone and MX41/AR cushion as the transducer of choice in AER measurement. There are compelling arguments for abandoning the practice in favor of insert earphones. The TDH-39 is an electrodynamic earphone with low electrical impedance. At high intensity levels, the TDH-39 (and most transducers) produces an electromagnetic field that results in stimulus artifact. This is a clinical disadvantage. Electromagnetic shielding of the earphone and part of the cable has been recommended (Coats, Martin, & Kidder, 1979; Elberling & Salomon, 1973) to eliminate electromagnetic artifact, but commercially available shielded earphones are far more expensive than unshielded earphones. The use of piezoelectric or electrostatic earphones, instead of the electromagnetic type, is also an effective but probably equally expensive means of eliminating stimulus artifact in AER recording (Hughes & Fino, 1980). However, with piezoelectric earphones, a larger voltage is required because of the high impedance. This may limit the maximum intensity level output.

When mounted in the standard sponge rubber MX41/AR cushion (shown in Figure 3.4), the TDH-39 or TDH-49 is a supra-aural earphone. That is, the earphone rests on the ear and also makes contact with the head. This is distinct from a circumaural cushion, such as the Pederson type, which encompasses the ear and rests entirely on the head. Although TDH-39 or TDH-49 earphones with the MX41/AR cushion occlude the ear and enclose a relatively small volume of air under the cushion, there is often a gap or space below the ear in the region of the jaw. This gap permits leakage of, primarily, low frequencies (250 Hz and lower). Removal of the earphone from the cushion, which was reported in early reports of ABR measurement of newborn and young children, may dramatically alter the acoustic characteristics of the stimulus and also reduce ambient noise attenuation. This practice is certainly not advised.

The TDH-49 earphone is externally identical to the TDH-39 earphone and is mounted in the same type of sponge rubber cushion (MX41/AR). Of these two earphones, the TDH-49 is better suited for AER measurement, at least with high-frequency or broad-spectrum (e.g., click) stimuli. The frequency response for the TDH-39 earphone is illustrated in Figure 3.5. *It is important to keep in mind, however, that insert earphones are generally best suited for auditory evoked response assessment, especially with children.* Practical differences between the two supra-aural earphones in ABR measurements are enumerated next. These differences among earphones were based on analysis of acoustic spectra within a 6 cc coupler (a hard-walled cavity). The acoustic spectra are further transformed (modified) by the human external ear and ear canal (Pickles, 1988). When measured with a probe-tube microphone in the ear canal located close to the tympanic membrane, characteristics of the stimulus, including the spectrum, are not the same as in the coupler. The intensity level differences between these two types of measurements (coupler versus real ear) are greatest for frequencies below 500 Hz and, importantly for ABR stimulation, in the 2000 to 5000 Hz frequency region (Cox, 1986).

Placement of the earphone cushion on the ear is a factor in AER measurement. Audiometric hearing threshold

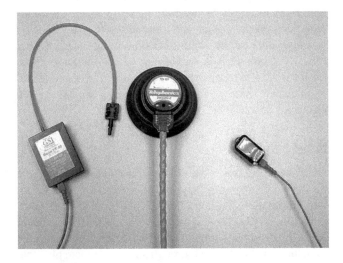

FIGURE 3.4.   An array of transducers for presenting acoustic signals in the measurement of auditory evoked responses. From left to right the transducers are insert earphone, supra-aural earphone, and bone oscillator.

Spectral Characteristics

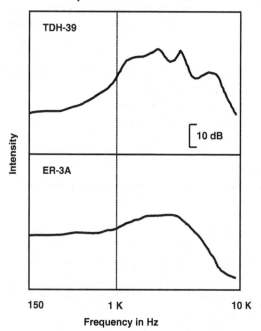

Temporal Characteristics

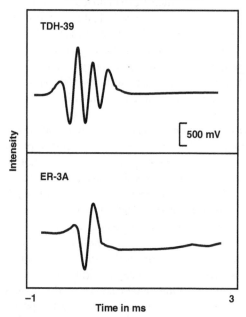

FIGURE 3.5. Temporal and spectral (frequency) responses for acoustic signals produced by TDH earphones versus Etymōtic ER-3A earphones.

standards and also AER intensity calibration on human ears assume that the earphone diaphragm is directly aligned with the external ear canal meatus and pressed against the pinna with no air leaks. In audiometric threshold assessment, care is taken to properly place the earphone and cushion on the external ear. The patient, who is sitting upright, is instructed not to move the headset. In AER measurement, test condi-

tions may fall short of this ideal. Even cooperative adult patients are often in a reclining position. The headband, in its usual coronal position, may not remain in place. This can cause earphone slippage. Head movements may produce changes in earphone position that can easily go unnoticed by the tester. With infants, the problems of precise earphone placement are compounded. The external meatus is smaller, head movement may be greater, and the headband (designed for adult head sizes) is often too large even when adjusted as tightly as possible. If the infant prefers to sleep on her or his side (versus supine), even an approximate placement for the earphone on the ear on which the head is resting may be impossible. In combination, these test problems conspire to reduce accuracy in acoustic stimulation in AER measurement.

One solution to the problem of stabilizing earphones on infant ears during ABR assessment was a specially designed rigid headset developed by Zubick, Fried, Thebeau, Feudo, and Strome (1983). Conventional audiometric earphones were mounted in a support unit, which was firmly attached to an adjustable bar. The bar, in turn, was connected to an extension, which could be secured to a bassinet. This device reportedly kept the earphones in the desired place and restricted head and body motion, reducing test time by 50 percent in most cases. Clark, Dybala, and Moushegian (1998) reported another investigation of the effects of earphone design on the ABR as documented with real ear measurements. The ear coupler typically used with the ALGO2 automated ABR screening device, a foam donut-shaped cushion that fits over the external ear of the infant, was substituted by probe tip couplers that are fit to insert earphone tubes for infant ABR measurement. The 35 dB nHL stimulus intensity level, and the click spectrum, delivered by the ALGO2 with the conventional foam couplers was significantly changed by the probe tip coupler. Importantly, real ear measurements confirmed markedly higher SPL values in infant ear canals with the probe tip design, and the levels in the ear canal varied depending on the depth of the probe tip within the ear canal. As Clark, Dybala, and Moushegian (1998) note, "The neonatal AABR results show that coupler type and placement can also produce inaccurate screening evaluations and erroneous conclusions."

Insert Earphones

Over twenty years ago, Mead Killion and associates reported the development of a new type of transducer for air-conduction stimulation (Killion, 1984; Killion, Wilbur, & Gudmundsen, 1985). The Etymōtic Research (ER) transducer is enclosed within a small box (one for each ear), and the acoustic signal is directed through a tube to a foam plug that is inserted into the outer portion of the external ear canal (as shown in Figure 3.6). The plug is the same type (E.A.R.) that is often used for ear protection. The Etymōtic ER-3A transducer and foam plug insert assembly has desirable acoustic characteristics, such as a wide and predictable frequency response. In fact, it was designed to mimic the acoustic characteristics of the standard audiometric earphone (TDH-39). Impedance of the insert earphones may be high (e.g., 300 ohms) or low (e.g., 10 or 50 ohms). *It is very important to use a set of insert earphones that is compatible with and selected by the manufacturer for your auditory evoked system.* When it is desirable to locate the evoked response instrumentation some distance from the patient, e.g., in the operating room, the stock cable for insert earphones with either impedance can be connected to an extension cable (e.g., 20 feet).

With insert earphones, there are a variety of options for coupling the insert transducer (see Figure 3.6) with the ear. For adults and older children, sound can be delivered to the ear via the acoustic tubing (see "C" in Figure 3.6) and a disposable polyurethane foam ear tip that is first compressed and then inserted into the external ear canal. Advantages of insert earphones in the measurement of auditory evoked responses are detailed below. The ear tips are available in two sizes (13 mm and 10 mm) (see "D" in Figure 3.6). For most male adult patients and some female adult patients, the larger size (13 mm and yellow) is a good fit. The smaller size (10 mm and beige) is appropriate for female adult patients and older children. *Take care in removing the ear tips from the silicone acoustic tubing to leave the little plastic connector ("nipple") within the tubing.* The connectors can easily be removed inadvertently with the ear tip and discarded. The next clinician to perform an auditory evoked response recording with insert earphones will, lacking the connector, be quite frustrated by the inability to attach an eartip to the acoustic tubing. The acoustic tubing for insert earphones should be inspected periodically for cracks and holes. If the integrity of the tubing is compromised, sound can escape and the intensity level of the stimulus is reduced. If biological calibration of the auditory evoked response stimuli (e.g., clicks or tone bursts) indicates reduced intensity levels, the clinician should immediately rule out a problem with the acoustic tubing. *Another warning—the length of the silicone acoustic tubing for insert earphones should never be modified (e.g., cut).* Shortening the length of the acoustic tubing will alter the time delay for presentation of the stimuli that evoke auditory evoked responses. When the user selects insert earphones as the transducer (and not supra-aural headphones or a bone oscillator), modern evoked response systems automatically adjust (decrease) latencies by a specific amount (e.g., 0.8 or 0.9 ms) to compensate for the time delay produced by the acoustic tubing. Cutting the acoustic tubing will reduce the actual time delay in the arrival of the stimulus to the ear and will produce a corresponding error in latency for auditory evoked responses.

Insert earphones can be used with infants (including neonates) and other younger children by coupling a special connector to the acoustic tubing (see "A" in Figure 3.6). The medial end of the connector (or adapter) is a narrow,

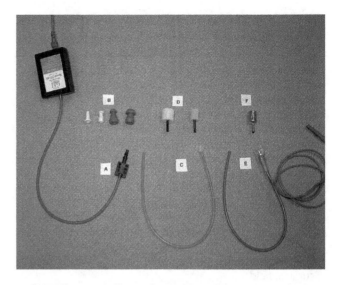

FIGURE 3.6. Options for coupling the acoustic tubing of insert earphones to the ear canal with pediatric and adult patients.

black, cone-shaped plastic device that fits into the bore (center hole) of rubber probe tips (see "B" in Figure 3.6). With these connectors, available also from manufacturers of auditory evoked response equipment, it's possible to attach probe tips used typically for aural immittance measurements with tip sizes ranging from very small (a thin layer of rubber) to very large probe tips. Rubber probe tips used with insert earphones can be discarded (some are disposable) or cleaned for reuse with an appropriate hospital-approved disinfectant. Of course, despite their many clinical attributes, insert earphones are of no value in patients with aural atresia who lack an external auditory canal. Clinicians who perform auditory evoked response assessments in children should have, in addition to the insert earphones, a set of supra-aural (e.g., TDH) earphones that are compatible with the instrumentation for such cases.

The Etymōtic ER-3A offers at least twelve potential clinical advantages over conventional audiometric earphones, as summarized in Table 3.3. Some of the advantages will now be highlighted. The problem of stimulus artifact extending into the region of early AER components, such as the ECochG AP component or the ABR wave I component, is essentially eliminated by the time delay introduced by the tubing. This feature of the ER-3A is illustrated in numerous waveforms throughout this book. The length of the Etymōtic ER-3A tubing (about 280 mm) produces an acoustic travel time from the transducer to the insert of about 0.9 ms. Recall that the speed of sound is 350 meters/second or 1100 feet/second. Electromagnetic energy generated by the ER-3A transducer can be removed from the recording electrode, which is located on the earlobe or the mastoid of the stimulated side. In fact, it is good clinical technique to extend the tubing and place the transducer as far from the ear

TABLE 3.3. A Dozen Clinical Advantages of Insert Earphones in Auditory Evoked Response Measurement

---

- Increased interaural attenuation of acoustic signal
- Increased ambient noise reduction (patient is essentially wearing sound-attenuating ear protection)
- Reduction of ear canal collapse (in infants)
- Increased patient comfort
- More precise placement in infants with small and soft ear tips, versus hand-held imprecise placement with supra-aural earphones
- Aural hygiene and infection control (insert cushions are disposed after single patient use)
- Insert earphones can be used as TIPtrode electrodes
- Insert cushion and tubing can be sterilized for intraoperative use
- Nonsterile portion of the earphone can be placed outside surgical field
- Flat frequency response (versus supra-aural earphones)
- Reduced transducer ringing with transient (click) signals
- Reduced stimulus artifact by separating the transducer box and the electrode (extend tube from ear and keep insert transducer box away from electrode wires)

(and electrode wires) as possible (see Chapter 7). In contrast, the TDH-39 earphone is essentially resting on the earlobe electrode. As a result, the use of TDH earphones can be associated with substantial stimulus artifact that encroaches on the wave I component of the ABR and precludes accurate identification and analysis. Stimulus artifact need not be a problem for the ER-3A.

Two precautions should be stated at this point. First, the travel time delay of the stimulus must be considered. Although the time delay is constant (0.9 ms), AER analysis time period for commercially available evoked systems is initiated at the time of the stimulus trigger, not when the stimulus reaches the ear. Therefore, absolute AER latency values are lengthened by 0.9 ms and need to be corrected by subtracting this time from the wave component latency. For example, an ABR wave V latency with ER-3A stimulus presentation of 6.50 ms would be corrected to 5.60 ms (6.50 minus 0.90 = 5.60 ms). Current AER systems adjust latencies for the tube delay when the insert earphone transducer option is selected. Interwave latency values and all amplitude calculations are not affected by the tubing time delay factor. The second precaution, naturally, is that if ER-3A tubing is cut or replaced with tubing of another length, this stimulus time delay will be altered. Also, it is important to recognize that the acoustic characteristics of the stimulus produced by the Etymōtic ER-3A were shaped taking into account the effect of tubing with these dimensions (length and diameter). Any change in the dimensions will modify the acoustic spectrum of the stimulus. The manufacturer strongly recommends using the tubing supplied with the transducer.

Another advantage of the ER-3A earphone is related to the temporal waveform of the click stimulus. As shown in Figure 3.5, the ER-3A earphone has limited acoustic ringing, in comparison to TDH earphones. That is, the extra deflections in the temporal waveform after the initial earphone response to the rectangular electric pulse, clearly evident for the TDH earphones, are not observed for the ER-3A "tube phone."

Also, insert earphones are quite effective in preventing the collapse of ear canals. The pressure of supra-aural earphones and cushions can cause the cartilaginous outer portion of the external auditory canal to collapse and occlude the opening. This problem tends to be more prevalent in infants and in the elderly. The problem of infant ear canal collapse with supra-aural earphones is, however, not inevitable. Galambos and Wilson (1994) systematically compared absolute thresholds for ABRs recorded from thirty-one ears of twenty-eight infants with an insert earphone and with a supra-aural earphone design. Estimated thresholds never differed by more than 10 dB, leading the authors to conclude that the supra-aural earphone "rarely if ever collapses the ear canal to cause an artificial conductive hearing loss." The effect of ear-canal collapse and occlusion is a worsening of air-conduction hearing thresholds for high frequencies. For behavioral hearing threshold levels, the decrease is on the order of 10 to 20 dB in the 1000 to 8000 Hz region. Bone-conduction hearing thresholds are, of course, not affected. Collapsing ear canals attenuate the stimulus intensity actually reaching the cochlea. For AERs that depend on higher frequencies of click stimuli (ECochG and ABR), latency values can be increased and response thresholds elevated by this reduced intensity. In newborn auditory screening at an intensity level of 30 to 40 dB nHL, an unrecognized collapsing ear canal can lead to an erroneous screening failure.

In addition, the insert cushion reduces concern about possible crossover of the stimulus from the test ear to the nontest ear. The interaural attenuation of the head, the "sound insulation" created between ears by the head, is approximately 40 to 50 dB HL. When an air-conduction stimulus presented to one ear via a conventional earphone exceeds the interaural attenuation, it is possible that some of the stimulus energy will reach the other (nontest) ear. Stimulus energy may seep around the earphone cushion and travel via air to the other ear, but the real problem with cross over is bone-conducted energy. That is, the earphone makes contact with the head and, at moderate-to-high intensity levels, stimulus-related vibration is transmitted from the earphone to the skull. Then, the vibrations reach the contralateral cochlea via bone conduction (bone-conducted sound also reaches the ipsilateral [test ear] cochlea). Because transfer of energy from the earphone to the cochlea via bone conduction occurs at high signal intensity levels, the conductive component of a hearing loss theoretically cannot exceed about 60 dB HL. The ER-3A foam insert makes contact with only the cartilaginous portion of the external ear canal, not the

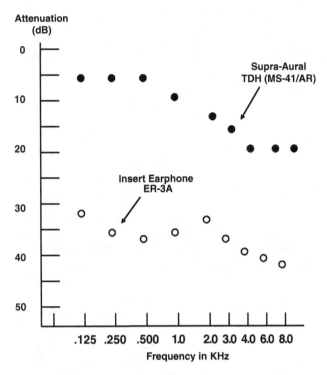

FIGURE 3.7. Sound attenuation levels for supra-aural earphones versus insert earphones as a function of signal frequency.

bony portion, and crossover may not occur until stimulus intensity reaches 70 dB or greater. That is, interaural attenuation is increased when the ER-3A insert earphone is used instead of the TDH earphones. The maximum increase in ER-3A interaural attenuation, relative to TDH earphones, is for frequencies of 100 Hz and below. Click-evoked ECochG and ABR measurements, however, are most dependent on higher frequencies. Reliance on the ER-3A earphones does not eliminate possible stimulus crossover or the need for masking in air-conduction AER measurement. This point is further discussed in the section on masking.

A related advantage results from the sound-attenuating properties of the ER-3A foam plug. As noted, this plug is the same type that is used to protect the ear from excessive environmental noise. It has been found to attenuate ambient noise in the AER test setting by approximately 30 dB (Figure 3.7). Also, the ER-3A stimulus-delivery arrangement ensures proper earphone placement, assuming that the probe cushion is securely fitted within the ear canal. A moderate amount of patient movement does not usually dislodge the insert. The slippage problem noted for the standard audiometric earphone/cushion is eliminated. A secure insert is particularly helpful for testing newborns. Not only is placement consistently precise, but also there are none of the difficulties associated with handholding the earphone or attempting to

present a stimulus to the downward-facing ear of a patient sleeping on her or his side. A practical clinical advantage is comfort. The conventional audiometric headset is rather inflexible and rather uncomfortable during extended use. When the standard headset is resting on earclip electrodes, patients may actually complain of pain over time. Patients seem to prefer the spongy insert plugs. In the interest of aural hygiene, it is necessary to begin each test session with a new set of the insert earplugs. Indeed, infection control is a real-world benefit of using disposable insert ear cushions in a clinical setting.

Systematic study of ER-3A earphones was conducted following their introduction as a clinical transducer option. Beauchaine, Kaminski, and Gorga (1987) compared the performance of Etymotic ER-3A insert earphones versus a circumaural earphone (Beyer DT48) in ABR measurement in ten normal-hearing adult subjects. Behavioral thresholds for a click stimulus were equivalent for the two earphone types (mean difference of 1.33 dB, with a standard deviation on the order of 5 dB). ABR thresholds were slightly elevated for the ER-3A versus the circumaural earphone (average of 10.63 versus 6.88 dB), but within the 5 dB intensity increment used in the study. As expected, ABR latency values increased with decreasing intensity for each earphone type, as did variability for latency. Wave V latency variability, however, appeared to be larger for the ER-3A. No explanation for this finding was offered. An absolute latency prolongation for wave V of 0.88 ms for the ER-3A (versus the circumaural) was consistent with the delay caused by the tubing (explained previously). Interpeak latencies (wave I–III, wave III–V, wave I–V) were comparable for the two earphones. Therefore, the authors state that only a simple latency correction to account for the tubing-related time delay is required to equate the ABR data for the two earphone types. Finally, the study was among the first to demonstrate the clinical feasibility of the ER-3A earphone with neonates.

Bone-Conduction Stimulation

A detailed discussion of theories on bone conduction of sound and principles and procedures for assessment of bone-conduction hearing is beyond the scope of this book. Information is available in numerous audiology texts. Briefly, the cochlea can be activated by sounds arriving via air or bone conduction. With the air-conduction route, sound (1) enters the external ear, (2) travels to the tympanic membrane through the external ear canal, (3) vibrates the tympanic membrane, which, in turn, (4) vibrates the ossicles and oval window, and (5) produces a traveling wave along the basilar membrane, which (6) activates the cochlea at the hair cells. The air-conduction route is an effective way of activating the cochlea because sound is amplified (energy is increased) by three factors: (1) the resonance properties of the ear canal, (2) the ratio of the area of the tympanic membrane versus the oval window, and (3) the lever action of the ossicular chain.

Bone-conduction hearing also results in activation of the cochlea, and, thereafter, hearing processes are presumably the same as for air-conduction stimulation. The mechanism of sound transmission to the cochlea via bone conduction is, however, not completely known. The work of von Békèsy (1960) and Tonndorf (1966), among others, suggests three probable bone conduction mechanisms that interact in some combination to activate the cochlea:

- Inertial bone conduction (in which the temporal bone is accelerated by a stimulus): As the temporal bone (including the bony cochlea) vibrates, the stapes footplate (the part of the ossicular chain nearest the cochlea) and cochlear fluids lag behind. Inertia of these two structures, in effect, produces both an in–out motion of the stapes footplate, similar to the air-conduction ossicular chain vibration, and a relative flow of cochlear fluid, both of which ultimately activate hair cells.
- Compressional bone conduction: Distortional vibrations of the temporal bone, when they arrive at the bony walls of the cochlea, produce traveling waves within the cochlea.
- Osseotympanic conduction: Vibrations in the temporal bone arriving at the walls of the bony portion of the external ear canal generate acoustic energy in the ear canal, which then eventually activates the cochlea via the aforementioned air-conduction route.

Although adequate bone-conduction stimulation can be presented anywhere on the head, including such unorthodox locations as the bony portion of the nose, the teeth, and the jaw, the two clinically most common vibrator placements are the mastoid bone (behind the lower part of the ear) and the frontal bone (forehead). Frontal placement produces more reliable threshold results, but mastoid placement is traditionally used, probably because it permits a higher effective intensity level to reach the cochlea. The expected decrease in the effective bone-conduction intensity level from mastoid to forehead placement for selected test frequencies are 15 dB at 500 Hz, 10 dB at 1000 Hz, 8.5 dB at 2000 Hz, and 6.5 dB at 4000 Hz. These values were derived from human studies with steady-state (versus transient) pure-tone stimuli. For a brief-duration (2.5 ms) tone burst of 2000 Hz, Boezeman, Kapteyn, Visser, and Snel (1983) found a mastoid-to-forehead decrement of 7 dB.

A factor that can influence bone-conduction thresholds, as measured with behavioral audiometry and also with AERs, is the occlusion effect. When a normal-hearing ear is covered (e.g., with an earphone), bone-conduction threshold levels for occlusion effect are relatively greater for lower frequencies (approximately 20 dB at 500 Hz and 10 dB at 1000 Hz) and negligible for higher frequencies. The difficulties and dangers in generalizing these types of data to bone-conduction stimulation of AERs with transients are reviewed next.

One bone-conduction vibrator shown in Figure 3.4 is a Radioear B-71. Other commercially available bone vibrators (e.g., Radioear B-70) have a similar external design. The clinician was alerted above to the importance of using insert earphones and supra-aural earphones with impedance that matched the specifications for the evoked response system (e.g., low or high). The same concern applies to bone-conduction oscillators (bone vibrator transducers), as they are available in low impedance (e.g., 10 ohms) or high impedance (e.g., 300 ohms) versions. Numerous authors note that bone vibrator output declines in the high-frequency region that is important for click stimulation (Mauldin & Jerger, 1979; Schwartz & Berry, 1985; Weber, 1983b; Yang, Rupert, & Moushegian, 1987). Output levels from three commercially available bone vibrators were compared with those of two air-conduction earphones (TDH-49 and a hearing-aid transducer plus insert plug) by Schwartz, Larson, and DeChiccis (1985). The air-conduction transducers produced a relatively flat frequency response, while each of the bone-conduction vibrators had energy predominantly in the 2000 Hz region, with maximum output not exceeding 35 dB HL. Of the three bone vibrators, the B-70 permitted greatest output. The preceding information on bone vibrators may not accurately reflect their potential for AER measurement (Gorga & Thornton, 1989). The reduction of bone-vibrator output for higher frequencies, when expressed in units of force, may not necessarily correspond to a diminished effective intensity level in this audiometric region. Bone-vibrator output is indeed reduced above 2000 Hz, but then so are behavioral hearing threshold levels. Consequently, effective output of the bone vibrator is actually greater in the higher frequency region. Bone oscillator placement in infants and young children is somewhat more challenging, due to smaller head dimensions and the design limitations of the typical headbands, than with older children and adults. Techniques for placement of the bone oscillator in pediatric AER applications, particularly ABR, are reviewed in Chapter 6.

Other problems shared by commercially available series of bone vibrators are excessive distortion and intersubject variability. The distortion, which is more pronounced with higher intensities, reduces or may even eliminate frequency-specific AER stimulation (Harder, Arlinger, & Kylen, 1983). The static force of bone-vibrator placement is another, often overlooked, factor in the effectiveness of bone-conduction stimulation. A force of 500 gm is generally preferred in audiometric bone-conduction measurement. Force of bone-vibrator placement is highly variable in clinical measurement and has not yet been systematically investigated in AER recording. Variability is due to inconsistencies in placement site and the pressure with which the vibrator is held to the skull and differences in skull impedance (Arlinger & Kylen, 1977). A predictable reduction in effective stimulus level occurs for forehead versus mastoid vibrator placement. Because of variations in skull impedance, it must be reemphasized that descriptions of the acoustic spectrum and intensity characteristics of bone vibrators, based on analysis with artificial mastoids, are probably not representative of the properties of the mechanical (vibration) stimulus actually activating the cochlea.

Furthermore, when interpreting bone-conduction ABR data, it is important to keep in mind that the actual characteristics of the stimulus reaching the cochlea for a given subject may be substantially altered by the transmission properties of the skull (Arlinger & Kylen, 1977). For example, there may be more acoustic radiation for some bone oscillators than for others. Acoustic radiation, which is air-conducted sound leakage from the bone vibrator, is undesirable because at higher test frequencies (e.g., 4000 Hz) a subject may actually hear the bone-conduction stimulus via air conduction at an intensity level better than his or her true bone-conduction threshold (Frank & Crandell, 1986).

Finally, as mentioned in the section on intensity, approximately 40 to 45 dB of effective intensity is lost in going from air to bone conduction. Therefore, if a bone vibrator is plugged into the earphone stimulus, jack of an evoked response system the actual output, even at a maximum attenuator dial or instrument intensity reading of 95 dB, will only be at most 45 to 50 dB nHL. Put another way, the intensity level (as indicated on the dial or the monitor screen) required for just detecting a bone-conduction click stimulus (0 dB nHL), at least in a young adult, is approximately 40 dB. Because the maximum equipment intensity reading is 95 dB, this leaves an effective range of only about 55 dB for bone-conduction stimulation. This intensity limitation applies as well to traditional bone-conduction pure-tone audiometry.

CONTRALATERAL MASKING IN AER MEASUREMENT

Masking, according to the ANSI (American National Standards Institute) standard on "Acoustical Terminology" (S1.1; ANSI, 1960), is "the amount by which the threshold of audibility of a sound is raised by the presence of another (masking) sound" (p. 46). In AER measurement, there are two broad clinical applications of masking. As already discussed earlier in this chapter, noise with specific frequency characteristics can be presented to the test ear, along with a stimulus to reduce or, one would hope, eliminate certain portions of the cochlea from contributing to the AER. Selective masking of certain frequency regions in the ipsilateral (stimulus) ear is one technique for enhancing the frequency specificity of a stimulus. Contralateral masking of the nontest ear, used more often clinically than ipsilateral masking in both conventional behavioral audiometry and AER measurement, is the focus of this discussion. Masking noise is presented to the nontest (nonstimulus) ear, in an attempt to ensure that the nontest ear does not contribute to the response. Before considering the use of masking in AER measurement, a few remarks about terminology are in order. Masking noise is generally described both by its effective intensity level in dB

and by its spectrum (frequency content). Broadband noise (BBN) is also referred to as "white noise," as an analogy to white light, which includes a wide range of wavelengths (and therefore colors). It is important to keep in mind that the effective frequency range of any broadband stimulus presented to an ear is, in fact, determined by the frequency response of the transducer, usually an earphone. The frequency response of most audiometric earphones begins to fall off for frequencies above 5000 to 6000 Hz and, therefore, so does the masking noise energy above this limit.

The spectrum of masking noise is often determined by filtering out energy in the undesired frequency region and by passing through energy at the frequencies of interest. Thus, a high-pass noise with a cutoff of 1000 Hz is derived from a broadband or white noise that is sent to a filter, which removes frequencies below 1000 Hz and which passes the frequencies above 1000 Hz. The cutoff is usually defined as the frequency at which the amplitude of the masker (or filtered noise) has decreased by a certain amount, such as by 3 dB (the 3 dB down point). A band-pass filter will remove both frequencies below a low-end cutoff (by means of a high-pass filter) and frequencies above a high-end cutoff (by means of a low-pass filter), resulting in a band of frequencies that pass through within these two cutoff points (e.g., 500 to 2000 Hz). Terminology used to describe filters may at first appear confusing. For example, a low-pass filter actually filters or eliminates high-frequency information, and the low-pass filter setting is actually the upper end of the frequency range that is passed. An understanding of such terminology is important in AER measurement, however, as it is also used in discussing the filters employed in recording and averaging evoked responses. Another masking principle in the measurement of auditory evoked responses should be noted at this juncture. The spectrum of the masking noise should be consistent with the signal used to evoke the response. For example, when an ABR is elicited with a broad-spectrum signal (e.g., a click), a broadband masking noise (e.g., white noise) is appropriate. On the other hand, with a tone burst signal (e.g., 1000 Hz), a narrowband masking noise (e.g., 500 to 1500 Hz) is most effective.

At least seven clinical questions are relevant in a discussion of masking and AER measurement:

1. Is masking ever necessary?
2. If so, what stimulus conditions suggest it?
3. How should masking be presented?
4. What kind of masking is best?
5. How much masking is enough?
6. Are there central auditory nervous system effects of masking that might influence AERs?
7. Are there measurement conditions for which masking is counterproductive?

These general issues are addressed as completely as possible. Next, findings from the relatively few published studies of masking and specific types of AERs are summarized.

Is Masking Always Necessary in the Measurement of AERs?

Perhaps the more appropriate question would be "Is masking ever needed in AER measurement?" Depending on the type of transducer used in the measurement of AERs, the intensity level at which air-conduction pure-tone signals first cross over from the test ear to the nontest ear may be as low as 40 dB. Clearly, interaural attenuation occurs at lower (fainter) intensity levels for supra-aural earphones (as low as 40 dB) than for insert earphones (usually greater than 60 dB). Interaural attenuation between subjects also varies as a function of test frequency. Interaural attenuation is relatively less for lower frequency pure-tone stimuli, at least with the long durations used in behavioral audiometry. In general, interaural attenuation for click stimuli is in line with that for high frequency pure-tone signals—that is, approximately 65 dB for the average adult subject (Chiappa, Gladstone, & Young, 1979).

The crossover of click signals, as assessed behaviorally, would appear to present the same clinical problem for AER measurement as pure-tone audiometry. There are, however, three methodologic differences between the two procedures that are relevant to decisions about masking. First, AERs are very time dependent, whereas stimulus and response timing is a minimal concern in behavioral audiometry. In behavioral audiometry, only the intensity level of the sound crossing over to the nontest ear is critical. In contrast, both the intensity level of the sound and the time it takes to cross over are factors in AER measurement, particularly for the shorter latency responses (ECochG and ABR).

Second, the intensity level of the click stimulus reaching the nontest ear is, of course, decreased by the amount of interaural attenuation for the subject. It might be instructive to consider a worst-case scenario for the problem of signal crossover for the ABR. Assuming there is total deafness in the test ear (a "dead ear") and there is normal hearing sensitivity, and a completely normal ABR, in the nontest ear, a very high intensity level click, such as 95 dB nHL, might be used. If so, one might expect that the click would stimulate the nontest ear at an intensity level of about 30 dB HL, i.e., 95 dB nHL minus 65 dB of interaural attenuation. An ABR would be elicited from the "good ear" with latency values corresponding to this intensity level (30 dB), plus the latency delay due to transit time from one ear to the other.

A third factor distinguishing AER measurement has to do with recording electrophysiologic versus behavioral responses in general. Distinct differences in behavioral versus ABR thresholds as a function of rate and duration have already been described in this chapter. Such differences are especially relevant to the discussion of masking. An ABR, for example, elicited by the air-conduction stimulus reaching the nontest ear will not have a wave I component when recorded with an electrode located on the test ("dead") ear side. An electrode located on the nontest ear, in dual channel recording, may show a wave I component, although at an effective intensity level of 30 dB, it would be unlikely. This concept is reviewed for ABR in more detail in Chapter 7. The main point is quite straightforward. A normal ABR, that is, a well-formed ABR with normal latencies for all wave components for a given high intensity level, cannot be recorded from a stimulus crossing over to the nontest ear. At best, in adults at least, the ABR resulting from crossover of the acoustic signal will be markedly delayed in latency and will lack a wave I component.

Masking is sometimes necessary in clinical AER measurement because responses reflecting auditory pathology, such as a waveform with only a markedly delayed wave V, may also fit the description of a response elicited by a signal that has crossed over from the test ear to the nontest ear. This important clinical principle was not always appreciated in early studies. Finitzo-Hieber, Hecox, and Kone (1979), for example, presented a patient with total unilateral impairment, who showed no ABR for a 90 dB click stimulus presented to the involved ear. According to the authors, "the results suggest that contralateral masking may not be needed for air-conducted brain stem evoked responses to click stimuli" (p. 1156) and added that "the ability to omit contralateral masking from the evaluation procedure simplifies and shortens the test procedure considerably" (Finizo-Hieber, Hecox, & Kone, 1979, p. 1157). Galambos and Hecox (1978) expressed a similar opinion.

Accumulated experience clearly indicates that when click stimuli are presented to a profoundly impaired ear at intensity levels exceeding 75 to 80 dB nHL, an ABR can be elicited from the contralateral (nontest) ear (Hatanaka, Yasuhara, Hori, & Kobayashi, 1990; Reid, Birchall, & Moffat, 1984; Rosenhamer, Lindstrom, & Lundborg, 1978; Smyth, 1985). Smyth (1985) convincingly demonstrated that in patients with unilateral hearing loss, the nontest ear must be adequately masked for valid interpretation of ABR findings. ABRs for click stimuli (TDH-49 earphone) were recorded from a normal-hearing control subject and four patients with unilateral hearing impairment: one with conductive impairment; one with a flat, severe sensorineural impairment with recruitment; one with a moderate-to-severe sloping sensorineural impairment without recruitment; and one with profound sensorineural impairment.

Smyth (1985) concluded that an auditory response due to signal crossover was a serious clinical concern in ABR measurement, although ABR latencies due to the crossover of stimulation to the nontest ear were almost always abnormal. Without the inclusion of masking, the degree of hearing impairment in the poorer ear could be underestimated, and the type of loss could be misinterpreted. For example, a retrocochlear lesion could be erroneously inferred from a grossly delayed response due to a profound cochlear deficit. Obtaining an ABR from the poorer ear for a single high-intensity stimulus level, referred to by Smyth (1985) as "single-shot data acquisition" (p. 29) is particularly suspect and essentially invalid. Smyth (1985) gave a "resounding yes" to the question of whether masking should be used. The answers to when and how masking should be employed clinically, she said, depend on characteristics of the evoked response system, stimulus conditions, and, importantly, the patient's audiometric configuration. This final point is reiterated often in this text. Whenever the patient's age and level of cooperation permit, pure-tone audiometry should precede AER assessment. Some authors go so far as to recommend use of contralateral ear masking routinely in every ABR measurement, to prevent any possibility of crossover (Chiappa, Gladstone, & Young, 1979; Hatanaka, Yasuhara, Hori, & Kobayashi, 1990; Levine, 1981). Masking is not always required in ABR measurement, however. A more clinically appealing approach is to mask the nontest ear whenever cross over of the signal from the test ear to the nontest ear is likely to occur. Clinical indications for masking are summarized next and are reviewed more thoroughly in Chapter 7.

If Masking Is Sometimes Needed, What Measurement Conditions Suggest the Need for It?

Contralateral masking of the nontest is indicated in AER measurement for any patient with a unilateral auditory impairment when an air-conduction stimulus is presented to the poor ear (at an intensity level exceeding 70 dB nHL) and the response has abnormal latency values and no distinct wave I component. These criteria are rather specific and are not met by the majority of patients undergoing AER assessment. For this reason, masking is not routinely required. Contralateral masking is not needed if (1) AERs are unequivocally normal bilaterally, regardless of the stimulus intensity; (2) there is no detectable response unilaterally or bilaterally; or (3) there is a clear and reliable wave I component for stimulation of the poorer ear. Otherwise, masking is generally indicated to rule out a contribution from the nontest ear to the auditory evoked response.

One must also consider the possibility that even a completely normal-appearing AER for very high stimulus intensities may actually contain components generated by the nontest ear, components due to crossover of the stimulus. That is, an ABR with markedly delayed wave V can be recorded from a normal nontest ear when a high-intensity stimulus is presented to a contralateral "dead ear." Indeed, Reid, Birchall, and Moffat (1984) found that with a click stimulus at 90 dB and no contralateral masking, there was a larger amplitude wave VI component than with 50 dB of contralateral masking. At lower stimulus intensity levels, the masking produced no change in wave VI amplitude. These authors speculate that at high unmasked stimulus intensity levels, the wave V due to crossover of the signal sums with wave VI in the ipsilateral (stimulus) ear, thus enhancing wave VI amplitude.

How Should Masking Be Presented?

The three main ways that masking can be presented are with conventional air-conduction earphones, with newer insert transducers, and with bone conduction. For each of these presentation modes, the spectrum of the noise used as a masker depends, in part, on the frequency response of the transducer. The crossover to the nontest ear of energy for moderate- to high-intensity stimuli associated with the conventional supra-aural earphone is the reason why masking is needed for air-conduction assessment. Yet, this problem may apply as well to the masking noise. That is, if a moderate- to high-intensity masking noise is presented with these earphones to the nontest ear, there is a chance that it will cross over and inadvertently mask the test ear. This is referred to as the "masking dilemma." It is a function of masking intensity level and the substantial physical contact or coupling between the supra-aural cushion and the skull.

One clinical exception to this generalization was cited earlier. Yang et al. (1987) found higher interaural attenuation (lower likelihood of crossover) for newborns whose cranial sutures remain flexible and open. Interaural attenuation may be considerably higher for insert transducers than for supra-aural earphones, especially for lower frequencies. Bone conduction masking, as in the SAL procedure (Jerger & Tillman, 1960), has some distinct clinical advantages, but it has rarely been adapted to AER measurement (Hicks, 1980; Webb & Greenberg, 1984). The SAL technique does show promise for estimation of bone conduction hearing with the sinusoidal signals used to elicit the auditory steady-state response (ASSR), as detailed in Chapter 8.

What Kind of Masking Noise Is Best?

For AERs elicited with click stimuli, a broadband masking noise presented to the nontest ear via air conduction is best. The click has a wide spectrum. Presumably, this same wide range of frequencies crosses over to the nontest ear, although there is little published evidence in support of this presumption (von Békèsy, 1960). The spectrum of the masking noise should at least equal or exceed the click spectrum. The preference for broadband noise for click-stimulated AERs contrasts with the routine and effective use of narrow bands of contralateral noise centered at pure-tone test frequencies in audiometry. Although narrowband noise maskers might conceivably be of value for AERs elicited by brief tone-pip stimuli, close analysis of the spectra of the stimuli would be needed first. As noted earlier, short-duration tonal stimuli may have considerable side bands and spectral splatter, which could contribute to the response, and which should be masked. Other types of noise applied sometimes in hearing science probably have no place in AER assessment. Finally, to ensure adequate masking, it is important that the transducer employed to deliver the noise has a frequency response equal to that used to deliver the click stimulus.

How Much Masking Noise Is Appropriate?

It is difficult, if not impossible, to provide an answer to this question, especially an answer that applies to all possible stimuli, patient conditions, and test settings. There are different approaches for determining appropriate masking in behavioral audiologic assessment. For AERs, masking noise presented to the nontest ear at 50 dB nHL is adequate for even the highest AER click stimulus intensity level (e.g., 95 dB nHL). With an interaural intensity level of 65 dB for the click, the effective intensity level of the crossed-over stimulus in the nontest ear is about 35 dB nHL. This intensity level will invariably be sufficiently masked by 50 dB nHL, even in an ear with normal hearing sensitivity.

The rationale for selecting a routine noise level of about 50 dB is provided by evidence from an eloquent set of studies on noise effects on the ABR conducted by Burkard, Hecox, and colleagues (Burkard & Hecox, 1983; Burkard, Shi, & Hecox, 1990a,b; Hecox, Patterson, & Birman, 1989). The relationship between an ipsilateral masker level and ABRs for different click intensities—that is, the overall effect of broadband noise on ABR—is increased latency and decreased amplitude for wave V. Assuming that the crossed-over click stimulus intensity in the nontest ear is, at most, 40 dB nHL in ABR testing (95 dB HL intensity level –55 dB interaural attenuation), the crossover response will be completely masked by 40 dB. An added 10 dB masker intensity is suggested for an extra safety margin. However, more masking is not necessarily better. Masking noise levels greater than 50 dB nHL, in unilateral impairment, should be used very cautiously because there is the possibility that the masking noise will cross over to mask the test ear.

Are There Effects of Masking on the Central Nervous System?

Central masking in conventional audiometry occurs when the hearing threshold level in one ear increases with the presentation of a masking sound, even of low intensity, to the contralateral ear. There is no direct interference between the two sounds—that is, the masker and the stimulus are both well within the limits of interaural attenuation (both less than 40 to 50 dB HL). Animal studies indicate that central masking is mediated in the caudal brainstem auditory centers and pathways. Therefore, it is reasonable to question whether a similar phenomenon affects AERs recorded in the presence of contralateral masking, that is, whether the masking noise is activating brainstem or even cerebral neurons in the same general anatomic regions in which the AER generators are located. Perhaps these neurons, if responding to noise, will be less likely to give rise to AERs.

There is no definite central masking effect in ABR measurement (Boezeman et al., 1983; Chiappa, Gladstone, &

Young, 1979; Prasher & Gibson, 1980a). Contralateral masking of the nontest ear, at low-to-moderate intensity levels (less than 70 dB HL), does not produce consistent alterations in ABR latency or amplitude. There is evidence that high-intensity contralateral noise crossing over to the test ear, or ipsilateral masking noise at a lower intensity, increases wave V latency and decreases wave V amplitude, but it has a less pronounced influence on wave I (Burkard & Hecox, 1983; Kramer & Teas, 1982; Lasky & Rupert, 1982). Rosenhamer and Holmkvist (1983) observed these contralateral effects and attributed them to central masking.

For Which Measurement Conditions Is Masking Contraindicated (Counterproductive)?

Routine masking for every patient undergoing AER assessment is not necessary and is probably not a wise test policy for three reasons:

- The masker becomes one more stimulus parameter that may be improperly set during AER assessment. An inappropriately high masker intensity level (greater than 70 dB nHL) presented to the ear contralateral to the stimulus ear may cross over and alter the AER in the test ear (Boezeman et al., 1983), perhaps leading to a false positive interpretive error.
- Another concern is that the masker will be presented to the same ear as the stimulus. Inadvertent ipsilateral masking can lead to a false positive AER outcome. For example, an ipsilateral broadband noise will usually artificially elevate AER threshold levels and may create nonpathologic ABR abnormalities. Also the ipsilateral masker may have little affect on ABR wave I but can produce an increase in wave V latency and a decrease in wave V amplitude. The resultant prolongation in the wave I to wave V latency interval and decrease in the V/I amplitude ratio are typical ABR signs of brainstem abnormality (Burkard & Hecox, 1983; Burkard & Voigt, 1989; Gott & Hughes, 1989).
- At high masking levels, the AER may be obliterated. For some evoked response systems, the masker is not automatically directed to the nontest (nonstimulus) transducer. If a masker is used, it is imperative that the masker is presented the opposite transducer when test ears are alternated. By avoiding the use of unnecessary masking this problem, too, is avoided.

ACQUISITION PARAMETERS

Analysis Time

In AER measurement, the analysis time should be long enough to encompass the response of interest under all test conditions. For the ABR evoked by click and high-frequency tone burst stimuli, a 15 ms analysis time (versus 10 ms) is recommended because there are many circumstances that will delay wave V, and the subsequent negative voltage trough that aids in wave V identification, up to or beyond 8 to 10 ms. Factors contributing to such a delay would include immature CNS function in children, neuropathology, low stimulus intensity, low-frequency tone burst stimulus, and peripheral hearing impairment. A 20 ms analysis time is required when an ABR is elicited with lower frequency tone burst stimuli (e.g., 1000 Hz or 500 Hz). With any ABR test protocol, a prestimulus baseline (for example, 10% of the entire analysis period) is useful to assess the amount of nonresponse noise in the waveform noise. The prestimulus averaging period can be selected from the collection parameters or configuration page when an ABR test protocol is first developed. For the ABR, a prestimulus baseline period of 1 or 2 ms (actually –1 or –2 ms) is appropriate. The prestimulus period is apparent in most of the ABR waveforms displayed in this book as a line occurring before the stimulus (in the negative time region).

A short analysis period for ECochG is useful to eliminate ABR components from the waveform (e.g., wave III and wave V) and to enhance resolution and detection of the components of interest, such as the summating potential (SP) and action potential (AP). For cortical AER measurement, appropriate analysis times range from 100 ms for the AMLR to as long as 700 ms (100 ms prestimulus and 600 ms poststimulus) for the later responses (e.g., ALR and P300).

Electrodes

ELECTRODE SITES. | A collection of general-purpose commercially available electrodes is shown in Figure 3.8. Many other electrode types available commercially can be found in catalogs of supplies distributed by various manufacturers of auditory evoked response equipment. Electrode types are discussed in the next section. Appropriate electrode sites can make the difference between recording a well-formed

response and not observing a response at all. Electrodes used for ECochG measurement are discussed further in Chapter 4, and in Chapter 7 for ABR. In AER measurement, and clinical neurophysiology in general, electrode sites are usually defined according to the International 10–20 system (Jasper, 1958). Electrodes used typically in AER measurement are labeled according to this system in Figure 3.9. There is a simple logic to the labels in the system. For example, electrodes containing the letter "z" are on the midline (anterior-to-posterior center of the head). The first letter of the label refers to the region of the brain over which the electrode is located, e.g., F = frontal, T = temporal, O = occipital, and P = parietal. The "C" electrodes are along the coronal line (corona = crown) from the vertex (middle top of the head) down each side to the ear canal. Cortical evoked responses are often recorded simultaneously with many electrodes located over the scalp.

There are several general principles relating electrode site and AER components. First, the closer the electrode is to

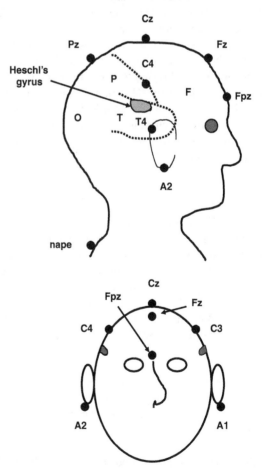

FIGURE 3.9. Electrodes locations labeled according to the International 10–20 system (Jasper, 1958) commonly used for auditory evoked response measurement.

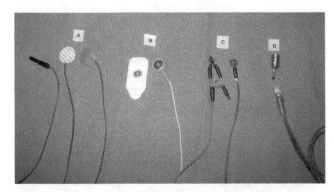

FIGURE 3.8. Electrodes commonly used for auditory evoked response measurement, including A. disposable electrode and cable, B. disposable electrode with snap-on cable, C. reusable metal disc electrode and ear clip electrode, and D. TIPtrode.

the anatomic generator, the larger the response. For example, the ECochG AP component recorded from the promontory (lateral wall of the cochlea) may be 20 times larger than the AP recorded from the earlobe or mastoid. Second, in recording far-field responses from sites equidistant from the generator, such as the ABR, the exact location of the noninverting electrode is not crucial. The response is essentially comparable when recorded anywhere along the midline from vertex (Cz) to forehead (Fz). For ABR recordings, inverting electrodes located on the earlobe are preferable to mastoid sites, because wave I tends to be larger (up to 30%) and the electrode picks up less electromagnetic artifact from bone vibrators with the typical mastoid placement than with electrodes located on the postauricular region. It is possible that wave V amplitude may be slightly reduced with earlobe placement of the inverting electrode. Either of these sites (mastoid or earlobe) is, however, active with reference to electrical activity arising from the auditory system (especially cochlea, eighth nerve, and lower brainstem) and is not properly termed a "reference" or "indifferent" electrode. If interactions among noninverting and earlobe electrodes are suspected, on the basis of waveform morphology and/or difficulty identifying waves beyond I, then a noncephalic electrode site (e.g., nape of the neck) is indicated. The nape of the neck can be identified as the bump in center of the upper back where the neck joins the shoulders. Third, for neurodiagnostic applications, the AMLR should be recorded with electrodes located over each temporal-parietal region (C4 over the right hemisphere and C5 over the left hemisphere). The traditional midline noninverting electrode site for AMLR (Cz or Fz) appears to reflect activity from each auditory cortical region (right and left) or the more prominent hemisphere, in the case of unilateral cortical dysfunction.

Electrode Types and Application

Electrode application is a technical factor that is extremely important for successful evoked response measurement. The overall objectives are (1) consistent placement among subjects, (2) anatomically accurate placement, (3) low inter-electrode impedance (less than 5000 ohms), (4) balanced inter-electrode impedance (difference between electrodes of less than 2000 ohms), (5) secure and consistent attachment throughout the test session, and (6) minimal discomfort and no risk to the subject. After acquiring experience in AER recording, each clinician will develop his or her own preferences for electrodes, supplies, and technique. The following discussion, naturally, reflects the author's clinical experiences and is not presented as the "right" or only way to apply electrodes.

TECHNIQUES FOR APPLYING SURFACE ELECTRODES. | There are two main techniques for metal disc or disposable electrode application. With one technique, the connection between the electrode and skin is enhanced by a conducting gel

or paste, and electrodes secured with tape or self-adhesive disposable electrodes are used. Included in the discussion of this technique are remarks about ear canal and tympanic membrane electrode placement. The other technique depends on collodion to secure the electrode and conduct neuroelectric activity. Since collodion is used less frequently by audiologists and by auditory neurophysiologists, the discussion of this electrode application approach is brief.

ELECTRODE APPLICATION. | A typical sample of supplies required for electrode application is shown in Figure 3.10. The electrode site is first prepared by scrubbing vigorously with one of several brands and variations of abrasive liquid substance designed for the purpose (e.g., NUprep[R] as shown by "A" in Figure 3.10). The mild abrasion removes the natural oils of skin and superficial layers of skin, thus improving inter-electrode impedance. Alcohol pads serve the function of removing natural oils, as well as makeup and other cosmetic substances, from the skin, but regular use of alcohol by clinicians in electrode application, without the protection of rubber gloves, tends to leave the skin on fingers dry and even cracked. In addition, neonatologists have questioned the safety of preparing with alcohol the skin of newborn infants as there is a risk, albeit slight, that the alcohol will be absorbed and diffused into the bloodstream. Dry skin preparation pads are also an option prior to electrode application. However, the abrasive surface is typically not sterile, prompting concerns about the possible introduction of infection to abraded skin, particularly if scratches or abrasions compromise the integrity of the skin.

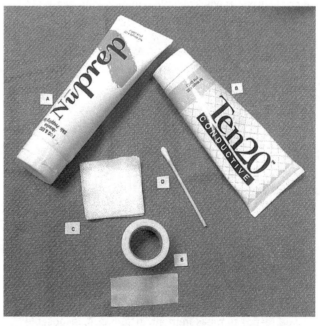

FIGURE 3.10. Supplies required for the application of electrodes used for clinical auditory evoked response measurement.

Before scrubbing an alert child or adult patient, it is good clinical manner to first describe briefly what is about to be done and to indicate that the scrubbing might be slightly uncomfortable. Of course, the same general explanation should be offered to the parent or caregiver of an infant before electrode application begins. In fact, it typically relieves the patient to learn that this is the "worst" part of the entire test. In routine clinical AER measurement, a small portion of mildly abrasive liquid is poured on a clean (not sterile) 2" × 2" or 4" × 4" gauze square (see "C" in Figure 3.10) and, with the index finger behind this part of the gauze, the electrode site is briskly rubbed (Figure 3.11). A cotton swab, (see "D" in Figure 3.10 and "A" in Figure 3.11) or an abrasive pad specially designed for electrode application, may also be used as an applicator. With a scalp site, the hair is first parted with the other hand. The earlobe site is prepared for electrode placement by grasping the earlobe between thumb and index finger with the gauze saturated with abrasive liquid, and then pulling downward briskly (see "D" in Figure 3.11). In preparing electrode sites around the eyes, it is important to keep the abrasive liquid from dripping into the eye. Excessive amounts of the liquid are wiped away with a clean portion of the gauze. Based on the observation of hundreds of students and neophyte auditory electrophysiologists applying electrodes prior to auditory evoked response mea-

surement, the author concludes that timidity is a common technical flaw. For children and adults alike, test time will be saved and frustration with high interelectrode impedance avoided by initially scrubbing the skin vigorously with ample liquid abrasive substance. Adults and older children having been duly alerted in advance to the clinician's intentions will invariably tolerate this approach without protesting, whereas infants and younger children are likely to squirm and cry no matter how gentle the scrubbing.

There are two relatively minor issues that should be noted regarding electrode site preparation. One question is whether each site should be prepared and the appropriate electrode affixed before moving on to the next site, or whether all sites should first be scrubbed and then the electrodes applied. One could probably find experienced clinicians who would endorse both approaches. My approach is to prepare (scrub) the relatively "easy" standard AER electrode sites in rapid sequence (i.e., Fz, Fpz, earlobes, and, as indicated, a noncephalic location). "Easy" in this instance refers to sites with flat surfaces and little or no hair. Then, each electrode is dabbed with paste, applied, and taped following the same sequence. For ABR recordings, electrode application at four sites, i.e., Fz (high forehead in the middle), A1, A2, and Fpz (middle of the low forehead) is relatively simple and straightforward. Electrodes on the forehead are secured after placement with

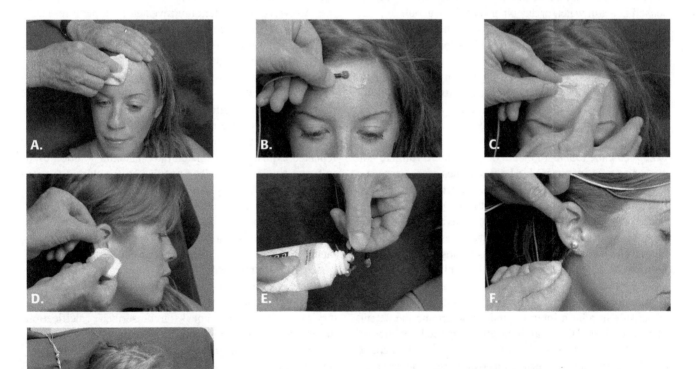

FIGURE 3.11. Steps in preparation of the skin and application of electrodes in ABR measurement and cleaning electrodes after data collection, including preparation of the scalp (A), placement of an electrode (B), securing an electrode with tape (C), preparation of skin at earlobe (D), application of electrode paste (or gel) to ear-clip-style electrode (E), placement of ear-clip-style electrode on earlobe (F), and a collection of recording electrodes in place (G).

short segments (1.5 to 2 inches) of tape (e.g., surgical tape or other medical-grade tape). Most clinicians experienced with auditory evoked response measurement have a preference for a specific type and material for the tape used to secure electrodes. Of course, tape is not necessary for the ear (inverting) electrodes with the earclip electrode design, and tape isn't required typically for any of the disposable electrodes used in ABR recording (as described below).

For electrode sites on hairy heads (e.g., hemispheric electrode sites for AMLR, or the Cz and Pz electrode sites for the ALR and P300 response), my approach is to prepare the scalp for one site, verify the location by keeping a finger in place, and then immediately apply the electrode with paste (*not* gel). Placing a cotton ball over the electrode that has just been applied to the skin with paste and pressing firmly for about 15 seconds will help to form a better and more durable connection. Then, one can move on to the next electrode site. Most electrode paste (as opposed to gel) actually adheres the electrode to the skin, although when possible tape should be used. Placing a second piece of tape on the electrode wire (lead) several inches from the electrode forms a "strain release" that helps to prevent electrode slippage (see "G" in Figure 3.11). This technique for electrode placement has several clinical advantages. It poses no risk to the patient and is relatively quick. Electrodes can be removed easily and the sites can be cleaned of paste or gel with an alcohol swab, diaper wipe, facecloth soaked in warm water, or any other suitable material.

Although there is little or no risk to the patient associated with ABR measurement, there is a remote possibility that the substances used to prepare electrode locations on the skin or to adhere electrodes to the skin will produce an allergic or other dermatologic reaction. Substances used for electrode preparation and placement (e.g., abrasive liquids, gel, cream, or paste) should be selected with regard to the manufacturer's recommendations for use with patients. For example, some brands of electrode paste and cream are not appropriate for infants. Other brands of these substances are specifically designed for use with certain types of patients (e.g., infants or persons who are highly allergic). The author many years ago had a very concerning experience following the application of surface disc electrodes with a severely burned child who was receiving massive doses of potentially ototoxic drugs to prevent potentially fatal infections. The child was very ill and unable to be evaluated behaviorally. He underwent an ABR assessment of auditory sensitivity at bedside in a burn intensive unit to determine the extent of hearing loss. Within an hour after I applied conductive paste to the electrode sides on the grafted skin, the patient developed an enormous hematoma (subdermal collection of blood) at each electrode site. As soon as ABR assessment was complete, I had left the hospital unaware of the complication associated with the electrode cream. Without relating all the worrisome details, the patient's attending physician was extremely upset at the child's unusual response to the electrode cream, fearing a systemic anaphylactic reaction

that might adversely affect the child's already unstable physical condition. Upon request by the physician, I attempted to determine from material printed on a tube of the paste the ingredients, but none were specified. I then called the manufacturer, explained the situation, and asked for a summary of the ingredients in the paste. The manufacturer, however, would not divulge the information. Fortunately, an hour or two later when I again made contact with the child's physician, the hematomas had resolved and there was no change in the child's health status.

The moral of this exciting little story is to always read closely fine print on any substance that will come into contact with a patient about appropriate precautions and contraindications. In the case of the severely burned patients, for whom the audiologic monitoring with ABR was essential for potential hearing preservation, I began to routinely apply electrodes for ABR measurement with alligator clips to skin graft staples placed in the proper locations (Fz, Fpz, and in each earlobe) by medical personnel. The new arrangement for electrode placement actually saved considerable time, yielded consistently acceptable interelectrode impedance (i.e., < 5 K ohms for absolute impedance and < 2 K ohms relative difference in impedance between any two electrodes in a pair). Most important, however, the alligator clip and skin staple arrangement eliminated all risk to the patient associated with electrode application.

A review of the literature revealed multiple references to dermatological reactions secondary to topical use of electrode paste (Johnson, Fitzpatrick, & Hahn, 1993; Mancuso et al., 1990; Wheeland & Roundtree, 1985; Wiley & Eaglstein, 1979; Zackeim & Pinkus, 1957; Zurbuchen, LeCoultre, Calza, & Halperin, 1996). Curiously, the original 1935 report of a skin reaction to calcium-based substances involved an Austrian ice cream maker who developed papules (a red elevated area on the skin) on his feet and legs after repeated exposure to a concentrated calcium solution used to freeze the ice cream. The papules on the skin of the ice cream maker more than seventy years ago were essentially the same problem I encountered with the burn patient during ABR measurement. In addition to the references cited, published in the English language, there are articles published in other languages. Much of the adverse experience with electrode paste was reportedly from EEG recordings in children, but there are a handful of papers describing skin reactions on the forehead and earlobes during measurement of auditory evoked responses. Focal (circumscribed) calcification in the dermis (skin), referred to as calcinosis cutis, can be caused by percutaneous (surface of skin) exposure to substances (e.g., fluids, solutions, gels, pastes) containing calcium or calcium chloride. Microabrasions, tiny scratches in the surface of the skin are, of course, purposefully produced in the conventional approach for preparing electrode locations by scrubbing the skin with a gritty substance. The skin reactions typically are evident within hours after the ABR. Factors contributing to adverse dermatological complications with electrode paste include the presence of calcium (calcium chloride), prolonged exposure to the substance (> 6 hours), and age (they are more likely in children).

The occurrence of calcinosis cutis during ABR measurement, although rare, can be minimized by thoroughly cleaning the skin immediately after the evoked response procedure to remove all traces of the conducting substance, avoidance of skin abrasion during preparation of electrode placement, and regular use of electrode conducting substances that do not include calcium as an ingredient. Aggressively abrading the skin before electrode placement also introduces the possibility of exposing the patient to risk of infection. The risk of infection is increased with the application of reusable electrodes that, while clean, are not sterilized. There is also a slight possibility of introducing infection via the percutaneous route with the use of commercially available abrasive pads, rather than a commercially available gritty liquid as the pads are, typically, not sterile.

The other question is whether electrode sites on children who require sedation for evoked response assessment (usually ABR or perhaps ECochG) should be prepared before or after the sedative is administered. Nuances of ABR measurement in infants and young children, including setup, electrode placement, and variations in the test protocol, are covered in Chapter 8 ("Frequency-Specific ABR and ASSR"). It seems logical to prepare the skin, and perhaps even attach the electrodes, before the child is sedated so as not to wake him or her with physical stimulation just before the assessment begins. This physical contact prior to or immediately after the sedative is administered, however, may agitate the child and reduce the likelihood of effective sedation. Also, a highly active child, even an infant, has an almost uncanny ability to grasp electrode wires and rip them off. In the process, hair may be painfully pulled and the child becomes more upset and active. On the other hand, waiting until the child has fallen asleep to prepare the skin permits accurate and complete electrode attachment if the child is adequately sedated. On the other hand, physical stimulation (especially scrubbing the skin prior to electrode placement on the earlobes) often arouses the child who is not completely asleep. In the final analysis, the question about when to prepare for electrode placement is based on clinical preference and clinical judgment at the time. Under ideal conditions (the child is to be given the full dose of sedative in a quiet test environment and has not shown prior sedation difficulty), I will aggressively prepare the electrode sites before sedation. Electrodes are then attached after sedation, with the child sleeping, with the expectation that the child will be aroused somewhat when the electrodes make contact with the skin. Of course, when children are to be anesthetized for ECochG and/or ABR measurement, electrode application can be completed after anesthesia is complete.

CONDUCTING PASTE, GEL, OR CREAM. | The foregoing discussion of skin preparation and electrode placement contained several references to the use of paste versus gel. Actually, three substances are available for application to the skin of nondisposable (i.e., reusable) types of electrodes. Advantages common to each of the substances include increased conductivity for evoked response activity and facilitation of lower inter-electrode impedance. The least viscous and most like liquid like substance is gel. Gel, easily squeezed onto the medial (skin side) surface of a disc electrode, is typically water-soluble. Some brands of gel are specially designed to avoid irritation to sensitive skin and staining of clothing. Electrode cream has properties similar to gel, and typically includes electrolytes adjusted to the pH of the skin. Adhesion of disc electrodes to the skin is most effectively accomplished with conductive paste. Typically white, electrode paste forms a relatively tight seal between the skin and the electrode to keep the electrode in place even without tape. Any of these three conducting substances is appropriate with disc electrodes, but the paste is particularly well suited for electrodes used on sites over the scalp (e.g., Fz, Cz, Pz, C3, and C4) for measurement of cortical auditory evoked responses.

COLLODION. | Application of electrodes with collodion is relatively time consuming, but results in firm and durable connections and minimizes artifacts. Preparation of the electrode site is done as described above. Then, the electrode is held on the location with an instrument (e.g., stylus) and collodion is spread around the rim of the electrode and onto adjacent skin. The collodion is left to dry (an air blower or hair blower hastens the drying). This secures the electrode. Conducting paste or gel is then injected into the hole in the center of the electrode. After testing, the electrode is removed (collodion dissolved) with acetone. A possible complication of collodion occurs when there is a leak in the tube. Collodion may then escape and be inadvertently dripped on the patient or clothing.

ELECTRODE REMOVAL (AFTER THE EVOKED RESPONSE PROCEDURE). | Alcohol preps are useful in removing electrode paste from the skin after testing, although a warmly moist washcloth, a paper towel, a piece of gauze, or commercially available disposable cloths designed for diaper changing work (perhaps with lotion) function equally well without irritating or drying the skin. Acetone, employed for cleaning up collodion, is somewhat hazardous and not advised for clinical use. In the neonatal or surgical ICU and OR, acetone would quickly erode plastic (e.g., plastic tubing used for arterial lines, nasogastric tubes, oxygen tubes). Reuseable electrodes should be cleaned with disinfectant soap and water, and then dried, immediately after use. An old toothbrush (sterilized and no longer used for oral hygiene) is handy for cleaning electrode paste, cream, and gel from the concave portion of disc electrodes. During cleaning, a finger should be used to support the electrode to minimize torsion and prevent breakage of the electrode lead (wire). Reusable metal electrodes should then be properly disinfected. With proper care, reusable disc electrodes will provide many months, and even years, of reliable service.

DISC ELECTRODES. | The conventional electrode design employed since the advent of clinical application of auditory evoked responses is the disc- or cup-type electrode ("C" in Figure 3.8). The electrode disc is available in adult or pediatric sizes (10 mm or 6 mm) and is made of a metal or metal alloy, such as gold, silver, or silver coated with silver chloride (AgCl). The disc has a hole in the center of the cup and is integrated with a lead or wire of 1.0 m or 1.5 m that ends with a DIN pin. Some disc electrode designs feature a reinforced molded hub near the disc to make it easier to apply to the skin and to prevent damage to the solder joint between the disc and electrode wire (Figure 3.8). Electrode wires are available in a variety of colors. The cost of reuseable metal electrodes is about $7 to $10 each. Extension cables are available to increase the distance from the electrode on the patient to the electrode box. It is important to keep in mind, however, that electrodes function like antennae in electrically hostile test environments, and longer electrode leads increase the likelihood of picking up unwanted electrical interference.

EAR CLIP ELECTRODES. | Ear clip electrodes are a variation of the disc or cup electrode design (see "C" in Figure 3.8). Two discs or cups are mounted in a spring-type device, then connected to a typical lead or wire ending in a standard DIN pin. Following preparation of the skin on both sides of the earlobe (as described above), a conducting substance (gel, cream or paste) is applied to both of the discs, and the clip is placed on the earlobe (see "D," "E," and "F" in Figure 3.11). Because the force of the spring maintains steady pressure of the disc against the skin, tape is not necessary. In fact, adhering paste is also not necessary, so gel is adequate as a conducting substance. Ear clip electrodes also are available in different metals (e.g., gold, silver, silver chloride), but they are always sold in pairs and with leads in two colors—red for the right ear and blue for the left ear. Depending on the vendor, a set of two ear clip electrodes costs about $50 to $60. Ear clip electrodes are cleaned with the same technique described above for the conventional cup electrodes. In the author's experience with this electrode design over the past twenty years, the ear clip electrode offers at least one-half dozen distinct advantages for routine clinical use: (1) amplitude for the AP component of the ECochG and ABR wave I is increased by about 30 percent with earlobe versus mastoid placement; (2) for bone conduction ABR recordings, earlobe (versus mastoid) placement increases the distance between the electrode and the bone vibrator, thus reducing electrical artifact; (3) consistently low inter-electrode impedance is enhanced by the firm pressure against the skin and by the doubling of surface area (i.e., two discs rather than one are connected to the lead); (4) tape is not required in applying the electrode; (5) if the electrodes are pulled off during recording, as they may be with restless children, replacement

is simple and reliable; and (6) with proper care the electrodes can be reused for literally hundreds of ABR recordings, resulting in low long-term cost.

DISPOSABLE ELECTRODES. | There are now a variety of designs for and manufacturers of disposable electrodes ("A" and "B" in Figure 3.8). Initially designed for use with newborn infants for universal hearing screening applications, disposable electrodes are relied upon by some clinicians for ABR recording in other patient populations. Skin preparation for application of disposable electrodes is not different to the foregoing description of the preparing for placement of disc electrodes. Commercially available disposable electrodes usually are made of foam or cloth and include within the center of the skin-side surface (recording area) a small quantity of conducting gel surrounded by adhesive glue-type substance. Disposable electrodes are available in several basic shapes (i.e., round, square, or rectangular) and are generally manufactured with silver/silver chloride gel within the recording area. There are two general disposable electrode designs. One is a single integrated design in which the electrode is connected to a lead or wire, with the entire piece discarded after use ("A" in Figure 3.8). The disc area is relatively small (about 20 to 25 mm), and the electrodes are sometimes manufactured in sets of three or four. The other design consists of individual disposable electrodes, shipped in sealed sterile enclosures, that include a snap in the center or off to one side. The disposable electrode is connected to a reuseable snap lead (wire) or alligator clip lead wire (see "B" in Figure 3.8). There are three obvious advantages of the disposable electrode design: (1) application to the skin without first applying a conducting gel, cream, or paste; (2) adherence to the skin without tape; and (3) the contribution to infection control offered by the disposable design. Disadvantages include cost for replacement ($.25 to $.75 per electrode) and limited selection of materials (e.g., not a variety of metal alloys) and design (e.g., no ear clip style). Each clinician will need to decide which general electrode design—reusable disc electrodes or disposable electrodes—is preferable given the evoked response to be recorded, the patient population to undergo recording, and the clinical application of the evoked response recording.

EAR CANAL ELECTRODES. | The most common type of ear canal electrode used clinically is the TIPtrode design (shown as "D" earlier in Figure 3.8), available for purchase from most manufacturers of evoked response instrumentation. The TIPtrode is a combination earphone and electrode consisting of a foam (polyurethane) insert ear cushion covered with gold foil. The TIPtrode is coupled to special acoustic tubing that connects the insert ear cushion to the transducer. The acoustic tubing (250 mm) includes an alligator clip design at the end that couples to the TIPtrode. Sound travels from the transducer down the acoustic tubing to the ear as with any insert earphone. Gold foil–covered TIPtrode cushions are available in two sizes—adult and pediatric (13 mm and 10 mm). The pediatric size is optimal for any patient with smaller ear canals, including women. The cost for one set of TIPtrodes is about $4.00 to $4.50. The gold foil covering the TIPtrode insert ear cushion is connected to a conventional electrode wire with an alligator clip device (refer to Figures 3.6 and 3.8). Bioelectric activity evoked to acoustic stimuli (e.g., components of the auditory evoked responses like ECochG components or wave I of the ABR) is conducted from the ear, auditory nerve, and other auditory structures to the TIPtrode via the walls of the external ear canal. The TIPtrode insert cushions are only used with one patient, whereas the acoustic tubing and alligator clips are reused.

For placement of ear canal electrodes, such as the TIPtrode, place a small amount of abrasive liquid onto a clean cotton swab (shown in Figure 3.12). With direct lighting, and after otoscopic inspection to verify that the ear canal is clear and a brief explanation of the procedure to the patient, the outer ear is gently pulled upward and backward. This maneuver tends to straighten and enlarge the outer portion of the ear canal meatus. Then, the walls of the outer portion of the ear canal are prepared by scrubbing vigorously with the cotton swab in a circular motion. Care is taken to keep the cotton within sight. The use of conducting gel or paste is not necessary with the TIPtrode. In fact, use of conducting gel is often counterproductive, as it often causes the TIPtrode to gradually slip out of the ear canal. In the author's experience, the technique just described will routinely produce inter-electrode impedance values well below the acceptable limit (5000 ohms) and comparable to impedance for other surface electrodes. In the interest of aural hygiene, ear canal electrodes, such as the TIPtrode, should only be used one time. Furthermore, the conducting property of the metal foil appears to dissipate with use, particularly in combination with abrasive liquids. Inter-electrode impedance for the TIPtrode is generally unacceptably high upon second application.

TYMPANIC MEMBRANE ELECTRODES. | As with the ear canal electrode type, it is important to first inspect the ear canal prior to insertion of tympanic membrane electrodes. Appropriate personnel should remove excessive cerumen or debris within the external ear canal before the electrode is placed. After preparing the tip of the electrode with a small amount of conducting gel, the electrode is slowly and carefully inserted into the ear canal. It is very important to use conducting gel rather than paste with the tympanic membrane technique. Within minutes after electrode application, conducting paste hardens and adheres to a surface. Clearly, it would be undesirable for the electrode tip to adhere to tympanic membrane as removal would be painful for the patient and would put the patient at risk for injury. During the insertion of the tympanic membrane electrode, the patient is instructed to report any sensation, including tickling, discomfort, or pain. At the least, the ear canal should be under direct lighting. Electrode insertion with the aid of a microscope is certainly appropriate, but not essential. The electrode is inserted until the patient reports a pressure sensation and/or hears a tapping sound. At that time, the clinician will often sense a slight resistance during insertion. Inter-electrode impedance is then measured. It is not uncommon for inter-electrode impedance to be rather high (> 5 to 10 kohms) following placement of the electrode, as the surface of the tympanic membrane cannot be prepared. The electrode lead is secured, with either tape or by insertion of a compressed foam plug.

SUBDERMAL NEEDLE ELECTRODES. | Subdermal electrodes offer the dual advantages of stability for long-term AER measurements and consistency in interelectrode impedance. They are well suited for special applications of AERs or non-auditory clinical neurophysiology, such as neurophysiologic monitoring during surgical procedures that put the auditory system or facial nerve at risk. The author's preference for needle electrodes is either a disposable or reusable subdermal stainless steel needle with a 12 mm uninsulated shaft and 0.4 mm diameter, a beveled tip, and a conventional cable length (1 meter). Subdermal needle electrodes are also constructed of platinum iridium, with the option of insulation along the shaft (uninsulated tip). Electrode cables for the disposable

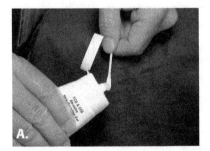
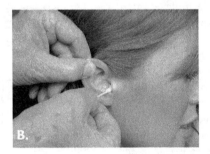
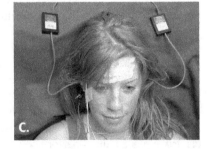

FIGURE 3.12. A figure showing the preparation for, and application of, a TIPtrode electrode used in clinical measurement of the ECochG and ABR, including application of abrasive substance on a cotton swab (A), preparation of the skin in the external ear canal (B), and electrodes and transducers in place (C). Note that the electrodes and transducers remain separated.

and reusable versions of the subdermal needles are available in a variety of colors. The value of color-coding placement of electrodes in auditory evoked response measurement is noted below. Disposable electrodes are sterilized and packaged individually, whereas reusable needle electrodes typically are purchased in packages of 5 or 10. *It is important to note that reusable subdermal needle electrodes must be sterilized before each use (e.g., gas sterilization is available in hospitals and medical clinics).* Needle electrodes can be used for an auditory evoked response recording when the patient is first anesthetized. Needle electrodes present at least three distinct advantages for routine use clinically in such cases. First, application is faster as there is little skin preparation. The skin at the electrode site should be wiped vigorously with an alcohol swab before the electrode is inserted almost horizontally under the skin, then the electrode lead (wire) is secured with a piece of tape. Second, needle electrodes tend to be more stable during prolonged auditory evoked response measurement than disc (surface) electrodes. And, finally, inter-electrode impedance is adequately low and invariably balanced, even though no valuable test time was consumed in scrubbing the skin. The two potential (and highly unlikely) health risks posed by needle electrodes are spread of disease by an unsterilized needle and needle breakage, i.e., a portion of the needle remains under the skin. Of course, placement of subdermal needle electrodes must be considered an invasive procedure. Although complications are very unlikely, subdermal needle insertion should always be done by appropriate medical personnel or by experienced nonmedical personnel with medical support readily available. Other types of needle electrode designs available commercially for auditory evoked response recording and used by some clinicians include longer (e.g., 25 mm) monopolar needles and disposable corkscrew electrodes.

TRANSTYMPANIC MEMBRANE ELECTRODE. | The specific technique for placement of transtympanic (TT) membrane electrodes varies depending on the type of needle that is used. The following description applies to the transtympanic placement of a subdermal needle electrode that was just described, rather than a longer needle electrode, as often reported in the literature and sometimes applied clinically. In the clinic, prior to insertion of the needle, the tympanic membrane is typically anesthetized with a Phenol (89%) swab. A microscope is used for viewing the tympanic membrane. The patient usually describes a burning or tingling sensation as the Phenol reaches the eardrum. In the operating room, when ECochG is applied during neurophysiologic intraoperative monitoring, the transtympanic membrane electrode placement is performed after the patient is under general anesthesia. A physician (e.g., otologist) places the needle electrode onto the promontory under an operating room microscope. The use of subdermal needle electrodes in transtympanic recording of the ECochG, including the tech-

nique for insertion, is described in Chapter 4, with clinical applications reviewed Chapter 5.

GENERAL ELECTRODE PLACEMENT. | The pin on any electrode lead wire is inserted into an electrode connection strip or box (see Figure 3.13). There are different types of electrode boxes. Some are relatively simple with receptacles for connectors for three or five electrodes (receptacles for a single channel of one noninverting, one inverting, and one common ground electrode) or two sets of noninverting and inverting electrodes with a common ground). Simpler electrode receptacles may be labeled with various symbols (e.g., A+, A- and C; G1, G2, and ground ["gnd"]; active, reference, and ground). Others are more sophisticated preamplifiers with electrode locations displayed on a head-shaped diagram and labeled according to the International 10–20 system

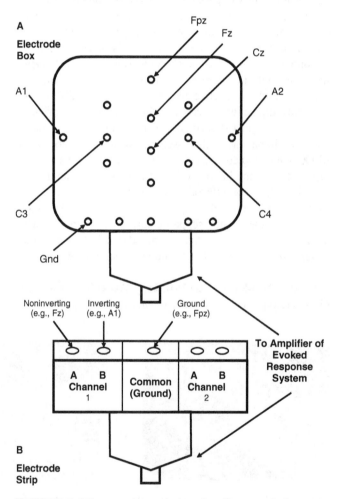

FIGURE 3.13. An electrode box for placement of electrodes in a variety of locations used in recording auditory evoked responses (A). An electrode strip with receptacles for noninverting and inverting electrodes for two recording channels and a ground electrode (B).

(Figure 3.9). With these devices, individual electrodes may be selected and changed via the computer keyboard. It is, of course, important to verify that each electrode wire pin is inserted in the proper slot before evoked response recording. A simple color-coding system is useful to facilitate consistently proper electrode placement. For ABR measurement, the author recommends the use of a different color for each site. Being among 10 percent of the male population that is color deficient (i.e., red-green "colorblind"), I always utilize the same primary colors for each of the electrodes, namely, a bright and light color (e.g., yellow or white) for the noninverting (Fz) electrode, red for the right earlobe or TIPtrode, blue for the left earlobe or TIPtrode, and a dull and dark color (e.g., gray, brown, or black) for the common (ground) electrode. The set of four reusable or disposable electrodes, each a different color, can be braided or tied loosely into a few knots to reduce the likelihood of electrical interference. Because the colors are so different, it's possible to verify which electrode site is plugged into which electrode box receptacle, even though the wires are braided or tied, and even in a darkened test room. Recall from the discussion above that it is possible to use one electrode for two channels, or to "link" any pair of electrodes (such as two earlobe electrodes) with "jumper cables" (short wires have a pin at each end and also a receptacle for an electrode pin at the top).

ELECTRODE ARRAYS. | The combination of two recording electrodes forms an electrode array or montage. For routine measurement of the ABR, a single-channel electrode array is recommended (Fz-Ai or ipsilateral earlobe). Under some clinical circumstances, such as bone conduction ABR measurement, the addition of a second channel (Fz-Ac or contralateral earlobe) is helpful for confident identification of wave I. The ipsilateral electrode array (Fz-Ai) combination of electrodes is most likely to produce clear waves I through V and to facilitate identification of wave I (present in the ipsilateral and absent in the contralateral arrays). Furthermore, digitally subtracting the contralateral array waveform from the ipsilateral array waveform yields a "derived" horizontal waveform (described and illustrated in Chapter 7). Use of a noncephalic inverting electrode, truly a "reference" electrode has definite electrophysiologic rationale and may, in some cases, contribute to the resolution or identification of selected wave components. As with any AER measurement strategy, a clinician should consistently utilize customary stimulus and acquisition parameters (for the facility) in initial recordings, but then modify these parameters as the need arises during the assessment to enhance the quality of AER waveforms.

Electrode sites used in AMLR measurement have undergone changes within recent years. Formerly, a midline (Cz or Fz) noninverting electrode site was used almost exclusively. Currently, the AMLR is recorded with multiple scalp sites for noninverting electrodes. What about the inverting electrodes? As just noted, some investigators continue to record AMLR with a two-channel array characterized by a common midline noninverting electrode and inverting electrodes on the ears ipsilateral and contralateral to the stimulus. Such an array is selected to enhance the different contributions to the waveform by the ipsilateral versus contralateral ear. With the multiple scalp electrode technique (noninverting electrodes at Fz, C5, and C6), on the other hand, an attempt is made to eliminate the ipsilateral versus contralateral ear contribution by "linking" these two electrodes. That is, the inverting electrode leads from each ear are usually plugged into a jumper lead connecting the amplifier inputs for each inverting electrode. The result is a "balanced reference" equalizing contributions of the ears to each of the scalp electrode arrays. Thus, differences among waveforms for the two or three scalp electrode arrays can be attributed to hemispheric, or CNS, factors, rather than contributions from the ear or differences in the orientation of the array with respect to the stimulus side.

Electrode Box

Electrodes are usually plugged into an electrode box that is connected to the amplifier with a shielded cable. Electrode boxes are available in different shapes and sizes (Figure 3.13). There may also be, at this stage, a preamplifier. An electrode box has minimally three receptacles (also called jacks), one each for the noninverting, inverting, and ground electrodes. This constitutes one recording channel. Most electrode boxes allow for at least two channel recordings with five or six electrode receptacles. The receptacles may be arranged in a single row, two or more rows, or in the shape of a head. Channels on electrode strips are sometimes indicated by numbers (e.g., Channel 1, Channel 2) or letters (A, B, C, . . .). Labels for the individual receptacles for each channel also vary. They may be color coded or referred to by polarity of the amplifier input (e.g., A+ for the positive voltage electrode in channel one, A– for the negative voltage inverting electrode in channel one, and C for the common [ground] electrode, with a similar format for the B or second channel). The term G (originating from the use of electrode grids) may be used to refer to electrode receptacles, so that G1 is the first electrode (noninverting), G2 is the second electrode (inverting), and so forth. Box type preamplifiers have electrode receptacles with the 10–20 International Electrode System labels (e.g., Cz, Fz, A1), while a few others on the electrode box are reserved for miscellaneous electrodes and given numbers or other labels (e.g., X1, X2).

For electrode boxes with receptacles for electrode placements at a variety of scalp locations (see Figure 3.13), the electrode sites to be used with a specific auditory evoked response recording are selected with evoked response system software. The protocol for a two-channel ABR might, for example, call for electrodes at Fz, A1, and A2 locations, and a ground (common) electrode. These labels would be selected from the collection parameters or settings page of the evoked response program. With electrode strips, the physical location of the electrode pin determines the actual electrode input (e.g., channel 1, + electrode). Each channel on the electrode strip has a receptacle for a noninverting ("positive" or "active") electrode. To avoid the need for placing two noninverting electrodes on the patient (one for each channel), the receptacles can be connected or linked with a short "jumper" cable consisting of both electrode pins and receptacles, i.e., male and female DIN connectors. The jumper cable is rather short (about 15 mm), with one end plugged into the noninverting electrode input (#1 or + input) for one channel, and the other end is plugged into the corresponding other input for the second channel. Then, the pin for a single noninverting electrode (e.g., at the Fz site high on the middle of the forehead) is inserted into one of the jumper cable receptacles (it doesn't make any difference which one). Jumper cables for linking electrodes can be purchased from most manufacturers of evoked response systems, and a few extra cables should always be available among evoked response supplies in a clinic. We will describe another application of the jumper cable in the review of auditory middle latency response (AMLR) measurement in Chapter 11 (see "Electrode Sites" in the section on "Acquisition Parameters").

Naturally, the first step in adequate amplification is plugging the electrodes in properly. Without careful attention to this task, however, mistakes are sure to occur. Troubleshooting guidelines, to prevent serious consequences from this technical error for specific types of auditory evoked responses, are described in subsequent chapters. Current evoked response systems permit keyboard control of electrode connections. With these evoked response systems, it is often possible for electrode switching (from one array to another) to be automated by simple programming. This feature can potentially eliminate some of the more frequent technical errors in AER assessment.

Electrophysiologic Amplification

Usually, the term *amplifier* suggests a device that increases the strength of a signal (acoustical or electrical). A simple example is found in every radio. Increasing the gain or amplification makes music or talking louder. *Gain* is technically defined as the ratio of the voltage of the signal at the output of the amplifier (after amplification) to the voltage delivered to the input. An amplifier is a crucial component of an evoked response system because AERs generated by the cochlea, eighth nerve, or brain are very small (as little as 1 millionth of a volt). The average amplitude for ABR wave V, for example, is about 0.5 microvolt (μvolt), i.e., one-half of one-millionth of a volt. AERs must, therefore, be amplified substantially before they can be processed by a signal averaging computer and displayed on an oscilloscope or computer monitor screen. As an example of AER amplification requirements, in ABR recording gain is typically set at X100,000. Since the amplitude of the output-to-input is expressed as a ratio, and amplification is usually expressed in order of magnitude of 10, gain is sometimes described in a logarithmic unit that reflects these characteristics, the dB (dB = X log 10 gain). A gain of 10 would, for example, be equivalent to 20 dB and the typical ABR gain of 100,000 would be 100 dB.

There are two characteristics of an amplifier that have a direct influence on successful AER recording. One is input impedance, simply defined as opposition to alternating current flow, specifically impedance across the amplifier inputs. Optimally, input impedance of the amplifier is comparable to or higher than the electrode impedance for AER recording. A serious problem develops when there is an imbalance in electrode impedance, with one electrode having higher impedance than another.

COMMON MODE REJECTION (CMR). | Common mode rejection is a vital function of the amplifier. It is also an important concept in understanding how relatively tiny AER voltages can be detected in the midst of a wide variety of other electrical signals, many with far greater amplitude. As a first step toward this understanding, several terms should be clarified. Two electrodes placed at different locations on the head (e.g., the high forehead in the midline [Fz] and an earlobe) will presumably each detect the same amount of electrical interference (electrical activity that does not include the response) that is in the region of the head (refer to Figure 3.14). This interference is common to, or the same for, each electrode. The differential preamplifier, which is a component of most evoked response systems, reverses polarity (positive or negative sign) of inverting electrode input voltage and adds it to noninverting electrode input. This is in effect a subtraction process. In this way, any activity that is the same as detected at each electrode is eliminated (rejected), as shown schematically in Figure 3.14. Therefore, one of the electrodes (amplifier inputs) is called the inverting electrode and the other is the noninverting electrode. This is the accurate, and preferred, terminology for describing electrodes, as noted previously in the discussion of electrode terminology.

If each electrode recorded exactly the same AER activity, then common mode rejection would subtract away the response. To demonstrate this point, record an AER with two electrodes (noninverting and inverting) placed next to each other, for example, both on the forehead. The result is nearly a flat line. All AER activity is detected similarly by each electrode and is eliminated by the common mode rejection process. However, with one electrode on top of the head and another located near the ear, the response detected by each is not the same but, in fact, very different. Early components of the ABR, in particular, are usually of opposite polarity. Subtracting the activity detected at the earlobe electrode from activity at the vertex electrode not only reduces noise interference, but it actually increases amplitude of some ABR components. However, if any AER activity as detected by the two electrodes is the same, it will be lost

Differential Amplification
(Noninverting and Inverting Electrodes)

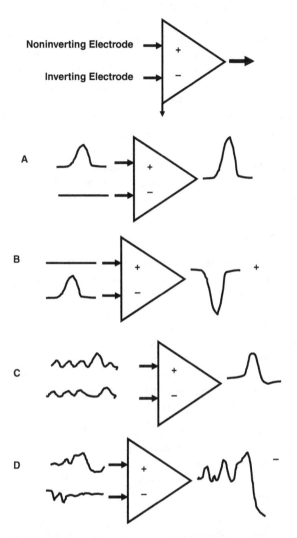

FIGURE 3.14. A schematic representation of the process of differential amplification that used in auditory evoked response measurement.

from the recording. With a cephalic electrode (located somewhere on the head) and noncephalic electrode combination, interference common to each is subtracted out, leaving only the response detected by the cephalic electrode. While there is no augmentation of early ABR components, which is a disadvantage, there is also no inadvertent rejection of portions of the response, which is a distinct clinical advantage. Recording far-field AERs with two relatively closely placed electrodes, each at the same end of the generator dipole, such as the vertex and forehead for ABR, is clearly not advised (see Chapter 7 for examples of this and numerous other technical faux pas in ABR recording). The effectiveness of common mode rejection is usually expressed in terms of a ratio of the amplifier output (the electrical activity that re-

mains after amplification) with only one input (i.e., without the benefit of the subtraction process) to the amplifier output when both inputs are the same. Usually the CMR ratio is more than 10,000, meaning that activity detected similarly by both electrodes, such as electrical interference, is more than 10,000 times smaller than the amplitude of activity detected by the noninverting electrode. The ratio is often expressed in decibels, which is a logarithmic value. A CMR ratio of 10,000 would be equivalent to a value of 80 dB. For example, a ratio of 10:1 is 10 dB, 100:1 is 20 dB, 1000:1 is 40 dB, and so forth.

ARTIFACT REJECTION. | A necessary feature in evoked response instrumentation is the capacity for viewing incoming electrical activity. The electrical activity detected by the electrodes is a combination of EEG, AER, and unwanted electrical interference, in a relatively "raw" state, before it is filtered or averaged. Even at this early stage, the input has been subjected to the common mode rejection process and to amplification. One might say that an AER is only as good as the raw EEG within which it is embedded. Ongoing, or at least periodic, inspection of the unaveraged electrical signal can provide clinically valuable information on subject state (quiet or active, awake or asleep) and the amount and type of electrical interference influencing the recording. With a little experience, the clinician can quickly differentiate quiet artifact-free EEG from EEG contaminated by general patient movement, neuromuscular artifact, electrical interference at 60 Hz, or another discrete frequency or high-frequency electrical interference. The clinician may be alerted to the presence of interference by the artifact rejection indicator; however, visual inspection of the raw incoming signal is a more effective approach for determining the type and, perhaps, the source of interference. This information can then guide attempts at reducing or eliminating the problem.

An artifact in AER recording is, by definition, electrical activity that is not part of the response and should not be included in analysis of the response. The artifact may be electromagnetic and generated from an external (nonpatient) source (e.g., earphones or an electrical device) or it may be electrophysiologic, originating from the patient, such as neuromuscular potentials related to patient movement. There are three main approaches for reducing the negative influences of artifact on AERs. The first, and best, is to determine the source of the artifact and eliminate it. For example, it might be possible, by process of elimination, to identify an X-ray view box as the source of serious electrical artifact that totally precludes AER recording. By turning off the view box, the artifact will disappear and test conditions are adequate. When excessive patient movement is the source of neuromuscular artifact, the patient may be given a sedative and fall asleep. Testing then proceeds without difficulty. Another approach for dealing with artifact is to modify test parameters, such as filter settings, electrode arrays, and number of sweeps. Practical guidelines for management of these sources of artifact in AER measurement are suggested in subsequent chapters. The third approach for minimizing the deleterious effect of artifact on AER recording is a technique known simply as artifact rejection. With earlier generations of signal averaging devices, the tester was required to constantly keep vigil over the ongoing EEG as displayed on an oscilloscope and manually pause the averaging process during periods of excessive artifact. This arrangement is not ideal because it necessarily occupies tester attention and time during the AER assessment session, time that could be devoted to record keeping, online inspection of the response, and analysis of AERs as they are signal-averaged. Also, in the time it takes the tester to determine the presence of artifact and pause the averaging process, artifact contamination of the response may have already begun.

Automatic artifact rejection is a feature on most evoked response systems. The simplest artifact rejection design is based on the sensitivity setting of the amplifier. Any signal detected by the electrodes that exceeds a designated preset voltage is not sent on to the signal-averaging device. This is an effective means of eliminating from the averaging process occasional very high-voltage sources of artifact. In theory, then, only relative pure signals (within an acceptable voltage range) are averaged. These are, of course, not necessarily AERs but are at least within a voltage region that AERs usually are found. To be effective clinically, an artifact rejection system must not permit any unwanted electrical signal to enter the averaging process. One way to accomplish this is to keep each analysis time period in memory, before it is sent on for averaging, in order to complete an artifact detection process. If no artifact is identified, the EEG (maybe including AER activity) is passed on to the signal-averaging device, but if artifact is present, the entire analysis time period (which was triggered by one stimulus) and maybe the preceding and following time periods are erased from memory.

Artifact rejection devices are very useful, but not an answer to every artifact problem. Two common clinical limitations are the inability to make progress with averaging because of almost continuous artifact rejection and the obvious contamination of an waveform that is being averaged with artifact despite the use of artifact rejection. Increasing the sensitivity of the amplifier (increasing amplifier gain) to solve the second problem will also increase the sensitivity of the artifact rejection process and perhaps create the first problem.

ALTERNATIVE TECHNOLOGY. | Conventional systems record AER with an interface module with a differential amplifier and a serial or USB port. The electrode lead wires are connected to the differential amplifier, and the computer is connected to a serial or USB port. This connection may introduce electrically conducted noises into the AER amplifier from the computer and the power line. In the Integrity™ system from Vivosonic Inc., communication between the interface module and computer is performed through a wireless interface module, the VivoLink™ employing Bluetooth® wireless communications. This eliminates the electrical path between the computer and AEP amplifier, and as a result eliminates introduction of electrically conducted noises from the computer and power line. In addition, it allows for convenient recording from a distance within the Bluetooth® range of about 30 feet (10 meters): The VivoLink™ can be placed in an infant's crib, bassinet, incubator, stroller, or car seat and the computer can be placed anywhere within a 10 meter radius. In the operating room, it can be placed on or near the operating table, while the operator performing the test—for example intraoperative monitoring—can be seated away from the operating table, even in another room, and not interfere with the crew performing the operation (Sokolov, Zhang, & Long, 2005).

Filter Settings

Filter settings are chosen to eliminate unwanted nonresponse activity (electrical and muscle interference or artifact) while preserving the actual response. A principle of filtering was stated earlier in Table 3.1. Filters, simply put, selectively remove part of the bioelectrical activity from the total bioelectrical activity plus electrical activity arising from sources outside of the brain. In AER measurement, filters reject electrical energy at certain frequencies and pass energy at other frequencies. An appreciation of four points is important for appropriate use of filtering in clinical AER measurement:

1. Why filtering is employed in recording AERs.
2. How the properties and performance of a filter are described.
3. The spectral composition of each type of AER.
4. How filtering can alter each type of AER.

Appropriate selection of a filter setting, then, requires an appreciation of the spectral characteristics of noise and signal (e.g., the auditory evoked response). The ECochG and ABR have spectral energy from just below 100 Hz up to 1000 Hz, or slightly higher frequencies. Thus, for measurement of these responses clinically, filter settings of 30 to 1500 Hz or 3000 Hz will effectively minimize general EEG activity (frequencies under 30 Hz) that do not contribute to the response while still preserving the spectral energy that forms the response. AMLR, in neurologically normal adults at least, has energy predominantly in the range of 20 to 40 Hz. The longer latency responses are dominated by low-frequency energy (below 30 Hz).

Analysis of the number of waves per second in the AER waveform is a handy way of estimating some of the frequency content of the response. For example, casual visual inspection of normal ABR waveforms reveals major waves approximately every 1 ms (e.g., 1000/second or 1000 Hz) plus a slow frequency wave with a frequency of about 100 Hz (one wave/second). The safest policy clinically is to filter as little as necessary, so as to reduce the possibility of filters contributing to distortion in the latency of components in the waveform, or even apparent components in the response that are really artifacts. Wider filter settings during data collection are desirable if evoked response instrumentation permits digital filtering after data collection, although with conventional artifact rejection options the averaging process may be slowed by the presence of unfiltered noise.

WHY IS FILTERING NECESSARY IN AER MEASUREMENT? | Filtering is a technique for enhancing detection of a signal (the AER) in the presence of background electrical noise. Noise here is defined simply as any electrical activity detected by the electrodes (from the patient or external sources) that is not auditory evoked response. Theoretically, noise with frequency content that is different from the frequency content of an AER can be filtered out of the raw electrical activity detected by the electrodes before the averaging process. It is more effective to average activity that is likely to include the response than unselected activity. The main objective of filtering is to reduce or eliminate from the averaging process nonresponse electrical activity with relatively well-defined and consistent frequency content. One example of this type of electrical noise is the normal EEG frequency region, which is below 30 Hz (including delta, theta, alpha, and beta EEG). Whenever appropriate, electrical energy in the region of 0.05 to 30 Hz is filtered out of AERs. This frequency region also encompasses electrodermal noise (0.01 to 5 Hz) and a portion of the frequency region of movement potentials (around 0.05 to 50 Hz). Another type of electrical noise targeted in routine AER filtering is neuromuscular (myogenic) activity. Electromyogenic noise may share a portion of the spectrum for some AERs (the 100 to 500 Hz region) and, therefore, cannot be entirely filtered out. However, it may also include frequencies of up to 5000 Hz. Low-pass filter cutoffs of 1500 or 3000 Hz minimize interference with AER measurement by activity in the higher frequency range.

PROPERTIES OF FILTERS. | Filter-related terms and concepts are illustrated in Figure 3.15. High-pass filters reject lower frequency energy and allows higher frequency energy to pass through. Low-pass filters function in just the opposite way. In combination, high- and low-pass filters can be set to pass a band of frequencies. A band-pass filter rejects energy below a certain cutoff and above a certain cutoff, passing energy for a band of frequencies within these two limits. Band-pass filtering is commonly employed in AER measurement. One essential property of a filter, then, is the frequency at which energy is rejected versus passed. This is often referred to as the cutoff frequency. There are two somewhat confusing terms in describing filters. The first is that the high-pass filter cutoff frequency is actually the lower frequency limit of the energy passed, whereas the low-pass filter cutoff frequency is the upper limit of energy passed. So, for a band-pass filter of 30 to 3000 Hz, the high-pass filter is from 0 to 30 Hz, the low-pass filter is from 3000 Hz

to some upper limit (e.g., 10,000 Hz). The term "cutoff" is also misleading because it implies an either/or function, a single frequency above or below which all energy is rejected or passed. For conventional analog filters that deal with input electrical activity in ongoing nondigital form, however, the cutoff frequency is simply where energy begins to be filtered (Figure 3.15).

A common definition for the cutoff frequency is that point at which electrical energy output from the filter is decreased by 3 dB (the 3 dB downpoint). The slope of an analog filter is an important feature, because it defines the sharpness of filtering. Filters in many evoked response systems, such as the standard-phase Butterworth filter, reject energy at a rate of 12 or 24 dB/octave. The important point here for clinical AER applications is that that energy will be passed for frequencies beyond the cutoff. A common clinical example of this limitation is experienced with attempts to eliminate bothersome 60 Hz power line interference. Selecting a high-pass filter cutoff of 100 Hz would seem be a solution to the problem, because 60 Hz is well below this cutoff. Unfortunately, 60 Hz energy will not be rejected (will be passed) with a filter slope of 12 dB/octave and interference

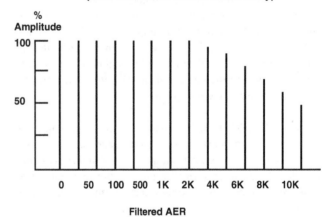

FIGURE 3.15. A schematic representation of the process used in filtering of electrophysiologic activity prior to the analysis of auditory evoked responses.

persists. It would appear that increasing the filter slope is a simple solution to this problem, that is, it would make the filter more precise. In fact, steeper slopes (e.g., 24, 48, or even 96 dB/octave) are possible for analog filters, but they cause greater distortion of the response. This point is discussed further in a later section. The optimal solution to this apparent dilemma is to digitally filter. Digital filtering permits very sharp filtering without associated distortion, particularly phase and latency distortion of the response.

60 HZ (CYCLE) NOTCH FILTERING. | Most evoked response systems provide the option for narrowband rejection, or filtering, of electrical activity in the region of 60 Hz. The objective is to selectively eliminate from the auditory evoked response 60 Hz power line interference without removing other frequencies from the response. Theoretically, then, a 60 Hz notch filter would be preferable to filtering out all frequencies below, for example, 75 Hz, which would include this interference. Such selective filtering is a questionable clinical practice for several reasons. First of all, harmonics of the electrical activity at 60 Hz interfering with AER measurement (occurring at higher frequencies) are not eliminated and may continue to contaminate the recording, limiting the effectiveness of the filtering technique. Second, any analog filtering will usually produce distortion of response phase (latency) and the purposely steep notch filter characteristics may actually cause more latency distortion than conventional band-pass AER filtering at the amplifier. Finally, for some AERs, such as the AMLR or ALR, even limited filtering around the frequency of 60 Hz will probably remove a substantial portion of the energy of the response and limit the inherent validity of the waveform.

THE SPECTRUM OF AERS. | Perhaps the most important issue in determining appropriate filter settings, and one sometimes overlooked, is the spectral composition of the AER being recorded. In the interest of filtering out unwanted electrical noise frequencies, it is possible to also eliminate part of the actual response. Clearly, "throwing the baby out with the bathwater" will not enhance AER recordings. How can the frequency composition of an AER be determined? The most accurate approach is spectral analysis of the response, made, for example, by performing a fast Fourier transformation (FFT) on an averaged waveform. Frequency content of the waveform can be assessed with an instrument designed for this type of analysis, a spectrum analyzer. Some commercially available evoked response systems also have software for AER spectral analysis.

Spectral characteristics of an AER can, without any equipment or special skills, be estimated by close examination and calculation of waveform changes over time. Examine a typical ABR waveform recorded with a relatively wide filter setting (30 to 3000 Hz). The major waves components (I, II, III, V, VI) occur at intervals of about 1 ms. Thus, the ABR would be expected to have energy in the region of 1000

Hz (1000 waves per second or 1 wave/ms). These sharper waves that occur more often appear to be superimposed on a slower wave that just about completes one cycle (it has its beginning and end) within a 10 ms time period. An event that occurs once every 10 milliseconds has a frequency of 100 Hz (100 cycles per second). Spectral analysis of the ABR also shows dominant energy in this general frequency region. Similarly, spectral composition of other AERs can be estimated by visual inspection of waveforms and extrapolation of the number of wave components per second. The AMLR wave components are found at approximately 25 ms intervals. An event occurring every 25 ms repeats itself approximately 40 times in a second, or at a frequency of 40 Hz. Clearly, the ALR and P300 have even slower frequencies. As a general rule, then, the most appropriate and effective filtering for each of these AERs preserves the frequency region of the response and excludes other frequency regions. Using band-pass filter settings from 0.1 to 50 Hz would be totally inappropriate for ABR recording since most of the response would be eliminated, but these settings would be quite adequate for ALR measurements. Conversely, a 30 to 3000 Hz filter setting is appropriate for ABR since it encompasses important frequencies in the spectrum while eliminating EEG frequencies and possible higher frequency (above 3000 Hz) artifact. This same filter setting would be very inappropriate for ALR, since the spectrum of response is primarily outside of the band-pass region (below 30 Hz) and would be rejected before the averaging process.

EFFECT OF FILTERING ON AERS. | The objective of filtering, as noted above, is to reduce the amplitude of unwanted electrical noise without altering the response that is measured. In clinical practice, however, this is probably accomplished only rarely. Often, the problem is too much rather than too little filtering. The reason for this tendency may be that excessive filtering offers a false sense of security in AER measurement. Electrical noise is often effectively eliminated with very restricted filter settings. The result is a smooth waveform that is appealing to the eye and deceptively easy to analyze. There are two potential dangers of severe filtering. First, important portions of the response are eliminated, rendering even the most meticulous waveform analysis invalid. Second, distortion products in the waveform caused by the filtering process can be mistaken for response components, perhaps the components that were removed by the filtering. Examples of these two dangers will be shown for selected AER waveforms in discussions to follow.

The second danger of filtering, response distortion, has been the topic of much investigation (Boston & Ainslie, 1980; Dawson & Doddington, 1973; Doyle & Hyde, 1981b; Glaser & Ruchkin, 1976; Lane, Mendel, Kupperman, Vivion, Buchanan, & Goldstein, 1974; Scherg & Volk, 1983). Analog filters, as just noted, produce rather complex alterations of both amplitude and phase (latency) of AERs. As a rule, all filtering reduces response amplitude. When amplitude of a component appears to increase with more filtering, the contribution of filter ringing effects must be suspected. Filtering may, however, produce shorter latency responses (create phase lead) or prolong response latency (phase lag), depending on whether the filter is high pass or low pass, the slope of the filter, and the frequency composition of the response. There are two additional complicating factors. One is that an AER may consist of components with different spectral content (low frequency or slow components and high frequency or fast components) that are, therefore, differentially affected by the same filter. The other is that, although the distortion effects of a filter become prominent as the cutoff frequency approaches the AER frequency component, distortion of the response can be demonstrated even when the filter cutoffs are well beyond (lower or higher than) the spectral limits of the response. The end result of these two types of filter effects can be misinterpretation of AERs.

Given these limitations of conventional analog filter in AER measurement, are there other options? Weiner filtering has been proposed as one alternative (Carlton & Katz, 1980; Doyle, 1975; Walter, 1969). Weiner filtering is theoretically more precise than conventional analog filtering. It's based on previously obtained information as to which frequencies contribute to the response and which frequencies are nothing but noise. The Weiner filter emphasizes the frequency regions that contribute to the signal (the AER) and that contain less noise. Other frequencies (with weak signal and strong noise) are suppressed. In this way, theoretically, the average square error of the noise is reduced and less averaging is needed to improve signal-to-noise ratio, or SNR (Møller, 1983c). Two assumptions underlying Weiner filtering are that the spectrum of the signal and noise are defined and that signal and noise are constant during the analysis period. As noted above, these assumptions are not always valid for clinical AER recordings. Nonetheless, the overall objective of Weiner filtering is to suppress the effects of noise and thereby reduce the signal averaging that is necessary to produce a quality response. The clinical usefulness of *a posteriori* Weiner filtering is not yet documented.

Another approach is the clinical application of time varying and adaptive filters to better separate signal from noise, and then to reduce or eliminate the noise components (Wastell, 1977; Woody, 1967). Hoke, Wickesberg, and Lutkenhoner (1984) propose a filtering approach described as time- and intensity-dependent that generates no significant phase or amplitude distortion. The concept of this technique is in some respects related to time varying and *a posteriori* Weiner filtering just noted, but it is adapted to the computer demands of ABR measurement. Short-time Fourier (spectral) analysis of 128 overlapping segments of an ABR within a time analysis period (e.g., 15 ms) is computed. Uniquely, filtering is customized on the basis of the specific ABR spectrum at different times and at different intensities, rather than on a fixed overall estimate of spectral characteristics throughout the analysis period and across intensities.

Ultimately, the best overall approach for AER measurement may be the routine use of digital zero phase shift filtering, either online (prior to the averaging process) or offline (after a response has been averaged with virtually no analog filtering). Either way the AER must be converted to a digital form first, and analog filtering typically needs to precede digital filtering to avoid aliasing errors. Aliasing can occur when the sampling rate is too low with respect to the upper frequency limit of the AER or the cutoff frequency of the low-pass filter. One problem with this approach is that information in the waveform is lost. In addition, low-frequency components that are not part of the response but, rather, a product of aliasing may appear in the waveform. Reports and examples of digital filtering of AERs are noted in the discussion below. A very important clinical implication of filter effects on all AERs relates to the collection and use of normative data. There must be consistency within a laboratory in the filter settings employed in collection of normative data versus routine clinical AER measurements. Similarly, interpretation of clinical AER latency and amplitude findings in the context of published normative data is valid only if filter class (e.g., active or passive), type (Butterworth, Bessel, Chebyshev), settings, and slope are equivalent. Kalman filtering, application of a relatively new type of filter in auditory evoked response instrumentation, is described toward the end of the chapter.

ALTERNATIVE FILTERING TECHNOLOGY. | Conventional ABR filtering is usually performed after the first stage of amplification in the differential preamplifier. In this arrangement, the first stage of the preamplifier is designed to amplify a broad-spectrum signal. This is why this stage is open not only to AER signals, but also to very low-frequency physiological signals coming from the ocular activity (EOG), brain activity (EEG), and cardiac activity (ECG). Since EEG and EOG can be more that 100 times the magnitude of ABR, great care must be taken to ensure that the input stage of the recording amplifier does not become saturated, which would distort the recorded signal, and subsequent filtering would not remove the created distortion (Bell, Smith, Allen, & Lutman, 2004). Moreover, the operator may not even recognize such signal distortion, because the so-called "ongoing EEG" on the recording equipment may display no significant artifacts. While a low front-end gain has the advantage of avoiding saturation, this arrangement has a significant disadvantage in its reduced common mode rejection ratio (CMRR) and consequent increased susceptibility to noise (Spinelli, Pallàs-Areny, & Mayosky, 2003).

The conventional arrangement of filtering after amplification may also result in signal contamination due radio frequency (RF) noise coming from cellular phones, wireless networks, and other high-frequency equipment (deJager et al., 1996). Electronic amplifiers—AER differential amplifiers being no exception—will demodulate (rectify) such high-frequency broadband signals due to their nonlinearity, causing an effective frequency shift of the radio frequency (RF) noise into the frequency range of AER. Once this occurs, no amount of low-pass filtering at the amplifier's output can remove the error. Moreover, common mode rejection, which is the major purpose of differential AER amplifiers, is typically ineffective for frequencies above 20 kHz (Kitchin, Counts, & Gerstenhaber, 2003).

An alternative approach, employed in the Amplitrode™, available as part of the Integrity™ system from Vivosonic Inc., is to filter the input signal prior to its amplification. Currently, the Amplitrode™ applies a high-pass 30 Hz filter, optimized for ABR measurement, and a low-pass RF filter prior to amplification. This technique eliminates contamination due to RF rectification as well as unwanted low-frequency physiological signals such as electro-oculography (EOG), electrocardiology (ECG), and most EEG from the measurement prior to amplification, reducing the risk of saturation in the first stage of the amplifier, thus making it possible to optimize the amplifier's gain.

Averaging

The heart of conventional evoked response systems is the signal averaging device. Techniques for averaging neurophysiologic signals introduced by Dawson in England in the late 1940s and refined by Clark and associates at MIT in the 1950s, ultimately made AER measurement clinically possible. From the outset, it is important to keep in mind that AERs can be recorded using techniques other than signal averaging. However, most of this section will be devoted to a discussion of signal averaging since it remains the commonest approach for detecting AERs in the presence of a background electrical noise. A straightforward explanation of principle of averaging was summarized in Table 3.1.

ANALOG-TO-DIGITAL CONVERSION IN AER MEASUREMENT. | After the raw EEG (which may include an AER) is amplified and filtered, it is converted from continuous analog activity to digital form. Voltage of the waveform over the course of the analysis period is sampled (measured) at a certain number of points and expressed in a number. The number of points can usually be determined, within some constraints, by the tester. Rarely are fewer than 256 sample points used. With current AER instrumentation, 512 or even 1024 sample points are typically used. The intervals between sample points are the same throughout the waveform. The more sample points used, however, the shorter the time interval between any two points. For a given time analysis period, for example 10 ms, sampling 256 points would produce a time interval, or time resolution limit, of about 0.04 ms. The time interval between sample points would be one-half this amount (0.02 ms) for twice as many sample points (512). A practical question, then, is how often does the waveform need to be sampled? With too few sample points (a low sampling rate), valuable information might be lost, especially in

determining the precise latency and amplitude of peaks. One guideline for answering the question is the Nyquist theorem: The sampling rate (or frequency) must be at least twice the highest-frequency within the signal spectrum. Another convention is to sample at a rate at least 2.5 times the low-pass cutoff frequency (high-frequency limit of the band-pass filter in AER measurement). This is a simple calculation. If the filter is set at 30 to 3000 Hz, the sampling rate should be 3000 × 2.5 = 7500/sec. If there are 256 sample points in 10 ms, then there are 25,600 sample points in 1 second, a value that exceeds the calculated minimum sampling rate. One clinical implication here is for that longer latency AERs, which are composed of lower frequency energy and recorded with lower band-pass filter settings, the sampling rate is much slower. Information in the waveform will be preserved even with relatively large intervals among the samples.

The measured voltage of the AER waveform is theoretically the same at any instant in time in reality in any one of the time "bins" sampled during the analysis period. During a summing (adding) process, the voltage will get larger. During an averaging process, a response is summed and then periodically divided by the number of stimuli presented. During this process, response will remain at an equivalent voltage. Nonresponse activity, randomly occurring electrical potentials arising from the patient or elsewhere, will not be linked to the stimulus. Within the same time bin just described, therefore, the background noise will have a different voltage for each stimulus. For some sweeps (stimulus presentations), voltage in this time bin will be positive, for others negative. Summing these random positive plus negative values gradually reduces the background activity voltage toward zero. A simple example helps to clarify this concept. A constant waveform (e.g., for an AER) can be thought of as a sequence of voltages (numbers) that may differ across the time period of analysis, but are all the same for a specific time sampled. Averaging a constant number in a time bin, such as three, will always yield this number. If in this time bin, EEG voltages are different for each sweep (random or evenly distributed across many sweeps), the average will approximate zero, just as the average of positive and negative sign numbers (e.g., +3, −1, −3, +2, etc.) when averaged result in zero. EEG noise is best described as a variable distributed randomly around a mean of zero. Standard deviation of the noise is approximately one-half the maximum amplitude from peak to peak. The basic concept in understanding signal averaging is the signal-to-noise ratio (SNR). The overall objective in any AER assessment is to detect a signal (the AER) in activity and the other patient and nonpatient sources of activity. The neural signal (AER) is usually closely time locked to the stimulus. In general terms, that is, if a repetitive stimulus is presented to the patient (same type, intensity, polarity and so on), each component of the response will occur at exactly the same time interval (latency) after the stimulus, while the random noise in which the signal is embedded will systematically cancel out. The signal-averaging computer within an evoked response system is triggered or initiated at the instant each stimulus is presented. A timing pulse ("sync pulse") sent from the signal-generator to the signal averaging unit of the system assures synchronization of the averaging process with stimulus presentation.

IMPROVING THE SIGNAL-TO-NOISE RATIO (SNR). | There are four major points to remember in clinical AER measurement for optimally applying signal averaging. The first is the mathematical relationship that describes how the AER is enhanced and noise is reduced during averaging. The SNR changes with averaging according to the following equation:

$$\text{SNR} = \frac{S = \text{signal amplitude}}{NR = \text{noise amplitude}} \times \sqrt{N} \text{ averages}$$

where SNR = signal-to-noise ratio, and N = noise.

As this equation indicates, there are three ways that the SNR can be increased (improved). Amplitude of the signal (AER) can increase, amplitude of the noise can decrease, or averaging can be increased (a greater number of sweeps). Each of these possibilities will be discussed separately below, but in reality the three usually interact clinically, and an overall objective in optimizing the measurement of AERs is to positively influence all three. Because the increase in SNR is related to the square root of the amplitude of the noise, considerable increments in the number of stimulus presented (and the responses averaged) beyond 1,000 to 2,000 yield diminished returns. That is, improvement of the SNR is much greater over the initial 1,000 (from the start of averaging to 1,000) than for the third increment of 1,000 sweeps (from 2,000 to 3,000). This does not imply, however, that averaging in ABR recording should never continue beyond 1,000 or 2,000 sweeps. The decision to stop the averaging process should not be based on an arbitrary or conventional number of sweeps but, rather, on a clinical or a statistical estimate of the adequacy of the response. Relatively few sweeps (e.g., 200) are quite adequate to produce a well-formed and reliable response. On the other hand, under noisy conditions, particularly near threshold where the response amplitude is smaller, more than 4,000 sweeps may be needed to detect a response. In short, the clinical principle governing the necessary number of sweeps is not intransitive. Averaging can be stopped as soon as a response can be confidently identified above the noise level. If a response is not apparent after the customary number of sweeps are completed, then averaging should be continued until there is little doubt that no response is present. Latency values do not differ for responses averaged for various numbers of sweeps, although latency variability from one averaged waveform to the next is reduced for larger numbers of sweeps. If AER recording involves a summation process, amplitude will progressively increase with additional sweeps and there will, therefore, be substantial difference in amplitude for 250 versus 2,000 sweeps. The

averaged AER shows less actual amplitude variation for few versus many sweeps, because of the averaging process, but amplitude will increase as background noise decreases. Initially, it may appear that the response amplitude is decreasing with additional averaging. This is, in fact, because noise contribution in the amplitude of the response is progressively reduced. In summary, then, the SNR increases as a function of N sweeps, but it is heavily dependent the level of background noise and the strength of the response.

Another point is simply an appreciation of the amplitude (magnitude or size) of the signal (the AER of interest). For ABR measurement, the optimal signal amplitude (of wave V) is usually 0.5 µvolts, and the filtered background EEG amplitude is about 10 µvolts, so that 1,600 sweeps are required to achieve a SNR of 2:1. The ALR recorded from a waking patient, in comparison, is on the order of 10 µvolts, while background EEG, filtered considerably less because the response is in the same frequency region, is about 40 µvolts. Only around 64 sweeps are necessary to reach the same SNR level (2:1) since the signal is relatively larger relative to the noise. Less averaging is required to confidently identify larger amplitude AERs. The AMLR Pa component normally has approximately twice the amplitude of ABR wave V. As a result, the signal-to-noise ratio is usually greater, and less averaging is required to obtain a clear and easily identifiable response. A total of 1,000 stimulus presentations is typically adequate, and under ideal measurement conditions (i.e., high stimulus intensity level, quiet but awake normal hearing subject) 512 sweeps or less produces a suitable waveform (Goldstein, Rodman & Karlovich, 1972; McFarland, Vivion, Wolf, & Goldstein, 1975). With appropriate adjustments in filter setting (e.g., opening up the low-pass filter cutoff to at least 1500 Hz), stimulus rate (no faster than about 7.1/sec), electrode placements, and analysis time, and the number of sample points, it is possible to obtain ECochG, ABR, and AMLR information simultaneously from the same waveform (Özdamar & Kraus, 1983; Scherg, 1982a). Also amplitude is directly related to stimulus intensity and usually less averaging is needed to produce a response for high versus low stimulus intensity levels. Amplitude is related to other factors, such as age and gender. More averaging may be needed in infants to acheive a given level of confident response identification because amplitude tends to be smaller than in adults. Since females have larger amplitude responses (at least ABR wave V) than males, less averaging would, theoretically, be required to reach an adequate response.

Finally, amplitude of the noise is an important factor. Reducing the overall amplitude of background noise in AER recording is the most effective means of enhancing the SNR. Limiting noise increases the efficiency and accuracy of clinical AER recordings more than simply averaging additional sweeps. A clinician can often effectively reduce noise from varied sources. Residual noise in an AER recording can be estimated in different ways. A final point, which is recognized but perhaps not fully appreciated clinically, is the possibility that AERs may not always be closely time-locked to the stimulus and, conversely, that background noise may sometimes not be stationary, normally distributed, or random and may include frequencies (i.e., rate of repetition) that are quite close to the stimulus presentation rate. Maximum SNR improvement in signal averaging occurs when AERs are perfectly related to stimuli and when noise is totally random. This is rarely the case. Slight latency variations in AERs for successive stimuli are normally expected and even greater desynchronization of responses can be characteristic some CNS pathology. Latency "jitter" may even be related to the stimulus. For example, slightly shorter ABR latency for rarefaction versus condensation stimuli introduces increased variability in the responses to alternating stimuli. Inconsistencies in measurement parameters during averaging can likewise contribute to response latency variability. An example would be changes in stimulus intensity resulting from the dubious practice of hand holding earphones. Also, noise encountered in AER recording is not always random but, rather, may occur regularly at a certain frequency (a certain number of times per second). As a consequence, complex interactions among stimulus rate, electrical noise, and AERs are not uncommon clinically. Probably the most well-appreciated problem is due to 60 Hz power line interference. This is sometimes referred to as 60 Hz (or cycle) hum, because if this electrical energy is converted or transduced to acoustic energy, it has a humming sound. If stimulus presentation rate is an even submultiple of 60 Hz (e.g., 10/second or 20/second), that is, can be evenly divided into 60, it is likely that some of the stimuli will be presented in phase (at the same time) that the 60 Hz noise appears in the response. Electrical interference at 60 Hz or harmonics of 60 Hz may be detected with the electrodes or even at one of the unshielded junctions of electrodes or electrode cables between the patient and the amplifier. Since some of the even number of stimuli are periodically time-locked with the electrical interference, the response during averaging appears to undulate, at times being dominated by the interference and then soon after appearing more like the desired response. Additional signal averaging is needed to reduce (but not eliminate) the effects of a 60 Hz artifact. A partial solution to the problem of interference by 60 Hz electrical activity is the routine use of odd stimulus rates (e.g., 21.1/second or 27.3/second) that are not evenly divided into 60 or harmonics (multiples) of this frequency. A simple demonstration of the effect, or presence, of interference at 60 Hz is to average EEG (just as if an AER were being recorded) without a stimulus (e.g., unplug the earphone cable) but with the stimulus rate set at 60 Hz. If interference at 60 Hz is a factor in AER measurement at the test session, it will be readily apparent.

STATISTICAL BASES FOR DETERMINING ADEQUACY OF AVERAGING. | It has been recognized for many years that statistical criteria can be applied in determination of response presence or absence. The criteria are established beforehand and offer the advantage of consistency and efficiency in response analysis. That is, if there is, based on statistical evaluation of AER data, a likelihood of 99.8 percent that a response is present, regardless of the number of sweeps, averaging can be terminated. On the other hand, if after a predesignated upper limit for number of sweeps (e.g., 12,000) this statistical criterion is still not met, averaging stops, and it is concluded that there is no response. Now, selected evoked response systems have the capacity for periodically subjecting AER waveforms to statistical treatment during the averaging process, to automatically and precisely determine when a sufficient number of stimuli have been presented and averaging can stop. Instrumentation for recording the auditory steady-state response (ASSR) relies on automated detection of the auditory evoked response, as described in Chapter 8. However, it is still quite common with most AER measurements for the clinician to base the decision to stop averaging on visual analysis of the averaged AER in the context of background noise.

WEIGHTED AVERAGING. | Conventional AEP recording requires the patient to be very quiet, i.e., lying down, relaxed, asleep, or even sedated, because muscular activity produces significant artifacts (EMG) in the frequency range of 50 to 500 Hz, i.e., well within ABR and ASSR frequencies. Their amplitude may be in excess of 100 μV RMS. For comparison, ABR amplitude is in the range of 0.1 to 1 μV and ASSR in the range of 10 to 50 nV. One technique for reducing the effects of EMG artifacts on ABR recordings is weighted averaging. Using this technique, recording periods that contain more artifactual noise are weighted less in the overall average than periods of relative quiet.

In the Integrity™ system from Vivosonic Inc., the relative weighting of recording periods is optimized based a technique known as Minimum Mean-Square Error filtering, or Kalman filtering (Li, Sokolov, & Kunov, 2001; Maybeck, 1979; Sokolov, Zhang, & Long, 2005). The technique estimates the error in each measurement based on the measurement variance and continuously updates this estimate. Using this information, the Kalman filter produces an estimate of the AER signal—for example, ABR—in which the probability of error in the amplitude estimate at each latency point is minimized. By reducing the effects of intermittent EMG noise, the Kalman filtering technique allows ABR to be recorded accurately during substantial muscular activity of the patient—for example, while the patient is moving, eating, sucking a bottle, or talking—despite strong EMG artifacts that may be in excess of 100 μV RMS. Clinically, this means that any of the aforementioned patient muscular activity will not force the clinician to cancel, postpone, or prematurely terminate the scheduled test.

Sweeps or Number of Stimulus Repetitions

There is no standard or invariably "correct" number of sweeps (stimulus repetitions) in AER measurement. Any AER recording is fundamentally a problem of detecting a signal (the AER) in the presence of noise (EEG and measurement artifact). The overall goal is to achieve an adequate signal-to-noise ratio (SNR), where the auditory evoked response is the signal and any other activity detected by the electrodes is the noise. When there is a larger signal and/or less noise, fewer sweeps (stimulus repetitions) are necessary, and vice versa. For a given level of noise, then, more repetitions will be needed for the typically smaller, short latency responses than for the larger, longer latency responses. Increasing stimulus intensity is perhaps the most important technique for increasing the size of the signal clinically, while adequate relaxation is most effective in minimizing noise. Under ideal test conditions, such as measurement of large amplitude promontory-recorded ECochG AP component under general anesthesia, only a handful of repetitions, or even just a single stimulus presentation, is required. A clear, well-formed ABR, and perhaps more often longer latency AERs, appears with one or two hundred sweeps at a high intensity level. Continuing the signal averaging process beyond the point at which a clear response is observed wastes precious clinical time. On the other hand, under poor measurement conditions or to accurately define AER threshold, it may be wise to continue the averaging process well beyond 1,000 to 2,000 repetitions to permit confident identification of a response or to conclude that there is no response.

RECORDING AERS

Test Strategies

The first logical step in developing an AER test strategy is to determine why testing is planned. This point was raised in the discussion of preparation at the outset of the chapter. Often the reason for testing is obvious or well known to the clinician. For example, if a clinician's attempts to assess the hearing of infants and young children with behavioral audiometry are unsuccessful and if an ABR is scheduled, the main objective of testing is to estimate auditory sensitivity. And if an adult patient presents with unilateral sensorineural hearing impairment and, perhaps, other unilateral audiologic or otologic signs and symptoms, the reason for AERs is likely to be neurodiagnostic assessment for cochlear versus retrocochlear pathology. Likewise, the rationale for certain applications of AERs, such as newborn auditory screening with ABR, are well defined in advance. The exact reason for others may not be as clear-cut. Reasonable questions to ask before or during an AER assessment are listed in Table 3.4.

There are various ways of verifying the major reason for an impending AER assessment, many of them founded on common sense. Four simple approaches are to (1) review the patient's medical chart or records for tentative diagnoses or impressions; (2) ask the referring health care professional; (3) ask the patient, or the patient's guardian or caregiver, or, if the reason(s) for testing are still unclear; (4) develop a

TABLE 3.4.   Questions to Consider Prior to or During AER Measurement

- What is the main objective of testing (see discussion earlier)? For example, is it to rule out a hearing impairment that could interfere with speech and language acquisition, to rule out retrocochlear dysfunction, or to evaluate brainstem or cerebral auditory function?
- What AER information is essential, and what approach will be used for evaluating this information? For example, minimally, the objective may be a replicable ABR wave V at 30 dB to rule out serious deficit in auditory sensitivity or replicable ABR waves I, II, III, and V to describe eighth nerve and brainstem status.
- What information is optimal? If testing proceeds as planned, with a quiet patient and no equipment problems, how will test time be spent and when will testing be terminated? With pediatric ABR assessment, this might involve a full latency intensity function, use of tone-burst stimuli, and, after ABR recording, tympanometry and acoustic reflex measurements bilaterally.
- Will more than one AER (e.g., ECochG, ABR, AMLR, ALR, and/or P300) be assessed, and, if so, what sequence will be followed?
- For a given AER, which specific test sequence will be followed? For example, which ear will be stimulated first, will test ears be alternated, or will data for all stimulus conditions be gathered first for one ear and then for the other ear?

comprehensive and adaptive test strategy based on observation of the patient and the customary reasons for AERs given by the person who referred the patient. That is, in carrying out the evaluation the clinician covers all logical bases and alters strategy in an ongoing fashion as information becomes available. Whenever possible, the clinician should be prepared to answer the question, Why is this patient being tested? Failure to appreciate the reason for conducting an AER assessment at the outset is one of the most common mistakes made by beginning clinicians and a important cause for unsuccessful AER application.

AER measurement in a clinical setting, with varied types of patients and test conditions, is far more challenging, and often frustrating, than data collection from young adult normal-hearing subjects in a laboratory setting under optimal test conditions. It is simply impossible to anticipate or describe each of the myriad test factors that may occur in AER measurement, even though proper clinical decisions in response to these factors contribute importantly to consistently successful AER measurement. Nonetheless, the clinician, especially the beginner, would probably benefit from some guidelines and suggestions on AER test strategy. What follows here, then, is a summary of typical approaches to different types of AER assessments. The author fully acknowledges the limitations of such a "cookbook" format for AER measurement guidelines. The inexperienced clinician following these step-by-step instructions can, perhaps, be compared to someone inexperienced in cooking who is following a recipe for the first time. With each example, the result may be adequate, but only simple recipes should be attempted at first, and even then mistakes are likely to be made. Consistently good results in recording various types of AERs come only with experience and a healthy dose of creativity. Continuing with this analogy, beginning cooks would be smart to try out their newly developed skills with friendly, sympathetic family members and friends. Similarly, beginning clinicians are advised to first record AERs from understanding normal subjects, rather than diverse types of patients with unknown auditory and/or neurologic diagnoses.

Assessment of Peripheral Auditory Function

ESTIMATION OF AUDITORY SENSITIVITY. | For estimation of auditory sensitivity in infants and young children, the AER techniques of choice are ABR and/or ASSR. The overall objective for the ABR is to determine the minimal intensity level at which a wave V can be reliably observed for each ear. An example would be hearing sensitivity in the speech spectrum region with frequency specific tone burst signals in a very young or a difficult-to-test (e.g., mentally retarded) child. For children with peripheral hearing loss, especially hearing loss in the range from moderate to profound, the ASSR offers distinct clinical advantages. For threshold estimation in malingering patients, recording the ASSR, or the AMLR with tone burst stimuli (500, 1000, 2000, and 4000 Hz), may be more precise and less time consuming.

DESCRIPTION OF COCHLEAR FUNCTION. | ECochG is the AER technique of choice for describing cochlear status and functioning. The overall objective is confident identification of SP and AP components. An example of clinical application is diagnosis of Ménière's disease. ECochG measurement strategies and clinical applications are summarized in Chapters 4 and 5.

DIFFERENTIATION OF COCHLEAR VERSUS EIGHTH NERVE DYSFUNCTION. | The AER technique of choice is combined a ECochG and ABR strategy. Otoacoustic emissions (OAE), of course, are also an important component of the diagnostic test battery. The overall objective is the confident identification of the ECochG AP component (ABR wave I) and ABR waves II, III, and V, even for patients with serious and asymmetric hearing sensitivity deficit. Two examples of clinical applications are the diagnosis of auditory neuropathy and the early identification of eighth cranial nerve dysfunction, e.g., an acoustic tumor.

Assessment of Auditory CNS Function

ASSESSMENT OF BRAINSTEM FUNCTION. | The AER technique of choice for evaluation of brainstem integrity is the ABR. The overall objective is confident identification of wave I, wave II, wave III, and wave V. For patients with serious hearing sensitivity deficit, one can follow the recording guidelines outlined above for differentiation of cochlear versus eighth nerve dysfunction. An example of a clinical application is confirmation of multiple sclerosis or a brainstem tumor.

MEASUREMENT OF THALAMIC AND CEREBRAL FUNCTION. | The AER techniques of choice are AMLR, ALR, P300, and computed evoked response topography if available. The overall objective is confident identification of the AMLR wave Pa for hemispheric and midline electrode arrays (for monaural stimuli), waves N1 and P2 of ALR, and the P300 wave complexes (for binaural stimuli). An example of a clinical application is identification of auditory processing disorder in a child or trauma-related cortical dysfunction.

Components of Efficient AER Assessment

Next to accuracy, speed is the most important ingredient in consistently successful clinical AER assessment. At the very least, prompt collection of necessary data contributes to patient comfort and satisfaction and a more efficient and profitable clinical operation. More importantly, however, speed is often essential in order to collect necessary data. This is especially true in the OR or ICU setting where only timely information is of value. AER findings are reported continuously in the OR, and immediately after testing in the ICU. In essence, old news is no news when decisions on patient management are being made on a minute-to-minute basis. With some pediatric evaluations, recording AERs quickly is almost as important and equally challenging. Usually, children remain sedated or sleeping naturally only for a short period. Furthermore, once awake, they are not likely to fall asleep again. The wisest approach to AER evaluations in these cases is to always collect top priority data, understanding that the child could wake up at any moment. The surest way for a clinician to develop speed in testing is to practice technique extensively with normal subjects prior to gathering clinical experience, but organization and discipline are also necessary. The following specific factors can contribute to more efficient use of test time for the beginner and experienced tester alike.

PREPARATION. | By definition, preparation should be complete before the AER assessment begins. That is, before a patient enters the test room or, for hospital settings, before the clinician arrives at the patient's bedside. Any preparation for an AER assessment after this point is a waste of both patient and clinician time. Preparation is largely a matter of planning and common sense, as demonstrated by the checklist for routine AER assessment displayed in Table 3.5.

PLANNING AND THINKING AHEAD. | Planning, like preparation, is to a large extent a matter of common sense and

TABLE 3.5. Checklist for Steps in Preparation before Auditory Evoked Response Measurement

General	Pediatric
• Adequate supplies are in the test area, including computer disks, data record worksheets, pens and pencils, abrasive liquid, gauze pads, conducting paste and gel, tape, tubephone insert cushions, TIPtrodes. • Electrodes (including several extra electrodes), electrode box/strip, located near patient head in test area. Disposable electrodes are an option. • Transducers (earphones, bone vibrator) are near the patient's head in test area. • Patient area is clean and ready, clean linen is on the bed, a chair for the tester is in place. Residue from previous testing is removed. • Space is available in the test room for gurney or stretcher if indicated. • Sterile electrodes are available if necessary. • Pieces of tape (for securing electrodes) are in a handy location. • Evoked response equipment has been turned on with current date/time entered. • Printer is turned on and loaded with paper. • Initial test program is loaded, or AER measurement parameters are set. • Patient biographical data is entered into evoked response system. • Adequate disk space is assured. • Proper stimulus and stimulus intensity has been verified with a listening check. • Equipment is ready for electrode impedance check. • Audiogram, patient medical chart, and other pertinent information is near the evoked response system.	• Chair is available for parent, guardian, or caregiver. • Indirect, incandescent (not fluorescent), soft lighting is available. • Pediatric tubephone (foam insert) cushions or electrodes are available if needed. • Sedation order is obtained, if required, with the proper dose drawn and in the medication in an appropriate dispenser (e.g., syringe, cup), and the nurse or other appropriate medical personnel is at test site. • Moist face cloth, towel, or paper towel is handy in case patient rejects sedation or vomits. • A cup of water is handy as "chaser" after sedation, if indicated. • A stethoscope is handy for assessing vital signs. • Emergency ("crash") cart handy in case of serious sedation-related complication. • Patient chart is available for documenting sedation and vital signs. • Referring physician's name and phone number are available in case of questions or sedation-related problems. • Immittance and otoacoustic emissions instruments are nearby for measurement of tympanometry, acoustic reflexes, and OAEs as indicated.

concentration on the task at hand. The clinician should have in mind a plan for the ideal test sequence, but also consider contingency plans in the not unlikely event that problems develop. Following a game plan is relatively straightforward when business is as usual. Experienced and well-prepared clinicians, however, are able to quickly adapt new strategies when things do not go as planned. It is advisable to always have a plan for what information one wants to obtain from the optimal AER evaluation—that is, the best case scenario—and also minimal information that one needs to obtain—i.e., the worst case scenario. Realistically, with some patients, especially with young children, it may be impossible to even begin testing. This problem, which is usually related to inability to sedate or an inadequate amount of sedation, is explored further in Chapter 8. The list of dos and don'ts in Table 3.6 is by no means presented as the best or only correct approach for AER evaluation. Rather, it consists of suggestions or guidelines directed mostly to beginning clinicians. Test protocols and procedures for specific AERs are described in subsequent chapters.

DATA RECORD KEEPING AND ONLINE ANALYSIS. | To utilize time most effectively, and to assure that replicable high quality data are acquired, it is extremely important for the clinician to consistently keep records and perform online data analysis during AER assessment. The record keeping is a matter of documenting what has been done, what is being done, and, usually, what is planned. Naturally, in clinical AER assessments, particularly with children or other difficult-to-test patients, plans are subject to change with little or no warning. Many software-based evoked response systems automatically document numerous measurement parameters (e.g., stimulus ear, intensity, rate, polarity, filter settings, number of sweeps and artifacts rejected, electrode montage, and so forth). In the author's experience, however, manually recording essential information about ongoing AER measurement for quick reference is often invaluable in many cases. This functions as a hardcopy backup to the information stored in the computer. It is vital for meaningful data analysis after testing for details such as patient biographical data, test date, or other important information to be entered

TABLE 3.6. Some Dos and Don'ts of Clinical AER Measurement for the Beginner

Do:	Don't:
• Verify that you are very familiar with the operation of the evoked response equipment and the location of all necessary peripheral devices (e.g., earphones, bone oscillator, electrodes) and supplies (e.g., abrasive liquid, conducting paste, tape, printer paper, etc.).	• Erase AER data during collection, unless it is clearly substandard or pure artifact.
• Write down important patient biographical data (including medical record number, sedative, and vital body signs), if appropriate, and AER information, in addition to entering it into the evoked response computer.	• Never simply "eyeball" AER latency or amplitude data to determine the presence or normality of a response. Calculate absolute and interwave latencies (in ms) and amplitudes (in μvolt) before making decisions on further testing or completion of testing.
• Always replicate waveforms, unless a clear-cut criterion for a response is met with a single waveform or well-formed waveforms are apparent in a latency-intensity function.	• Never wake a sleeping infant before first reviewing and verifying with preliminary analysis that all the important AER data are collected and interpretable.
• Whenever possible, continuously collect (average) AER data during a test session with as little wasted time between the end of one averaging period and the beginning of the next. Plan each step of the test in advance, rather than between periods of averaging.	• Remove electrodes and earphones before assuring replicable waveforms and adequacy of data.
• Always store all data as soon as possible, even if you're not sure it's important at the time of collection.	• Waste time recording, plotting, or discussing AER data without simultaneously collecting new data (e.g., don't sit in "neutral"), unless absolutely necessary.
• Analyze important evoked response data, at least in a preliminary fashion, to assure validity and completeness before the patient is disconnected and released.	• Leave electrodes or earphones on patient after recording is completed and the quality and validity of AER data has been been verified.
• Keep the patient awake whenever possible for AMLR, ALR, and P300 recordings, yet encourage sleep for ECochG and ABR measurement.	• Discuss, interpret, or comment indiscreetly on patient findings in his or her presence during testing. Always remain in strict compliance with HIPAA policies regarding PHI (patient health information). Joking and laughing during testing is likewise inappropriate and unprofessional.
• Plot latency data on latency-amplitude function as it is collected in ABR measurement for estimation of auditory sensitivity and verification of wave V.	• Have food or drink anywhere on or near an evoked response system.
• Remove electrodes and earphones (or stimulating electrodes for ENOG) as soon as AER measurement is definitely completed (the validity of data has been verified).	• Leave a patient unattended for extended periods in test area; never leave an infant or small child alone.
• Get in the habit of analyzing AER results during (NOT after) recording whenever possible.	• Turn power for the evoked response system off or on with electrodes on the patient and connected to the system. Always first unplug electrodes from the preamplifier box or strip, or disconnect the electrode cable from the evoked response device.
• Whenever possible, print waveforms during (NOT after) testing.	• Attempt to use AER system, or new or updated AER software, for the first time with a patient. Practice with the device first.
• Prepare report immediately after testing, NOT later in the day or on another day, whenever possible.	• Use nonsterile needle electrodes with a patient.
• Periodically monitor vital signs of sedated children.	
• Immediately troubleshoot equipment, especially inter-electrode impedance and earphone placement if the auditory evoked response deteriorates or disappears.	

into the computer. A few notes on events that occur during the assessment can also be extremely useful to the tester or others during offline (after testing) data analysis. Much of the tester's time during a typical AER assessment is spent in viewing data collection (the averaged response development). Of course, this time should be used for analysis of previously collected AER data and to plan the next logical step in the AER assessment. As the test proceeds, insights and ideas regarding the patient often come to mind during

this time and, if they are not written down, they may be forgotten. There is no substitute for diligent record keeping in auditory evoked response measurement.

After the Test

After the last AER has been recorded, and a brief review of collected data confirms that no further testing is required, an adult patient can be informed that the testing is completed and thanked for his or her cooperation. The first order of business is to gently remove the earphones and electrodes, taking care that the patient's hair remains intact. Excess electrode paste can be removed in a number of ways. Alcohol swabs are effective, but in conscious patients may cause a slight stinging or burning sensation and leave the skin very dry. A moist paper towel is adequate, although considerable scrubbing may be required. Clinical experience with infants, older children, and also adults has shown that prepackaged moist cloths (actually designed for use after a child's diaper is changed) are effective in wiping away excess electrode paste, without drying or irritating the skin. These can be conveniently purchased in many grocery or drug stores (baby supplies section). Finally, adult outpatients appreciate access to a mirror and even a sink in order to freshen up before returning to the waiting room or leaving the test area.

Rarely is it necessary to provide to the patient a detailed verbal description or interpretation of the findings. In fact, it is quite appropriate in most cases to simply state that the recordings are stored in the computer and will be analyzed carefully later in the day. Following the analysis of results, a written report will be prepared and sent to the physician or the referral source. The patient is entitled to a copy of the report, upon request. Report writing is discussed below.

This same general approach is appropriate for the parent of a child undergoing AER assessment, with several exceptions. A sedated and sleeping child must be aroused and examined before dismissal (see the discussion on sedation earlier in this chapter and in the next chapter). Also, if there is no question that the AER findings are normal, parents appreciate receiving the news immediately, rather than waiting anxiously for the official report to arrive in the mail. Counseling the parents of a newly identified hearing-impaired child is an extremely important clinical duty. If this counseling is the tester's responsibility in a clinical facility, it must be done with care, compassion, and understanding. There are certain fundamental guidelines to follow. Guidelines on proper counseling techniques are beyond the scope of this discussion.

ELECTRODE CLEANING. | If disposable electrodes are not used, the best time to clean reusable electrodes is immediately after the recording session is finished, the electrode paste is removed from the patient, and the patient has been counseled and dismissed. Disposable electrodes, of course, eliminate this task. Warm water, disinfectant soap, and a toothbrush (or another soft brush) are usually adequate for cleaning disc electrodes, including ear clip types. Electrodes are then dried immediately with a paper towel and placed near the equipment in their customary storage place. Also, immediately following an AER assessment or just before an assessment begins, it's good practice to clean earphones, probe assemblies, electrode cables, and other components of the evoked response system that will come into contact with the patient. Commercially available germicidal disposable

cloths (e.g., SaniCloth Plus®) work very well for this purpose. Representatives from the infectious disease prevention office in a medical center will have good recommendations on disinfecting practices that are effective and pose no risk to the patient. There are many ways of storing electrodes, but it is preferable to allow them to dangle freely from a rack, hook, or other hanger on or near the evoked response system. This facilitates thorough drying after cleaning and reduces the chance of tangled cables. Delaying the cleaning task may lead to later inconveniences and wasted time, as well as shorten longevity of the electrodes due to oxidation. Conducting gel and paste is far easier to remove from electrodes when it is still moist. Within 10 to 15 minutes after testing, the paste will dry and harden, making it difficult to remove. Gel does not harden within hours after testing. If the brief time necessary to clean the electrodes is not available immediately after the test, they can be soaked in a container of water (cup, emesis basin, or bowl) and cleaned later. This practice is not advised, however, because a subsequent AER assessment might be delayed while the electrodes are first located and then cleaned.

Manufacturers may recommend using disposable electrodes for all AER measurements. However, when reusable electrodes are used, they must be disinfected after every use. A mild disinfecting detergent can be used in addition to warm water during cleaning, or the electrodes may be soaked in a hospital-approved liquid disinfectant. Long-term soaking, however, will almost certainly limit the life of the electrode. Electrodes, but not their cables, can be placed in boiling water. Disinfecting electrodes and all parts of evoked response equipment making contact with the patient or the tester's hands after patient contact (e.g., earphones, electrode cables) is particularly important following AER assessment of a patient in isolation (for infection). Obviously, disposable electrodes and insert ear cushions (plugs) eliminate these concerns. Potentially reusable probe tips often coupled to adapters and used in pediatric applications of AERs, such as hearing screening or pediatric diagnostic measurement with ABR, are adequately cleaned by soaking overnight in a hospital-approved disinfectant liquid (e.g., Cidex). Sterilization of electrodes is not necessary after routine AER assessment, but it is good clinical practice after contact with a patient in isolation and essential before electrode use in an operating room in which there will be a surgical field. Sterilization of subdermal needle electrodes is always necessary before their repeated use with a patient. Manufacturers recommend sterilization with gas (Eto). Wet or dry autoclave sterilization is also acceptable, but temperatures must not exceed 140 degrees centigrade (284 degrees Fahrenheit). The routine disposal of needle electrodes after a single use is another viable clinical option.

OFFLINE WAVEFORM AND DATA ANALYSIS. | ECochG analysis is described in Chapter 4, whereas ABR waveform analysis is discussed in detail in Chapter 7. Absolute latency and amplitude are routinely determined for waves I, III, and V, and sometimes waves II and IV as well. Then, relative latency values, interwave latencies (e.g., between waves I and III, waves III and V, and waves I and V), and relative amplitude measures (e.g., the wave V/wave I amplitude ratio) may be calculated either manually (by moving a cursor onto each of the two waves or subtracting the latency of the first wave from the second wave) or automatically by the evoked response system.

For most evoked response systems, time zero in the analysis period is the default onset of the stimulus. Positioning the cursor on the precise moment of stimulus onset (indicated by deviation of data points from baseline at the first portion of the stimulus artifact) should produce a 0 ms latency display. When one cursor is used to mark waves, the latency displayed is actually the time interval between stimulus onset and the wave. A prestimulus baseline period is very useful in ABR measurement, with data points occurring before the stimulus indicated as negative latency values (e.g., −1.5 ms). A prestimulus baseline period that is 10 percent of the total analysis time is suggested. Latency calculations are straightforward when each wave is clearly recorded with a distinct peak. A suitable test protocol can greatly enhance the likelihood of recording a well-formed and reliable ABR waveform. Realistically, however, ABR waveforms have peaks that are not always clear-cut. There may be multiple small peaks superimposed on a larger wave component, or there may be a prominent "shoulder," particularly in the wave IV–V complex, following the peak. There will probably never be a "standard" interlaboratory approach for latency interpretation. However, within a laboratory or facility, there must be consistency in criteria used by those analyzing and interpreting AER waveforms. Details on analysis for each type of AER (e.g., ECochG, ABR, AMLR, ALR, and P300) are discussed in subsequent chapters.

REPORTING RESULTS. | Patient reports are a vital component of the evoked response assessment. Thorough, even flawless, clinical evoked response measurement is perhaps satisfying to the clinician, but of purely academic value unless the results are communicated clearly, accurately, and promptly to the appropriate persons. AER findings usually contribute to patient management. Clinical decisions based, in part, on AERs vary substantially. ECochG outcome may contribute to diagnosis of Ménière's disease and may lead to a specific medical or surgical course of therapy. Early identification of serious hearing impairment in an infant with ABR may prompt aggressive audiologic management and thereby have a profound impact on the child's communication and life in general. Early identification of retrocochlear pathology in an adult with ABR may prompt aggressive neuro-otologic surgical management and contribute to preservation of hearing or, perhaps, preservation of the function of the facial cranial nerve. The application of AERs in neuromonitoring of patients in the OR or ICU may impact on audiologic or

neurological outcome, and even survival. The common and essential link throughout each of these examples of AER applications is an accurate, complete, and understandable report of results. The extent of and demand for reports varies considerably from one facility or clinical setting to the next. One must always keep in mind requirements of third-party payers, as well as professional colleagues, in developing a policy for AER reports.

With current software-based evoked response systems, it is usually possible and rather simple to document in a written printout the biographical data and measurement parameters, as recommended by the American EEG Society Committee. The Committee also offers guidelines for a written and signed report interpreting evoked response findings. Components of the report are (1) the object of the testing; (2) a brief summary of clinical history; (3) the type of evoked response(s) recorded; (4) relevant medications the patient was taking either therapeutically or specifically for the test; (5) a description of waveforms, including wave latency and amplitude data; and (6) the clinical importance of evoked response abnormalities ("alterations") whenever possible. The Committee states that copies of recorded waveforms could either be included with the written report, or supplied upon request.

LETTER FORMAT. | Although the report for each patient should describe his or her unique findings, there are certainly some relatively consistent features of all reports. Furthermore, when AER results are unequivocally normal, a "form letter" report approach is appropriate. A form letter approach is not advised if the results are in any way atypical or abnormal. This is not to say that standard features of the report cannot be stored on a computer for retrieval as the framework upon which the rest of the report is built.

OFFLINE WAVEFORM MANIPULATIONS

Optimally, the quality of AER waveforms is improved by altering test parameters or conditions before or during data collection. With this adaptive approach, the clinician first notices that AER waveform quality is less than optimal and responds by altering the customary test protocol in an attempt to improve quality. If this is not possible, or the result is inadequate, waveform quality can sometimes be improved after data collection is complete. Any processing of AER data after it has been collected, and stored on disk, is referred to as *offline* versus *online* processing. Three offline processing or manipulation techniques for AER waveforms often employed with commercially available instrumentation are digitally adding and subtracting, smoothing, and filtering of AER waveforms.

Adding, Subtracting, and Inverting Waveforms

With many clinical evoked response systems, one waveform can be either digitally added or subtracted from another waveform. These same systems usually feature an option for inverting polarity of a waveform, i.e., turning it upside down. Instructions for such functions that are specific to a piece of equipment are described in the manual supplied by the manufacturer. In effect, the voltage recorded (and stored) at each data point (e.g., 256, 512, 1,024 total data points) in one waveform is either added or subtracted from the corresponding data point in the other waveform. Therefore, two waveforms that are almost identical will appear unchanged when added. Subtracting one from the other produces what appears to be a flat line because the voltage recorded at each data point is essentially subtracted from itself. Actually, multiple waveforms (more than 2), and waveforms from different patients, can be added or subtracted. Adding a series of waveforms from different patients or from the same patient results in a "grand average" for the group. Similarly, reversing polarity of a waveform is accomplished by changing the sign of the voltage at all data points. For example, if the voltage at exactly 5 ms is +0.37 μvolt, with inversion of polarity it becomes –0.37 μvolt. When this process is applied to all data points, the waveform becomes totally inverted. AER peaks that are customarily plotted upward flip downward and vice versa. A clinical application of the inverting feature is cited below in a discussion of mistakes involving electrode placement or usage.

WAVEFORM ADDITION. | When two waveforms recorded with different stimulus polarities (one waveform with rarefaction and one with condensation stimuli) are added, stimulus artifact is reduced or eliminated. This is because the artifact occurs in opposite directions (upward versus downward going) in each of the waveforms. The result of adding voltages at each data point that are opposite in sign (negative in one and positive in the other) is to approximate zero voltage. The same principle holds for any artifact that is of opposite polarity in the two waveforms.

Multiple replicated AER waveforms for certain stimulus and acquisition conditions (e.g., all recorded with click stimuli presented to the same ear, at the same intensity level) when added create a waveform that is actually the result of the combined number of sweeps (stimulus repetitions). That is, if four waveforms averaged from 1,000 stimuli, all are added together, the resulting waveform is based on a total of 4,000 sweeps. Digital addition of waveforms can thus be a powerful technique for enhancing the signal-to-noise ratio. Clinically, it's generally a better use of time, and statistically preferable, to first record two or even more waveforms for a given set of measurement parameters with a relatively modest number of sweeps, assess repeatability, and then add the waveforms together for latency and amplitude calculation, rather than recording a single waveform for the total number of sweeps. Artifact is less likely to contaminate the final outcome. Another advantage of first replicating waveforms and then adding them together is that atypical waveforms (those with an unusually great amount of noise) can be de-

leted from the grand average (not included in the adding process). With continued averaging over a large number of sweeps, these noisy AER data would of course be included and would serve to contaminate the waveform. Deletion of noisy runs is a simplified version of the highly sophisticated mathematical signal-to-noise enhancement and AER analysis techniques.

WAVEFORM SUBTRACTION. | ABR waveforms recorded simultaneously with an ipsilateral (i) and a contralateral (c) electrode array (Fz-Ai and Fz-Ac) can be used to derive a horizontal electrode array. Briefly, vector theory predicts, and clinical study confirms, that subtraction of the contralateral (Fz-Ac) recording from the ipsilateral (Fz-Ai) recording yields a horizontal (Ac-Ai) waveform. The validity of this technique is easily proved by then subtracting derived horizontal waveform from a waveform actually recorded, simultaneously, with an ear-to-ear electrode array. The result is a flat line, indicating that the two horizontal waveforms (actual and digitally derived) were equivalent. One obvious implication of digital subtraction, therefore, is the availability of AER data for three channels from only two channel recordings. The clinical advantages of a horizontal electrode array include enhanced identification of waves I and wave III. An ABR recorded with an horizontal electrode array is also less susceptible to electrical artifact.

By subtracting a no-stimulus waveform (just background activity) from an AER waveform to an adequate stimulus, it is theoretically possible to produce a waveform lacking much of the nonstimulus, or ongoing, EEG noise that typically characterizes AERs. Spectral analysis of the waveform resulting from the subtraction process confirms a reduction of low-frequency background brain activity. Although appealing, this approach is not routinely applied clinically. One problem is that the two waveforms (no-stimulus versus stimulus) are not stimultaneously recorded and, therefore, arise from somewhat different EEG environments.

SMOOTHING. | Smoothing is a digital process that, as the term implies, removes small irregularities in waveforms and produces a smoother waveform. High-frequency noise (electrical or muscular in origin) causes many tiny spikes that are often superimposed on the major components in an AER waveform. With three-point smoothing, a common method, voltage at an actual data point in the waveform is replaced by the average of voltages for this data point plus the two adjacent data points (one earlier and one later). Actually, smoothing is a moving average that may include more than three nearby data points. Minor AER waveform "wrinkles" are thus "ironed out." A single waveform can be repeatedly smoothed without producing serious latency distortions. When excessive high-frequency artifact interferes with wave component identification, multiple smoothing may be useful. With repeated smoothing, however, amplitude of small wave components may be reduced because in the smoothing process, actual peaks are treated the same as high-frequency noise peaks. Also, although smoothing improves the appearance of waveforms and ease of latency and amplitude analysis, rarely do wave components become apparent after smoothing that could not be detected beforehand.

FILTERING. | Filtering is an important factor in AER measurement. Offline digital filtering (after data collection) may be useful in enhancing waveform quality, particularly when electrical activity above or below the frequency range of the response is present in the waveform. Large amplitude, slow wave activity (lower frequency activity), evident with a filter setting of 30 to 3000 Hz, may be minimized with digital filtering at 150 to 3000 Hz, which essentially removes this low-frequency component and facilitates identification of an apparent wave V in the waveform. As a rule, however, such filtering should be done as a last resort in AER recording. Filtering may produce undesirable effects on ABR waveforms if the low-frequency energy contributes critical information for the identification of components. Filtering can, therefore, serve to enhance waveforms but it can also deteriorate waveform quality.

AER MEASUREMENT PROBLEMS AND SOLUTIONS

Some factors that may cause problems in AER measurement or interpretation are easily identified, even before the assessment begins. The effect on these factors (e.g., age, gender, body temperature, hearing loss) on AER latency, amplitude, or morphology can then be estimated, and perhaps corrected, before response interpretation. Other measurement problems, such as electrical or muscular artifact, produce characteristic deviations in waveform appearance. There are a finite number of such problems, as reviewed (along with solutions) in subsequent chapters for ECochG (4), ABR (7), AMLR (11), ALR (12), P300 (13), and electroneuronography (15). The specific problem must first be analyzed and identified. Then, once recognized, the source of the problem is sought out and, hopefully, the problem is corrected or eliminated. At the very least, deleterious effects on AER waveform are minimized. In some cases, however, these types of problems cannot be minimized, and they preclude valid AER measurement. A final group of measurement problems may have multiple causes. Some are due to operator errors, others mechanical failure, and still others result from a certain characteristic of the subject. Examples of these latter problems are absence of response components (waves), poor waveform morphology, or even elimination of the entire response.

Troubleshooting is the term used to describe the process of identifying measurement problems, determining their cause, and, whenever possible, finding an adequate and feasible solution. Troubleshooting requires a rational, logical approach to problem solving and is a skill that improves

with experience. As a rule, the first time a certain problem is encountered, the clinician may take some time to find a solution or may not be able to solve the problem independently. Troubleshooting in these instances may involve a trial-and-error solution method, or even telephone calls to other more experienced clinicians. The next time this same type of problem interferes with AER measurement, however, the clinician is able to apply prior experiences and to find a timely solution.

Subject Characteristics

The many effects of subject characteristics on ECochG and ABR are reviewed in detail in Chapters 4 and 7. The effect of one or more subject characteristics must be considered whenever the quality of AER recordings is suboptimal, or at least poorer than expected. By keeping in mind a few general principles of subject characteristic effects, the clinician can often promptly determine whether a specific characteristic should be suspected or can be safely ruled out as a cause of poor AER outcome. These generalizations are as follows:

- Age: Young age (in children) affects all AERs except ECochG, whereas advancing (beyond 50 years) primarily affects P300.
- Gender: Male versus female differences are important mostly for ABR.
- Body temperature: Hypo- and hyperthermia (low and high body temperature) exerts the greatest effect on short latency AERs.
- State of arousal: The effect of subject state is greatest on longer latency AERs.
- Muscular artifact: Movement artifact can interfere with any AER recording, but it is prominent with measurement of the AMLR.
- Hearing sensitivity: Hearing loss may influence any AER, but high-frequency hearing deficits especially affect ECochG and ABR recordings.
- Drugs: Drugs that influence the CNS (e.g., sedatives, anesthetic agents) exert the greatest effect on longer latency, cortically generated AERs and have virtually no influence on ECochG and ABR.

Electrical Interference

Since AER measurement involves detection of minute (several μvolts or less) electrical events within the ear, auditory nerve and brain with electrodes typically located on the surface of the scalp, it is not really surprising that electrical interference can be a major problem. Surface electrodes are just as likely to detect extraneous electrical activity outside of the head as stimulus-related activity within the head. In fact, the unwanted extraneous electrical activity may be far more prominent. Fortunately, when each electrode in a pair detects similar electrical artifact, that is, artifact that is of similar amplitude and phase), then it will largely be cancelled out (rejected) by the differential amplifier. A problem arises, however, if such electrical artifact is detected mostly by just one of the electrodes in the pair.

Another factor contributing to electrical interference in AER recording is the amount of amplification required in processing the responses. Before the electrophysiologic activity of less than a millionth of a volt can be processed and analyzed with an evoked response system, it must be amplified up to 100,000 times. Amplification not only increases the problem with extraneous electrical activity detected by the electrodes, but it also introduces electrical noise to the auditory evoked response waveform from the amplifier circuit. Of course, circuitry for various brands of evoked response systems differs in the amount of noise produced during amplification. Finally, transducers that produce acoustic stimuli necessary to evoke an AER are electromagnetic devices that can, in fact, be a source of electrical artifact. Again, the amount of electrical interference varies among transducer types.

STIMULUS ARTIFACT. | Among electrical interference problems, stimulus artifact is probably the easiest to isolate and solve. This discussion is limited to electrical artifact produced by acoustic stimulus transducers. Artifact problems associated with electrical stimulation used in electrically evoked responses and electroneuronography (ENoG) and are reviewed in Chapter 15. Acoustic transducers (various types of earphones) produce electromagnetic fields. That is, they generate electrical activity. Very often, the acoustic transducer generating the stimulus for an AER is located close to an electrode recording the AER, and stimulus-related artifact would seem to be unavoidable. These undesirable interactions between electrical activity from earphones and recording electrodes can be reduced or eliminated with some common sense precautions.

Early investigators of AERs recommended electromagnetic shielding of earphones with a layer or two of special metals (Coats, 1984; Elberling & Salomon, 1973). The shielding is designed to contain the electromagnetic energy and insulate adjacent electrodes from its effects. Shielding of earphones is expensive, may produce unwanted changes in the acoustic properties of the transducer, and is not really a practical alternative for most clinicians. Shielding also is not an alternative with bone-conduction transducers (oscillators or vibrators).

The best general technique for reducing stimulus artifact is to put as much distance as possible between the transducer (earphone) and cables and the recording electrodes. The tubing for insert electrodes permits this distancing, and the time delay from the transducer (box in the figure) and earplug creates a delay between the stimulus and early components of the ABR (e.g., the AP or wave I component). For any kind of transducer, wires leading to the earphone that carry an electrical signal and aren't completely insulated should be remote from electrode leads. These two types of wires should

not make contact or be draped over one another at any point along their course. One simple method of avoiding such contact is to extend electrode leads in one direction (e.g., up toward the top of the head) and the earphone transducers (for inserts) and cables in another direction (e.g., downward toward the chest), or vice versa. Since electrode leads may function somewhat as antennae in picking up unwanted electrical activity (from the air), shorter leads are desirable. Ideally, there would be no distance between the electrode and the amplifier. The typical electrode lead, which is 1 meter (about 3 feet), may be adequate in most settings but specially constructed shorter leads (2 feet or less) are helpful in reducing artifact in especially noisy test environments. Braiding (intertwining) electrode leads also tends to reduce the likelihood of electrical interference. Tracking a specific electrode from one end to the other, for a color-deficient tester, is particularly difficulty when a group of electrodes are braided.

With a conventional supra-aural audiometric earphone (TDH-39 or TDH-49), the earphone is often resting on a mastoid or earlobe electrode. At high intensity levels, stimulus artifact may create a serious problem because stimulus-related waves extend into the time frame of the ABR. There is an additional problem with evoked response instrumentation if an automatic display gain option is selected. The size of waveform displayed on the screen is adjusted on the basis of the largest peaks so that a fixed portion of the screen (e.g., one-third) is filled. If the stimulus artifact is large, the remainder of the waveform (the actual response) may be scaled down excessively, sometimes appearing as a flat line. Some evoked response systems offer a blocking feature in which the display in the time period of the stimulus (around 0 ms) can be eliminated. Display scaling is therefore determined by the actual response waveform, rather than by stimulus artifact. This technique does not, however, actually solve the artifact problem and may actually contribute to other problems with measurement or analysis. The most effective means of reducing stimulus artifact with supra-aural earphones is to rely on alternating polarity stimuli. The artifact produced by each of the two polarities is opposite in direction and when averaged (summed) is mostly cancelled out (the positive plus negative voltages when added approach zero voltage). The obvious limitation of routine use of alternating polarity stimuli is that a single polarity (rarefaction) is preferable in most patients. One way around this dilemma is to first record replicated responses with each polarity (rarefaction and condensation) and then, if excessive stimulus artifact is present, to digitally add waveforms for the two polarities.

Optimally, alternating polarity stimuli are presented, but waveforms are separately averaged in one channel for rarefaction clicks and another channel for condensation clicks. Some evoked response systems have this capacity. The process can also be implemented by adapting the P300 program for some evoked response systems. That is, instead of frequent versus rare tone burst stimuli with a rare stimulus probability of 20 percent (as in P300 measurement), the condensation and rarefaction clicks are presented with a 50 percent probability. The process of adding and subtracting waveforms was described above. The effect is a set of waveforms essentially produced by alternating stimuli. Stimulus artifact should be minimal. This approach, of course, is not necessarily time effective nor ideal clinically since averaging a response to both polarities doubles test time and might not have been required, and the adding process must be done offline, precluding ongoing analysis of data.

Perhaps the most effective method for reducing stimulus artifact is use of insert earphones (e.g., Etymōtic Research ER-3A). Electrical activity is generated from the cable leading from the plug to the box and by the box that houses the transducer. Then, an acoustic signal travels down the plastic tube to the insert cushion. The objective, then, is to keep the earphone cable and box as far away from electrode leads as possible. The plastic tube is not a source of electrical activity and will not produce stimulus artifact, even it is resting on an electrode lead. Insert earphones contribute to reduced stimulus artifact in two ways. The transducer (box) can be positioned away from electrode leads. The more the transducer is separated from the electrode, the less likely the artifact. Also, the plastic tube produces a time delay between stimulus and response. As manufactured by Etymōtic, the length of tubing produces a delay of 0.8 or 0.9 ms. Even if stimulus artifact is present, the delay virtually eliminates any interference with identification of early AER components (e.g., ECochG SP or AP components, or ABR wave V). Other advantages of the tubephones (e.g., comfort, less ringing, prevention of collapsing ear canals), and some associated precautions (e.g., accounting for the time delay in absolute latency calculations, lack of an interaural attenuation advantage) were reviewed earlier.

ELECTRICAL NOISE AND ARTIFACT. | Electrical power in the United States is supplied with a frequency of 60 Hz. The power line frequency in Europe is 50 Hz. Any electrical outlet or electrical device may produce electrical noise with a frequency of either 60 Hz or of harmonics of this frequency (e.g., 120 Hz), or much higher frequencies that are not multiples of 60 Hz. Examples of the numerous sources of 60 Hz electrical noise (also referred to as line noise) in a clinical setting include electrical wiring in a test area, fluorescent lights, X-ray viewing boxes, power transformers, copy machines, conveyer belts, escalators, elevators, whirlpools in physical therapy, electrical machinery, patient video monitors, blood pressure transducers, computers, heating blankets and incubators, EKG (electrocardiogram) equipment, and operating room microscopes. Even the evoked response system itself, especially the monitor, can produce excessive electrical artifact in AER measurements if positioned close to the recording electrodes. From this partial list of electrical interference suspects, it is clear that some test settings are inevitably quieter electrically than others. The ideal test environment is a relatively isolated area (none of the devices listed are on a floor above or below, nor in any nearby room), with new preferably dedicated wiring (no other equipment or devices are on the same lines) in which AER recording is done with the patient in a radio-frequency (RF) shielded room. At the other extreme of the electrical noise continuum is the typical newborn or surgical ICU or operating room (OR) that is filled with the above-noted electrical devices (many of them life supporting), has electrical wiring that supplies a variety of machines and functions, and is adjacent to other trouble spots, such as an X-ray department. Electrical interference may be extremely unpredictable, as well as elusive. That is, at one test session there may be so much interference that AER recording is impossible, yet at some other time in the same setting there is electrically silence. Electrical interference may be highly unpredictable. That is, during the course of a 6-minute test session, significant electrical interference may appear and then disappear. Serious electrical artifact may appear in one electrode channel but not in another simultaneously recorded channel and then, inexplicably, the artifact problem may appear in the opposite channel. Although this is an extremely frustrating feature of electrical interference, it does suggest that one possible solution is simply to "wait out the storm."

A rather consistent observation regarding electrical interference and electrode arrays deserves mention at this point. In very noisy environments, considerably less electrical interference is typically found for a horizontal (ear-to-ear) recording array for the ABR than for electrode arrays consisting of one electrode on the forehead or vertex. Typically, waveforms recorded with a forehead noninverting electrode are characterized by excessive high-frequency artifact, although the actual frequency of the artifact is different in each case. Yet the Ac-Ai electrode array often is remarkably clean. As noted above, if the same electrical interference were present at each of the electrodes in these four pairs, it would be minimized by differential amplification (cancelled by subtracting the inverting from the noninverting input). The figures, however, suggest that the electrical interference is different as detected by the forehead (or vertex) electrode versus ear electrodes. With differential amplification, the artifact is therefore not rejected at the amplifier and persists in the Fz-to-ear array. The artifact is apparently common to the two ear electrodes and is largely rejected at the amplifiers. A practical implication of these patterns is that electrical interference in conventional electrode arrays (ipsilateral or contralateral) that precludes meaningful waveform interpretation might be minimized by digital subtraction of the contralateral waveform from the ipsilateral waveform (as described above). This, in effect, subtracts the activity (including interference) at the forehead (or vertex) site from itself, leaving the ear-to-ear electrode array.

There are two fundamental approaches to dealing with 60 Hz, or any other, electrical artifact. The first, and most effective, is to determine and eliminate the source. The other approach, which is often really a last resort, is to attempt to minimize the effect of the artifact on AER measurement. The following is a general discussion of this topic. Problems encountered more frequently in specific test environments, such as the newborn ICU, OR, or surgical ICU are noted in Chapters 6 and 10. Møller (1987) provides a detailed and highly informative discussion on localizing sources of electrical interference and reducing their effects on evoked response recordings. Although his focus is electrical interference in the operating room, the troubleshooting principles he describes are equally valuable for any test setting. According to Møller (1987), unwanted electrical noise interferes with evoked response equipment and recordings via four pathways: (1) Unshielded electrodes and electrode leads act as antennae in picking up airborne activity from nearby sources, (2) activity may be transmitted to the patient from other electrode leads (not used in evoked response measurement) connected to other electronic devices (e.g., EKG or heart monitors) and then on to the evoked response equipment, (3) evoked response electrodes pass through magnetic fields and conduct magnetic energy on to the evoked response equipment, and (4) power line electrical activity enters the evoked response system amplifiers and appears in waveforms.

Various sources of electrical interference and some techniques for reducing the effects on evoked responses are detailed for ECochG and ABR in Chapters 5 and 7, respectively. Detection of specific sources of unwanted electrical activity in a test area is not always possible, but should be attempted, particularly if the problems are consistently encountered and evoked responses are routinely recorded in the setting. The overall objective in this situation is a systematic and, hopefully, permanent remedy for the electrical interference problems rather than spending time during each test session attempting to circumvent the interference. Møller (1987) provided instructions for constructing simple antenna-type devices for detecting sources of electrical and also magnetic interference. A length of wire (for electrical interference) or a wire loop (for magnetic interference) can be plugged into one input of the differential amplifier (the positive or negative electrode input) for the evoked response system. The other input is grounded. The amplifier output is sent to an oscilloscope or loudspeaker, rather than to the evoked response system. The clinician then places the antennae near suspected sources of electrical interference and notes the presence of electrical activity on the oscilloscope or via the loudspeaker. With this "ghost-busting" technique, it is often possible to pinpoint sources of electrical interference and, sometimes, to determine frequency characteristics of the interference. Knowledge of the electrical activity waveform for different electrical devices might be useful in solving future artifact problems.

The alternative to eliminating the source (s) of electrical interference is to manipulate the test protocol so as to minimize the effect on AER recordings. Manipulation of electrode configuration was noted above. Electrical interference is more likely if the interstimulus interval (the stimulus rate) is even divided into 60 (60 Hz). An odd stimulus rate (e.g., 21.1/sec) reduces the likelihood of an interaction. Electrical interference at 60 Hz may interact with some stimulus rates to produce undulations (waxing and waning) in the appearance of electrical artifact in the waveform. Adjusting the stimulus rate slightly often minimizes the contamination of the waveform by this electrical interference. The extent of electrical artifact may fluctuate also with the number of sweeps. It is sometimes possible to manually stop averaging at a point of relatively waveform clarity. Altering filter settings is usually a futile technique for reducing excessive electrical interference. The use of a notch filter at 60 Hz is rarely helpful because harmonics (higher multiples of 60 Hz) are still passed into the averaging process. As noted above, the frequency of unwanted electrical interference may fall well within the frequency region of the AER being recorded. Furthermore, notch filtering produces undesirable filter ringing and response latency distortion. In short, notch filtering is to be avoided. With electrical interference at 400 Hz, for example, it is impossible to filter out the artifact without eliminating important spectral content of the ABR, ranging from below 100 Hz to over 1000 Hz. Other possible methods of reducing the effects of electrical interference artifact on AER recordings involve manipulation of the test environment rather that test protocol. Simple and routine precautions, such as either braiding a set of electrode leads (wires) or tying the electrode wires into several loose knots, will often minimize or even eliminate some types of electrical interference from averaged auditory evoked response waveforms.

As reviewed earlier in this chapter, conventional AER measurements are made with patient-mounted passive electrodes that are connected to lead wires. The leads are, in turn, electrically coupled to the inverting and noninverting inputs and the ground of a differential preamplifier. The length of each lead wire is typically in excess of 1 m. Electric and magnetic fields from surrounding electrical wiring, and various equipment in the measurement environment, contaminate the AER measurement by inducing electrical currents and generating voltages in the lead wires. The amount of contamination from the electric field increases with the length of the leads, while the amount of contamination from magnetic fields is proportional to the area of the three loops formed by the inverting, noninverting, and ground leads (Ferree, Luu, Russell, & Tucker, 2001). Another significant extraneous source of noise is motion artifact—i.e., the noise induced in lead wires as a result of their movement through a magnetic field (Bell, Smith, Allen, & Lutman, 2004).

An alternative arrangement that reduces the effects of electric and magnetic fields on AER measurements is the Amplitrode™ (Figure 3.16), available as part of Integrity™ system from Vivosonic Inc. The Amplitrode™ integrates an AER preamplifier and clip that snaps directly onto the ground electrode, thus eliminating the ground lead wire completely. Furthermore, since the preamplifier is mounted directly on the patient's head, the inverting and noninverting

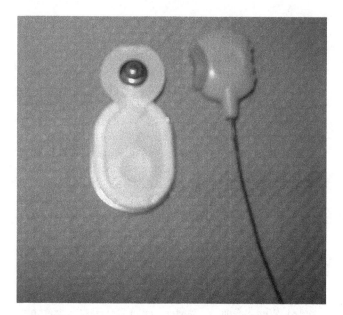

FIGURE 3.16. The Amplitrode™ combination electrode and amplifier.
Courtesy of Vivosonic.

signal lead length and corresponding loop areas are minimized, while the leads themselves are electrically shielded (Kurtz & Sokolov, 2005; Metting Van Rijn, Kuiper, Dankers, & Grimbergen, 1996).

ELECTRICAL SAFETY. | Concern for patient safety and comfort should always be foremost in the minds of clinicians carrying out evoked response measurements. Electrical safety is an important consideration in recording AERs, as well as electrically stimulated evoked responses. Isolation transformers contribute to patient safety. As emphasized throughout the book, an evoked response system should never be turned on or off with the patient connected to the device with electrodes. Electrodes should be removed from the electrode box or preamplifier before power is changed to the system.

Measurement Problems and Solutions

Some measurement problems are common to all AERs, and troubleshooting procedures tend to be fairly consistent among AERs. That is, many of the items in a troubleshooting checklist are the same for all AERs. For any of the AERs,

selected problems solutions are identical, because basic equipment malfunction or misuse inevitably produces the same constellation of symptoms. At the same time, other problems that appear to be quite similar often differ in the extent with which they affect AERs. For example, profound hearing impairment can account for absence of any AER. Certain anesthetic agents, on the other hand, can account for absence of the AMLR or ALR, but not the ECochG or ABR. Also, stimulus artifact within the first millisecond or two after the stimulus can interfere with ECochG and ABR analysis, but is of no concern with later latency responses. A detailed discussion for specific AERs is offered in subsequent chapters. The symptom-oriented format was chosen because it most closely resembles clinical reality. Because of the common effect of some problems on AERs, there is a certain degree of redundancy in the problems and solutions listed in the series of tables. The beginner is advised to purposefully make as many of these mistakes as possible, in a controlled setting, before venturing into clinical AER measurement. The least threatening way to follow through on this recommendation is for the clinician, with plenty of time and behind closed doors, to prepare him- or herself, or a good friend, for each type of AER. The first objective is to obtain a high-quality normal response. Then, by systematically altering the measurement parameters or purposefully committing technical errors, such as leaving an electrode unplugged, using an inappropriate filter setting, and so forth, the clinician can view firsthand many of the symptoms that are listed in the tables. A "mistake-making session" can also be valuable laboratory assignment in workshop or a graduate level course on AERs.

CONCLUDING COMMENTS

The objective of the foregoing review was to introduce the reader to principles important in recording auditory evoked responses in general. Principles, protocols, and procedures of specific auditory evoked responses are discussed in more detail in subsequent chapters. However, the clinician who understands principles that are common to all AERs will readily learn the techniques and strategies that are essential for recording each specific type of AER and, in all likelihood, auditory evoked responses that are discovered and applied clinically in the future.

4

Electrocochleography
Protocols and Procedures

For more than sixty years, ECochG has been investigated clinically with frequency-specific stimulation (Fromm, Nylen, & Zotterman, 1935; Perlman & Case, 1941). Major developments in ECochG were reviewed from a historical perspective in Chapter 1. Numerous studies have also been conducted in animal models (e.g., Ruben, Elberling, & Salomon, 1976), and technical aspects of stimulus generation for ECochG are explained in detail elsewhere (Eggermont, Odenthal, Schmidt, & Spoor, 1974; Ruben et al., 1976). Different techniques for eliciting frequency-specific AERs (e.g., shaped tone bursts, derived responses) are described later in this chapter, in reference to ABR. Each of the major ECochG components (CM, SP, and AP) is differentially affected by stimulus frequency. The CM waveform closely resembles the waveform of a pure-tone stimulus of a single polarity and, therefore, is altered distinctly and predictably by frequency. The CM can, as demonstrated in classic studies by Wever and Bray (e.g., 1930) in an animal model, be recorded from anywhere within the cochlea or on the surface of the cochlea. With clinical application of ECochG, it is very important to keep in mind the long-recognized principle that CM, as typically recorded in the time domain with an electrode located outside of the cochlea (e.g., promontory or external ear canal), arises only from the basal turn of the cochlea, primarily from outer hair cells, regardless of the tone frequency (Dallos, 1973; Hoke, 1976; Sohmer, Kinarti, &

Gafni, 1980). There is some clinical evidence that analysis of frequency and phase components of the CM might permit detection and localization of more apical site of hair cell activity in normal and pathologic ears (Euler & Kiessling, 1983). Because the CM follows polarity of a click stimulus, summing or averaging the response to stimuli of alternating polarity (rarefaction and condensation) will generally cancel out the CM (Yoshie, 1971). This process is specifically employed clinically to eliminate interference of CM in recording the SP and AP.

The SP is a direct current (DC) shift receptor potential reflecting cochlear electrical activity in response to acoustic stimulation (Tasaki et al., 1954). The SP follows the envelope of the stimulus. The SP is, therefore, clearly influenced by stimulus duration (as noted in a following section) but not markedly influenced by stimulus frequency. While the ECochG AP component is most often generated by click stimuli clinically, it is possible to obtain highly frequency-specific information. There are numerous reviews and original research papers on this topic (Eggermont et al., 1974; Ruben et al., 1976; Teas, Eldridge, & Davis, 1962; Terkildsen, Osterhammel, & Huis in't Veld, 1975). Perhaps the most effective and relatively simple frequency-specific ECochG technique is to stimulate the response (e.g., AP) with tone-burst stimuli of different frequencies and to record the response with a promontory electrode (Aran, 1971; Eggermont, 1974; Eggermont et al., 1974; Naunton & Zerlin, 1976; Odenthal & Eggermont, 1974; Yoshie, 1971). The only major stimulus-related constraint is, of course, that the onset of the signal must be abrupt, with a rise time of less than about 5 msec.

ELECTRODE TYPE AND LOCATION

Electrode location is the single most important ECochG measurement factor. The electrode site influences or interacts with other acquisition parameters (e.g., amplification, signal averaging), as well as stimulus parameters (e.g., intensity, rate, and polarity). For this reason, the discussion

---

Abbreviations used in this chapter:
ABR = auditory brainstem response
AP = action potential
CM = cochlear microphonic
DC = direct current
ECochG = electrocochleography; electrocochleogram
SP = summating potential
TM = tympanic membrane
TT = transtympanic

of electrode type and location in ECochG will precede the review of other test parameters. Virtually all of the initial clinical studies of ECochG were conducted with a noninverting electrode, often a silver ball, placed on the promontory (on the medial wall of the middle ear space) or on the round window, typically in patients with perforated tympanic membranes or following surgical exposure of the middle ear (Lempert, Wever, & Lawrence, 1947; Perlman & Case, 1941; Ruben, Bordley, & Lieberman, 1961; Ruben, Sekula, & Bordley, 1960). Round window ECochG techniques still were applied clinically, especially for estimation of hearing sensitivity in children with severe-to-profound hearing loss in the assessment of cochlear implant candidacy (Aso & Gibson, 1994). Subsequent investigators, in the late 1960s, having the benefit of signal averaging of responses, demonstrated the clinical feasibility of nonsurgical transtympanic needle insertion for electrode placement (Aran & LeBert, 1968; Sohmer & Feinmesser, 1967; Yoshie, Ohashi, & Suzuki, 1967). Since the promontory electrode site is very near the ECochG generators (the cochlea and eighth nerve), the ECochG recorded with this electrode array is a near-field response, and the SP and AP components are typically large and easy to detect, even at low intensity levels and with minimal averaging. Amplitude is, for example, on the order of ten times larger than recordings made from the TM, twenty times larger than ear canal (e.g., TIPtrode) recordings, and as much as fifty times larger than mastoid recordings. The result is accurate, ear-specific and, potentially, frequency-specific electrophysiologic assessment of auditory thresholds without the need for masking. The clinical limitation of the technique, however, is clear. Reliance on a TT electrode renders ECochG an invasive procedure that cannot be carried out independently by most nonsurgeon clinicians. There is some evidence that the round window ECochG technique produces responses that differ from and are superior to those recorded with a TT needle promontory placement (Aso & Gibson, 1994). However, in a study of ECochG in the diagnosis of Ménière's disease, Krueger and Wagner (1997) found no significant differences in the SP/AP ratio between these two recording techniques.

The invasiveness and technical difficulty of the conventional TT electrode ECochG technique was, in fact, a major reason why, in the mid-1970s, clinicians quickly turned to ABR as the electrophysiologic measure of choice for assessment of peripheral auditory status. The growth in ABR clinical popularity took place despite the publication of series of papers by an international collection of investigators in the late 1960s and early 1970s describing the first generation of ear-canal electrodes for ECochG recording (Coats & Dickey, 1970; Cullen, Elis, Berlin, & Lousteau, 1972; Elberling & Saloman, 1971; Khecheniashvili & Kevanishvili, 1974; Yoshie, Ohashi, & Suzuki, 1967). Some of these electrode techniques, unfortunately, still involved placement of a needle in the ear canal wall or TM and were potentially as painful and invasive as the TT approach. Electrode-related factors

now are responsible in part for a renewed clinical interest in ECochG measurement. As early as 1974, Coats described recording an ECochG with a specially designed, commercially available ear-canal electrode. This electrode type is sometimes referred to as an "eartrode." Designed and first described in ECochG recording by Coats (1974), it consists of a butterfly arrangement of soft plastic wings with a silver ball (0.5 mm diameter) at the end of one and a thin wire leading to a 2 mm pin connector. The two wings are squeezed together with a pair of tweezers, and then the electrode is inserted into the ear canal. The wings expand when released, and the silver ball makes contact with the ear canal wall. This electrode type is available in three sizes (adult, small adult, pediatric). Other authors later described a similar electrode design (e.g., Schoonhoven, Fabius, & Grote, 1995). The electrode design has several clinical disadvantages that have probably limited clinical application. First, because of the limited electrode area making contact with the skin (just the silver ball), impedance is characteristically high, even under ideal conditions. Use of the ear-canal electrode, therefore, in combination with relative low impedance disc electrodes can result in marked impedance imbalance and increased noise in recordings. Second, the recommended test protocol calls for irrigation of the external ear canal with alcohol in preparing the skin for improved electrical impedance. This process is time consuming and may be uncomfortable for the patient. Third, insertion of the electrode to the ideal depth within the ear canal (near the tympanic membrane) requires manual skill and minor instrumentation (forceps). Laceration of the external ear canal wall can occur. Finally, some patients experience discomfort with the electrode resting against the ear canal wall during testing and also with removal of the electrode after testing.

A variety of other ear-canal electrode designs have been reported over the years. Humphries, Ashcroft, and Douek (1977) described ECochG recording with a silver ball electrode, also located near the TM. Montandon, Megill, Kahn, Peake, and Kiang (1975) carried out ECochG recordings as an office procedure with a silver foil disc placed in the external ear canal. Durrant, Burns, and Ronis (1977) and Walter and Blegvad (1981) recorded the ECochG AP (ABR wave I) with an electrode type consisting of silver chloride wire wrapped in cotton, soaked in a saline solution (saltwater is a good electrical conductor), and covered with electrode paste. This electrode is also mounted on a V-shaped plastic device that is squeezed together between the thumb and forefinger, inserted into the ear canal to within 5 mm of the annulus of the tympanic membrane and then allowed to expand. Electrode contact with the ear-canal wall is adequate. The electrode can reportedly be consistently inserted without the use of instruments, and there is little or no discomfort to the unanesthetized patient.

Harder and Arlinger (1981) also recorded relatively larger ECochG AP component amplitude with a specially constructed ear-canal electrode in comparison to the

ECochG recorded with electrode placement. The electrode shown in this paper appears as an elongated stirrup, with the head of the stirrup directed into the ear canal as close as possible to the annulus of the TM. An electrode cable soldered to the foot of the electrode leads to the amplifier. The body of this device is acrylic, but the surface is very pure silver (99.9%, according to the authors). As with the other ear canal electrodes just described, the skin on the canal wall must first be prepared, preferably with the use of an otomicroscope. Following ear-canal preparation, electrode impedance ranges from 1000 to 8000 ohms. Lang, Happonen, and Salmivalli (1981) also described a specially designed ear-canal electrode: A steel wire is attached to a metal electrode frame (almost rectangular-shaped). The tip of the wire is a spherical silver electrode, coated with conductive gel. This flexible insulated wire cable leads away from the electrode. When the frame is placed against the tragus of the ear and the skin in the sideburn area anterior to the ear, the electrode at the tip of the wire extends about 2 mm into the ear canal and presses against the lower posterior wall. According to the authors, a technician can easily place the electrode, and average impedance is 20,000 ohms (ranging from 7 to 43,000 ohms). For a variety of practical reasons (e.g., difficulty in placement and discomfort), this electrode style is not longer commonly used for ECochG measurement.

In the 1980s and into the 1990s, other ear-canal electrode designs were introduced and became commercially available (e.g., Nishida, Komatsuzaki, & Noguchi, 1998; Nowosielski, Redhead, & Kattula, 1991). The common objective of these electrode types is to facilitate analysis of the SP and AP components. When recorded with ear canal electrodes, wave I can be confidently identified, even though it remains undetectable with other surface-inverting electrode sites, such as the mastoid or earlobe (e.g., Musiek & Baran, 1990). This introduction of commercially available ear-canal electrodes has contributed to a marked increase in clinical investigation of ECochG in assessment of auditory threshold levels and diagnosis of varied otologic pathologies, especially Ménière's disease (Ferraro, Murphy, & Ruth, 1986; Yanz & Dodd, 1985).

TIPtrode

The TIPtrode is shown in Figure 4.1. For placement of the TIPtrode, the author applies a small amount of abrasive liquid (e.g., NuPrep®) onto a clean cotton swab. With direct lighting, the outer ear is pulled upward and backward. TIPtrode preparation was illustrated in Figure 3.12. This maneuver tends to straighten and enlarge the outer portion of the ear canal meatus. Then, the walls of this outer portion of the ear canal are prepared by scrubbing in a circular motion with the cotton swab. Care is taken to keep the cotton within sight. Aural immittance measurement and/or otoscopic inspection of the ear canal is strongly advised prior to preparation of the

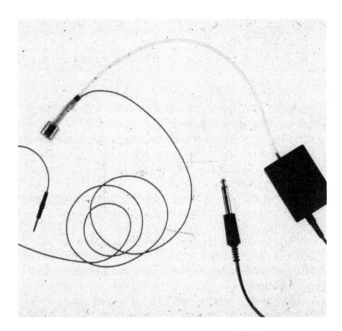

FIGURE 4.1. Photograph of TIPtrode, a combination insert transducer and external-ear-canal electrode.

ear-canal walls or insertion of ear-canal electrodes. Conducting gel or paste is not necessary with TIPtrodes.

In the author's experience, the technique just described will routinely produce interelectrode impedance values well below the acceptable limit (<5000 ohms). It is likely that residual abrasive liquid on the ear-canal walls is a factor. Application of gel or paste to ear-canal electrodes may, in fact, contribute to electrode slippage during testing. In the interest of aural hygiene, ear-canal electrodes, such as the TIPtrode, should only be used one time. Furthermore, the conducting property of the metal foil appears to dissipate with use, particularly in combination with abrasive liquids. Interelectrode impedance for the TIPtrode is generally unacceptably high upon second application. Steps in the application of the TIPtrode are summarized in Table 4.1.

TYMPANIC MEMBRANE ELECTRODES. | Cullen et al. (1972) successfully recorded ECochG with a twisted wisp of cotton soaked in saline, attached to the end of an electrode wire, and placed on the lateral surface of the TM. Clinical evaluation of electrodes that are inserted into the ear canal or placed on the lateral surface of the tympanic membrane have since been described by numerous other investigators (e.g., Arsenault & Benitez, 1991; Campbell, Faloon, & Rybak, 1993; Durrant, 1990; Ferraro, Blackwell, Mediavilla, & Thedinger, 1994; Ferraro & Ferguson, 1989; Haapaniemi et al., 2000; Laureano, McGrady, & Campbell, 1995; Matsuura et al., 1996; Ruth & Lambert, 1989; Stypulkowski & Staller, 1987). The motivation for development of the tympanic membrane (TM) electrode technique, along with other extra-tympanic electrode designs, is the well-appreciated indirect relationship

TABLE 4.1. Summary of the Steps Taken in the Placement of the TIPtrode

Details are provided in the text. The TIPtrode is shown in Figure 4.1.

- Use an adult-size TIPtrode for most adult patients; use pediatric-size TIPtrode for women with smaller external ear canals and for children.
- Attach a TIPtrode insert cushion (foam plug covered with gold foil) onto the TIPtrode tubing.
- Secure an alligator clip onto the gold foil on the stalk of the insert earphone cushion.
- Verify that the insert tubing color (red or blue) matches the proper transducer (for right or left ear).
- Apply the noninverting electrode at either the Fz (high midline forehead) location or on the opposite earlobe, and the common (ground) electrode on the Fpz (midline low forehead) location. The noninverting electrode can be a TIPtrode.
- Plug all electrode wire pins into the proper inputs on an electrode strip or pre-amplifier head-box (right or left inverting electrode).
- Apply abrasive gel (e.g., Nu-Prep) onto a clean cotton swab.
- Explain to the patient that you will be gently cleaning the outer portion of the ear canal.
- While pulling the pinna upward, backward, and slightly outward, and with a circular movement, gently but firmly ream out the outer portion of the external ear canal, observing the patient for possible discomfort.
- Compress tightly the TIPtrode plug.
- Insert the TIPtrode plug into the ear canal deeply, if possible until the lateral portion reaches the tragus.
- Verify that the patient is comfortable.
- Repeat the same process for the other ear.
- Check interelectrode impedance; verify impedance is < 5000 ohms.
- Begin ECochG recording.

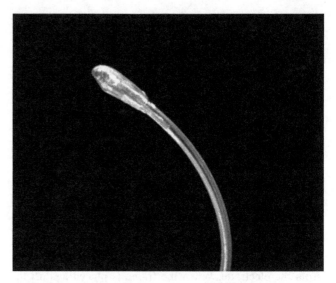

FIGURE 4.2. Photograph of tympanic membrane electrode (the gel-covered silver wire at the end of the electrode that makes contact with the tympanic membrane).

between amplitude of the AP component and distance of the recording electrode from the cochlea and eighth nerve. In the words of Stypulkowski and Staller (1987, pp. 304, 305), this electrode was designed to "maximize response amplitudes while minimizing clinical preparation, cleansing and insertion requirements." The electrode consists of a small gauge silver wire enclosed within a flexible silastic tube and connected to a soft foam sponge at the tip. The sponge is filled with conductive gel. A solid gel remaining within the sponge may be used to eliminate residue on the eardrum after testing (Ferraro & Ferguson, 1989). Another design, similar to the Cullen et al. (1972) electrode, substitutes a cotton wisp for the sponge and saline for the gel. The tube is fed down the ear canal until the electrode at the tip actually makes contact with the TM. Earphones can be placed over the bent outer portion of the flexible tube. A TM electrode type (approved for use with patients by the U.S. Food and Drug Administration, or FDA) is commercially available from Bio-Logic Systems (Figure 4.2).

As with the ear-canal electrode type, it is important to first inspect the ear canal prior to insertion of TM electrodes. Prior to placement of the electrode, cerumen and other debris within the ear canal should be removed by a trained health care professional. After preparing the tip of the electrode with saline or conducting gel, the electrode wire and the sheath (silastic tubing) surrounding it are slowly and carefully inserted into the ear canal. The patient is instructed to report sensations during the process, including any discomfort or pain. At the least, the ear canal should be under direct lighting. Electrode insertion with the aid of a microscope is certainly appropriate. The electrode is inserted until the patient reports a pressure sensation and/or slight resistance is met. Interelectrode impedance is then measured. Confirming electrode placement on the TM under microscope is recommended. The TM electrode lead is secured, with either tape or a foam plug. Steps in application of the TM electrode are summarized in Table 4.2.

TRANSTYMPANIC (TT) MEMBRANE ELECTRODE. | There is abundant clinical evidence that a TT placement of a needle on the promontory yields optimal ECochG recordings. The TT ECochG technique was among the first described (see the historical overview in Chapter 1), and it continues to be the strategy of choice in clinical practice for high-quality recordings of the CM, SP, and AP. Dozens of authors enthusiastically recommend the TT electrode technique, citing multiple clinical advantages. First and foremost, the amplitude of ECochG components recorded with the TT electrode technique is on the order of 15 to 25 μV, and typically from ten times to over forty times larger than for ECochG recordings with ear-canal electrode placements (e.g., Schwaber & Hall, 1990; Wuyts, van de Heyning, van Spaendonck,

TABLE 4.2. Summary of Steps in ECochG Measurement with a Tympanic Membrane (TM) Electrode Technique

The tympanic membrane electrode design is illustrated in Figure 4.2.

- Follow general test protocol for preparation, patient instruction, and test parameters.
- Closely inspect the ear canal for debris and any evidence of pathology.
- Apply all electrodes (discs) except the tympanic membrane electrode and plug these other electrode pins into the appropriate electrode box receptacles.
- Instruct the patient on the proposed procedure, and ask him or her to report whatever sensation he or she feels (e.g., tickle, discomfort, coughing reflex, pain, pressure).
- Ask the patient to report when he or she senses that the electrode is resting on the TM.
- Have the patient turn onto his or her side with the test ear upward (employ the force of gravity as you insert the electrode).
- Apply conducting gel to the TM end of the electrode, if recommended by the manufacturer.
- Begin inserting a clean TM electrode gradually into the ear canal.
- Continue to insert the TM electrode as you question the patient on his/her sensations and as you note any changes in the "feel" of the electrode.
- Once you and/or the patient sense that the electrode is resting on the TM, secure the electrode lead temporarily with a finger.
- Grasp a compressed foam insert plug, or TIPtrodeTM, perhaps with bayonet forceps, and insert into the ear

canal. Pediatric-sized foam inserts fit best with women and other persons with small ear canals.
- Allow the foam insert earplug to expand against the electrode lead.
- Tap the electrode lead very gently and ask the patient to report any sensation. He or she should hear a sound associated with the tapping if the electrode is resting on the TM.
- Plug the acoustic tubing from the ER-3A transducer into the stalk tube of the insert earplug (or TIPtrode).
- Plug the tympanic membrane electrode pin into the appropriate electrode box receptacle.
- Immediately verify electrode impedance for all electrodes.
- Don't be alarmed if the impedance for the TM electrode is excessively high (>20 K ohms).
- Begin presenting stimulation to tympanic membrane electrode ear.
- Inspect waveform for AP component in the 1.5 to 2.0 ms region.
- AP amplitude should exceed 1.0 µV, even in mild-to-moderate hearing loss.
- If a reliable AP component is not observed, withdraw the TM electrode and reinsert as described above.
- If no AP is observed on the second attempt, remove TM electrode and inspect closely for any evidence of damage. Replace if condition is in doubt.
- Proceed with ECochG measurement and analysis.

& Molenberghs, 1997). In comparison to other techniques, published clinical experience with the TT electrode approach also confirms enhanced reliability, confidence in waveform analysis, and, for the diagnosis of Ménière's disease, optimal test performance (sensitivity and specificity). The diagnostic value of the TT electrode approach will become apparent as the literature on clinical applications of ECochG is reviewed in the next chapter.

A needle electrode, designed for electromyography (EMG), can be used to record ECochG with the TT approach. Earlier papers on the TT ECochG technique describe the use of rather long (>50 mm) needle electrodes that extend from the promontory past the pinna, and sometimes secured partly by placement through the tragus of the external ear (e.g., Aran & LeBert, 1968; Sohmer & Feinmesser, 1967; Yoshie, Ohashi, & Suzuki, 1967). Other authors describe the use of a "doughnut shaped headset" (e.g., Wuyts et al., 1997) with cross-lines for stabilization of the needle within the ear canal. However, a shorter subdermal needle offers some clear clinical advantages for ease of insertion and simplicity in stabilization (Schwaber & Hall, 1990). Relatively short subdermal needles offer a simpler option for TT ECochG

(Schwaber & Hall, 1990). Teflon-coated needles are available in different lengths (20 to 60 mm), each having 0.8 mm of the tip exposed, i.e., the tip is not coated with Teflon (Figure 4.3). The cable and connector pin design is the same as those for other electrode types. The subdermal needle electrode is also suitable for promontory ECochG recording and, in fact, is more convenient than longer needle electrode designs used in early reports of ECochG clinical application. The specific technique for placement varies depending on the type of needle that is used. The following description is summarized in Table 4.3. It applies to the TT placement of a subdermal needle electrode, rather than a longer needle electrode. The use of a steel electrode that is coated with Teflon for insulation, except for the tip, is usually recommended (Wuyts et al., 1997). The insulation reportedly isolates detection of electrical activity to the promontory region and eliminates the possibility of extraneous signals detected from other anatomic sites, e.g., the tympanic membrane. In the author's experience, however, an uninsulated steel subdermal electrode yields high-quality ECochG recordings, with no apparent electrical contamination (Hall, 1992; Schwaber & Hall, 1990).

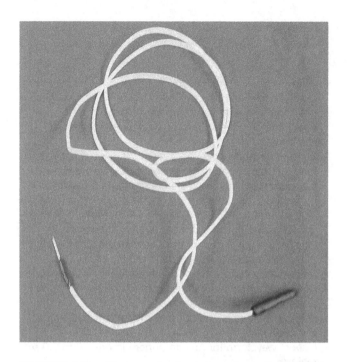

FIGURE 4.3. Photograph of subdermal needle electrode for transtympanic placement (a 14-inch noninsulated shaft is on the left and the conventional electrode pin is on the right).

The needle is inserted by skilled (e.g., otologic) personnel through the eardrum (posterior and inferior quadrant) and placed on the promontory, typically with either local or general anesthetic (Bath, Beynon, Moffatt, & Baguley, 1998; Roland, Yellin, Meyerhoff, & Frank, 1995; Schwaber & Hall, 1990; Wuyts et al., 1997). There are published reports of TT membrane electrode placement without local anesthesia (Beynon, Clarke, & Baguley, 1995), although patients describe discomfort associated with the technique. Local anesthesia of the tympanic membrane probably does not affect sensation of pain at the promontory, the actual electrode site. However, with the application of local anesthesia to the tympanic membrane, most patients undergoing TT needle placement on the promontory do not complain of discomfort (e.g., Haapaniemi et al., 2000).

In the clinic, electrode placement is usually done with the tympanic membrane *anesthetized.* A variety of local anesthetic agents have been described, among them iontophoresis (e.g., Roland et al., 1995), combinations of phenol, menthol, and even cocaine (Bath et al., 1998). Sensation of the TM can be easily reduced with a phenol (89%) swab (Schwaber & Hall, 1990; Johannson et al., 1997), 10 percent lidocaine (Wuyts et al., 1997), or a 2 percent xylocaine solution (Densert et al., 1994). The phenol is applied to the TM under microscope immediately before the ECochG pro-

TABLE 4.3. Summary of Steps in ECochG Measurement Using a Transtympanic (TT) Membrane Electrode Technique

The transtympanic membrane needle electrode design is illustrated in Figure 4.3.

- Follow general test protocol for preparation, patient instruction, and test parameters.
- Apply all electrodes (discs) except the transtympanic electrode and plug into the appropriate electrode box receptacles. In the operating room, only subdermal needle electrodes are used, rather than disc electrodes.
- Under microscope, apply anesthetic (e.g., phenol) to the region of the tympanic membrane that will receive the needle. See the chapter text for a review of options for local anesthetic agents. A local anesthetic for the tympanic membrane is needed only for measurement of ECochG in the clinic setting. For intraoperative monitoring applications of EcochG, the transtympanic needle is placed after the induction of general anesthesia.
- Grasp with bayonet forceps a short, stainless steel, uninsulated, subdermal needle electrode at the needle end of the electrode wire (cable). Subdermal needle electrodes (see Figure 4.3) are available from most manufacturers of evoked response systems.
- Insert the tip of the needle through the inferior posterior portion of the tympanic membrane and place against the promontory.
- Secure the electrode wire temporarily with a finger.
- Grasp a compressed foam insert plug, or TIPtrode™, with bayonet forceps and insert into the ear canal.

- Allow the foam insert earplug to expand against the electrode wire.
- Plug the acoustic tubing from the ER-3A transducer into the stalk tube of the insert earplug (or TIPtrode).
- Plug the transtympanic needle electrode pin into the appropriate electrode box receptacle.
- Immediately verify interelectrode impedance for all electrodes. In the operating room, before neurophysiologic monitoring with ECochG, it is important to verify interelectrode impedance while the electrodes remain accessible, before the surgical field is prepared and disinfected, and before the patient is draped for surgery.
- Transtympanic electrode impedance should be about 12 K ohms or lower, and impedance for other electrodes should be less than 5 K ohms.
- Before surgery begins (i.e., before the opening) initiate stimulation to the test ear (the ear with the transtympanic electrode) to verify that there are no technical problems.
- Inspect the waveform for an AP component in the 1.5 to 2.0 ms region.
- AP amplitude should be robust (as high as 10 μV even for patients with mild-to-moderate hearing loss).
- Proceed with ECochG measurement and analysis.

cedure is performed. Some patients report a burning sensation as the phenol contacts the TM. Iontophoresis is another anesthetic technique reported for TT ECochG recordings (Ramsden, Gibson, & Moffat, 1977). With iontophoresis, a low level of direct electrical current is applied within the external ear canal to enhance the effectiveness of the anesthetic agent. The technique produces adequate anesthesia, but is time consuming. British investigators have described the reduction of discomfort during TT electrode ECochG with the use of an anesthetic "EMLA" cream (Bath et al., 1998). Anesthetic ingredients of the cream include lignocaine and prilocaine. In a systematic study of discomfort with twenty-four patients, the authors confirmed that the cream "provides a quick, simple technique ideal for reducing the level of discomfort experienced with TT ECochG," adding that the cream was contraindicated for patients with perforated TMs. Indeed, one formal investigation has confirmed that patients report less discomfort with TT electrode ECochG than with the noninvasive TM electrode technique (Haapaniemi et al., 2000).

A microscope is used for inspecting and viewing the TM during electrode placement. The patient usually describes a mild burning or tingling sensation as the phenol reaches the TM. Keep in mind that for TT membrane electrode placement in the operating room, the patient is already under general anesthesia at this point in the procedure. The promontory electrode is placed by a physician (e.g., otologist) under a operating room microscope. The insulated portion of the sterile subdermal needle electrode (between the shank and the wire) is grasped with bayonet forceps and the electrode is directed down the external auditory canal. The needle is then inserted through the inferior–posterior portion of the TM to rest on the promontory. In the clinic, patients do not report pain and rarely describe discomfort during insertion of the TT needle.

After TT electrode placement, the electrode lead (wire), extending from just lateral to the TM membrane, is secured temporarily by hand against the wall of the ear canal. The physician or assistant then grasps a compressed foam ear insert or TIPtrode with the bayonet forceps and places it within the ear canal in the customary fashion (Figure 4.4). It is important to note that the foam ear insert is sterile for intraoperative use. At the conclusion of ECochG recording, the foam insert is removed first, and then needle electrode is removed by pulling gently and slowly outward. The preceding promontory electrode placement procedure requires less than one minute in the operating room and less than three minutes in the clinic. Although the TT electrode technique is clearly invasive, it is as noted above well tolerated by patients, and associated medical problems and complications are atypical. As evident from the listing of papers in Table 4.4, numerous clinical investigators record with success ECochG with the transtympanic needle technique. In a formal retrospective review of the medical records for 205 patients who underwent TT ECochG recording, Ng, Srireddy, Horlbeck, and Niparko (2001) reported that one case of a nonhealed persistent perforation with acute otitis media was attributed to the TT technique. Another two patients developed otitis media with intact tympanic membranes, and three patients described ear pain for up to five days. These authors concluded from their chart review and patient survey that complications from the TT electrode technique were infrequent and patient acceptance was good.

SUBDERMAL NEEDLE ELECTRODES. | When ECochG is recorded in the operating room during intraoperative neurophysiologic monitoring, subdermal needle electrodes are often used for all locations (e.g., noninverting, inverting, and ground), rather than disc electrodes. Subdermal electrodes offer the advantages of a secure attachment to the patient during lengthy surgical procedures and neurophysiologic monitoring sessions and consistently lower impedance. Insertion of subdermal needle electrodes may appear more difficult than it really is. To begin with, the electrodes should be sterilized and in good condition (sharp and not bent irregularly or rusted). The skin at each proposed electrode site is prepared by scrubbing vigorously with a fresh alcohol swab. Then the electrode is removed from its packaging, grasped firmly between the thumb and index finger at the junction between the cable and the needle, and fully inserted at a sharp angle (less than 20 degrees from the skin). Appropriate lengths of tape should be handy to secure the electrode to the skin and prevent torsion. Needles are sometimes purposefully bent at a 90-degree angle before insertion to prevent slippage after insertion. If this technique is used, electrode needles must be inspected very carefully before each application. The two main health risks posed by needle electrodes are spread of disease by an unsterilized needle and needle breakage, with a portion remaining under the skin. Subdermal needle insertion should always be done by appropriate medical personnel or by experienced nonmedical personnel with medical support readily available.

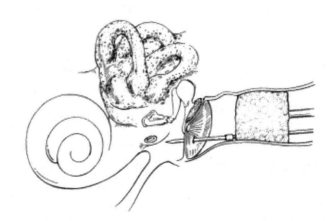

FIGURE 4.4. Illustration of the placement of a subdermal needle through the inferior–posterior quadrant of the tympanic membrane. The tip of the needle rests on the promotory, and the electrode lead is held in place within the external ear canal by a foam insert earphone cushion. Adapted from Schwaber & Hall, 1990.

TABLE 4.4. Summary of Clinical Studies Utilizing the Transtympanic (TT) Electrode ECochG Measurement Technique

STUDY, YEAR	ELECTRODE TYPE(S)	DIAGNOSIS	COMMENTS
Schwaber & Hall, 1990	TT, EAC	Varied	ECochG up to ten times larger than TIPtrode ABR wave I with severe hearing loss TT ECochG useful in intraoperative monitoring TT ECochG more reliable; analysis easier
Aso, 1990	TT	Ménière's, other	Normal normative data for TT ECochG values
Gibson, 1991	TT	Ménière's, other	Improved diagnosis with 1000 Hz tone burst
Hohmann, 1992	TT	Tumor	TT ECochG technique valuable intraoperatively
Marangos, 1992	TT	Varied	TT ECochG valuable diagnostic tool
Moffat et al., 1992	TT	Ménière's, other	ECochG useful in diagnosis of bilateral MD
Orchik, Shea & Ge, 1993	TT	Ménière's, other	TT ECochG sensitive to Ménière's disease
Campbell et al., 1993	TM, TT	Chinchilla	Compared TIPtrode, TM, and TT electrodes TT electrode produced superior ECochGs
Dornhoffer & Arenberg, 1993	TT	Ménière's	
Densert et al., 1994	TT	Ménière's	Normative TT ECochG data
Roland et al., 1995	TT, TM	Normal	TT ECochG superior to TIPtrode
Schoonhoven et al., 1995	TT, EAC	Varied	TT ECochG amplitude twice larger than EAC; both TT and EAC techniques useful clinically
Deans et al., 1996	TT	Normal	ECochG affected by location of TT electrode
Negri et al., 1996	TT	Normal	TT compared to ear canal ECochG techniques
Schoonhoven et al., 1996	TT, EAC	Varied	TT ECochG useful in estimating hearing loss
Krueger & Wagner, 1997	TT	Ménière's	No difference in SP/AP ratio for TT vs. round window electrode site
Krueger & Storper, 1997	TT	Ménière's	Normative TT ECochG data
Ge, Shea, & Orchik, 1997	TT	Ménière's	Larger CM in Ménière's disease other SNHL
Dornhoffer, 1998	TT	Ménière's	Normative TT ECochG data
Sass, Densert, & Arlinger, 1998	TT	Ménière's	Recording technique described normal
Conlon & Gibson, 1999	TT	Ménière's	ECochG useful in detecting bilateral MD
Konradsson, Carlborg, Grenner, & Tjernstrom, 1999	TT	Ménière's	Hyperbaric effect studied with ECochG
Noguchi et al., 1999	TT	SNHL	Both TT and ear-canal electrodes useful
Haapeniemi et al., 2000	TM, TT	Ménière's	TT vs. TM ECochG 4 to 6 times larger TT electrode caused less discomfort TT ECochG more reliable; easier analysis
Ng et al., 2001	TT	Varied	Infrequent complications (only one perforation); good patient acceptance
Hoffer et al., 2001	TT	Ménière's	Study of gentamicin treatment effectiveness
Ghosh, Gupta, & Mann, 2002	TT, TM	Ménière's	Normal differences in normal SP/AP ratio for TT vs. TM

Comparative ECochG Findings with Different Electrode Types and Locations

There is a substantial accumulative clinical experience with each the three general types of electrodes—extra-tympanic, TM, and TT. In addition, some investigators have conducted studies comparing data collected from the same normal subjects using combinations of two or more types of electrodes, including extra-tympanic versus TT electrodes (Elberling, 1976; Negri et al., 1996; Roland, Yellin, Meyerhoff, & Frank, 1995; Schoonhoven, Fabius, & Grote, 1995; Schwaber & Hall, 1990) and tympanic membrane versus TT electrodes (Haapaniemi et al., 2000; Ruth & Lambert, 1989). It bears repeating that the term "extra-tympanic" encompasses a broad range of electrode types and locations, ranging from surface electrodes rather far removed from the cochlea (e.g., the mastoid or earlobe) to the TIPtrode located laterally in the cartilaginous portion of the external ear canal, to needles placed into the skin at the medial extreme of the internal ear canal, near the annulus (e.g., Negri et al., 1996).

Some general conclusions are clear from these investigations. Selected ECochG properties are equivalent among the three electrode types. For example, there are no differences in latency values among the three different electrode approaches. ECochG amplitude is invariably larger for the TT needle electrode located on the promontory than for the tympanic membrane electrode site (a four- to sixfold increase), and at least ten times greater for the TT electrode than for the ear canal (e.g., TIPtrode) electrode site. The amplitude differences among the three electrode types for ECochG components are illustrated in Figure 4.5, and the relative SP/AP ratio varies as a function of electrode placement. Normal expectations for the SP/AP ratio with each electrode design are summarized in the appendix. As the electrode site approaches the cochlea (e.g., ear canal to promontory sites), amplitude for the AP component increases more than the amplitude for the SP component. The result of this differential effect of electrode site on SP versus AP amplitude is a decrease in the upper limit for normal SP/AP ratio as the electrode site approaches the cochlea. To produce comparable signal-to-noise ratios, up to five times more signal averaging is required for the extra-tympanic electrode ECochG than for the transtympanic technique. Sensitivity and specificity for cochlear disorders is consistently greater for the TT electrode ECochG technique than for the extra-tympanic techniques. Even for the TT electrode technique, differences in ECochG findings have been associated with variations in the exact site of needle placement on the medial wall of the middle ear (Deans, Hill, Birchall, Davison, Fitzgerald, & Elliott, 1996). However, there is also evidence (e.g., Hall, 1992; Krueger & Wagner, 1997) of comparable ECochG absolute and relative amplitude for the SP and AP components with electrode locations on the promontory versus other adjacent sites (e.g., medial and lateral locations around the round window niche).

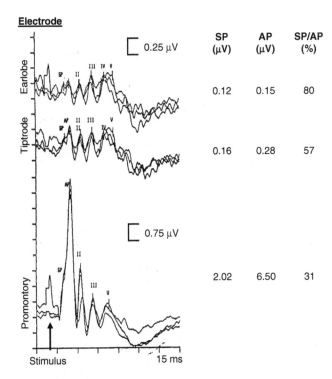

FIGURE 4.5. Examples of ECochG waveforms recorded with three electrode types (TIPtrode, tympanic membrane electrode, and transtympanic needle electrode). Note the increase in amplitude as the electrode location approximates the cochlea. Also evident is the effect of electrode location on the SP/AP ratio.

Patient acceptance and comfort varies among the electrode techniques. As expected, the TIPtrode technique is generally well tolerated. Differences in patient tolerance and satisfaction reported for the TM versus TT electrode approaches might deviate from expectations of some clinicians. In a direct comparison of these two electrode techniques, Haapeniemi et al. (2000) found that patients were more satisfied with the TT electrode technique, as it was painless (when applied with appropriate local anesthesia) in comparison to the TM electrode. Specific differences in ECochG components that are associated with these electrode types (e.g., amplitude, latency, reliability, and variability) are described in more detail in later sections of this chapter and, for patient populations, in the next chapter.

STIMULUS PARAMETERS

Transducer

The advantages of insert earphones cited for auditory evoked response measurement in general (see Table 3.3 in Chapter 3) apply as well to ECochG recording. At least three advantages of insert earphones in the measurement of ECochG are particularly noteworthy. First, because the

ECochG components occur early in the waveform (within the first 2 or 3 milliseconds), waveform analysis can be enhanced by separation of the transducer box from the electrode site (via the insert tube) and elimination of stimulus artifact within this time frame. Stimulus artifact may be indistinguishable from ECochG components, especially the CM and AP, and it can serious interfere with their confident identification. Second, insert earphones contribute to the quality of recordings for each of the three major ECochG electrode options. The TIPtrode electrode is an insert earphone cushion covered with gold foil and coupled via an electrode lead to a preamplifier. The TM electrode and the TT electrode lead wires within the ear canal can be effectively held in place and secured with insert earphone cushions, as illustrated in this chapter. Third, insert earphones offer a clear advantage over conventional supra-aural earphones for intraoperative monitoring with ECochG during otologic surgical operations. The tubes and insert cushions are necessarily within the surgical field for patients undergoing surgical procedures requiring intraoperative monitoring (e.g., acoustic tumor removal or vestibular nerve section). Both components can be sterilized prior surgery and placed in the surgical field before the area (ear and mastoid region) is bathed with a liquid disinfectant, and the insert cushions (earplugs) can be discarded after surgery. As illustrated in Figure 4.6, placement of insert earphones does not interfere with access to the postauricular area during otologic surgical procedures.

Type

Click signals are most commonly used in clinical ECochG measurement, regardless of the application (e.g., the enhancement of the wave I component of the ABR, intraoperative monitoring, diagnosis of Ménière's disease). As with ABR measurement, the click is produced with a 0.1 ms (100 μsec) electrical pulse. ECochG can be elicted with tone burst signals (Campbell, Faloon, & Rybak, 1993; Ferraro et al., 1994; Ge & Shea, 2002; Laureano, McGrady, & Campbell, 1995; Orchik, Shea, & Ge, 1993; Schoonhoven, Fabius, & Grote, 1995; Schoonhoven, Prijs, & Grote, 1996). ECochG measurement with tone burst signals is often applied in the diagnosis of Ménière's disease (e.g., Campbell, Harker, & Abbas, 1992; Margolis, Ricks, Fournier, & Levine, 1995; Orchik, Shea, & Ge, 1993). There is some evidence that the diagnostic value of ECochG is relatively higher for a 1000 Hz tone burst signal frequency (e.g., Conlon & Gibson, 1999, 2000; Gibson, 1991; Sass, 1998; Sass, Densert, Magnusson, & Whitaker, 1998). The confident detection of ECochG components produced by tone burst signals, particularly for lower frequencies, is significantly greater for TM and TT electrode recordings than with ECochGs recorded from more distant electrode sites (e.g., the ear canal). The clinical application of tone-burst stimulation in ECochG measurement is further described in Chapter 5.

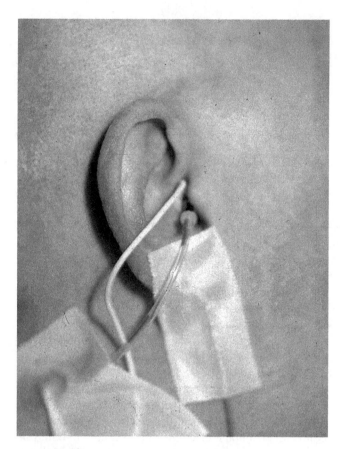

FIGURE 4.6. Placement of the transducer of the ER-3A insert earphone out of the surgical field during intraoperative neurophysiologic monitoring with ECochG. The insert earphone secures the lead for the transtympanic needle electrode.

Duration

An abrupt-onset stimulus is required for generation of the ECochG AP component, and only the onset portion of the stimulus contributes to the response. Shorter duration stimuli are most effective in producing the ECochG AP, and the response is not detected with stimulus rise times of 10 ms or greater. The dependency of ECochG AP on stimulus duration characteristics is, in many aspects, the same as for ABR. Therefore, general concepts of rise/fall and plateau times for both responses are presented in the ABR discussion that follows. One duration characteristic of the ECochG AP component, however, deserves special mention. The ECochG AP (the same electrophysiologic component as ABR wave I) is essentially an onset response. That is, it is produced by a stimulus with rapid rise time (onset). The subsequent duration of the stimulus has no appreciable effect on the response (Gorga, Beauchaine, Reiland, Worthington, & Javel, 1984).

In contrast, the ECochG SP component is dependent in stimulus duration. Stimulus duration, like stimulus frequency, differentially affects ECochG components. The CM and SP can be generated with a wide range of stimulus rise/

fall times and can persist throughout the extent of tonal stimulus duration. At one extreme, CM and SP activity is easily recorded with a very abrupt (0.1 msec) click stimulus. A single polarity (vs. alternating polarity) must be used to detect the CM. At the other extreme, CM and SP components can be generated both by stimuli with relatively long rise times and by tone bursts of extended duration. Measurement of ECochG with long-duration (e.g., 50 ms) tone burst signals is typically reported in the diagnosis of Ménière's disease (e.g., Densert, Arlinger, Sass, & Hergils, 1994). The SP appears as a shift in baseline electrical activity that directly reflects stimulus duration (Figure 4.7). In fact, a clinical technique for clarifying the presence of the SP, and distinguishing SP versus AP components of the ECochG, is to extend the duration of a tone-burst stimulus to, for example, 10 ms or longer. This technique is described in the discussion of ECochG analysis techniques below. The SP persists for the duration of the stimulus, whereas the AP appears only immediately following stimulus onset. The distinctly different effect of stimulus duration on SP versus AP is well recognized in clinical ECochG application (e.g., Dauman, Aran, Charlet de Sauvage, & Portman, 1988).

ECOCHG EVOKED WITH STIMULUS OFFSET. | Eggermont and Odenthal (1974a) produced a clear ECochG AP by the offset of a long duration (20 ms) tone-burst stimulus. The rise/fall times of this stimulus were brief (0.33 ms). Interestingly, the offset ECochG AP was clearest for stimulus intensities below about the region of 65 dB. The offset ECochG threshold was from 15 to 20 dB higher (worse) than that for the onset response.

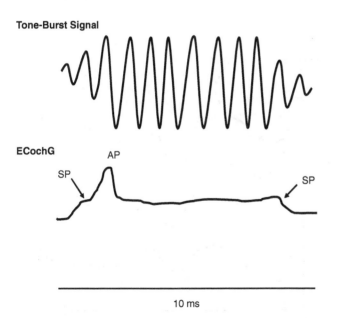

FIGURE 4.7. Effect of stimulus duration on the SP and AP components of the ECochG. Note the presence of the SP component throughout the stimulus duration, in contrast to the AP only at stimulus onset.

Intensity

Basic information on physiology and anatomy of ECochG, important for understanding the effects of intensity, was presented in Chapter 2. The receptor potentials of the cochlea include the SP component, reflecting DC (direct current) activity, and an AC (alternating current) component (the CM component). Because they are receptor potentials, neither the generation of the CM nor the SP involves a synapse. Therefore, the latency of neither really changes with stimulus intensity. That is, each potential is generated within the cochlea as soon as the cochlea is activated by an acoustic stimulus, before the first synapse (hair cell to eighth-nerve afferent fibers). The onset of the CM can, in fact, be used as a stimulus onset marker in ECochG measurement. Amplitude of both the CM and the SP does increase with intensity. The CM is the AC potential that follows closely the vibratory pattern of the basilar membrane, including the amplitude and the phase of its displacement (Dallos, 1973; Davis, 1958), and its amplitude directly reflects stimulus amplitude.

Higher stimulus intensity levels produce greater basilar membrane displacement and proportionally greater CM activity. As noted previously, evidence of CM waveform in the ECochG recording can be minimized or eliminated with the use of alternating polarity stimuli. CM cancellation with stimulus polarity reversal is, however, most effective only for lower stimulus intensity levels (Peake & Kiang, 1962), at which amplitude is equivalent for each polarity, and phase is exactly reversed. At higher stimulus intensity levels, CM cancellation may be incomplete because of slight differences or distortions in phase and amplitude of the response for one polarity versus the other. The phase differences are presumably due to distortion in production of the CM within the cochlea. An understanding of the relation between the CM and stimulus intensity is useful in auditory neuropathy. By definition, the ABR cannot be detected in auditory neuropathy. Although the ABR has no value in estimating auditory sensitivity, the CM may serve this purpose.

The SP is the DC cochlear potential (Dallos, Schoeny, & Cheatham, 1972; Honrubia & Ward, 1969), which unlike the AP component and the CM, is typically recorded only at high intensity levels (Davis, 1958; Davis, Deatherage, Eldredge, & Smith, 1958). Inner hair cells play an important role in the generation of the SP (Dallos, 1973; Durrant et al., 1998). There is experimental evidence of a relationship between the amplitude of the AP (scala media negative) to the RMS (root mean square) SPL of a tonal stimulus (Davis, 1958). The normal human SP is first detected at a click intensity level of about 92 dB SPL (approximately 62 dB nHL), then amplitude gradually increases as click intensity level increases (Chatrian, Wirch, Edwards, Lettich, & Snyder, 1984; Eggermont, 1976a,b; Eggermont & Odenthal, 1974a,b).

Chatrian et al. (1984) described the relationship of amplitude versus intensity for an ECochG recorded from the ear canal using a power function:

$$\log SP \text{ amplitude in } \mu V = b \log \text{ click SPL} + \log k$$

where *b* is the exponent of the logarithmic function and *k* is the intercept of the function.

The power function was found by these authors to be a more representative model of the stimulus intensity-versus-amplitude relation for their group of 10 subjects than a similar logarithmic function. There was pronounced variability between subjects, however, both in the SP amplitude at any given intensity level and in the amplitude-versus-intensity slopes, so neither function adequately described the amplitude-versus-intensity function for all subjects. SP variability extended, naturally, to the SP/AP relation as well, and to changes in the SP/AP relation with intensity. Absolute SP amplitude varied, depending on measurement parameters, especially the recording electrode sites. For example, with an external auditory meatus electrode, average SP amplitudes at high intensity levels (80 to 100 dB HL) were in the order of 0.39 μV (Coats, 1981) to 0.56 μV (Chatrian et al., 1984). These values are in contrast to 6.0 μV (Eggermont, 1976a) to 10.0 μV (Gibson, 1982) with a promontory electrode site. Chatrian et al. (1984) found a similarity between their SP input–output function average power function exponent (0.46) and a power function (0.51) calculated from raw data published by Eggermont (1976a). In both studies, despite methodological differences, there was a tenfold increase in SP amplitude for each increase of 20 dB in stimulus intensity.

There is abundant experimental and clinical evidence that amplitude of ECochG AP increases and latency decreases as stimulus intensity is increased. Almost forty years ago, researchers (e.g., Yoshie, 1968) recognized clinically that the input–output curve (i.e., stimulus intensity is the input and the ECochG AP component is the output) appears to have two segments. The amplitude growth curve (intensity-versus-amplitude function) is shallow up to approximately 60 dB HL, then much steeper for higher intensity levels. These two segments are often referred to as the low (L) and high (H) portions of the ECochG AP amplitude growth functions. The input–output curve takes on a somewhat different shape when plotted on a logarithmic amplitude scale. These rates of amplitude change as a function of intensity are quite consistent among normal-hearing individuals, even though the absolute amplitude at any given intensity may vary from person to person and depending on recording technique, especially electrode site. Rate of amplitude change in normal subjects is on the order of 0.5 to 1.0 percent for intensity levels up to 60 dB, then increases to 1.03 to 3.0 percent above 60 dB. Numerous investigations and years of clinical experience have shown that latency of ECochG AP systematically decreases as stimulus intensity increases. The latency shift as a function of intensity is relatively greater for low stimulus frequencies. One factor in the latency-versus-intensity relationship is the site

of cochlear activation. Higher intensity levels activate more basal (high-frequency) portions of the cochlea, while lower intensity levels activate more apical portions. The time delay from stimulus onset is shorter for basal versus apical cochlear activation because travel time along the basilar membrane is less. This factor is involved in both intensity-versus-latency and frequency-versus-latency interactions. Schoonhoven, Fabius, and Grote (1995) extended ECochG measurement to include analysis of input–output functions in the diagnosis of sensorineural auditory dysfunction.

Another factor is synaptic delay. This delay is less with high than with low stimulus intensity levels. The latency changes due to synaptic delay are equivalent for all stimulus frequencies. One important principle of ECochG measurement, especially for audiometric assessment, is evident from these comments. Frequency specificity in ECochG generation is greatest for lower intensity levels and is reduced for higher stimulus intensity levels.

Rate

CM and SP components of ECochG remain relatively stable over a wide range of stimulus rates. In contrast, latency of the AP component increases and amplitude decreases as stimulus rate increases (Mouney, Berlin, Cullen, & Hughes, 1978; Wilson & Bowker, 2002). As signal rate increases, the SP/AP ratio increases due to the relative decrease in amplitudes for the AP versus the SP component. At signal rates approaching 100 sec, the AP is minimal and detection of the remaining SP is enhanced. These relationships between signal rate of presentation and ECochG amplitude values are illustrated in Figure 4.8. The mechanism for the rate-related

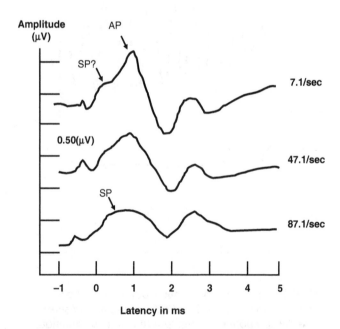

FIGURE 4.8. Effect of stimulus rate on ECochG components (CM, SP, and AP).

changes in AP component latency and amplitude may be due to desynchronization at the cochlear level and perhaps an adaptation phenomenon at the synapse between hair cells and auditory nerve afferents (Eggermont, 1974). In any event, inclusion of a fast signal rate into the clinical ECochG test protocol is useful for confirmation of the SP component and accurate calculation of SP amplitude.

Polarity

Signal polarity has a marked and differential influence on the three ECochG components (Figure 4.9). The effect of stimulus polarity on responses from the cochlea and the eighth nerve was demonstrated experimentally with studies employing single unit recordings (Anderson, Rose, Hind, & Brugge, 1971; Burkard & Voigt, 1989; Coats et al., 1979; Gerull et al., 1985; Kiang, 1965; Møller, 1983; Peake & Kiang, 1962; Pfeiffer, 1974; Pfeiffer & Kim, 1972; Teas et al., 1962). Clinically, signal polarity effects are evident with averaged ECochG recordings. The CM component is recorded for single polarity signals (rarefaction or condensation), with the waveform (direction of the CM changes) approximately 180 degrees out of phase for one polarity versus the other. With an alternating polarity signal (rarefaction and condensation polarity signals presented in alternate sequence), the CM is mostly cancelled out. The SP and AP ECochG components are more readily detected when the CM is cancelled in this way. It is important to keep in mind, however, that only ECochG components elicited with single polarity signals are true electrophysiologic responses, whereas the waveform produced by alternating polarity signals is really derived from two individual responses (Sass et al., 1998). Each of these

responses to a signal polarity can be influenced by differences in noise content, and signal averaging.

In normal ears, rarefaction polarity signals presented at moderate or high intensity levels produce AP latency values that are shorter by a modest amount than those elicited by condensation polarity signals (e.g., 0.1 to 0.2 ms). The AP latency difference for the two signal polarities is considerably, and statistically, larger (e.g., 0.6 or 0.7 ms) in Ménière's disease, but not for patients with other cochlear disorders (Levine, Margolis, Fournier, & Winzenberg, 1992; Margolis et al., 1995; Sass et al., 1998). With an alternating polarity signal, the AP components at slightly different latency values are partially cancelled. As a result, the AP (ABR wave I) amplitude is relatively smaller with alternating polarity signals. This enhancement of wave I amplitude underlies the rationale for utilizing rarefaction polarity click signals in the ABR test protocol.

Published evidence supports the practice of recording ECochG with rarefaction and condensation polarity click signals, and perhaps tone bursts, for the diagnosis of Ménière's disease (Johannson, Haapaniemi, & Laurikainen, 1997; Margolis et al., 1992; Orchik, Ge, & Shea, 1998; Sass et al., 1998; Sparacino, Milani, Magnavita, & Arslan, 2000). For example, Sass et al. (1998), using a TT electrode ECochG technique, found that the sensitivity of the rarefaction versus condensation difference alone was 37 percent in the diagnosis of Ménière's disease. In contrast, sensitivity of the SP/AP ratio was 83 percent. Specificity was 100 percent for the SP/AP ratio alone. Combining the SP/AP ratio with the polarity difference analysis produced a sensitivity of 87 percent. Given the ease of analysis of the AP latency for signals with rarefaction versus condensation polarity versus identification of the SP and calculation of the SP/AP ratio, this analysis technique can make an important contribution to the diagnosis of endolymphatic hydrops and Ménière's disease. Cochlear pathophysiologic mechanisms for the polarity effects are reviewed for specific disorders in Chapter 5. Sparacino et al. (2000) reported a mathematical algorithm for describing in auditory disorders even small differences in CM and AP findings for rarefaction (negative) and condensation (positive) polarity click signals.

Stimulus intensity level is also an important factor in polarity effects on ECochG. At lower intensity levels (40 dB and below), polarity does not influence either latency or amplitude of the AP component. Polarity effects are more prominent for narrowband than for wideband (click) stimuli. Polarity reversal of high-frequency (above 4000 Hz) stimuli, with relatively short wavelengths, has little effect on the auditory response. With single-slope click stimuli (e.g., a rapid onset but very gradual offset), AP latency is considerably earlier (0.6 ms) for rarefaction versus for condensation polarities (Gerull et al., 1985).

This complex interaction among stimulus polarity, intensity, and frequency is the subject of much speculation in the literature (e.g., Burkard & Voight, 1989). Møller (1986) conducted a study of the effect of click spectrum and polarity on the ECochG AP and wave II components (in the

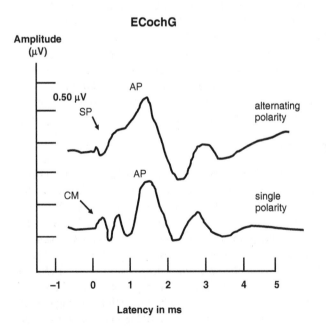

ECochG

FIGURE 4.9. Differences in the effect of click stimulus polarity (single polarity, e.g., rarefaction, condensation, and alternating polarity) on the three ECochG components (CM, SP, and AP).

rat) and concisely summarized the literature in the context of his findings. The amplitude-versus-intensity function, and, to a lesser extent, the latency-versus-intensity function, each have two segments. The first segment (intensity levels of 40 dB and below), for which rarefaction and condensation stimuli produce responses with comparable latency and amplitude values, is actually produced mainly by the high frequency portion of the broadband click. This is because low-frequency cochlear units have a higher threshold. The second segment appears as stimulus intensity level is increased (above 40 dB) and reaches the threshold for the low-frequency components, when the rarefaction polarity begins to produce its characteristic larger amplitude and shorter latency responses. High-frequency stimuli, as just noted, are typically associated with minimal polarity effects. There is evidence that the diagnostic sensitivity of ECochG, particularly in Ménière's disease, can be enhanced by analysis of the SP amplitude, the SP/AP amplitude ratio, or AP latency for responses elicited with rarefaction versus condensation click signals (Ge & Shea, 2002; Orchik, Ge, & Shea, 1998; Sass et al., 1998). This evidence argues for the routine measurement of ECochG with single-polarity signals. Current clinical evoked response systems permit the presentation of alternating polarity signals, with ongoing separate storage and later retrieval of the responses produced by each polarity. Thus, without increasing test time, it's possible to analyze each of the ECochG components (CM, SP, and AP) for each polarity condition (rarefaction, condensation, and alternating).

Bone-Conduction ECochG

Stimulus-related artifact is a major problem in recording ECochG because the artifact may extend well into the time period of the response and may obscure the individual components of the response. Kylen, Harder, Jervall, and Arlinger (1982) and Harder, Arlinger, and Kylen (1983), citing the limitations of conventional bone vibrators and placement techniques (such as placement on intact skin over the mastoid bone), assessed the performance of a piezo-ceramic accelerometer, the A21T, attached to the mastoid process with a modified bone screw. Data with these two types of bone vibrators and placements were reported for cadavers and for patients. Although mounting the B-72 vibrator to the skull with a screw reduced distortion of the skull vibration pattern, the authors still found excessive distortion for high-frequency stimuli and excessive electromagnetic stimulus artifact. Performance of the high mechanical impedance A21T vibrator, screw-fixed to the mastoid bone, was superior. The authors stated that the screw-fixed technique for placement caused only minor discomfort and created no safety problems. Minimum distance between screw tip and sigmoid sinus was 4mm.

Monaural versus Binaural Stimulation

Although effects of monaural versus binaural stimulation have been studied mostly for ABR and AMLR, as reviewed in the following subsections, there is evidence that ECochG is also subject to these effects. Prasher and Gibson (1984) recorded the ECochG from thirty subjects, using a TT needle electrode resting on the promontory. Stimuli were clicks presented via TDH-39 earphones. For 87 percent of the subjects, the peak-to-peak amplitude of the AP component was diminished for binaural versus monaural stimulation. Magnitude of the binaural amplitude decrease varied considerable among subjects, ranging form 0 percent (no change) to 75 percent, with an average (mean) decrease of about 30 percent. This mean reduction in AP amplitude for the group corresponded to the effect of a stimulus intensity attenuation of 20 dB. Despite these distinct amplitude changes, AP latency remained equivalent for monaural versus binaural stimulation. The efferent auditory system presumably plays a role in these findings. Efferent system activation by electrical stimulation produces both an inhibitory effect on the eighth-nerve AP (Galambos, 1956) and an enhancement of the CM. This is, by no means, a complete explanation.

ACQUISITION PARAMETERS

Analysis Time

An analysis time in the range of 5 to 10 ms is typically used for ECochG measurement. With a minimum of 512 data points distributed across this period, temporal resolution (the time interval between any two consecutive sample points) is 0.02 ms or better (a shorter interval) that is more than adequate to define response waveform. A relatively brief 5 ms analysis time may be preferable for recording the ECochG, because potentially larger amplitude and later latency brainstem components (e.g., ABR wave V) are eliminated from analysis. If the clinical objective, however, is combined recording of ECochG and ABR, then a 10 ms or even 15 ms analysis time is appropriate. Latency of the ECochG AP component is prolonged for low-frequency tonal stimuli (e.g., a 500 Hz tone burst) presented at reduced effective intensity levels (close to normal threshold or to patients with peripheral auditory deficits). In these instances, an analysis time of greater than 5 ms is required to ensure that the entire response is visible.

Filter Settings

Since the CM component reflects stimulus polarity and frequency, it contains energy in the region of the stimulus. Filter settings should be sufficiently wide to encompass these frequencies and avoid any distortion of CM phase. The SP presents a unique problem in filtering. Since it is a DC potential, theoretically the SP is best recorded with little or no high-pass filtering. In fact, band-pass filter settings of 3 or 10 to 1500 or 3000 Hz are typically described in reported ECochG test protocols. Clinically, extending the high-pass filter setting to such extremes as 0.1, 1, 3, 5, or even 10 Hz may introduce irrelevant EEG activity and substantial patient-related artifact and may preclude rapid data collection. There is clinical evidence that a distinct SP component can be recorded with high-pass filter settings in the range of 10 to 30 Hz, and even 100 Hz (e.g., Durrant & Ferraro, 1991; Ferraro & Durrant, 1989), with no detectable change in the SP/AP ratio. For ECochG applications that rely on SP measurement (e.g., diagnosis of Ménière's disease), extending the high-pass filter setting to below 100 Hz is certainly preferable but not essential.

Amplification

NUMBER OF SWEEPS (NUMBER OF STIMULUS REPETITIONS). |
The amount of averaging (i.e., the number of sweeps or repetitions of the stimuli) necessary for defining a reliable ECochG waveform and adequate signal-to-noise ratio depends, of course, on the noise level during recording and the size of the response (signal). Therefore, electrode type is a critical factor. The ECochG recorded with a true near-field electrode (TT) placement on the promontory, or even a tympanic membrane electrode site, typically produces a robust ECochG with large amplitude (2 to over 10 µV), in comparison to an extra-tympanic (ear canal) electrode site (less than 1 µV. This point was clearly indicated in Figure 4.5.

ECochG Recording Problems

Although the list of general problems that may develop in ECochG recording is long, many can be solved with opti-mal electrode placement. ECochG activity arising from the cochlea and distal (cochlear end) eighth nerve is best measured with a near-field technique, with the electrode near the electrical field (dipole) generating the recorded response. Therefore, as the recording electrode approaches the cochlea, response amplitude increases substantially. For a normal ear, ECochG SP or AP components detected with a promontory electrode (resting on the outer wall of cochlea) are from ten to even twenty times larger than those detected with an electrode located in the ear canal. The large amplitude the near-field ECochG response serves to overcome various measurement problems encountered clinically. Response reliability (repeatability), often poor with ear-canal electrodes, is typically excellent with the promontory electrode site. With a promontory (or TM) electrode, ECochG is usually identified confidently even from patients with serious hearing impairment, whereas these patients usually do not show a clear response with a more distant electrode site. Finally, because the near-field response is so much larger, the signal-to-noise ratio is corresponding smaller. The clinical advantage is that far fewer sweeps (stimulus repetitions) are required to detect a response. These and other problems and solutions are summarized in Table 4.5.

TABLE 4.5. Troubleshooting in ECochG Measurement

SYMPTOM	POSSIBLE PROBLEMS	POSSIBLE SOLUTIONS
No response	No stimulus	Perform listening check Verify correct transducer Verify test ear
	Improper electrode Severe hearing loss Inadequate stimulus	Verify electrode array Obtain audiogram Increase stimulus intensity
Small response	Distant electrode	Use TT or TM electrode
Large early waves	Excessive CM	Use alternating stimulus polarity
Early artifact	Stimulus interference	Use alternating stimulus polarity Use insert tube-phones Keep transducer away from electrode Use shielded earphones Reduce stimulus intensity Keep transducer cord away from electrodes
Small or absent AP		Increase stimulus intensity Increase stimulus rate to distinguish SP vs. AP Lengthen tone-burst duration Use TT or TM electrode Lower high-pass filter setting
Small or inconsistent AP		Increase stimulus intensity Decrease stimulus rate Use TT or TM electrode Use additional sweeps
Electrical artifact	Check electrode impedance	Change stimulus rate Increase distance between patient and electrical devices Lower low-pass filter setting (e.g., from 3000 to 1500 Hz)

AN ECochG TEST PROTOCOL AND STRATEGY

Test Protocol

STIMULUS PARAMETERS. | Even though clinical research of ECochG dates back to 1930, and clinical application to the 1940s, there is no standard test protocol. Guidelines for clinical measurement of ECochG are summarized in Table 4.6. *Transducer type* is optional. Insert earphones are certainly not required, but the many advantages noted in Chapter 3 are all pertinent for evoking cochlear responses. There are two added advantages on insert earphones specific to ECochG measurement. One is the option of adapting the insert earphone to serve as a TIPtrode. The second advantage applies to ECochG measurement with either a tympanic membrane electrode or a transtympanic needle electrode. With the tympanic membrane electrode (see Figure 4.2), the insert earphone cushion can be used to secure the silastic tube against the ear canal wall and the end of the TM electrode against the TM. The insert earphone cushion also secures the lead (wire) for the transtympanic electrode (see Figure 4.3) against the external ear canal wall and maintains the tip of the needle at the promontory.

TABLE 4.6. Guidelines for Electrocochleography (ECochG) Test Protocol

PARAMETER	SUGGESTION	RATIONALE/COMMENT
Stimulus		
Transducer	ER-3A	Permits TIPtrode usage
		Secures transtympanic electrode wire
Type	Click	Produces robust response
		Evaluates cochlear function in basal turn
		Tone bursts can be used
Duration	0.1 ms	0onset response
		Longer tone burst duration to verify SP component, e.g., 2–10–2 cycle duration
Polarity	Alternating	For recording SP component (cancels out CM)
	Single polarity	When recording CM component (rarefaction and condensation separately)
Rate	7.1/sec	Low rate enhances the N1 (AP) component
		Very rapid rate is useful for SP delineation (e.g., >91/sec)
Intensity	70 to 90 dB nHL	Produces robust response (no SP for intensities below about 50 dB)
Masking	None	Never necessary
		Detectable response always is generated by test ear
Presentation	Ear	Monaural
	Mode	Air conduction
		Bone conduction may be useful in selected patients with conductive hearing loss
Acquisition		
Electrodes (options)*	TT-Ac	Very large amplitude (4 to 20 μV)
		Standard stainless steel subdermal needle for promontory site
	TM-Ai	Noninvasive, but AP rarely exceeds 0.6 μV; TIProde for EAC
	IEAC-Ac	Noninvasive and large amplitude ECochG (normally >1.0 μV)
	Fpz ground	Convenient and used for ABR
Filter	10–1500 Hz	Encompasses response
		Lower high-pass filter cutoff if possible for SP definition
Amplification	×75,000	Adequate for large response
Analysis time	5 or 15 ms	Shorter time for ECochG
		Longer time for ECochG/ABR and multichannel ECochG
Sweeps	<50 to >1500	<50 for promontory electrode
		>1500 for EAC electrode

* Options ranked according to relative effectiveness in producing a clear response; TT = transtympanic; EAC = external auditory canal; A=earlobe; i = ipsilateral to stimulus; c = contralateral to; TM = tympanic membrane

The *type of stimulus* is also optional. Clicks are by far the most commonly reported stimulus for eliciting the ECochG, but the response can also be evoked with tone burst stimuli, as noted in the discussion of stimulus parameters. Brief *stimulus duration* is essential for producing the synchronous firing of afferent auditory nerve fibers required for generating compound action potentials. *Stimulus polarity* is also a critical parameter for ECochG measurement. Alternating polarity stimuli are required to detect a clear SP and, therefore, for ECochG applications that rely on analysis of amplitude ratio for the SP versus the AP, e.g., diagnosis of Ménière's disease. Single-polarity stimuli—rarefaction and condensation—are required to elicit the CM response. Detection of a clear CM is an objective in the identification of auditory neuropathy. The choice for stimulus polarity, therefore, depends on the clinical application of the ECochG measurement. As a rule, slower *stimulus rate* is associated with larger ECochG amplitude. However, with a near-field electrode technique (e.g., transtympanic electrode), the response is typically robust and faster rates still produce adequate amplitudes for ECochG components. A very fast stimulus rate (e.g., 91.1/sec) is useful in differentiating the SP and the AP components. As stimulus presentation rate increases, amplitude of the action potentials (the AP component) gradually decreases. In contrast, SP amplitude remains unchanged. As shown in Figure 4.8, at very fast stimulus rates the SP becomes more prominent relative to the AP component. *Stimulus intensity* is typically high in ECochG measurement as the goal is to generate a clear and highly reliable response. However, in patients who cannot be assessed behaviorally and who lack a clear and reliable ABR wave V, it is possible to estimate auditory threshold with ECochG components, particularly the AP component.

ACQUISITION PARAMETERS. | The importance of the location and *type of the electrode* in ECochG measurement has been repeatedly emphasized in this chapter. ECochG quality—amplitude, morphology, and repeatability—is superior with transtympanic membrane placement of a needle on the promontory. Placement of a silver ball electrode in the round window niche is equally effective, but certainly not as convenient, for detection of the best possible ECochG. The TM electrode design offers the optimal noninvasive approach for recording a clear and easily detectable ECochG. Lacking medical support and personnel, the TM electrode is the ideal option for recording ECochG from adults undergoing diagnostic assessment. The TM electrode usually permits confident identification of all ECochG components. The TIPtrode is the least useful option and, some would argue, not even worthy of the label "an ECochG electrode." Although adequate for detection of the AP component (the ABR wave I) in all patients except those with severe high-frequency hearing loss, the TIPtrode really is not sufficient for consistently confident detection of the SP component even for patients with modest degrees of sensorineural hearing loss. Finally,

the *number of sweeps* required in ECochG measurement is highly dependent on the signal-to-noise ratio, and mostly on the magnitude of ECochG components. As few as 50 to 100 sweeps are needed to detect an unequivocal response when a very large ECochG is recorded with a transtympanic membrane electrode, whereas 2,000 or more sweeps might be needed before an AP component emerges in attempts to record the ECochG with the TIPtrode electrode option.

A general ECochG strategy is summarized as follows:

- If it is feasible, obtain and analyze the patient's audiogram. Assess low- and high-frequency hearing status. Determine the suspect ear, if possible. Decide on the most appropriate inverting electrode type (e.g., ear canal, tympanic membrane, transtympanic needle).
- Set up the equipment, and then instruct and prepare the patient.
- Apply scalp and inverting electrodes and verify impedance.
- For transtympanic (TT) electrode by a physician, anesthetize the eardrum for TT promontory electrode placement with a phenol solution (Schwaber & Hall, 1990), iontopheresis anesthesia (Roland et al., 1995), or a cream anesthetic (Bath, Beynon, Moffat, & Baguley, 1998). Place the TT electrode while visualizing the tympanic membrane under the microscope. Insert the compressed cushion (earplug) into the ear canal and attach the tubing to the transducer box. Verify the TT electrode impedance.
- For tympanic membrane (TM) electrode, the electrode can be inserted into the ear canal and placed on the TM without anesthesia. Insert the cushion (earplug) into the ear canal and attach the tubing to the transducer box. Verify TM electrode impedance. Recheck impedance to assure proper TM electrode placement. Note that TM electrode impedance is typically very high. It is appropriate to proceed with ECochG recording even when impedance is too high to be established. Adequate TM electrode placement is then verified by the presence of ECochG components with expected amplitude values in the recording.
- Record replicated (at least three separate runs) responses at a high (80 to 95 dB HL) click stimulus intensity level.
- Verify that the ECochG components are reliably recorded. For diagnosis of Ménière's disease, then calculate the SP and AP latency and amplitude, and calculate SP/AP amplitude ratio, from the sum of waveform replications. Compare the SP/AP ratio to normative data collected with equivalent measurement parameters and also compare the inter-ear symmetry of the ECochG SP/AP ratio for the patient.

A combined ECochG and ABR test protocol can be useful clinically. A two-channel (ipsilateral and contralateral) ABR is recorded with a brief analysis time (10 ms), stimulus polarity (alternating or separate averages for condensation and rarefaction polarity clicks), and slow rate (7.1/sec). The filter settings of 10 to 3000 Hz are appropriate for ECochG and ABR. The waveform in channel one is recorded with a noninverting electrode on the forehead (Fz) and an inverting transtympanic needle electrode on the promontory. In channel one, amplitude of the AP (wave I) is high (over 5 μvolts). However, because of this large amplitude of the AP (wave I), the waveform display must be reduced, and wave V is barely detected. In channel two (F_z–TIPtrode), the display gain can be increased because the amplitude of ABR wave I and wave V is equivalent. Thus, wave V is clearly detected. Three replications of at least 500 sweeps are obtained for each ear. ABR waveforms recorded in the ipsilateral electrode array are assessed for reliability, a copy of one is made, and then the three replications are summed (leaving each original waveform intact). Replicated waveforms are superimposed. Absolute latency and amplitude data for waves I, II, III, IV, and V, interwave latencies, and the wave V/I amplitude ratio, are calculated for the summed waveform.

For ECochG analysis, a horizontal electrode array may be useful in enhancing the AP component (Hall, 1992; Yellin & Chase, 1991). A horizontal array waveform can be derived by subtracting from a waveform recorded with the ipsilateral electrode array the corresponding waveform recorded with the contralateral electrode array. A copy of one of these waveforms is made. The repeatability of the SP and AP components is carefully evaluated. Then, these derived horizontal waveforms are summed. SP and AP analysis (latency, amplitude, the SP/AP amplitude ratio) is made from the summed waveform. Finally, replications are overlaid, and all waveforms are plotted.

Analysis of ABR and ECochG data for the ear stimulated first can be made while waveforms are averaged for the second ear, so that a report may be prepared immediately following data analysis, using the word processing feature of the evoked response system.

Interelectrode Impedance

In order to successfully record AERs on a consistent basis, measurement conditions should always be optimized before and throughout testing. Interelectrode electric impedance, opposition to alternating current flow between one electrode and another, is an important technical factor. It is easily measured with most commercially available evoked response systems. A small electrical current is applied automatically to one of the electrodes, and the amount of current reaching the second electrode is determined. From these data, interelectrode impedance is calculated. With some evoked response systems, the impedance test module is manually set for each possible pair of electrodes and interelectrode impedance is read directly from a meter. The tester must, for this type of evoked response impedance testing system, specifically rearrange electrodes at the switch box to measure all electrode combinations, including the ground electrode. Software-based systems facilitate impedance measurement. The tester presses the appropriate help key or enters the designated keyboard command and simply reads the automatically determined impedance values for all electrodes in all recording channels. Often, testing cannot proceed until a certain criterion for interelectrode impedance is met. Electrode impedance in each of the above examples is measured with alternating current because the electrical properties of this signal are more similar to evoked responses than direct current and also because direct current may polarize electrodes.

Electrode impedance should be measured before an AER recording session begins, and then during testing whenever there is reason to suspect a change in electrode impedance, such as increased electrical artifact or excessive patient movement. Low and balanced electrode impedance contributes to higher quality AER recordings by limiting internal noise of amplifiers, reducing the effects of externally generated electrical interference (noise), and maintaining higher common mode rejection ratios. Excessive electrical interference can be one of the most frustrating problems in AER measurement and, at the worst, may totally obliterate an AER, invalidate data, and preclude further assessment. The convention for maximum desirable interelectrode impedance is 5000 ohms (5 K ohms). Naturally, the tester attempts to keep impedance below this limit (in the range of 1000 to 5000 ohms) by using good electrode application technique. Unusually low impedance (less than 1000 ohms) is not necessarily desirable, as it may reflect a direct connection between two closely spaced electrodes and may lead to a short circuit at the amplifier input. The major determinant of interelectrode impedance that can be directly influenced by the tester is the integrity and extent of contact between an electrode and the skin. While low absolute impedance for each electrode is preferable, balanced impedance among electrodes is also an important factor. An electrode with high impedance in combination with an electrode with low impedance can create in electrical imbalance at the input to a differential amplifier (described earlier in this chapter) and lead to excessive interference from sources of electrical artifact.

The conventional guideline for acceptable balance in impedance among electrodes is for the interelectrode impedance to be within $\pm$ 2 K ohms. Every attempt should be made to keep impedance differences between electrode combinations within this range. Electrodes with relatively higher impedance should be removed and reapplied after the skin is again prepared. Sometimes, the electrode impedance can be lowered by simply pressing on the electrode for several moments, moving it slightly to better approximate the area of skin that was prepared, adding a little more conducting paste, or securing the electrode snugly with additional tape. If repeated attempts to reduce overall high electrode impedance fail, but each electrode is intact and there is at least balanced impedance among electrodes, the testing can proceed.

Experimental evidence (Eccard & Weber, 1983) and clinical experience indicates that AERs can be successfully recorded, under some environmental conditions, even with electrode impedance values of 10,000 ohms or higher, if there is interelectrode balance. The input impedance of the physiological amplifier determines the upper limit for electrode impedance in AER recordings.

Because of differences in design, particularly available surface area, optimal expected impedance values vary among electrode types. As reported by Ferraro, Murphy, and Ruth (1986), average impedance for the "eartrode" ECochG electrode is about 20 K ohms, while for the ear-canal TIPtrode type or a surface electrode on the mastoid, the impedance is typically less than 5 K ohms. High impedance values were associated with a TM electrode design described by Ruth and Lambert (1989). Electrode impedance, however, is not consistently correlated with ECochG AP amplitude nor do high electrode impedance values preclude successful ECochG measurement.

If electrodes, cables, or pins show signs of damage or excessive wear, or impedance remains high for an electrode even after conscientious preparation of the skin, then one must consider the possibility of a break in the electrical conduction capacity of the electrode. Measurement of interelectrode resistance (opposition to direct current flow presented by the structures between two electrodes) is useful in assessing the integrity of an electrode. A simple test for verifying electrode integrity can be conducted by plugging the electrode pins in the usual way, placing the electrodes in water (using a cup, an emesis tray, etc), and then checking impedance. If the electrode is intact, interelectrode impedance should be very low (0 or 1 kohms).

ECochG WAVEFORM ANALYSIS AND INTERPRETATION

The test protocol dictates which ECochG components (CM, SP or AP) will be recorded. The CM is best detected with single-polarity (rarefaction or condensation) signals, whereas the SP and AP are clearer with either alternating-polarity signals or the mathematical summing of the responses for each of the single-polarity signals. ECochG components almost always occur within the first two to three milliseconds after a transient acoustic stimulus, such as a click or tone burst. That is, latency of the response is relatively consistent. Response morphology and amplitude are, however, highly dependent on a variety of measurement parameters such as stimulus intensity, rate, and polarity, and electrode location. Following is a discussion of each of these three general ECochG analysis strategies: (1) calculation of the amplitude of the major components and, in the diagnosis of Ménière's disease, a comparison of the relative amplitudes for the SP and AP components, i.e., the SP/AP ratio; (2) latency analysis for the AP component and, for diagnosis of Ménière's disease,

a comparison of the latency difference for the AP component evoked with signals of rarefaction versus condensation polarity; and (3) calculation of the duration of the SP and AP complex and, in a variation of this analysis approach, calculation of the area under the SP and AP components. For clinical applications of ECochG, the calculations made with each of these three analysis approaches are compared to normative data, collected with an equivalent test protocol. Normative data for one of the techniques—analysis of ECochG amplitude—are displayed in the appendix. The application of analysis techniques in auditory pathologies and the subject and pathologic factors influencing ECochG outcome (e.g., degree of hearing loss, duration of disease, status of symptoms) are reviewed in Chapter 5.

Latency Analysis

Calculation of the absolute latency of components of any auditory evoked response is a fundamental analysis strategy. For all clinical applications of ECochG, one of the initial steps in waveform analysis is the identification of a reliable AP component and, using a cursor to mark the peak, manual measurement of the AP latency (refer to Figure 4.10). In normal ears, latency is slightly shorter for AP components evoked with rarefaction versus condensation signals. There is some evidence that this normal latency difference associated with signal polarity is more pronounced for persons with Ménière's disease and absent or even reversed for persons with other etiologies for cochlear hearing loss.

Amplitude Analysis

An ECochG waveform and labeling schema is shown in Figure 4.10. Typically, the peak in SP and AP amplitude in μV is calculated from a baseline. The use of a prestimulus period of averaging (e.g., 1 to 2 ms) facilitates determination of a stable waveform baseline for these measurements. Some authors (e.g., Ge & Shea, 2002) describe measurement of the SP amplitude from the baseline to the notch between the SP and AP peaks, rather than the actual peak of the SP. With tone-burst signals of extended duration, the SP amplitude can also be measured from a point on the SP plateau after the AP to the pre- or post-SP baseline. Early investigators of ECochG as a diagnostic procedure in Ménière's disease (e.g., Coats, 1981) noted the large intersubject variability in the absolute amplitude of SP and the AP components. The SP/AP ratio was considered a more repeatable and the SP/AP ratio, stated either as a decimal (e.g., 0.4) or a percent (e.g., 40%), is then calculated by dividing the SP amplitude by the AP amplitude. For the application of ECochG in diagnosis of Ménière's disease, the most common analysis approach is the calculation of SP and AP amplitude (in μV) from a common baseline, and then the calculation of the SP/AP ratio (see Figure 4.10). When the ECochG components are large and noise is minimal, the ECochG analysis and calculations can be made from a single averaged waveform.

ECochG Analysis

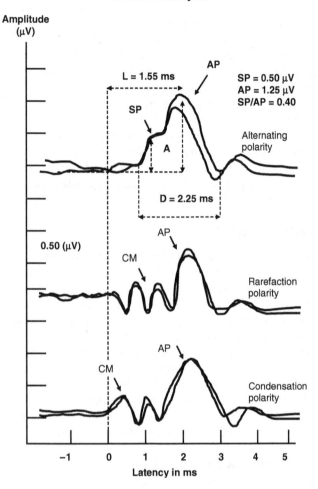

ECochG in Ménière's Disease

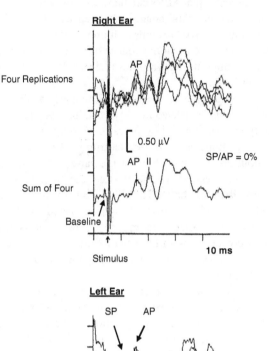

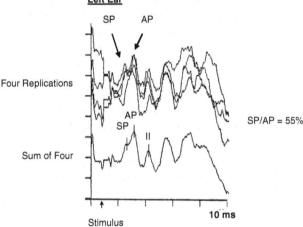

FIGURE 4.10. Schematic diagram an ECochG waveform illustrating the calculation and analysis of amplitude for the SP, CM, and AP components, including definition of the baseline and duration measures, the latency of the AP component, and the duration of the ECochG complex.

FIGURE 4.11. Replicated ECochG waveforms and a summed waveform. Reliability of separate waveforms is first verified. The amplitude and latency calculation and analysis is performed for ECochG components in the summed waveform.

The confident analysis of ECochG waveforms is improved by performing latency and amplitude calculations on the sum of two or more waveforms, after each is first averaged separately (Figure 4.11).

Duration Analysis

Beginning with the earliest published reports of ECochG in the diagnosis of Ménière's disease, duration or width of the SP and AP components in combination has been offered as a measurement parameter for ECochG, especially for diagnosis of Ménière's disease (Ferraro & Tibbils, 1999; Ge & Shea, 2002). The duration analysis technique is illustrated in Figure 4.10. Based on a literature review, this analysis strategy is apparently not utilized in other clinical applications of ECochG. The time in ms is determined from the beginning to the end of the SP/AP complex. The initial

width measurement point is the deviation from baseline of the leading edge of the SP/AP wave complex. A straight line from the baseline preceding the SP/AP complex is extended out in time (to the right). The width of the SP/AP portion of the waveform, in ms, is defined from the onset to the point where the waveform returns to the baseline. The suspected mechanism underlying the prolongation in the SP/AP width, at least in Ménière's disease, is slowed velocity of the traveling wave within the cochlear secondary to restricted basilar membrane movement with increased loading in endolymphatic hydrops (Ferraro & Tibbils, 1999). Preliminary evidence suggests that ECochG sensitivity in the diagnosis of Ménière's disease may also be enhanced by analysis of the SP/AP area measure, especially in patients whose diagnosis was categorized as probable (as compared to definite).

Area under the Curve

A third ECochG analysis strategy involves calculation of the area encompassed by the SP/AP waveform complex, or the "area under the curve." The product of this calculation is essentially a combination of the data from the amplitude and width analysis approaches. Indeed, one motivation for the development of this analysis approach is an appreciation that the SP/AP ratio is characterized by less than optimal sensitivity (60 to 65%) in the diagnosis of Ménière's disease. Perhaps because the area under the ECochG curve could not be calculated with some clinical ECochG systems, relatively few investigators have employed this promising technique (Ferraro & Tibbils, 1999; Ge & Shea, 2002; Morrison, Moffatt, & O'Connor, 1980).

Nonpathologic Factors in ECochG Analysis

STIMULUS FACTORS. | As expected, AP latency decreases slightly and amplitude increases markedly as stimulus intensity is increased. The SP is not observed at lower intensity levels (usually below 60 dB peSPL). A monophasic (rarefaction or condensation) stimulus polarity, as opposed to an alternating stimulus polarity, produces a CM component and perhaps latency differences in the SP and AP components. Increasing stimulus rate eventually reduces AP amplitude, whereas the SP characteristically remains unchanged. Extending duration of a tone-burst stimulus likewise produces a correspondingly extended SP waveform that can be distinguished from the AP component near the onset of the stimulus. ECochG morphology also changes dramatically for click versus tone-burst stimuli, and also for low- versus high-frequency tone-burst stimuli.

ABNORMAL PATTERNS. | Assuming that the normal ECochG waveform has a robust AP component, immediately preceded by a distinct yet relatively small amplitude SP component, there are two general types of abnormal ECochG waveforms. When the AP is of small amplitude, or not reliably recorded, the SP is almost never observed. Most manipulations of measurement parameters used to enhance ABR wave I amplitude are equally valuable in recording a more distinct ECochG. Among them, increasing stimulus intensity, decreasing stimulus rate, and moving the recording electrode closer to the cochlear are characteristically effective in producing a larger response. The most common cause of a reduced ECochG response clinically is cochlear pathology with associated sensory hearing impairment, particularly affecting the higher frequency region (above 1000 Hz). With the second type of abnormal ECochG waveform, there are clear SP and AP components, but SP amplitude is atypically large in comparison to AP amplitude. This finding is associated with Ménière's disease (endolymphatic hydrops). The actual criteria for interpretation of an enlarged SP/AP relation depend on test parameters, especially electrode site as noted throughout this chapter and the next chapter as well.

ECochG Electrode Problems

Although the list of general problems that may develop in ECochG recording is long, many can be solved with optimal electrode placement. ECochG activity arising from the cochlea and distal (cochlear end) eighth nerve is best measured with a near-field technique. The concept of near- versus far-field electrophysiologic recording was explained in Chapter 2. Therefore, response amplitude increases substantially as the recording electrode approaches the cochlea. For a normal ear, SP or AP components of the ECochG as detected with a promontory electrode (resting on the outer wall of the cochlea) are from ten to even twenty times larger than those detected with an electrode located in the ear canal. The large amplitude the near-field ECochG response serves to overcome various clinical measurement problems. Response reliability (repeatability), often poor with ear-canal electrodes, is typically excellent with the promontory electrode site. With a promontory or TM electrode site, ECochG components are usually identified confidently even from patients with serious hearing impairment, whereas these patients usually do not show a clear response with a more distant electrode site. Finally, because the near-field response is so much larger, the signal-to-noise ratio is corresponding smaller. The clinical advantage is that far fewer sweeps (stimulus repetitions) are required to detect a response.

Effect of Electrode Location on ECochG

Electrode location is the most important measurement factor influencing ECochG outcome. There are clear clinical advantages and disadvantages associated with major electrode types and locations, as summarized in Table 4.7. In studies published initially in the 1960s, ECochG recordings were conducted with a noninverting electrode, often a silver ball, placed on the promontory (on the medial wall of the middle ear space) or on the round window. Typically, the ECochG was recorded from patients with perforated tympanic membranes or following surgical exposure of the middle ear (Lempert, Wever, & Lawrence, 1947; Perlman & Case, 1941; Ruben et al., 1960, 1961). With the advent of signal averaging in the late 1960s, subsequent investigators demonstrated the clinical feasibility of nonsurgical TT needle insertion for electrode placement (Aran & LeBert, 1968; Sohmer & Feinmesser, 1967; Yoshie, Ohashi, & Suzuki, 1967). Since the promontory electrode site is close to the ECochG generators (the cochlea and eighth nerve), the ECochG recorded with this electrode array is a near-field response, and the SP and AP components are typically large and easy to detect, even at low intensity levels and with minimal averaging. Amplitude is, for example, on the order of ten times larger than recordings made from the TM, twenty times larger than ear-canal

TABLE 4.7. Clinical Advantages and Limitations of Electrode Techniques in Different ECochG Clinical Applications

ELECTRODE LOCATION (TYPE)	PREFERRED APPLICATIONS	ADVANTAGE(S)	DISADVANTAGE(S)
Ear canal (TIPtrode)	Enhancement of ABR wave I Detection of CM in auditory neuropathy	Noninvasive Patient comfort	Small amplitude Low reliability for SP Limited value in hearing loss
Tympanic membrane	ECochG in Ménière's disease	Noninvasive Fair amplitude	Requires technical skill Some patient discomfort
Promontory (trans-tympanic needle)	ECochG in Ménière's disease Intraoperative monitoring	Large amplitude Very reliable Stable placement	Invasive technique Requires local anesthesia Requires medical personnel

(e.g., TIPtrode) recordings, and as much as fifty times larger than mastoid recordings. The result is accurate, ear-specific electrophysiologic assessment of auditory thresholds without the need for masking. The clinical limitation of the technique, however, is clear. Reliance on a TT electrode renders ECochG an invasive procedure that cannot be carried out by most nonsurgeon clinicians.

The invasiveness and technical difficulty of the conventional transtympanic electrode ECochG technique was, in fact, a major reason why, in the mid-1970s, clinicians quickly turned to ABR as the electrophysiologic measure of choice for assessment of peripheral auditory status. The growth in ABR clinical popularity took place despite the publication of series of papers by an international collection of investigators in the early late 1960s and early 1970s describing the first generation of ear-canal electrodes for ECochG recording (Coats & Dickey, 1970; Cullen, Ellis, Berlin, & Lousteau, 1972; Elberling & Saloman, 1973; Khecheniashvili & Kevanishvili, 1974; Yoshie, Ohashi, & Suzuki, 1967). Some of these electrode techniques, unfortunately, still required the insertion of a needle into the ear-canal wall or the TM and were potentially as painful and invasive as the transtympanic approach.

The effect of the inverting electrode site on the ECochG waveform is clear when recordings are made simultaneously with TT and ear canal (TIPtrode) electrode designs (shown in Figure 4.5). For each of five patients, the AP component was more easily identified and more reliable with the TT electrode design. With the TT electrode design, AP amplitude is often 5 μV or more, even for persons with hearing loss of 50 dB HL or greater. With the TIPtrode design, however, the AP component is typically less than 0.5 μV, even in normal-hearing persons. Therefore, a distinct and reliable AP can be detected with as few as 25 to 50 stimulus presentations (sweeps) for the TT electrode approach, whereas for the TIPtrode electrode up to 2,000 or more sweeps may be required for confident identification of the AP component. Speed of ECochG data collection is particularly important for intraoperative monitoring applications.

Differences in ECochG amplitudes are also clearly apparent with TT versus tympanic membrane TM recordings. In a study of patients with suspected Ménière's disease Haapaniemi et al. (2000), for example, reported that amplitudes of the AP component were four to six times larger for the TT electrode design. The average amplitude of the AP component was 14 to 19.5 μV for the TT electrode, in comparison to 2 to 3.7 μV for the TM electrode. Similarly, SP amplitude values ranged from 3.5 to 5.8 μV for the TT electrode versus 0.8 to 1.6 μV for the TM electrode. As expected, the SP/AP ratio was lower with ECochG recordings from the TT electrode in comparison to the TM electrode.

The focus of this discussion has been on the inverting electrode site. Various noninverting electrode locations are reported, including the mastoid or earlobe ipsilateral to the stimulus or earlobe, the contralateral mastoid or earlobe, the forehead and the nasion. Recording ECochG with noninverting and inverting electrodes located on the same side (ipsilaterally) may yield slightly smaller AP amplitude. An inverting electrode site ipsilateral to the stimulus is clearly active, since it is routinely used to record ABR wave I. A horizontal electrode array for the noninverting and inverting electrodes (e.g., contralateral-to-ipsilateral ear canals) is therefore preferable, even though early ABR waves (II, III, IV) may be apparent in the ECochG waveform. Use of a Fz or Cz site for the noninverting electrode, with the inverting electrode on the ear ipsilateral to the stimulus, or the conventional ABR electrode array, is an alternative, although not typically employed for ECochG recording.

Waveform polarity may become inverted as the second electrode site is relocated with respect to the cochlea. With an electrode array consisting of a noninverting electrode on the vertex or forehead and an inverting electrode near the ear (mastoid, earlobe, or external ear canal, tympanic membrane, or even promontory), the AP component is positive in voltage (plotted upwards). It cannot be properly referred to as "N1." However, if the noninverting electrode is relatively close to the cochlea and the inverting electrode is relatively far away (e.g., vertex or opposite ear), a negative-going AP (an "N1") will be recorded. A negative-going waveform format is often utilized in recording and reporting ECochGs (e.g., Ferraro & Tibbils, 1999; Sparacino et al., 2000). Consistent with the convention for recording major components as positive waves for ABR, AMLR, and later cortical AERs, the author records ECochG components in the positive-upward format, and ECochG components are plotted with positive upward in this text. Reversing the noninverting and inverting electrodes in the pair will simply invert the polarity of the waveform.

RELIABILITY. | Reliability is a basic feature of test performance. In the literature, reliability is also referred to as response repeatability and reproducibility. As with other clinical audiologic procedures, test reliability for ECochG has been inadequately studied. Reliability is clearly higher when ECochG is recorded with TT versus ear-canal electrodes, especially at lower stimulus intensity levels and/or in patients with hearing loss. However, more detailed information on reliability is needed as diagnostic significance may be attached to changes in ECochG over time and before versus after treatment. One of the few formal investigations of ECochG intra- and intertest reliability was reported by a group of Swedish investigators (Densert et al., 1994). Intratest reliability was defined for multiple runs (averaged waveforms) within a single ECochG measurement, whereas intertest measurements were made before and after replacement of all recording electrodes at the same test session. ECochG was recorded with a TT technique from 17 normal subjects and 26 patients diagnosed with Ménière's disease using click and tone-burst (1000, 2000, and 4000 Hz) stimuli presented at slow (10/second) and faster (90/second) rates. Notably, the authors noted "the majority of patients reported the presence of aural fullness at the time of investigation." ECochG response parameters analyzed included absolute amplitudes for the SP and AP components, the SP/AP ratio, and the width of the SP/AP complex. Predictably, intratest reliability was consistently higher (variability lower) than intertest reliability, and variability was greater (reliability lower) for patients with Ménière's disease than normal subjects. Also, consistent with earlier reports (Margolis et al., 1992), variability was substantially greater for ECochG recorded with tone burst signals in comparison to clicks. The smallest variability was noted for the SP/AP ratio and the width measure, whereas repeatability was higher for the SP measure and especially with tone-burst stimulation. Less than 35 percent of the intertest variability could be accounted for by electrode replacement. Other factors, such as biological fluctuations, interelectrode impedance, slight differences in electrode location within a region (promontory, round window, TM, or ear canal), and the method used for calculation of response parameters, contributed importantly to intertest variability.

Margolis et al. (1992) reported intrasubject versus intersubject reliability findings in normal subjects and patients with Ménière's disease for latency and amplitude of the SP and AP components and for the SP/AP ratio. ECochG was recorded with a tympanic membrane electrode. As expected, intersubject variability was greater than intrasubject variability. However, AP latency was characterized by remarkably low intersubject variability with a range for 13 normal subjects of only 2.07 to 2.34 ms. Intersubject variability was much greater for AP amplitude than latency at all signal intensity levels. Also, perhaps not as expected, differences in AP latency for rarefaction, condensation, and alternating polarity signals for normal subjects were not statistically significant, and intrasubject reliability was lower for the SP/AP ratio than it was for AP amplitude.

Schwaber and Hall (1990) examined differences in variability of ECochG SP and AP components recorded with an external ear canal (TIPtrode) versus transtympanic membrane (TT) technique. The authors' simplified TT ECochG technique was described earlier in this chapter. Three groups of subjects were studied: (1) five patients assessed diagnostically for Ménière's disease in a clinic setting, (2) five patients with Ménière's disease monitored with ECochG while undergoing endolymphatic sac decompression surgery, and (3) five patients monitored with ECochG and ABR while undergoing surgical removal of an acoustic neuroma. Amplitude for the AP component and the SP/AP amplitude ratio was analyzed for three replications of waveforms recorded simultaneously with the two electrode types. With data from each ECochG waveform replication (1, 2, and 3), variability in absolute amplitude and in the SP/AP ratio was calculated using the following equation:

$$\frac{(AP1 - AP2) + (AP2 - AP3) + (AP1 - AP3)}{\text{mean AP amplitude}} \times 100$$

Variability for the SP component could not be assessed because it could not be confidently detected with the TIPtrode electrode for two of the clinic patients, two of the patients undergoing endolymphatic sac surgery, and all five of the patients undergoing acoustic tumor removal. Variability for both ECochG response parameters is clearly lower (reliability higher) for the TT electrode type.

Analysis Time Period

An analysis time in the range of 5 to 10 ms is typically used for ECochG measurement. With the customary minimum of 256 or 512 data points distributed across this period, temporal resolution (the time interval between any two consecutive sample points) is 0.04 ms or better (a shorter interval), which is more than adequate to define a response waveform. An analysis time of 5 ms may be preferable for recording the ECochG, because potentially larger amplitude and later latency brainstem components (e.g., ABR wave V) are eliminated from analysis. If the clinical objective, however, is combined recording of ECochG and ABR, then an analysis time of 10 ms or even 15 ms is appropriate. Latency of the ECochG AP component is prolonged for low-frequency tonal stimuli (e.g., a 500 Hz tone burst) presented at reduced effective intensity levels (close to normal threshold or to patients with peripheral auditory deficits). In these instances, an analysis time of greater than 5 ms is required to ensure that the entire response is visible.

The Relation between Onset of Stimulus and Analysis Time

Commercially available evoked response systems have an option for altering the relationship between stimulus onset and the initiation of analysis. With this option, averaging can begin before or after the stimulus is presented, as well as the conventional synchronous triggering of averaging with stimulus presentation. Some systems offer a fixed pre- or poststimulus time period option (e.g., 10% of the entire analysis time will be devoted to one or the other selection). Other systems allow the tester to specify the amount of analysis time to be allotted to the pre- or poststimulus period. Use of a prestimulus period of data collection (averaging) is a handy technique for assessing the level of EEG activity unrelated to the stimulus. Response-related electrical activity does not begin until after the stimulus is presented. The prestimulus baseline activity reflects the state of patient activity more accurately than a no-stimulus average because it is based on simultaneously recorded EEG. That is, the prestimulus baseline reflects the patient's activity level during the AER recording. A prestimulus baseline time that is approximately 10 percent of total analysis time is usually an appropriate selection. Delaying the averaging process until a brief time after stimulus presentation can effectively reduce or eliminate stimulus artifact from the waveform and prevent the evoked response system from locking up in the artifact rejection mode due to stimulus-related electromagnetic activity. If insert earphones and sound delivery tubes are used for stimulus presentation, however, this function of poststimulus delay is not required.

One must remember that the amount of analysis time available for averaging the response is reduced when the prestimulus baseline time is employed. The response analysis time is equal to the total analysis time minus the prestimulus baseline time. For example, with an ABR analysis time of 15 ms and with a 10 percent prestimulus baseline time, averaging the response (poststimulus) occurs over a 13.5 ms period. Clearly, a total analysis time of 10 ms is not advised if a pre- or poststimulus baseline is employed. Selection of a pre- or poststimulus time exceeding the total analysis time is not permitted by commercially available systems. Also, latency cursors for evoked response systems automatically account for pre- or poststimulus times and will also correct for the time delay caused by insert earphone sound delivery tubes (about 0.9 ms for the ER-3A tube, i.e., when averaging began, not when the stimulus was presented) as zero time.

STIMULUS FACTORS. | As expected, AP latency decreases slightly and amplitude increases markedly as stimulus intensity is increased. The SP is not observed at lower intensity levels (usually below an intensity level of 60 dB peSPL). A monophasic (rarefaction or condensation) stimulus polarity, as opposed to an alternating stimulus polarity, produces a CM component and perhaps latency differences in the SP and AP components. Increasing stimulus rate eventually reduces AP amplitude, whereas the SP characteristically remains unchanged. Extending duration of a tone-burst stimulus likewise produces a correspondingly extended SP waveform that can be distinguished from the AP component near the onset of the stimulus. That is, the AP occurs only following the beginning of the stimulus, whereas the SP persists throughout the stimulus presentation. ECochG morphology also changes dramatically for click versus tone-burst stimuli, and also for low- versus high-frequency tone-burst stimuli.

ABNORMAL PATTERNS. | Assuming that the normal ECochG waveform has a robust AP component, immediately preceded by a distinct yet relatively small amplitude SP component, there are two general types of abnormal ECochG waveforms. One is little or no response under typical clinical measurement conditions. When the AP is of small amplitude, or not reliably recorded, the SP is almost never observed. Most manipulations of measurement parameters used to enhance ABR wave I amplitude are equally valuable in recording a more distinct ECochG. Among them, increasing stimulus intensity, decreasing stimulus rate, and moving the recording electrode closer to the cochlear are the characteristically effective in producing a larger response. The most common cause of a reduced ECochG response clinically is cochlear pathology with associated sensory hearing impairment, particularly affecting the higher frequency region (above 1000 Hz). With the second type of abnormal ECochG waveform, there are clear SP and AP components, but SP amplitude is atypically large in comparison to AP amplitude. This finding is associated with Ménière's disease (endolymphatic hydrops). The actual criteria for interpretation of an enlarged SP/AP relation depend on test parameters, especially electrode site, as just noted.

Age

INFANCY AND CHILDHOOD. | A clear ECochG N1 component is normally recorded as early as 27 weeks conceptional age. In comparison to adult values, latency is prolonged and amplitude reduced (Stockard, Stockard, & Coen, 1983). The discovery that ECochG could be reliably recorded from normal-hearing infants and young children contributed to the early interest in the application of ECochG in the "objective" assessment of hearing function in this population (Cullen, Ellis, Berlin, & Lousteau, 1972; Eggermont, 1976a,b; Ruben, Bordley, & Lieberman, 1961; Yoshie, 1973). Still, the relationship among ECochG, young age, and stimulus parameters in human subjects is not well studied. A major reason for the relative scarcity of research is probably the requirement of an invasive recording technique (TT needle electrode) or specially designed electrodes that were not commercially available. Application of the TT technique in children requires deep sedation or general anesthesia (Aran & Charlet de Savage, 1976; Eggermont & Odenthal, 1974a,b; Naunton & Zerlin, 1976; Yoshie, 1973), whereas local anesthesia of the TM is adequate for cooperative adults. Virtually all of the electrophysiologic studies of the development of cochlear function are experimental and based on animal models.

The main objective of most ECochG studies was to assess the relation between ECochG and behavioral hearing threshold levels, rather than to examine waveform characteristics (e.g. CM, SP, and AP) as a function of age. Thresholds for ECochG and behavioral testing may be within ± 10 dB in normal hearing subjects, hearing-impaired children, and adults with high-frequency sensorineural loss when TT recordings are made (Eggermont, 1976a,b; Eggermont & Odenthal, 1974a,b; Naunton & Zerlin, 1976; Spoor & Eggermont, 1976a,b; Yoshie, 1973). Accuracy of hearing threshold estimation with ear-canal electrode placement ECochG is poorer for persons with low-frequency hearing loss. In any event, with the availability of ABR there is now little clinical demand for the evaluation of hearing sensitivity with ECochG. The new generation of noninvasive tympanic membrane electrodes, however, may well encourage renewed interest in ECochG clinical study of the developing auditory periphery.

A clinical investigation by Schwartz, Pratt, and Schwartz (1989) provided evidence that CM and SP components can be consistently recorded even in preterm newborn infants. ABR was recorded from both ears of 20 newborn infants with ages of conception ranging from 35 to 38 weeks (a full-term birth occurs at 40 weeks). Responses were detected with conventional cup electrodes located on the vertex (non-inverting) and both the stimulus ipsilateral and contralateral earlobes (inverting). A CM and SP component appeared in composite waveforms for 40 ears of 20 newborn infants for single-polarity (rarefaction or condensation) click stimuli. As expected, when the waveforms for rarefaction and condensation stimuli were added together, the CM was eliminated and the SP remained. Detection of the CM component in infants is now a primary objective in the diagnosis of auditory neuropathy, as discussed in Chapter 5.

ADVANCING AGE IN ADULTS. | In contrast to the extensive literature on age and gender influences on ABR, there is little written about the effect of these factors on ECochG. One study by Chatrian et al. (1985), although quite thorough, yielded a confusing set of findings. That is, age-related differences were observed, but not consistently for each response parameter. SP detection level (in dB) was positively correlated with age (higher intensity was required to detect a response in older subjects), whereas SP amplitude decreased as a function of age (only for the left ear). There was a strong negative correlation between AP amplitude and age and, as a result, a positive correlation between the SP/AP ratio and age. With advancing age, amplitude of the AP component decreases relatively more than amplitude of the SP component. Therefore, the SP/AP ratio increases with age.

Chatrian et al. (1985) recorded no significant difference between male versus female adults for detection of the SP, the SP onset time, SP peak latency, or for the duration of the SP/AP complex. SP amplitude, on the other hand, was significantly larger for females than males but, curiously, only for the left ear. As an aside, a significantly larger average SP was produced with right- than left-ear stimulation. Significantly larger AP amplitude was consistently recorded for females versus males, yet the SP/AP ratio was equivalent between sexes. Coats (1986) similarly reported a generally greater SP amplitude, and especially AP amplitude, for women versus men, and for right- versus left-ear stimulation.

Advancing age influences auditory system functioning, including activity of the cochlear and eighth nerve. Therefore, it would not be unreasonable to expect age-related changes in CM, SP, and AP components of the ECochG. This issue has not, apparently, been systematically investigated. Two likely reasons for this lack of research are the requirement, until recently, of an invasive recording technique and the fact that clinical demands for ECochG (e.g., intraoperative monitoring and Ménière's disease) are infrequent among the elderly. It is important to keep in mind, however, that an unselected population of older subjects would be expected to have high-frequency sensorineural hearing deficit (presbycusis) and, as a consequence, show an altered ECochG. For example, the click-stimulated ECochG AP component is dependent on high-frequency hearing and would, therefore, probably be characterized by an increase in latency and reduction in amplitude in the average older subject.

BODY TEMPERATURE

Body temperature is, obviously, a characteristic feature of every patient. If normal temperature (37 degrees centigrade or 98.6 degrees Fahrenheit) is verified at the time of testing, then there is no need to further account for temperature in the interpretation of AER data. Temperature exceeding ± 1 degree from this value (i.e., below 36 degrees centigrade or above 38 degrees) must be considered as a possible factor in AER outcome. Patients at risk for temperature aberrations include those with infection (high temperature) and those in a coma or under the effects of alcohol or anesthesia (low temperature).

The effect of low body temperature (hypothermia) on the ECochG was investigated extensively for a variety of animal models (see Hall, Bull, & Cronau, 1988, for review). Clinically, most reports of ABR in hypothermia describe changes observed during open-heart surgery. Alterations in auditory electrophysiology related to low body temperature are summarized as follows. In vitro depolarization in membrane potentials (a decrease) is recorded in supporting cells (Hensen's) of the organ of Corti (Santos-Sacchi, 1986). CM amplitude is reversibly reduced, while CM latency shows little or no change (Butler, Konishi, & Fernandez, 1960; Coats, 1965; DeBrey & Eggermont, 1978; Kahana, Rosenblith, & Galambos, 1950). Variable changes during hypothermia are found for the summating potential (Butler, Konishi, & Fernandez, 1960; Manley & Johnstone, 1974). Basilar membrane traveling wave transit time is increased (DeBrey & Eggermont, 1978).

Lowered temperature also produces a reversible reduction in eighth nerve compound action potential (ECochG N1 component and ABR wave I) amplitude and a reversible increase of N1 (wave I) latency (Kahana, Rosenblith, & Galambos, 1950). An initial effect of hypothermia may be the selective loss of auditory sensitivity for high-frequency signals, as estimated electrophysiologically (Manley & Johnstone, 1974). Also, synaptic transmission is delayed and axonal conduction velocity is decreased.

ATTENTION AND STATE OF AROUSAL

Muscular and movement artifact is a major source of unwanted noise in the recording of AERs and can seriously reduce the signal-to-noise ratio. Therefore, it is customary during clinical measurement of the shorter latency responses (ECochG and ABR) to encourage natural sleep or induce medically a drowsy or sleep state. In addition, AERs are relied on as a measure of auditory sensitivity in patients who, for a variety of causes, are lethargic, in a stupor, generally unresponsive behaviorally, or even in coma. The effect of state of arousal increases progressively as latency of the AER increases. Unlike most subject characteristics, state of arousal often can be manipulated and, for this reason, should be appreciated by the tester. The optimal subject state of arousal for each AER varies substantially. For example, a deeply sleeping subject is ideal for measurement of short-latency responses such as the ECochG, whereas subject attention or at least an awake state is required for later responses.

Most available clinical evidence indicates no difference in ECochG waveforms recorded in the awake versus natural sleep state for moderate-to-high stimulus intensity levels (Amadeo & Shagass, 1973; Jewett & Williston, 1971;

Osterhammel, Shallop, & Terkildsen, 1985; Picton et al., 1974; Sohmer & Student, 1978) or for low intensity stimuli close to auditory threshold. Sleep state is best verified and quantified by EEG recordings interpreted by an experienced electroencephalographer. Even extremely reduced states of arousal, such as narcolepsy (Hellekson et al., 1979) and metabolic coma (Hall, 1988; Hall, Hargadine, & Kim, 1985; Hall, Huangfu, & Gennarelli, 1982; Starr, 1976; Sutton et al., 1982) have no serious effect on ECochG latency or amplitude). The independence of ECochG/ABR and state of arousal constitutes a major advantage for clinical evaluation of peripheral and central auditory function of a wide variety of patients.

Muscle/Movement Artifact

In comparison to later latency AERs, the ECochG components occurring within 2 or 3 ms period after a stimulus are minimally affected by muscle activity. A quiet patient state contributes to less background noise and facilitates detection of even a small amplitude response. Random movement related artifact confounds ECochG interpretation, especially identification of the SP component. The SP often appears as a hump on the upward slope of the AP. False identification of the SP is more likely when excessive movement artifact is present in the waveform, particularly without strict criteria for reliability. The author is unaware of publications specifically addressing the effect of muscle artifact in ECochG measurement.

CONCLUSIONS

For assessing cochlear function, regardless of the actual clinical objective, the AER technique of choice is ECochG. The overall objective is confident identification of CM, SP, and/or AP components. The specific procedure to be followed, particularly the electrode type that is used, will vary depending on a variety of factors, e.g., the diagnostic objective, hearing status, age of the patient (infant versus adult), and the availability of medical support. Although patient comfort is a factor to be taken into account in the decision regarding electrode type (Beynon, Clarke, & Baguley, 1995), most patients will gladly tolerate some discomfort for procedures that are likely to contribute to the diagnosis of their disorder. Two specific examples of the clinical application of ECochG are diagnosis of auditory neuropathy and Ménière's disease. The application of ECochG in these and other patient populations is reviewed in the next chapter.

5

CHAPTER

ECochG
Clinical Applications and Populations

Nowadays, ECochG is not just for the diagnosis of Ménière's disease. Although the diagnostic value of ECochG in Ménière's disease is well appreciated, other clinical applications of ECochG in other clinical populations are more common and, perhaps, of more interest to some audiologists (see Table 5.1). ECochG can certainly be applied independently as an electrophysiological measure of auditory function in specific diseases and pathologies. The disease-specific application of ECochG is perhaps best illustrated by its use in Ménière's disease, but, as delineated in this chapter, ECochG may also contribute to the diagnosis of other clinical entities. More commonly, however, ECochG is recorded in combination with the ABR with the goal of describing of the extent (degree) and anatomic site of auditory dysfunction or

TABLE 5.1. Common Clinical ECochG Applications

APPLICATION	RATIONALE
Enhancement of ABR Wave I	ECochG maximizes the AP amplitude. A clear wave I is very important in neurodiagnostic ABR recordings. Wave I permits calculation of interwave latency values (minimal influence by peripheral hearing status).
Diagnosis of Auditory Neuropathy	Detection of cochlear microphonic (CM) confirms outer hair cell function. CM may be present in patients without OAEs. Detection of summating potential provides evidence of inner hair cell function. Detection of ECochG AP provides evidence of integrity of inner hair cells (IHCs) and synapse communication between IHCs and afferent auditory fibers (spiral ganglion).
Diagnosis of Ménière's disease	Ménière's disease is characterized by abnormally large EcochG SP component. Repeatable SP and AP are recorded; AP amplitudes are calculated from a common baseline. The SP/AP ratio is calculated. Patient's SP/AP ratio is compared for the ear suspected of Ménière's involvment vs. the opposite ear. A patient's SP/AP ratio is compared for the ear suspected of Ménière's involvement vs. normative data.
Intraoperative Monitoring	ECochG parameters maximize the AP (wave I) amplitude. A clear wave I is very important in intraoperative ABR recordings. The AP (wave I) component is a measure of peripheral (cochlear) status. A large wave I (e.g., > 5 μV) can be recorded quickly (<1 minute) in patients with serious hearing loss. Wave I permits calculation of interwave latency values. Interwave latencies are not seriously influenced by peripheral hearing status. Transtympanic technique (Schwaber & Hall, 1990) is optimal for the intraoperative application of ECochG.

in monitoring status of the auditory system. And, as noted in the preceding chapter, the concepts and principles underlying ECochG measurement can be incorporated into ABR test protocols to enhance the detection of a component (e.g., ABR wave I in severe hearing loss or during intraoperative monitoring) or to differentiate among sites of auditory dysfunction, as in the diagnosis of "auditory neuropathy." I encourage the reader to approach this chapter with open mind and broad perspective, guided by the rather general question, How can ECochG contribute to the audiologic assessment of my patients?

ASSESSMENT OF PERIPHERAL HEARING LOSS

Estimation of Auditory Threshold

Prior to the emergence of ABR as a clinical procedure, ECochG was the technique of choice for electrophysiological assessment of auditory function. As early as the 1960s, Ruben and colleagues at Johns Hopkins Medical Center applied ECochG in the estimation of auditory thresholds in children who could not be properly assessed with behavioral audiometry (Ruben, Bordley, & Lieberman, 1961). ECochG was also applied in pediatric assessment around the world by other investigators during the 1970s (e.g., Aran, 1971; Eggermont & Odenthal, 1974a; Yoshie, 1973). With the growing popularity of ABR in the late 1970s and throughout the 1980s, ECochG was largely abandoned as a procedure in the pediatric audiology test battery. The shift from ECochG to the ABR in clinical settings was particularly rapid in the United States where audiologists, rather than physicians, are typically responsible for hearing assessment of children. Interestingly, ECochG is now once again a part of the pediatric audiologic test battery due to its newly discovered value in the diagnosis of "auditory neuropathy." This topic is reviewed in a later section of the chapter.

The ECochG recorded with a transtympanic (TT) needle technique continues to be applied selectively for assessment of auditory sensitivity in children, at least by clinical investigators located outside of the United States (Aso & Gibson, 1994; Bellman, Barnard, & Beagley, 1984; Conti, Arslan, Camurri, et al., 1984; Dauman, 1991; Ferron, Ouellet, Rouillard, & Desgange, 1983; Prijs, 1991; Ryerson & Beagley, 1981; Schoonhoven, Lamore, de Laat, & Grote, 1999). The use of an invasive TT placement of an electrode near the round window for recording ECochG, reminiscent of the approach taken years ago by Ruben, Bordley, and Lieberman (1961), is also still suggested by some authors (Wong, Gibson, & Sanli, 1997) for pediatric audiology assessment. Based on their experiences for a series of 198 children, Wong et al. (1997) compare favorably the surgical difficulty and degree of invasiveness of the placement of either a straight or a "golf club" (an iron, not a wood) shaped electrode through

a myringotomy into the round window niche to the insertion of ventilation tubes (grommets). On the average, differences between behavioral thresholds and ECochG estimations of threshold were less than 6 dB at 500, 1000, 2000, and 4000 Hz.

Among invasive techniques, TT ECochG measurement is more commonly reported in children. The following reviews of two of these papers highlight pediatric application of the TT electrode ECochG technique. Inadequacy of behavioral audiometry findings is the common rationale for performing ECochG in children. René Dauman also offers two other arguments for the application of ECochG in selected pediatric populations. For young children (between the ages of about 4 months and 4 to 5 years), sedation is generally required even for ABR measurement. For some of these children (e.g., children with developmental disabilities) conscious sedation is inadequate and general anesthesia is required. ECochG is certainly feasible under general anesthesia. Also, peripheral auditory dysfunction (middle and/or inner ear) is the most common etiology for hearing impairment in children. ECochG is well suited for assessment of peripheral hearing loss. Dauman (1991) described TT ECochG findings for 65 children aged 0 to 3 years who could not be fully assessed behaviorally and who required general anesthesia for ABR measurement. Whenever possible, ECochG findings were compared with the outcome of behavioral audiometry conducted before or on the day of the ECochG assessment. As expected, behavioral audiometry findings were "doubtful" or "not possible" for children aged 0 to 6 months and for children with abnormal developmental levels. Based on the findings of the study, Dauman reported that the analysis of ECochG provided information on the type of hearing loss (conductive versus sensory versus neural) and on the slope of the hearing loss. ECochG was especially useful in the estimation of the degree of hearing loss with neural dysfunction when the ABR could not be detected and, therefore, wave V was not available as an index of auditory threshold. Test time with tone burst signals was quicker for ECochG than ABR, as the ECochG AP component recorded with the TT electrode technique was relatively larger than the ABR components. A significant disadvantage of the ECochG technique was inadequate assessment of low-frequency hearing sensitivity. And, of course, it was necessary to combine ABR measurement with the ECochG to provide information on brainstem auditory function.

Schoonhoven and colleagues at Leiden University Medical Centre and Effatha Institute for Deaf Children in The Netherlands demonstrate the value of the TT ECochG technique in children with severe hearing impairment (Schoonhoven et al., 1999). In this selected population, the severity of the hearing loss precluded confident estimation of residual hearing with the ABR. ECochG was evoked with tone bursts at octave frequencies of 500 to 8000 Hz. The subjects were a series of 126 children in the age range of 0 to 6 years with reliable behavioral estimation of hearing loss.

The majority of children were aged 1 to 2.5 years. Most of the children in the 4 to 5 year age range had questionable behavioral audiometry findings due to mental retardation. Schoonhoven et al. (1999) report scatter plots showing on the relationship between behavioral and ECochG estimations of auditory threshold, as well as some case reports. There was a tendency for behavioral estimations of auditory thresholds to be worse than thresholds predicted by ECochG findings. The average error for ECochG versus behavioral thresholds estimations was 18 dB. The authors speculated on possible explanations for this trend. One was the possibility that the behavioral thresholds overestimate actual hearing loss. This was unlikely as the subjects were well trained in behavioral audiometry and yielded reliable findings. Another possible explanation is that electrophysiological threshold estimation for some of the subjects was made with preneural ECochG components, whereas the behavioral estimations of threshold were, of course, dependent on neural auditory function. The authors raise the possibility that auditory deprivation in preschool years would be associated with inadequate development of the central auditory nervous system. ECochG measurements did produce other interesting findings. Despite the degree of hearing loss in the series of children, a CM was recorded in almost all of the ears. Also, an ECochG recorded with the transtympanic technique could be identified in the majority of children for whom no ABR could be detected. The logical explanation for this discrepancy is that the ECochG is a near-field response, with large amplitude, whereas the ABR is a far-field response with considerably smaller amplitude. Because the ECochG amplitude was larger, and higher signal intensity levels were possible for tone-burst versus click signals, frequency-specific estimations of auditory thresholds were often obtained. The frequency-specific information on auditory threshold was very useful in the development of a rehabilitation strategy and, especially, for hearing aid fitting.

Each of these papers illustrates the value of ECochG measurements, or at least the inclusion of ECochG principles, in the electrophysiological assessment of infants and young children. The papers also confirm the impressive quality of ECochG recordings made with the near-field TT needle electrode technique, even when detection of an ABR is precluded by the severity of hearing loss. ECochG in pediatric assessment can maximize the likelihood of defining accurately the site of lesion and the extent of auditory dysfunction and providing a "cross-check" (Jerger & Hayes, 1976) to behavioral audiometry and the ABR.

Assessment of Neoplastic Retrocochlear Auditory Dysfunction

ENHANCEMENT OF THE ABR WAVE I (ECOCHG AP) COMPONENT. |
Perhaps the most common example of the application of ECochG principles in clinical audiology is for the enhancement of the ABR wave I in patients with significant

sensorineural hearing loss. The overall objective of the electrophysiologic assessment in these cases is differentiation of cochlear versus neural auditory dysfunction. The etiology for neural dysfunction is typically an "acoustic tumor," i.e., a vestibular schwannoma, within the internal auditory canal that with growth will impinge on the auditory nerve. A patient usually presents with a unilateral, or an asymmetric bilateral, high-frequency sensorineural hearing loss. A this point in the clinical process the loss is described as "sensorineural" because the sensory versus neural auditory function (or dysfunction) has not yet been differentiated. An ABR recording with a mastoid or, preferably, earlobe inverting electrode site often fails to yield a clear and reliable wave I component, due to the degree of hearing loss and the difficulty presenting a stimulus that is sufficiently above hearing threshold to generated a detectable wave I (Figure 5.1). ECochG measurement involves, with the appropriate electrode locations, a near-field recording of activity generated in the cochlea and distal (cochlear) end of the auditory nerve. Locating the inverting electrode closer to the cochlea enhances the ECochG action potential (AP), i.e., the ABR wave I. The wave I (AP) is a peripheral "marker" for the calculation of interwave latencies. The interwave latencies, reflecting only neural activity (versus middle ear or cochlear function), provide a relatively stable index of retrocochlear neural transmission time. The analysis and interpretation of the ABR is affected and confounded by cochlear (sensory) hearing loss, without a clear ABR wave I (ECochG AP component). That is, due to the hearing loss a delay in absolute ABR latencies (e.g., wave I, wave III, or wave V) for the ear with poorer hearing cannot be attributed confidently to retrocochlear auditory dysfunction, as delays in absolute latency would result also from a moderate to severe cochlear hearing loss. When a clear and reliable ABR wave I (ECochG AP component) is recorded, and subsequent interwave latencies are analyzed, then auditory dysfunction distal to the generator of wave I (within the middle ear and cochlear) is taken out of the equation.

Multiple modifications of the ABR test protocol will increase the likelihood of recording a clear and reliable wave I component, as discussed in Chapter 6. Some of these changes in test protocol, such as slowing the stimulus rate, are essentially incorporated in the conventional ECochG measurement approach. The following discussion focuses on the application of ECochG electrode techniques in ABR measurement for the purpose of increasing wave I amplitude. There is ample evidence that the use of a TIPtrode electrode technique and, of course, the TT promontory electrode approach, will enhance detection of the ECochG AP and ABR wave I component in patients with sensorineural hearing loss, including acoustic neuromas (Bauch & Olsen, 1990; Hall, 1992; Musiek & Baran, 1990; Tanaka et al., 1999). Often, the AP (wave I) will emerge with the use of a TIPtrode even when the component was not detected with a surface electrode on the earlobe or mastoid. A clear ECochG

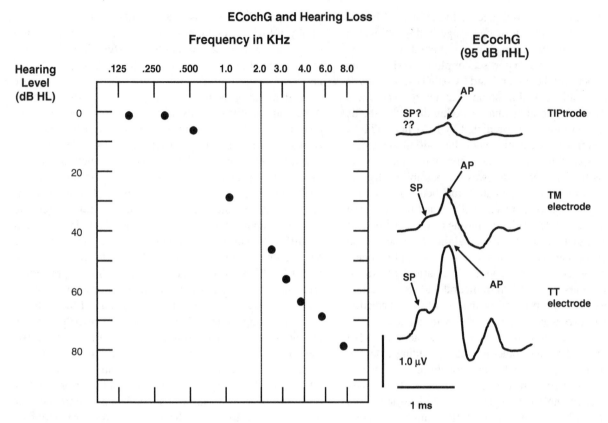

FIGURE 5.1. The enhancement of the ABR wave I component when recorded with different ECochG electrode locations. A larger wave I amplitude permits more accurate analysis and interpretation in neurodiagnostic applications of ABR, e.g., in high-frequency sensorineural hearing loss.

can certainly be detected with a TT needle electrode located on the promontory, even in the absence of an ABR as recorded with surface electrodes (e.g., Hall, 1992; Schwaber & Hall, 1990).

"AUDITORY NEUROPATHY"

Background

Electrocochleography (ECochG) plays an important role in the detection and diagnosis of what is commonly called "auditory neuropathy." This clinically challenging auditory problem is discussed in this chapter; reference to ABR findings in "auditory neuropathy" are also found in Chapter 9. The initially unexpected and rather paradoxical combination of audiologic test findings now commonly referred to as "auditory neuropathy" was first recognized in the late 1980s. The term is enclosed within quotation marks here and throughout this section of the chapter because it is, as discussed below, not really accurate anatomically, and certainly not consistent with the definition of "neuropathy" as used by neurologists. In published reports, otoacoustic emissions (OAEs), often entirely normal, were recorded in patients with very abnor-

mal pure tone hearing threshold and/or no detectable ABR. In the early to mid-1990s, as more audiologists gained access to equipment for measurement of OAEs in the clinical setting, this essential pattern of audiologic test findings was reported repeatedly, especially with infants and young children at risk for neurological dysfunction. The ABR findings, and in some cases the outcome for pure tone and speech audiometry, were consistent with severe-to-profound sensorineural hearing loss. However, OAEs—often robust and with amplitudes entirely within the normal region—argued strongly against a typical sensory (cochlear) hearing loss.

Neurologist Arnold Starr and colleagues apparently coined the term "auditory neuropathy" in 1996 (Starr et al., 1996). The reader may recall that Dr. Starr was among the earliest clinical investigators of the ABR, reporting ABR findings in a variety of neuropathologies in the 1970s (see Chapters 1 and 7 for more information). Of course, the clinical entity that most clinicians refer to as "auditory neuropathy" did not first develop as a disorder, or spread as an epidemic, as recently as the 1980s. The finding of absent ABRs and/or very poor speech audiometry performance in persons with normal or near-normal pure-tone audiograms, has been occasionally reported for decades (e.g., Chisin,

Perlman, & Schmer, 1979; Davis & Hirsh, 1979; Hallpike, Harriman, & Wells, 1980; Hildesheimer, Muchnik, & Rubenstein, 1985; Kraus et al., 1984; Starr et al., 1991; Stockard & Stockard, 1983; Worthington & Peters, 1980). "Auditory neuropathy" is, therefore, not a new clinical entity but, rather, a newly appreciated pattern of findings. With the benefit of hindsight provided by an appreciation of the nature of "auditory neuropathy," retrospective review by many experienced clinicians of ABR and other audiologic findings recorded in the 1970s in children at risk for neurological dysfunction revealed patterns of findings compatible with those of "auditory neuropathy." Along with colleagues who since the 1970s have applied behavioral and electrophysiologic audiologic techniques clinically in children, the author has identified former patients with the unmistakable audiologic hallmarks of "auditory neuropathy." That is, patients with a robust CM with no subsequent ABR, abnormal pure tone audiometry with very poor word recognition performance and, unfortunately, the unexpected failure to obtain benefit with amplification. To the chagrin and disappointment of many talented audiologists in the years before "auditory neuropathy" was appreciated, children with this constellation of auditory findings often inexplicably rejected hearing use. With the "discovery" of "auditory neuropathy," the conventional approach for pediatric audiologic diagnosis changed abruptly and, of course, so did audiologic management of some infants and young children.

Definition of "Auditory Neuropathy"

The meaning of the term "auditory neuropathy" has undergone changes since it was first introduced. In fact, the meaning of the term has expanded and been distorted to the point where, for most patients diagnosed with "auditory neuropathy," it is no longer an accurate descriptor for the pathologic process, the clinical course, or even the onset of the disorder. Arnold Starr, Terrence Picton, Yvonne Sininger, Linda Hood, and Charles Berlin coined the term "auditory neuropathy" and stated that it was "due to a disorder of auditory nerve function" (Starr et al., 1996, p. 741). Most of the initial patients identified by these authors with "auditory neuropathy" showed clinical neurological findings of "elevated or impaired deep tendon and/or ankle reflexes" that "suggested some form of peripheral neural disease" (Berlin, Hood, & Rose, 2001, p. 226). Confirming the suspicion, one of the patients met criteria for the diagnosis of Charcot-Marie-Tooth disease. That is, the group of researchers at the time described the entity as auditory *peripheral nerve* pathology, involving "auditory nerve dendrites, auditory neurons in the spiral ganglion, and/or axons of the auditory nerve between the cochlea and the pontine brainstem." However, in some publications, these authors also include within the category of "auditory neuropathy" cochlear abnormalities involving the tectorial membrane, inner hair cells and the synapse between inner hair cells, and the afferent fibers of

the eighth nerve as neuropathy. In the words of this group of authors,

> a set of salient features distinguishes these patients from the majority of patients with sensorineural hearing loss or other described syndromes. The symptoms always seen in presumed "auditory neuropathy" are: (1) mild-to-moderate elevation of auditory thresholds to pure-tone stimuli by air and bone conduction, (2) absent or severely abnormal ABRs to high-level stimuli, *including absence of wave I*, (3) present otoacoustic emissions that do not suppress with contralateral noise, (4) word recognition ability poorer than expected for pure-tone hearing loss configuration, (5) absent acoustic reflexes to both ipsilateral and contralateral tones at 110 dB HL, and (6) absent masking level differences. (Sininger, Hood, Starr, & Berlin, 1995, p. 10)

In the years since the classic paper by Starr et al. (1996), the above rather invariant description of "auditory neuropathy" has undergone substantial revision with the perspective of clinical experience with untold hundreds of patients accumulated independently by investigators around the world. Also, since the mid-1990s, one group of researchers (Berlin, Hood, and colleagues) have qualified the phrase by adding the word "auditory dys-synchrony" (i.e., auditory neuropathy/dys-synchrony), in recognition of one of the variations in auditory findings (e.g., Berlin, Hood, & Rose, 2001; Berlin, Hood, Morlet, Rose, & Brashears, 2003). Based on comprehensive audiologic assessment of large series of patients with "auditory neuropathy" (AN), coupled with pathophysiologic studies of selected patients, Starr et al. (2004) suggested that "AN with involvement of the ganglion cells, axons, and proximal dendrites be designated as a proximal AN or type I AN" and, further,

> We suggest that the clinical picture of AN accompanying disorders of distal components of the auditory periphery (terminal dendrites, inner hair cells, synapses) be designated as a distal AN or type II AN to be distinguished from proximal or type I AN due to primary degeneration of the auditory nerve. The latter may or may not be accompanied by the presence of a peripheral neuropathy. (p. 424)

Beginning in the mid-1990s, clinical researchers around the world began observing similar patterns of auditory findings, particularly, preservation of OAEs and CMs in patients with no detectable ABR. Despite its inherent inaccuracy, the term "auditory neuropathy" was not used "senso stricto" (Rapin & Gravel, 2003) but, rather, with increasing frequency to describe this rather superficial pattern of auditory findings, even though the underlying pathological processes and subsequent medical diagnoses varied greatly among patients. The term "auditory neuropathy" was, and continues to be, applied by authors and research groups in textbooks and peer-reviewed journals to patients who lack any clear evidence of neural auditory dysfunction. There are dozens of examples in the literature of the loose use of the term "auditory neuropathy." For instance, Deltenre et al. (1997)

describe with "auditory neuropathy" three newborn infants with varied medical findings but who "shared the same major anomaly of their click-evoked BAEPs; no neural component could be identified, although they exhibited a prominent early fast oscillation identified as an isolated microphonic potential" (p. 17). Rance et al. (1999) reported one of the first relatively large series of infants and young children (N = 20) with a variety of etiologies, hyperbilirubinemia being the most common, who were collectively described with the diagnosis of "auditory neuropathy." And Madden et al. (2002) state "the pathophysiology of AN has been suggested to involve an abnormality of the peripheral auditory system localized to the inner hair cells, to the eighth cranial nerve, or to the synapse between them" (p. 1027). With this broad usage of the term, "auditory neuropathy" encompasses a spectrum of auditory disorders from isolated inner hair cell abnormalities to variations of "nontumor, noncochlear" hearing impairment reported previously before OAEs were regularly applied clinically (e.g., Cacace, Parnes, Lovely, & Kalathia, 1994; Hallpike et al., 1980; Hildesheimer, Muchnik, & Rubenstein, 1985; Kraus et al., 1984; Stockard, 1983; Worthington & Peters, 1980).

As experience with "auditory neuropathy" has accumulated, therefore, stark contradictions in the term have become apparent. The patterns of findings in some patients with "auditory neuropathy" appear to be more consistent with severe inner hair cell dysfunction than eighth-nerve dysfunction. The absence of an ABR, including wave I, and the concomitant preservation of CM activity and/or OAEs—implying outer hair cell integrity—could be explained by totally nonfunctional inner hair cells and/or by a breakdown in the synaptic transmission from the base of the inner hair cells to the afferent fibers of the eighth nerve, perhaps due to deficiency in the neurotransmitter glutamate. Abnormalities or even absence of inner hair cells may have a genetic basis in experimental animals (mouse) and humans (e.g., Steel & Bock, 1983). Of course, abnormal inner hair cell function is really a "sensory" hearing loss and, in the presence of normal synaptic and neural function, incompatible with the term "auditory neuropathy." Another inherent inconsistency in the term "auditory neuropathy" is the occurrence in many patients of nervous system pathology that extends beyond the auditory pathways. Of course, pathology beyond the auditory nervous system is entirely consistent with the conventional term *peripheral neuropathy*. Other regions and functions of the brain may be involved in patients with "auditory neuropathy," including visual, somatosensory, and motor pathways and centers. Patients included in the "auditory neuropathy" category often present with a pattern of diagnostic findings consistent with a "poly-neuropathy," and with obvious neurological dysfunction, e.g., developmental delay or cerebral palsy. The term "*auditory* neuropathy" in such cases is misleading and inaccurate, as it implies that the disorder is limited to the auditory system.

Inappropriate use of the term "auditory neuropathy" has been clearly exposed and elucidated by Drs. Isabelle Rapin and Judy Gravel (e.g., Rapin & Gravel, 2003, 2006), two well-respected clinical researchers (a neurologist and audiologist, respectively). Rapin and Gravel (2003) emphasize the accurate definition of the term *neuropathy*—pathology in peripheral nerves.

> To neurologists, the term *neuropathy* has a precise connotation: it refers to pathology of peripheral nerve fibers rather than pathology in their neuronal cell bodies of origin (referred to as a neuronopathy or ganglionopathy). Neuropathies can be divided into three broad types, demyelinating, axonal, and mixed. (Rapin & Gravel, 2003, p. 710)

Of course, there are some published reports of "auditory neuropathy" in well-defined neurological disease, such as the neurodegenerative disorder Friedreich ataxia (e.g., López-Diaz-de-León et al., 2003; Satya-Murti, Cacace, & Hanson, 1980). Rapin and Gravel (2003, 2006) explain that peripheral nerves, such as the eighth cranial nerve, are enclosed by myelin from Schwann cells, whereas the myelinization of neurons within the central nervous system (from the cochlear nucleus to more rostral auditory centers) is by oligodendroglial cells. Rapin and Gravel (2006) make a clear distinction between the anatomic nature and the pathologic processes of Schwann cells versus oligodendroglial cells. In addition, these authors review features of two general types of neuropathies—primary demyelinating neuropathies and primary axonal neuropathies. The former is characterized by asynchronous activity if there is a mixture of demyelinated and normal axons within the nerves. Eventually, prolonged demyelination will lead to marked dysfunction and, finally, death of the axon. Rapin and Gravel (2003, 2006) point out, however, that the term "auditory dys-synchrony" is not appropriate to describe this form of neuropathy. The authors summarize the seriousness of the inappropriate application of the term "auditory neuropathy" as follows:

> From a biologic point of view, the indiscriminate use of the term neuropathy for disorders of the spiral ganglion cells and their axons myelinated by Schwann cells as well as for those of the central auditory pathway myelinated by oligodendroglial cells is as inappropriate as not making a distinction between *conductive* and *sensorineural* hearing loss. Therefore, we propose that: (1) hearing impairments due to disorders of the hair cells be referred to as *sensory hearing losses;* (2) those which through comprehensive behavioral, electrophysiological, and pathologic investigation can be specifically attributed to pathology of the spiral ganglion cells and their VIIIth nerve axons be referred to as *auditory neuropathies;* and (3) that disorders of the central auditory pathway (brainstem, thalamus, and cortex) be referred to as *central hearing losses*. (Rapin & Gravel, 2006, p. 149)

Unfortunately, despite the accuracy and logic of these arguments, it is doubtful that the widespread and admittedly indiscriminate use of the term "auditory neuropathy" will abate any time soon. The classification of auditory dysfunction in children and adults into three simple categories (sensory, neural, or central) based on the findings for comprehensive diagnostic assessment, however, is a reasonable expectation.

Anatomic Sites and Physiologic Mechanisms

As the term is typically used, "auditory neuropathy" is not a unitary or homogeneous disorder but, rather, a collection of auditory abnormalities with distinctly different sites of dysfunction, diverse etiologies and causes, variations in patterns of auditory findings, and, in most cases, correspondingly different management strategies. This final statement warrants emphasis. The response to a common clinical question, What do you do for a patient with auditory neuropathy? must be another two-part question, that is, Where in the auditory system is the dysfunction, and what was the pattern of auditory findings? Management of "auditory neuropathy" is reviewed below. The presumed relations among these multiple aspects of "auditory neuropathy" are summarized in Table 5.2. Of course, information on "auditory neuropathy" is constantly updated and modified as clinical experience with patients accumulates and formal investigations are completed and published. Information found in Table 5.2 is, therefore, not necessarily all supported by experimental evidence and is certainly subject to change. It is offered as a starting point for the clinician faced with the challenge of detecting, diagnosing, and managing patients with "auditory neuropathy."

Sites of dysfunction identified in patients diagnosed with "auditory neuropathy" include inner hair cells in the cochlea (e.g., Amatuzzi et al., 2001; Rea & Gibson, 2003), disruption in neurotransmission across the synapse between the inner hair cells and the afferent fibers in the distal end of the auditory portion of the eighth nerve (Starr et al., 2004), abnormalities within the spiral ganglion cells within the distal auditory nerve, very few myelinated fibers within the auditory nerve (Starr, Picton, & Kim, 2001), and dysfunction within the auditory brainstem (Doyle, Sininger, & Starr, 1998).

Depending on the specific site and extent of auditory dysfunction, patients with "auditory neuropathy" may experience highly divergent auditory sensations. Some children develop normal speech and language function, presumably reflecting reasonably intact perception of essential features and information in speech. Others reportedly perceive a very distorted and abnormal quality of sound with no measurable speech perception skills. The extreme of auditory dysfunction may be illustrated by patients who have no activation of the auditory cortex with sound stimulation, as documented by positron emission topography (PET) imaging (e.g., Lockwood, Berlin, Hood, Burkard, & Salvi, 1999).

Suspected Sites of Dysfunction

A finding of normal OAE and/or CM activity, or at least some evidence of cochlear integrity, coupled with neural dysfunction within the caudal auditory system, is an essential component of the definition of "auditory neuropathy." As noted by Starr et al. (2003), two basic mechanisms are suggested for the auditory dysfunction characteristic of "auditory neuropathy"—an impairment in the synchrony of auditory nerve firing and a reduction in neural input. Both of these pathophysiologic processes affect behavioral and electrophysiological auditory findings. However, there is considerable variation in the specific site of dysfunction

TABLE 5.2. Summary of the Relation between Specific Anatomic Sites of Dysfunction and Characteristic Patterns of Auditory Dysfunction

Combinations of multiple sites of dysfunction are associated with varied patterns of auditory findings. The pattern of findings compatible with a strict definition, that is, *senso stricto* (Rapin & Gravel, 2003) of auditory neuropathy are in bold.

Key: − = normal; +/− = variable; + = abnormal

ANATOMIC SITE OF DYSFUNCTION	OAES	ECOCHG CM	SP	AP	ABR I	V	ACOUSTIC REFLEX	BEHAVIORAL AUDIOMETRY Pure Tones	Speech
Outer hair cells (OHCs)	+	+	−	+/−	+/−	−	−	+/−	+/−
Inner hair cells (IHCs)	−	−	+	+	+	+	+	+	+
Synapse (IHC – auditory afferents)	−	−	−	+	+	+	+	+	+
Spiral ganglion cells	**−**	**−**	**−**	**+**	**+**	**+**	**+**	**+/−**	**+/−**
Auditory nerve	**−**	**−**	**−**	**+/−**	**+/−**	**+**	**+**	**+/−**	**+**
Auditory brainstem									
pons	−	−	−	−	−	+	+	+	+
midbrain	−	−	−	−	−	+	−	+/−	+

for "auditory neuropathy" and the associated patterns of audiologic findings. Patterns of audiologic findings associated with different sites of dysfunction within the auditory system were summarized in Table 5.2. Only dysfunction of the spiral ganglion cells and the auditory nerve would be appropriately called "auditory neuropathy." Behavioral audiometry findings in the diverse collection of disorders known as "auditory neuropathy" may range from normal pure tone thresholds or to auditory thresholds associated with varying degrees of hearing impairment (Rance et al., 1999). Patients with "auditory neuropathy" have, in common, reasonably intact outer hair cell function within the inner ear, combined with dysfunction of retrocochlear auditory structures that is not secondary to a mass lesion, such as an acoustic tumor. Starr et al. (2004) infer from the benefit obtained from cochlear implantation of selected patients with "auditory neuropathy" that the site of lesion for "auditory neuropathy" be localized to distal regions of the auditory nerve (dendrites, inner hair cells, or their synapses) rather than at the proximal auditory nerve (ganglion cells or axons)" (p. 423).

Berlin et al. (2001) described in a series of 100 patients with "auditory neuropathy" six categories based not so much patterns of test findings but, rather, communicative outcome and other nonauditory characteristics:

1. Children with absent ABR but otherwise normal hearing abilities who develop speech and language and communicate effectively. As older children or adults, their only auditory deficit is difficulty understanding speech in background noise.
2. Children who initially have clear OAEs and CMs. In time, these auditory responses disappear and the patient's behavior is consistent with a severe-to-profound hearing loss. Curiously, however, hearing function occasionally appears to be improved.
3. For a similar category of patients who behave as severely hearing impaired most of the time, OAEs eventually disappear but CM activity remains.
4. Patients who consistently have no evidence of ABR and whose behavior is consistent with profound hearing impairment (deaf).
5. Children who are apparently normal at birth but later are diagnosed with "auditory neuropathy" as part of a more general peripheral neuropathy (e.g., Charcot-Marie-Tooth disease) and develop problems with hearing, speech, and language.
6. Adults who simply have no ABR, if they undergo an ABR assessment by chance, despite otherwise normal auditory and language function. Berlin et al. (2001) speculate that category 6 is the adult version of category 1.

As the term is commonly, albeit incorrectly, used clinically, "auditory neuropathy" may be first identified in the neonatal period or later in childhood. "Auditory neuropathy" present from birth is likely to be secondary to perinatal disease, e.g., especially hyperbilirubinemia or, less often, asphyxia. However, as Rapin and Gravel (2003) point out after a brief review of the literature, "kernicterus is rarely if ever attributable to the spiral ganglion cell or its axon but rather to pathology in the central auditory pathway, so that the term 'auditory neuropathy' is a misnomer" (p. 716). Patients with a later onset of "auditory neuropathy" are at risk for peripheral neuropathies (e.g., Charcot-Marie-Tooth disease) and may show other neurological deficits (e.g., dysarthria of speech or general motor abnormalities). A firm diagnosis may never be made in patients who appear to develop the characteristics of "auditory neuropathy" later in childhood or in early adulthood.

Patterns of Auditory Findings

ECOCHG. | ECochG measurement is really essential for the diagnosis of "auditory neuropathy," and to monitor cochlear status over time in patients with "auditory neuropathy." OAEs are also very useful in the detection and diagnosis of "auditory neuropathy" in infants. There are several disadvantages, however, to reliance on OAEs for monitoring cochlear status over time in this patient population and for detection and diagnosis of "auditory neuropathy" in older children. Since the earliest descriptions of "auditory neuropathy," authors have noted the gradual disappearance of OAEs in some children (e.g., Starr et al., 2001). The precise mechanism(s) responsible for the loss of OAEs is not known. Middle ear dysfunction, a rather common and easily explained reason for absent OAEs in older children with "auditory neuropathy," can be confirmed by other audiologic procedures (e.g., tympanometry) and clinical examination.

The classic ECochG finding in "auditory neuropathy" is a clear and often very robust CM for single-polarity stimuli, with no subsequent AP and no ABR waves. A rather obvious, yet representative, example of the CM component of the ECochG in "auditory neuropathy" is shown in Figure 5.2A. At first glance, one might confuse the peaks and valleys in the periodic CM waveform with very distinct ABR waves, e.g., wave I, wave II, wave III, and wave V. The peaks would appear highly repeatable if superimposed for two separate averaged waveforms. The CM of the ECochG can be quickly and confidently differentiated from ABR waves with two simple manipulations of the test parameters. First, ECochG recording can be repeated with click stimuli of the opposite polarity (e.g., rarefaction and then condensation). The CM waveform is, as shown in top portion of Figure 5.2A, perfectly inverted by the change in stimulus polarity. Repeatable and robust OAEs are a characteristic feature of "auditory neuropathy" at diagnosis, as shown in Figure 5.2B. Importantly, an ABR waveform remains essentially identical for both rarefaction and condensation polarity click stimuli. That is, polarity of the ABR peaks does not invert when polarity of the stimulus is changed from rarefaction to condensation. The presence of waveforms that are out of phase for rarefaction versus condensation clicks can be confirmed when a flat line results from digitally adding them together. On the other hand, digitally subtracting the CM waveforms evoked by stimuli of opposite polarity increases the amplitude of the responses. If the waveforms remain with digital addition, then the waveform is likely to be an ABR, rather than the CM component of the ABR. The cancellation of the CM with addition of the waveforms for the two stimulus polarities highlights a potential pitfall in detection of "auditory neuropathy" with the ABR. If the ABR is recorded with alternating polarity stimulation, during the averaging processing the CM for rarefaction and condensation polarity stimuli are consistently cancelled, and the result is simple background electrical activity, that is, no ABR. The absence of an ABR for maximum stimulus-intensity levels could easily be misinterpreted as consistent with a profound hearing loss when, in fact, the outer hair cells are normal. This point is reviewed in more detail in a discussion of the ABR in "auditory neuropathy" (Chapter 9).

The value of ECochG in the detection and diagnosis of neural hearing loss (aka "auditory neuropathy") in children and adults is confirmed by several formal investigations (e.g., Rea & Gibson, 2003; Santarelli & Arslan, 2002; Starr et al., 2001), published case reports, and extensive unpublished clinical experiences. Gary Rance and Australian colleagues recorded the CM component of the ECochG from 20 infants and young children (aged 1 to 49 months) who showed no evidence of an ABR. Electrodes were placed on the vertex or high forehead (noninverting) and the earlobe or mastoid ipsilateral to the stimulus (inverting). The CM component was evoked with single-polarity click stimuli (two runs of

rarefaction and two runs of condensation clicks) presented at a rate of either 12 or 30/second and an intensity level of 95 to 100 dB nHL. Stimuli were delivered via Etymōtic insert earphones, minimizing stimulus artifact. To verify the validity of the CM component, the acoustic tubing was clamped with each subject. This maneuver eliminated the CM, thus differentiating cochlear activity from stimulus artifact. Presence of a CM component was defined by an 180 degree reversal in the polarity of the response waveform associated with a change in the polarity of the stimulus. Rance et al. (1999) identified a clear CM component for at least one ear in all 20 subjects (bilaterally in 18 subjects), with amplitude ranging from 0.5 to 1.2 μV.

Starr et al. (2001) described findings for ECochG (SM and SP), ABR, and OAEs recorded from 33 patients with "auditory neuropathy" ranging in age from 4 months to 64 years. In this study, however, the authors did not utilize a true ECochG test protocol. Rather, ECochG and ABR were evoked concomitantly with click stimuli at an intensity level of about 80 dB nHL and recorded with a scalp (mastoid) electrode, rather than a near-field electrode (e.g., tympanic membrane or transtympanic placement). Although average ECochG amplitudes were small (<0.5 μV) for all subjects (due to the use of scalp electrodes versus tympanic membrane or promontory electrodes), Starr et al. (2001) reported larger than normal CM amplitudes for patients with "auditory neuropathy" in comparison to a control group, and speculated that a disorder of the efferent nervous system (olivo-cochlear bundle) and subsequent hyper-polarization of the outer hair cells might be related to the augmentation in receptor potentials underlying the CM. Interestingly, Starr et al. (2001) raise the possibility that cochlear dysfunction

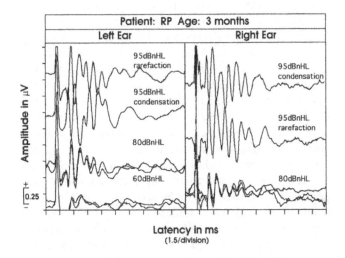
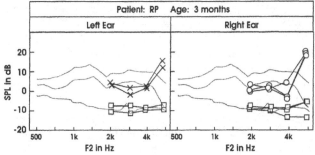

FIGURE 5.2. Cochlear microphonic (CM) characteristic of auditory neuropathy (A, in left portion of the figure) recorded from a 3-month-old infant with robust OAEs (B, in the right portion of the figure) and no evidence of an ABR. Immediately after birth, the child was airlifted to an NICU at a major medical center for management of multiple health problems.

may be a factor in "auditory neuropathy" stating, "We are unable to distinguish whether the alterations of cochlear hair cell functions are a cause or a consequence of disordered auditory nerve activity in these patients" (p. 97). Close analysis of the three components of the ECochG—CM, SP, and AP—in patients with suspected "auditory neuropathy" offers a possible approach for differentiating between outer hair cell, inner hair cell, and spiral ganglion (or synaptic) auditory dysfunction. Data for these three ECochG components were not systematically compared in the study. Citing the likely enhancement of ECochG amplitudes if recordings were made with an electrode closer to the cochlea, the authors noted the inability in their study to make any firm conclusions about SP data because it wasn't detected in approximately half of the subjects. Starr et al. (2001) also comment on the value of SP as an indicator of inner hair cell function in "auditory neuropathy" based on evidence from animal investigations (e.g., Durrant, Wang, Ding, & Salvi, 1998; Zheng, Ding, McFadden, & Henderson, 1997).

The combination of normal OAEs and CM activity in children with sensorineural hearing impairment, as documented by the AP component of the ECochG or by ABR, may be more common that suspected. It is important for readers to appreciate that published ECochG findings in infants and young children include those obtained with high-quality transtympanic and other near-field ECochG techniques. Rea and Gibson (2003) recorded ECochG and ABR using a round window technique in a consecutive series of 464 children ranging in age from 2 to 82 months, including 342 children with bilateral congenital hearing loss. OAEs were also measured in a subgroup within the series. The authors concluded that up to 40 percent of children in the intensive care nursery showed evidence of intact outer hair cell activity and inner hair cell dysfunction. Inner hair cells appear to be more susceptible to damage secondary to hypoxia than previously suspected. Inner hair cell abnormalities due to hypoxia, plus genetic etiologies, appear to account for a substantial portion of hearing impairment in the at-risk infant population. A test protocol that combines OAEs with ECochG and ABR is effective for differentiation of inner versus outer hair cell dysfunction and sensory versus neural dysfunction. Reliance on OAEs alone in the intensive care nursery population, however, will result in an unacceptably high proportion of false negative findings, i.e., normal findings in children with inner hair cell or neural auditory dysfunction.

Is there always agreement in findings for the CM and OAEs? It is clear that OAEs reflect acoustic energy in the external ear canal secondary to outer hair cell motility (movement), whereas the CM component is electrical activity generated mostly by the receptor potential arising from the apical portion of the outer hair cells. Although the inner hair cells may, at least in some animal species, play a role in the production of the CM (e.g., Dallos & Cheatham, 1976), the contribution is probably very modest. Disassociation of findings for OAEs and the CM have been reported in the literature, with the CM remaining in some patients who no longer show detectable OAEs (e.g., Hall, 2000; Rance et al., 1999). In other words, the mechanisms underlying generation of the receptor potential (an early step in a sequence of events leading to outer hair cell motility) versus actual outer hair cell motility appear to be differentially affected by pathophysiologic processes. Typically, the OAEs are abolished by even minor insults to the outer hair cells or relatively subtle middle ear dysfunction, whereas the CM is present with mild to moderate degrees of hearing loss and, with very high click stimulus intensity levels, in the presence of middle ear abnormalities (e.g., Rance et al., 1999; Sohmer, Kinarti, & Gafni, 1980).

PURE-TONE AUDIOMETRY. | Audiologic characteristics of "auditory neuropathy," in addition to ECochG findings, are summarized in Table 5.3. Pure-tone thresholds vary widely in "auditory neuropathy." Some subjects have hearing sensitivity within normal limits, for example, 8 of the 20 subjects in the study reported by Rance et al. (1999). However, most children with "auditory neuropathy" have hearing loss ranging in severity from mild to profound (including no response at equipment intensity limits). Some children with "auditory neuropathy" have fluctuating hearing loss (Madden et al., 2002; Sininger et al., 1995), including 5 out of 20 in the series reported by Rance and colleagues (1999). In general, hearing loss in "auditory neuropathy" is characterized by a flat configuration (similar degree of hearing loss across audiometric frequencies), or a rising pattern, i.e., greater for low frequencies (e.g., Rance et al., 1999; Sheykholeslami, Kaga, & Kaga, 2001; Sheykholeslami, Murofushi, Kermany, & Kaga, 2003; Shivashankar, Satischandra, Shashikala, & Gore, 2003; Starr et al., 1996). Interestingly, there is little connection between the degree of hearing loss in "auditory neuropathy" and speech perception. Exceptionally poor word recognition scores are often found in children with normal hearing sensitivity for pure-tone stimuli. In contrast, on rare occasions a child with "auditory neuropathy" will demonstrate relatively good speech perception. This latter finding has important implications for the possible role of amplification in the management of children with "auditory neuropathy" (Rance et al., 1999), as noted later in this section. In developing a management plan for patients with "auditory neuropathy," one must appreciate the possibility of spontaneous improvement in hearing status over time. Madden et al. (2002), for example, reported significant audiological improvements in 50 percent of their series of infants and young children (N = 22) with "auditory neuropathy," especially those with the diagnosis of hyperbilirubinemia. For patients with etiologies associated with potential spontaneous improvement in hearing sensitivity, it would be wise to defer certain management options, e.g., cochlear implantation, until hearing status is stable. According to data provided by Madden et al. (2002), "Children achieved a stable audiogram by a mean age of 18 months . . . with clinically meaningful

TABLE 5.3. General Auditory Characteristics of Patients with Auditory Neuropathy

Specific patterns of auditory findings depend on the site and extent of auditory dysfunction.

- OAEs are present, at least initially, and often robust and of normal or greater than normal amplitude.
- Contralateral and ipsilateral suppression of OAEs (transient and distortion product) with masking sound is typically lacking.
- The ECochG cochlear microphonic (CM) is clearly recorded (often in the ABR waveform) with single polarity stimuli (e.g., rarefaction or condensation clicks).
- The ECochG summating potential (SP) may be detected or absent, depending on the site of auditory dysfunction.
- The compound action potential (AP) of the ECochG is usually not present, even under ideal measurement conditions (e.g., near-field recording electrode and high stimulus intensity level).
- ABR is absent (no response even at maximum stimulus intensity levels), or markedly abnormal (only wave I is present).
- Acoustic reflexes are usually not present.
- Hearing thresholds as measured behaviorally range from entirely normal to profound hearing loss.
- Word recognition is unusually poor, even with good hearing sensitivity.
- Marked deficits on speech audiometry measures of auditory processing, especially in the presence of background noise, even with good hearing sensitivity.
- Masking level differences (MLDs) show no release from masking.
- Electrically elicited compound action potentials (ECAP) and auditory brainstem response (EABR) are normal (see Chapter 15).

---

improvement (i.e., the decision for cochlear implantation) occurring by a mean age of 12 months" (p. 1028).

SPEECH PERCEPTION. | A characteristic finding of "auditory neuropathy" is inordinately poor speech perception in relation to the degree of hearing impairment, even word recognition scores that are nil (0 percent) in persons with normal pure tone thresholds (Starr et al., 1991; Zeng et al., 1999). Marked deficits in temporal processing of speech are usually cited as the explanation (e.g., Zeng et al., 1999). However, speech perception may be relatively good in some patients with "auditory neuropathy" (e.g., Rance et al., 1999; Shivashankar et al., 2003), a finding that once again has positive implications for hearing aid use, as noted below. Even when syllable or word recognition performance is not markedly impaired, scores are further depressed on more difficult measures of speech perception, such as dichotic listening tasks and speech perception in background noise (e.g., Shivashankar et al., 2003).

ACOUSTIC REFLEXES. | Acoustic reflexes are typically abnormal (absent) in "auditory neuropathy" (e.g., Rance et al., 1999; Sheykholeslami, Kaga, & Kaga, 2001; Sheykholeslami et al., 2000; Shivashankar et al., 2003; Starr et al., 1996, 2004).

VESTIBULAR ABNORMALITIES. | Most investigations of "auditory neuropathy" do not include formal assessment of vestibular function. Sheykholeslami et al. (2000) performed a battery of vestibular procedures, including a clinical test of stability, ENG, a rotation test, and vestibular evoked myogenic potentials (VEMP) with three adult patients with normal findings for OAE and ECochG recordings. The authors reported evidence of abnormal vestibular results for some procedures (e.g., Romberg, Mann, and stepping tests, caloric stimulation, vestibular evoked myogenic potential, or VEMP), but normal findings for other tests (e.g., saccades, smooth pursuit eye movements, optokinetic nystagmus). Sheykholeslami et al. (2000) conclude that involvement of the vestibular branch of the eighth cranial nerve can be a feature of auditory neuropathy.

Etiologies for "Auditory Neuropathy"

RISK FACTORS. | The prompt identification, and thorough assessment, of "auditory neuropathy" is facilitated by heightened vigilance in selected patients. The literature clearly confirms that some patients are more likely to present with "auditory neuropathy." For example, Madden et al. (2002) reported that two-thirds of their series of 22 patients "had a complicated perinatal course." Diseases and etiologies associated with "auditory neuropathy" are summarized in Table 5.4. Not surprisingly, children with neurological disease or dysfunction, or who later are found to have neurological abnormalities, are at greatest risk. From this list, it's clear that a sizable proportion of children who are diagnosed with "auditory neuropathy" are admitted to an intensive care nursery for medical problems that are well known as risk factors for hearing loss, such as prematurity, hypoxia (asphyxia as documented by respiratory distress syndrome, mechanical ventilation, and/or a low APGAR score at 3 or 5 minutes), and hyperbilirubinemia (e.g., Amin et al., 2001; Chisin, Perlman, & Sohmer, 1979; Deltenre et al., 1997; Madden et al., 2002; Rance et al., 1999; Starr et al., 1996). Among these, the most consistently reported risk factor is hyperbilirubinemia. Bilirubin levels in children with "auditory neuropathy" vary considerably (from as low as 5 mg/dL [84 µmol/L] up to criterion for exchange transfusion) (Madden et al., 2002; Stein, Barth, Eichmann, & Mehdorn, 1996). Indeed, there is a sizable body of literature documenting the pathology and dysfunction of retrocochlear structures (Shapiro & Conlee, 1991) and the relation between retrocochlear auditory dysfunction and serious sensorineural hearing impairment in hyperbilirubinemia (Chisin et al., 1979; Perlman et al., 1983; Vohr et al., 1989), sometimes with reversal of the ABR-documented hearing impairment over time (Hall et al.,

TABLE 5.4. Diagnoses and Clinical Entities Associated with the Clinical Entity Described in the Literature as "Auditory Neuropathy"

Perinatal Diseases

- Hyperbilirubinemia
- Hypoxic insults
- Ischemic insults
- Prematurity

Neurological Disorders

- Demyelinating diseases
- Hydrocephalus
- Immune disorders, e.g., Guillain-Barre sydrome
- Inflammatory neuropathies
- Severe developmental delay

Neurometabolic Diseases

Genetic and Hereditary Etiologies

- Family history
- Connexin mutations, e.g., GJB3 (D66del)
- Otoferlin (OTOF) gene
- Nonsyndromic recessive auditory neuropathy
- Hereditary motor sensory neuropathies (HMSN), e.g., Charcot-Marie-Tooth syndrome
- Leber's hereditary optic neuropathy
- Waardenburg's syndrome
- Neurogenerative diseases, e.g., Friedreich's ataxia
- Mitochondrial disorders, e.g., mitochondrial enzymatic defect

Other

- Delayed visual maturation

1985a; Ito, 1984; Thoma, Gerull, & Mrowinski, 1986; Wennberg et al., 1982).

Family history is a strong predictor of "auditory neuropathy," as up to one-half of patients have either a family history of hearing loss or a genetically determined disease associated with the diagnosis of "auditory neuropathy" (e.g., Sininger & Oba, 2001; Starr et al., 1998; Wang, Hsu, & Young, 2003). Related to family history as a risk factor are hereditary disorders (e.g., Friedreich's ataxia and Charcot-Marie-Tooth disease) that now are clearly associated with later onset of "auditory neuropathy" (e.g., Berlin, Hood, Hurley, & Wen, 1994; Doyle, Sininger, & Starr, 1998; Starr et al., 1996). Neurometabolic and mitochondrial diseases also account for some infants with "auditory neuropathy" (e.g., Corley & Crabbe, 1999; Deltenre et al., 1997).

It is wise clinical policy to include measurement of OAEs, the CM of the ECochG, and ABR in the test battery for any patient with a history of one or more of these factors. OAEs or ABR in isolation are insufficient to alert the clinician to possible "auditory neuropathy." Since OAEs and the CM are, by definition, normal in "auditory neuropathy," reliance on either or even both measures will fail to detect "auditory neuropathy." That is, OAEs and the CM are insensitive to "auditory neuropathy." If only the ABR is recorded, a problem will be detected but, without the information on cochlear function provided by OAEs and the CM, the abnormal ABR is not specific to "auditory neuropathy." Rather, an absent ABR is also characteristic of severe-to-profound sensory hearing loss.

Keep in mind that a final medical diagnosis may not be available when the first audiologic signs of "auditory neuropathy" are recorded. In fact, when the audiologic assessment is first completed, often during the neonatal period, there may be no suspicion of neurological dysfunction. The audiologic evidence of "auditory neuropathy" may precipitate the referrals to medical specialists and centers that will ultimately lead to a definitive diagnosis. Rarely will a child with "auditory neuropathy" be found otherwise entirely normal after a comprehensive diagnostic workup, including neurological, neurometabolic, and neuroradiologic studies.

Not all patients with "auditory neuropathy" have risk factors or associated neuropathology. There are recurring anecdotal cases, often unpublished, or case reports of children with the combination of normal OAEs and an absent ABR discovered by routine newborn hearing screening in the well-baby nursery setting (e.g., Dunkley et al., 2003). Sheykholeslami, Kaga, and Kaga (2001) reported "isolated and sporadic auditory neuropathy" in five patients without evidence of "a generalized neuropathologic process." Common findings for each of the subjects were normal OAEs and ECochG CM components, abnormal pure tone hearing thresholds, poor word recognition scores, and absent ABRs. None of the patients in the study had cranial or peripheral neuropathy, other deficits on neurological examination, family history or the suggestion of a hereditary pattern, or serological abnormalities.

GENETIC FACTORS. | The literature clearly confirms that genetic factors are important in the diagnosis of "auditory neuropathy" (e.g., Leonardis et al., 2000; Madden et al., 2002; Rodriguez-Ballesteros et al., 2003; Starr et al., 1998, 2003, 2004; Varga et al., 2003; Wang et al., 2003). According to data reported by Madden et al. (2002), a genetic factor is involved in one-third of children with "auditory neuropathy." Jutras and colleagues (Jutras, Russell, Hurteau, & Chapdelaine, 2003) reported audiologic findings consistent with "auditory neuropathy" in two siblings with a family history of Waardenburg's syndrome. Wang et al. (2003) described a general audiologic pattern consistent with "auditory neuropathy" (normal OAEs absent ABRs) in 12 patients from four Chinese families. Investigations in East European Roma (Gypsy) families initially provided the most compelling evidence of hereditary neuropathies involving the auditory system (e.g., Butinar et al., 1999; Kalaydijieva et al., 1998; Kovach et al., 2002). These hearing deficits, including "auditory neuropathy" in patients with Charcot-Marie-Tooth disease and autosomal recessive sensorimotor neuropathy, are associated with mutations in the MPZ gene (Starr et al., 2003). Starr et al. (2003) conducted a detailed genetic, psychoacoustic, and neurophysiologic investigation of a family from Costa Rica with acquired mild-to-moderate hearing loss. The authors also conducted a neuropathologic examination of one family member by biopsy (at age 70 years) and postmortem examination (at age 77 years). The neuropathologic studies showed reduction in spiral ganglion cells (1,161 in one ear and 1,548 in the other ear versus about 23,000 in a normal eighth nerve) and loss of auditory nerve fibers and abnormal amounts of myelin on surviving nerve fibers, in the presence of essentially intact outer and inner hair cells and sensory epithelium of the vestibular organs (Starr et al., 2003). Starr et al. (2004) reported a comprehensive investigation of auditory function in 72 people within a kindred characterized by an inherited autosomal dominant pattern of hearing loss. Audiologic assessment included basic measures (audiogram, DPOAEs, word recognition), psychoacoustic studies (gap detection, temporal integration, frequency discrimination), and auditory electrophysiology (ABR and cortical auditory evoked responses). Data were also reported for three family members with cochlear implants.

INFLUENCE OF BODY TEMPERATURE. | Starr et al. (1998) reported that the audiologic deficits (e.g., degree of hearing loss and marked abnormalities of the ABR) for some patients with "auditory neuropathy" were produced by elevation of body temperature by 1 to 2 degrees. In this study, two of the three subjects (age 3 and 6 years) were siblings, and the other subject was an unrelated child (age 15 years). Selected auditory findings (e.g., pure-tone thresholds, acoustic reflexes, ABR) were abnormal even in the afebrile state, although the abnormalities worsened significantly with increased temperature. OAEs, however, were consistently normal regardless of body temperature. Some measures of auditory function (e.g., pure tone audiometry, word recognition, ABR) were dramatically improved, although not normal, when the subjects were normothermic (afebrile). The mechanism proposed for the changes in auditory findings is a temperature related "reduction of neural input accompanying the development of conduction block in demyelinated fibers" (Starr et al., 1998, p. 1616).

How Common Is "Auditory Neuropathy"?

The exact prevalence of "auditory neuropathy" is not known. Information on the likelihood of "auditory neuropathy" in various patient populations (e.g., newborn infants), would contribute to rather fundamental clinical decisions, such as which technique—OAE or ABR—should be utilized to screen newborn infants for hearing impairment, or when

OAE measurement should be included in the pediatric test battery. It is now clear that audiologists in tertiary medical facilities (major medical centers that offer the "last resort" for sophisticated hearing health care) encounter "auditory neuropathy" regularly, for example, audiologists who are responsible for hearing assessment of NICU graduates and children suspected of hearing loss who are referred from physicians and other audiologists for a definitive diagnosis prior to management. Although exact statistics are not yet available, several recent papers provide general estimates. An estimated 11 to 15 percent of children with hearing loss may show the pattern of findings consistent with "auditory neuropathy" (e.g., Davis & Hirsch, 1979; Kraus, Özdamer, Stein, & Reed, 1984). Rance et al. (1999) found the pattern of absent ABR and normal outer hair cell function (verified by the ECochG cochlear microphonic) in twelve children of 5,199 who were screened. The proportion with the "auditory neuropathy" pattern was 0.23 percent of their at-risk infants. Of the 109 children with permanent hearing impairment, however, the proportion was 11 percent (one in nine cases). Vohr, Carty, Moore, and Letourneau (1998) reported 5 children with hearing impairment out of a total of 111 who had initially passed a TEOAE screening. Two of these infants had the diagnosis of "auditory neuropathy." In an investigation of a combined OAE and ABR hearing screening technique, Hall, Smith, and Popelka (2004) reported one child with the diagnosis of "auditory neuropathy" in a series of 300 well babies. As implied above by the reference to "auditory neuropathy" among children admitted to the well baby nursery versus NICU, the likelihood of "auditory neuropathy" varies with the patient population. "Auditory neuropathy" is a rare finding among healthy newborn infants or older children (preschool or school age) undergoing routine hearing screening. However, among children at risk for hearing impairment and undergoing a sedated ABR (e.g., those with severe language delay and difficult to test with behavioral audiometery), the author (Hall, 2003) has found that approximately 10 percent have auditory findings consistent with "auditory neuropathy."

In a study of "auditory neuropathy "in 123 school-age children (age 7 to 18 years) with hearing impairment (in Hong Kong), Tang et al. (2004) estimated that 2.4 percent had "auditory neuropathy." Berlin et al. (2000) reported some evidence of OAE activity in 10 percent of 1,000 school age children with severe-to-profound hearing loss.

CAN "AUDITORY NEUROPATHY" APPEAR IN OLDER CHILDREN AND ADULTS? | Starr and colleagues (Starr, Picton, Sininger, Hood, & Berlin, 1996) first applied the term "auditory neuropathy" to describe ten patients who developed neurological signs and symptoms of peripheral nerve abnormalities, including neural auditory dysfunction presumably involving the spiral ganglion cells and auditory portion of the eighth cranial nerve. Age at the onset of hearing loss ranged from 2 years to 30 years. At the time the article was written, only

one patient (a 4-year-old boy) was under the age of 15 years. Auditory findings included the presence of OAEs and/or CM and markedly abnormal ABRs. Other auditory procedures administered included pure-tone and speech audiometry, acoustic reflexes, auditory middle latency, late and P300 evoked responses (plus somatosensory and visual evoked responses), masking level difference (MLD), gap detection, and tone decay tests. Audiometric configurations were varied in the ten patients, with five showing decreased low-frequency pure-tone hearing thresholds, two a high-frequency loss, and three a flat configuration. All but two of the patients in this series met criteria for demyelinating peripheral neuropathy characterized by clinical examination ("loss of deep-tendon reflexes and elevated vibratory threshold"), a chronic and progressive course, abnormal nerve conduction studies, and, with some patients, with formal diagnoses such as hereditary sensorimotor neuropathy (HSMN) or Charcot-Marie-Tooth disease. Importantly, in the series of patients reported by Starr et al. (1996), auditory dysfunction was typically identified years before peripheral neuropathy was suspected or diagnosed.

Somehow, in the years following this initial report, the term "auditory neuropathy" was broadened and distorted to include a variety of etiologies (e.g., hyperbilirubinemia) far removed from the diseases producing true peripheral neuropathies. That is, the label "auditory neuropathy" was applied indiscriminately to most patients, particularly children, with an absent or very abnormal ABR in the presence of normal OAEs. As use or application of "auditory neuropathy" expanded, incorrectly and inappropriately, diverse sites of dysfunction were described, including brainstem auditory pathways and even sensory structures (e.g., inner hair cells). Of course, sensory and central auditory dysfunction is not compatible with the term "neuropathy." And, ironically, despite the lack of any infants in the patient series reported in original paper by Starr et al. (1996), the term "auditory neuropathy" became associated with neonatal onset, rather than a progressive deficit later in childhood. The answer to the question "Can "auditory neuropathy" appear in older children and adults?" is, therefore, almost always "yes." Indeed, when the pattern of a very abnormal ABR and normal OAEs is found in an infant, one should not immediately apply the label "auditory neuropathy."

Detection and Assessment

DETECTION. | An approach for detection of "auditory neuropathy" is shown schematically in Figure 5.3. Because OAE measurement is now the standard of care in pediatric hearing assessment (e.g., Joint Committee on Infant Hearing, 2000a,

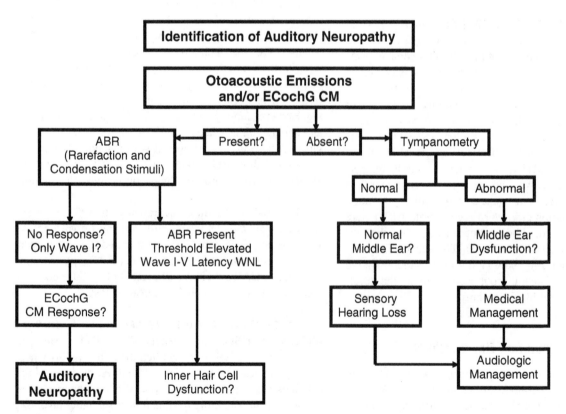

FIGURE 5.3. Flowchart for detection or identification of "auditory neuropathy" showing the pivotal role of OAEs and/or the cochlear microphonic (CM) component of ECochG.

b), OAEs typically play the initial, and pivotal, role in the detection of "auditory neuropathy." If there is no evidence of OAEs or CM (right side of flowchart in Figure 5.3), then the diagnostic effort is directed to ruling out middle ear pathology and, if middle ear function is normal, defining the degree of sensory hearing impairment. Confirmation of middle ear dysfunction leads to recommendations for medical referral and possible management (e.g., for middle ear disease). On the other hand, if middle ear dysfunction is ruled out, a sensory (cochlear) hearing loss is presumed and audiologic management follows (e.g., hearing aid selection and fitting). OAE presence, in the context of abnormal ABR findings, raises the suspicion of "auditory neuropathy" (left side of flowchart in Figure 5.3). An appreciation of a basic ECochG concept is important at this stage in the assessment of possible "auditory neuropathy." The cochlear microphonic (CM) is recorded with single-polarity (rarefaction or condensation) click stimuli, not with alternating-polarity stimulation (e.g., Berlin et al., 1998). Confirmation of outer hair cell integrity in suspected "auditory neuropathy" is dependent on the presence of a CM, as well as OAEs. This point is explained further below in a review of ECochG findings in "auditory neuropathy."

DIAGNOSTIC ASSESSMENT. | As schematically depicted in Figure 5.4, the finding of normal OAEs or some evidence of OAEs, plus an abnormal neurodiagnostic ABR, is followed by more precise electrophysiologic evaluation. This diagnostic assessment could be conducted immediately upon first evidence of an "auditory neuropathy" pattern. An alternative approach is to defer the assessment, and management other than audiologic monitoring, until two to three months after the initial detection of a possible "auditory neuropathy" pattern, because it appears that some forms of "auditory neuropathy" are transient, or reversible. Madden et al. (2002), for example, reported that 50 percent of their series of patients (N = 22) "showed audiologic evidence of a spontaneous improvement in their hearing. This occurred 1 to 15 months after their diagnosis, with a mean improvement time of 5.8 months . . . children with jaundice were more likely to have a profound initial hearing loss but showed a greater tendency to improve spontaneously and to end with a better hearing outcome" (p. 1028). I have also documented in infants with history of, for example, hypoxic insults (asphyxia), meningitis, and hyperbilirubinemia, a complete return of ABRs and/or resolution of ABR abnormalities from the initial assessment to a follow-up assessment two to three months later.

A formal diagnostic test battery for "auditory neuropathy" consists of an "all-star" collection of auditory procedures, each carefully selected to assess a very specific site within the auditory system or a circumscribed auditory function. Evaluation of "auditory neuropathy" requires a finely tuned diagnostic approach, utilizing all available techniques for selectively assessing the function, whenever possible, of specific structures. Atypical, or expanded, test protocols are

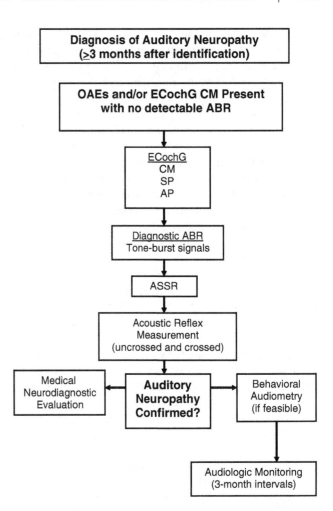

FIGURE 5.4. Flowchart for diagnosis of "auditory neuropathy" showing the pivotal role of OAEs and/or the cochlear microphonic (CM) component of ECochG.

followed for each procedure in order to maximize diagnostic information on auditory status. For example, ABRs are recorded with rarefaction and condensation stimulus polarities to differentiate sensory versus neural responses (e.g., Berlin et al., 1998). Measurement of multiple electrophysiological responses from the auditory periphery is especially important to differentiate clearly between outer versus inner hair cell dysfunction. For example, one might question the need for including both OAEs and the CM of the ECochG in the test battery, as both are electrophysiological measures of outer hair cell function. There are at least two reasons why OAEs and CM are complementary, rather than redundant. CM is thought to reflect receptor potentials (see Chapter 2 for a review of cochlear physiology underlying ECohG) produced at the apical end of outer hair cells when they are activated mechanically. OAEs reflect outer hair cell motility that results, in part, from electromechanical events subsequent to the receptor potentials. Conceivably, then, CM might be recorded in the absence of OAEs if receptor potentials remained intact yet the complex mechanisms involved in active processes (motility) were disrupted. Second, measurement of OAEs is dependent on outward propagation of energy from the cochlea through the middle ear to the ear canal. Subtle middle ear dysfunction may essentially obliterate OAE detection without affecting CM recordings. Third, CM generation is not entirely dependent on outer hair cells. There appears to be some inner hair cell contribution to the CM, although considerably less than the contribution by activity due to outer hair cells (Dallos & Cheatham, 1976). In contrast, the cochlear summating potentials appear to be primarily generated by inner hair cells (Zheng et al., 1997). A subpattern of auditory findings can be inferred from these fundamental distinctions in generation of the CM versus OAEs. CM may be recorded in patients with no detectable OAEs, including some with behavioral evidence of hearing sensitivity deficits. As evidence of this point, Rance et al. (1999) found that about half of their series of 20 patients with "auditory neuropathy" had CM activity, but no OAEs. Without CM measurement, "auditory neuropathy" might not have been diagnosed for these patients.

Although each desired or diagnostically indicated audiologic procedure may not be feasibly performed with every patient, the major objective of the assessment should be met, namely the differential evaluation of cochlear, eighth nerve, and central auditory nervous system function with electrophysiological and behavioral procedures requiring synchronous and less time-dependent activity. The ultimate goal of the diagnostic process is behavioral definition of hearing status with pure-tone and speech audiometry.

Diagnosis in "auditory neuropathy" is challenging in part due to the complexity of this clinical entity. Clinical presentations are highly variable, as "the effects of neuropathy on auditory function appear to be idiosyncratic" (Rance et al., 1999). In most cases, the diagnostic process in "auditory neuropathy" is ongoing, often for years, until hearing status is completely described electrophysiologically and behaviorally, medical diagnosis is reached, and effective medical and audiologic management is initiated. Deficits in speech perception and understanding, and probably a collection of psychoacoustic auditory functions, are a characteristic finding in "auditory neuropathy," if patients survive and are followed until their age and health status permits sophisticated speech audiometry. For some patients, it is likely that changes in medical and/or audiologic status will continue throughout childhood, requiring corresponding alterations in the management plan. And, sadly, a proportion of infants with "auditory neuropathy" will not thrive or even survive due to widespread and serious disease processes.

Management

Management of "auditory neuropathy" is extremely challenging. Some of the considerations in assessment, and subsequent management, are depicted in the flowchart in Figure 5.5. At the very least, a team approach is necessary,

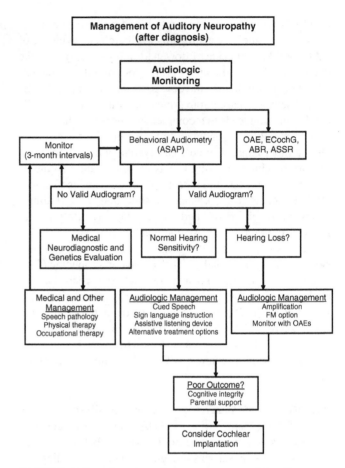

FIGURE 5.5. Flowchart for management of "auditory neuropathy." Details of management are reviewed in the text, and summarized in Table 5.5.

involving medical and nonmedical professionals, including representatives from audiology, speech pathology, medicine (otolaryngology, pediatrics, neurology), genetics, and sometimes occupational and physical therapy.

During the first months after detection of "auditory neuropathy" in infants and young children, the most prudent management strategy is to monitor audiologic status periodically until a pattern of findings emerges. Most audiologists, along with some parents and primary care physicians, will be frustrated by this apparent delay in management. In the past, an abnormal or absent ABR with, perhaps, no response to behavioral signals, unquestionably triggered prompt audiologic intervention, especially amplification. Experience has clearly shown, however, that subsequent audiologic assessment for some children with this initial pattern will show normal hearing sensitivity, or audiometric contraindications to amplification. Hearing aid fitting would, in such children, be inappropriate and, possibly, harmful. When hearing aids are fit, cautiously and with low gain, outer hair cell integrity can be verified regularly with OAE.

Although amplification may be withheld, other management steps can and should be initiated, as summarized

TABLE 5.5. Management Options for Children with "Auditory Neuropathy"

The relationship between the pattern of auditory dysfunction and presumed site of dysfunction is summarized in Table 5.2.

OPTION	COMMENT
Auditory	
Monitoring of auditory function	Regular monitoring with electrophysiologic and, as feasible, behavioral procedures is essential for documentation and complete definition of auditory status. Long-term management is dependent on evidence of permanent hearing loss based on valid behavioral audiometry findings.
Hearing aid	Although amplification is rarely of benefit to children with auditory neuropathy, a trial period with conservative hearing aid fitting (mild gain) and close monitoring of tolerance and responsiveness to sound is reasonable before decisions are made for other long-term options (e.g., cochlear implant). Cochlear function should be monitored closely with OAEs. Unilateral hearing aid fitting may be indicated to minimize risk to hearing status.
Assistive listening device	Assistive listening technology is a conservative and usually helpful management approach.
Cochlear implant	Communicative benefit with cochlear implantation is proven, particularly for children with hearing loss by behavioral assessment and who are intact cognitively.
Nonauditory	
Neurodevelopmental evaluation	Evaluation is necessary to document neurological and developmental status, and the possible need for more detailed neurodiagnostic evaluation and possible medical management.
Genetic counseling	Auditory neuropathy can be associated with family history of hearing loss and with hereditary factors.
Speech reading	Supplementing auditory information with visual cues enhances the communication of children with very poor auditory processing.
Cued Speech	Supplementing auditory information with visual cues enhances the communication of children with very poor auditory processing. Information on Cued Speech is available at the website: www.cuedspeech.mit.edu.
Sign language	It is very important for children with auditory neuropathy to develop language function, and a practical form of communication, pending decisions regarding long-term management of auditory neuropathy. See websites for American Sign Language (ASL) and Signing Exact English (S.E.E.). Information on baby signing, simple signs for basic needs and wants, is available from the Baby Signs Institute (www.babysigns.com).
Speech and language treatment	All children with auditory neuropathy require comprehensive speech and language evaluation, and the majority will require therapy.
Family counseling	Families of children with auditory neuropathy may experience marked frustration with their inability to communicative effectively with the children.
Parent support groups	See website www.auditoryneuropathy.tripod.com.
Psychological counseling	Children and adults with auditory neuropathy may experience marked frustration with inability to communicate effectively.

in Table 5.5. These include referral for comprehensive neurological, developmental, and communication evaluation, and perhaps neuroradiological studies. A child development center is ideal for this multidisciplinary diagnostic effort. Other appropriate referrals include genetics and otolaryngology. Speech-language evaluation, with intensive treatment, is certainly indicated. Cued speech may also be an effective management strategy (Berlin et al., 1998). Alternative forms of communication, such as sign language, should probably be considered only if responsiveness to auditory stimulation fails to develop with remediation efforts. Assistive listening devices to enhance, but not amplify, speech signals may also be appropriate in some cases. In children with "auditory neuropathy," it would be quite reasonable to implement a management approach appropriate for a child with a peripheral (sensorineural) hearing loss, but without amplification initially. Perhaps the most well appreciated and least controversial management option is close, careful, and long-term monitoring of auditory status. In most cases, the complete picture on hearing status and a clear direction for multidisciplinary management is apparent only after audiologic assessment is conducted over a period of months or, in some case, years, and valid behavioral measures of hearing are obtained.

HEARING AIDS. | Should children with "auditory neuropathy" ever be managed purposefully with hearing aids or cochlear implantation? Professional opinions are split on this basic audiologic management approach. Early papers on "auditory neuropathy" suggested that amplification provided little or no benefit and posed a risk to cochlear (outer hair cell) integrity (e.g., Berlin, 1999; Starr et al., 1996). For example, Berlin (1999) stated, "We do not recommend hearing aids unless or until the cochlea degenerates . . . We are fitting hearing aids only when children no longer show OAE. . . . if outer hair cells are present and presumably working, hearing aids are not appropriate physiologically" (p. 311). Most audiologists, however, recommend a conservative trial period with amplification to determine possible increased responsiveness to sound (e.g., Fabry, 2000; Madden et al., 2002; Rance et al., 1999). According to this viewpoint, hearing aids are indicated especially for children with two audiologic characteristics, that is, behavioral evidence of an abnormal audiogram coupled with relatively less deficit in speech perception or aided benefit with speech perception. Rance et al. (1999), for example, ". . . recommend that some form of amplification be attempted in all pediatric neuropathy cases in which the behavioral thresholds are abnormal" (p. 249). This approach is confirmed by experiences reported Madden et al. (2002), who comment, "Patients in our study [N = 22] with significant and persistent hearing loss have responded well to conventional rehabilitation with amplification [16 of the 22 children, or 73 percent] and cochlear implantation" (p. 1029). Strategies for management of "auditory neuropathy" are clearly evolving with the accumulation of clinical experience and with analysis of data on relatively long-term communicative outcome associated with different courses of management. There is little doubt that before the pattern of "auditory neuropathy" was recognized, some children were unwittingly managed with both hearing aids and cochlear implants. Among these children are those who did not obtain benefit from, or simply rejected, amplification. Presently, careful documentation of long-term outcome of children with "auditory neuropathy," related to different management strategies, is lacking. Reported experiences suggest that, with evidence of hearing loss by audiometry, careful introduction of mild-gain amplification may be associated with improvement in speech and language development. With marginally more optimism than implied by the earlier quote in this section, Berlin, Hood, and colleagues, who have collected considerable experience with pediatric "auditory neuropathy" noted in 1998 that:

So far we have seen no compelling evidence that hearing aids will help these children, but we are trying them cautiously with some patients whose parents are amenable, on the outside possibility that these problems are related to displaced or pathologic tectorial membranes and that increased displacement of the cochlear partition may lead to more productive shearing forces in the organ of Corti. (Berlin et al., 1998, p. 45)

With or without amplification, cochlear status should be monitored periodically with OAEs, keeping in mind that over time OAEs may disappear spontaneously in "auditory neuropathy" or with the development of middle ear dysfunction secondary to otitis media. Disappearance of OAEs, especially, at all frequency regions, does not necessarily imply excessive amplification. In these children, ECochG measurement to record a CM for documentation of cochlear status is helpful if it can be performed periodically and without sedation.

In summary, conservative (e.g., mild gain) amplification is a reasonable and justifiable management option pending the availability of behavioral audiologic findings, or with behavioral audiometry evidence of a hearing loss, and prior to the initiation of other forms of treatment (e.g., cochlear implants). The benefits of amplification for stimulation of the auditory and language portions of the intact brain in infants and young children (before 6 months of age) are now quite clear (e.g., Yoshinago-Itano, Sedley, Coulter, & Mehl, 1998). Also, for infants with the typical pattern of auditory findings associated with "auditory neuropathy" who will be considered for cochlear implant candidacy, a period of hearing aid use with close monitoring of responsiveness and cochlear status will meet requirements for cochlear implantation in young children. Early intervention with amplification also provides family members with a daily reminder of the importance of oral communication efforts and the assurance that steps are being taken to maximize communication in their child.

COCHLEAR IMPLANTS. | Thinking about cochlear implants in children with "auditory neuropathy" has changed considerably during the past ten years. Soon after "auditory neuropathy" was first described and audiologists were faced with developing management strategies for a problem about which they knew very little, cochlear implants were far down on the list of options. Frankly, it seemed inconceivable that insertion of a device into a cochlea with normal outer hair cells was an appropriate recommendation. If a child had neural dysfunction characterized by auditory dys-synchrony and obtained no apparent benefit from sound stimulation, including amplification, then a cochlear implant would seem to be contraindicated. Initial experiences with cochlear implantation appeared to confirm this opinion. For example, after an early experience with a cochlear implant in a child with "auditory neuropathy," Miyamoto et al. (1999), remarked, "Although cochlear implantation may offer significant benefits to subjects with 'auditory neuropathy,' caution should be exercised when considering this technology. As with conventional hearing aids, less than optimal results may be seen" (p. 185). It is relevant to the discouraging outcome of the patient reported in this paper to note some specifics of the case. The child, a 5-year-old boy at the time of implantation, had lost hearing progressively. He had other neurological deficits, including severe visual impairment, and was subsequently diagnosed with Friedreich's ataxia. Skepticism persisted into the late 1990s, as typified by Berlin's statement, "whether implantation will become a treatment of choice for "auditory neuropathy" remains to be seen. . . . However, our current understanding of auditory physiology suggests that implantations might be at best only marginally successful if the underlying pathophysiology is a loss of myelin or a loss of neural elements" (p. 312). Recognizing the likelihood of different mechanisms for "auditory neuropathy," Berlin continues "if, on the other hand, the underlying problem is an absence of inner hair cells . . . biochemical, or in some other way connected to deficits in transmitter substances, or even related to a disruption in the linkage between outer and inner hair cells as suggested by Berlin (1999), then electrical stimulation of residual nerve fibers should ultimately be effective after suitable training and organization of the coding and feature extraction system of the cochlea and CNS" (p. 312).

Nonetheless, despite reservations by audiologists and otolaryngologists alike, and perhaps because there were precious few other management options available, some children with "auditory neuropathy" were implanted with surprising benefit. Successful communicative outcome with cochlear implantation of young children with "auditory neuropathy," apparently present from birth, led to a dramatic shift in opinion on cochlear implants as a viable management technique (e.g., Mason et al., 2003; Rance et al., 1999; Shallop et al., 2001; Trautwein, Sininger, & Nelson, 2000). In fact, there is longstanding evidence that auditory fibers are more highly synchronized when activated by electrical stimulation than by acoustic stimulation (e.g., Goldstein & Kiang, 1958). Factors contributing to a good prognosis for effective communication with a cochlear implant include, as summarized in Table 5.5, are (1) a hearing loss based on behavioral audiometry, (2) integrity of the spiral ganglion and eighth nerve fibers, (3) intact cognitive function, (4) family support, and (5) implantation in young children. Audiologic indicators of good prognosis of cochlear implantation in auditory neuropathy include severe hearing loss by pure tone audiometry, essentially absent speech recognition ability, and the characteristic features of the disorder (OAEs present and ABR absent). The presence of a robust electrical compound action potential (ECAP) confirms stimulation of the auditory afferent fibers following cochlear implantation and is also a good prognostic indicator (e.g., Shallop et al., 2001). Among children grouped within the broad "auditory neuropathy" category, therefore, the best cochlear implant candidates are those who in fact have inner hair cell impairments and who, in reality, have a sensory hearing loss and not a neuropathy. In

the words of Jon Shallop and colleagues of the Mayo Clinic, "We conclude that multichannel cochlear implants may provide an effective solution to the documented sensorineural hearing loss in some cases of auditory neuropathy" (Shallop et al., 2001, p. 561). Mason et al. (2002) at the University of Virginia concur that "greater confidence and enthusiasm for cochlear implantation in appropriately selected patients with "auditory neuropathy" are gained through experience . . ." (p. 45). Two factors that can be viewed as indicators of poor prognosis for cochlear implants, or actual contraindications, include evidence (e.g., neuroradiologic or neurophysiologic) of severe auditory nerve dysfunction or aplasia (absence) and older age with no language development.

OTHER MANAGEMENT OPTIONS. | Despite the debate and confusion on management of "auditory neuropathy" with hearing aids and, to a lesser extent, cochlear implants, there is consensus on the value of maximizing visual cues with formal instruction in, for example, cued speech (see Table 5.5). Efforts to develop language as early as possible would be logical, particularly while awaiting more definitive or stable evidence of auditory function by behavioral or electrophysiological assessment. Berlin (1999) expressed concerns, stating,

> I recommend management with cued speech instead of sign language or hearing aids. ASL or similar sign language does not relate to either English phonology or syntax; therefore, if a child's language learning periods are occupied with a system that does not generalize easily to spoken or written English, that child may be put at a disadvantage when and if normal hearing is developed or if a cochlear implant is chosen." (p. 312)

Rather than embarking on extensive instruction of child and family with a formal sign language system, there appears to be value in assisting the family in the development of a modest number of simple signs for communication of basic wants and needs. There is increased interest among parents and educators in "baby signing" for normal hearing infants, as evidenced by books for laypersons (e.g., *Baby Signs: How to Talk with Your Baby before Your Baby Can Talk* [Linda Acredolo, Susan Goodwyn, Douglas Abrams, New York: McGraw Hill]; *My First Book of Sign* [Pamela J. Baker, Washington, DC: Gallaudet University Press]) and the Baby Signs Institute (website www.babysigns.com). Baby signing can be included in the overall effort to enhance practical communication and coupled with cued speech, assistive listening devices, and amplification.

It is fitting to conclude this review with a passage from the conclusion of the article by Rapin and Gravel (2003):

> We object on scientific grounds to the use of the term "auditory neuropathy" when the main site of pathology is in the brain stem or more centrally in the auditory pathway. Loose use of the term "auditory neuropathy" is confusing, likely to be anatomically incorrect, and engenders imprecision rather than

emphasizing the strong need for comprehensive behavioral, electrophysiological, and pathologic investigation. . . . Therefore, we urge that the term "auditory neuropathy" senso stricto be reserved for demonstrable involvement of the spiral ganglion cells or their processes, and not be used for pathologies of uncertain or mixed locations." (p. 724)

MÉNIÈRE'S DISEASE AND ENDOLYMPHATIC HYDROPS

Ménière's disease is a pathologic process involving the inner ear. Although Ménière's disease has been extensively studied experimentally and clinically, the precise pathophysiology remains poorly understood. In 1861, a French physician, Prosper Ménière, described four classic symptoms of the disease. The symptoms are (1) *vertigo* (a true spinning sensation), (2) hearing loss, (3) *tinnitus* (described by patients as roaring, buzzing, or other sounds in the ear), and (4) a feeling of "fullness" in the ear. These symptoms are episodic, periodically decreasing and increasing over the course of months or even years (see Table 5.6). Fluctuating hearing loss is an example of the episodic nature of the disease. Vertiginous attacks may be very sudden and debilitating, accompanied

TABLE 5.6. Criteria Used in the Diagnosis of Ménière's Disease

---

Certain Ménière's disease

- Definite Ménière's disease, plus histopathologic confirmation

Definite Ménière's disease

- Two or more definitive spontaneous episodes of vertigo lasting 20 minutes or longer
- Audiometrically documented hearing loss on at least one occasion
- Tinnitus or aural fullness in the treated ear
- Other causes excluded

Probable Ménière's disease

- One definitive episode of vertigo
- Audiometrically documented hearing loss on at least one occasion
- Tinnitus or aural fullness in the treated ear
- Other causes excluded

Possible Ménière's disease

- Episodic vertigo of the Ménière type without documented hearing loss, or
- Sensorineural hearing loss, fluctuating or fixed, with dys-equilibrium, but without definitive episodes
- Other causes excluded

Source: Adapted from Committee on Hearing and Equilibrium. *Otolaryngology-Head and Neck Surgery 113:* 181–185, 1995.

by nausea and/or vomiting, and lasting from a few minutes to hours.

A typical component of Ménière's disease is excessive pressure of fluid within the *scala media* (the middle of three divisions or compartments of the inner ear) that produces distention of the boundaries of the scala media (Reissner's membrane). The fluid in this compartment is *endolymph,* and the disease is often called *endolymphatic hydrops.* The hydrops (increased pressure) may also be found within portions of the vestibular labyrinth (utricle, saccule, semicircular canal ampulla).

A review of the many theories on the cause of Ménière's disease and modes of treatment are far beyond scope of this book. A common treatment of the most bothersome symptom (vertigo) is sedatives or anti-vertigo medication, in combination with diuretic medication and dietary salt restriction.

Ménière's disease produces sensory hearing impairment. Initially, in evolution of the disease in a patient, there is only low-frequency hearing deficit (a *rising* audiometric configuration). Hearing sensitivity is often within the normal region for test frequencies above 2000 Hz. With progression of the disease and the extent of hearing loss, the audiogram generally becomes flat (equivalent degree of hearing loss across audiometric frequencies). There are, however, occasional reports of total return of normal hearing. A low-frequency hearing loss, and a rising audiogram configuration, usually reflects a conductive hearing loss. Ménière's disease is an exception to this rule. Typically the apparent hearing impairment is unilateral, although bilateral evidence of hearing deficit is found in about 10 to 20 percent of patients. In addition, almost one-half of the patients who initially exhibit unilateral Ménière's disease will later develop bilateral hearing involvement. ECochG abnormalities may be recorded in the apparently uninvolved ear of patients with unilateral Ménière's disease (e.g., Podoshin, Ben-David, Pratt, Fradis, & Feiglin, 1986). Indeed, ear-specific information on the presence of Ménière's disease is potentially one of the main clinical advantages of ECochG. Finally, there are infrequent reports of the application of ECochG in the diagnosis of children with endolymphatic hydrops and Ménière's disease (e.g., Mizukoshi, Shojaku, Aso, Asai, & Watanabe, 2001) and, at the other end of age span, in the diagnosis of elderly patients with Ménière's disease (Mizukoshi, Shojaku, Aso, Asai, & Watanabe, 2000).

By far, the most studied and well-known clinical application of ECochG is the diagnosis of Ménière's disease. Space does not permit a review of each, or even most, of the hundreds of publications on ECochG in Ménière's disease. Selected published papers on the topic are listed in Table 5.7. Early clinical papers in the late 1970s and early 1980s, and subsequent clinical investigations ongoing to the present, confirm that the characteristic ECochG feature associated with Ménière's disease is a large SP amplitude relative to the AP amplitude (Coats, 1981; Gibson, Moffat, & Ramsden, 1977; Goin, Staller, Asher, & Mischke, 1982; Kitahara,

TABLE 5.7. Summary of Studies of ECochG in the Diagnosis of Ménière's
Disease (MD), Arranged Chronologically

STUDY, YEAR	N	STIMULUS	ELECTRODE	COMMENTS
Mori et al., 1990	35	click	EAC	No correlation between negative SP and ENG results.
Mori et al., 1990	47 ears	click; TB	EAC	Positive SP most likely with 8000 Hz tone burst.
Aso et al., 1991	168	click	??	Effects of glycerol and endolymphatic sac surgery.
Gibson, 1991	80	click; TB	TT	Tone burst increased sensitivity to MD.
Ohashi, Ochi, Okada, & Takeyama, 1991	24	click	??	Serial ECochG recordings in MD showed no change.
Campbell, Harker, & Abbas, 1992	10	click; TB	TM	SP/AP ratio did not differentiate MD vs. normals.
Moffat et al., 1992	40	click	TT	ECochG diagnosis of MD in contralateral ear of 35% of patients with unilateral MD.
Dornhoffer & Arenberg, 1993	15	click	TT	Sensitivity of SP/AP ratio = 73%.
Chen & Wong, 1993	22	click	TT	Sensitivity = 59%; specificity = 92% in MD.
Kitaoku et al., 1993	15 (normal)	click	EAC	Examined normal ECochG changes with glycerol.
Lajtman, Marinovic, Krpan, & Gasparovic, 1993	??	click	EAC	Increase in SP amplitude in MD.
Kitaoku, 1994	??	click	EAC	Changes in ECochG during glycerol test.
Matsuura et al., 1996	??	click	TM	Significant increase in SP/AP ratio in MD; demonstrated the value of contralateral recordings.
Filipo et al., 1997	185	click	??	
Johansson et al., 1997	5	click	TT	Condensation vs. rarefaction latency differences.
Zhang, Ji, & Jiang, 1997	70	click	TT	ECochG in MD, NIHL, ototoxicity, and sudden onset.
Arakawa, 1998	29 ears	click; TB	EAC	Examined enhanced negative SP and SP/AP ratio.
Orchik et al., 1998	84	click	TT	Enhanced SP/AP ratio correlated with duration of MD.
Sass et al., 1998	61	click, TB	TT	Normative findings; click vs. tone burst differences.
Conlon & Gibson, 1999	3000	1K Hz TB	TT	High percentage of patients with apparent unilateral MD have contralateral disease.
Gamble et al., 1999	??	click	EAC	Salt loading increased SP/AP ratio.
Konradsson et al., 1999	16	click	TT	Documentation of hypobaric effects with ECochG.
Conlon & Gibson, 2000	??	click; TB	TT	Sensitivity of negative SP and SP/AP ratio about 85%.
Anft, Jamali, Scholz, & Mrowinski, 2001	29	click	??	ECochG findings consistent with MD in 62%.
Mizukoshi et al., 2001	6	click	??	ECochG value in pediatric MD.
Camilleri & Howarth, 2001	70	click	??	Abnormal ECochG predicts benefit from sac surgery.
Ghosh et al., 2002	20	click	TT; EAC	EAC is feasible but not as sensitive as TT ECochG.

Takada, Yazawa, & Matsubara, 1981; Schmidt, Eggermont, & Odenthal, 1974). Sensitivity of the SP/AP ratio in the diagnosis of Ménière's disease is typically in the range of 30 to 65 percent (Ferraro, Arenberg, & Hassanein, 1985; Goin et al., 1988; Margolis et al., 1992; Pou et al., 1996), although some investigators have reported higher average sensitivity statistics (Sass et al., 1998). Another response parameter applied in the diagnosis of Ménière's disease is the width of the ECochG complex, i.e., the combined duration of the SP and the AP components. A variety of factors appear to influence sensitivity of ECochG in diagnosis of Ménière's disease. The likelihood of a positive (large) SP/AP ratio in Ménière's disease is, for example, higher with certain patient characteristics, e.g., whether the patient is experiencing symptoms, a late versus early stage of the disease, the degree of hearing loss, and measurement factors, e.g., tone burst versus click signals.

Diagnosis

ECochG has been applied more in suspected Ménière's disease than in any other single cochlear pathology (Coats, 1981; Coats & Alford, 1981; Coats, Jenkins, & Monroe, 1984; Dauman, Aran, Sauvage, & Portmann, 1988; Dauman & Charlet de Sauvage, 1984; Eggermont, 1979; Ferraro, Arenberg, & Hassanein, 1985; Gibson, Moffat, & Ramsden, 1977; Gibson, Prasher, & Kilkenny, 1983; Goin et al., 1982; Kansaki, Oushi, Yokobori, & Ino, 1982; Kumagami, Nishida, & Baba, 1982; Mori, Asai, & Sakagami, 1990; Podoshin, Ben-David, Pratt, Fradis, & Feiglin, 1986). The fundamental ECochG analysis technique used by most of these investigators was the calculation of amplitude of the SP and AP components. Then, ECochG analysis involves an evaluation of these two values, usually calculation of amplitude for the SP and AP components, and also an assessment of the relationship between these two values, usually the calculation of a simple amplitude ratio.

An international collection of investigators has provided clinical evidence that ECochG can contribute to the diagnosis of Ménière's disease and endolymphatic hydrops. Typically, SP amplitude recorded from ears with endolymphatic hydrops is enhanced in comparison to the SP amplitude recorded from normal ears. Beginning in the late 1970s and early 1980s, investigations of ECochG in Ménière's disease were reported independently by researchers from at least four different countries, including Japan (Yoshie, 1976), the Netherlands (Eggermont, 1976a,b; Odenthal & Eggermont, 1976), Great Britain (Gibson, Moffat, & Ramsden, 1977), and the United States (Brackmann & Selters, 1976; Coats, 1981). A common, though not consistent, finding among these studies was abnormally enlarged SP amplitude in persons with diagnosed Ménière's disease. However, there continues to be disagreement as to the clinical usefulness of this observation. To a large extent, this is because of characteristically high variability of absolute SP amplitude, even in nor-

mal ears. Except for persons showing extreme SP amplitude values (extremely small or extremely large), there tends to be a disappointing overlap in measurements among normal versus pathologic ears (Coats, 1981; Goin et al., 1982). The ratio of the SP amplitude to the AP amplitude within a patient is a more stable ECochG measure. Other factors, such as the recording site (electrode placement), stimulus type and rate, and the definition of disease (mentioned previously), contributed to the differences among these studies.

ECOCHG ANALYSIS IN MÉNIÈRE'S DISEASE. | Three general ECochG analysis approaches have been employed. The most popular is a calculation of the ratio between SP and AP amplitude. This technique was shown in Figure 4.11. Amplitude of the SP and AP components in microvolts is measured from a common baseline. An SP/AP ratio is calculated these individual amplitude values. Eggermont (1976b) was among the first to use the SP/AP ratio, mainly in an attempt to reduce measurement variability. The problem of intersubject variability that plagued absolute SP amplitude appears to occur also with AP/AP amplitude ratio. The overlap of ECochG data among groups can be appreciated when SP and AP findings are displayed graphically (see Figure 5.6) as reported originally by Goin et al. (1982) and Coats (1981), and later others. For example, if a normal upper limit for the SP/AP ratio were 2 standard deviations above the normal average for the SP/AP ratio, one would be hard pressed to identify accu-

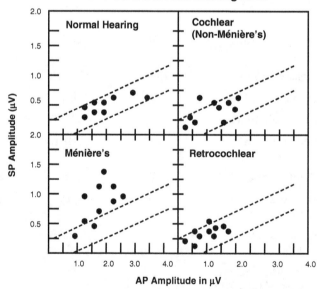

FIGURE 5.6. Distribution of amplitude data for SP and AP components of the ECochG relative to normative data for normal subjects, and patients with three categories of sensorineural hearing loss (cochlear non-Ménière's disease, Ménière's disease, and retrocochlear pathology).
Adapted from Goin, Staller, Asher, & Mischke, 1982.

rately the patients with Ménière's disease among those with other cochlear pathology or even retrocochlear pathology.

In contrast to the inherent imprecision of ECochG data for identification of individual patients, however, Goin et al. (1982) found the SP/AP ratio a useful diagnostic measure in separating groups of patients. These authors reported statistically significant differences in the SP/AP ratio for patients with Ménière's disease versus other groups of patients, a finding supported by the results of an investigation by Gibson, Prasher, and Kilkenny (1983). Gibson and colleagues reported a range in SP/AP ratios of 10 to 63 in normal ears. This would suggest excessive variability. However, for cochlear pathology that was not due to Ménière's disease, the range was only 0 to 29 (with a mean SP/AP ratio of 13). In contrast, Ménière's patients produced SP/AP ratios ranging from 29 to 89 (mean of 51). Thus, a ratio of 29 was an effective lower cutoff for Ménière's disease, according to these data. It is important to recognize that both Coats and Goin (and Goin's colleagues) used broadband click stimuli and an ear-canal recording electrode, whereas Gibson, Prasher, and Kilkenny (1983) used a TT electrode. The relation between amplitude for the SP and AP components is sometimes shown in a graph (refer again to Figure 5.6). Most persons with normal hearing, of course, have relatively larger absolute values for the SP and AP components, and SP/AP ratios that fall within the normal range (indicated in the figure by the diagonal dashed lines). Patients with cochlear hearing loss that is not due to Ménière's disease and patients with retrocochlear hearing loss also tend to have SP/AP ratios within normal limits, although absolute amplitudes may be smaller due to the degree of hearing impairment. The characteristic feature of Ménière's disease (shown in Figure 5.6) is enhanced SP amplitude relative to AP amplitude, as indicated by the symbols falling above the upper diagonal dashed line. One must keep in mind that measurement techniques vary considerably among studies. The differences in protocols, especially electrode location, will have a pronounced influence on ECochG waveform and on the absolute amplitudes for the SP and AP components and their relative amplitudes (e.g., ratio).

The normally high variability in absolute SP amplitude would appear to detract from clinical usefulness. Coats and colleagues (Coats, Jenkins, & Monroe, 1984) also correctly pointed out that the SP/AP ratio varies considerably as AP amplitude changes, i.e., in normal ears, as the AP increases the ratio decreases. Coats therefore developed and applied more sophisticated data analysis techniques to normalize the SP versus AP relation and to reduce measurement variability (Coats, 1981, 1986). Normal SP and AP values are used to develop a log-transformed plot, with the upper 95 percent confidence limit indicated with a least squares fit line. Others (e.g., Goin et al., 1982) have likewise produced scatter plots for SP and AP amplitude in normal subjects, patients with Ménière's disease, and patients with other cochlear pathology (see Figure 5.6 above). With the inclusion of lines indicating some definition of an upper limit for expected

data, such as +2 SEM (standard error of the mean) limits of normal, these plots are quite easy to apply clinically. A patient's ECochG data are simply compared graphically to normal expectations. However, the plot must be constructed with measurement parameters that are used in a clinical facility. These specifically include electrode type and location and stimulus factors employed in ECochG measurement.

Another general ECochG analysis technique is measurement in milliseconds of the combined width of the SP and AP components, i.e., the duration of the SP/AP complex (Aran & LeBert, 1968; Booth, 1980; Brackmann & Selters, 1976; Gibson & Beagley, 1976a,b; Gibson, Moffat, & Ramsden, 1977; Podoshin, Ben-David, Pratt, Fradis, Feiglin, 1986) (illustrated in the previous chapter in Figure 4.11). Prolongation of the duration of this wave complex is found in up to two-thirds of patients with Ménière's disease (Gibson, Moffat, & Ramsden, 1977). Podoshin et al. (1986), for example, calculated the duration of AP component as the latency difference between shoulders on the wave. These authors found average AP durations of 0.96 ms for normal subjects, 1.16 msec for the nonaffected ear of 24 patients with unilateral Ménière's disease, and 1.33 msec for the affected ear. The difference in duration was significant in ECochG findings between normal and Ménière's disease ears, but not between the two ears of these patients with apparently unilateral involvement. A total of 58 percent of the patients with Ménière's disease had abnormal ECochG duration findings. Nonetheless, variability in this response parameter is a serious clinical limitation (Coats, 1981; Goin et al., 1982), and ECochG width has not gained widespread clinical use.

The third analysis approach reported in Ménière's disease in comparison of latency of the AP component for rarefaction versus condensation polarity signals (Johannson, Haapaniemi, & Laurikainen, 1997). In normal ears, the ECochG AP component (and ABR wave I) has a shorter latency for rarefaction versus condensation polarity signals. Some authors have reported that the difference in AP latency values as a function of signal polarity may be greater than normal for patients with Ménière's disease (Gibson, 1991; Johannson et al., 1997; Levine, Margolis, Fournier, & Winzenburg, 1992; Margolis, Rieks, Fournier, & Levine, 1995). Also, there is some suggestion that this latency difference for different signal polarities can differentiate Ménière's disease from other cochlear disorders (Johannson et al., 1997).

Other ECochG response parameters have also been analyzed in Ménière's disease, often with conflicting conclusions. Odenthal and Eggermont (1976) cited four characteristic findings, in addition to relatively large SP amplitude, including steep amplitude–intensity functions (input–output curves), relatively longer response latency values near threshold and normal latency–intensity functions. Brackmann and Selters (1976) found ECochG waveform morphology most useful in diagnosis of Ménière's disease. In contrast to Odenthal and Eggermont (1976), they noted shorter response latency at threshold in Ménière's disease. However, two-thirds of their Ménière's patients produced an abnormal waveform morphology, mainly multiple or very broad peaks. The problem with this observation was difficulty in quantification of the abnormality.

POLARITY OF SP IN MÉNIÈRE'S DISEASE. | Conventionally, the SP is described as a "hump" on the leading slope of the AP (as shown in Figure 4.11). The polarity or direction of the deflection is the same as that of the AP. With an electrode array consisting of a noninverting electrode relatively close to the cochlea, (e.g., the promontory) and an inverting electrode relatively distant (e.g., the contralateral earlobe), the SP and AP have negative polarity. With a typical ABR electrode array (noninverting electrode on the forehead or vertex and inverting electrode on the earlobe, within the ear canal, or even on the promontory), these potentials are positive in voltage.

Two measurement conditions, however, sometimes produce a divergence in polarity for SP versus AP components of the ECochG in both normal subjects and patients with Ménière's disease. Under these conditions, the SP is positive in voltage when the AP is negative in voltage, and vice versa. One condition is a high-frequency tone-burst stimulus, such as 4000 or 8000 Hz (Dauman, Aran, Charlet de Sauvage, & Portmann, 1988; Kansaki et al., 1982). Dauman et al. (1988) consistently observed a positive-voltage SP, as opposed to a negative-voltage AP, for an 8000 Hz stimulus in Ménière's disease, whereas Kansaki et al. (1982) described this finding in 38 percent of their 42 cases. The second condition is an electrode location within the middle-ear cavity. A positive SP is more likely to be recorded as the electrode is placed closer to the oval versus the round window.

Factors Influencing ECochG in Ménière's Disease

It is beyond the scope of this book to provide a full discussion of the myriad combinations of measurement and pathophysiologic factors influencing ECochG recording in Ménière's disease. Among the important factors that must be kept in mind, however, are the site of the recording electrode, the stimulus characteristics, the definition of Ménière's disease, and the degree of hearing loss. These factors are now reviewed with reference to Ménière's disease. The effects of stimulus and acquisition factors on the ECochG, in general, were reviewed in Chapter 4.

ELECTRODE TYPE AND SITE. | This very important factor in ECochG recording was reviewed in some detail in Chapter 4, and guidelines for the application of different electrode types were summarized in Chapter 4 (in Tables 4.1 through 4.3). The exact point of electrode placement relative to the cochlea, and even specifically within the middle-ear cavity (on the medial wall), is particularly crucial in determining the morphology of ECochG waveform. Amplitude of the SP and AP also depends on the proximity of the electrode to

the cochlea. As the recording electrode is located closer to the promontory, amplitude of the AP increases relative more than amplitude of the SP component.

For over twenty-five years, investigators have described the application of extratympanic electrode ECochG techniques in the diagnosis of Ménière's disease (Chung, Cho, Choi, Hong, 2004; Coats, 1981; Ghosh, Gupta, & Mann, 2002; Mori, Asai, Doi, & Matsunaga, 1987; Pappas, Pappas, Carmichael, Hyatt, & Toohey, 2000; Roland, Rosenbloom, Yellin, & Meyerhoff, 1993; Roland, Yellin, Meyerhoff, & Frank, 1995; Ruth & Lambert, 1989). There are a variety of electrode designs for securing an electrode within the external ear canal. Some actually are modestly invasive, involving insertion of a needle electrode subdermally into the wall of the external ear canal (e.g., Ghosh, Gupta, & Mann, 2002). Other electrode placements described by authors as "extratympanic" involve placement of the electrode at the annulus of the tympanic membrane, rather than more laterally within the external ear canal (e.g., Noguchi, Komatsuzaki, & Nishida, 1999; Schoonhoven, Fabius, & Grote, 1995). Extratympanic electrodes are noninvasive and are relatively easy to apply, hence the clinical popularity of the TIPtrode design (e.g., Pappas et al., 2000; Roland, Yellin, Meyerhoff, & Frank, 1995). Those two features are attractive to audiologists performing ECochG in the diagnosis of Ménière's disease. However, when the extratympanic electrode technique is compared with TM and TT ECochG electrode techniques, the advantage of noninvasive placement is offset by substantial drawbacks. Disadvantages of the ear-canal electrode placement include markedly smaller amplitude for all ECochG components, lower reliability and greater variability in calculations of the SP and AP, a high degree of inter-interpreter variability, and relatively weaker test performance (sensitivity and specificity) in the diagnosis of Ménière's disease. Importantly, because ECochG component amplitude is lower with extratympanic membrane electrodes, at least one out of ten patients will have no apparent response, thus precluding the diagnostic usefulness of ECochG in a proportion of persons with Ménière's disease (Chung et al., 2004).

Tympanic membrane (TM) ECochG electrode designs offer a compromise between extratympanic and TT ECochG measurements. Although the TM ECochG technique is not as simple as the extratympanic (ear-canal) electrode placement, response amplitude is considerably greater. Mostly audiologists have described ECochG findings in Ménière's disease using the tympanic membrane technique (Hall, 1992; Margolis et al., 1992; Margolis, Ricks, Fournier, & Levine, 1995; Pou, Hirsch, Durrant, Gold, & Kamerer, 1996; Ruth & Lambert, 1989). Despite the invasive nature of the technique, the literature strongly supports the application of TT ECochG measurement in Meniere's disease (e.g., Aso, 1990; Aso, Watanabe, & Mizukoshi, 1991; Conlon & Gibson, 2000; Ge & Shea, 2002; Gibson, Moffat, & Ramsden, 1977; Gibson, Prasher, & Kilkenny, 1983; Hall, 1992; Orchik, Ge, & Shea, 1998; Orchik, Shea, & Ge, 1993; Ruth &

Lambert, 1989; Sass, 1998; Schwaber & Hall, 1990). The TT technique is most useful in the diagnosis of Ménière's disease because it produces robust ECochG components in virtually all patients, regardless of degree of hearing loss. This, in turn, contributes to highly reliable responses and increased diagnostic accuracy.

STIMULUS PARAMETERS. | Stimulus parameters, of course, exert an important influence on ECochG outcome. Because a brief stimulus onset is essential, high-intensity acoustic clicks are most often used for clinical ECochG measurement. If a tone-burst stimulus with abrupt onset (one or two stimulus cycles) but prolonged plateau (e.g., 10 ms) is presented, however, it is still possible to record a distinct AP, as well as a SP component that extends throughout the stimulus duration. Thus, prolongation of tone-burst duration permits confident SP identification. This technique reported by Dauman and colleagues (Dauman, Aran, & Portmann, 1986; Dauman, Aran, Charlet de Sauvage, & Portmann, 1988) was illustrated in Chapter 4. According to some investigators, the use of tone burst stimuli in Ménière's disease may yield information not available with reliance only on click stimuli. As noted by Margolis et al. (1992), "The exclusive use of alternating polarity clicks is not adequate to reveal the nature of these abnormalities [ECochG patterns in hydropic ears]" (p. 8).

For click stimuli, and relatively low-frequency tone bursts (2000 Hz and below), the SP is in the same direction (same polarity) as the AP. For higher frequencies, such as 4000 and especially 8000 Hz, the SP is in the opposite direction of the AP (Dauman et al., 1988; Kansaki, Ouchi, Yokobori, & Ino, 1982; Kumagami, Nishida, & Baba, 1982). There is not necessarily intrasubject correlation between the amplitude of the negative versus the positive SP components for these stimulus conditions. With tone bursts, low-frequency stimuli appear to produce abnormal ECochG findings more often than high-frequency tone bursts or clicks, at least among Ménière's patients with a rising-configuration audiogram (Dauman et al., 1988; Eggermont, 1979; Kansaki et al., 1982; Koyuncu, Mason, & Saunders, 1994; Ohashi, 1983). The SP/AP ratio increases directly as stimulus frequency increases, up until 4000 Hz and above. Rate of stimulation is also a factor to consider. The SP/AP ratio decreases as rate of stimulation is increased.

DISEASE STATE. | The incidence of abnormally large SP amplitude in Ménière's disease has been reported to be between 60 and 65 percent (e.g., Coats, 1981; Gibson, Moffat, & Ramsden, 1977; Goin, Staller, Asher, & Mischke, 1982), implying of course that more than one-third of patients with this inner-ear pathology have normal ECochG findings. Ferraro, Arenberg, and Hassanein (1985) provide evidence that ECochG is influenced by the status of the disease on the test date. All 45 subjects who were without symptoms showed a normal ECochG SP/AP ratio (0.5 or less), as re-

corded with an *extratympanic* electrode. However, among the 10 subjects with symptoms, hearing loss and aural fullness were the strongest predictors of an abnormal ECochG, whereas tinnitus and vertigo were not strong predictors of ECochG outcome. The authors recommend that, whenever possible, ECochG be measured when the patient is experiencing typical symptoms of Ménière's disease. Margolis et al. (1995) described changes in the SP and AP relationship with progression of the symptoms of Ménière's disease.

Gamble, Meyerhoff, Shoup, and Schwade (1999) described an innovative approach for increasing the sensitivity of ECochG in the diagnosis of Ménière's disease. A group of 43 patients carefully selected to meet criteria for "inner ear fluid imbalance" were given an "oral salt challenge" of four 1 gram tablets on three consecutive days before ECochG measurement with a TIPtrode electrode technique. Findings for the experimental group were compared with those for a control group of 13 normal subjects. The upper limit for normal SP/AP amplitude ratio was 37. Among the experimental group, 90 percent had repeatable ECochG waveforms. Before the salt challenge, all experimental patients had SP/AP ratios <0.37, whereas after the administration of sodium chloride 23 percent of the ears showed an SP/AP ratio exceeding 0.37. Also, in the experimental group the SP/AP ratio increased from 0.21 in the baseline (unchallenged) condition versus 0.30 in the salt load condition. This difference from the baseline to salt loading condition was statistically significant. The difference was also statistically different (p = 0.0003) from the very modest SP/AP change in the control group before and after salt loading. Perhaps most clinically relevant for the diagnosis of Ménière's disease, for 38 percent of the experimental patients, ECochG measurement with salt loading was useful in identifying an "active" ear that could then be considered for medical treatment. Ge and Shea (2002) described CM amplitude data for more than patients (2,421 ears) for a TT ECochG technique. There was significantly larger CM amplitude in Ménière's disease (36.98 μV) in comparison to a group of subjects without Ménière's disease (16.31 μV).

DEGREE OF HEARING IMPAIRMENT. | Degree of hearing impairment in Ménière's disease may be a factor in ECochG outcome. Using a TT (transtympanic) technique, Gibson, Prasher, and Kilkenny (1983) reported an average SP/AP ratio of 0.35 (ranging from 0 to 0.59) in patients with hearing loss in the 2000 to 4000 Hz region of 40 dB or less. This was comparable to normal subjects (an average SP/AP ratio of 0.25, with a range of 0.10 to 0.63). Also, patients with hearing loss of greater than 40 dB in this frequency region showed SP/AP ratios ranging from 0.29 to 0.89 (average of 0.51). Dauman, Aran, Charlet de Sauvage, and Portman (1988), while confirming enhanced SP in Ménière's disease, offered conflicting data. They found no correlation between SP amplitude and either duration of symptoms or auditory thresholds for lower or higher audiometric frequencies. Findings by Mori, Asai, and Sakagami (1990) and Asai and Mori (1989) are also relevant to the discussion. These investigators examined the relations among SP, AP, and hearing threshold levels in 46 patients with unilateral Ménière's disease. ECochG was recorded with a silver ball electrode placed in the ear canal within 3 mm from the tympanic annulus. AP amplitude decreased as hearing impairment increased, whereas SP amplitude did not vary systematically as a function of hearing thresholds. Thus, as the degree of high-frequency hearing impairment increased, the SP/AP ratio tended to increase correspondingly. The change was not due to abnormal enlargement of the SP component; it was due to the diminished AP amplitude expected with greater high-frequency hearing deficit. In a follow-up paper, several of these same authors also described the effect of fluctuating hearing impairment (a characteristic finding in Ménière's disease) on ECochG in 8 patients (Asai & Mori, 1989). AP amplitude decreased as hearing thresholds in the 2000 to 8000 Hz frequency region increased. Changes in hearing thresholds for lower frequencies (250 to 1000 Hz) had no effect on AP amplitude. In contrast, SP amplitude showed no alteration as a function of either high- or low-frequency hearing sensitivity. Consequently, changes in low-frequency hearing status generally did not influence the SP/AP ratio, whereas the ratio was decreased when high-frequency hearing sensitivity worsened. Animal investigation with experimentally induced endolymphatic hydrops revealed increased amplitude for SP but not AP in early stages of the pathophysiologic process, associated with integrity of hair cells and auditory neurons (Horner & Cazals, 1988; van Deelen et al., 1988). Then, with progression of the disease process (and histopathology) and increased hearing loss, both the SP and AP amplitudes were diminished. According to some clinical studies, abnormally enhanced SP findings, particularly for lower frequency stimuli, are most likely to be recorded in early Ménière's disease with average hearing loss of less than 50 dB, whereas AP amplitude decreases as disease-related hearing loss increases (e.g., Dauman et al., 1988; Eggermont, 1979). Using a TT ECochG technique, however, Ge and Shea (2002) described data for a large series of patients (2,421 ears). For example, these authors reported a statistically significant increase in the SP/AP ratio as the stage of Ménière's disease progressed, with 71 percent showing an abnormally large ratio in Stage 1 (hearing loss <25 dB), 83 percent in Stage 2 (hearing loss 26 to 40 dB), 85 percent in Stage 3 (hearing loss 41 to 70 dB), and 90 percent in Stage 4 (hearing loss >70 dB) of the disease. The proportion of subjects with an abnormally large SP/AP ratio increased also as a function of the duration of the disease (from 43 percent for duration less than one year to 100 percent for disease duration greater than thirty years). Ge and Shea (2002) also commented on the diagnostic value of a shift in AP latency, as well as the SP/AP amplitude ratio.

ECochG AND PATHOPHYSIOLOGY OF MÉNIÈRE'S DISEASE. |

The relation between ECochG abnormalities and underlying pathophysiology in Ménière's disease is a topic of speculation. Increased endolymphatic (i.e., intralabyrinthine) pressure alters mechanical properties of the cochlea. Normally, there is some asymmetry in the vibration of the basilar membrane, which is thought to produce the SP. Vibratory asymmetry is greater with increased endolymphatic pressure, and, therefore, the SP is larger (Dauman, Aran, Sauvage, & Portmann, 1988; Ferraro, Arenberg, & Hassanein, 1985; Gibson, Prasher, & Kilkenny, 1983; Morrison, Moffat, & O'Connor, 1980).

ECochG IN MONITORING EFFECTIVENESS OF TREATMENT. |

ECochG measurement before, during, and after surgical or other medical therapy for Ménière's disease may be useful in documenting the effectiveness of the treatment. This clinical application is, of course, based on the assumption that ECochG is a valid index of Ménière's disease. A number of investigations have provided evidence in support of ECochG documentation of the effectiveness of treatment for endolymphatic hydrops. Although some authors have reported that medical therapy (e.g., glycerol or mannitol) or surgical therapy (e.g., endolymphatic sac decompression with or without insertion of a shunt), which relieves cochlear fluid pressure, may decrease or normalize the SP/AP ratio, others (e.g., Aso, 1990; Schwaber & Hall, 1990), have not confirmed this treatment effect with the ECochG .

Glycerol is a hyperosmolar drug that has been used in the diagnosis of Ménière's disease. It is thought to diminish the expansion of the endolymphatic sac and temporarily to relieve the endolymphatic hydrops underlying Ménière's disease. A positive glycerol test outcome, one that is consistent with Ménière's disease, is improvement in hearing immediately after ingestion of the drug. There is clinical evidence of a strong correlation between enlarged SP amplitude and a positive glycerol test and, in addition, a reduction of SP amplitude with glycerol (Coats & Alford, 1981; Dauman et al., 1988; Morrison, Moffat, & O'Connor, 1980). A positive-voltage SP (i.e., the divergent SP vs. AP voltage pattern described previously) is apparently not correlated with glycerol test results (Kansaki et al., 1982).

In a relatively recent report, Kimura, Aso, and Watanable (2003) described the effects of glycerol tests on ECochG in an attempt to monitor the progression of patients from atypical to definite Meniere's disease, an investigative approach taken years earlier by Futaki, Kitahara, and Morimoto (1977). Atypical Ménière's disease is characterized by some (but not all) of the features of Ménière's disease. The subjects with definite Ménière's disease (N = 352) and atypical Ménière's disease (N = 319) were drawn from a sizable pool of patients (N = 1,569) with various peripheral otologic pathologies. A TT electrode technique was used to record ECochG at an early stage of the disease. The 99th percentile for the SP/AP ratio in a group of normal hearing subjects (N = 29) at an intensity level of 100 dB SPL was 37 percent. The authors reported that the likelihood of a positive ECochG finding with the glycerol test was not statistically different for definite Ménière's disease and other pathologies, e.g., syphilitic labyrinthitis and contralateral endolymphatic hydrops. Also, there was no difference in ECochG findings with the glycerol test for patients with atypical Ménière's disease versus definite Ménière's disease. However, the authors did find in a retrospective analysis of data that the frequency of positive ECochG outcomes was significantly higher for patients with atypical Ménière's disease who later progressed to definite Ménière's disease than for those patients who showed no progression to Ménière's disease. That is, ECochG findings appeared to be useful in predicting which patients would progress to definite Ménière's disease.

As noted previously, the two major forms of surgical management for Ménière's disease are vestibular nerve section (for debilitating vertigo) and endolymphatic sac decompression, with or without insertion of a drainage shunt. There is disagreement in the literature regarding ECochG patterns and endolymphatic sac decompression. Some investigators found that ECochG has value in predicting the outcome of treatment for Ménière's disease. Morrison et al. (1980) reported better postoperative otologic status for patients without ECochG abnormalities (increased duration of the response) than for those with apparently normal ECochG before surgery. The inference was that patients with ECochG abnormalities had reached a stage of pathology that was no longer reversible with surgical therapy.

On the other hand, Gibson, Moffat, and Ramsden (1977) came to the opposite conclusion. Their patients with longer duration SP/AP complexes preoperatively tended to experience greater benefit (less vertigo) from surgery. Reported changes in ECochG recorded before versus after endolymphatic sac decompression include a reduction in the width (duration) of the response and diminished SP amplitude and/or SP/AP ratio (Coats, Jenkins, & Monroe, 1984; Goin et al., 1982; Morrison, Moffat, & O'Connor, 1980). For the most part, the changes were recorded over a considerable time period after the surgery (from several months to more than a year). Arenberg, Gibson, Bohlen, and Best (1989), Booth (1980), Bouchard and Bojrab (1988), and Staller (1986) have actually monitored cochlear status intraoperatively with ECochG. Arenberg, Kobayashi, Obert, and Gibson (1993) reported for 56 percent of 23 patients with Ménière's disease a reduction in the SP/AP ratio after endolymphatic sac decompression relative to a preoperative baseline measurement. On the other hand, Staller (1986) and Schwaber and Hall (1990) found no consistent intraoperative or pre- versus postsurgical (endolympatic decompression and shunt) change in the SP/AP complex, including the SP/AP ratio.

OTHER PATHOLOGIES

Perilymph Fistula

ECochG has been specifically investigated in patients with suspected or confirmed perilymph fistula in an attempt to find an objective and ear-specific test for this rather elusive and hard-to-diagnose otologic disorder (Arenberg, Ackley, Ferraro, & Muchnick, 1988; Aso & Gibson, 1994; Gibson, 1992; Meyerhoff & Yellin, 1990; Sass, Densert, & Magnusson, 1997). Gibson (1992) manipulated intrathoracic pressure to enhance the clinical symptoms of perilymph fistula during ECochG measurement. Briefly, for the raised intrathoracic pressure test, patients were instructed to hold their breath for up to about 20 seconds and to slowly and consistently press down on their diaphragm. Repeated ECochG recordings were made before, during, and after the intrathoracic pressure test. ECochG data were collected from a series of 78 patients who were confirmed by surgical exploration to have the diagnosis of perilymph fistula.

Sass et al. (1997) described ECochG findings for a TT technique for three cases of perilymph fistula. The diagnosis was confirmed or "strongly suggested" upon surgical exploration. The criterion for an abnormal ECochG SP/AP ratio was 0.41. In summary, the authors reported that baseline changes in the three patients were similar to those for patients with endolymphatic hydrops. During the raised intrathoracic pressure test, the ECochG components (SP and AP) for the three patients were unstable in comparison to stable responses recorded from a group of patients with Meniere's disease. The authors interpreted this pattern of findings for the three patients as consistent with the diagnosis of perilymph fistula.

Consistent with the lack of consensus about the demographics, diagnosis, and management of perilymph fistula in general, disagreement exists also regarding the diagnostic value of ECochG in perilymph fistula (Aso & Gibson, 1994; Gibson, 1992). Conclusions derived from studies of ECochG in perilymph fistula are limited due to small numbers of subjects, ambiguity in criteria for surgical or other diagnostic strategies for verification of the disease, inconsistency in ECochG findings, and questions about statistical approaches for data analysis.

Lyme Disease

Selmani, Pyykko, Ishizaki, and Ashammakhi (2002) applied ECochG measurements clinically in attempt to differentiate patients with Ménière's disease from those with Lyme disease. They stated, as their rationale, the similarities in the clinical presentation of patients with each of these pathologies. ECochG was recorded using a TT electrode from 91 patients with Meniere's disease and 11 with the diagnosis of Lyme disease. The symptoms of vertigo, tinnitus, and sensorineural hearing loss were common to both groups, including all patients with Ménière's disease and

54 percent (six out of eleven) of the patients with Lyme disease. ECochG findings were consistent with endolymphatic hydrops (enlarged SP/AP ratio) for 71 percent of the patients with Ménière's disease and 45.5 percent of the patients with Lyme disease. Based on their findings, the authors recommended that patients with Lyme disease undergo complete assessment for possible endolymphatic hydrops, to include ECochG.

Sudden Onset Hearing Loss

Filipo, Cordier, Barbara, and Bertoli (1997) reported enhancement of the ECochG SP/AP ratio in sudden onset sensorineural hearing loss. These investigators compared ECochG findings for 185 patients with Meniere's disease and 117 patients with sudden onset hearing loss. They interpreted the findings as evidence that endolymphatic hydrops was a pathophysiologic process underlying sudden onset hearing loss.

INTRAOPERATIVE NEUROPHYSIOLOGIC MONITORING

ECochG principles and procedures can play an important role in neurophysiologic monitoring during surgical operations putting the auditory system at risk. Ongoing intraoperative ECochG recording can provide minute-to-minute, and sometimes close to real-time, information on cochlear status. ECochG components recorded with the transtympanic needle electrode technique are typically of large amplitude, often more than 10 μV, as noted in Chapter 4 and elsewhere in this chapter. Muscle artifact, i.e., myogenic interference, is rarely a factor in the operating room since the patient is anesthetized. Often, if the facial (seventh cranial) nerve is not risk and is not monitored neurophysiologically, the patient will be chemically paralyzed, further reducing the possibility of muscle interference with ECochG recordings. Sources of electrical interference, e.g., microscopes, cautery devices, and other electrical devices (laser and ultrasound machines, ultrasound), are commonplace in the operating room. However, even with these multiple sources of electrical interference, the signal-to-noise ratio (SNR) is adequate for confident ECochG analysis because the promontory electrode placement near the cochlea results in a robust response of large amplitude. ECochG also provides reasonably site-specific information on auditory function. The generators of the ECochG components are well defined. Site-specificity is a clear advantage in the operating room where ongoing documentation of cochlear status is highly desirable. Recorded in combination with the ABR, a sensitive neurophysiologic index of neural integrity, ECochG permits consistent feedback on the functional status of the auditory system from the cochlea to the upper brainstem. This anatomic territory is at greatest risk during most neuro-otologic surgical procedures, e.g., acoustic tumor removal and vestibular nerve sectioning.

Since the mid-1980s, ECochG and ABR have been applied clinically in monitoring functional integrity of the cochlea, eighth cranial nerve, and auditory brainstem during surgical procedures. Although various surgical operations put these auditory regions at risk, the majority of surgical operations are carried out within the posterior fossa. Two of the most common are vestibular nerve section and eighth-nerve tumor removal. Clinicians involved in AER neuromonitoring in the OR may find themselves also monitoring facial nerve responses because many surgeries endangering the integrity of the auditory system also put the facial nerve at risk. Attempts to preserve hearing and facial nerve function during surgical removal of mass lesions are, of course, influenced by a variety of factors, in addition to neurophysiological monitoring, among them the size of the tumor, the age and general health status of the patient, the surgical approach used to access the tumor, and the skill and experience of the surgical team.

Intraoperative monitoring in the OR can be extremely challenging. The test environment contains multiple potential sources of electrical interference and limits ready access to the subject. A common OR layout showing possible locations of auditory evoked response instrumentation and other essential personnel and equipment is displayed in Figure 5.7. Electrical interference can be generated by numerous devices shown in the figure, including the microscope, the laser, the bipolar coagulator, the X-ray view box, and other devices that might be brought into the room in support of surgery. The source of electrical interference detected by evoked response systems in the OR may, of course, be located outside of the room, e.g., an adjacent room or even one floor above or below the room. Furthermore, during intraoperative neurophysiologic monitoring, subject characteristics are generally not stable. Rather, moment-to-moment alterations in neurophysiologic status, and therefore auditory evoked response patterns, must be expected and anticipated. These neurophysiologic alterations may result from surgical manipulations; from the drugs used to induce and maintain anesthesia; from changes in body temperature, blood pressure, and blood gases; and from other physiologic factors. Clearly, the tester must differentiate between these two general causes of AER alteration, namely, those that are related to surgery versus all other causes. Limited test time contributes to the clinical challenge of intraoperative monitoring. In the OR, test time is an ever-present measurement factor. Not only must quality AER data be recorded under unfavorable conditions, these data must be recorded over a time span of only several seconds and then immediately analyzed and interpreted. Finally, the interpretation may have a very serious impact on surgical decisions and, ultimately, patient outcome. Whether a patient's hearing, facial-nerve integrity, or even life is preserved may hinge, to a large extent,

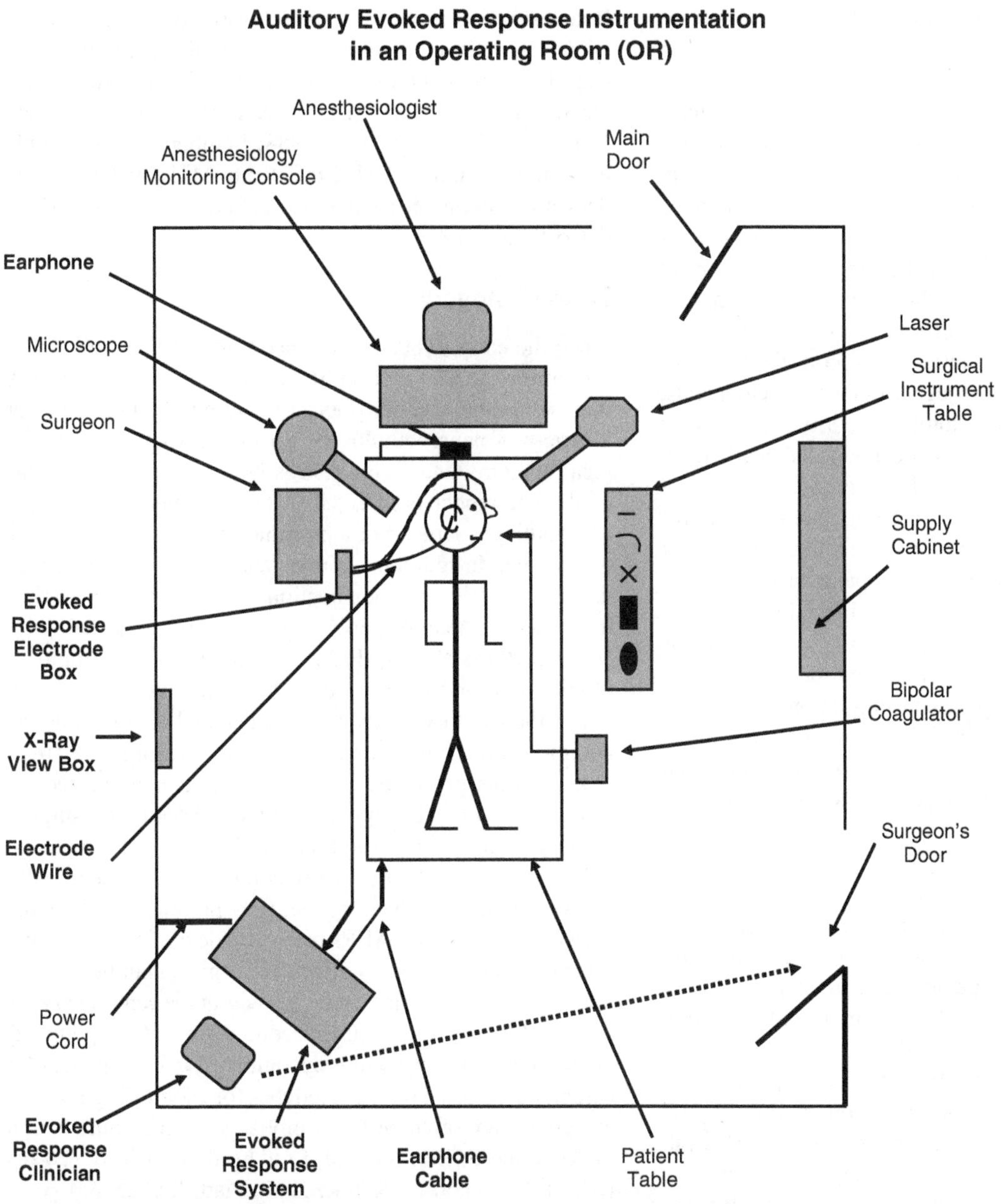

**Auditory Evoked Response Instrumentation
in an Operating Room (OR)**

FIGURE 5.7. Typical layout for an operating room (OR) showing the location of the evoked response equipment and operator (lower left corner) and some of the many electrical devices that can be sources of artifact in the test setting.

on prompt and accurate interpretation of intraoperative ER findings.

Rationale for Intraoperative Monitoring

AERs, particularly ECochG and ABR and also a technique for neurophysiologic recording of facial nerve function, are now routinely applied in intraoperative neuromonitoring. The two major and related clinical applications are monitoring of peripheral nervous system (i.e., cranial nerve) function and central nervous system function and

to preserve hearing. Evidence has accumulated since the early 1980s that sensory evoked responses, in general, can provide an early indicator of changes in neurophysiologic status of the peripheral and central nervous system during surgery. Changes in evoked responses may be due to various physiologic or surgical factors, such as hypotension, hypoxia, and compression or retraction of nerves or brain tissue. Early detection of a significant alteration in neurophysiologic status can potentially lead to effective medical or surgical correction of the problem and reversal of the pathophysiologic process. The ultimate goal of monitoring, of course, is prevention of avoidable permanent neurologic and, in the case of AERs, neuro-otologic dysfunction.

A second and more specific reason for increased intraoperative application of AERs is preservation of hearing during posterior fossa surgery. Since the mid-1980s, advances in microsurgical techniques have contributed to an effort on the part of neuro-otologists and neurosurgeons to leave the auditory pathways functionally intact during surgical removal of tumors in the region of the auditory nerve and brainstem. AERs, because they provide information on the functional status of these anatomic structures, can contribute importantly in this effort. As a consequence of these developments, auditory neurophysiologists, audiologists, or technicians may find themselves called on to provide a new and challenging AER clinical service in an atypical test setting.

The focus of this chapter is the rationale for monitoring with ECochG auditory function during different types of surgical procedures. The various intraoperative applications of ABR are discussed in Chapter 10, and facial nerve monitoring is covered in Chapter 15. Intraoperative monitoring is often a challenging clinical activity. Therefore, this chapter and the other two include practical suggestions for preparing for intraoperative neurophysiologic measurement, along with discussion of common technical problems encountered during neuromonitoring in the OR and possible solutions.

Historical Perspective

The earliest reports on intraoperative monitoring, in the 1970s, described assessment of spinal cord integrity with SSER during various orthopedic and neurosurgical procedures, such as removal of spinal cord tumors and correction of scoliosis (Nash, Loring, Schatzinger, & Brown, 1977). Beginning in approximately 1980, clinical application of AERs in intraoperative monitoring was reported mostly by anesthesiologists, neurosurgeons, and neurologists (Daspit, Raudzens, & Shetter, 1982; Friedman, Kaplan, Gravenstein, & Rhoton, 1985; Grundy, Jannetta, Procopio, Lina, Boston, & Doyle, 1982; Grundy, Lina, Procopio, & Jannetta, 1981; Hardy, Kinney, Lueders, & Lesser, 1982; Hashimoto, Ishiyama, Totsuka, & Mitzutani, 1980; Kalmanchev, Avila, & Symon, 1986; Levine, Ojemann, Montgomery, & McGaffigan, 1984; Little, Lesser, Leuders, & Furlan, 1983; Lumenta, Kramer, & Bock, 1986; Møller & Janetta, 1984; Raudzens, 1982; Raudzens & Shetter, 1982; Schramm, Mokrusch, Fahlbusch, & Hochstetter, 1985; Zappulla, Greenblatt, Kaye, & Malis, 1984). A major objective of this research effort was to evaluate the clinical feasibility and value of monitoring status of the peripheral and central nervous system intraoperatively with multimodal ERs. These many publications included data on the use of AERs, primarily ABR, for monitoring eighth-nerve status during posterior fossa surgery with the ultimate goal of preserving hearing status. A few years later, audiologists, notably Michael Dennis, Paul Kileny, Roger

Ruth, Gary Jacobson, and Dan Schwartz, reported extensive clinical experience in intraoperative monitoring with AERs, and also experience in monitoring facial nerve status during surgical procedures (Dennis & Earley, 1988; Jacobson & Tew, 1987; Kileny, 1985, 1988; Lambert & Ruth, 1988; Rosenblum, Ruth, & Gal, 1985; Ruth, Mills, & Jane, 1986; Schwartz, Bloom, & Dennis, 1985; Schwartz, Bloom, Pratt, & Costello, 1988).

Types of Surgery

Since the early 1980s, experience with intraoperative neuromonitoring of function in the eighth nerve, auditory brainstem, and seventh (facial) nerve has accumulated for a variety of neuropathologies. Specific information on surgical anatomy and techniques is beyond the scope of this book. The reader is directed to texts on neurological and neurootologic surgery, or appropriate sources accessible via the Internet. In addition, a journal and multiple textbooks are devoted entirely to the application of SERs (sensory evoked responses) in neurophysiologic monitoring in the OR (e.g., Møller, 1996; Nuwer, 1986). Intraoperative neurophysiologic monitoring can be useful during any procedure in which the auditory pathways (cochlea, eighth cranial nerve, auditory brainstem, or cerebrum) or the facial nerve are at risk. In some procedures, such as vestibular nerve section or removal of cerebellopontine angle (CPA) tumor, surgery directly involves vital auditory and facial nerve structures. Other neurological surgery procedures do not specifically involve the auditory system, but they put nearby structures at risk. In these cases, AERs may provide clinically valuable information on secondary effects of surgical manipulation of neural tissue or vascular structures within the central nervous system. Examples of such procedures are fifth (trigeminal) cranial nerve microvascular decompression or removal of a cerebellar tumor. These procedures for monitoring secondary effects are often best accomplished with a combination of ABR and SSERs (Gentili, Lougheed, Yasashiro, & Corrado, 1985; Jacobson & Tew, 1987; Piatt, Radtke, & Erwin, 1985).

Mechanisms for Intraoperative Alterations of AERs

Sensitivity of AERs to dynamic intraoperative pathophysiology is the fundamental reason for their use in monitoring. However, as Grundy (1983) pointed out, it is not easy to establish a clear cause-and-effect relationship in the OR, at least with clinical data. A variety of innocuous and common intraoperative events may affect auditory electrophysiologic recordings, such as irrigation, opening of the dura, changes in core body temperature, and focal tissue temperature. Anatomic or technical problems more peripherally (e.g., blood or irrigation fluid in the middle or external ear, problems with electrodes or the earphones), may also conspire to adversely affect intraoperative AER findings. The three major pathophysiologic processes responsible for intraoperative changes in AERs are (1) ischemia secondary to or unrelated to hypotension, (2) blood gas abnormalities (hypoxia and hypercarbia), and (3) mechanical alteration of neural structures (including compression, distortion, stretching, or transection of a nerve). It is important to remember that during intraoperative monitoring, an AER alteration can only be attributed to pathophysiology, after the possible effect(s) of technical factors have been ruled out. Also, more than one mechanism may simultaneously contribute to the AER alteration. Practical guidelines for considering technical factors, such as body temperature, equipment problems, and anesthesia, are presented in a later section of this chapter.

ISCHEMIA. | The brain and the ear require a constant adequate supply of blood for normal functioning. *Ischemia* results from inadequate blood flow to neural tissue. In brain ischemia, neurons are deprived of necessary amounts of oxygen and glucose (a primary source of metabolic energy). Mechanisms include occlusion, severing, or vasospasm of the internal auditory artery. With decreased blood flow, cochlear hair cells or neurons undergo metabolic changes leading to dysfunction. These initial alterations in function can be detected at an early stage, while they are still reversible, by electrophysiologic techniques (Colletti, Fiorino, Carner, & Tonoli, 1997a; Møller, 1996). Persistent ischemia will eventually produce irreversible, structural neuronal damage. Among the different causes for the development of brain ischemia intraoperatively are *hypotension* (reduced blood pressure), surgery-induced compression of vital blood vessels, and pressure directly on cranial nerve or other structures within the central nervous system that prevents adequate perfusion of neural tissue with blood. Appropriate and timely intervention may result in a reversal of the pathophysiologic process. Common examples of such intervention would include medical management of hypotension and the surgeon's removal or repositioning of retractors compressing vascular or neural structures.

BLOOD GAS ABNORMALITIES. | Alterations in blood gases are probably the least likely cause for intraoperative changes in AERs. Laboratory analysis of blood samples is periodically obtained during the course of an operation by the anesthesiology staff, and oxygen saturation can be monitored continuously. Medical measures are taken, as indicated, in ensure the proper proportion of oxygen, carbon dioxide, and pH. Inadequately low arterial pressure of oxygen (PaO_2) levels in hypoxia may impair neuronal and cochlear function. There are different mechanisms for hypoxic insult, but the common component is low PaO_2.

MECHANICAL ALTERATION OF NEURAL STRUCTURES. | Perhaps the most common cause of ER alterations, and the one of primary interest intraoperatively, is some type of mechanically induced disruption of auditory system or seventh-nerve function. The eighth cranial nerve is quite vulnerable to damage intraoperatively because it is surrounded by a relatively thin layer of myelin, especially at the distal and proximal ends, in comparison to the protection offered to other cranial nerves (e.g., facial nerve) by more dense amounts of myelin. Heating, compression, and stretching of the eighth cranial nerve are not uncommon consequences during surgical maneuvers. Stretching may be more traumatic when the nerve is pulled medially, i.e., toward the brainstem and away from the cochlea, rather than in the other direction (Colletti, Fiorino, Carner, & Tonoli, 1997a; Matthies & Samii, 1997; Sekiya, Iwabuchi, Kamata, & Ishida, 1985). The exact pathophysiologic processes contributing to abnormalities of AERs are varied. Possibilities would include desynchronization of neural activity, a block in neural conduction, or biochemical and microvascular disturbances in neuronal function (Lenarz & Sachsenheimer, 1985). Naturally, these alterations will be detected only during the intraoperative period when auditory (or facial nerve) structures are being manipulated.

It is crucial to keep in mind that other intraoperative events, such as saline irrigation within the surgical field, may also produce neurophysiologic changes (e.g., due to reduced focal temperature). In contrast, other AER changes due to systemic factors (e.g., hypothermia or hypotension) theoretically can occur at any time during surgery, from induction of anesthesia to closing. It is advisable, then, for the tester to be informed of the surgeon's activities throughout the case and to remain especially vigilant during manipulations such as retraction of structures (e.g., cerebellum), dissection of tumor, or sectioning of the vestibular portion of the eighth cranial nerve.

COCHLEAR INTEGRITY. | In addition to these three major physiologic processes affecting intraoperative ER changes, the integrity of the cochlea is, of course, essential when AERs are applied in neurophysiologic monitoring. That is, if serious cochlear impairment develops intraoperatively, AERs may be markedly altered or even abolished, even if neural integrity is maintained. Surgery-related disruption or destruction of blood vessels supplying the cochlea (mainly the internal auditory or labyrinthine artery) may produce "cochlear ischemia" and sensory hearing impairment. As reviewed in Chapter 2, the cochlea and eighth nerve receive their blood from the vertebrobasilar arterial system, and specifically from the AICA (anterior inferior cerebellar artery) and one of its branches, the internal auditory artery. Interruption of blood supply via these vessels, particularly the internal auditory artery, typically produces sensorineural auditory dysfunction and will be reflected by AER abnormalities (Levine et al., 1984; Sabin, Prasher, Bentivoglio, & Symon, 1987; Sekiya et al., 1985).

Obvious damage to the blood vessels is not necessary to trigger this mechanism for cochlear deficit. Mechanical stimulation of the blood vessels—directly or indirectly through tumor manipulation—may lead to vasospasm and subsequent interruption of blood to the cochlea and eighth nerve. In 1959, Perlman, Kimura, and Fernandez showed in animal experiments that the cochlea could survive up to 5 minutes of interruption in blood supply. The CM and AP disappeared within 30 seconds but returned after blood supply was reinstated. Other mechanisms for cochlear damage resulting from surgery are direct trauma to the labyrinth or to the endolymphatic duct.

Intraoperative ECochG Protocol

A test protocol for intraoperative neurophysiologic monitoring of the auditory system really combines measurement parameters for ECochG and ABR, as summarized in Table 5.8. Specific stimulus and acquisition parameters in the ECochG test protocol were reviewed in detail in the Chapter 4, including each of the settings and options appropriate for recording ECochG intraoperatively. The emphasis in this chapter is the application of ECochG during surgeries putting the ear and auditory nerve at risk. The discussion will continue for ABR in Chapter 9.

Intraoperative Monitoring with ECochG

In the twenty-plus years since neurophysiologic monitoring was first described, a rather substantial literature has accumulated on the intraoperative application of ECochG and ABR for hearing preservation. Despite some promising findings (e.g., Arenberg et al., 1993; Gibson, 1991; Krueger & Storper, 1997), most investigations of other intraoperative applications of ECochG (e.g., documentation of changes in the SP/AP ratio during endolymphatic surgery or vestibular nerve section in patients with Meniere's disease) failed to produce evidence of value either for surgical decisions or in predicting postoperative outcome (e.g., Bojrab, Bhansali, & Andreozzi, 1994; Hall, 1992; Schwaber & Hall, 1990). The following review is limited to selected papers, mostly published in recent years, on the exclusive or primary application of ECochG during surgery for the purpose of hearing preservation. The use of ABR alone, or a combined ECochG and ABR technique, in intraoperative monitoring for hearing preservation is discussed in Chapter 10.

When conventional auditory evoked response techniques are applied in the operating room, using a far-field recording approach with scalp electrodes, there are unacceptable delays (e.g., several minutes or more) before latency and amplitude data are available for analysis. Each of the response components is relatively small in amplitude (usually less than 1 μV), and often not clearly detected in patients with

TABLE 5.8. Test Protocol for Intraoperative Monitoring with a Two-Channel Combined ECochG and ABR Approach

PARAMETERS	ECOCHG (CHANNEL 1)	ABR (CHANNEL 2)
Stimulus		
Transducer	ER-3A with TIPtrode	same
Type	click	same
Rate	21.1/sec (variable)	same
Polarity	rarefaction	same
Intensity	85 to 95 dB nHL	same
Masking	none	as indicated
Mode	monaural	same
Acquisition		
Electrodes		
Noninverting		
Site	Fz	same
Type	subdermal needle	same
Inverting		
Site	ipsilateral promontory	ipsilateral ear canal
Type	subdermal needle	TIPtrode
Ground		
Site	Fpz	same
Type	subdermal needle	same
Analysis time	5 or 15 ms	15 ms
Pre-stimulus time	1 ms	same
Gain	× 75,000	× 100,000
Filters		
High pass	30 Hz	30 or 100 Hz
Low pass	1500 Hz	1500 or 3000 Hz
Sweeps	< 500	as indicated

moderate-to-severe sensorineural hearing loss. Confident detection and analysis of evoked responses is related to the signal-to-noise ratio (SNR), as reviewed in Chapter 3. For the surface-recorded ABR, SNR is characteristically small for two reasons. As just noted, the signal (the response) is of modest amplitude. In addition, electrical noise levels in the operating room environment are often quite high due to multiple sources of artifact (e.g., electrical instruments, microscope, etc.). Consequently, considerable time (minutes) must be spent in signal averaging to obtain an adequate SNR and to permit confident response analysis. Of course, it is very important to consistently record clear and reliable responses, given the importance and often irreversible decisions made intraoperatively by the surgeon on the basis of changes in electrophysiologic measures (e.g., changes in latency). Damage to the auditory system may be inadvertently caused by surgical manipulations during the delay created by the need for ongoing signal averaging. Recognition of the serious problem caused by recording delays has prompted rather creative investigation of alternative monitoring strategies, including the use of TT placement of needle electrodes on the promontory (e.g., Schwaber & Hall, 1990), direct eighth nerve recordings (e.g., Cueva, Morris, & Prioleau, 1998), monitoring of the cochlear microphonic (Noguchi, Komatsuzaki, & Nishida (1999), and even intraoperative measurement of distortion product otoacoustic emissions (e.g., Cane, O'Donoghue, & Lutman, 1992; Morawski et al., 2004). The initial two ECochG techniques will now be reviewed briefly. The clinical application of OAEs is beyond the scope of this book.

ECochG measurement with needles placed in a transtympanic fashion on the promontory has been conducted for over fifty years, as noted in Chapter 1 and in the discussion of Ménière's disease in this chapter. Details on the technique, including electrode options and placement and stabilization of the needle, were provided in Chapter 4. The application and value of TT ECochG recording in the operating room is well established by independent investigations conducted around the world, and dates back to the late 1980s (e.g., Hall, 1992; Hohmann, 1992; Lenarz & Ernst, 1992; Ojemann, Levine, Montgomery, & McGaffigan, 1984; Schlake et al., 2001; Schwaber & Hall, 1990; Symon et al., 1988; Yokoyama, Nishida, Noguchi, & Komatsuzala, 1996; Zappia, Wiet, O'Connor, & Martone, 1996). Amplitude of the AP component of the ECochG is robust (well over 1 μV and as high as 30 μV) because the technique yields a near-field recording of activity from the cochlea and distal auditory nerve. A typical ECochG waveform recorded with the TT electrode technique is shown in Figure 5.8. Due to the high SNR produced by the large amplitude ECochG recorded with the TT electrode technique, a clear response can often be detected with less than 100 stimulus presentations (sweeps). With a typical stimulus presentation rate of 21.1/sec, therefore, a response can be obtained in less than 10 seconds. When the TT electrode lead is secured within

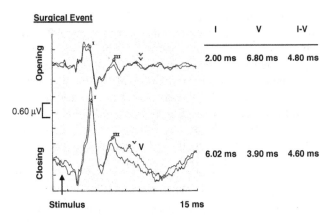

FIGURE 5.8. ECochG waveform recorded in the operating room with a transtympanic membrane electrode technique (Fz-to-promontory) showing highly favorable signal-to-noise (SNR) and, therefore, very brief recording time (less than 5 seconds).

the external ear canal by an insert earplug (as described in Chapter 6), electrode placement is highly stable. Intraoperative ECochG recordings over the course of hours show no electrode-related changes in latency or amplitude (e.g., Hall, 1992; Schwaber & Hall, 1990). Qualitative (waveform morphology) and quantitative (response amplitude) differences in waveforms for the TT electrode versus extratympanic electrode are clearly apparent when intraoperative ECochG recordings are simultaneously with each technique, as illustrated in Figure 5.9. At this point, it is important to recall that the presence of a clear and consistent AP component in the ECochG in isolation does not necessarily assure normal hearing. There is long-standing appreciation that dam-

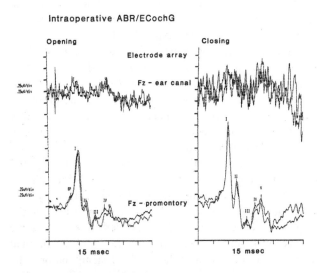

FIGURE 5.9. Waveforms recorded simultaneously during intraoperative monitoring with a combined ECochG (promontory inverting electrode) and ABR (TIPtrode inverting electrode) technique.

age to the eighth cranial nerve somewhere between the distal portion (e.g., spiral ganglion) that generates the AP (ABR wave I) and the proximal end (e.g., root entry zone near the brainstem), even complete sectioning of the nerve, may spare the AP yet result in total loss of hearing postoperatively (e.g., Hall, 1992; Kanzaki, Ogawa, Shiobara, & Toya, 1989; Levine et al., 1984; Ruben, Hudson, & Chiong, 1963; Silverstein, Wazen, Norrell, & Hyman, 1984; Symon et al., 1988). Impairment in eighth nerve function secondary to injury within the medial portion of the nerve will, however, be detected with the DENM technique, or a combination TT ECochG and ABR monitoring technique.

Another technique introduced to enhance the efficiency and quality of intraoperative neurophysiologic monitoring involves documentation of eighth (cochlear) nerve integrity directly, that is, with an electrode located on the nerve rather than in a far-field location. The technique has been described as "direct eighth nerve monitoring, or DENM" (e.g., Danner, Mastrodimos, & Cueva, 2004) and also as cochlear nerve action potential, or CNAP (e.g., Tucker, Slattery, Solcyk, & Brackmann, 2001). DENM or CNAP is a really a variation of the ECochG technique. First demonstrated by some of the early investigators of intraoperative monitoring of the auditory system (e.g., Møller & Jannetta, 1981, 1984; Silverstein, McDaniel, & Norell, 1985), and then about a decade later by authors of papers on techniques for preservation of auditory function with neurophysiologic monitoring (e.g., Colletti & Fiorino, 1994; Dornhoffer, Helms, & Hoehmann, 1995; Roberson, Senne, Brackmann, Hitselberger, & Saunders, 1996; Wazen, 1994; Zappia, Wiet, O'Connor, & Martone, 1996). The electrodes used by these investigators for direct monitoring from the auditory nerve were custom made and usually consisted of either a smooth silver ball or a wick (e.g., cotton or Teflon wool) connected to a very thin wire leading to an electrode box. During intraoperative monitoring for surgery to remove an acoustic tumor (vestibular schwannoma), the electrode is typically placed on a segment of the nerve between the tumor and the brainstem, or the porus acousticus. A retrosigmoid surgical approach best exposes the nerve for placement of the electrode. The main advantage of monitoring activity of the cochlear nerve directly with an electrode placed on the nerve rather than the more conventional recording approach with an electrode located on the promontory or a more remote location (e.g., earlobe) is the size of the response (up to 50 μV or more) and, therefore, the possibility of real-time (almost immediate) functional information on nerve integrity. The clear value of providing real-time data on nerve status to the surgeon is the opportunity for early detection of negative changes in function and, with an alteration of the surgical technique or a delay in further surgical manipulations, the preservation of nerve integrity and hearing (Cueva, Morris, & Prioleau, 1998). Direct nerve recordings also offer the advantage of a high degree of site specificity, that is, rather exact anatomic information on integrity of the eighth

cranial nerve. Mechanisms for intraoperative changes in auditory physiology, and causes of pathophysiologic processes, were reviewed in a previous section. According to Cueva and colleagues (1998) practical limitations to direct cochlear nerve monitoring include "difficulties with maintaining electrode position and action potential fluctuation with cerebrospinal fluid pulsating in the operative field have discouraged many surgeons from using this modality routinely" (pp. 202–203).

The feasibility of direct neurophysiologic recordings from the cochlear nerve is facilitated by the development of commercially available (FDA-approved) electrodes specially designed for the purpose (see Figure 5.10). The distal (nerve) end of the electrode, shaped like the letter C, is positioned around the nerve bundle. The inner (concave) surface of the electrode consists of a conductive metal (platinum). An insulated wire runs through an arm used to position the electrode on the nerve, and continues on to an electrode pin. When used for intraoperative monitoring with an ECochG and/or ABR test protocol, the cochlear nerve electrode is the inverting electrode, with a noninverting electrode placed in the customary position (e.g., Fz) and a ground electrode on either the low forehead (e.g., Fpz) or some other convenient site (e.g., shoulder). Other test parameters are as summarized in Table 5.8 for an ECochG intraoperative monitoring approach. The electrode is stabilized when it is clipped to surgical drapes with a tab attached to the electrode wire. The opening in the "C" allows the electrode to break loose from the nerve without damage to the nerve in the event of inadvertent movement. Details on surgical placement of the "atraumatic, self-retaining electrode" design are available in published articles (Cueva, Morris, & Prioleau, 1998; Ruckenstein, Cueva, & Prioleau, 1997) and the manufacturer's literature (AD-TECH Medical Instrument Corporation).

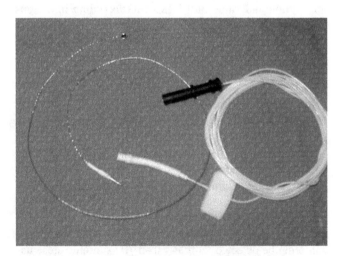

FIGURE 5.10. Electrode specially designed for direct eighth nerve monitoring intraoperatively (Electrode courtesy of AD-TECH Medical Instrument Corporation).

With this electrode design, amplitudes of 5 up to 70 μV are recorded, depending on hearing status (Cueva, Morris, & Prioleau, 1998). Danner, Mastrodimos, and Cueva (2004) studied in 77 patients undergoing surgical removal of vestibular schwannomas (ranging in size from 0.5 to 2.5 cm) the effectiveness of neurophysiologic monitoring for hearing preservation with the DENM versus conventional ABR techniques. The likelihood of hearing preservation was, as expected, a factor of tumor size, but also related to the monitoring approach. With ABR monitoring intraoperatively, hearing preservation was accomplished with 41 percent of the patients with small (1 cm or less) tumors and only 10 percent of patients with larger (1 to 2.5 cm) tumors. In contrast, with the DENM technique for neurophysiologic monitoring, hearing was preserved for 71 percent of the patients with small tumors and 32 percent for large tumors. The differences in hearing preservation rates for the two monitoring approaches were statistically significant. As an aside, facial nerve monitoring was associated with preservation of function in 94 percent of the cases. Battista, Wiet, and Paauwe (2000) also found evidence of higher hearing preservation rates during surgical removal of cerebellopontine angle (CPA) tumors with DENM monitoring (40 percent) versus conventional far-field ABR (17 percent) and even the TT ECochG (18 percent) techniques.

Drugs

SEDATIVES AND HYPNOTICS (DEPRESSANTS). | A substantial number of drugs can affect CNS activity and, consequently, may influence AERs. The following section is limited to the effects of commonly administered drugs that influence central nervous system function. These are controlled drugs—that is, they can be acquired only with a prescription. Sedatives are the first drugs on a continuum of CNS depressants—drugs that reduce CNS activity. They reduce diminish physical activity and calm the patient. Sedatives and hypnotics cause drowsiness or sleep and, therefore, may be used to quiet patients for AER measurement. Although sedatives and hypnotics facilitate the onset and maintenance of sleep, the patient can be easily aroused with stimulation. At the other end of the continuum of the depression of CNS activity is anesthesia, discussed below. Sedatives commonly used in ABR measurement, such as chloral hydrate, are discussed in detail in Chapter 8. Sedatives are often classified as either long acting (e.g., diazepam and librium) or short acting (lorazepam). Controlled drugs are further divided into schedules, depending on their effect and the penalties for illegal possession. Schedule I drugs (e.g., marijuana, LSD, heroin) are not for clinical use, but only for research purposes. Schedule II controlled drugs can only be obtained with a written (versus telephoned) prescription that cannot be refilled. Examples of Schedule II drugs that may be encountered clinically and may influence AERs are pentobarbital, secobarbital, methylphenidate (Ritalin®), synthetic narcotics (meperidine, or Demerol®) and opium narcotics (e.g., morphine). Schedule IV drugs (a prescription must be rewritten after six months or five refills) also fall within this general category. Among them are benzodiazepines, such as diazepam (Valium®), lorazepam (Ativan®), chlordiazepoxide (Librium®), and chloral hydrate.

Accumulated clinical experience and published reports confirm that *chloral hydrate* does not affect ECochG or ABR (Mokotoff, Schulman-Galambos, & Galambos, 1977; Palaskas, Wilson, & Dobie, 1989; Sohmer & Student, 1978).

Morphine (morphine sulfate), an alkaloid derived from opium, is a narcotic analgesic (pain reliever). The other main type of analgesic is a non-narcotic drug (e.g., aspirin). In addition to analgesia, morphine produces drowsiness and changes in mood. The suspected site of action is the limbic system (hippocampus, amygdala), and it does not affect the major sensory pathways. An IV agent, it is used (in relatively high doses) as a sedative in acute brain injured patients in the intensive care unit. Morphine does not appear to exert an influence on ECochG or ABR (Hall, 1988; Samra, Krutak-Krol, Pohorecki, & Domino, 1985).

Meperidine is an IV opioid analgesic, like morphine, which has no apparent effect on early or late latency AERs (Pfefferbaum, Roth, Tinklenberg, Rosenbloom, & Kopell, 1979).

Anesthetic Agents

During the past twenty-five years, an increasing number of papers have described the application of AMLRs during surgical procedure as an index of the depth of anesthesia. An appreciation of the effects of anesthetic agents on AERs is essential for any clinician involved in neurophysiologic intraoperative monitoring during surgery. Anesthesia is defined as loss of sensation (partial or complete), with or without loss of consciousness, that may be drug-induced or due to disease or injury. The following discussion will be limited to general anesthesia that affects the brain and produces loss of sensation and consciousness. Local anesthesia of nerves serving a specific anatomic region may be used in AER measurement. An example would be phenol (89 percent), which effectively numbs the tympanic membrane for transtympanic needle ECochG recordings. The ECochG response is, of course, not affected.

Depth or stage of general anesthesia may be described according to different schema. According to one description, there are three stages. In stage one, the patient is first excited until voluntary control is lost (hearing is the last of the senses to become nonfunctional). The corneal reflex is still present in the second stage of anesthesia, although loss of voluntary control persists. The third stage of anesthesia is defined as complete relaxation, deep regular breathing, and a sluggish corneal reflex. There are four stages of anesthesia according to another schema, including: (1) analgesia (no feeling), (2) delirium, (3) surgical anesthesia, and (4) CNS depression at the level of the medulla. From these terms, it is clear that the patient should be maintained in stage 3 during surgery.

Stages 1 and 2 represent inadequate anesthesia, while anesthesia is excessive in stage 4.

Before anesthesia, drugs are administered to decrease anxiety, relieve pre- and postoperative pain and provide amnesia for the perioperative period. Examples of these drugs are benzodiazepines (e.g., Valium), conscious sedatives (e.g., Versed), barbiturates, and neuroleptics. There are three major components to anesthesia. The purpose of the first component, induction, is to produce a rapid loss of consciousness. Drugs used to induce anesthesia include benzodiazepines, barbiturates, narcotic analgesics, etomidate, ketamine, and inhalation agents. The second, and longest lasting, component is maintenance of anesthesia. The purpose of this phase, which persists throughout surgery, is to produce a stable state of loss of consciousness and loss of reflexes to painful stimuli. Among the drugs often administered to during maintenance of anesthesia are inhalational agents (gases), narcotic analgesics, ketamine, muscle relaxants, and antiarrhythmic agents. Finally, anesthesia must be reversed so the patient will wake up and return to the preanesthetic state. This is achieved with opioid antagonists and anticholinesterase agents.

Anesthetic agents are often categorized according to their mode of administration. Some are intravenous (IV) agents, infused directly into the bloodstream via a line inserted into a vein (at the wrist or ankle). Examples of IV agents are barbiturates (thiopental/Sodium Pentothal, methohexital/Brevital, thiamylal), benzodiazepines (diazepam/Valium, midazolam), etomidates (amidate), opioid analgesics (morphine, fentanyl, meperidine), neuroleptics (droperidol + fentanyl), and dissociative anesthetic agents (ketamine). With IV anesthetics, there is fast action and fast recovery. The brain receives one-tenth of the dose within 40 seconds following IV administration. Other anesthetic agents are administered as a gas by inhalation. Inhalational agents, in contrast to those administered IV, are slower acting and are measured by partial pressure (tension) in the blood (brain). One commonly used inhalational agent is nitrous oxide, a gaseous anesthetic that is a good analgesic and induction agent, but has a low anesthetic potency. Others are called volatile anesthetics (e.g., halothane, isoflurane), which are potent even at low concentrations.

Anesthetic agents produce differential effects on AERs. ECochG components, which are dependent on the end organ (cochlea) and eighth nerve, are not seriously influenced by anesthesia. The ABR is generated by the eighth cranial nerve and by primary (lemniscal) sensory pathways within the brainstem. The ABR is influenced some categories of drugs (e.g., enflurane and halothane), although generally the effect is not great. In contrast, so-called "extralemniscal" AERs (e.g., AMLR, ALR), which involve multisynaptic nonlemniscal pathways, are highly sensitive to the effects of anesthetic agents on the central nervous system. These responses are also affected to a greater degree by sedatives, such as chloral hydrate. Unfortunately, much of the information on the relationship between the anesthesia and these latter AERs was obtained from animal experiments versus clinical experience (Pradhan & Galambos, 1963; Smith & Kraus, 1987).

HALOGENATED INHALATIONAL AGENTS. | Among the most common anesthetic agents used clinical in various types of surgery are the halogenated inhalational drugs, such as desflurane, enflurane, halothane, isolfurane, and sevoflurane. Drugs in this category differ, however, in their effects on the EEG and auditory evoked responses. In general, coincident with effects on anesthetic depth and overall CNS activity, the halogenated inhalational agents depress the EEG and produce increases in latency and decreases in amplitude. ECochG is not affected.

FENTANYL. | Fentanyl is a popular narcotic analgesic. It is a synthetic opioid that is eighty times as potent as morphine. Fentanyl is used exclusively as an anesthetic, as opposed to morphine, which is used as a sedative. Fentanyl has no apparent effect on ECochG or ABR (Samra, Lilly, Rush, & Kirsh, 1984).

SUFENTANIL. | Sufentanil is a narcotic anesthetic that is ten times more potent than fentanyl, but provides a greater margin of safety (especially in animal research) because is produces less hemodynamic stress than fentanyl.

Neuromuscular Blockers (Chemical Paralyzing Agents)

These drugs produce paralysis by interrupting transmission of neural impulses at the skeletal neuromuscular junction. Examples of neuromuscular blockers used in the operating room and intensive care unit are pancuronium (Pavulon), Metocurine, succinylcholine, and curare. All AERs can be reliably recorded during chemically induced muscle paralysis with such agents as Pavulon, Metocurine, and succinylcholine (Hall, 1988; Hall, Hargadine, & Allen, 1985; Hall, Mackey-Hargadine, & Kim, 1985; Harker, Hosick, Voots, & Mendel, 1977; Kileny, 1983; Kileny, Dodson, & Gelfand, 1983; Smith & Kraus, 1987). Waveforms are, in fact, often enhanced in patients under the influence of chemical paralysis due to the lack of muscle-related noise or artifact.

CONCLUDING COMMENTS

ECochG measures contribute to the diagnostic assessment of diverse patient populations—children and adults—and are clearly useful in Meniere's disease. The clinician who understands the principles of ECochG, and incorporates them into routine clinical practice, will enhance add diagnostic power to the electrophysiologic test battery and improve the quality and accuracy of other evoked responses, especially the ABR.

6

CHAPTER

ABR Parameters, Protocols, and Procedures

The reader is referred to information in Chapter 3 for an overview of stimulus features and their relation to AERs in general. Transducer types and their influence on auditory evoked responses were also reviewed in Chapter 3 and will not be dealt with again in this chapter. The early latency auditory evoked responses (e.g., ECochG and ABR) are best generated with very brief (transient) stimuli having an almost instantaneous onset. In fact, the ECochG and ABR are primarily "onset responses." The rapid onset of the transient stimulus generates synchronous firing of numerous auditory neurons. Portions of the stimulus other than the onset contribute little or nothing to the response. Therefore, extremely brief clicking sounds, produced by electrical signals with an abrupt onset and a duration of only 0.1 ms (100 microseconds), are by far the most commonly used signals for ABR measurement. When this almost instantaneous electrical impulse is converted (transduced) into a sound by an earphone (transducer), the resulting acoustical signal (click) is longer in duration. The duration of the temporal acoustic waveform of the signal may persist for a millisecond or more, depending on the characteristics of the transducer (i.e., earphone). The acoustical click stimulus may actually be one of several somewhat different acoustic signals produced by clearly distinctive electrical signals, including a rectangular voltage electrical pulse, diphasic square-wave pulses, triangular waves, a single period of a high-frequency haversine or half-sine wave, chirps, and others.

An abrupt signal, such as a rectangular electrical pulse, has a very broad spectrum and, when delivered to a transducer, produces an acoustic signal encompassing a wide range of frequencies (refer to Figure 6.1). The cochlea, therefore, is stimulated by a broad sound spectrum, and hair cells are, potentially, activated throughout a wide region of the basilar membrane. The frequency content of the stimulus actually generating the AER for a given subject, however, depends on a variety of factors, such as (a) stimulus intensity, (b) the electroacoustic properties of the transducer, (c) ear-

canal and middle-ear properties affecting sound transmission, and (d) the integrity of the cochlea. The ABR evoked by highly transient stimuli, such as clicks, cannot be used to define hearing sensitivity or cochlear status at audiometric frequencies or, really, within frequency regions. Frequency-specific information is, of course, available from ABR recordings and is, in fact, necessary in pediatric applications of the ABR. Because it is so important for clinical measurement of ABR in infants and young children, a separate chapter is devoted to the topic of frequency-specific ABR measurement. Tone-burst stimuli are not discussed in detail in this chapter but, instead, in a separate review (in Chapter 8) of protocols and procedures for measurement of frequency-specific ABR and auditory steady-state response (ASSR). What follows herein is a review of the background information required to understand the rationale for selection of the specific stimulus and acquisition parameters used to record

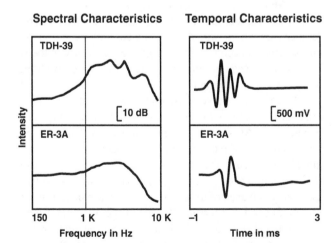

FIGURE 6.1. Temporal and spectral characteristics of a click signal presented with insert and supra-aural earphones.

optimal ABR waveforms under different clinical and patient conditions and for varying clinical applications. The chapter culminates with a synthesis of the information in the form of a clinically proven ABR test protocol that offers a starting point for successful measurement of the ABR in children and adults. Introduction of the protocol is followed by a summary of the important steps in conducting a clinical ABR assessment of auditory function. After the best-possible ABR is recorded, the waveform must be analyzed and the findings interpreted in the context of other audiologic findings, medical history, and perhaps nonaudiologic diagnostic findings. The important topic of ABR analysis and interpretation, and troubleshooting that is inevitable in clinical application of ABR, is covered in Chapter 7.

STIMULUS PARAMETERS

Type of Stimulus

The ABR, as typically measured clinically with 0.1 ms click signals, is generated by higher frequencies in the click spectrum, at least in normal ears. An ABR evoked by moderately intense (e.g., 60 dB nHL) click signals that are delivered with conventional audiometric earphones, for example insert (ER-3A) earphones, reflects activation of the high-frequency region of the cochlea, roughly from 1000 though 8000 Hz. There is lack of agreement among investigators regarding the frequency region most important for generation of the ABR—that is, whether the ABR reflects activation of the 1000 to 4000 Hz region, 4000 to 8000 Hz region, or just frequency regions of the cochlea above 2000 Hz, above 3000 Hz, or above 4000 Hz (Balfour, Pillion, & Gaskin, 1998; Bauch & Olsen, 1986; Coats, 1978; Coats & Martin, 1977; Eggermont & Don, 1980; Gorga, Reiland & Beauchaine, 1985; Gorga, Worthington, Reiland, Beauchaine, & Goldgar, 1985; Hoke, Lutkenhoner, & Bappert, 1980; Jerger & Mauldin, 1978; Kileny, 1981; Kileny & Magathan, 1987; Møller & Blegvad, 1976; Stapells, 1989). It is likely that differences among the studies in both methodology and subject characteristics account for the reported variability in the relationship between minimum response level for click stimuli and pure tone audiogram.

More apical (lower frequency) regions of the cochlea are also activated by the click, but these regions do not contribute to the ABR, at least in normal hearers. There are two reasons for this. First, the response to cochlear activation has already occurred in the higher frequency regions by the time the traveling wave has traversed the basilar membrane from the base to the apex of the cochlea to activate hair cells in this region. Second, the leading "front" of the traveling wave is more gradual (less abrupt) when it reaches the apical region and, consequently, the traveling wave is not as effective in generating synchronous firing of many eighth-nerve afferent fibers over a concentrated portion of the basilar membrane. Instead, smaller numbers of afferents sequentially fire over a more dispersed stretch of the basilar membrane. In persons with an impairment of auditory sensitivity for the higher frequency region, ABR generation may not necessarily follow this pattern. In addition, it is likely that the portion of the cochlea contributing to the ABR may vary as a function of response components (e.g., wave I vs. wave V) and stimulus intensity. For example, wave I appears to reflect more basal activation, whereas wave V may reflect activity from a more apical region. Also, at high stimulus intensity levels, there is spread of activation toward the apex, whereas at lower intensity levels, activation is limited more to the basal region. These points are important for meaningful clinical interpretation of the ABR.

In considering stimuli for clinical ABR measurement, it is important to keep in mind two general principles. First, the frequency specificity of a stimulus (i.e., the concentration of energy in a specific frequency region) is indirectly related to duration (Burkard, 1984; Gabor, 1947; Gorga, Reiland, & Beauchaine, 1985; Harris, 1978). With very brief stimuli, energy tends to be distributed over more frequencies, whereas stimuli with longer duration (including rise/fall times and plateau time) are spectrally constrained. Second, there is generally a direct relationship between duration of the response and duration of the stimulus. That is, slower (longer latency) responses are activated best by slower (longer onset and duration) stimuli, whereas faster (shorter latency) responses require faster (shorter onset and duration stimuli).

Although the ABR can be most effectively elicited with click signals, their lack of frequency-specificity is a major drawback for clinical electrophysiological assessment of auditory function in infants and young children and, particularly, for estimation of auditory sensitivity a different frequency regions. Currently, the use of tone-burst signals is the preferred technique for frequency-specific estimation of auditory function. The demand for an electrophysiologic technique for estimation of auditory sensitivity has increased markedly with the emergence of universal newborn hearing screening (UNHS). Newborn infants who do not pass hearing screening must be followed closely during the first few months after birth. If the hearing screening failure is confirmed, then diagnostic audiometry is indicated. A critical component of the diagnostic process is estimation of auditory sensitivity at different frequencies within the range of 500 to 4000 Hz. For the infant, hearing sensitivity within this frequency region is important for speech perception and for speech and language acquisition. Timely, accurate, and frequency-specific estimation of auditory sensitivity within the first two to four months after birth is an essential prerequisite for optimal audiologic management of infants with hearing impairment. The information on auditory sensitivity is critical for successful hearing aid fitting. Given the importance in audiology today of electrophysiologic frequency-specific estimation of auditory sensitivity in infants and young children, a separate chapter of the book is devoted to this topic.

Details on the use of tone-burst signals for ABR measurement and in the electrophysiologic estimation of auditory sensitivity—"the electrophysiologic audiogram"—are reviewed in Chapter 8.

Duration

Synchronous firing of many neurons, which is a general physiologic underpinning of the ABR, is very dependent on an abrupt stimulus onset. The two practical consequences of this principle are that (1) the ABR is not heavily dependent on stimulus duration (Gorga et al., 1984; Hecox, Squires, & Galambos, 1976) and (2) an almost instantaneous onset (almost always 0.1 ms or 100 μsec) click stimulus is routinely used in clinical ABR recordings, although click durations as short as 20 μsec (Coats, 1978; Coats & Kidder, 1980) and as long as 400 μsec (Yamada, Yagi, Yamane, & Suzuki, 1975) have been reported. For many clinical applications, the default stimulus duration is typically 0.1 ms.

Appreciation of the spectral characteristics of the click has traditionally been important for accurate interpretation of ABR in audiologic assessment, but not for neurodiagnostic or neurologic evaluation. Studies of the effects of stimulus duration on ABR have yielded mixed and rather unimpressive results (Beattie & Boyd, 1984; Funasaka & Ito, 1986; Gorga et al., 1984; Hecox, Squires, & Galambos, 1976). One of the earliest reports by Hecox, Squires, and Galambos (1976) described alterations in the ABR to changes in the duration (on time) and interburst interval (off time) of white-noise-burst stimuli in six normal-hearing female subjects. These investigators found an increase in ABR wave V latency (0.5 ms) and decreased amplitude as duration was increased from 0.5 to 30 ms, but these changes were not observed when the stimulus off time was lengthened (i.e., with a longer recovery period). On the basis of this observation, the authors concluded that the wave V component of the ABR was strictly an onset response, that is, the ABR changes were due to response recovery processes, not to duration. Gorga et al. (1984) estimated ABR and behavioral thresholds for 2000 Hz tone-burst stimuli (with 0.5 ms rise/fall times) ranging in duration from 1 to 512 ms. They demonstrated that stimulus duration does not affect ABR threshold for normal or hearing-impaired subjects, whereas behavioral thresholds decreased (improved) on the order of 10 to 12 dB per decade of time for normal subjects. Subjects with sensorineural hearing impairment showed less change in behavioral threshold with increased stimulation duration (5 dB per decade of time). The findings of this study are consistent with psychophysical data on temporal integration.

In another study of click duration on ABR in normal-hearing subjects, Beattie and Boyd (1984) analyzed latency for wave I, wave III, and wave V at durations of 25, 50, 100, 200, and 400 μsec. There were no latency differences within the region of 25 to 100 μsec, but latency did increase by about 0.10 ms (100 μsec) with an increase in duration from 100 to 200 μsec and by 0.20 ms over the duration range of 100 to 400 μsec. Notably, the interstimulus interval for the signal rate of 10.1 clicks/second was approximately 100 ms, an adequate recovery time. The longer duration stimuli (200 and 400 μsec) lacked the spectral energy around 4700 Hz that was present in shorter duration stimuli, which might have contributed to the subtle latency differences. Duration of the stimulus and amplitude of the spectrum are systematically related. Although the click has a broad spectrum, at certain frequencies, there is reduced energy. As Gorga and Thornton (1989) point out, these points of reduced energy (or "zeros") occur at frequencies equal to integer multiples of 1 divided by the duration. For a 100 μsec click, reduced energy occurs every 10,000 Hz, whereas for a 200 μsec click, the reduced energy occurs every 5000 Hz. Beattie and Boyd (1984) acknowledge that the apparently duration-related latency effects, though small, may combine with other stimulus parameters. The duration of 100 μsec was recommended because at shorter durations stimulus intensity in dB HL was reduced (by 13 dB at 25 μsec), thereby reducing maximum effective intensity in clinical measurement.

Funasaka and Ito (1986) investigated the effect of 3000 Hz tone bursts with durations of 5, 10, 20, and 30 ms on ABR. Subjects were 20 young adults. Rise/fall times were constant at 1 ms. Interstimulus intervals ranged from 80 to 140 ms. As stimulus duration was lengthened, there were increases in latency and amplitude of waves V and VI. Wave III latency remained unchanged, but amplitude decreased. The authors argue that these effects are not a function of the recovery process limitation. Instead, the duration differentially affects the slow wave (frequency) component of the ABR and not the fast component.

ABR latency increases directly with stimulus rise times, beginning with instantaneous (0 ms) onset stimuli, at least for normal-hearing subjects (Hecox, Squires, & Galambos, 1976; Kodera et al., 1977; Salt & Thornton, 1984a,b; Suzuki & Horiuchi, 1981). When rise time exceeds 5 ms, identification of earlier ABR wave components, such as wave I, becomes difficult. The physiologic basis for this general effect is a reduction in the amount of neural units that fire synchronously (Spoendlin, 1972). Also, because the traveling wave is slower, there is an increased contribution of the more apical regions of the cochlea to the ABR (Kiang, 1975). An additional possible factor is activation of more basal cochlear regions by the increased proportion of spectral energy in higher frequency regions for briefer versus longer stimuli.

Selected studies of rise/fall time and ABR are now briefly abstracted. Salt and Thornton (1984a, b) evaluated the effect of click-stimulus rise time, along with polarity, in 8 normal-hearing subjects and found a slight, but unspecified, increase in latency as rise time was increased from 170 to 580 μsec. Suzuki and Horiuchi (1981) recorded ABRs in eight normal female hearers for tone pips (bursts) of 500 and 2000 Hz at different intensities (15 to 50 dB HL). Rise/fall times were several values in the range of 0.5 to 5 ms for the

2000 Hz stimulus and 1 to 10 ms for the tone-burst stimulus at 500 Hz. Stimuli had linear envelope shapes and, importantly, constant-onset slopes. Only the initial past of the stimulus was involved in eliciting the ABR, except at very low intensity levels at which later portions were involved. For the 2000 Hz stimulus, the response was completely generated by the first 0.5 ms portion of a higher intensity (50 dB) stimulus, and longer stimuli had no effect on the response. However, at lower intensity levels, signals with a rise time of 0.1 ms generated a completely developed response (minimal latency and maximum amplitude). Results at 500 Hz were less consistent, perhaps because neural units, according to the authors, begin to respond to individual components of the stimulus.

STIMULUS OFFSET ABR. | Basic studies of the auditory CNS have provided evidence of a variety of functional neuron types (Tsuchitani, 1983). Two of these types are onset neurons, which fire only at the onset of a stimulus, and offset neurons, which fire only at the offset of a stimulus (when the stimulus is turned off). As typically recorded, ABR is thought to reflect synchronous firing of onset neurons. For a click stimulus with the conventional duration of 0.1 milliseconds, stimulus onset and offset occur almost simultaneously, and identification of any offset contribution to the response is impossible. Over the years, papers have sporadically appeared describing AERs generated by the offset portion of stimuli. Early work in this area was conducted with the ALR (Rose & Malone, 1965). An offset ALR resembling the onset ALR was recorded in all subjects showing an onset response and it was not systematically affected by stimulus frequency or rise/fall time. Prolonged stimulus duration of 850 to 1500 ms was required to elicit the offset response (Rose & Malone, 1965).

Studies of ABR measurement with offset stimuli are not conclusive and, in fact, the existence of a true offset ABR is somewhat controversial (Antonelli & Grandori, 1984; Brinkmann & Scherg, 1979; Grandori, 1979; Kodera, Yamane, Yamada, & Suzuki, 1977; Laukli & Mair, 1985; Perez-Abalo, Valdes-Sosa, Bobes, Galan, & Biscay, 1988; Radionova, 1989). The offset ABR is generally less distinct than the onset response. A long-duration stimulus (tone burst or noise burst) is necessary to separate in time the offset response from the onset response, yet with a tone burst of 15 to 20 ms, the offset ABR may be obscured by the AMLR generated by stimulus onset.

Clinical studies, conducted with modest numbers of normal-hearing subjects, suggest that in comparison to onset responses, the offset responses (a) are not as robust (70 to 80% smaller amplitude) or as reliably recorded, (b) have a higher (poorer) threshold (by 10 to 20 dB), and (c) may be reversed in polarity (showing downward peaks) with white-noise-burst stimuli (Brinkmann & Scherg, 1979; Kodera et al., 1977). The offset response is recorded with a stimulus of extended duration (e.g., 10 ms duration or longer) to prevent

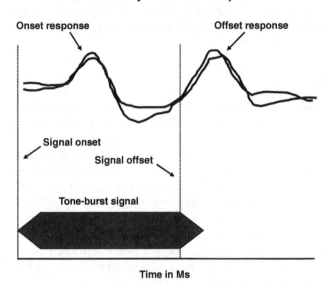

FIGURE 6.2. Diagram of auditory brainstem responses evoked by onset and offset portions of a 2000 Hz tone-burst signal.

overlapping with the invariable onset response. The problem with this method, at least when rise/fall times are very brief (less than 5 ms) is interference of offset identification by AMLR activity. There is also some concern in human investigations that what is thought to be an offset response is, in fact, produced by acoustic transducer ringing that follows stimulus onset (Brinkmann & Scherg, 1979). In short, offset ABRs are poorly understood, at best. More normal descriptive research is needed on the relationship of stimulus parameters, such as intensity, duration (rise/fall time, plateau), presentation rate, the type of stimulus (noise versus tone burst), and response acquisition parameters (e.g., filtering) to offset ABRs. Nonetheless, with careful stimulus selection, including stimuli characterized by no ringing artifact, it is possible to record a reliable ABR for the offset of tonal stimulation, as illustrated in Figure 6.2 (Van Campen, Hall, & Grantham, 1997). The stimulus depicted in this figure is a 2000 Hz tone burst with onset–offset times of 0.5 ms and a duration of 10 ms. An ABR appears at the onset of the stimulus and also following the offset.

SUMMARY. | Click duration does not have a marked influence on ABR latency or amplitude. There is no latency change for stimulus durations ranging from 0.25 to 100 μsec, and an increase in latency of 0.2 ms, at most, can be expected for durations ranging from 100 through 400 μsec. Nonetheless, click duration should be routinely specified and used in a consistent manner in clinical ABR measurement. A complete discussion of stimulus duration, although seemingly straightforward, actually leads to concerns about the possible effects of related stimulus characteristics. For example, duration directly influences frequency content of the stimulus and to the audibility of the stimulus. Duration effects also interact with the envelope of the rising portion of the stimulus and whether the onset slope is constant or variable. Finally, current understanding of stimulus duration effects is limited to data obtained from young, normal-hearing subjects. There is no published study of click duration in older subjects and/ or in those with hearing impairment, even though these and perhaps other subject characteristics might be expected to interact with duration.

Other Stimulus Types

FILTERED CLICKS. | In addition to clicks and tone bursts, miscellaneous additional types of acoustic stimuli have been reported in ABR measurement, often in animal models rather than in patients (e.g., Møller & Jho, 1989). Although none of these stimuli enjoy widespread clinical application yet, some are worth noting. For example, filtered clicks are produced when a wide-spectrum click (e.g., the usual unfiltered or raw click resulting from delivering a rectangular electric pulse to a transducer) is passed through a set or series of filters to produce transient stimuli, with energy centered at desired frequencies (Arlinger, 1981; Davis & Hirsh, 1976; Klein & Teas, 1978). ABRs (Lehnhardt, 1982) and later latency AERs (Arlinger, 1977; Lehnhardt, 1971; Spoor, Timmer, & Odenthal, 1969) have been elicited with chirps or linear frequency ramps. These stimuli consist of a sweep through a defined frequency range (e.g., 1200 to 1700 or 4200 to 4700 Hz) over a defined period of time (e.g., 10 ms). The sweep frequencies can be rising or falling. Intensity level is determined at the center frequency of the ramp.

PAIRED CLICKS. | Ernest Moore and colleagues (Davis-Gunter, Lowenheim, Gopal, & Moore, 2001; Moore et al., 1992) describe another component of the ABR—a I^l potential—evoked by presentation of two closely spaced click stimuli (0.1 ms duration). As the reader may recall from the historical overview in Chapter 1, Dr. Moore was one of the first investigators to report the identification of reliably recorded auditory evoked responses in the time period immediately following the ECochG, what we now clearly recognize as the ABR. With the paired-click stimulus paradigm, the presentation of a "standard" click is followed soon by a second click. The time difference (delta t) between the two clicks in the pair is manipulated, with interstimulus intervals ranging from 4.0 ms down to only 0.1 ms. As stated by Davis-Gunter et al. (2001), "These time intervals were chosen to be shorter than, encompass, as well as exceed the duration of the absolute (1.0 ms) and relative (4 to 5 ms) refractory periods of the VIIIth nerve" (p. 53), and then the authors cite the experimental findings on auditory physiology of Eggermont and Odenthal (1974b). The first click, of course, generates combined (ensemble) action potentials (AP) in the distal portion of the auditory nerve, the ABR

wave I. If the second click is presented before the auditory nerve fibers have fully recovered from firing (during their refractory period), it presumably will not generate an AP. The second click will, however, produce excitatory postsynaptic potentials (EPSPs) that are reflected within the activity measured as an ABR. To isolate and identify the EPSP activity, the authors utilize a derived response technique, i.e., the waveform for the first (standard) click is subtracted from the waveform for pair of clicks. In theory, the derived response (the difference wave) consists of only EPSP activity. When Davis-Gunter et al. (2001) performed the paired stimulus and derived response analysis technique with three normal-hearing adult subjects, the authors identified two waves—I^0 and I^l—appearing before the conventional wave I. As reported previously (Moore et al., 1992), the average latency for wave I^l was 0.97 ms, whereas conventional wave I latency was 1.83 ms. The authors speculate "that peaks I^0 and I^l represent the summating potential and the generator potential, generated by the cochlea and VIIIth nerve dendrites, respectively" (Davis-Gunter et al., 2001, p. 50).

PLOPS. | In a study of novel stimulation and analysis techniques, Scherg and Speulda (1982) recorded ABRs with conventional clicks (100 µsec square-wave pulses) and with Gaussian-shaped impulses centered around 1000 Hz, referred to by the authors as "plops." Stimuli were presented separately for three polarity modes (alternating, rarefaction, and condensation), via a TDH-39 earphone. The envelope of the acoustic waveform for the plop, as depicted in a figure in the paper, resembled that of a click, but it lacked the ringing (and added frequency components) of the click waveform. It appeared, from data presented in a table, that absolute latency values for wave I, wave III, and wave V were greater for the "plop" versus the click, while other ABR parameters (absolute amplitude of wave V and interwave latencies) were similar for the two stimuli types. A latency delay for a stimulus with a center frequency of 1000 Hz versus a click is expected because the click activates a more basal region of the cochlea.

CHIRPS. | There is consensus that the ABR evoked by conventional click stimulation is dominated by activation of the basal region of the cochlea, mostly frequencies above 2000 Hz. Attempts to enhance the contribution of other regions of the cochlea to ABR generation include the generation of rather unique types of stimuli, such as "chirps" and sophisticated recording techniques, such as "stacked ABR." The *chirp stimulus* is designed mathematically "to produce simultaneous displacement maxima along the cochlear partition by compensating for frequency-dependent traveling-time differences" (Fobel & Dau, 2004). Several groups of authors since 2000 have reported detailed technical descriptions and mathematical models for chirp stimuli (e.g., Dau, Wagner, Mellert, & Kollmeier, 2000; Fobel & Dau, 2004; Wegner & Dau, 2002). In theory, the chirp will optimize synchronization across a broad frequency region at high and low intensity levels, yielding a more robust ABR than the conventional click stimulus. A detailed explanation of the model of cochlear biomechanics and the mathematical functions important in the rationale for and generation of chirps is far beyond the scope of this discussion.

The article authored by Fobel and Dau (2004) provides a useful source of information on the topic. Fobel and Dau (2004) designed two chirp stimuli for elicitation of the ABR. One—referred to as the O-chirp—was derived from previously published group-delay data (Shera & Guinan, 2000) from stimulus frequency OAEs (the term "O" chirp refers to the derivation from an OAE stimulus). The other stimulus—referred to as the A-chirp—was designed with reference to data (Gorga, Kaminski, Beauchaine, & Jesteadt, 1988) demonstrating the relationship between tone burst frequency and ABR latency (the term "A" chirp refers to the derivation from ABR data). ABRs generated by these two chirp stimuli were compared also to a previously developed type of chirp (Dau et al., 2000)—the M-chirp—based on a model (the "M" refers to "Model") for producing a flat-spectrum stimulus. Fobel and Dau (2004) recorded ABRs from 9 normal-hearing adult subjects with the different chirp stimuli, and with conventional click stimuli. Since the frequency composition of the chirp stimuli covered a range from 0.1 to 10,000 Hz, durations for the chirp stimuli were remarkably long in comparison to clicks. Duration for the O-chirp was 13.52 ms, whereas duration for the M-chirp was 10.32. For the A-chirp, however, duration varied as a function of stimulus intensity, from 12.72 ms at 10 dB SL (sensation level) to 5.72 ms at 60 dB SL. Fobel and Dau (2004) reported no difference in the ABRs evoked with O- and M-chirp stimuli at any of the intensity levels. Each of the chirp stimuli, however, evoked ABRs with larger amplitude values than those elicited by conventional click stimuli. Among the three types of chirps, the A-chirp produced the most robust ABR waveforms, and it "is particularly effective at very low [intensity] levels where wave-V amplitude is about three times as large as for the click" (Fobel & Dau, 2004, p. 2221). The authors speculate on the potential benefits of the A-chirp for clinical application of ABR, especially for estimation of auditory thresholds.

TONE BURSTS. | Tone bursts are now regularly used in clinical ABR measurement for estimation of auditory sensitivity for discrete frequency regions, especially in infants and young children. The minimum response level for the wave V component of the ABR evoked by tone-burst stimuli is recorded within 10 dB or the behavioral threshold for a comparable pure-tone frequency for the majority of patients with sensory hearing loss, with over 90 percent of patients yielding a difference within ±20 dB (e.g., Balfour, Pillion, & Gaskin, 1999; Gorga, Kaminski, Beauchaine, & Jesteadt, 1988; Stapells, Gravel, & Martin, 1995; Stapells, Picton, & Durieux, 1994). The clinical application of tone-burst stim-

uli for electrophysiological estimation of pure-tone hearing thresholds is discussed in Chapter 8. What follows here is a brief mention of other, primarily research, uses of tone-burst stimulation of the ABR. As noted in the section below on stimulus polarity, differences in the ABRs evoked by tone-burst stimuli in different frequency regions shed light on the mechanisms of cochlear physiology and, in particular, the cochlear response to rarefaction versus condensation stimulus polarity. A number of investigators have examined with ABR the forward masking phenomenon (e.g., Burkard & Hecox, 1987; Kramer & Teas, 1982; Lasky & Rupert, 1982). Walton, Orlando, and Burkard (1999) utilized tone-burst maskers and probe signals in an investigation of the recovery from forward masking as a function of age in adults. Using the forward masking paradigm, the authors found an age difference in the latency shift of wave V with short intervals (e.g., 16 ms) between the masker and the probe for higher tone-burst frequencies (e.g., 4000 and 8000 Hz), but not for a lower frequency (1000 Hz). Recovery from masking, that is, baseline latency values for the ABR, was always complete under all stimulus conditions and age groups with an interval of at least 64 ms between masker and probe signal.

MODULATED TONES. | There are also descriptions of AER generation with stimuli that are frequency modulated (Eggermont & Odenthal, 1974b; Lehnhardt, 1971) and with stimuli that are amplitude modulated (Eggermont & Odenthal, 1974b; Kuwada, Batra, & Maher, 1986; Milford & Birchall, 1989; Møller, 1987b; Rees, Green, & Kay, 1986). Amplitude modulated (AM) and frequency modulated (FM) sinusoidal signals are discussed further in reference to the auditory steady-state response (ASSR) in Chapter 8. Legendre sequences and maximum length sequences (MLS) of pulse trains have also been described in stimulation of ABR (Burkard, Shi, & Hecox, 1990a, b; Eysholdt & Schreiner, 1982). Although these techniques may potentially increase efficiency of ABR data collection and reduce test time, clinical confirmation is lacking.

STIMULUS TRAINS. | Tietze (1980) reported two clever techniques for simultaneous stimulation and recording of the ABR and ALR. The methodological problem in simultaneously recording these two AERs is that the ABR requires stimuli with rather abrupt onset (e.g., 2 to 4 cycles), a similarly brief duration, and short interstimulus intervals (e.g., 25 ms), whereas the ALR is best elicited with stimuli having relatively leisurely rise/fall times (e.g., 8 to 30 ms), plateau durations (30 to 500 ms) and interstimulus intervals of approximately 2.5 seconds. With one technique, trains of tone pips are presented with an interval of 2.5 seconds between each train. Each train has the effect of a single stimulus unit in eliciting the ALR. However, within each train, individual tone pips at intervals of 25 ms serve as the stimuli for the ABR. The second technique is similar. The individual tone pips continue to serve as the ABR stimuli, and between each group of tone pips, a tone burst of a slightly lower intensity level is inserted, to evoke the ALR. Because the ALR is a larger amplitude response (i.e., a more robust signal), fewer stimuli must be averaged to obtain a stable waveform. As a consequence, although relatively few trains of tone pips versus numerous individual tone pips are presented per given unit of time, the number of stimuli averaged is equally adequate for the ABR and ALR.

Trains with multiple stimuli (20, 56, and more), often presented at very rapid rates, are also used to evoke the ABR in an attempt to minimize test time (e.g., Burkard et al., 1990; Hamill, Hussing, & Sammeth, 1991; Henry et al., 2000; Mitchell, Kempton, Creedon, & Trune, 1996, 1999; Thornton & Slaven, 1993). A significant reduction in the time required to evoke the ABR would contribute, at least in pediatric populations to the clinical feasibility of estimating auditory status for each ear with multiple frequency-specific stimuli. Several such techniques, including "maximum length sequence (MLS)" and "chained stimuli" are mentioned in the review of ABR analysis (Chapter 7). Maximum length sequence (MLS) is defined mathematically as "a quasi-random binary sequence represented by a train of +1s and −1s. In its audiological application it may be represented by +1s and 0s or by clicks and silences" (Thornton & Slaven, 1993). One undesirable outcome often associated with the rapid presentation of a train of stimuli (clicks or tone bursts) is a reduction in the response amplitude and prolongation of latency, presumably secondary to adaptation within the auditory system. Modification of the stimulus-train techniques may minimize the impact on response latency and amplitude (e.g., Mitchell et al., 1999). Since the early 1980s, claims of important savings in test time and increased test efficiency with stimulus-train techniques are cited regularly in many papers on the technique. Nonetheless, even though techniques such as the MLS have been offered as features with commercially available evoked response systems, stimulus-train strategies are still not widely incorporated into the clinical ABR test battery.

NOISE STIMULI. | Noise signals, presented alone or in the presence of click or tone-burst stimuli, are often described in the clinical ABR literature. Reasons for incorporating noise as the stimulus, or with the stimulus, vary among studies of the ABR and include investigation of fundamental auditory phenomenon (e.g., temporal response properties of the cochlea and auditory nerve) or more clinically applicable objectives (e.g., achieving greater frequency specificity for clinical assessment of infants and young children). Noise stimuli used to measure gap detection, a psychophysical procedure for assessing temporal auditory processing, or temporal resolution, are also effective as stimuli for generation of the ABR (Poth, Boettcher, Mills, & Dubno, 2001; Werner, Folsom, Mancl, & Syapin, 2001). An ABR is evoked by an initial noise burst with a duration of >15 ms, and then within milliseconds a second noise burst is presented as a stimulus for

a second ABR. The silent interval—the gap—is usually varied over the range of 0 ms to over 100 ms. A basic assumption underlying the electrophysiological measurement of gap detection is that the ABR for the second of the two noise bursts will be unchanged if the silent gap is fully processed by auditory system—that is, the gap is equal to or exceeds the interval required for temporal resolution. Normative data are collected for the ABR evoked by a noise burst presented following another noise burst, i.e., the normal gap detection threshold is defined. Changes in the latency of ABR wave V, or absence of an ABR, for a stimulus presented after a silent gap that is detected by normal subjects, i.e., a gap duration that is long enough to not interfere with the ABR, are associated with deficits in temporal auditory processing. Normal changes in the ABR with shorter gap durations include latency prolongation and amplitude reduction. A detectable ABR is present in young normal subjects with gap durations as short as 8 ms, whereas the ABR may not be present when the silent gap is a short as 4 ms (Poth et al., 2001).

Werner et al. (2001) investigated application of the ABR as an electrophysiological measure of temporal processing with a gap detection method. Subjects were 35 young normal adult subjects and 30 infants, ten who were 3 months old and 20 who were 6 months old. Stimuli were a pair of 15 ms bursts of broadband noise separated by silent gaps ranging in duration from 0 to 125 ms. In one experiment, Werner et al. (2001) found that gap detection thresholds determined with ABR (2.4 ms) were on the average similar to those obtained with conventional psychophysical methods (2.9 ms). In another experiment, the authors recorded for subjects with sloping high-frequency sensorineural hearing loss higher gap detection thresholds (longer thresholds for silent gaps) with both the ABR (12.7 ms) and the psychophysical techniques (10.7 ms). In contrast, data recorded from infants revealed a difference in the gap detection thresholds as measured with the electrophysiological versus psychophysical methods. Temporal resolution was immature for infants (longer silent gaps were required for detection) as measured with the psychophysical method, whereas developing age did not influence ABR gap threshold. According to Werner et al. (2001), these findings "suggest that it is not immaturity at the level of the brainstem that is responsible for infant's poor gap detection performance" (p. 748).

Poth et al. (2001) described the use of broadband noise with silent gaps as a stimulus for investigating auditory temporal processing with the ABR. The electrophysiological study of gap detection using noise bursts was a clinical follow-up to experiments conducted by the authors with various animal models (e.g., Boettcher, Mills, Swerdloff, & Holley, 1996). Stimuli consisted of 50 ms broadband noise bursts interrupted by a silent period varying in duration from 4 to 64 ms. This ABR stimulus paradigm is comparable to the stimuli used in psychophysical measurement of temporal resolution. Poth et al. (2001) reported that ABR amplitudes were reduced, and in a group of older subjects (> 60 years), the proportion of subjects yielding measurable responses was diminished. In other words, longer gaps of silence were required for generation of a normal ABR for older subjects.

STIMULATION OF "STACKED ABR." | Dr. Manny Don and colleagues at the House Ear Institute developed the "stacked ABR" technique with the goal of detecting with greater accuracy and sensitivity than convention click stimuli retrocochlear auditory dysfunction, particularly small acoustic tumors (Don, Masuda, Nelson, & Brackmann, 1997). The technique is an outgrowth of previous investigation by the authors and others of the effects of ipsilateral high-pass masking on "cochlear response times," i.e., traveling wave distance and velocity along the basilar membrane (Don & Eggermont, 1978; Don, Ponton, Eggermont, & Masuda, 1993, 1994; Donaldson & Ruth, 1993; Eggermont, Brown, Ponton, & Kimberley, 1996). Discussion of the stacked ABR technique could logically be included here in the review of stimulus parameters, in the following chapter on ABR analysis techniques, in the discussion about frequency-specific ABR techniques (Chapter 8), or even in the summary of clinical applications of ABR in adult patient populations (Chapter 10). The following is an overview of the method for deriving stimuli within different frequency regions utilized in the stacked ABR technique. Clinical performance of the stacked ABR technique in retrocochlear auditory pathology and other clinical entities (e.g., Ménière's disease) is reviewed in Chapter 10. To more completely appreciate the derived-band technique in stacked ABR for assuring that stimuli are frequency-specific, the reader may find useful the information on ipsilateral masking strategies presented in the introduction to Chapter 8.

As noted in Chapter 3 and earlier in this chapter, the click stimuli used to evoke the ABR include energy from a wide frequency region, yet the response is mostly generated by stimulus-related activity for the high-frequency region of the cochlea and, correspondingly afferent fibers in the eighth cranial (auditory) nerve serving this region. Development of the stacked ABR technique was motivated by appreciation that small acoustic tumors often have negligible impact on functional integrity of high-frequency neural fibers and, therefore, little or no influence on the click-evoked ABR. Even when an acoustic tumor does impinge on high-frequency neural fibers with resulting disruption in their capability to fire synchronously, an ABR may still be generated by frequencies in another portion of the broadband click spectrum. In either case, the result is a normal ABR in a patient with an acoustic tumor—i.e., a false-negative diagnostic outcome. To circumvent this limitation of conventional click stimuli, the stacked ABR technique calls for the use of bands of ipsilateral masking to derive a series of ABRs, each generated by cochlear activity within a designated frequency region and, therefore, activity of a tonotopically defined set of nerve fibers.

Measurement of the stacked ABR begins with conventional click stimuli of 0.1 ms duration and rarefaction polarity, presented at interstimulus intervals of 22 ms and an intensity level of 93 dB peak-to-peak SPL. Then, bands of pink noise are presented ipsilaterally at levels sufficient to mask the ABR evoked by the click stimulus. High-pass masking noise with five different low-frequency cutoffs (8000, 4000, 2000, 1000, and 500 Hz) is sequentially presented with the click stimulus. A total of 6 ABR waveforms are thus obtained—one for the conventional click and then one waveform generated by a different frequency region, i.e., only frequencies above 8000 Hz, then only for frequencies above 4000 Hz, and so forth. In other words, with each change in the cutoff for the ipsilateral masking, more of the lower frequency region is masked and its contribution to the ABR removed. Once the ABRs are recorded, ABRs for different frequency regions are derived by digitally subtracting the ABR waveform for one ipsilateral masking condition from the ABR waveform generated by the previously recorded condition. The ABRs for each of the derived bands reflect activity of the cochlea region and auditory nerve fibers that serve the frequencies within the band, with characteristic frequencies of 11,300 Hz, 5700 Hz, 2800 Hz, 1400 Hz, and 700 Hz. Wave V latencies of the ABRs for each of the derived bands vary predictably. The derived band with the highest characteristic frequency (11,300 Hz) produces the ABR with the shortest wave V latency, and wave V latency is progressively longer for subsequent lower frequency bands.

After the ABRs for each frequency region are derived, they are aligned according to wave V latency, that is, lower frequency ABR waveforms are shifted to the left until wave V latencies for all bands are the same as the wave V latency for the 11,300 Hz band. The term "stacked ABR" is therefore quite appropriate as the result of the manipulation of ABR waveforms according to wave V latency produces a stacking of waveforms. Each waveform represents ABR energy generated by stimulation of a band of frequencies. If all of the frequency bands are normally represented in the overall ABR—that is, the cochlea and the auditory nerves are functionally intact within each frequency region—then adding them together should result in an ABR equivalent in amplitude to the click-evoked ABR. If, however, an acoustic tumor is affecting neural integrity within one or more of the frequency regions, the amplitude sum of the five individual stacked ABRs will be less than the amplitude of the click ABR. The influence of an acoustic tumor on the auditory nerve, therefore, is inferred by a reduction in summed amplitude of the stacked ABRs versus normal expectations (the "standard" ABR for the conventional unmasked click). Clinical application of the stacked ABR technique in detection of small acoustic tumors is discussed in Chapter 10.

SPEECH STIMULI. | Ample evidence now exists confirming the feasibility of generating an ABR and a frequency-following response (FFR) with speech stimuli. Nina Kraus and colleagues at Northwestern University have published a series of articles describing in detail characteristics of the ABR and FFR evoked by speech sounds (King, Warrier, Hayes, & Kraus, 2002; Russo, Nicol, Musacchia, & Kraus, 2004; Wible, Nicol, & Kraus, 2005). These researchers further introduce the application of speech-evoked ABR and FFR as a tool for investigating the neural representation of speech processing at the brainstem and for documenting neural plasticity with auditory training. The 40 ms speech stimulus (/da/) in each of the studies just cited was a synthetically generated stop consonant (/d) and shortened vowel (/a/) consisting of a fundamental frequency and five carefully defined formants. For details on the composition of the speech stimulus and other technical aspects of the procedure for recording and analyzing speech-evoked ABRs, the reader is referred to the original publications, available in PDF format from Dr. Kraus at the Northwestern University website. The speech stimuli were typically presented via insert earphones with alternating polarity at an intensity level of 80 dB SPL and in trains of four stimuli with an interval of 12 ms between the offset of one train and the onset of a consecutive train. Subjects were distracted during the ABR recording by watching a videotape of a movie or cartoon with a low-intensity sound track.

The ABR waveform evoked by the speech stimulus (/da/) consisted of an initial segment within 10 ms that contained the typical positive ABR peaks (e.g., wave III and wave V, and sometimes wave I) and a negative wave (labeled wave A) that resembled the SN10 wave. After the transient portion of the ABR, there was within the next 30 to 40 ms a complex FFR waveform—the "sustained response"—that contained two rather stable waves, referred to as peak C (latency of about 18 ms) and peak F (latency of about 40 ms). As noted by Russo et al. (2004), "The defining feature of the sustained portion of the response is its periodicity, which follows the frequency information contained in the stimulus" (p. 2023). Analysis of the waveform included calculations of interpeak latency intervals, and the amplitude, slope, and area of individual peaks. The speech-evoked ABR was recorded in quiet (no background noise) and also in the presence of noise to evaluate speech processing in an adverse listening condition. The authors of the above-noted papers describe five analysis techniques for extracting speech stimulus related information from the complex FFR waveform: (1) calculation of root mean square (RMS) amplitude, (2) calculation of the amplitude for a spectral component evoked by the fundamental frequency of the stimulus, (3) calculation of the amplitude for a spectral component evoked by the first formant frequencies of the stimulus, (4) correlations of the stimulus-to-noise response, and (5) correlations between the ABR and FFR recorded in quiet versus noise. An additional waveform analysis technique ("wavelet-denoising") was required to identify speech-evoked peaks in the noise condition. Russo et al. (2004) aptly summarize the exciting implications of this line of investigation as follows:

The ability to quantify a brainstem response elicited by speech sounds provides a powerful tool for research and clinical use. The speech-evoked brainstem response faithfully reflects many acoustic properties of the speech signal. In the normally perceiving auditory system, stimulus timing, on the order of fractions of milliseconds, is accurately and precisely represented at the level of the brainstem. (p. 2027)

Clinical applications of speech-evoked ABR measurement are reviewed in Chapter 9.

Intensity

Intensity is clearly a critical variable influencing ABR latency and amplitude, and it is among the measurement parameters manipulated most often in clinical application of the ABR. A series of ABR waveforms for decreasing intensity levels is shown in the left portion of Figure 6.3. The salient features of the effect of intensity on wave V latency in this series of waveforms become more clearly apparent when latency values are plotted as a function of intensity (Figure 6.4). The latency–intensity function for wave V is the most common graphic display of clinical ABR data. The dotted

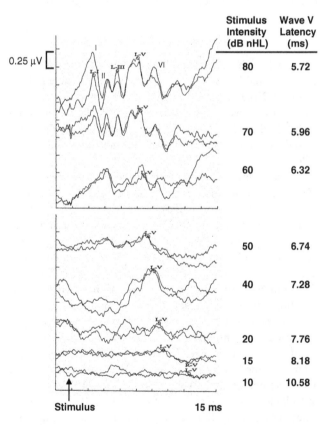

Stimulus Intensity (dB nHL)	Wave V Latency (ms)
80	5.72
70	5.96
60	6.32
50	6.74
40	7.28
20	7.76
15	8.18
10	10.58

FIGURE 6.3. Auditory brainstem response waveforms as evoked with signals of descending intensity levels. Note the increase in wave latency with decreased signal intensity level and the disappearance of the wave I component before the wave V component.

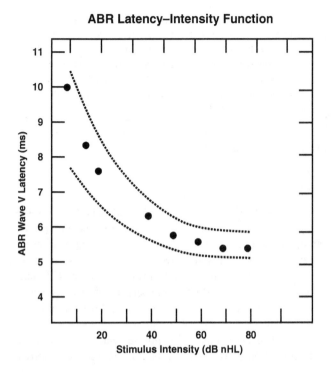

ABR Latency–Intensity Function

FIGURE 6.4. Example of a latency–intensity function for the ABR wave V. Waveforms were shown in Figure 6.3.

lines enclose the mean wave V latency values for a group of young normal-hearing males and females (±2.5 standard deviations). Note that this normal region encompasses a wider latency range as intensity decreases, reflecting more variability in the ABR at lower stimulus intensity levels. Standard deviations for normal wave V latency are usually about 0.20 ms at 70 dB and 0.30 ms at 30 dB. For low to moderate intensity levels, there is normally a systematic and rather abrupt shortening of latency values (up to 0.50 or 0.60 ms of latency per 10 dB of intensity, or 0.06 ms/dB) for wave V up to approximately 60 dB nHL. A wave V, even in normal hearers, is generally not detected visually at intensity levels below 10 dB nHL. At these apparent ABR threshold levels, normal wave V latency is 7.5 to 8.0 ms or more. For intensities from 60 to 95 dB nHL, the slope of the latency–intensity function is more gradual, producing a rate of change of only about 0.10 to 0.20 ms/10 dB. Indeed, as intensity is increased at the highest click signal intensity levels, there is little decrease in wave V latency. Overall, the latency–intensity slope is on the order of 0.38 ms/10 dB (Gorga, Worthington, Reiland, Beauchaine, & Goldgar, 1985; Hecox & Galambos, 1974; Pratt & Sohmer, 1977). Because the latency-intensity function has a bend at about 60 dB, it is not linear. According to Picton, Stapells, and Campbell (1981), the latency–intensity function can be calculated with the following power function:

$$\log 10 \text{ (V latency in ms)} = -0.0025 \text{ (click intensity in dB)} + 0.924$$

At high intensity levels (75 to 95 dB nHL), wave V latency is normally in the region of 5.5 to 6.0 ms (Coats, 1978; Hecox & Galambos, 1974; Picton, Woods, Baribeau-Braun, & Healey, 1977; Starr & Achor, 1975; Wolfe, Skinner, & Burns, 1978; Yamada, Yagi, Yamane, & Suzuki, 1975; Zöllner, Karnahl, & Stange, 1976). As noted previously, wave V latency increases by about 2 ms over the range from high intensity levels (e.g., 80 dB) to threshold levels (e.g., 20 dB). That is, over this intensity range absolute latency increases from about 5.5 ms to 7.5 ms. At high signal intensity levels, it's possible to identify wave I and wave III (and even wave II, wave IV, and wave VI). In normal hearers, at high intensity levels (>80 dB nHL) for the click signal, wave I latency is about 1.5 ms, wave III is about 3.5 ms, and, as just noted, wave V is in the 5.5 ms region. Interwave latency values are approximately 2.0 ms for both the wave I to III interval and the wave III to V interval. Added together, this results in an average wave I to V interval on the order of 4.0 ms. Subject factors, such as gender or body temperature, may influence interwave latency values.

Although wave V can be detected for intensity levels down to 10 dB, and even lower, the lowest level at which wave I and wave III are usually visible in adult normal-hearing subjects with conventional recording techniques is about 25 to 35 dB nHL. Partly, this is because wave V normally has relatively larger amplitude. In addition, however, the rate of decrease in amplitude with decreasing intensity is more rapid for the earlier waves. The smallest amplitude that can be reliably detected visually is usually about 0.05 μV, but this is heavily dependent on the amount of background noise in the recording. On the average, at high intensity levels, the amplitude of wave V is 0.50 μV and for wave I it is 0.25 to 0.35 μV, producing a normal wave V:I amplitude ratio of 1.50. At low signal intensity levels, wave I latency is around 3.5 to 4 ms (versus the wave V latency at 7.5 to 8 ms). It would appear, then, that the wave I to V latency interval of about 4.0 ms generally holds constant across this range of stimulus intensity levels for normal subjects. While this is sometimes the case, the increase in latency with decrease intensity may not be precisely parallel for wave I versus wave V, or among waves in general (Pratt & Sohmer, 1976; Starr & Achor, 1975). A greater (increased) latency shift with declining intensity may occur for wave I than for wave V in normal adults, resulting in a net shortening of the interval between wave I and wave V latency by about 0.20 ms, or even more at lower intensity levels (Stockard, Stockard, Westmoreland, & Corfits, 1979). The clinically important wave I to V latency intensity interval may also be influenced by subject characteristics (such as age, in children), by stimulus parameters other than intensity, by audiogram configuration, and, of course, by retrocochlear and brainstem auditory dysfunction.

ABR amplitude, even for wave V at very high intensity levels, rarely exceeds 1.0 μV. As intensity level is decreased, amplitude for all wave components steadily diminishes.

As with latency, the trend is usually not linear (Hecox & Galambos, 1974; Jewett & Williston, 1971), although some researchers have reported an essentially linear relationship (e.g., Starr & Achor, 1975; Wolfe et al., 1978). In addition, intensity-related amplitude changes are characteristically more variable than latency changes for subjects at all ages (e.g., Hecox & Galambos, 1974; Jewett & Williston, 1971; Lasky, 1984; Lasky, Rupert, & Walker, 1987).

There are well-recognized interactions among stimulus intensity, rate, duration, and frequency. The preceding comments have pertained mostly to the influence of intensity on ABR latency and amplitude for click signals. Gorga, Kaminski, and Beauchaine (1988) described latency–intensity functions for tone-burst stimuli (cosine^2 gating functions) at frequencies from 250 Hz through 8000 Hz. Data were for 20 normal-hearing subjects. Latency was shorter for high versus low frequencies. Also, latency clearly decreased as intensity increased for all test frequencies. Intersubject variability was greater for lower than for higher frequencies. It appeared that the latency–intensity slopes were steeper for lower frequency stimuli. That is, the decrease in latency with intensity was greater for low than for high frequencies. Gorga and colleagues (1988) suggested that this convergence in functions among test frequencies at the highest intensity levels for low frequency stimuli was related to spread of activation to higher frequency regions. Ten years earlier, Klein and Teas (1978) reported similar latency trends for filtered click stimuli (octave frequencies 500 to 8000 Hz) as a function of intensity. Characteristics of the ABR evoked by tone-burst signals are described in more detail in Chapter 8.

PHYSIOLOGIC EXPLANATIONS FOR THE LATENCY–INTENSITY FUNCTION. | There are several explanations for the decrease in latency and increase in amplitude as intensity of a click stimulus increases. Even though a click contains energy across a broad frequency region, the site of ABR generation along the basilar membrane is, in part, related to intensity. Very high intensity levels activate the cochlea near the base. The site of cochlear activation then moves progressively toward the apex for lower intensity levels. At the lowest intensity levels (i.e., normal threshold), the portion of the cochlea representing frequencies 1000 to 2000 Hz generates the ABR. This apical shift in the primary place of stimulation along the basilar membrane produces roughly a 1 ms latency increase (Picton et al., 1981). Because wave V latency increases from 5.5 to 8 ms, a change of 2.5 ms, there must also be another mechanism in the intensity–latency function. One theory is that postsynaptic excitation potentials reach threshold faster for higher intensity levels, and therefore synaptic transmission time decreases.

The latency decrease with increasing transient (tone-burst or click) stimulus intensity is due to a progressively faster rising generator potential within the cochlea and a similarly faster development of excitatory postsynaptic potentials, or EPSPs (Møller, 1981). Compound AP latency is directly dependent on how quickly the generator potential and EPSPs increase and reach the threshold for firing. Higher intensity stimuli may also bring into play nonlinear activity within the cochlea and widening of tuning curves. These stimuli produce a shift in the place of maximal cochlear excitation along the basilar membrane toward the base. Travel time from the oval window to this more basal site is, of course, shorter and, therefore, so is compound AP latency.

One explanation of the physiologic mechanism underlying ABR, which takes into account stimulus intensity, frequency, and rate parameters, might be referred to as the "dual structure" or the "fast versus slow component" theory (Davis, 1976b; Klein, 1983; Maurizi, Paludetti, Ottaviani, & Rosignoli, 1984; Suzuki, Hirai, & Horiuchi, 1977; Suzuki, Kobayashi, & Takagi, 1985). The ABR can be viewed as a broad, slow wave (i.e., slow component) upon which the characteristic wave components I through VI or VII (i.e., fast component) are superimposed. Spectral analysis of ABR suggests that the dominant energy around or below 100 Hz forms the slow component, and the energy peaks around 500 Hz and 900 Hz contribute mainly to the fast component (Hall, 1986; Kevanishvili & Aphonchenko, 1979; Suzuki, Sakabe, & Miyashita, 1982). Presumably, slow-versus-fast components do not share the same neural generators (Davis, 1976a; Klein, 1983). As stimulus (click) intensity is increased, amplitude of the slow component reaches a plateau in the 40 to 50 dB region, but the fast components (waves I through V at least) show the characteristic steady amplitude increase discussed previously (Takagi, Suzuki, & Kobayashi, 1985).

One way of viewing this phenomenon is to think in terms of an amplitude ratio (slow-to-fast component amplitude). Intensity, therefore, produces an increase in the ratio of fast-to-slow components. The consequence of this dual component view for clinical ABR application is apparent. Namely, auditory threshold estimation, at low intensity levels, is dependent mainly on analysis of the slow component.

There are several theories on the physiologic basis for the two-segmented compound (whole nerve) AP with an increase of stimulus intensity. One theory is that there are two sets of primary fibers, a low- and a high-sensitivity population. The other viewpoint maintains that the slow-growing portion of the input–output function (at lower stimulus intensity levels) reflects activity in the sharp tip portion of the tuning curves, and the rapidly growing portion of function for higher stimulus levels reflects recruitment of higher frequency neural units on the "tail" of the tuning curves (Özdamar & Dallos, 1976).

RELATION BETWEEN ABR AMPLITUDE AND LOUDNESS. | One concept that is relevant in this discussion is the possible relationship between ABR amplitude–latency parameters and the behavioral perception of loudness. Intensity is a physical property of sound, and loudness is the perceptual correlate of intensity. Loudness is a subjective estimation of the strength of the stimulus. As an aside, there is a comparable correspondence between frequency (another physical property of sound) and the perception of pitch. Pratt and Sohmer (1977) attempted to correlate latency and amplitude for ABR and other AERs with psychophysical magnitude estimates of click stimuli. Amplitude, but not latency, was correlated with loudness estimation. In a follow-up study, Babkoff, Pratt, and Kempinski (1984) essentially replicated the earlier research and also reanalyzed the original results with a correction for the nonlinearity of the latency–intensity function. The second set of data and reanalysis showed closer agreement between electrophysiologic and psychophysical parameters, but did not alter the original conclusions. Similarly, Darling and Price (1990) failed to find a clear connection between ABR and the perception of loudness. On the other hand, Thornton and colleagues (Thornton, Farrell, & McSporran, 1989; Thornton, Yardley, & Farrell, 1987) describe a clinical protocol for estimating loudness discomfort level (LDL) with ABR wave V latency versus intensity data. Also, in a group of adult subjects (18 to 65 years), Serpanos, O'Malley, and Gravel (1997) "established a relationship between loudness and the ABR wave V latency for listeners with normal hearing, and flat cochlear hearing loss" (p. 409), whereas there was poor correlation between behavioral and electrophysiological intensity functions for patients with sloping sensorineural hearing loss.

AGE. | The latency–intensity change in newborns is in the range of 30 to 40 μsec/dB (Despland & Galambos, 1980; Hecox, 1975; Lasky & Rupert, 1982). Age is also a determinant in the stimulus intensity level required for generating a just-detectable ABR. Among infants, there is some rather dated evidence that ABR threshold declines with age (Lary, Briassoulis, de Vries, Dubowitz, & Dubowitz, 1985; Lasky, Rupert, & Walker, 1987). These authors reported a distinct reduction in the ABR threshold (on the order of 10 to 30 dB), even within the interval from 2 hours after birth to 50 hours after birth. ABR latency and amplitude values at these two times post-birth, when corrected for the threshold differences, were comparable. These studies did not, however, address several possible factors in the ABR threshold decrease with age, including imprecision in the placement of supra-aural earphones, collapse (closure) of the ear canal secondary to earphone cushion pressure on the cartilaginous portion, maturational changes in middle ear status, the likelihood of residual vernix caseosa in the external ear canal, and even mesenchyme in the middle ear space in the hours following birth. The latter two possible factors would essentially create a slight conductive hearing loss that could elevate thresholds and extend latencies for the ABR in newborn infants.

CALIBRATION AND VERIFICATION OF STIMULUS INTENSITY. | Techniques for calibration of stimulus intensity levels in general were reviewed in Chapter 3. The approach used most often to verify and monitor stimulus intensity levels in clinical settings—collection of normative data for each stimulus type from a small group of normal hearers—is applied also for ABR. The resulting description of intensity level in dB nHL is referenced to average normal hearing threshold levels for different stimuli (e.g., air-conduction clicks and tone bursts, and bone conduction clicks) in a specific clinical test setting with the measurement conditions encountered with patients. Admittedly, there are weaknesses inherent within the common strategy of establishing "biologic norms" for a specific clinic and verifying that ABR latency and amplitude data as a function of stimulus intensity are consistent with published databases for larger numbers of subjects carefully selected with regard to auditory and neurological status and age. The most serious constraint, by far, is the application of these normative data from adult subjects to clinical ABR measurement in infants and young children. The flaw in this approach is readily apparent. For a given acoustic stimulus generated by an earphone, either a supra-aural or insert transducer and cushion, the effective intensity level at the tympanic membrane will vary as a function of ear-canal acoustic characteristics, especially size. The ear-canal volume enclosed under the earphone is likely to be many times larger for an adult subject than for an infant, and the effective intensity level correspondingly higher for the infant than for the adult. Technology for measurement and monitoring of stimulus intensity levels within the ear canal obviously exists and is consistently applied during data collection with certain audiologic procedures, e.g., otoacoustic emissions. McCall, Chertoff, and Ferraro (1998) provided evidence that even for adults "in-situ calibration" of click stimuli affected ABR latencies and amplitudes, and even threshold estimation with the ABR wave V. The time has clearly come for routine in-the-ear calibration of acoustic stimuli used to evoke the ABR, and other auditory evoked responses.

Rate

NORMAL ADULTS. | Beginning with the earliest studies on ABR in human subjects (Jewett, Romano, & Williston, 1970; Jewett & Williston, 1971), numerous investigators have described the effect of stimulus rate on ABR in normal-hearing adults (Burkard, Shi, & Hecox, 1990a; Chiappa, Gladstone, & Young, 1979; Don, Allen, & Starr, 1977; Eggermont & Odenthal, 1974b; Fowler & Noffsinger, 1983; Hyde, Stephens, & Thornton, 1976; Paludetti, Maurizi, & Ottaviani, 1983; Picton et al., 1974, 1981; Pratt & Sohmer, 1976; Salamy, McKean, & Buda, 1975; Sand, 1986; Sininger & Don, 1989; Suzuki, Kobayashi, & Takagi, 1985; Terkildsen, Osterhammel, & Huis In't Veld, 1975; Thornton & Coleman, 1975; van Olphen, Rodenburg, & Vervey, 1979; Weber & Fujikawa, 1977; Yagi & Hughes, 1975; Yagi & Kaga, 1979; Yoshie, 1973; Zöllner, Karnahl, & Stange, 1976). There is general agreement that stimulus repetition rates up to approximately 20/second have little effect on ABR, but above

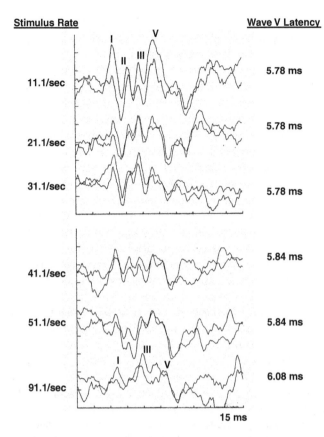

Stimulus Rate   **Wave V Latency**

11.1/sec   5.78 ms

21.1/sec   5.78 ms

31.1/sec   5.78 ms

41.1/sec   5.84 ms

51.1/sec   5.84 ms

91.1/sec   6.08 ms

15 ms

FIGURE 6.5. The effect of changes in stimulus rate on the ABR waveform (left portion) and on wave V latency (right portion).

this level, ABR latency generally increases and amplitude decreases as rate increases. These trends are illustrated in Figure 6.5.

Changes are not the same for each wave component. Wave V amplitude appears to show less decrement with increasing rate (from a relatively slow rate, such as 8 to 10/sec, to a rapid rate, such as 80 to 90/second) than earlier components and also than ABR wave VI. At the higher rate, then, amplitude for wave V has typically decreased about 10 to 30 percent relative to original amplitude, whereas wave I decreases to about 50 percent of its original amplitude. A clinical implication of these observations is that, for threshold estimation, higher stimulus rates permit collection of the largest quantity of data in the smallest amount of test time.

Latency prolongations with faster stimulus rates occur for all wave components, but they may be somewhat greater for later than for earlier waves. From about 20 to 80 clicks/second, for example, a wave V latency shift usually of 0.4 to 0.6 ms is expected (Gerling, 1989; Paludetti, Maurizi, & Ottaviani, 1983; van Olphen et al., 1979; Yagi & Hughes, 1975; Yagi & Kaga, 1979), although shifts in normal subjects of as little as 0.25 ms to over 1.0 ms have been reported (Don, Allen, & Starr, 1977; Gerling, 1989; Weber & Fujikawa, 1977). Because of this variability, a cutoff for the upper limit

of normal values of, for example, three standard deviations, may be a shift as large as 1 ms or more. The average amount of wave V latency shift with rate increases to 80/second is equivalent to the latency change observed when stimulus intensity is decreased by 15 to 25 dB (Don, Allen, & Starr, 1977; Weber & Fujikawa, 1977). In adults, rate-associated changes in wave V are independent of stimulus intensity. That is, latency shifts at increased rates are essentially constant for different intensity levels.

There is some evidence that, over this same range of rates, wave I latency shifts by 0.4 to 0.5 ms (Paludetti et al., 1983; Terkildsen et al., 1975; Zöllner et al., 1976), although others have reported no rate effect for wave I (Hyde et al., 1976; Jewett & Williston, 1971; Pratt & Sohmer, 1976; Thornton & Coleman, 1975; Yoshie, 1973). According to still other investigators (Buchwald & Huang, 1975; Eggermont & Odenthal, 1974b; Fowler & Noffsinger, 1983; Yagi & Kaga, 1979), the effect of rate increases from 5 signals/second to 90/second on wave I latency is about 0.23 ms. Difficulty identifying with confidence ABR wave I and precise determination of latency might have contributed to these discrepancies. Because both peripheral and central ABR components are similarly affected by rate, interwave latencies generally do not vary significantly as a function of rate.

Although ABR wave components I and V usually do not become indistinct with increased rate in normal subjects, waves II, III, and IV may become less identifiable or may even disappear at higher stimulus rates, such as 80 to 100 signals/second (Don, Allen, & Starr, 1977; Fowler & Noffsinger, 1983; Paludetti et al., 1983; van Olphen et al., 1979). Techniques that are useful for enhancing these components at slower rates, such as increasing the stimulus intensity level or using alternative electrode arrays, are of value also for higher rates. As discussed in Chapter 2, the latencies of ABR waves (after wave I) are a product of both axonal and synaptic transmission times. Of course, more synapses may be involved for each successive ABR wave (e.g., II, III, IV, and V). Therefore, increasing stimulus rate (especially to 100 stimuli/second and higher) will result in progressively longer latencies for the later ABR waves. Also, this anatomic mechanism for the influence of rate on ABR latency plays an important role in relatively greater effect of stimulus rate on the ABR of infants. That is, maturation of the ABR is a factor in the interaction between stimulus rate and ABR latency (e.g., Ponton, Moore, & Eggermont, 1996).

There are discrepant findings on the interactive effects of rate and advancing age in adults. Harkins (1981a) noted no difference in latency values at high stimulus rates for young (mean age 25 years) adults, but amplitude tended to be reduced in the elderly group. Response variability was comparable for both age groups. Weber and Fujikawa (1977), on the other hand, found that rate effects increased directly with advancing age. Finally, variations in adult ABRs, particularly the wave IV and V complex, can result from interactions among stimulus rate, intensity, and polarity (Gerling, 1989).

INFANTS AND YOUNG CHILDREN. | There is a direct relationship between maturity of the CNS and the effect of rate on ABR. Stimulus rate has a more pronounced influence on ABR latency for premature than term neonates, for younger children (under age 18 months) than older children, and for older children (up to age 13 years) than adults (Cox, 1985; Despland & Galambos, 1980; Fujikawa & Weber, 1977; Jiang, Brosi, & Wilkinson, 1998; Pratt, Ben-David, Peled, Podoshin, & Scharf, 1981; Schulman-Galambos & Galambos, 1975; Starr, Amlie, Martin, & Sanders, 1977; Stockard et al., 1979; Stockard, Stockard, & Coen, 1983). In these studies, changes in ABR latency as a function of signal rate is often expressed in units of 10 µsec per decade (of rate). Despland and Galambos (1980) stated that the slope of the latency-versus-rate function declined from about 270 µsec/decade of rate in the 30-week gestational age preterm infant to about 110 µsec/decade in the term infant. These slopes are both considerably steeper than the linear latency-versus-rate slope in adults (approximately 35 to 40 µsec/decade in rate). Lasky (1984) essentially confirmed this development-versus-rate pattern with data for subjects distributed equally among age groupings, as summarized in Table 6.1. The latency-versus-rate slopes are steeper for the 60 and 80 dB intensity levels than at 40 dB. The slope at 80 dB is generally about 130 µsec/decade for neonates versus 70 µsec/decade for adults. The much greater increase in ABR latency values, and diminished amplitude values, with increased stimulus rate for infants versus adults are reflected in progressively steeper slopes for the latency–rate functions, particularly for later ABR waves (Jiang, Brosi, & Wilkinson, 1998). Still, a reliable ABR can be recorded from term, and also preterm, neonates for stimulus rates up to the 455/sec rate and even the 909.1/sec rate used in the maximum length sequence (MLS) recording technique (e.g., Jiang, Brosi, & Wilkinson, 1998; Weber & Roush, 1993).

As a rule, the rate effect is greatest for wave V. This results in a combined effect of young age and rate on the wave I to V interval. Prolonged neural transmission in younger subjects, due to incomplete myelinization and reduced synaptic efficiency, is suggested as a general neurophysiologic basis for these age–rate–latency interactions (Hecox, 1975; Jiang, Brosi, & Wilkinson, 1998; Lasky, 1984; Pratt & Sohmer, 1976; Pratt et al., 1981). Slow rates may be necessary to obtain age-independent AERs. Lasky and Rupert (1982) found no ABR latency difference for 40-week term infants between signal rates of 3/second versus 10/second. Preliminary data for 32-week infants, however, suggested that wave V latencies were less for a 5/second than for a 10/second stimulus rate. As noted previously, stimulus rate in the adult can be increased to at least 20/second with no resulting effect on ABR latency or amplitude. These age–rate–ABR interactions, along with the possible influence of even more factors (e.g., stimulus intensity and polarity), must be considered both in developing a normative database, in establishing clinical ABR protocols, and in interpreting ABRs clinically.

RATE-RELATED ABR FINDINGS IN AUDITORY PATHOLOGY. | Some investigators have suggested increased stimulation rate as an effective technique for detecting subtle auditory neuropathology (Don et al., 1977; Stockard, Stockard, & Sharbrough, 1978), presumably because the nervous system is stressed beyond its functional capacity. Pratt et al. (1981) speculated that the sensitivity of high-rate ABRs to neuropathology was specific to white versus gray matter. In support of this contention, abnormal latency shifts or disappearance of later waves at very rapid stimulus rates have been reported in various types of peripheral and CNS pathology, including eighth-nerve tumors (Daly, Roeser, Aung, & Daly, 1977; Fowler & Noffsinger, 1983), epidermoid tumor of the fourth ventricle (Yagi & Kaga, 1979), head injury, hypoxia (Hecox, Cone, & Blaw, 1981), mixed CNS diseases (Fowler & Noffsinger, 1983; Pratt et al., 1981), and multiple sclerosis (MS) (Fowler & Noffsinger, 1983; Jacobson, Murray, & Deppe, 1987; Pratt et al., 1981; Robinson & Rudge, 1977). Other authors confirmed a relatively greater degree of abnormality for the faster stimulus rates in neuropathology. However, they generally found that abnormal ABRs also were recorded at the conventional rate (Elidan, Sohmer, Gafni, & Kahana, 1982).

Mechanisms for the excessive latency shifts with increased rate in auditory pathology, when they occur, are proposed but not yet confirmed. For example, Yagi and Kaga (1979) note that the abnormal rate-related latency changes may have an essentially different basis than normal latency shifts, citing data from experimental studies of induced axon demyelination or neuron synapse disorders (McDonald & Sears, 1970; Saha, Bhargava, Johnson, & McKean, 1978). Other authors, however, describe comparable degrees of latency shift at high stimulus levels for ABR waves in auditory pathologies, such as cochlear impairment of various etiologies (Fowler & Noffsinger, 1983) and different neuropathologies (Chiappa, Gladstone, & Young, 1979; Terkildsen et al., 1975).

TABLE 6.1. Summary of the Effect of Increases in the Rate of Click Stimuli on Latency of the Auditory Brainstem Response Wave V for Adults versus Infants

Data shown are the increase in ABR wave V latency for each increase of 10 stimuli per second, e.g., from 30/sec to 40/sec.

| GROUP | LATENCY CHANGE IN µSEC/DECADE | |
	Mean	Standard Deviation (SD)
Adults	71	20
Infants		
40 weeks	166	53
36 weeks	219	38
32 weeks	245	68

PHYSIOLOGIC BASES OF RATE EFFECTS. | Several investigators have speculated on possible neurophysiologic mechanisms underlying the divergent effect of increased rate on ABR latency versus amplitude. One physiologic explanation offered for the overall rate effect is a cumulative neural fatigue and adaptation, and incomplete recovery, involving hair cell–cochlear nerve junctions and also subsequent synaptic transmission. The effect of rate would, by this theory, be additive as the number of synapses increased (from wave I through wave V). Why then is amplitude less affected than latency? Pratt and Sohmer (1976), Terkildsen et al. (1975), and Suzuki, Kobayashi, and Takagi (1985) have attempted to reconcile this discrepancy, theorizing that adaptation may not be precisely uniform for all neurons. This would result in desynchronization of the response and prolonged latency. Temporal summation would remain adequate for amplitude preservation. The role of divergence and convergence of auditory neurons from lower to higher order auditory neurons has also been implicated (Pratt & Sohmer, 1976).

According to a number of investigators (Davis & Hirsh, 1976; Klein, 1983; Maurizi, Paludetti, Ottaviani, & Rosignoli, 1984; Suzuki, Hirai, & Horiuchi, 1977; Suzuki, Kobayashi, & Takagi, 1985), the ABR consists of two major spectral components—a slow component (energy at frequencies of 100 Hz and below) and a fast component (energy mostly at frequencies in the regions of 500 and 900 Hz). This dual nature of the ABR is easily appreciated by inspecting the typical ABR (recorded with wide filter settings). The ABR is a slow wave on which the fast components (waves I through VII) are superimposed. There is a physiologically based distinction in the effects of stimulus rate, intensity, and frequency on these fast-versus-slow ABR components. Suzuki, Kobayashi, and Takagi (1985) recorded ABRs for signal rates of 8/second up to 90.9/second, then performed power spectral analysis, and then digitally separated the ABR waveforms into a slow component (0 to 400 Hz) and fast component (400 to 1500 Hz). Slow-component amplitude was relatively constant across this range of stimulus rates, whereas amplitude of ABR waves I through V (the ABR fast component) decreased. Latency of each component increased with rate. Interestingly, slow component amplitude, which did decrease very slightly with increasing rate, paradoxically showed an amplitude increase at a rate of 40 Hz. These authors point out that the differential effect of rapid stimulus rate on ABR latency (an increase) versus amplitude (essentially no change) reported by others may be explained by this dual nature of the ABR. ABR amplitude is especially resistant to rate effects when stimulus intensity is maintained below about 50 dB.

Polarity

NORMAL EARS. | For the first decade of ABR clinical research and application, considerable attention was given to other stimulus characteristics, and polarity was rarely specified in publications. Some investigators, however, reported significantly shorter ABR wave V latency values for rarefaction than for condensation unfiltered clicks in most normal hearers for some wave components (Emerson, Brooks, Parker, & Chiappa, 1982; Kevanishvili & Aphonchenko, 1981; Maurer, Schafer, & Leitner, 1980; Ornitz & Walter, 1975; Stockard et al., 1979), although the magnitude of the difference is small (average of about 0.2 ms). Other investigators, however, noted that 15 to 30 percent of normal subjects may show the opposite polarity pattern—that is, shorter latency values for condensation than for rarefaction clicks (Borg & Löfqvist, 1982; Coats & Martin, 1977; Hughes, Fino, & Gagnon, 1981; Pijl, 1987; Stockard et al., 1979). The results of other studies failed to demonstrate a clear and consistent polarity effect on ABR latency (Beattie, 1988; Don, Vermiglio, Ponton, & Eggermont, 1996; Fowler, 1992; Terkildsen, Osterhammel, & Huis in't Veld, 1974), a finding explained by the dominance in generation of the ABR by high-frequency cochlear activity and neural responses (Don & Eggermont, 1978; Fowler, 1992). There is no consensus on which of the ABR wave components are most affected or most consistently affected. That is, selected waves, such as waves I and V, may have shorter latencies for rarefaction clicks, whereas another wave, such as wave III, may have shorter latency for condensation clicks.

Perhaps the most consistent polarity-related ABR finding is shorter latency for wave I (on the average about 0.07 ms) for rarefaction clicks, but a condensation click advantage still occurs in some subjects. Relatively shorter latency for click stimuli of rarefaction polarity is consistent with mechanical effects of polarity on cochlear physiology. Recall from the review of basic principles of stimulus polarity, in Chapter 4, that activation of auditory (eighth cranial nerve) fibers is mostly caused by upward movement of the basilar membrane secondary to rarefaction polarity stimulation (e.g., Brugge et al., 1969), and not for stimuli during the condensation polarity phase (producing downward movement of the basilar movement). The same trend with polarity is seen for amplitude of ABR wave I, but it is more variable. Subject age and signal rate also may influence these wave I polarity effects. A greater wave I latency difference for rarefaction versus condensation clicks was reported for neonates (0.13 ms) than the value just noted for adults (Stockard et al., 1979). With rapid click rates (e.g., 80/second), an even longer latency for wave I (on the order of 0.35 ms) is recorded for condensation versus rarefaction signal polarity. Stockard and Stockard (1983) provided an example of marked wave I differences for condensation versus rarefaction click stimuli in a 9-month-old. Because wave I was 180 degrees out of phase between the two stimulus polarities, adding the waveforms for the alternating polarities abolished the wave I response. Of course, the presence of a wave I component versus cochlear microphonic (CM) activity must always be confirmed when polarity of ABR components are entirely out of phase for rarefaction and condensation click signals.

There is evidence from some early studies that the largest polarity-related latency differences are found for waves IV and VI. These later ABR waves may receive greater low-frequency contribution than others, at least wave I and wave III (Burkard & Voigt, 1989). Again, phase effects are greatest for lower frequencies. An even greater rarefaction-versus-condensation latency advantage was found for click stimuli with more low-frequency energy (Coats et al., 1979; Salt & Thornton, 1984a; Scherg & Speulda, 1982) and for rarefaction-versus-condensation unfiltered single-slope clicks, with a steep onset but a very slow offset portion (Gerull et al., 1985). With the single-slope click, amplitude was twice as large for the rarefaction than for the condensation polarity. Other investigators, in contrast, found no consistent latency difference for responses to the two polarities in normal hearers (Kevanishvili & Aphonchenko, 1981; Rosenhamer, Lindstrom, & Lundborg, 1978; Ruth, Hildebrand, & Cantrell, 1982; Terkildsen, Osterhammel, & Huis in't Veld, 1975).

In contrast, Hughes, Fino, and Gagnon (1981) reported longer latencies for rarefaction than for condensation clicks, as traditionally defined. Upon close inspection of the entire acoustic waveform for the stimuli presented with piezo-electric earphones, however, these investigators noted that a higher amplitude component of the opposite polarity followed the initial component with which the stimulus polarity was labeled (e.g., condensation or rarefaction). Data from this study also provided more evidence of inconsistencies inherent in polarity effects on different wave components. Hughes et al. (1981) reported that the range of latency change with polarity inversion was many times larger for wave III (0.82 ms) than for wave I (0.16 ms) or wave V (0.32 ms).

Other investigators also have found waves I through V variably influenced, in both the latency and amplitude parameters, for rarefaction versus condensation clicks (Kevanishvili & Aphonchenko, 1981). Waveform analysis may be confounded considerably by polarity. Studies showing decreased latency for wave I (but not wave V) with rarefaction versus condensation clicks confirm that the wave I to wave V interwave latency value may vary with polarity (Maurer, Schafer, & Leitner, 1980). That is, interwave latencies tend to be shorter for condensation clicks. As an aside, this is further evidence that the wave I to V latency interval is not a pure measure of "brainstem transmission time." Amplitude of wave I can be larger for rarefaction clicks than for condensation clicks. Without a similar enhancement for wave V, the wave V-to-I amplitude ratio is reduced.

Emerson, Brooks, Parker, and Chiappa (1982) summarized stimulus polarity ABR data for a relatively sizable series of subjects. There were 45 subjects who had normal hearing and CNS status and 600 patients with various pathologies. The distribution of pathologies was not indicated, although MS was prominent. For the normal group, wave I had significantly shorter mean latency (0.05 ms) for rarefaction clicks, while the mean polarity difference for waves III and V (0.02 ms for each) was not significant. As a result

of this differential polarity effect for wave I versus wave V latency, I-to-V latency intervals were slightly (and again significantly) greater for rarefaction stimuli. Rarefaction stimuli contributed to a clearer separation of the wave IV versus wave V components. The polarity difference was slightly larger for female than for male subjects. In no normal subject did wave V disappear on the basis of a polarity inversion. In normal hearers, click polarity does not appear to influence ABR detection level (Sininger & Masuda, 1990).

In addition to the foregoing investigations of click polarity and the ABR, polarity effects have been studied for frequency-specific stimuli, including tone bursts and frequency bands derived with ipsilateral masking techniques (e.g., Don et al., 1996; Fowler, 1992; Gorga, Kaminski, & Beauchaine, 1991; Schoonhoven, 1992). Findings suggested an apparent influence of polarity that was indirectly related to stimulus frequency—that is, smaller polarity effects for higher frequency stimuli and larger effects for lower frequency stimuli.

AUDITORY SYSTEM PATHOLOGY. | Borg and Löfqvist (1982) conducted a comprehensive study of stimulus polarity. The stimulus in this study was a 2000 Hz haversine pulse presented at an intensity level of either 75 or 35 dB nHL and at a rate of 20/sec. Data were collected for sixty-five normal ears, twenty ears with conductive hearing impairment, twenty-nine with steep-sloping high-frequency loss, and 17 with retrocochlear auditory dysfunction. For normal ears, latency of wave V was on the average 0.1 ms shorter for rarefaction versus condensation clicks, but 30 percent of the ears showed the opposite effect. Recall that, with the ½-wavelength rule, a 0.25 ms difference would be expected for a 2000 Hz stimulus. Comparable polarity differences for wave V latency were found in the ears with conductive hearing impairment. Rarefaction clicks produced progressively shorter latencies as wave V latency increased and also as the frequency decreased, beginning at the frequency at which the hearing loss began. These findings for ears with high-frequency (presumably cochlear) impairment were not observed with stimulation of ears with retrocochlear pathology.

In the series of 600 patients with largely undescribed pathology studied by Emerson et al. (1982), there were twenty patients for whom detection of wave V was dependent on click polarity. Pathology among these twenty patients included MS, brainstem tumor, head injury, and primary lateral sclerosis. No wave V was recorded for seventeen of the twenty patients with rarefaction clicks and for three of the twenty with condensation clicks. Curiously, seven patients were retested at lower intensity levels and then showed a reliable wave V component. Only five of the twenty patients were assessed by audiometry. Two apparently had normal hearing and three showed abnormal audiometric findings. These waveforms were recorded from a normal-hearing adult undergoing routine clinical ABR assessment. Neither single polarity (condensation or rarefaction) produced a clear and reliable ABR for both ears. The relation of polarity effects to stimulus frequency is probably the best explanation for the pronounced influence of click stimulus polarity on ABRs recorded from persons with high frequency sensory hearing loss is probably explained best by. As stated by Fowler (1992) "The normal high-frequency neural dominance that obscures phase-dependent low-frequency effects is removed by the hearing loss, and the lower-frequency phase-dependent responses are uncovered" (pp. 172, 173).

SUMMARY. | Clearly, as revealed by the foregoing discussion and other published reviews (Don et al., 1996; Fowler, 1992; Gorga et al., 1991; Schoonhoven, 1992), the literature on stimulus polarity and the ABR is characterized by inconsistencies and, to some extent, conflicting findings. Findings are at variance in part because of differences in experimental methodology, such as subject selection criteria and test protocols ad (including potential interactions of polarity with other factors, such as stimulus intensity and rate). Age is also a factor influencing the effect of polarity on ABR latency and amplitude, as noted in the discussion of nonpathologic factors on ABR (Chapter 7). The lack of a clear polarity effect for ABR wave V, generated well beyond the afferent fibers in the auditory nerve, is explained by other intervening variables that influence its latency. As noted by Don et al. (1996), "The underlying variability that affects peak latency of wave V compromises any polarity effect even when using absolute measures" (p. 465). Furthermore, even polarity-related latency differences for ABR wave I are not consistently documented. One explanation offered for the inconsistent effect of click polarity on ABR wave I is the major contribution of high- versus low-frequency regions of the cochlea to the response and the difficulty of detecting small phase shifts occurring in specific frequency regions. However, consistent polarity effects are not even demonstrable for ABR wave I when frequency-specific recordings are made with tone burst stimuli or with the derived band technique (e.g., Don et al., 1996; Fowler, 1992; Gorga et al., 1991; Schoonhoven, 1992). Variability—neural variability (e.g., "relative heights and domination of peaks in the in post stimulus time histograms," Don et al., 1996, p. 465) and individual subject response variability—appears to be the prominent factor contributing to the confusing literature on polarity and the ABR. Recommendations for clinical selection of stimulus polarity are, likewise, divergent. Some authors have advocated alternating polarity because the stimulus-related electromagnetic artifact and the CM artifact associated with each polarity (and thus also alternating in polarity) is effectively canceled out during averaging (Davis, 1976a; Terkildsen et al., 1975). The signal-to-noise ratio (SNR) is thus improved, and wave I is more easily and confidently identified, especially at high stimulus intensity levels.

However, without documentation of stimulus polarity calibration for AER instrumentation, there is no assurance that a specific-polarity electrical signal (selected by the appropriate knob or keyboard command) will be delivered to the patient with the same polarity. Simply alternating the terminals (or cables) on a earphone (supra-aural or insert) will reverse polarity of the acoustic waveform—that is, diaphragm movement will be in the opposite (and unintended) direction. Also, there still remains a possibility of physiology-based polarity reversal from the diaphragm to the inner ear. Any single flaw in this sequence may produce an effective stimulus polarity that is opposite to the desired polarity. The use of alternating polarity stimuli in AER measurement would appear to offer a simple solution because it makes no difference which polarity is first and which is second, and there would at the least be no doubt as to the stimulus polarity conditions. For earlier latency AERS, however, alternating polarity stimulation presents some serious clinical disadvantages. As noted in Chapter 4, manipulation of stimulus polarity is an important measurement strategy for detection of the SP component (with alternating polarity) versus the CM component (with separate polarities). The impact of stimulus polarity of ABR was discussed earlier in this section.

Others recommend reliance on rarefaction polarity stimuli in routine clinical applications (Chiappa et al., 1979; Kevanishvili & Aphonchenko, 1981; Rosenhamer et al., 1978; Schwartz & Berry, 1985; Schwartz, Morris, Spydell, Brink, Grim, & Schwartz, 1990; Stockard et al., 1978, 1979; Stockard & Stockard, 1983). One overall reason is evident from the previous discussion. Namely, rarefaction polarity actually activates, or depolarizes, hair cells within the cochlea and produces responses of shorter latency and greater amplitude, whereas condensation polarity stimuli may produce hyperpolarization of cochlear hair cells or may produce the opposite cochlear effect (Peake & Kiang, 1962). Increased diagnostic sensitivity of rarefaction clicks is inferred from the higher proportion of abnormal findings with this polarity than with condensation. Another reason in support of single rarefaction polarity stimuli is that the latency differences between responses to each polarity, when combined into a response for alternating stimulus polarity, increase variability or "jitter" of the response. Conceivably, with alternating polarity stimuli, out-of-phase responses could be added together to produce responses with reduced amplitude or even an artificially abnormal or absent response in a normal subject (Maurer et al., 1980).

Variations on this recommendation include the use of rarefaction as the polarity of choice, with alternating polarity as an option, as needed for clarification of waveform morphology (Stockard & Stockard, 1983), or the routine use of both rarefaction and condensation (separate waveforms for each) whenever time permits (Emerson et al., 1982). The separate use of rarefaction and condensation appears to be supported by those investigators who have reported a substantial minority of patients yielding a clearer response for condensation versus rarefaction clicks. The experiences of Hoult (1985), based on ABR clinical data obtained from 703 ears with each polarity are instructive in this regard. There were no age or gender interactions with polarity. Rarefaction clicks generated a clear response significantly more often than condensation clicks. However, of the total group, 39 subjects showed a clearer response with one polarity on one ear and the other polarity on the other ear. An additional 18 ears yielded a response classified as abnormal for one polarity and yet normal for the other polarity.

The optimal clinical test protocol is probably stimulation with each polarity separately. This might involve measurement of AERs first for rarefaction polarity stimuli and then for condensation polarity stimuli. With current evoked response systems it is often possible to present stimuli with alternating polarity and then to analyze separately the waveforms for each of the polarities. In this way, test conditions (subject state, number of stimulus repetitions, measurement artifact) are apt to be equivalent for each stimulus polarity. Again, waveforms for the two single polarities can later be added if an alternating polarity mode is desired. Anticipating the recommendations for stimulus polarity in ABR measurement summarized at the end of this chapter, the selection of rarefaction polarity is a good starting point in ABR measurement with air-conduction stimuli. However, the experienced clinician will promptly manipulate polarity if the initial choice does not produce an optimal, or expected, ABR waveform.

Bone-Conduction Stimulation in ABR Measurement

Stimulation of the ABR with bone conduction is not only feasible. Bone-conduction ABR measurement is an essential component of the test battery for auditory assessment of infants and young children. Comparison of threshold estimations based air- versus bone-conduction stimulation permits objective documentation of the degree of air-bone gap, and differentiation among conductive, sensorineural, and mixed hearing losses, even in patients who cannot be properly evaluated with behavioral audiologic techniques (e.g., Campbell, Harris, Hendricks, & Sirimanna, 2004; Gorga, Kaminski, Beauchaine, & Bergman, 1993; Hall, 1992; Muchnik, Neeman, & Hildesheimer, 1995; Stuart & Yang, 1994; Stuart, Yang, Stenstrom, & Reindorp, 1993; Yang & Stuart, 2000; Yang, Stuart, Mencher, Mencher, & Vincer, 1993; Yang, Stuart, Stenstrom, & Green, 1993). Evidence in support of bone conduction ABR as a clinically viable technique in infants dates back to the 1980s (Hooks & Weber, 1984; Stapells & Ruben, 1989; Stuart, Yang, & Stenstrom, 1990; Yang, Rupert, & Moushegian, 1987). Hooks and Weber (1984) assessed forty premature infants with both air- (TDH-49 earphone) and bone-conduction (Radioear B-70A vibrator) click stimuli. In thirty-six out of forty infants, a mastoid bone-vibrator placement was used, and forehead placement was used in the remainder. A significantly larger proportion of infants showed an ABR for a stimulus-intensity level of 30 dB nHL for bone conduction (93%) than for air conduction (73%).

Similar bone- versus air-conduction statistics were found at a 45 dB intensity level. Because of technical problems (mostly excessive stimulus artifact), two subjects had an interpretable ABR for air but not for bone conduction. Contrary to expectations for adult subjects, latencies for ABR wave I, wave III, and wave V were shorter (by about 0.30 to 0.45 ms) for bone-conduction stimuli than for air-conduction stimuli. These authors (and later Yang et al., 1987) speculate that the earlier bone-conduction latencies are due to the pattern of cochlear development in the newborn. In the immature cochlea, responsiveness to low-frequency stimuli develops initially in the basal regions, which are the place for high-frequency responsiveness in the adult cochlea (Rubel & Ryals, 1983).

In the study by Yang et al. (1987), ABRs with bone conduction signals were recorded from three sets of patients: adults, 1-year-old children, and healthy neonates tested between 24 and 72 hours after birth. Stimuli (0.1 ms rarefaction clicks at 30/second) were delivered with a Radioear B-70A bone vibrator at intensity levels of 15, 25, and 35 dB nHL. ABR results for three vibrator surface placements were analyzed: (1) on the frontal bone (midline forehead), (2) on the occipital bone (1 cm lateral the ipsilateral occipital protuberance), and (3) on the temporal bone (superior postauricular area). Spectra for the bone vibrator versus the TDH-39 earphone were described, and other pertinent measurement data (e.g., head coupling pressure for the vibrator, acquisition parameters) were provided. The data reported by Yang et al. (1987) clearly emphasize the importance of bone oscillator placement on effective intensity level, on ABR latency, and, indeed, for successful measurement of bone conduction ABRs. In a follow-up study of the variability of the ABR for bone conduction stimulation in newborn infants, Yang et al. (1993) found no significant difference in the test–retest variability between air- and bone-conduction click stimuli. For clinical ABR measurement in infants, Stuart, Yang, and Stenstrom (1990) recommend placement of the bone vibrator in a superior and posterior region of the temporal bone. The same authors in other papers (Stuart & Yang, 1994; Yang, Stuart, Stenstrom, & Hollett, 1991) also emphasize, based on data collected from neonates, the importance of the pressure with which the bone vibrator is coupled to the skull, and of an appropriately low cutoff for the high-pass filter (30 Hz) for successful bone-conduction ABR measurement. ABR wave V amplitude is markedly diminished (by up to 50%) even with a modest reduction in low frequency energy produced by a high-pass filter setting of 100 or 150 Hz. The evidence on specific techniques generated by these investigations, and others, is incorporated into the test protocol for bone conduction recommended toward the end of this chapter.

Some of the important findings of the Yang et al. (1987) study were as follows. Latencies varied as a function of (1) air- versus bone-conduction stimulation, (2) vibrator placements for bone conduction, and, as expected, (3) age. In adults, wave V latency was shortest for air-conduction stimulation. The temporal-bone placement yielded the next shortest latency values, while frontal and occipital bone placement latency values were longer and comparable. As noted, effective stimulus intensity for a brief duration stimulus is decreased by about 7 dB (Boezeman et al., 1983) when the vibrator is moved from the mastoid to the frontal bone. The latency pattern in the Yang et al. (1987) study varied somewhat for 1-year-old infants, in that frontal versus occipital bone placements were associated with different latencies. A remarkable finding of this study was the very unique latency versus placement pattern observed for the neonates. For temporal bone placement, wave V latency was markedly shorter than for the other two bone-vibrator locations and was slightly shorter than even the air-conduction latency values. Even the specific site of bone vibrator placement on the temporal bone is an important factor (Stuart, Yang, & Stenstrom, 1990). The relation of bone- versus air-conduction latency in neonates confirms the observations of Hooks and Weber (1984). A substudy of masking and the bone-conduction ABR by these investigators showed that it is wise to presume an interaural attenuation value of 0 dB in adults, 15 to 25 dB in 1-year-old children, and as much as 25 to 35 dB in neonates. Interaural attenuation is highest in neonates because the temporal bone has not yet become fully fused with other regions of the cranium, and, therefore, there is no direct route for transmission of the energy from the stimulus from the temporal bone where the bone-conduction oscillator is placed to the cochlea on the side contralateral to the stimulus.

The wave V latency difference between air- versus bone-conduction stimulation reported by Yang et al. (1987) in their adult subjects was on the order of 0.5 ms. Mauldin and Jerger (1979) studied bone- versus air-conduction ABRs in four normal-hearing adults and eleven patients with conductive hearing impairment. Notably, air-conduction stimuli were presented binaurally with TDH-39 earphones, and forehead placement was used for bone-conduction stimulation (with a B-70A vibrator and no masking). On the average, bone-conduction wave V latency was 0.46 ms greater than wave V for air conduction for intensity at equal sensation levels; therefore, the authors recommended correcting bone-conduction wave V latency values clinically (subtracting 0.50 ms) before comparing these findings to air-conduction latencies. Both air- and bone-conduction ABR thresholds and estimations of the air-bone gap were highly correlated with respective behavioral hearing thresholds and air-bone gap values in the high-frequency region. The closest association between ABR versus behavioral threshold was for a high-frequency pure-tone average, the PTA2 (1000 + 2000 + 4000 Hz / 3). The PTA1 is the traditional three-frequency pure-tone average (500, 1000, and 2000 Hz). Analysis of the spectrum of the bone vibrator in this study showed energy mostly below 2500 Hz. Early investigators of bone conduction ABR (e.g., Don & Eggermont, 1978; Mauldin & Jerger, 1979; Suzuki et al., 1977) found that an air-conduction stimulus with energy primarily in this frequency region (2500 Hz) pro-

duces an ABR wave V latency that was also approximately 0.50 ms greater than for a wide-spectrum click. The air- versus bone-conduction latency difference, they conclude, is a product of the spectral difference in stimuli. However, this may not be a sufficient explanation and later findings argued against a latency difference for ABRs evoked by air- versus bone-conduction stimulation, presuming equivalent intensity levels for each mode of stimulation (Hall, 1992; Stuart, Yang, & Green, 1994; Stuart et al., 1990; Yang et al., 1987; 1991).

Using a 2000 Hz tone pip presented via a B-71 bone vibrator and a TDH-39 earphone to 22 adult subjects, Boezeman et al. (1983) found a somewhat greater average air- versus bone-conduction discrepancy (0.88 ms), but variability was substantial (standard deviation of 0.43 ms). These authors also attempted to replicate stimulus conditions used by Mauldin and Jerger (1979) and confirmed the contribution of the more limited spectrum for bone- versus air-conduction stimuli to the latency shift. For example, shifting the filter cutoff from 20,000 to 2000 Hz (i.e., simulating the limited frequency response of the bone vibrator) produced a latency increase of 0.325 ms. Still, the finding of a bone- versus air-conduction difference at 2000 Hz argues against the dominance of a transducer effect, because frequency responses are not substantially divergent at this frequency. Stuart, Yang, and Green (1994) described a clear difference in ABR thresholds for air versus bone conduction in newborn infants as a function of test time after birth. The authors compared air- and bone-conduction ABR thresholds recorded from twenty term infants within 48 hours after birth with the same ABR measures recorded between 49 and 96 hours after birth. In the "younger" group of infants, air-conduction ABR thresholds were, on the average, 14.5 dB nHL, whereas the average bone-conduction ABR threshold was 1.8 dB nHL. In comparison, in the older postpartum group the average air-conduction threshold was 3.8 dB HL and the average bone-conduction threshold was 1.5 dB nHL. The age-related difference in air-conduction thresholds was highly significant, but there was no difference in the bone-conduction thresholds for the two groups. Stuart, Yang, and Green (1994) speculate that the elevated air-conduction thresholds soon after birth are secondary to residual birth fluid in the middle ear space that resolves over the next few days.

These same authors also compared a psychophysical cancellation procedure with ABR measurement in order to determine the accuracy of air-bone gap estimation with ABR (Boezeman, Kapteyn, Feenstra, & Snel, 1985). With the cancellation procedure, a subject adjusts the level and phase of an air-conduction pure-tone signal until it cancels the perception of a bone-conduction pure tone. Boezeman et al. (1985) analyzed data for twenty-four patients with primarily conductive hearing impairments, although some had sensorineural components to the loss ("mixed hearing impairment"). Transducers were a TDH-39 earphone and a Radioear B-71 bone vibrator. In comparison to the cancellation technique data, ABR underestimated air-bone gap. The stated reason was the effect of recruitment on the ABR (by a sensorineural component of the hearing impairment) but not on the cancellation method, which only estimates magnitude of air-bone gap.

Cornacchia, Martini, and Morra (1983) conducted a study of ABR for bone-conduction signals in infants and young adults. The age of the infants was reported as 16 to 20 months. Alternating clicks were presented to the forehead via bone conduction with a Radioear B-70A vibrator. Acoustic output of the click produced by the bone vibrator showed an energy peak in the range of 1000 to 2000 Hz, whereas the spectrum of the other transducer used (a TDH-39 earphone) was flat up to 6000 Hz. As expected, ABR latencies in general were greater for adults than for infants. Bone-conduction wave V latency values (at 60 dB nHL) were an average of 0.59 ms greater than air-conduction values for adults and 0.67 ms greater for infants. Another interesting finding was the convergence of wave V latency values for adults versus children with decreasing intensity of the air-conduction but not the bone-conduction stimuli. That is, bone-conduction latency–intensity functions were parallel for adults and infants. For air-conduction stimuli, however, there was an adult-versus-infant wave V latency difference of 0.58 ms at high intensity levels, but a difference between adults versus infants of only 0.08 ms at 20 dB nHL. These authors also comment on the importance of skull impedance differences between adults and infants as a factor in bone conduction ABR measurement. In contrast, however, Gorga et al. (1993) found parallel wave V latency–intensity functions for adults (n = 20) versus infants (n = 1120) over the range from 20 to 80 dB HL, and offered compelling evidence that these two stimulation modes can be compared clinically with confidence.

There is clinical evidence that bone-conduction ABR assessment can be useful in circumventing the masking dilemma associated with behavioral pure-tone hearing assessment, even in patients with maximum conductive hearing loss due to aural atresia (Hall, Gray, Brown, & Tompkins, 1986; Jahrsdoerfer & Hall, 1986; Jahrsdoerfer, Yeakley, Hall, Robbins, & Gray, 1985). The main premise underlying this clinical application is that a wave I component observed from an electrode located on or near the ear ipsilateral to the stimulus confirms contribution of the stimulated ear to the response, regardless of whether masking is presented to the nontest ear. Analysis of the waveform simultaneously recorded with an electrode on the ear contralateral to the stimulus is also helpful. If, in the contralateral waveform, there is no peak corresponding to the ipsilateral wave I (in the same latency region), one has further assurance that the presumed ipsilateral component is indeed ABR wave I. The characteristic patterns of ABR waveforms associated with these two electrode arrays for bone-conduction stimulation are illustrated in Figure 6.6.

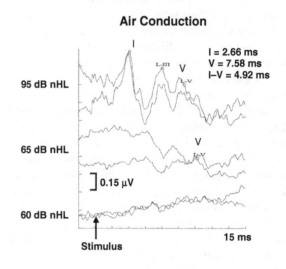

Air Conduction

95 dB nHL

I = 2.66 ms
V = 7.58 ms
I–V = 4.92 ms

65 dB nHL

0.15 μV

60 dB nHL

Stimulus

15 ms

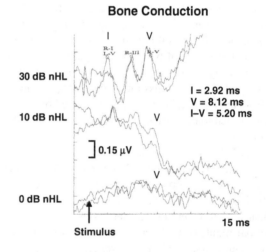

Bone Conduction

30 dB nHL

10 dB nHL

I = 2.92 ms
V = 8.12 ms
I–V = 5.20 ms

0.15 μV

0 dB nHL

Stimulus

15 ms

FIGURE 6.6. ABR waveforms for air- versus bone-conduction stimulation in a child with conductive hearing loss. The presence of a reliable wave I in the ipsilateral recording array confirms ear-specific bone-conduction stimulation.

Tone-burst stimuli presented by bone conduction can certainly be used for frequency-specific estimation of sensory hearing status. Stapells and colleagues, and others, have clearly demonstrated the accuracy of frequency-specific estimation of cochlear status with bone-conductive tone-burst stimuli (Foxe & Stapells, 1993; Nousak & Stapells, 1992; Stapells & Oates, 1997; Yang & Stuart, 2000). In addition, Hofmann and Flach (1981) demonstrated clinical differentiation of type of hearing loss with ABRs evoked by air- versus bone-conduction stimulation with tone-burst stimuli of 1000, 2000, 4000, and 8000 Hz. The authors confirmed that ABR with frequency-specific bone-conduction stimuli was clinically useful in assessing inner-ear status in infancy, and in older children, results were comparable for behavioral-versus-ABR bone-conduction thresholds. Nonetheless, in clinical practice bone-conduction ABR measurement is often conducted exclusively for click stimuli, rather than frequency-specific stimuli (i.e., tone bursts). The common clinical reliance on only click stimuli is, in some cases, due to test time constraints imposed by the pressing need for other audiologic information, such as ear- and frequency-specific thresholds for air-conduction stimuli. Decisions regarding management, including amplification, may be more dependent on the degree and configuration of air-conduction hearing loss than on frequency-specific estimations of air-bone gap. The tendency for limiting bone-conduction stimulation to clicks is also a reflection of the clinical necessity of generally differentiating conductive versus sensory hearing loss, rather than documenting the specific degree of conductive hearing loss component across the audiometric frequency region. In other words, in the audiologic assessment of an infant, objective and unequivocal documentation that the hearing loss is conductive will prompt referral for medical consultation and possible management, regardless of the extent of the conductive hearing loss at individual frequencies.

In summary, bone-conduction stimulation in clinical ABR measurement is underutilized (Campbell et al., 2004; Hall, 1992; Hall, 2004). The apparent reluctance of clinicians to adapt this approach to auditory assessment with ABR probably developed for at least four practical reasons (Campbell et al., 2004; Hall, 1994). First, the maximum effective intensity level of about 55 dB nHL for bone-conduction stimulation, which typifies clinical bone vibrators, is a limiting factor. For ABR recording with air-conducted stimuli at intensity levels below 40 to 45 dB nHL, a normal-hearing adult typically has a distinct wave V component, but not waves I and III. With bone-conduction stimulation in normal-hearing adults, waves I and II are recorded only at the upper limits for stimulus intensity level. Furthermore, because the minimal intensity level required to produce an air-conduction ABR, even the relatively large wave V, is around 15 to 20 dB greater than hearing threshold level (in the 1000 to 4000 Hz region), the effective range of intensity for the bone-conduction ABR is on the order of 30 to 40 dB (55 dB maximum minus the 20 dB ABR threshold) and, therefore, rather small. A greater maximum intensity level is possible with special vibrators, such as the Bruel & Kjaer Mini Shaker type 4810, but its size and the necessity of being hand-held preclude its routine clinical use.

Understandably, difficulty generating a clear ABR waveform with normal adult subjects may have led some clinicians to assume that bone-conduction ABRs would not be clinically feasible or useful for assessing sensorineural hearing sensitivity in infants and young children (Kavanaugh & Beardsley, 1979). In fact, in normal-hearing infants and young children, who tend to have better than average sensorineural hearing sensitivity in the frequency range of 1000 to 4000 Hz, in comparison to adult standards, the dy-

namic intensity range for bone-conduction ABR stimuli may be substantially larger (Hall, 1992). In addition, a distinct wave I component can often be consistently recorded with a bone-conducted stimulus in these younger subjects.

A second practical reason for reluctance to use a bone-conduction method with ABR assessment is that electromagnetic energy radiating from the bone vibrator can cause serious stimulus artifact in ABR recordings. This is intensified when the mastoid is used for both bone-vibrator placement and as a site for the inverting electrode and when the stimulus is a single-polarity click (rarefaction or condensation). Two simple modifications in the protocol for bone-conduction ABR measurement can minimize these problems. Use of an earlobe or ear-canal location for the inverting electrode, versus a mastoid location, reduces stimulus artifact associated with mastoid placement of the bone vibrator. Stimulus artifact is further reduced when the ABR is evoked with bone-conduction clicks with alternating polarity, rather than a single polarity (rarefaction or condensation).

A third possible reason for clinicians' reluctance to regularly record bone-conduction ABR is their appreciation that conductive hearing impairment is usually greatest for audiometric frequencies in the region of 1000 Hz and below, whereas the click-evoked ABR is dependent on stimulus energy mostly in the 1000 to 4000 Hz region (noted previously in the section on frequency in this chapter). This discrepancy suggests that the analysis of air- versus bone-conduction ABR will underestimate the predominantly lower frequency deficit produced by some middle-ear pathologies, such as otitis media or otosclerosis (Campbell et al., 2004; Stapells, 1989; Stapells & Ruben, 1989). In clinical practice, the main diagnostic value of bone-conduction ABR is not precise and frequency-specific estimation and comparison of the audiometric thresholds for air- and bone-conduction signals are not used. Rather, the goal is to verify with an electrophysiologic measure that the hearing loss is either conductive (normal bone-conduction thresholds) or mixed (bone-conduction hearing loss and even greater air-conduction hearing loss), and not a sensory hearing loss. A secondary goal is to provide a general estimation of the degree of conductive component contributing to the hearing loss. There is considerably less error in threshold estimation with middle-ear pathologies, such as congenital aural atresia, that typically produce a flat configuration hearing impairment throughout the audiometric frequency region, i.e., relatively similar hearing thresholds at different audiometric frequencies. This later category of middle-ear pathologies poses a more serious communicative handicap because hearing loss can be moderate to severe (40 to over 60 dB HL) throughout the speech frequency region of 500 to 4000 Hz.

Finally, the masking dilemma and the need for contralateral masking is cited in discussions of problems associated with bone-conduction ABR measurement (Weber, 1983b). This concern applies as well to behavioral audiometry. In serious bilateral conductive hearing impairment, the intensity level of an air-conducted stimulus must sometimes be increased well above the interaural attenuation level of the adult skull, leading to potential crossover of the acoustic energy to the nontest ear. The likelihood that the acoustic signal will cross over from the test ear to the nontest ear is considerably higher for supra-aural earphones than it is with insert earphones. As noted in the discussion about transducers, earlier in this chapter, with conventional supra-aural earphones interaural attenuation can be as slow as 40 to 50 dB, whereas interaural attenuation is usually over 60 dB with insert earphones. With bilateral conductive hearing loss, the intensity level of noise necessary to adequately mask the nontest ear may also exceed the interaural attenuation of the head, and it can cross back over (via bone conduction) to mask the test ear. In adult patients, the head offers little (10 dB or less) or no interaural attenuation for bone-conduction stimulation with commercially available vibrators placed against the skin (Harder, Arlinger, & Kylen, 1983). Therefore, a stimulus presented via bone conduction to one mastoid may equally activate each cochlea.

Since the early years of ABR application in clinical populations, clinicians assumed without question that the nontest ear must be routinely masked when the ABR was evoked by either air conduction or bone conduction (e.g., Weber, 1983b). As in pure-tone audiometry, masking was applied to rule out a contribution to the response from unintended stimulation of the better-hearing nontest ear. Consensus was lacking, however, about the intensity level at which an air-conduction click stimulus will cross over to the nontest ear and evoke an ABR (Finitzo-Hieber, Hecox, & Cone, 1979). The demand for masking in ABR measurement is not equivalent to behavioral audiometry. That is, the presence of a clear wave I component within the normal latency region from the electrode array ipsilateral to the stimulus, or a wave V of normal latency, is strong evidence that the ABR is not due to stimulation of the nontest ear. Masking is not necessary to verify that activation of the test ear is producing the response. As indicated previously, the likelihood of obtaining ear-specific bone-conduction ABR data is enhanced in infants due to incomplete fusion of the temporal bone with portions of the skull.

Thus, although each of the foregoing arguments has some validity, bone conduction ABR recording is clinically feasible and often extremely valuable in electrophysiologic auditory assessment. Furthermore, modifications of test protocol can minimize some of these technical limitations. Fortuitously, bone-conduction ABR measurement is successful most often with newborns and very young children, as opposed to adolescent and adult patients (Campbell et al., 2004; Hall, 1992; Hall, Gray, Brown, & Tompkins, 1986; Stapells & Ruben, 1989; Yang, Rupert, & Moushegian, 1987). A practical protocol for successful measurement of bone conduction ABR is presented toward the end of this chapter.

SENSORINEURAL ACUITY LEVEL (SAL) WITH ABR. | The SAL test was developed to circumvent some of the technical limitations of conventional bone-conduction audiometry (Jerger & Tillman, 1960). Briefly, in the SAL test, bone-conducted noise is presented to the forehead, and the patient's hearing threshold levels are assessed by air conduction. Air-conduction threshold levels in the presence of the bone-conducted masking noise are compared to those obtained in quiet (without noise). The degree of conductive hearing impairment (the air-bone gap) is directly related to the amount of shift in air-conducted thresholds produced by the noise. A pure sensorineural loss of 40 to 50 dB or more will produce no shift because the noise will not be perceived. For subjects with normal hearing or, particularly, for subjects with conductive hearing loss (and intact sensorineural hearing), the noise will produce a shift (worsening) of thresholds.

Several investigators have adapted the SAL technique to ABR assessment of conductive hearing impairment (Hicks, 1980; Webb & Greenberg, 1984). Hicks (1980), using click stimuli, studied SAL ABR for 15 normal subjects and 4 patients with conductive, sensorineural, or mixed hearing losses. ABR threshold levels were determined monaurally for air-conduction stimulation. A high-pass noise (1200 Hz cutoff) was presented with a bone vibrator (forehead placement) and was increased in intensity until it just masked out the air-conduction ABR recorded at 5 dB above ABR threshold intensity. An approximate estimate of sensorineural (bone-conduction) threshold could be determined by subtracting 15 dB from the amount of noise needed to just mask both the ABR threshold and the 5 dB above threshold. The author claimed that the main advantages of the SAL ABR technique versus conventional bone conduction ABR measurement were the ease of calibration and minimal or no contribution from the nontest ear. The technique is based on the assumption that crossover of the signal to the nontest ear is rarely a concern in ABR measurement. This is not necessarily a valid assumption.

The SAL approach with ABR was taken one step further by Webb and Greenberg (1984). Subjects in this study were 10 normal hearers, as well as these same normal-hearing subjects with an artificial conductive impairment (occluding one ear canal with a sound-attenuating plug), 10 subjects with sensorineural impairments, and 8 subjects with mixed hearing impairments. Stimuli were tone pips of 1000, 2000, and 4000 Hz, as well as clicks. A bone-conduction broadband noise intensity level of 29 dB nHL (on the average) was needed to just mask the ABR in normal subjects and those with the induced conductive loss. For subjects with sensorineural hearing impairment, approximately 50 dB nHL of noise was needed to mask the ABR. Bone-conduction thresholds estimated with the ABR SAL technique using click stimuli corresponded within ±10 dB of behavioral bone-conduction thresholds for 100 percent of the normal subjects, 90 percent of the induced-conductive subjects, 60 percent of the sensorineural subjects, and 28 percent of the mixed loss patients. Slightly better correspondence was noted for the tone-pip stimuli in the sensorineural and mixed loss groups. The authors conclude that their method was a reliable predictor of bone-conduction threshold. A maximum bone-conducted nose level of 55 dB effective masking limited the extent of sensorineural loss that could be assessed to about this level. The SAL approach for electrophysiologically estimating the air-bone gap has also been used with the ASSR, as reviewed in Chapter 8.

Binaural Stimulation in ABR Measurement

Binaural interaction in the ABR is the topic of a large volume of published research, even though binaural interaction is not yet measured clinically. The persistent interest in the binaural interaction component (BIC) of the ABR is probably a reflection of the importance of binaural phenomena in auditory processing, and the possible relationship of the BIC for the ABR to psychophysical measurement of binaural fusion and sound lateralization with interaural differences in time and intensity (e.g., Furst, Levine, & McGaffigan, 1985; McPherson & Starr, 1995). Another likely factor driving the ongoing interest in the BIC is its anatomic substrate in the caudal brainstem, specifically the olivary complex (superior and medial superior olive), and the possibility of probing this anatomic region objectively with the ABR or important auditory centers higher in the brainstem (e.g., inferior colliculus) with the FFR (Caird, Sontheimer, & Klinke, 1985; Smith, Marsh, & Brown, 1975). Numerous terms are actually used to refer to normal differences in ABR waveforms for monaural versus binaural stimulation, including binaural interaction, summation, augmentation, enhancement, or advantage. The binaural difference wave is sometimes denoted as the "β-wave" (e.g., Brantberg, Fransson, Hansson, & Rosenhall, 1999). The term *binaural interaction*, quantified in ABR recordings by the binaural interaction component, is used here. The term *binaural interaction* encompasses each of the concepts, but it does not restrict the effect to a simple increase in response amplitude, as implied by the others. For many years, there has been interest in psychophysical study of binaural auditory phenomena. The fundamental question is, Are two ears better than one, and, if so, how are they better? A major objective of this research is to determine the role of binaural hearing in sound localization and in the perception of speech within noise. Often, the paradigm involves manipulating time of arrival of a sound to one ear versus to the other ear (interaural time differences) and/or the intensity level of a sound reaching one ear versus the other ear (interaural intensity or level differences), using psychoacoustic test procedures.

Variations on the general theme of binaural interaction research include investigations of the phenomenon in other auditory evoked responses, including the frequency-following response, or FFR (Krishnan & McDaniel, 1998; Parthasarathy & Moushegian, 1993). Krishnan and McDaniel (1998),

for example, found a "robust" BIC for the FFR, with amplitude that decreased as a function of the interaural intensity difference until the intensity difference between ears reached 20 dB and no binaural component was observed. Binaural interaction has also been investigated for cortical auditory evoked responses, including the AMLR and the ALR (e.g., McPherson & Starr, 1993, 1995; Suzuki, Kobayashi, Aoki, & Umegaki, 1992).

CHARACTERISTICS OF THE ABR FOR BINAURAL STIMULATION. | One manifestation of binaural interaction in ABR recording, an enhancement of the amplitude of components of the response for binaural versus monaural stimulation, was recognized by early experimental (Jewett, 1970) and clinical (Blegvad, 1975; Starr & Achor, 1975) investigators. For example, the average normal human subject shows wave V amplitude values for binaural stimuli that range from 30 percent to as much as 200 percent greater than those for monaural stimuli (Ainslie & Boston, 1980; Barratt, 1980; Blegvad, 1975; Davis, 1976a; Gerull & Mrowinski, 1984; Hall, 1981; Prasher, Sainz, & Gibson, 1982; Starr & Achor, 1975; van Olphen, Rodenburg, & Vervey, 1978; Wrege & Starr, 1981). Put another way, the binaural wave V amplitude is up to twice the monaural amplitude, resulting in a typical binaural-to-monaural wave V amplitude ratio of around 1.50 to 2.00. However, there is substantial variability in this response parameter among normal subjects and among ABR studies of binaural interaction. For example, some authors reported no statistically significant difference between wave V latency values for monaural versus binaural stimulation (Dobie & Norton, 1980; Hosford-Dunn, Mendelson, & Salamy, 1981), whereas other investigators found a smaller wave V for binaural versus monaural stimulation (e.g., McPherson & Starr, 1993). Latency of the difference wave is also a topic of some disagreement. Most papers report shorter wave V latency values for the binaural than for the monaural condition (Brantberg et al., 1999; Kelly-Ballweber & Dobie, 1984; Levine & Davis, 1991; Woods & Clayworth, 1985) or variable differences among subjects (Decker & Howe, 1981).

When the ABR waveform for right-ear stimulation is added (usually digitally) to the waveform for left-ear stimulation, the resultant summed waveform should minimally approximate in amplitude and latency the waveform actually recorded for binaural stimulation, according to most investigators. This process is illustrated in Figure 6.7. Replicated waveforms for right-ear and left-ear stimulation are added digitally (A + B) to yield a derived ("calculated" or "predicted") binaural response waveform. This summed monaural waveform can then be compared in latency and amplitude with the actual waveform for binaural stimulation. If there is an effect unique to the binaural stimulus condition, then the binaurally stimulated ABR should differ from the summed monaural responses. This results in a binaural difference (BD) waveform. Unfortunately, the process of

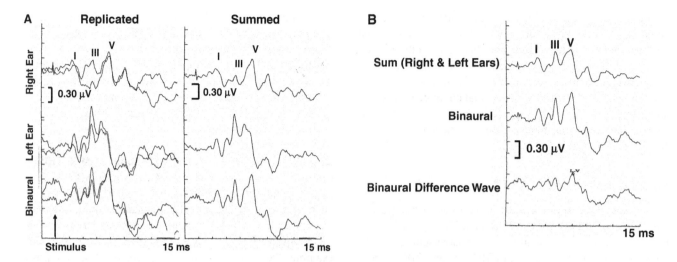

FIGURE 6.7. Calculation of the binaural difference (BD) wave by addition of the waveforms produced by separate stimulation of the right and left ears (A), and then the subtraction of this waveform from the waveform for binaural stimulation (B). Waveforms were recorded from a young normal-hearing female subject using insert earphones.

subtracting the summed monaural responses from the binaurally evoked response introduces noise into the binaural interaction waveform, adversely affecting the signal-to-noise ratio (Stollman et al., 1996). Application of sophisticated methods for objective detection and statistical confirmation of binaural interaction activity within the waveform appear to effective in enhancing the amplitude of the typically small BIC (e.g., Brantberg et al., 1999; Stollman et al., 1996). One method for statistical verification of the BIC or "β-wave" is the Fsp method now commonly used for automatic detection of the ABR in newborn hearing screening. Another promising analysis approach is a measurement of the area under the "β-wave" curve, or A_β (e.g., Brantberg et al., 1999).

Consistent evidence of a difference in some parameter of the actual binaural waveform versus the derived binaural (summed monaural) waveform would prove the existence of a true binaural interaction in the ABR. The existence of binaural interaction in ABR is, however, controversial. Subtraction of the derived binaural (summed monaural) waveform from the actual recorded binaural waveform should, if there is no difference between the two, yield an essentially flat line, that is, zero voltage across time. Differences in the predicted or derived binaural data (summed monaural waveforms) versus actual binaural data consist of smaller wave V amplitude and shorter wave V latency for the actual binaural waveform than for the predicted binaural waveform. As shown in Figure 6.7, this subtraction process usually does not produce a flat line. Instead, it produces another waveform with a component with a latency value approximately in the wave V region, the BD waveform, which is thought to reflect binaural interaction. The BD waveform typically consists of two positive (P1 and P2) and two negative (N1 and N2) peaks in the 4 to 6 msec region, within ±1 ms of

ABR wave V. The major peak (negative) usually occurs at a latency value slightly greater than for ABR wave V. BD peak amplitude is extremely modest, usually no more than 10 to 20 percent of the wave amplitude (i.e., 0.25 to 0.05 μV). There is no binaural interaction for the first three waves (I, II, and III) of the ABR, as evidenced by the essentially flat line in the early portion of the BD waveform.

The BD waveform has generated more interest than simple analysis of the monaural and binaural waveforms (Dobie & Norton, 1980; Furst, Levine, & McGaffigan, 1985; Hosford-Dunn, Mendelson, & Salamy 1981; Kelly-Ballweber & Dobie, 1984; Wilson, Kelly-Ballweber, & Dobie, 1985; Wrege & Starr, 1981), because it is assumed to be clinical evidence of binaural interaction, reflecting selective activation of brainstem neurons to binaural stimulation. The ultimate aim of the rather intense study of the BD waveform in normal subjects is to develop a valid and clinically usable electrophysiologic index of binaural processes, such as localization, lateralization, and fusion. An additional potential clinical benefit of the technique could be precise information on the site of certain auditory CNS pathologies.

In contrast to these collective reports in support of the BD as a characteristic ABR finding, however, are clinical data implying that the apparent binaural interaction is minuscule at best. These other data suggest that the BD is often not detected even in normal subjects. When present, it may be a product of confounding factors in ABR recording, such as slight measurement variations in monaural versus binaural waveforms, crossover of the acoustic stimulus at high intensity levels, inadvertent differences in effective intensity level for monaural versus binaural stimuli, or subtle right versus left brain stem asymmetry (e.g., Ainslie & Boston, 1980; Decker & Howe, 1981b). Neither Ainslie and Boston's nor

Decker and Howe's somewhat disparaging papers on binaural interaction are cited as references in several otherwise comprehensive reports on the topic by Furst, Levine, and McGaffigan (1985), Kelly-Ballweber and Dobie (1984), and Wilson, Kelly-Ballweber, and Dobie (1985). Furthermore, Ainslie and Boston (1980) clearly concluded that there is no significant binaural interaction in the ABR when factors such as stimulus crossover are controlled, yet this study is cited by others (e.g., Kelly-Ballweber & Dobie, 1984; Wilson, Kelly-Ballweber, & Dobie, 1985) as evidence in support of a binaural interaction in the ABR.

PHYSIOLOGIC BASIS OF BINAURAL INTERACTION. | Binaural interaction mechanisms in the auditory brainstem were investigated and demonstrated long before the emergence of ABR (Hall, 1965). The anatomic origin of BI as detected by ABR, however, is open to speculation (Jones & Van der Poel, 1990; Levine & Davis, 1991; Rawool & Ballachanda, 1990). The results of animal experiments have confirmed binaural-stimulus-related activity within certain structures within the auditory brainstem. In addition, the effects of experimentally induced lesions in specific auditory structures and pathways have shed light on ABR BI components (Fullerton & Hosford, 1979; Gardi & Berlin, 1981; Smith, Marsh, & Brown, 1975). The major anatomic regions of interest within the brain in this research are the medial nucleus of the trapezoid body, the lateral superior olive, the medial superior olive, and the inferior colliculus. There is no consensus, however, regarding which specific structures mediate the ABR changes observed with interaural time and intensity differences in animals. Furthermore, the anatomic source of the ABR BI component within the brainstem is unknown.

Factors Influencing Binaural Interaction in the ABR

Evaluation of binaural interaction in ABR is not as straightforward as it may at first appear. A variety of factors appear to contribute to the confusion regarding the ABR binaural interaction, including subject characteristics, the number of subjects investigated, the number of stimulus repetitions (sweeps), acquisition parameters (stimulus intensity level, stimulus rate, filter settings, location of recording electrodes), and the protocol used for waveform analysis. As an example of the effects that multiple and diverse measurement conditions might exert on findings for investigations of binaural interaction, one study appeared to implicate sleep as a factor in diminished binaural difference wave amplitude (Suzuki et al., 1992). Clearly the relative intensity of the stimulus for the right versus left ear—the interaural intensity difference (IID)—and interaural time differences are two very critical factors. Unfortunately, it is extremely difficult to evaluate published findings on binaural interaction, or to draw from these data firm conclusions about the clinical value of the phenomenon, because of the differences in methodology among studies. Factors that have been specifically investigated in these studies are now described.

STIMULUS INTENSITY LEVEL. | There are discrepancies among studies in the definition of intensity for monaural versus binaural stimuli. In the Decker and Howe (1981) study, for example, behavioral hearing thresholds were first determined for right ear, left ear, and binaural stimuli, and then ABR waveforms were recorded at a constant SL, such as 60 dB SL, above these individual thresholds. The rationale for this approach, articulated by Decker and Howe (1981), is to reduce variables related to the stimuli and highlight neurophysiologic differences. At a fixed SPL (sound pressure level) for the intensity of stimuli presented to each ear—that is, without the SL correction—binaural stimulus intensity, because of summation within the CNS, is approximately 5 dB greater than monaural stimulus intensity. Therefore, the actual binaural recording might show intensity-related shorter latencies than the summed monaural (derived binaural) recording, which, in turn, contributes to the difference wave when the one version of binaural waveform is subtracted from the other. Furst et al. (1985) reported stimulus intensity in dB SL (60 dB SL), referenced to the individual's threshold for the click. Presumably, intensity was referenced to the monaural threshold, although this was not stated.

The customary definition of intensity among studies is dB SPL (Ainslie & Boston, 1980; Dobie & Norton, 1980), dB HTL (according to ANSI, 1969), or dB nHL (Levine, 1981). With this approach, ABRs are recorded for monaural and binaural stimuli at selected fixed intensity levels, such as 50, 70, 90, and 110 dB SPL. The corresponding average dB SL value for the subjects is generally stated for each level, but no attempt is made to ensure that a fixed SL for each subject is used for each condition (monaural and binaural). This may be an important limitation, since Conijn, Brocaar, and van Zanten (1990) showed that binaural ABR thresholds were on the average 5.5 dB better (lower) than mean monaural ABR thresholds. In short, monaural sensation level appears to be a critical factor in generation of the BI component (Spivak & Seitz, 1988).

RIGHT VERSUS LEFT EAR ASYMMETRY. | Some investigators report equal amplitude and latency values of ABR waves for right versus left monaural stimulation (Ainslie & Boston, 1980; Woods & Clayworth, 1985). In contrast, Levine and McGaffigan (1983) found evidence of differences in ABR waveforms for stimuli presented to the right versus the left ear in a group of 32 neurologically and audiologically normal adult subjects. The most consistent right-versus-left-ear ABR asymmetry, observed in all recording electrode arrays, consisted of significantly greater amplitude for wave III. These ear differences were generally comparable for right-versus left-handed subjects. There was no stimulus ear difference for the eighth-nerve ABR component, wave I. These authors speculate on the relevance of this ABR evidence of brainstem asymmetry to well-recognized anatomic and functional cerebral asymmetry.

Decker and Howe (1981), in one part of their study, described "auditory tract preference" during binaural stimulation in four of eight normal subjects. For these subjects, there were no asymmetries in the right and left monaural waveforms. As proof of this, subtraction of the right-ear waveform from the left-ear waveform yielded a flat line. Rather than summing the monaural waveforms and subtracting the sum (predicted binaural response) from the actual binaural response, they subtracted each monaural response sequentially from the actual binaural response. In so doing, they discovered that the binaural waveform sometimes was identical to one of the monaural waveforms, the preferred auditory tract. Subtraction in this case produced a "null difference trace." Further subtraction of the other slightly different waveform produced the so-called binaural difference trace. Another possible source of the BD waveform, based on this study, is the artificial latency shift and variability created by adding asymmetric monaural waveforms.

There is a practical concern in calculating and comparing ABR amplitude for binaural versus monaural stimulation. Namely, from which of the two monaural waveforms should amplitude data be entered into the calculation? This is not a problem if the waveforms are entirely symmetrical, but often, there are interaural amplitude differences. Surprisingly, this question is not addressed in reports describing binaural interaction. One option is to average amplitude for the two ears. Another is consistently to use either the larger or the smaller of the amplitude values across all tests.

INTERAURAL STIMULUS TIME AND INTENSITY DIFFERENCES. |

There are numerous psychophysical studies of the effects of stimulus intensity and time of arrival on binaural auditory perceptions, such as localization of sounds. When there is a slight time (e.g., within 1 ms) or intensity (5 dB or less) advantage for a click signal arriving at one ear, the perception is a single sound coming from the direction of the lead or louder ear. As the lead-time or loudness imbalance increases, the sound seems to move toward the advantaged ear. Many investigators have applied ABR in electrophysiologic assessment of either or both of these factors in binaural auditory function (Arslan, Prosser, & Michelini, 1981; Brantberg et al., 1999; Furst et al., 1985; Gerull & Mrowinski, 1984; Jones & Van der Poel, 1990; McPherson & Starr, 1993, 1995; Prasher, Sainz, & Gibson, 1982; Wrege & Starr, 1981). Interaural time and/or intensity differences may produce alterations in later ABR waves (VI and VII), but the BI component may be a more sensitive index of these stimulus parameters.

Furst et al. (1985) found a correlation between the first major peak in the ABR BI component and perceptions of interaural time and intensity differences, as measured psychophysically. The BI component was recorded when subjects perceived a binaural click stimulus as fused. That is,

even though sets of click stimuli were presented to each ear separately, the subject heard only a single set. When the difference in click arrival time between ears (interaural time difference) exceeded 1 ms, the click was perceived as moving to the leading ear, and the BI component was no longer observed. As intensity of the clicks presented to one ear versus the other was varied, the perception of the click moved toward the ear without attenuation (greater intensity), and BI component amplitude decreased. When the interaural intensity difference was above 30 to 35 dB, a BI component was no longer recorded, and the subject perceived only a monaural stimulus (in the ear with the greater intensity level).

BINAURAL INTERACTION WITH BONE-CONDUCTION STIMULATION. | Setou and colleagues at the University of Tokyo have explored binaural interaction with bone-conduction stimulation in normal subjects (Setou, Kurauchi, Tsuzuku, & Kaga, 2001) and children with serious conductive hearing loss due to aural atresia (Kaga, Setou, & Nakamura, 2001). The authors describe a binaural interaction wave or component with bone-conduction stimulation in normal hearing subjects and patients with conductive hearing loss. The BI component appeared as a "sharp negative wave" at about the same latency as the wave IV–V complex for monaurally evoked ABRs. As the authors note, "the crossover effect is an important problem" in calculating BI with bone-conduction stimulation.

INTERAURAL ATTENUATION AND ACOUSTIC SIGNAL CROSSOVER. | With monaural stimulation, masking of the contralateral (nontest) ear can effectively eliminate the possibility of stimulus crossover that occurs when stimulus intensity exceeds the subject's interaural attenuation. Masking is not possible with the binaural presentation mode because a stimulus must be delivered to each ear. In all but one study (Ainslie & Boston, 1980), circumaural earphones (usually conventional audiometric TDH-39 or TDH-49 earphones) were used as transducers. There is, with these earphones, a chance that the stimulus could cross over from one ear to the other, or probably from each ear to the opposite ear, at high intensity levels. Energy crossing over from one ear to the other could contribute to the BD waveform. This concern is repeatedly expressed in reports of ABR binaural interaction (Ainslie & Boston, 1980; Furst et al., 1985; Levine, 1981; Wilson et al., 1985). Stimulus crossover, in effect, leads to a double stimulation of each ear, first with the original stimulus and then with delayed stimulation (within a few milliseconds) by the crossed-over sound. Consequently, the binaural difference waveform confounded by stimulus crossover has a relatively large component appearing after the usual BI components (Levine, 1981).

The possibility of contamination of findings by stimulus crossover must be considered for the numerous clinical studies of ABR binaural interaction that delivered stimuli at intensity levels of about 60 dB nHL or greater (Arslan et al., 1981; Debruyne, 1984; Decker & Howe, 1981; Dobie & Norton, 1980; Fowler & Leonards, 1985; Furst et al., 1985; Kelly-Ballweber & Dobie, 1984; Levine, 1981; Prasher & Gibson, 1980a,b; Wilson et al., 1985). A suspicion of the contamination of ABR findings by stimulus crossover from the test to the nontest ear is heightened when BI effects are most apparent for high- versus low-intensity stimuli (Levine, 1981; Wilson et al., 1985). Most investigators of ABR BI have stated an awareness of the problem of stimulus crossover. Some argue that the possibility of crossover contamination can be eliminated as a major factor in their findings and support their contention with data. Levine (1981), in describing the results of the 1981 study, clearly stated that BI was observed most consistently for the highest stimulus intensity levels (58 dB nHL) and was evident for some subjects (6%) for stimulus intensity level of less than 51 dB. He later discusses potential stimulus crossover effects at length. Analysis of the stimulus waveform recorded from the contralateral ear canal with a probe microphone, along with click-stimuli interaural attenuation characteristics in subjects with unilateral profound hearing impairment, clearly showed that crossover could be a factor in BI with stimulus intensity levels of 50 dB or greater. Levine (1981) concluded that:

> Consequently, at high intensity levels the BD will have a component that results from ACT [acoustic cross talk] rather than from neural interaction. This point is very important in any study of binaural interaction . . . attenuating the air-conducted ACT markedly reduces BD, albeit incompletely. (p. 389)

Other researchers have modified their test protocols in an attempt to reduce the likelihood of crossover effects. For example, Furst et al. (1985) presented a broadband masking noise of about 25 dB SL to the contralateral (nontest) ear during monaural stimulation, reportedly to avoid crossover contribution to BI. This, however, does not solve the problem of stimulus crossover during binaural stimulation, and it also introduces a potentially important difference in test conditions for monaural versus binaural stimulation.

In fact, Ainslie and Boston (1980) found that BI with the masked test protocol was significantly different than with no masking. The authors inferred from this observation that crossover definitely contributes to BI, as it is usually recorded. They went on to carry out the BI stimulus paradigm with insert earphones versus conventional TDH-39 earphones. With the insert earphones, there was no significant BI. Ainslie and Boston (1980) conclude that BI observed by others "are due primarily to acoustic cross-talk in the monaural stimulus condition" (p. 300). To eliminate the possibility of acoustic or bone-conduction stimulus crossover, Levine (1981) cautions that the intensity level for stimuli presented to one ear should not exceed the behavioral threshold levels of the opposite (nontest) ear by more than 50 dB. Routine use of insert tube earphones would appear to be the most effective means of reducing the likelihood of BI contamination by stimulus crossover.

STIMULUS FREQUENCY. | Binaural interaction wave latency and amplitude values are clearly affected by stimulus frequency and type. Shorter binaural interaction waves are recorded for click stimuli than for tone bursts (e.g., Parthasarathy & Moushegian, 1993). Fowler and Leonards (1985) evaluated BI in 24 normal-hearing subjects and 5 patients with severe high-frequency hearing impairment, using 1000 Hz and 4000 Hz tone bursts. The 1000 Hz stimulus at the highest intensity level (100 dB SPL) was associated with a larger BI component. The BI appeared in the ABR wave V and VII latency region. BI morphology was comparable for normal-hearing versus hearing-impaired persons for the 1000 Hz stimulus, even when there was an abnormal ABR or no ABR for the 4000 Hz stimulus. Wilson et al. (1985) studied BI with ABR, using filtered click stimuli with center frequencies of 500, 2000, and 8000 Hz. Although there was no important amplitude difference for BI among stimuli, the BI waveforms were more distinct relative to background noise for the two higher frequency stimuli. A BI component was also found for a 1000 Hz tone-burst stimulus presented to one ear and a 3000 Hz tone burst presented to the other ear.

STIMULUS RATE. | The effects of increased stimulus rate on the BI were consistent with known rate effects on the ABR in general, according to Wilson et al. (1985). That is, with increasing rate, ABR latency increased significantly for monaural, binaural, predicted (derived) binaural, and BI wave components. The effect of rate on response amplitude for these stimulus conditions was not statistically significant. Fowler and Broadard (1988) reported more reliable and robust BI components at a fast rate (50/sec) versus slower rates (10/second or 25/second). Levine (1981) reported greater BI amplitude for slow click rates (10 to 30/second) than for faster rates. He recommended using a slower click rate in BI measurement in order to minimize the likelihood of acoustic stapedius reflex influence on the BI.

STIMULUS POLARITY. | Consistent with expected rate effects on the ABR, Wrege and Starr (1981) reported shorter BI latencies for rarefaction than for condensation click stimuli. Wilson et al. (1985) also found shorter BI latencies for rarefaction versus condensation clicks but no amplitude differences in ABR recordings from guinea pigs, but they did not study human subjects. According to Rawool and Ballachanda (1990), latency values are also shorter for binaural stimulation with out-of-phase click stimulation (rarefaction to one ear and condensation to the other ear).

RESPONSE AVERAGING AND ACQUISITION. | The possible importance of differences in the number of stimuli averaged for monaural versus binaural conditions, or the sequence in which data for these conditions are gathered, is not known. In the majority of studies, an equal number of stimulus repetitions (usually either 1,024 or 2,048) are presented for each monaural and the binaural condition. An exception was the study by Fowler and Leonards (1985), in which, for each condition (two monaural and binaural), three replicated waveforms were each averaged for 4,000 stimuli; these were added before the usual binaural interaction paradigm was followed. Thus, the composite responses for each condition were based on 12,000 stimuli. Routine presentation of equal numbers of stimulus repetitions for each condition is logical because the summed monaural response (predicted binaural waveform) and the actual binaural are then produced with equivalent numbers of stimulus repetitions. Furst, Levine, and McGaffigan (1985) repeatedly (about 25 times) interleaved (alternated) sequences of 256 click presentations for each of the three stimulus conditions until the response for each condition was averaged for a total of 6,400 stimuli, in most instances. The interleaving approach for stimulus presentation was used in order to equally distribute any changes in the subject state or EEG during the testing.

FILTER SETTINGS. | The most commonly used band-pass filter settings in studies of binaural interaction are 1, 10, 20, or 30 Hz to at least 3000 Hz (Ainslie & Boston, 1980; Furst, Levine, & McGaffigan, 1985; Gerull & Mrowinski, 1984; Levine, 1981; Wilson, Kelly-Ballweber, & Dobie, 1985), or slightly more restricted filter settings of 100 or 150 to 3000 Hz (Arslan, Prosser, & Michelini, 1981; Decker & Howe, 1981; Fowler & Leonards, 1985; Kelly-Ballweber & Dobie, 1984). Analysis of the spectral composition of the binaural difference waveform apparently has not been evaluated, but it would provide practical information. If there were normally a substantial low-frequency contribution to this component, it is possible that by filtering with a somewhat higher high-pass cutoff frequency, the amplitude of the component might be reduced. This would perhaps account for the inconsistent presence of the binaural interaction (BI) component even under otherwise optimal measurement conditions. In fact, however, Fowler and Broadard (1988) reported larger and more reliable binaural interaction components with a high pass filter setting of 150 Hz versus 30 Hz.

ELECTRODE ARRAY. | The inverting electrode in ABR recordings for monaural stimuli is usually located on the mastoid or earlobe ipsilateral to the ear stimulated. The inverting electrode site is an important factor in measuring BI with ABR, and it cannot be selected arbitrarily. Early waves (II and III) may be out of phase for ABRs recorded with the inverting electrode on the earlobe (or mastoid) ipsilateral versus contralateral to the stimulus (Ainslie & Boston, 1980). A wave I is not observed with an inverting electrode array involving the ear contralateral to the stimulus, and wave V amplitude recorded with the contralateral electrode array is about two-thirds of that recorded with an ipsilateral electrode array. Wave V latency differences for ipsilateral versus contralateral electrode arrays may also occur (e.g., Woods & Clayworth, 1985). Because the ABR recorded for binaural

stimuli includes both the waveform for the conventional electrode array (with an electrode on the ear ipsilateral to the stimulus) and the waveform for the contralateral electrode array (which is also the stimulus-ipsilateral array for the opposite ear), a binaural enhancement of about 67 percent for wave V amplitude would be expected, strictly on the basis of electrode effects, even with no true BI. Indeed, different investigators have independently reported a binaural advantage on the order of 60 to 75 percent (Ainslie & Boston, 1980; Blegvad, 1975; Davis, 1976a; Hall, 1981; van Olphen et al., 1978).

There is no convention for inverting electrode placement with binaurally stimulated ABRs. Ainslie and Boston (1980) reported that binaurally stimulated responses were similar when recorded with right- versus left-ear electrodes. Some investigators suggest that a noncephalic electrode, which is essentially neutral and equivalent for monaural and binaural stimulation, is preferable to mastoid placement. Sites used for this electrode in binaural ABR studies include the laryngeal prominence (Kelly-Ballweber & Dobie, 1984; van Olphen et al., 1978), the inion (Arslan et al., 1981), and the nape of the neck (Decker & Howe, 1981; Fowler & Leonards, 1985; Furst et al., 1985; Gerull & Mrowinski, 1984; Levine, 1981; Wilson, Kelly-Ballweber, & Dobie, 1985). This practice is well advised because it essentially renders the inverting electrode inactive and, incidentally, also reduces PAM (post-auricular muscle) contamination of the AMLR in BI detection. A more recent report suggests that the BI wave amplitude distribution varies also as a function of noninverting electrode site (Jones & Van der Poel, 1990).

SUBJECT CHARACTERISTICS. | Whether subject age exerts an important influence on BI, as measured with ABR, is open to question. Hosford-Dunn, Mendelson, and Salamy (1981) successfully recorded BI components from healthy full-term neonates. Although ABR latency, including that of the BI component, showed the expected age-related prolongation, the overall morphology and amplitude of the BI component was comparable for newborns versus adults. On the other hand, in another comparison of BI for the ABR in infants versus adults, Jiang and Tierney (1996) found "a marked difference between the neonatal and adult BI wave forms," with smaller BI for wave VII in the infants. Although Jiang and Tierney (1996) attributed this finding to immaturity in neonates of the neuronal responses generating the later ABR waves, the authors reported no difference between adults and newborn infants in the response of the BI to changes in stimulus intensity and rate. At the other end of the age spectrum, Kelly-Ballweber and Dobie (1984) found no significant difference in BI components for younger (31 to 49 years) versus older (64 to 76 years) adult subjects. The effect of peripheral auditory status on BI has not been evaluated specifically, but Kelly-Ballweber and Dobie (1984) implied that the BI was observed less consistently in patients with high-frequency impairment. There are no systematic investigations of the effect on BI of other subject characteristics, such as gender, body temperature, state of arousal, and drugs.

ACOUSTIC STAPEDIAL (MIDDLE-EAR) REFLEX. | There is general consensus that the acoustic stapedial reflex has little or (probably) no effect on ABR differences for monaural versus binaural click stimulation, at least at relatively slow presentation rates. Levine (1981) closely examined the possible influence of acoustic reflex activity on the ABR BI. Arguing against acoustic reflex activity as a factor, he noted that contraction of the middle ear muscles in response to acoustic stimulation attenuates mostly low-frequency energy. The ABR, however, is normally elicited by higher-frequency components in the click spectrum. Also, attenuation takes place at the level of the middle ear, before cochlear activation, so all ABR components should be affected. These arguments remain speculative.

CLINICAL APPLICATION OF ABRS FOR MONAURAL VERSUS BINAURAL STIMULATION. | As noted at the outset of this discussion, there is general agreement that monaural stimulation is preferable to binaural stimulation for neurodiagnostic applications of ABR (Chiappa, Gladstone, & Young, 1979; Prasher & Gibson, 1980a,b; Prasher, Sainz, & Gibson, 1982; Rosenhamer & Holmkvist, 1983; Stockard et al., 1978). The sensitivity of ABR to various pathologies is reduced with binaural stimulation, because a normal response can be observed if there is at least unilateral auditory brainstem integrity. Given the rather extensive investigation of binaural interaction in normal subjects, it is surprising that there are only a handful of clinical studies comparing ABRs for monaural versus binaural stimuli. Lack of the normally expected ABR amplitude enhancement for binaural versus monaural stimulation has been reported for patients with varied disorders, including multiple sclerosis, or MS (Prasher, Sainz, & Gibson, 1982) and spasmodic dysphonia (Hall, 1981). The proposed basis for this finding in MS is an asymmetry in the ABR latencies (and phase characteristics) for stimulation of one ear versus the other, which eliminates neural summation of the response. Hausler and Levine (1980) found marked ABR abnormalities for monaural stimulation in 18 of 29 patients with MS, ranging from waveforms with good morphology but interwave latency delays to waveforms with no components after wave I. These authors, however, found no correlation between monaural ABRs and the patients' ability to discriminate interaural intensity differences. Binaural ABRs were not recorded. Hall (1981) reported a decreased binaural-to-monaural amplitude ratio for wave III, but not for wave V, in 7 patients with spasmodic dysphonia, when compared to data for an age- and gender-matched control group. He speculated on a possible impairment in binaural interaction in the caudal brainstem in this patient population.

Whether measurement of BI with ABR, or other AERs, has potential clinical value is not known, but there is reason to be skeptical. The BI component, even in audiologically and neurologically normal subjects and under ideal recording conditions, is of very modest amplitude (0.10 to 0.20 μV or less) and rather elusive. The BI is frequently not reliably observed in patients with peripheral hearing impairment, even of a mild degree. Also, as noted previously, the validity of the ABR BI as a reflection of neural function versus a product of stimulus crossover is open to question for some measurement conditions. Although clinical research should be undertaken to test the usefulness of BI in various patient populations, it is not likely to fulfill initial expectations as an electrophysiologic index of auditory functioning in anatomically discrete brainstem regions.

MASKING LEVEL DIFFERENCE OF ABR. | Fowler and Leonards (1985) found a distinct ABR BI effect for a 4000 Hz stimulus. They point out that by psychoacoustic measurement, the MLD is typically negligible at this frequency, and, therefore, ABR BI and MLD are perhaps dissimilar phenomena. Kevanishvili and Lagidze (1987) were unable to show an MLD effect by ABR, although a release from masking was observed for later latency AERs. In contrast, Hannley, Jerger, and Rivera (1983) and Noffsinger, Martinez, and Schaefer (1982) demonstrated a relationship between ABR wave III (not wave V) and MLD in patients with MS.

ACQUISITION PARAMETERS

Analysis Time

Under certain test conditions and with certain subject characteristics, major components of the ABR (I, III, and V) are observed within a 5.5 to 6 ms period after stimulus presentation. These conditions include a high intensity level for a click or high-frequency tone-burst stimulus, presented at a reasonably slow rate (30/second or below) by air conduction via conventional earphones to a subject who is normal audiologically and neurologically, especially a young adult female. If one or more of these conditions are not met, ABR wave V may exceed 6 ms. Five commonly cited clinical explanations for prolongation of ABR latency values are (1) insert earphones with stimulus delivery tubes producing a acoustic travel time delay of 0.9 ms (and no correction), (2) severe conductive hearing impairment, (3) immature CNS in a newborn infant, (4) stimulus intensity level near auditory threshold, and (5) severe auditory brainstem dysfunction. Naturally, these causes for ABR latency delay are not mutually exclusive and may be additive. For example, ABR wave V latency for a newborn at 35 dB nHL may normally be about 8 ms. Add to this a 1 ms prestimulus baseline period (described below), a low-frequency tone-burst stimulus, plus another 1 ms prolongation due to neurologic immaturity or a mild conductive hearing impairment, and wave V will be well outside of the 10 ms range. Although it is certainly possible to utilize various analysis times within a laboratory, depending on test conditions and subject characteristics, this practice can contribute to errors in test protocol and confusion in the analysis of results.

For routine clinical ABR assessment, a minimal analysis time of 10 ms is necessary and recommended by the majority of manufacturers of evoked response systems. An analysis time of 15 ms, however, is recommended because it encompasses ABR latencies for virtually all patients, including infants and patients with hearing loss, while still permitting adequate time resolution with as few as 256 data points.

RELATIONSHIP BETWEEN ONSET OF STIMULUS AND ANALYSIS TIME. | Evoked response systems have an option for altering the relationship between stimulus onset and the initiation of analysis. With this option, averaging can begin before or after the stimulus is presented, as well as the conventional synchronous triggering of averaging with stimulus presentation. Some systems offer a fixed pre- or poststimulus time period option (e.g., 10% of the entire analysis time will be devoted to one or the other selection). Other systems allow the tester to select the analysis time to be allotted to the pre- or poststimulus period. Use of a prestimulus period of data collection (averaging) is a handy technique for assessing the level of EEG activity unrelated to the stimulus. Response-related electrical activity does not begin until after the stimulus is presented. The prestimulus baseline activity reflects the state of patient activity more accurately than a no-stimulus average because it is based on simultaneously recorded EEG. That is, the prestimulus baseline reflects the patient's activity level during the time the AER is being recorded. A prestimulus baseline time that is approximately 10 percent of total analysis time is usually an appropriate selection. For ABR, then, the prestimulus time would be about 1 to 2 ms (assuming a 15 ms analysis time). Delaying the averaging process until a brief time after stimulus presentation can effectively reduce or eliminate stimulus artifact from the waveform and prevent the evoked response system from locking up in the artifact rejection mode due to stimulus-related electromagnetic activity. If insert earphones and sound delivery tubes are used for stimulus presentation, however, this function of post-stimulus delay is not required.

One must remember that the amount of time available for averaging the response is reduced when the prestimulus baseline time is employed. The response analysis time is equal to the total analysis time minus the prestimulus baseline time. For example, with a 15 ms ABR analysis time and a 10 percent prestimulus baseline time, averaging the response (poststimulus) occurs over a 13.5 ms period. Clearly, a total analysis time of 10 ms is ill-advised if a pre- or poststimulus baseline is employed. Selection of a pre- or poststimulus time exceeding the total analysis time is not permitted by commercially available systems. Also, latency cursors for most evoked response systems automatically account for pre- or poststimulus times, but may not automatically correct for the time delay caused by insert earphone

sound delivery tubes (about 0.9 ms for the Etymotics ER-3A tube).

RELATIONSHIP BETWEEN STIMULUS RATE AND ANALYSIS TIME. | As a rule, the upper limit for rate of stimulation with an evoked response system is governed by the analysis time. For facial nerve or somatosensory stimulation, rate may also be limited by stimulus intensity, i.e., the strength of electrical shock in milliamperes (mA). Analysis time and rate are inversely related such that rapid rates are not permitted for long analysis times. As analysis time increases, maximum stimulus rate (stimuli/sec) decreases. For some evoked response systems, there is no way to override this limitation. Other systems, however, provide a warning that more than one stimulus will be delivered within the analysis time and then permit the tester to proceed. The maximum stimulus rate per analysis time can be easily calculated for transient stimuli, such as clicks. For a 10 ms (0.01 or 1/100 second) ABR analysis time, maximum stimulus rate is 100/sec, and for a 15 ms analysis period the maximum allowable stimulus rate would be 67/second. In order to carry out ABR measurement at rapid stimulus rates, it may be necessary to adjust acquisition parameters and temporarily use a shorter analysis period (e.g., 10 ms) and also to avoid use of the pre- or poststimulus baseline period option.

Electrodes

Literature on the topic of electrode effects in ABR measurement is reviewed here. Students or other readers who are inexperienced in auditory evoked response principles, protocols, and procedures will benefit from the detailed general review of electrodes found in Chapter 3, including the many types of electrode designs now available commercially, and the impact of electrode types and sites on AER measurements. The topic of electrodes in ECochG measurement, also relevant for some applications of the ABR, was covered in Chapter 4.

WAVE I ENHANCEMENT. | The primary clinical advantage of the ear canal and TM electrode types in ECochG recording, namely increased AP amplitude, is equally applicable for ABR wave I. In fact, it appears that the time has come when combined ECochG and ABR recording of this wave component is clinically feasible, without additional test time, patient discomfort, or evoked response equipment or supplies (Ferraro & Ferguson, 1989). The diagnostic value of ABR is largely dependent on analysis of interwave latencies, especially the wave I to V interval. The use of an ear-canal electrode for routine ABR measurement is endorsed, particularly for these frequent instances when a clear wave I is required clinically (Ferraro, Murphy, & Ruth, 1986). When recorded with an ear-canal electrode, wave I may be more distinct at high intensity levels and detected at lower intensity levels. There are, in addition, significant differences in wave I amplitude among the various ear-canal electrode types. As demonstrated by Yanz and Dodds (1987), Wave I amplitude is further enhanced with the TM flexible tube design electrode.

There are, then, a number of different clinical ear-canal electrode options. Which one is preferable for clinical ABR measurement? The insert earphone and electrode combination, the TIPtrode, is best suited for routine clinical use. The TIPtrode electrode type will resolve detection of wave I in most patients. A practical approach is to initially use either the regular insert "tube phone" with an earlobe electrode or the TIPtrode electrode type and then, in patients showing no clear wave I, to employ a TM electrode. Clinical data show that the TIPtrode electrode type leads to confident identification of wave I in the majority of patients with moderate sensory hearing loss. Another alternative when the TIPtrode and manipulation of measurement parameters fail to reveal a clear wave I, especially in the operating room environment, is to carry out the simplified transtympanic promontory ECochG technique described in Chapter 4.

THE CONVENTIONAL ELECTRODE ARRAY. | In clinical practice, ABRs are usually recorded with the noninverting electrode located in the midline on the forehead (the Fz site) or on the vertex (Cz), and with the inverting electrode on the earlobe of the stimulus side (ipsilateral to the stimulus), as shown in Figure 6.8. This "ipsilateral electrode montage" is entirely adequate for most ABR applications in adults (e.g., Hall, 1992) and children, including infants (e.g., Stuart, Yang, & Botea, 1996). For adults, wave V amplitude is marginally larger when recorded with a noninverting electrode at the vertex site than with a forehead noninverting electrode site. Amplitude of ABR wave V tends to be slightly less (decreased by no more than 0.1 μvolt) for an electrode on at a high forehead versus vertex location (Starr & Squires, 1982; van Olphen, Rodenburg, & Vervey, 1978) Starr and Squires (1982) found that wave I is actually largest over a frontal midline location, such as forehead. In addition, the forehead site for the noninverting electrode produces a more robust wave V with infants. Moving the noninverting electrode from vertex to forehead results in a modest wave I amplitude decrement, according to van Olphen, Rodenburg, and Vervey (1978). However, studies of ABR topography indicate that the precise location of the noninverting electrode, at least along the midline (the sagittal plane), is not a major factor in the response (Martin & Moore, 1977; McPherson, Hirasugi, & Starr, 1985; Picton et al., 1974; Starr & Squires, 1982; Streletz, Katz, Hohenberger, & Cracco, 1977; van Olphen, Rodenburg, & Vervey, 1978). An ABR can be recorded from rather unorthodox anterior locations, such as the tip of the nose or the nasopharynx, confirming that these sites are active. Responses from posterior midline sites, such as the inion, are characteristically small.

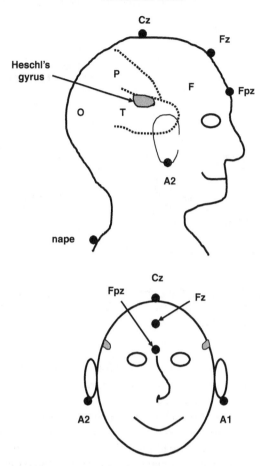

Auditory Brainstem Response (ABR) Electrode Sites

FIGURE 6.8.   Electrode sites used typically in clinical ABR measurement in ipsilateral and contralateral arrays. Either the Cz or Fz site can be used for the noninverting electrode in clinical measurement of the ABR.

Curiously, there may be intersubject differences, even among adults, in the effect of electrode site on ABR amplitude. This may be related to differences in skull thickness from one subject to the next. Furthermore, the differences in amplitude that exist between electrode sites equidistant from the far-field generators of the ABR within a subject are perhaps due to irregularities in thickness of the skull and corresponding electrical resistance. Change in placement of the electrode along the midline produces no other significant differences in latency or amplitude. In a coronal plane, amplitudes for waves II through V are, according to most investigators, greatest at the vertex and diminish systematically to very low values as the mastoid is approached (Starr & Squires, 1982; van Olphen, Rodenburg, & Vervey, 1978). In these studies, the vertex to mastoid amplitude decrease is most pronounced for wave V. Hashimoto et al. (1981), however, found maximum wave V amplitude and shortest amplitude with an electrode located over the frontal area

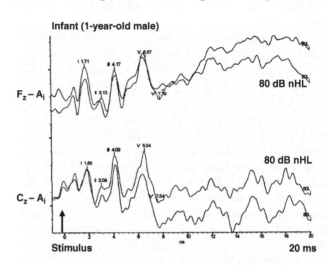

FIGURE 6.9. ABR waveforms recorded simultaneously from an adult (left panel) and an infant (right panel) with a noninverting electrode on the vertex and a noninverting electrode on the forehead.

contralateral to the stimulus (with a noncephalic reference site). Responses were not assessed from this specific electrode location in the other studies cited.

There are three main clinical advantages to placement of the noninverting electrode at the hairline of the forehead near the Fz site, instead of at the vertex (see Figure 6.9). First, it eliminates problems associated with preparing the skin and securing an electrode with tape on the scalp where there is usually hair. Second, in some patients a vertex electrode site is not technically optimal or clinically feasible. With neonates, vigorous scrubbing at the fontanel (the soft portion of the skull in the vertex area) is best avoided. Brain-injured patients often have an intracranial pressure monitor or bandages on the top of the head. A high forehead location, therefore, contributes to consistency in electrode placement across subjects. Normative data for a clinical facility should, of course, be collected with these, and other, electrode considerations in mind. According to data reported by Starr and Squires (1982), the forehead site is in most subjects associated with larger wave I amplitude than more posterior locations along the midline (e.g., Cz). For adults, the high forehead (Fz) noninverting electrode site is associated with slightly larger amplitude wave III and smaller amplitude for wave V, in comparison to a vertex (Cz) noninverting electrode. Among infants, however, this pattern of amplitude for wave III and wave V is reversed.

With this conventional bipolar array, both the noninverting electrode (vertex or forehead site) and the inverting electrode (earlobe or ear canal ipsilateral to the stimulus) are active with respect to electrophysiologic activity in the head (cephalic activity), such as AERs (Barratt, 1980; Hughes,

Fino, & Gagnon, 1981; Rossini, Gambi, Marchionno, David, & Sollazzo, 1980). The dipole sources of AERs are located between the two electrodes. Some generators (e.g., the eighth nerve) are located closer to the inverting (mastoid or earlobe) electrode, while others (e.g., nucleus of lateral lemniscus or inferior colliculus) are closer to the noninverting (vertex or forehead) electrode. The response recorded with the conventional array, then, is highly dynamic and varies as a function of time and generator site. There may be unpredictable interactions among portions of the response conducted simultaneously from each of the two electrodes.

NONCEPHALIC ELECTRODE RECORDINGS. | There are compelling neurophysiologic reasons for considering a noncephalic electrode array in ABR measurement. A number of investigators have demonstrated that there is no detectable ABR when recordings are made between two electrodes located off the head, including the thorax, nape of neck, side of neck, laryngeal prominence, or ankle, confirming that these sites are essentially neutral for this response (Barratt, 1980; Hughes, Fino, & Gagnon, 1981; Picton, Hillyard, Krausz & Galambos, 1974; Starr & Squires, 1982; Stockard, Stockard, & Sharbrough, 1978; Terkildsen & Osterhammel, 1981; Terkildsen, Osterhammel, & Huis in't Veld, 1975; van Olphen, Rodenburg & Vervey, 1978). Although no electrode site on the body is totally inactive when volume conducted responses are recorded, the terms "reference electrode" or "indifferent electrode" are entirely proper in discussing noncephalic sites, in contrast to the inappropriate use of these terms in referring to mastoid or earlobe inverting electrode sites. The vertex or forehead to noncephalic electrode arrangement is sometimes referred to as a vertical array (Hall et al., 1984; Starr & Squires, 1982).

Differences in the contribution of each electrode in the conventional electrode array (the top waveform in Figure 6.10) to the ABR are vividly demonstrated by comparing simultaneous recordings made from a mastoid to noncephalic electrode pair versus a vertex to noncephalic electrode pair (Barratt, 1980; Hughes, Fino, & Gagnon, 1981; Starr & Squires, 1982; Streletz, Katz, Hohenberger & Cracco, 1977; Stuart, Yang, & Botea, 1996; Terkildsen & Osterhammel, 1981; Terkildsen, Osterhammel, & Huis in't Veld, 1977). An ABR waveform recorded with a mastoid to noncephalic electrode array consists only of earlier latency ABR components (I, II, III, IV) while all components are observed with the vertex to noncephalic array. Importantly, some of these early latency wave components (through wave IV) shared by the two arrays are out of phase by 180 degrees—that is, opposite in polarity. Wave I, for example, is of negative polarity when recorded with a mastoid to noncephalic array but of positive polarity when recorded with a vertex to noncephalic array. With differential amplification, as noted earlier in this chapter, amplitude of these components would be enhanced. There is an additive effect of the two active electrodes (vertex and mastoid or earlobe). Similarly, components that are in phase for the two arrays (e.g., wave II)

might be effectively cancelled out and complex alterations of amplitude and morphology, such as extra peaks, might occur for wave components that are partially out of phase for the two arrays (e.g., wave V). Waves IV and V are recorded as small positive polarity waves with a mastoid to noncephalic array and as larger positive voltage waves with the vertex to noncephalic electrode pair. Differential amplification of the inputs from the mastoid and vertex electrodes (the voltage difference), therefore, results in a reduction in recorded amplitude for waves IV and V with the conventional array. Waves VI and VII are primarily recorded by the vertex electrode in the conventional electrode array. These interactions among electrode arrays and phase have complicated the correlations between surface electrodes versus depth electrode recordings of response generators using surface versus depth electrode recordings (Møller, 1985). The most accurate measure of brainstem activity is derived from the vertex to noncephalic recording.

There are, as implied earlier, distinct differences in the latencies of ABR wave components and amplitudes between vertex to mastoid or earlobe versus vertex to noncephalic electrode arrays (see Figure 6.9). Recording ABRs simultaneously for three channels with noninverting electrodes on the vertex, the stimulus ipsilateral ear, and the stimulus contralateral ear, each paired with a noncephalic inverting electrode is a handy way of assessing the activity of each noninverting site in the conventionally measured ABR (see Hughes, Fino, & Gagnon, 1981).

As illustrated in Figure 6.10, the three most pronounced ABR differences observed in the noncephalic versus conventional electrode array are wave V amplitude enhancement (larger amplitude), separation of wave IV versus V, and a more distinct wave VI component (Hall et al., 1984). Amplitude of wave V may be 50 percent larger in the noncephalic waveform than it is with the conventional array, and wave V is more clearly separated from IV in the wave IV/V complex. The result is more confident and accurate identification and latency calculation for wave V (and in turn the I to V latency interval) in patients with CNS pathology (Hall et al., 1984). The augmentation of wave V amplitude with a noncephalic electrode array in infants (e.g., Hall, 1992; Katbamma, Metz, Adelman, & Thodi, 1993; Stuart, Yang, & Botea, 1996) is especially appealing because it enhances the accuracy of estimations of auditory threshold. There is some evidence that wave II may also be more prominent in a vertex to noncephalic waveform than with the conventional array (Starr & Squires, 1982). If this were a consistent finding, it might have important implications for identification and localization of pathology of the eighth cranial nerve with ABR. As discussed in Chapter 7, the ABR wave I to II interval is a potentially valuable response index in evaluating suspected eighth-nerve pathology. Unfortunately, it has been of limited practical value because of the inconsistency of wave II in conventionally recorded ABRs. One potential drawback to this approach, however, is the relatively smaller amplitude

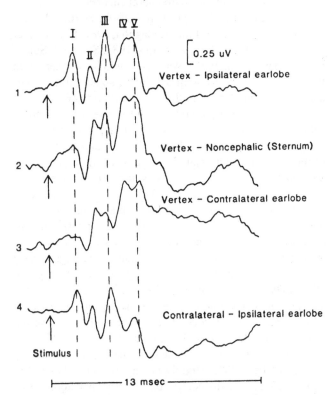

FIGURE 6.10. ABR waveforms recorded with four different electrode arrays (ipsilateral, contralateral, vertical, and horizontal).

and greater variability in the latency for wave I as recorded with a non-cephalic versus conventional electrode array (McPherson, Hirasugi, & Starr, 1985).

A vertex (or forehead) to noncephalic electrode array is heartily endorsed and recommended for clinical ABR recording by a host of auditory neurophysiologists (Barratt, 1980; Hall et al., 1984; Hashimoto et al., 1981; Hughes, Fino, & Gagnon, 1981; McPherson, Hirasugi, & Starr, 1985; Møller, 1985; Rossini et al., 1980; Starr & Squires, 1982; Streletz et al., 1977; Terkildsen & Osterhammel, 1981)

The use of a noncephalic inverting recording electrode is crucial if abnormal ABR waveforms recorded clinically with surface electrodes are interpreted for the purpose of neurodiagnosis, such as site-of-lesion localization. A noncephalic far-field ABR recording is most consistent with the intracranial (near-field) recordings used to define generators (Møller, 1983, 1985). There are distinct differences between ABR waveforms recorded with surface electrodes in the conventional electrode array versus intracranial electrodes referenced to a noncephalic site. Noncephalic recordings should be routinely considered for accurate and confident definition of ABR components in clinical assessments for reasons stated above and illustrated below.

A reasonable question at this point is where the noncephalic electrode should be located. Commonly used sites are the nape of the neck, on either side of the neck, and on the thorax (chest), specifically at the sternum. Among these three general sites, the thorax appears to be least active with respect to intracranial neurophysiologic activity. A major problem with electrode placement anywhere in the chest or shoulder area, however, is electrical interference from the heart (EKG). Amplitude of heart electrophysiologic activity is substantially greater than for AERs and occurs in the lower end of the AER spectrum. Therefore, it cannot be effectively filtered out without degrading the auditory response. The solution to this technical problem is a balanced noncephalic reference in which two electrodes, one placed over the clavicle and one placed directly behind it, on the back over the scapula, are linked. This balanced sterno-vertebral (SV) reference electrode arrangement was introduced by Stephenson and Gibbs (1951) and described further by Lehtonen and Koivikko (1971). Each electrode in the pair detects EKG (the heart is located between the two) exactly out of phase from the other and consequently the EKG is cancelled out and does not interfere with AER recording. Noncephalic electrodes are also apt to detect myogenic activity from large muscle groups and to reduce the effectiveness of common mode rejection.

Despite the foregoing argument for considering a noncephalic inverting electrode site, a clear ABR with major wave components is clearly recorded at a high stimulus intensity level for most normal subjects and many patients with the conventional electrode array.

IPSILATERAL VERSUS CONTRALATERAL ELECTRODE ARRAYS. | Waveforms recorded simultaneously from a normal subject

with the convention array just described, and with three other electrode arrays, were shown in Figure 6.9. The sites for noninverting and inverting electrode pairs for all four arrays were illustrated in Figure 6.8. A contralateral inverting electrode array is most often used, in addition to the ipsilateral array, for ABR measurement with bone-conduction stimulation. Ipsilateral versus contralateral recordings have been extensively studied in attempts to determine the generators of the ABR, to define expected differences in respective wave components (Hughes, Fino, & Gagnon, 1981; McPherson, Hirasugi, & Starr, 1985; Mizrahi, Maulsby, & Frost, 1983; Prasher & Gibson, 1980a; Rosenhamer & Holmkvist, 1982; Stockard, Stockard, & Sharbrough, 1978), to assess developmental effects on ABR, and to develop ear-specific techniques for assessing air- versus bone-conduction auditory status in patients with severe conductive hearing impairments (Hall et al., 1984; Jahrsdoerfer & Hall, 1986). The most distinctive difference between ABR waveforms recorded from a contralateral array (inverting electrode on stimulus contralateral mastoid, earlobe, or ear canal), in comparison to the conventional or ipsilateral array (inverting electrode on stimulus ipsilateral earlobe or mastoid), is the typical absence a wave I component (see Figure 6.9). Although at first glance, there may appear to be a wave I in the contralateral channel waveform, upon closer scrutiny the positive voltage wave I is not present but the negative voltage trough immediately following the latency region for wave I (sometimes referred to as "I neg") does remain in the contralateral channel.

There are other differences in waveforms recorded for the two arrays (Hughes, Fino, & Gagnon, 1981; Rosenhamer & Holmkvist, 1982; Starr & Squires, 1982; Stockard, Stockard, & Sharbrough, 1978). Wave II is definitely observed in the contralateral array with amplitude significantly larger and latency longer than in the ipsilateral array (Kato et al., 1995). This wave II pattern is found in over 85 percent of subjects. In view of evidence (Møller, 1981, 1983, 1985) that ABR wave II arises from the proximal (brainstem) portion of the eighth nerve in man, the larger wave II amplitude for the contralateral recording array is unexpected. One would expect larger amplitude for an ABR recorded from the closer stimulus ipsilateral electrode. The explanation may be related to dipole orientation of the ABR and in phase relationships of very early latency waveform peaks as detected by the inverting (e.g., earlobe) versus noninverting (e.g., vertex) electrodes in the ipsilateral array (Hughes, Fino, & Gagnon, 1981). That is, in the ipsilateral recording array, there is a small negative deflection just before the expected latency for wave II, which, when added to the response from the vertex electrode, decreases overall amplitude.

Wave III amplitude is somewhat smaller, and the latency for wave III and IV is slightly but significantly shorter (by about 0.15 ms) for the contralateral versus ipsilateral array. This relationship is also observed in about 85 percent of subjects. There are published reports of latency and amplitude differences for wave V that are related to electrode array.

Hughes, Fino, and Gagnon (1981), in comparing ipsi- versus contralateral recordings, noted a tendency for wave V latency to be longer and amplitude smaller in the contralaterally recorded waveform. Starr and Squires (1982), isolating responses from ipsi- versus contralateral mastoids with a noncephalic (seventh cervical vertebra neck electrode) array found that wave IV occurred from 0.1 to 0.5 ms earlier ipsilaterally and wave V occurred from 0.0 to 0.6 ms later contralaterally. Because of the shorter wave III as recorded with the contralateral array, the wave III–V latency interval is typically longer for contralateral recordings. The larger amplitude for wave III in the ipsilateral versus contralateral waveform is presumably due to the out-of-phase relationship between the response recorded from the ipsilateral inverting electrode versus vertex noninverting electrode. With differential amplification, the voltage difference between the two electrodes is greater at any point in time that one electrode detects a negative voltage and the other a positive voltage. As noted, wave IV latency may be altered by as much as 0.36 ms for ipsilateral versus contralateral waveforms. This, in turn, can affect the morphology of the IV/V wave complex. There may be a fused wave IV/V complex in the ipsilateral waveform while a separate wave IV versus V can be distinguished in the contralateral waveform. Fusion of waves IV and V is a normal waveform variant with conventional array recordings, but it is almost never observed with the contralateral array (Hughes, Fino, & Gagnon, 1981; Mizrahi, Maulsby, & Frost, 1983; Starr & Squires, 1982; Stockard, Stockard, & Sharbrough, 1978). Latency variability is reduced in part because wave V is more distinct. Latency can therefore be calculated more accurately for the contralateral array. The average intertrial difference in the wave I–V interval (an index of test–retest repeatability) is significantly less for contralateral (0.08 ms) than ipsilateral (0.30 ms) ABR recordings. Variations in ABR waveform morphology, and their potential influence on ABR analysis, are discussed further in the next chapter.

There are four additional noteworthy clinical implications of the differences between ABRs recorded with an ipsilateral versus contralateral electrode array. First, differences may vary somewhat as a function of stimulus polarity (rarefaction versus condensation), according to Hughes, Fino, and Gagnon (1981). The differential effects of polarity on ABR recordings for other electrode arrays have not been reported. Second, spectral composition of the ABR and the influence of filter settings is a factor in evaluating responses recorded with different electrode arrays. For example, wave I consists of relatively high-frequency energy, whereas wave V receives a greater contribution from lower frequencies. The differences in waveforms for ipsilateral versus contralateral electrode arrays might vary as a function of filter setting. Restricting the high-pass filter cutoff (e.g., from 30 to 300 Hz) would affect the wave V component, without having a serious effect on the earlier components recorded with the ipsilateral (earlobe) array. Conversely,

limiting the low pass setting—for example, a reduction from 3000 Hz to 1000 Hz—would exert a relatively greater influence on the early components (ipsilateral array) than wave V.

Third, longer latencies for wave II and shorter latencies for waves III and IV for the contralateral versus ipsilateral electrode arrays have been suggested as evidence that wave II arises from a structure(s) ipsilateral to the stimulus, and waves III and IV are generated from brainstem regions contralateral to the stimulus (Hashimoto, Ishiyama & Tozuka 1979; Hughes, Fino, & Gagnon, 1981; Kevanishvili & Aphonchenko, 1981; Oh, Kuba, & Soyer, 1981; Prasher & Gibson, 1980a). The value of ipsilateral versus contralateral recording in localizing ABR dipole sources and in identifying and lateralizing brainstem pathology is still unclear. Finally, the wave V/I amplitude ratio used clinically is actually a relationship between amplitude for a wave recorded by both vertex and mastoid electrodes (wave I) versus a wave recorded by only the vertex electrode (wave V). A more consistent ratio might be obtained with a vertex to noncephalic recording array. Finally, newborn infants typically have a well-formed ABR with the ipsilateral electrode array but little or no evidence of ABR activity with the contralateral array (e.g., Hall, 1992; Katbamma et al., 1993). Purposeful reliance on the contralateral electrode array for detection of ABR in infants, or inadvertent dependence on only the contralateral electrode array due to a technical mistake (stimulation of the wrong ear or analysis of the wrong electrode combination), can lead to gross misinterpretation of ABR findings. The most obvious and serious outcome would be a conclusion that the ABR is abnormally absent, when in fact it was entirely normal (Hall, 1992).

On the basis of observed differences in recordings for ipsilateral versus contralateral arrays, there is the possibility that the response for each array reflects activity within the brainstem on the side of the inverting electrode. That is, if the inverting electrode is active it detects the ABR in the ipsilateral array. However, it is now well established that responses are also recorded without an inverting electrode at the mastoid/earlobe site or anywhere on the head, and that the noninverting vertex electrode is definitely active with respect to brainstem auditory activity. Furthermore, the vertex electrode cannot distinguish between electrical activity arising from one side of the brainstem versus the other (Barratt, 1980; van Olphen, Rodenburg, & Vervey, 1978).

HORIZONTAL ELECTRODE ARRAY. | With this array, the noninverting electrode is typically located on the stimulus contralateral earlobe, mastoid, or ear canal while the inverting electrode site is the stimulus ipsilateral mastoid, earlobe, or ear canal (refer to Figure 6.9). Waveform components recorded with a reversal of the two electrode positions are reversed in polarity, but otherwise unchanged. The responses from individual electrode sites are isolated when recorded with an electrode at the side referenced to a noncephalic electrode, as described above.

When this is done for the two electrode sites in the horizontal array, waves I and III are negative in polarity at the ipsilateral mastoid and positive in polarity at the contralateral mastoid (Starr & Squires, 1982). The additive effect of the opposite polarity components is enhancement of amplitude. This is the basis of the somewhat greater amplitude for early components (I and III), sometimes noted with horizontal versus conventional ipsilateral electrode arrays.

Wave I is prominent in the horizontal recording, although in normal subjects not necessarily easier to define than with the conventional electrode array (Ruth, Hildebrand, & Cantrell, 1982). For patients with peripheral auditory pathology, the horizontal array may appear to provide an advantage in detection of wave I (Hall et al., 1984). Wave II and the following negative trough ("II neg") are not always clearly observed in the horizontal recording and when present typically have a shorter latency than when recorded conventionally. Theoretically, the horizontal electrode array is oriented in the same plane (parallel to) the dipole for wave III and, therefore, should yield greater amplitude for this component than the conventional or even noncephalic arrays, which have a more vertical orientation. In fact, wave III may have relatively larger amplitude when recorded with the horizontal electrode array than for other arrays, but it appears broadened, and latency is consistently longer. In the horizontal recording, the wave IV/V complex actually appears as a single component with a latency between that expected for waves IV and V and with reduced amplitude. Adult subjects often fail to show a true wave V with this array (Hall et al., 1984; Ruth, Hildebrand, & Cantrell, 1982; Starr & Squires, 1982).

The waveform recorded with the horizontal electrode array can also be derived by subtraction of the waveform for contralateral array from the waveform for the ipsilateral array, as depicted in Figure 6.11. These ipsilateral and contralateral electrode pairs form "diagonal" arrays, as seen before in Figure 6.8, which resemble the sides of a triangle. The base of the triangle is the horizontal electrode array. The subtraction process removes the contribution of the electrode shared by each diagonal array (the vertex or forehead electrode) leaving as noninverting and inverting electrodes the stimulus ipsilateral and stimulus contralateral electrodes from each array. This process is represented algebraically as follows:

$$(Fz + Ai) - (Fz + Ac) = Ai - Ac,$$

where Ai and Ac = the ipsilateral and contralateral earlobe electrodes respectively.

Evidence that subtraction of the contralateral from ipsilateral electrode arrays yields the equivalent of a horizontally recorded waveform is shown in Figure 6.11. That is, the actual and derived horizontal waveforms appear similar for normal subjects and patients with CNS pathology (head injury). Another subtraction process, this time of the real horizontal from the derived horizontal waveform (or vice versa) yields an essentially flat line. This confirms equivalency of the waveforms. The practical implication of this observation

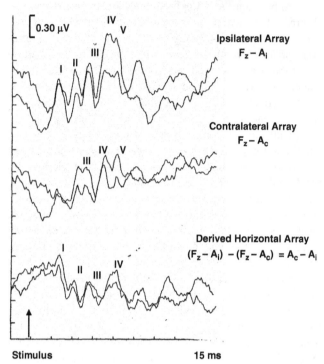

FIGURE 6.11. Derivation of a horizontal electrode array waveform by subtracting the waveform recorded with a contralateral array from a waveform recorded with an ipsilateral electrode array.

is that devoting an evoked response system channel to recording in the horizontal array is not necessary if the equipment has capacity for digital subtraction of waveforms and if ipsi- versus contralateral electrode arrays are used.

APPLICATIONS OF MULTIPLE ELECTRODE ABR RECORDING TECHNIQUES. | Which electrode arrays should be used? The conventional electrode array is relied on almost exclusively, perhaps because clinicians seem to be understandably reluctant to deviate from an ABR recording approach that yields adequate responses from many patients. There is a good argument for using the conventional electrode array, if ABRs are recorded for only one channel. Major components are usually observed, and the clinically important early waves (especially wave I) are enhanced because of the opposite phase relationship between inverting and noninverting electrodes. Since most evoked response systems have two-channel capacity, routine ABR recording simultaneously with two channels is clinically feasible and, it would appear, of clinical value.

What two channels should be used routinely in recording the ABR? Some authors have suggested the conventional electrode array plus a vertex (forehead) to noncephalic electrode array (Hughes, Fino, & Gagnon, 1981). Others propose, rather uniquely, that one channel be devoted to a vertex to noncephalic recording and the second channel to a horizontal array (Terkildsen & Osterhammel, 1981). A two-channel ipsi- versus contralateral recording protocol has also been recommended to facilitate identification of wave I (Hood & Berlin, 1987; Ruth, Hildebrand, & Cantrell, 1982; Stockard, Stockard, & Sharbrough, 1978). An added advantage of this latter two-channel recording technique is the possibility for deriving a horizontal waveform by subtracting the contralateral from the ipsilateral waveform, as just described.

MULTIPLE ELECTRODE ABR PATTERNS IN NEONATES. | The patterns of ABR waveforms recorded with multiple electrode techniques in adults are not necessarily characteristic of those found in infants (Hecox & Burkard, 1982; McPherson, Hirasugi, & Starr, 1985). Hecox and Burkard (1982) reported a statistically significant interaction among electrode array, ABR waveform, and age in the developing infant. Waveforms recorded with horizontal and with conventional (referred to by the authors as vertical) arrays were compared for infants less than 8 months of age versus adults. Wave I was equivalent for each array and each age group. As expected, adults showed a clear wave V for the conventional recording array but little or no wave V for the horizontal waveform. In contrast, infants showed a distinct wave V for the horizontal array that was, in fact, relatively greater in amplitude than for the conventional array. McPherson, Hirasugi, and Starr (1985) confirmed this observation and noted that wave V in the infant horizontal recording had a significantly shorter latency.

There is some evidence that infants yielding a well-formed ABR with the conventional (ipsilateral) recording array do not typically show a recognizable ABR waveform in the contralateral electrode array (Edwards, Buchwald, Tanguay, & Schwafel, 1982; McPherson, Hirasugi, & Starr, 1985), at least through wave V. Although McPherson, Hirasugi, and Starr (1985) did observe an apparent wave V in neonates with the contralateral recording array, its latency was significantly prolonged relative to the conventional waveform. Other investigators confirm that the contralateral ABR waveform recorded from newborn infants varies substantially in latency and amplitude from that of adults (Edwards et al., 1982). McPherson, Hirasugi, and Starr (1985) conducted one of the more comprehensive studies of multielectrode ABR recordings in adults versus neonates. As expected, wave component latency of all arrays was greater for neonates than for adults. Furthermore, latency differences in waves among the electrode arrays (i.e., conventional, contralateral, noncephalic, and horizontal arrays) were greater for neonates than adults. One finding with obvious clinical implications was that waveform morphology and component latency values were equivalent for a nasion to noncephalic versus a vertex (Cz) to noncephalic recording. With the nasion noninverting electrode site, morphology was somewhat more variable and the IV component and the following negative voltage trough were not consistently identified. The clinical practice of using forehead

(versus vertex) noninverting electrode placement for ABR assessment on neonates is apparently justified by these findings.

Another clinically relevant observation made by McPherson, Hirasugi, and Starr (1985) is their observation of additional or unusual components that defy traditional labeling in multielectrode waveforms from adults or neonates. These authors, for example, refer to component "x," which was seen between the usual waves I and II, and a "y" peak located between waves II and III. The "y" component appeared to obliterate the traditional wave II in the infant. Since the "y" peak was minimal in adults, the traditional wave II usually remained prominent. The "x" component similarly influenced adjacent traditional waves.

Averaging

Conventional (mean) averaging is invariably utilized clinical to extract and enhance auditory evoked responses embedded within background neurogenic and neurologic activity. Principles important in understanding signal averaging were discussed in Chapter 3. As noted by Özdamar and Kalayci (1999), "mean averaging assumes that recorded single sweep responses contain a stationary signal superimposed on a randomly occurring noise. Therefore, the synchronous summation of responses improves the signal component while reducing noise" (p. 253). Although conventional averaging clearly has stood the test of time as an effective technique, it is not without limitations. Over the years, the primary assumption of conventional averaging, namely, that in clinical settings with real patients the response remains constant and time locked to stimuli and noise is always "stationary and random" (e.g., Özdamar & Kalayci, 1999), has been repeatedly challenged by electrical engineers, physicists, and basic hearing scientists. Clinicians have also been well aware that a little substantial artifact during ABR measurement, perhaps due to brief and unexpected patient movement, can immediately contaminate minutes of good signal averaging, complicating or even precluding confident analysis of the waveform. As early as the 1980s, various innovative ABR measurement, processing, and analysis strategies were offered as alternatives to conventional averaging or improvements in signal averaging, among them weighted averaging, a Bayesian version of weighted averaging (Elberling & Wahlgreen, 1985), Wiener filtering (Doyle, 1975), adaptive filtering (Vaz & Thakor, 1989), and median averaging (Özdamar & Kalayci, 1999; Yabe, Saito, & Fukushima, 1993). Preliminary data on the latter approach to ABR acquisition—median averaging—was promising. Although findings were reported for only four normal-hearing adults, the technique was reportedly feasible, reliable, and less susceptible to the effects of extraneous (non-ABR) activity (artifact), especially for small numbers of sweeps (signal averages). Any novel signal-processing technique introduced for ABR measurement must undergo rigorous clinical trials by clinicians with diverse patient populations (patients with normal and abnormal auditory function from infancy to elderly adults) and in adverse test environments (e.g., NICU) before it can be considered a viable and better alternative to existing conventional signal averaging.

The person who is just beginning to record the ABR in a clinical setting often asks: "How much averaging is required in ABR measurement, or how many stimulus repetitions (sweeps) should I present before analyzing the ABR?" Evidence-based answers to that logical and very practical question are given at the end of this chapter, in the discussion of the ABR test protocol, and in the review of ABR in the auditory assessment of infants and young children in Chapter 8. The simple answer to the question is "the amount of averaging (the number of sweeps) that produces an adequate signal-to-noise ratio for confident identification of major ABR waves—no more and no less." Invariably using the same amount of signal averaging for all patients and under all measurement conditions is ineffective, inefficient, and often inadequate. For example, at a high intensity level with quiet normal-hearing persons, rigid reliance on 2,000 stimulus repetitions (sweeps) will waste valuable test time because the ABR will be clearly identified with one-tenth the number of stimulus presentations. Beattie, Zipp, Schaffer, & Silzel (1992) confirmed experimentally with ten normal-hearing adult subjects a high degree of confidence in identification of the ABR for 500 sweeps, with little or no change in the identifiability, reliability, latency, and amplitude of wave I, wave III, and wave V with further averaging. The unequivocal identification of major ABR waves with minimal signal averaging is readily apparent in Figure 6.12. Averaging beyond 250 to 500 sweeps for a high intensity level in a cooperative normal-hearing subject is a total waste of time. In the ABR assessment of auditory function in infants sleeping naturally, severely restricting unnecessary signal averaging to only the number of sweeps required to first detect the response will minimize test time. By limiting the amount of signal averaging to the bare minimum, but always replicating waveforms, the author can perform in less than 20 minutes of test time a combined neurological ABR analysis and frequency-specific estimation of auditory thresholds with ABR using click stimuli and tone bursts (at least 4000, 1000, and 500 Hz). In contrast, with stubborn adherence to a fixed number of sweeps (e.g., 2,000) and with no other changes in the test protocol, the total time required for the ABR assessment would exceed 40 minutes. Most unsedated children will grow restless and untestable before the 40-minute ABR is completed.

Filters

A review of the methodology of investigations reported in the literature attests to the diverse combinations of filter settings used clinically in ABR measurement. High-pass filter cut off frequencies ranging from 5 to 500 Hz, while low-pass filter frequencies from 1000 to 8000 Hz are reported. According to manufacturer recommendations in evoked response system manuals and these published reports, the largest propor-

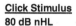

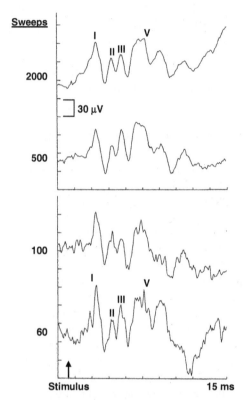

FIGURE 6.12. The influence of signal averaging, i.e., the number of stimulus repetitions or sweeps, on the ABR waveform for click stimulation at a high intensity level. The impact of signal averaging is generally more pronounced at low stimulus intensity levels.

tion of clinicians appear to record ABRs with settings of 100 or 150 Hz for high-pass and 1500 or 3000 Hz for low-pass filters. Less restricted settings of 10 or 30 to 3000 Hz are employed and strongly endorsed by a substantial minority of authors. Also, over the years there has been a trend toward more open settings, particularly for the low-frequency end of the spectrum, as investigators with accumulated clinical experience have come to appreciate the deleterious effects of restrictive filtering.

Beginning with the earliest papers on human ABR (Jewett & Williston, 1971), numerous reports have described effects of analog filtering (e.g., Boston & Ainslie, 1980; Cacace, Shy, & Satya-Murti, 1980; Doyle & Hyde, 1981a; Elberling, 1979; Hyde, 1985; Kevanishvili & Aphonchenko, 1979; Laukli & Mair, 1981; Osterhammel, 1981; Suzuki & Horiuchi, 1977). Results of these studies will now be briefly summarized. For illustrative purposes, ABR waveforms recorded simultaneously from a young normal subject for various combinations of high-pass and low-pass filter settings are depicted in Figure 6.13.

HIGH-PASS ANALOG FILTERING. | Changes in high-pass filter settings exert pronounced effects on the ABR. As the cutoff

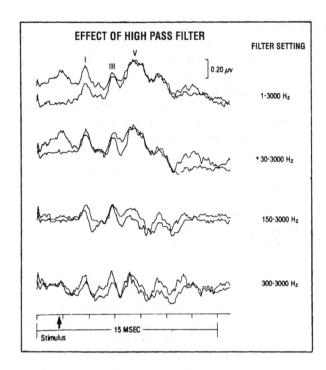

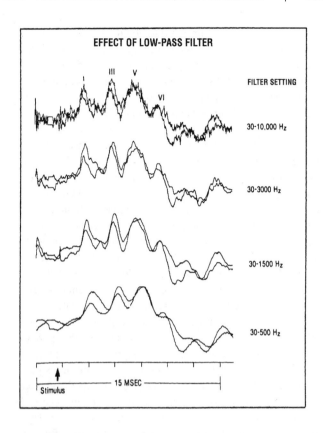

FIGURE 6.13. Waveforms recorded with various high- and low-pass filter settings from a normal adult subject.

is increased from a very low value (e.g., 0.05 Hz) up to a restricted setting of 500 Hz, ABR amplitude, especially for the wave V component, is reduced by up to about 50 percent and latency progressively decreases (Cacace, Shy, & Satya-Murti, 1980; Chiappa, Gladstone, & Young, 1979; Laukli & Mair, 1981; Stockard, Stockard, & Sharbrough, 1978). The latency decrease is attributed by Laukli and Mair (1981) to filter related deflection of wave peaks onto the following wave component, which results in an invalid calculation of waves latencies, i.e., too early. Latency distortion is usually greater for wave V than wave I. This is actually one of the complications of analog filter effects. Since different ABR peaks may receive different frequency contributions, they will often not be uniformly affected by conventional analog filtering. Filtering techniques that produce a phase shift that is linear across frequencies and the same for all peaks are suggested as a partial solution to this problem (Doyle & Hyde, 1981a). At least a constant phase correction could then be applied to compensate for the filter effect.

Amplitude changes are most pronounced as the high-pass filter cutoff is manipulated from 100 to 300 Hz. With this filtering, the slow-frequency component upon which the major waves (I, III, V) are superimposed is rejected, yet peak identification is not typically compromised for ABRs evoked by click stimuli and recorded from normal subjects. Complete loss of an ABR wave V may, however, result from increasing the high-pass filter cutoff (e.g., to 300 Hz or higher) when recording an ABR for low-frequency stimuli, such as 500 Hz tone bursts (Bauch, Rose, & Harner, 1980; Hyde, 1985; Kileny, 1981; Maurizi, Ottaviani, Paludetti, & Lunga-

rotti, 1986) or from neurologically impaired patients, particularly infants (Hall, Brown, & Mackey-Hargadine, 1985). An unrestricted high-pass filter setting (no higher than 30 Hz) is essential for consistent recording of the slow negative wave in the 10 ms region (SN10). Some investigators have applied the SN 10 component in frequency-specific ABR measurement of auditory threshold (e.g., Davis & Horsh, 1979). The SN10 is not apparent in waveforms recorded with high-pass filter settings of 150 or 300 Hz.

The effect of high-pass filtering is most pronounced for waveforms abnormally dominated by low-frequency energy. An ABR evoked by low-frequency tone-pip stimuli is one example of this type of waveform. Restrictive high-pass filter effects on ABR morphology have contributed to controversy regarding the clinical usefulness of tonal stimuli and differences between tonal and click-generated ABRs (Kileny, 1981; Maurizi, Paludetti, Ottaviani, & Rosignoli, 1984, 1986). Filter effects are generally negligible so long as the cutoff frequencies, particularly for high-pass filters, do not intrude on the ABR spectrum (Doyle & Hyde, 1981a; Kevanishvili & Aphonchenko, 1979; Osterhammel, 1981).

LOW-PASS ANALOG FILTERING. | The effects of changes in low-pass filter settings (Figure 6.13) have received relatively less research attention. In general, decreasing the cutoff frequency from a very high value (e.g., 10,000 Hz) to 3000 Hz actually eliminates noise and thereby enhances waveform analysis without distorting ABR latency or amplitude. This is not unexpected, since ABR contains virtually no spectral energy above 2000 Hz. Further reduction of the low-pass filter cutoff from 3000 to about 1500 Hz produces an increase in absolute latencies of major components (I, III, V) and produces a smoothing effect on the waveform. Sharp (high-frequency) peaks of ABR components are rounded off and the proportion of multipeaked or notched waves is reduced. Interwave latency values are not affected.

DIGITAL FILTERING. | Since 1980, investigators have endorsed routine clinical application of digital filtering (Domico & Kavanagh, 1986; Doyle & Hyde, 1981a,b; Fridman, John, Bergelson, Kaiser, & Baird, 1982; Møller, 1983). Digital filtering clearly improves detection of AERs in noise without the distortion of latency associated with analog (electronic) filtering. Now digital filtering is a feature of some commercially available evoked response systems. Among the advantages of setting a high-pass cutoff (of, for example, 100 Hz with 36 dB/octave slope) with digital filtering versus the conventional analog approach are reduction of baseline shift, electrical interference, and muscular artifact without corresponding amplitude reduction at low intensity levels or latency distortion. With most commercially available evoked response systems featuring digital filtering as a feature, however, the filtering is possible only offline, after the AER has been averaged and after artifact rejection. Before digital filtering becomes accepted clinically, instruments will need to be designed that permit online digital filtering during AER recording and before artifact rejection (Kavanagh, Domico, Franks, & Han, 1988). Other new and innovative processing strategies for improving the quality of AER recordings involve the development of amplifiers that can be located at the electrode site, rather than a meter or more away from the electrodes, and filter algorithms (e.g., Kelman filtering) that may offer important advantages for improving signal-to-noise ratio in clinical ABR measurement. These technologic advances in AER instrumentation and measurement were described in this Chapter 3.

RECOMMENDATIONS. | Although a high-pass filter setting of 100 or 150 Hz is suggested by some investigators (Ruth, Hildebrand, & Cantrell, 1982; Stockard, Stockard, & Sharbrough, 1978), a setting in the 10 to 50 Hz region is recommended for routine clinical applications, especially for threshold assessment and newborn auditory screening (Arlinger, 1981; Elberling, 1979; Hall, 1986; Kavanagh, Harker, & Tyler, 1984; Osterhammel, 1981; Schwartz & Berry, 1985). Low-frequency energy may not be vital for accurate interpretation of ABR in neurodiagnosis. Low stimulus intensity levels used in threshold assessment tend to shift the dominant ABR energy toward the lower end of the spectrum. Restrictive high-pass filtering for this application is therefore contraindicated (Elberling, 1979; Takagi, Suzuki, & Kobayashi, 1985). Low-pass filter setting should be no lower than 1500 Hz to produce clinically acceptable waveforms. A setting of 1500 Hz (versus a higher frequency) is clinically appealing because the major peaks in the waveform are often quite clean and relatively uncluttered by high-frequency energy. In comparison to a somewhat higher setting of 3000 Hz, however, the 1500 Hz limit

still imposes latency shifts (prolongations) on ABR components and may reduce accuracy of peak latency calculations. Under good recording conditions, then, a 3000 Hz low-pass filter cutoff frequency is probably preferable. A low-pass filter setting of 3000 Hz is therefore recommended (Laukli & Mair, 1981; Schwartz & Berry, 1985; Stockard, Stockard, & Sharbrough, 1978). A band-pass analog filter from 30 to 3000 Hz, then, will have negligible latency effects on ABR yet contribute to suppression of two major forms of measurement-related artifact (EEG and electromyogenic activity) in clinical ABR recordings.

A CLINICAL PROTOCOL FOR ABR MEASUREMENT

Findings of basic and applied ABR research accumulated over the past thirty-five years, in combination with clinical experience with literally millions of patients, provide clear guidelines for clinical test parameters and protocols. A protocol for clinical measurement of the ABR is displayed in Table 6.2. Several general comments regarding clinical protocols for ABR measurement are in order. The likelihood of recording an optimal ABR is highest with a well-proven protocol, and parameters must be manipulated during assessments to record the best possible response. A inflexible "cookbook" approach to ABR measurement, with rigid adherence to the same test parameters in every patient, simply doesn't work in the clinical setting. Unexpected patient findings and unpredictable test problems demand flexibility in the test protocol. The experienced clinician has the ability to recognize measurement problems and immediately implement adequate solutions and to modify the test protocol based on online analysis of findings. With this approach to ABR assessment, satisfactory and often optimal recordings are possible with most patients and in most test settings. At least nine test parameters must be selected by users of current evoked response systems, including stimulus type, polarity, intensity level, masking (and if so, the level and type), repetition rate, the number of repetitions (sweeps), filter settings (high- and low-pass filters), the analysis time (and the start time relative to the stimulus), and electrode sites.

Stimulus Parameters

Transducer options include earphones (insert or supraaural), bone oscillators, and loudspeakers. *Transducer type* is optional. Insert earphones are certainly not required, but the many advantages noted in Chapter 3 are all pertinent for evoking cochlear responses. The *type of stimulus* is also optional. Clicks are by far the most commonly reported stimulus for neurodiagnostic ABR assessment. Brief *stimulus duration* is essential for producing the synchronous firing of afferent auditory nerve fibers required for generating compound action potentials. However, the ABR can also be evoked effectively with tone-burst stimuli, as discussed more in Chapter 8. *Stimulus polarity* is in most patients not a critical parameter for ABR measurement. Stimulus polar-

TABLE 6.2.   Guidelines for a Test Protocol for Clinical Measurement of the Auditory Brainstem Response (ABR)

PARAMETER	SELECTION	RATIONALE/COMMENT
Stimulus Parameters		
Transducer	Insert earphone	There are a dozen good reasons (see Table 3.3)
		Bone conduction is also feasible
Type	Click	Optimal, but tone bursts also feasible (see Chapter 8)
Duration	0.1 ms (100 μs)	Best for transient (synchronous firing) onset
Polarity	Rarefaction	Larger amplitude and shorter latency than condensation
		Change polarity if waveform is suboptimal
Rate	> 20/sec, e.g., 27.3	Faster rate saves time
		Slow the rate as needed to enhance the response
		An odd number reduces chance of interaction with 60 Hz
	> 90/sec, e.g., 91.1	High rate may be increase likelihood of detecting retrocochlear dysfunction in neurodiagnostic ABR
Intensity	Variable in dB nHL	High for neurodiagnosis
		Perform latency–intensity function for threshold estimation
Repetitions	Variable	As many or few signal presentations as needed for an adequate signal-to-noise ratio (SNR)
		Repetitions are another term for sweeps (see below)
Masking	Rarely needed	Only if ABR is abnormal and no wave I is detected
Mode	Monaural	Ear-specific information is typically desired clinically
Acquisition Parameters		
Electrodes		
Noninverting	Fz	A high forehead site is preferred to the vertex
Inverting	Ai	Ipsilateral earlobe; a TIPtrode is sometimes indicated
Ground	Fpz	A low forehead site is convenient for the common electrode
Filters		
HP (high pass)	30 Hz	Low frequencies contribute importantly to the ABR, and are essential for detection of an ABR from infants
LP (low pass)	3000 Hz	1500 Hz if there is excessive high-frequency artifact
Notch	none	Avoid, as the notch removes important low-frequency energy in the ABR spectrum
Amplification	100,000	× 100,000 is equivalent to sensitivity of ± 25 or 50 μV
Analysis time	15 ms	Encompasses ABR in all cases (except low-frequency tone-burst signals)
Prestimulus baseline	−1 ms	Information on response quality
Sweeps (# stimuli)	Variable	Whatever is needed for good SNR

ity should be changed (e.g., from rarefaction to condensation) whenever the ABR waveform recorded is suboptimal. The overall objective in selecting stimulus repetition rate in ABR measurement is to present stimuli as fast as possible without affecting waveform quality or repeatability and the latency and amplitude of ABR components. For most patient populations, increasing stimulus rate up to 30 per second has minimal impact on ABR waveform. There is an interaction between stimulus rate and effective stimulus intensity. As the presentation of stimuli increases from a slow rate (e.g., 11/sec) to a very fast rate (e.g., 99/sec), the influence of temporal integration produces a decrease of about 10 dB SPL in behavioral threshold for the stimulus.

Acquisition Parameters

The number of electrodes and electrode locations in ABR measurement are rather straightforward, as reviewed in Chapter 3 and in this chapter. The *number of sweeps* required

in ABR measurement is highly dependent on the signal-to-noise ratio, on both the magnitude of ABR components and the amount of measurement noise arising from diverse sources (e.g., electrical, myogenic). As few as 100 to 200 sweeps are needed to detect an unequivocal response when a very large ABR is recorded from a normal-hearing and very quiet (e.g., sedated) patient at a high stimulus intensity level, whereas 2,000 or more sweeps might be needed to confidently detect an ABR for a restless patient, a patient with hearing impairment, and/or a stimulus intensity levels approaching auditory threshold. Filtering of electrophysiologic activity during ABR measurement is ongoing with analog filters within the hardware of the evoked response system, whereas digital filtering after data collection is now possible with evoked response software. Nonlinear filtering distorts the phase of ABR activity, producing latency changes (usually increases) in ABR components. Factors contributing to the amount of phase, or latency, distortion include the slope or rolloff per octave of the filter skirt.

ABR Analysis and Interpretation

Fundamental principles in AER identification, description, and measurement are summarized in Chapter 3. The reader with little or no experience in AER measurement is advised to first review this information. Most ABR waveforms are plotted in the time domain—that is, the amplitude of ABR components (almost always μvolt) is displayed over time (almost always in milliseconds, or ms). This is such a convention in ABR measurement that one might reasonably ask whether there is any other way a waveform can be displayed. There is another approach for describing ABR data. The ABR can be plotted also in the frequency domain, with amplitude (expressed in μvolts, μvolts^2, or dB), or phase (expressed in radians or degrees) displayed as a function of frequency (in Hz). Spectral composition of the ABR, the frequency response of the waveform, is revealed with this plotting approach.

In the time domain, ABR waveforms are, simply put, a sequence of peaks (amplitude of greater voltage) and valleys (amplitude of less voltage) occurring within a specific time period (the analysis period or epoch). Morphology of a waveform is the pattern or overall shape of these waves. Usually, morphology is described with reference to an expected normal appearance for the AER. For example, if an ABR waveform does not fit the clinician's expectation of normal appearance or two ABR waveforms recorded in sequence are not highly reliable, even though wave component latency and amplitude values may be within normal limits, morphology is often judged "poor." In routine clinical AER measurement, morphology currently remains a rather subjective analysis parameter.

Basic steps in ABR analysis are illustrated in Figure 7.1. Latency is the time interval between stimulus presentation, really the onset of the stimulus, and the appearance of a peak or valley in the ABR waveform. Latency of ABR waves is expressed in milliseconds (ms). Latencies calculated for any waveform depend on the analysis criterion used to precisely define each component, that is, where the peak is marked. Peak voltage (the very highest amplitude on the

wave) is used for some waves and by some clinicians. However, other clinicians do not always define ABR waves by the peak. Instead, some other portion of the wave, such as the shoulder, is used for selected components. Among audiologists, this is a common clinical practice for definition of ABR wave V. The ABR wave V often appears combined with ABR wave IV—the wave IV/V complex—and a clear peak is not apparent. In such cases, latency is calculated at toward the end of the combined wave IV and V complex. Latency is an *absolute* measure calculated from the stimulus onset to some point on or near the peak of an ABR component, as illustrated by the horizontal arrows in Figure 7.1. Interwave latencies are *relative* measures calculated as the time between two different ABR waves. As illustrated in Figure 7.1, latency intervals commonly calculated between waves include the wave I to wave III, the wave III to wave V, and the wave I to wave V latencies. Latency varies indirectly with stimulus intensity. That is, as stimulus intensity is decreased the absolute latency of ABR waves increases, and waves with relatively smaller amplitudes (e.g., wave I and wave III) gradually disappear. Each of these two trends is evident from the waveforms in Figure 7.1. Interwave latencies represent general indices of transmission times along the auditory pathways, from the eighth (auditory) nerve to the midbrain and beyond. Specifically, interwave latencies reflect delays associated with either axonal conduction time along neuron pathways and/or synaptic delay between neurons (e.g., Ponton, Moore, & Eggermont, 1996).

Amplitude is the second major response parameter typically analyzed. Although amplitude is usually described in μvolts, different techniques are used for calculating amplitude for ABR waves, sometimes within a single waveform. One common technique is measurement of the voltage difference between the peak and the preceding trough the peak of a wave. This is typically the approach used for determining amplitude for ABR wave I, as shown in Figure 7.1, and for wave III. Another clinically popular approach is calculation of the peak and following trough, typically used in determin-

ABR Waveform Analysis

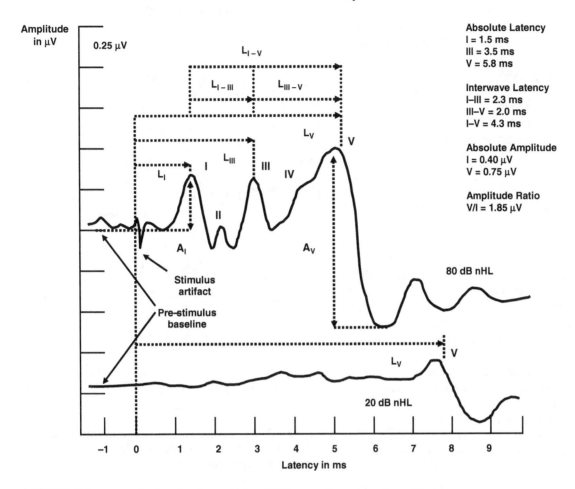

FIGURE 7.1. Steps in the simple analysis of ABR wave latency and amplitude.

ing wave V amplitude, also illustrated in Figure 7.1. A third approach, calculation of the difference in amplitude between peak voltage of the wave and some measure of a baseline voltage, is rarely applied in analysis of ABR waveforms. This approach is, however, commonly used in calculating the ratio of two wave components, such as the ratio of amplitude for the ECochG summating potential and action potential, or in calculating the absolute amplitudes of later latency auditory evoked responses, e.g., AMLR, ALR, and P300 response, as described in subsequent chapters. The most commonly calculated relative amplitude measure in ABR analysis is the wave V to wave I ratio. Normally the value is at least 1.0, or considerably larger (as shown in Figure 7.1).

A final fundamental concept in ABR waveform analysis is the direction of response polarity—that is, which way is up? Polarity of an ABR is dependent on the electrode location relative to the generator of the response and, of course, which electrode is plugged into the positive and negative voltage inputs of the differential amplifier. The clinician can record major waves of any ABR as negative or positive

in voltage depending on which electrodes are plugged into which amplifier inputs. For most ABR recordings, the electrode located at a high forehead (or vertex) site are plugged into the positive (noninverting) voltage input of the amplifier, and the electrode located near the ear (e.g., earlobe) is plugged into the negative (inverting) amplifier input. With this approach, the resulting, and familiar, ABR waveform is characterized by positive voltage peaks (e.g., wave I, wave III, and wave V) plotted upward and the negative voltage troughs plotted downward. This convention for plotting waveform polarity is not followed consistently, however, as some investigators in Canada, Scandinavia, Israel, and the United States (e.g., Picton, Terkildsen, Sohmer, and Møller, respectively) show these characteristic waves plotted "upside down," that is, with positive voltage downward.

One must keep in mind that the ABR waves do not adequately describe all underlying neurophysiologic activity produced by the stimulus. As emphasized in Chapter 2, the relation between ABR waves and anatomic generators is complex and not entirely understood. Electrodes located on the scalp and ear are insufficient to resolve all auditory regions (nerve pathways and nuclei) that are activated with acoustic stimulation, due to the inherent imprecision of far field evoked response measurements. Different ABR components, reflecting activity of different anatomic structures, may occur within a single ABR wave. In addition, there is variability in the temporal relation between ABR waves and the caudal-to-rostral arrangement of potential anatomic generators due to differences in the number of synapses and differences in direct versus indirect ascending pathways within the auditory brainstem.

CONVENTIONAL ABR WAVEFORM ANALYSIS

Nomenclature

Beginning with the first descriptions of the human ABR, independently by Jewett and Williston (1971) and Lev and Sohmer (1972), different schema have been used to denote wave components. Initially, wave components were labeled by Roman numerals, positive (P) and negative (N) voltage indicators plus Arabic numerals, and simply with Arabic numbers. There are inconsistencies, as noted above, in vertex polarity (negative or positive), and even in the sequence of wave components. For example, with the Roman numeral labeling system as introduced by Jewett and Williston (1971), vertex positive waves are plotted upward. However some investigators, as noted previously, display waves with Jewett Roman numeral labels and negativity plotted upward. As typically recorded, there is often no clear distinction between wave IV and wave V in the ABR waveform. Probably for this reason, some investigators (Lev & Sohmer, 1972; Thornton, 1975) have labeled the wave IV–V complex with the number 4 and have labeled what is conventionally referred to as wave VI with number 5 (or P5 or N5). In this book, nomenclature prevailing in the United States and most other countries will be used in description of ABR waveforms—namely, wave I through wave VII are labeled with Roman numerals, and voltage positive activity is plotted upward.

Normal Variations

There are myriad normal ABR variations. In fact, ABR waveforms among individuals are quite distinctive, much like fingerprints. That is, rarely are identical ABR waveforms recorded from any two persons. The normal variability in ABR morphology among subjects is illustrated in Figure 7.2. There may, in addition, be differences in waveforms between ears for a single person. ABR waveforms in multiple birth newborn infants (twins, triplets, quadruplets) may even have distinctly unique waveforms under the same recording conditions. Subtle differences in waveforms among patients are not important clinically, so long as there are clear and consistent criteria for distinguishing a normal response from

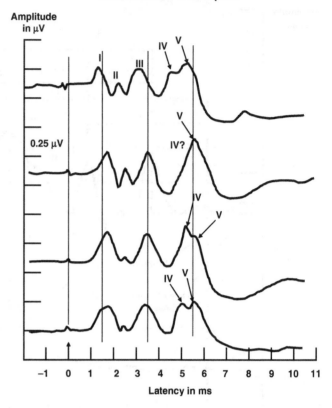

FIGURE 7.2. Examples of ABR waveforms recorded from normal subjects showing variations in the morphology (appearance), especially for wave V.

an abnormal response. As noted in the introduction to this chapter, latency and amplitude criteria are traditionally relied on in ABR analysis. Classification of waveforms is most straightforward when based only on the latency values for major components. The various ABR components are largely time-dependent, each occurring within a limited time period following the stimulus. Latency values are remarkably consistent among audiologically and neurologically normal persons. However, even a latency analysis approach becomes difficult when identification of components is obscured, either because of normal variability, poor reliability, or the effects of auditory pathology. ABR analysis based on response amplitude is often problematic because amplitude normally tends to be highly variable. Finally, due to normal variability in ABR waveforms, analysis of morphology (versus latency and amplitude) rarely permits confident differentiation of normal versus abnormal findings.

Response Reliability and Analysis Criteria

The "textbook" normal ABR has clear and repeatable wave components. Waves I through V are each unequivocally present in two or more repeated waveforms recorded with the same stimulus and acquisition parameters. Repeatability of at least two ABR waveforms recorded in succession with the same measurement conditions (e.g., stimulus with no change intensity, rate, and polarity in one ear) is a typical prerequisite for waveform analysis. An exception to this definition of and requirement for reliability occurs in pediatric applications of the ABR when waveforms are successively recorded at different intensity levels, and repeatability is determined for waveforms for two stimulus intensities. Strategies for ABR measurement in children, including details of response analysis, are reviewed in Chapter 8. Different terms are used to refer to consistency or repeatability in ABR waveform appearance and response parameters including reliability, reproducibility, and replication. The basic concept is simply that two or more averaged waveforms, when superimposed, are very similar. Ideally, the two waveforms are almost indistinguishable, except for slight differences in background activity or noise. In this case, even the inexperienced clinician can assess repeatability of the waveforms at a glance. As a rule, only waveforms (minimally two) that meet criteria for repeatability can be considered responses. While there are occasional exceptions to this policy, the clinician is well advised to routinely attempt replication of ABR waveforms. Put very simply, "If the waveform does not repeat, your ABR recording is not complete" or "If the waveforms do not replicate, you must investigate." No single factor contributes more to confidence and accuracy in ABR analysis than waveform repeatability, so every effort should be made to manipulate measurement conditions to, in turn, enhance the repeatability of ABR waveforms. Techniques for improving ABR morphology and repeatability and, specifically, ongoing manipulation of stimulus and acquisition parameters and sometimes subject status during ABR recording to optimize ABR waveforms, were reviewed in the previous chapter.

As Hoth (1986) points out, two sources of uncertainty in recording AERs are variability or error within the response and measurement variability or error. There is in AER measurement the assumption that the response is perfectly time-locked to the stimulus and background noise is minimal and "stationary," that is, randomly distributed (a Gaussian distribution). According to this assumption, sequential averaged waveforms will be essentially identical. Flaws in the assumption that AER recordings are invariability time-locked to stimuli are reviewed in some detail for the mismatch negativity (MMN) response in Chapter 14. For ABR recordings the assumption is often approached under optimal measurement conditions (e.g., ABR assessment of a very quiet normal subject at a high stimulus intensity level). Sources of variability in all AERs have been identified by accumulated clinical experience, along with systematic study of specific factors affecting measurement. Clinically, it is extremely difficult to analyze AER waveforms that are contaminated by excessive artifact. The presence of large amplitude, relatively low-frequency artifact, usually related to patient movement, may seriously interfere with, or preclude, accurate identification of AER components. During the course of a test session, at least in a relatively relaxed normal subject, muscle (electromyographic, or EMG) activity decreases significantly as signal averaging progresses. Since muscle activity is considered noise in an AER recording, it will decrease with increased averaging. The noise level in an evoked response recording is inversely proportional to the square root of the number of samples (stimulus repetitions or sweeps). Because the ABR signal-to-noise ratio is the magnitude of amplitude for ABR waves divided by the amount of noise during measurement, a reduction in noise with averaging will result in a larger signal-to-noise ratio (SNR). Small amplitude, high-frequency artifact, whether electrical or myogenic in origin, can interfere with precise estimation of the wave component peak and, therefore, influence accuracy of latency calculations (Ogleznev, Zaretsky, & Shesterikov, 1983).

Other sources of variability in AER measurement, in order of their importance, are differences in the responses between subjects, between ears, from one test session to another (separated by days or longer intervals), and from one run to the next. Response latency and amplitude may change also during extended test sessions, lasting hours. Poor reliability of response amplitude is a well-appreciated problem in AER measurement (Chiappa, Gladstone, & Young, 1979; Edwards, Buchwald, Tanguay, & Schwafel, 1982; Rowe, 1978). Amplitude is highly influenced by EEG activity level and muscle artifact, as well as by measurement parameters such as stimulus intensity and filter settings. Amplitude ratios of, for example, wave V/I, vary with subject characteristics and stimulus factors. Greater amplitude for wave I than for wave V (a small V/I ratio) may be a normal finding in young children (Gafni, Sohmer, Gross, Weizman, & Robinson, 1980). Immature neurological development, reflected by reduced synchronization of neural firing and incomplete myelinization, is suggested as a basis for this phenomenon (Gafni et al., 1980). A reduced wave V/I amplitude ratio may also be due to specific test conditions. An example would be the use of a TIPtrode electrode that enhances wave I amplitude without similarly affecting wave V amplitude.

A second source of uncertainty in AER analysis involves, in Hoth's (1986) words, the "measuring device." Clinically, this usually means the tester, including analysis criteria used by the tester. There are reports of high agreement between and within interpreters in ABR analysis. Two interpreters using common criteria will be consistent in judging an ABR as normal or abnormal in over 95 percent of cases (Rossman & Cashman, 1985) and a single interpreter will render the same judgment on repeated analysis of waveforms approximately 80 percent of the time (Kjaer, 1979). Interpreter agreement is decreased for waveforms that are less repeatable. Repeatability, in turn, tends to decline as hearing loss increases. Nonetheless, the experienced clinician with a good understanding of the impact on the ABR waveform of manipulation of measurement parameters will for the majority of patients succeed in recording repeatable waveforms.

Due to sources just noted, there are often obvious differences between sequentially recorded AER waveforms. Some criteria, therefore, must be employed for determining whether waveforms are indeed reliable (i.e., repeatable, replicated, or reproducible). A full description of criteria for determining reliability of waveforms would be very lengthy. This is, without doubt, an aspect of AER analysis that is most influenced by the clinician's experience. Methods for determining AER repeatability, or, conversely, sources of variability, have been the topic of systematic investigations, in part because they are essential for automated analysis of waveforms (Don, Elberling, & Waring, 1974; Edwards et al., 1982; Elberling & Don, 1984; Hoth, 1986; Mason, 1988; Schimmel, Rapin, & Cohen, 1975; Wong & Bickford, 1980). Automated AER analysis is reviewed later in this chapter. Furthermore, a discussion of techniques for enhancing the quality of ABR waveforms should logically be included in a review of analysis criteria. It is academic to debate whether techniques for waveform enhancement should be employed only after analysis criteria fail to confirm a repeatable response or whether optimal measurement conditions should first be attempted, and then the waveform analyzed. Clinically, one employs whatever test approach or strategy is necessary to arrive at confident interpretation of reliable and valid AER data.

How does a clinician know which wave component is which? That is, before the clinician closely analyzes latency and amplitude of, for example, wave V of the ABR, how can he or she be certain that it is wave V? For the "textbook normal" AER waveform, confident identification and preliminary analysis of each component is quite easy. Waves are clearly larger in amplitude than background noise in the waveform and labeled according to their sequence and approximate latency. Wave V, for example, is the fifth repeatable wave and has a latency that is within ±2.5 standard deviations of the average normal wave V latency value. Clinically, problems in wave identification can arise for a variety of reasons and occur singly or in combination. One or more of the wave components expected in the normal waveform may not be present. Amplitude of some presumed waves may barely exceed the amplitude of background activity present throughout the waveform, including a prestimulus baseline period. Some, or even none, of the waves may fall within expected latency regions. A special problem, stimulus artifact, may be encountered in identification of wave I. That is, a sequence of peaks are recorded within the latency period expected for wave I. These peaks may be very reproducible. Clearly, only one of these peaks can be wave I. It is risky, and possibly inaccurate, to simply select the peak among these that has the most typical wave I latency. There are numerous techniques for both enhancing the real wave I and also reducing stimulus-related artifact. Problems in wave identification and analysis, and potential solutions, are addressed later in this chapter.

A clinically useful criterion for reliability is a maximum limit on the acceptable time difference (in milliseconds) between latencies of peaks for the same wave component on two separate waveform averages or runs. This criterion may vary among wave components (for example, wave I versus V), or it may depend on response acquisition parameters (for example, the number of sample points or the rate of data sampling). One such criterion for wave V latency reliability is 0.2 ms. More strict reliability criteria (accepting less latency difference between waveform peaks) may be appropriate with certain measurement conditions, such as slow click rates and high intensity levels that usually produce more clear-cut responses. A problem exists with application of this peak-dependent approach clinically—namely, a wave component may be unequivocally present, yet latencies calculated for each run exceed the criterion limit because of morphologic variations. Such run-to-run differences may result from spontaneously occurring fluctuations in the number or shape of wave peaks in a subject (Edwards et al., 1982) or technical factors, such as earphone slippage or movement artifact.

Stockard, Stockard, and Sharbrough (1978) also addressed the question of how many waveforms should be averaged before a response is confidently analyzed. They employed a criterion for interwave latency values. To be considered a reliable response, wave I–III, III–V, and I–V latency differences between averaged waveforms (two separate runs) should not exceed 0.8 ms (80 μsec). Failure to meet this criterion requires a change in measurement conditions, such as increasing the stimulus intensity or inducing a more relaxed subject state. These authors provide a similar criterion for amplitude reliability. The wave V/I amplitude ratio differences between runs should not exceed 5 percent. Stockard, Stockard, and Sharbrough (1978) add that if waveforms meet these reliability criteria, then latency and amplitude values are calculated from the summation of the responses.

Calculation of a wave V to wave I (V/I) amplitude ratio is an attempt to limit the variability inherent in absolute amplitude measures. Amplitude ratio of ABR wave V/I was recommended by numerous early investigators of the ABR as a clinically useful parameter for analysis (Chiappa, Gladstone, & Young, 1979; Rowe, 1978; Starr & Achor, 1975; Stockard, Stockard, & Sharbrough, 1977). Actual criteria for abnormality vary, but a wave V/I ratio, for high intensity monaural click stimuli, of less than 0.5 (i.e., wave V is less than one-half as large as wave I) is a conservative lower normal cutoff (Starr & Achor, 1975). A wave V/I of less than 1.00, but greater that 0.5, is found in about 10 percent of normal subjects. Even this finding, in isolation, is not considered a strong ABR sign of auditory dysfunction by most authors.

Although infinite normal variations in ABR waveforms are possible, some normal patterns recur and can be categorized. These are now reviewed.

The Art of "Peak Picking"

"Picking the peak," that is, consistent and accurate selection of the single representative data point on a waveform that will be used in labeling the wave and calculating latency and amplitude values, is an important clinical skill. There are two fundamental approaches to this type of wave analysis, as illustrated in Figure 7.1. One is to select as the peak the point on wave component that produces the greatest amplitude. In waveforms with sharply peaked components, this selection is simple and unequivocal. Although intuitively appealing, this approach can present analysis problems. One problem occurs when the point of greatest amplitude clearly does not best represent the wave. Perhaps the most frequent example of this limitation, even in normal subjects, is found with patterns of the wave IV–V complex that do not have two actual peaks (i.e., one for wave IV and another for wave V). These patterns are illustrated further in the discussion on "Fused Peaks" on page 218. With a prominent wave IV and relatively minor wave V pattern, selecting the maximum amplitude as the peak essentially substitutes wave IV latency for wave V latency. The clinical consequences of this type of waveform misinterpretation would include calculation of an unusually short latency on the suspect ear, a significant interaural latency difference for wave V and the wave I–V latency interval, and possibly the presumption that the nonsuspect ear is abnormal.

Another problem with defining peaks on the basis of maximum amplitude arises when the top portion of the wave is rounded or even a plateau, rather than sharply peaked. This morphology may occur spontaneously, or it may be the result of a restricted low-pass filter setting. An apparent solution to this problem is to take as the peak the point at which lines extended from the two slopes of the wave intersect. Several disadvantages of the technique are readily evident. First, the point of intersection of the two lines does not correspond to an actual peak. Also, slight variations in either the leading or following slope may produce important variations in the arbitrarily defined "peak."

The second fundamental "peak picking" approach is to select the final data point on the waveform before the negative slope that follows the wave. This point may be the final peak, or a plateau or shoulder in the downward slope. This technique virtually eliminates the incorrect selection of wave IV versus V, but introduces its own problems. Some waves have multiple shoulders on the downward slope, caused by background activity. Other waves have shoulders that are extremely subtle and ill defined. The initial solution to these intricacies in waveform morphology, again, is to adhere to consistent analyses criteria. There is a one further complication in ABR peak peaking. A set of criteria may be legitimately used in analysis of some wave components within the waveform, but not for others. Thus, as seen in Figure 7.1, the maximum amplitude (midpoint) may be selected as the wave peak for certain components, such as wave I and wave III, while the shoulder is selected for other components.

Within a laboratory or clinical facility, this apparent complexity, confusion, and uncertainty in ABR interpretation can be minimized by specifying which of these two fundamental waveform analysis approaches—wave peaks or shoulders—must be applied with each major wave component by all persons interpreting ABR waveforms. And, as emphasized in the previous chapter, optimizing waveform morphology and repeatability during ABR recording by modifying the test protocol is very effective for minimizing confusion in ABR interpretation.

Extra Peaks

A normal variant in AER morphology is when selected peaks are reliably recorded, but smaller in amplitude, than the major components in an ABR waveform. Inspection of waveforms illustrated throughout this text will reveal numerous examples of extra peaks. Edwards et al. (1982) carefully tallied up the number of peaks occurring between major ABR waves in a group of 10 normal subjects. They consistently showed repeatable peaks between successive waves in the wave II through V region (between waves I and II, between waves II and III, and so on). Approximately 25 percent of the waveforms for the subjects in their study had one or more extra peaks. Extra peaks, especially in the early portions of ABR waveforms, may be partially related to the conventional high forehead-to-earlobe (or vertex-to-ipsilateral mastoid) electrode array used for ABR recording. McPherson et al. (1985) associated an extra component between waves I and II (referred to by them as "x") and another component between waves II and III (referred to as "y") when the ABR was recorded with an electrode on the mastoid ipsilateral to the stimulus. These extra components were most prominent in ABRs recorded from newborn infants (McPherson et al., 1985).

A *bifid* wave I component, that is, a wave I with two closely spaced peaks, is sometimes observed in ABR waveforms. The latency separation between the two peaks is generally less than 0.5 ms, thus ruling out the possibility that the second peak is actually wave II. Factors that may increase the likelihood of recording a bifid wave I component are high stimulus intensity level, mastoid or earlobe electrode site, and, possibly, stimulus polarity. Slightly different wave I latencies are sometimes recorded with rarefaction versus condensation clicks. With an alternating click stimulus in which theoretically each polarity contributes to the averaged response, a shorter latency peak in a bifid wave I may be generated by one polarity (most often rarefaction) while the second peak is generated by the opposite polarity (typically condensation). Chiappa, Gladstone, and Young (1979) similarly reported that 3 of their 52 normal subjects (5.8 percent) showed a bifid wave III component. Based on an inspection of ABR waveforms from one of these subjects, the wave III was generally poorly formed in comparison to wave V.

Ambiguities in accurate peak identification of wave V are, without doubt, the most common and most troublesome. Two such problems, the fusion of waves IV–V and the combination of a diminished wave V plus prominent wave VI, are addressed later in the chapter. Multiple-peaked wave V components present a third major problem. Typically, with this waveform variation there are two or more distinct peaks superimposed on a broad wave within the expected latency region for wave V. The problem is that selection of one of the peaks results in a normal interpretation while selection one or more of the other peaks yields an abnormal interpretation. The first step in solving this dilemma is application of consistent analysis criteria. For example, if the analysis convention for wave V is to calculate latency from the point of the shoulder preceding the large negative slope, then this criterion should be applied in analysis of the multiple-peaked component. This is a reiteration of the axiom stated above: The first principle of waveform analysis is to achieve repeatability of waveforms. Manipulations of stimulus and acquisition parameters are often very useful for resolving confusion in identification of the true wave V.

A related normal variation in ABR morphology is an unusually prominent wave VI that closely resembles the characteristic wave V. In some cases, wave V appears as a relatively minor hump on the initial slope leading to the wave VI, rather than a distinct wave component. The clinical problem presented by the prominent VI is similar to the bifid wave configuration just noted for waves I and III. If the earlier component is taken as wave V, the response is interpreted as normal, but if the apparent wave VI is reported as wave V then there is a markedly abnormal wave I to V latency interval. Minor extra peaks falling between major waves are curious, but not a concern or a factor in AER interpretation.

Fused Peaks

Fused peaks are, technically, two peaks combined into a single wave complex. Both peaks are distinct yet one of the peaks usually dominates. The peaks most often fused in normal ABR waveforms are IV and V (Chiappa, Gladstone, & Young, 1979; Rowe, 1978; Stockard & Rossiter, 1977). In these cases, wave IV usually appears as a hump or short plateau before wave V, or, conversely, wave IV is a distinct peak and is followed by a shoulder or plateau. Examples of these variations of the wave IV–V complex were illustrated in Figure 7.2. If there is single peak in the expected latency region for waves IV–V, it is typically labeled as wave V, and the wave IV is presumed missing. Wave IV is often not observed in normal ABR waveforms. Edwards et al. (1982), for example, found that about 50 percent of their subjects showed no wave IV. This was a consistent finding within subjects. That is, waveforms for selected subjects showed a clear wave IV and V on some runs and did not on others. Chiappa, Gladstone, and Young (1979) provided a thorough discussion of normal wave IV–V relationships and delineated six patterns for this wave complex. Examples of normal variations in wave IV and wave V patterns were shown in Figure 7.2. Fusion of waves IV and V is more likely in cochlear pathology (Borg & Löfquist, 1982) than in normal hearers.

Stimulus and acquisition parameters also influence fusion of ABR waves. Stimulus polarity can cause changes in wave component latency. Because wave V latency may be different for rarefaction versus condensation stimuli, configuration of the wave IV/V complex may vary with polarity (Borg & Lövquist, 1982). Electrode array, which exerts a very prominent effect on waveform morphology, is discussed separately in a following section. There is some evidence, at least in normal adult subjects, that differentiation of wave IV versus wave V is poorer (a fused complex is more likely) when high-pass filter settings are extended below 150 Hz. Put another way, raising the high-pass setting from 5 or 30 Hz to about 150 Hz appears to resolve separate waves IV and V (McPherson, Hirasugi, & Starr, 1985). This strategy for resolution of the wave IV and wave V complex is, however, not advisable with infants because the ABR is dominated by low-frequency energy. Increasing the high-pass filter setting for infants will reduce ABR amplitude and, in some cases, may remove the response itself.

Missing Peaks

Peaks often missing in normal ABR waveforms include wave IV, as just noted, and waves II and VI. These patterns are illustrated in Figure 7.3. In waveform "A," waves I, III, and V are repeatable and well formed. Absolute and interwave latency values are within normal limits. Amplitude of each of these components is also within normal expectations (note

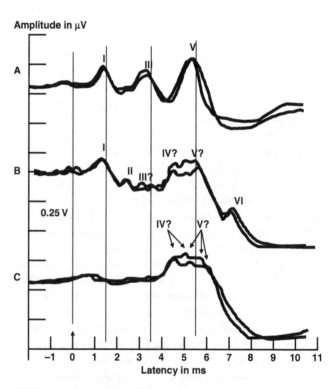

FIGURE 7.3. ABR patterns with missing waves.

the amplitude marking of 0.25 μv in the figure) and in the proper relationship (wave V/I amplitude ratio is greater than 1.00). By conventional latency and amplitude criteria, this can be classified as a normal ABR. There is no evidence, however, of waves II, IV, or VI. Waveform "B" shows a distinct wave I and a wave IV–V complex and also evidence of waves II and VI. There is a small deflection in the ABR waveform in the wave III latency region, but it is no larger in amplitude than the background activity observed elsewhere in the waveform. The wave IV–V complex, in contrast to the pattern in waveform "A," is not sharply peaked but, rather, consists of multiple minor humps. At least three different sites on the wave could be selected for latency calculation, including the peak, a slight shoulder following the peak, and a repeatable small plateau on the slope after the peak. Waveform "C," also recorded from a normal-hearing subject, has only a clear wave V. Even a wave I is not observed. Again, even for the presumed wave V, latency could be calculated from one of several peaks, depending on which sweep (run) was used or from a shoulder following these peaks. As noted above, well-defined criteria for "peak picking" are required for consistency in ABR interpretation of these types of waveform. Such criteria include both consistency between clinicians and consistency for a single clinician for ABR interpretation among patients, or even from one ear to the other. In waveform "C," there appears to be a wave I, wave II, and wave III, but they are not reliably recorded.

Although each waveform in Figure 7.3 serves to illustrate a problem of missing waves, the examples also suggest another facet of ABR recording. When selected waveform components differ markedly in amplitude, the level of background activity during recording differentially affects the components and the number of sweeps used to average the waveform. For waveforms "B" and "C," it is likely that waves I, II, and III, at the least, would have clearly emerged with additional averaging or more quiet recording conditions. High-frequency background activity obscures a possible wave III in "B" while in "C" considerable lower frequency artifact (perhaps movement-related), which is evident in the prestimulus baseline period, precludes identification of early waves (I, II, and III).

Kjaer (1980) reported that one or more of these ABR waves (II, III, IV, VI) were not identified for up to 6 percent of 40 normal subjects between the ages of 13 and 48 years. Some clinicians would maintain that, by definition, absence of waves I or V implies an abnormality. Whether an absent wave III yet a normal wave I-to-V latency interval, is normal or abnormal is debated. On the one hand, some authors describe wave III latency as very stable (Edwards et al., 1982; Kjaer, 1980). However, clinical experience shows that wave III is occasionally absent in normal subjects. Before reaching this conclusion, one must carefully determine that subjects are normal audiologically and neurologically. Relatively minor peripheral hearing deficits in the high-frequency region, including interoctave audiometric test frequencies

(3000 and 6000 Hz) and other frequencies in that region, can influence ABR waveform morphology. Without careful audiometric assessment, this factor in ABR interpretation may go undetected. Missing peaks for waves II, III, and IV are not unexpected in some otherwise normal subjects, such as newborn infants.

The Wave I–V Latency Interval

The latency intervals between wave components (I–III, III–V and I–V) are relied on extensively in clinical application of the ABR Interwave latencies are often referred to as an index of "brainstem transmission time (BTT)" or "central conduction time" (Elidan, Sohmer, Gafni, & Kahana, 1982; Fabiani, Sohmer, Tait, Gafni, & Kinarti, 1979). Interwave latencies may also be described as interpeak latencies, abbreviated IPLs. This concept is probably valid for some nonauditory sensory evoked responses, such as the somatosensory evoked response, because latency of the peripheral component or time marker (Erb's point potential) is essentially invariant, except for predictable effects of stimulus intensity, the subject's physical dimensions, and the subject's age. For a variety of reasons, ABR interwave latency values are not a pure or consistently accurate measure of neural transmission through the auditory brainstem. Factors influencing the wave I–V latency interval may be related to stimulus and acquisition parameters and to peripheral and central auditory dysfunction. For accurate interpretation of ABR interwave latency data in neurodiagnostic assessment, it is very important to consider such factors. As an example, calculations of I–V latency may, in part, be affected by changes in wave V morphology as a function of stimulus rate in certain populations. In a study of neonatal ABRs, Lasky (1984) noted that there was no difference between wave V latencies calculated from the peak versus shoulder at slow repetition rates, but for fast rates wave V latency was considerably longer when determined from the shoulder. Discrepancies among studies of ABR and rate may in part be attributed to such differences in response analysis technique.

Electrode Arrays

The electrode array used in ABR recording is an important measurement parameter to consider in waveform analysis. Electrode options, locations, and arrays were introduced in Chapter 3, and the rather extensive literature on this topic was reviewed in the previous Chapter 6.

ABNORMAL ABR PATTERNS

There is virtually no limit to the ways that ABR waveforms can be altered in pathology of the peripheral and/or central auditory system. Whereas normal variations are typically rather subtle, abnormal ABR findings range from subtle latency aberrations to total absence of a detectable response. Naturally, ABR abnormalities are not mutually exclusive—that is, waveforms recorded in a test session from a single patient may demonstrate a variety of abnormalities. Furthermore, with certain ABR clinical applications, such as intensive care unit or operating room monitoring, ABR abnormalities may be highly dynamic, varying from day to day or moment to moment. Various schema for categorizing abnormalities have been described for the purpose of discussing patient findings and providing instruction in ABR interpretation (Chiappa, 1983; Jacobson, 1985; Starr & Achor, 1975; Stockard, Stockard, & Sharbrough, 1980). Without exception, these techniques for categorizing waveforms rely on analysis of response component latency and, to a lesser extent, amplitude. Since these techniques are currently not applied routinely in clinical settings, the following discussion will be limited to conventional latency and amplitude analysis. A danger in any attempt to categorize or grade AER abnormalities is that description of severity or extent of abnormality becomes diluted. That is, distinct differences in waveforms between or among patients, which may have clinical significance, can be lost within any one category. The clinician must always maintain a flexible and open-minded approach in interpreting ABR waveforms, considering both obvious abnormalities and more subtle alterations. The following discussion is presented with this limitation in mind.

Abnormalities in Absolute Latency Patterns

The most common absolute latency abnormality is a delay in wave I, plus an equivalent delay in subsequent wave components. In combination, this pattern implies peripheral auditory dysfunction. Slightly increased wave I latency suggests a high-frequency sensory (cochlear) deficit. For sensory deficits that are moderate to severe or more serious (greater than 50 dB in the 1000 to 4000 Hz region), however, there may be no detectable wave I with the conventional electrode array. A substantial wave I delay is a characteristic finding in conductive or mixed (middle ear) deficits. A wave I may be recorded even in maximum conductive hearing losses (60 dB or more), in contrast to sensory hearing impairment that has a more pronounced effect on the morphology and even presence of wave I. There are, of course, exceptions to these general patterns for ABR absolute latency, such as extremely delayed wave I latency in patients with normal middle ear function or, conversely, a normal or even slightly shortened wave I latency in some sensory hearing loss configurations.

Absolute ABR latency is also greatly affected by subject characteristics and stimulus/acquisition parameters, even in persons with normal auditory functioning. These factors must be known for meaningful interpretation of an ABR waveform. For example, before interpreting absolute or interwave latencies, the clinician must know the age and gender of the patient and take into account stimulus characteristics and acquisition parameters.

Abnormalities in Relative (Interwave) Latency Patterns

Selected abnormal ABR waveforms, based on latency criteria or obvious changes in waveform morphology, are displayed in Figure 7.4. Each waveform, including a normal waveform ("A") shown for comparison, was recorded with the same stimulus and acquisition parameters. Stimuli were 0.1 ms clicks, of alternating polarity, presented at a rate of 21.1/sec and an intensity level of 85 dB nHL monaurally via ER-3A insert earphones. The response was recorded with an analysis time of 15 ms and a 10 percent prestimulus baseline period. The ABR activity was detected with an Fz-to-Ai (ipsilateral earlobe) electrode array, amplified X100,000, and filtered with settings of 30 Hz to 3000 Hz (6 dB/octave). Depicted in Figure 7.4 are ABR waveforms recorded with a scale of 0.15 μvolt (noted at the top of the figure). Interwave (I–III, III–V, and I–V) latency values are indicated on the right portion of the figure. For a group of young adults (males and females) and the above-noted measurement parameters, upper limits (+2.5 standard deviations) of the normal range for these measures are: I–III, 2.55 ms; III–V, 2.40 ms; I–V, 4.60 ms. These seven waveforms, of course, only represent a sample of the myriad abnormal patterns that may be encountered clinically.

In waveform B, both the wave I–III and the III–V latency intervals are within normal limits yet the wave I–V latency interval is prolonged slightly beyond normal limits. In such cases, precise definition of wave peaks and calculation of wave latency values is essential. A minor inconsistency or error in calculation of wave latency could easily mean the difference between a normal and abnormal interpretation. Before classifying a slight overall interwave latency prolongation like this as abnormal, especially if the finding was bilateral, it would be important to have some information about the patient. Given the expected effects of age and gender, for example, this slight latency prolongation would be of more concern if recorded from a young female than from an older male. This waveform, if bilaterally symmetrical, would be considered normal if recorded from an infant. Likewise, if there were even mild hypothermia (one or two degrees below normal body temperature of 37° centigrade), this latency prolongation might not be viewed as abnormal.

Waveform C (see Figure 7.4) is a "textbook" example of a delay in the wave I–III latency interval. Identification of major peaks and calculation of the abnormal latency prolongation are unequivocal. The wave I–III latency delay, as expected, contributes to a wave I–V latency abnormality. If this abnormality were unilateral, it would be a characteristic ABR reflection of tumor-related auditory dysfunction in the region of the eighth cranial nerve and lower brainstem (the cerebellopontine angle). Bilateral ABR I–III latency

Abnormal ABR Patterns Based on Analysis of
Latency, Amplitude, and/or Morphology

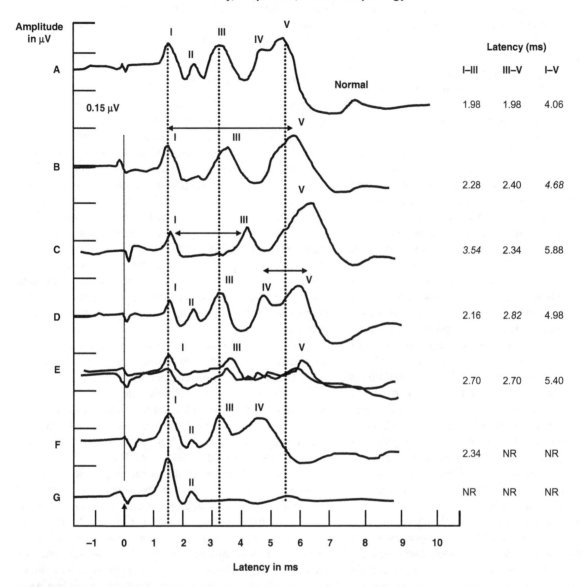

	Latency (ms)		
	I–III	III–V	I–V
A	1.98	1.98	4.06
B	2.28	2.40	*4.68*
C	*3.54*	2.34	5.88
D	2.16	*2.82*	4.98
E	2.70	2.70	5.40
F	2.34	NR	NR
G	NR	NR	NR

FIGURE 7.4. Examples of seven ABR waveforms with different patterns of morphology, ranging from normal (waveform A) to markedly abnormal (waveform G). Each waveform is described in the text.

prolongation is consistent with brainstem (pons) dysfunction or, less often, bilateral eighth nerve dysfunction, as found in neurofibromatosis I or in von Recklinghausen's disease. More precise localization of the site of dysfunction would be possible wave I–II, and wave II to III latency intervals could be determined.

The III–V latency interval is abnormally prolonged in waveform D, even though all components from wave I through V are reliably recorded and well formed. Notice that the prolongation is mainly due to an extended wave IV to V latency separation. This finding suggests a rostral brainstem (pons-midbrain) auditory dysfunction. It is often bilateral. If

observed in a patient with hydrocephalus, increased intracranial pressure, or other dynamic neuropathology, the wave III–V delay would indicate supra-tentorial compression of the upper brainstem, a very serious finding.

Waveform E (Figure 7.4) shows markedly abnormal interwave latencies and, in addition, generally poor morphology. The prestimulus baseline period suggests relatively stable background activity. Poor repeatability of subsequent (poststimulus) activity may, therefore, reflect asynchronous neural function and neuropathology. As with waveform B, other factors must be considered. The magnitude of the latency delay cannot be accounted for by subject age and gender factors, but documentation of body temperature in a seriously ill patient would be necessary to properly interpret the ABR. An overall latency delay, particularly if recorded bilaterally, confirms significant auditory brainstem dysfunction, but does not contribute to further localization of the pathology. In an apparently healthy person, multiple sclerosis would be a possible explanation for this ABR finding.

The sequence of waves seen in waveform F (Figure 7.4) is quite unusual. Measurement conditions appear excellent. There is minimal background activity in the ABR waveform, implying electrical and movement artifact are not a problem. A well-formed wave I confirms adequate peripheral auditory functioning. Distinct waves III, IV, and V are not observed. Rather, a poorly formed wave III–IV complex is present. The latency interval between wave I and the final peak in this complex is only 3.78 ms, and the wave III to IV/V complex is just over 1 ms. Here, again, information on subject characteristics is helpful for confident interpretation of the response. One must conclude that wave V is missing.

Bilateral waveforms characterized by only wave I and wave II, with no subsequent components (waveform G in Figure 7.4) are invariably a sign of severe brainstem dysfunction. The presence of clear waves I and II rules out serious peripheral auditory deficit. In most unconscious adult patients, the finding of only an ABR wave I and II bilaterally is incompatible with survival. Patient medical status is important for interpretation of this finding. If the patient is alert and oriented, a demyelinating disease (e.g., multiple sclerosis) affecting the brainstem might be suspected. If this pattern is observed unilaterally, with a normal response on the opposite side, it is most consistent with cerebellopontine angle pathology. When recorded in infants, the pattern may reflect severe hypoxic-ischemic brain insult and is not always consistent with brain death.

There are numerous and varied possible explanations for the total absence of an ABR. Initially, it is important to rule out technical problems (inadequate stimulus, improper electrode pairs, and so forth). The most obvious explanation for an absent response is a severe-to-profound hearing impairment. This conclusion can be confirmed in some patients by other auditory measures (impedance or behavioral audiometry). Infrequently, patients with no apparent ABR will have evidence of longer latency AERs. Pathology producing desynchronous neural dysfunction can produce an absent ABR yet not seriously affect these later AERs. As early as 1980, some authors, furthermore, describe the finding of no detectable ABR despite neurologic and apparent audiologic integrity (Worthington & Peters, 1980). This pattern would now be referred to as auditory neuropathy (see Chapters 5 and 9).

Fowler and Noffsinger (1983) describe the proportion of subjects showing identifiable waves I, III, and V among groups (N = 14 each) of normal hearers, cochlear-impaired patients, and patients with retrocochlear (eighth nerve and/or brainstem) lesions. Normal hearers were more likely to have a wave I component than subjects in the other two groups.

Waves III and V were more often identified in the normal-hearing and cochlear-impaired subjects than those with retrocochlear lesions. Although wave I latency was equivalent among groups, wave V latency was, as expected, significantly greater for patients with retrocochlear pathology.

Abnormal Amplitude Patterns

As noted above, ABR amplitude is generally more variable and more susceptible to the effects of movement artifact and fluctuations in background EEG activity than latency. Because of these characteristics, it is often difficult to determine with confidence whether a patient's ABR amplitude value is within the expected normal range or outside of this range. Absolute amplitude of each ABR component is typically so variable that defining the normal range as ±2.5 standard deviations around the average normal value encompasses virtually any amplitude value that will be recorded clinically, from normal subjects or patients with confirmed auditory pathology. This is obviously a serious clinical limitation, since general neurophysiology principles would suggest that amplitude offers information on auditory function not available from latency.

In an attempt to account for the inherent variability of amplitude and extract from it some clinically meaningful information, many investigators have relied on an analysis of the ratio of wave V/I amplitude. The wave V/I amplitude ratio was noted above. The amplitude ratio (wave V and wave I are from the same waveform) is calculated only after waveforms have met criteria for reliability. Actually, some investigators (Stockard, Stockard, & Sharbrough, 1978) include as a criterion for reliability the amplitude difference between two successive ABR averaged waveforms. There is general consensus that an amplitude ratio of less than 0.5 is abnormal. That is, wave V amplitude is unusually small, less than one-half of wave I amplitude. Normally, wave V is from one to two times larger than wave I. Even this ABR analysis technique is not without constraints. A major limitation, of course, is that not all ABR waveforms include a clear wave I. Also, the ratio may be abnormally reduced when wave I is unusually large, even if wave V amplitude is at expected amplitude. Also, it technically does not fulfill conventional criteria for a reduced wave V/I amplitude ratio. That is, the waveform is characterized by a small wave V relative to a normal-sized wave I. The pattern may, however, be found in infants and adults with varied neuropathology. Recall that inverting electrode types that enhance wave I will normally produce a decreased wave V/I amplitude ratio.

Figure 7.5 shows ABR waveforms typically recorded from patients with specific pathologies. A normal ABR waveform (A) is presented as a reference for expected or optimal ABR latency, amplitude, and morphology. An ABR from a person with conductive hearing loss is represented in waveform B. Waveform morphology is good, with a high degree of reliability for each ABR component including wave I. The

**Normal and Abnormal ABR Waveform Patterns
(Stimulus intensity = 80 dB nHL)**

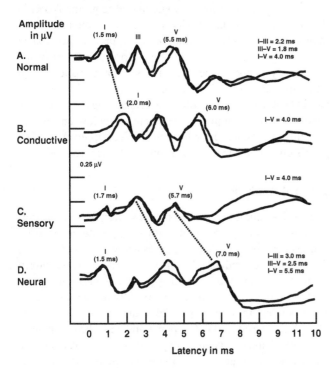

FIGURE 7.5. A normal auditory brainstem response (ABR) waveform and waveforms representing three different types of hearing loss, i.e., conductive, sensory (cochlear), and neural (retrocochlear).

distinctive feature is a delay in the absolute latency for each of the ABR waves, beginning with wave I. Interwave latency values are well within normal limits. The conductive hearing loss effectively reduces stimulus intensity level reaching the cochlea. The waveform resembles a normal ABR evoked by a stimulus after the intensity level has been reduced, in this case by the degree of the conductive hearing loss component. However, once the stimulus reaches the normal cochlea, a normal-appearing ABR is generated.

A high-frequency sensory (cochlear) hearing loss is represented by waveform C. The characteristic features of the ABR for sensory hearing loss include a small and poorly formed wave I component, slightly delayed in latency. Interwave latency values, however, are within normal limits. As stimulus intensity level is decreased, wave I disappears. Then, as the click-stimulus intensity level approaches auditory threshold within the 1000 to 4000 Hz region, wave V latency increases sharply. Waveform D is a classic example of a retrocochlear pathology in the cerebellopontine angle, e.g., an acoustic tumor. Wave I is clearly present and of normal latency. The most obvious abnormality is a delay in the latency between wave I and wave III, i.e., the response parameter reflecting transmission of the auditory signal along the eighth cranial nerve from the cochlea to the lower brainstem.

A useful adjunct to the visual inspection in ABR analysis is the examination of the latency–intensity function for ABR wave V in comparison to the audiogram. The general categories of latency–intensity functions in normal hearing, conductive hearing loss, and sensory hearing loss are illustrated in Figure 7.6. Published clinical experience confirms the complexity of the relationship between ABR latency and auditory dysfunction. The patterns shown in Figure 7.6 are certainly not invariant. Other ABR findings in various auditory and central nervous system disorders, including conductive hearing loss, sensory hearing loss, retrocochlear auditory dysfunction, and brainstem pathology affecting the auditory system, are presented and discussed in Chapters 9 and 10.

OTHER ABR ANALYSIS TECHNIQUES

Although relatively simple calculation of ABR component latency and amplitude, as reviewed above, is relied on almost exclusively in clinical applications, there are a wide range of more sophisticated techniques for AER analysis. With advances in evoked response instrumentation, one would

**ABR Wave V Latency Intensity Function in
Conductive versus Sensory Hearing Loss**

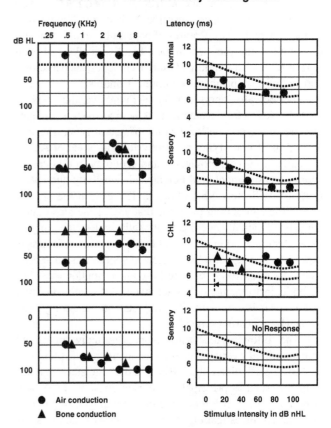

FIGURE 7.6. ABR latency-intensity functions associated with audiograms representing conductive and sensory hearing loss.

expect that these sophisticated analysis techniques would be applied in clinical ABR measurement (Hall & Rupp, 1997). Multidimensional analysis, measurement of area under the curve, principal component analysis, and, in general, systematic investigation of multivariate approaches for quantitative analysis of event-related auditory evoked responses date back to at least the 1960s (e.g., see Donchin, 1966, 1969; Donchin & Heffley, 1978, for reviews). The motivation for extending AER analysis beyond simple visual inspection of the waveform then, as now, was to develop a more refined, sensitive, objective, and precise index for assessing the deviations of waveforms from normal expectations. To be sure, mathematically and statistically based strategies are now utilized in analysis of the ASSR—a response closely related to the ABR—and of cortical evoked responses, such as the MMN response. In general, however, ABR analysis in the typical clinical setting remains dependent almost entirely on manual calculations of two simple response parameters in the time domain, namely, latency and amplitude.

Three rather sophisticated techniques applied in ABR analysis are spectral analysis, multidimensional analysis, specifically with three-channel Lissajous trajectory (3CLT) techniques, and automated data collection/analysis (machine scoring) of responses. Also, topographic mapping of with multiple electrode arrays is commonly done with cortical evoked responses, e.g., the AMLR, ALR, and P300 evoked response. Recent papers describe ABR dipole localization methods, which share features of both multidimensional and topographic analyses techniques. Finally, analysis of each type of AER with a variety of other techniques, such as cross-correlation and principal component analysis (PCA), has been periodically reported in the literature over the years.

Motivation for development of these analysis techniques includes more precise localization of neural generators and definition of underlying neurophysiologic bases of AERs, increased accuracy, efficiency, and economy in clinical response measurement, and heightened sensitivity and specificity of AERs to CNS pathology. There is, at the present time, little compelling evidence that any of the techniques, applied individually or collectively, fully achieve these objectives. Documentation of clinical feasibility and usefulness is especially needed. However, selected approaches have been adapted successfully for specific clinical applications. For example, instrumentation for automated ABR data collection and analysis is commercially available and commonly used for newborn hearing screening.

The following discussion is an admittedly superficial and simplified overview of selected techniques for analysis of AERs, particularly the ABR. Multivariate statistical approaches, such as principal component analysis (PCA) and cross-correlation averaging, are only mentioned in passing, even though investigation of their uses in AER analysis has continued for about thirty years. Due to advances in computer technology, increased clinical application of such mathematical and computer-intensive techniques is now

feasible. The Fsp technique (e.g., Don, Elberling, & Waring, 1984; Elberling & Don, 1984, 1987) for verifying the presence of an electrophysiologic signal (e.g., the ABR) in the midst of nonsignal activity (e.g., noise) is the most common statistical analysis technique incorporated into clinical evoked response systems and clinical practice. Most of the other analysis approaches have not yet made the leap from laboratory to clinic. Reference to additional information would be essential for adequate understanding of most of the sophisticated techniques to be discussed below and would certainly be needed prior to their clinical application. The papers cited in the text are one source of this information.

Spectral Analysis

The earliest studies of evoked response frequency (spectral) composition were carried out with steady-state, as opposed to transient, visual evoked responses and were based on Fourier analysis techniques (Regan, 1966). The ABR waveform elicited by a series of repetitive stimuli is periodic, or repetitive, and composed of one and usually more frequencies, corresponding in some way to the frequency of the stimulus. The ASSR, introduced in Chapter 1 and described with more detail in Chapter 8, is an example of this type of response. By means of Fourier analysis, these discrete frequencies contributing to the steady-state response can be identified, verified statistically, and quantified. That is, the amplitude (or strength) of each frequency in the response is determined. The phase of each frequency can also be calculated. Within recent years, there has been renewed interest in Fourier analysis of auditory steady-state responses (ASSRs). Indeed, frequency and phase analysis is, as reviewed in Chapter 8, a common approach with the ASSR.

Most AERs are typically generated with a transient or very brief stimulus. The response is aperiodic. That is, it is not repetitive but, rather, one response waveform is produced for each stimulus. Electrical activity within the response is time-locked to multiple discrete stimuli and is averaged. The averaging process occurs over time (in the time domain). Waveform analysis consists of calculation of the latency between stimulus and wave components and the amplitude of the components. Even casual visual inspection of an AER waveform, such as the ABR, shows that it typically consists of prominent sharp, closely spaced peaks (occurring frequently) riding atop (superimposed on) more gradual widely spaced peaks (occurring less frequently). The presence of the rounded (versus peaked) waves depends mostly on the low-pass filter setting used to record the response. Also, depending on the low-pass filter setting, there may also be numerous (very frequent) tiny spikes or background noise in the waveform. By means of fast Fourier transform (FFT) techniques, it is possible to deconvolute, decompose, or separate out the relative contribution of major frequencies within the response waveform after it has been digitized. In this way, AERs are displayed in the frequency domain.

The audiologist who measures frequency response characteristics of acoustic transducers or hearing aids will be familiar with this analysis concept. In these examples, peak amplitude (or phase) of a signal is plotted across a range of frequencies after the signal passes through the electronic device of interest. FFT may produce more than simple graphs of either the phase or amplitude of a response over a range of frequencies. For example, instead of directly displaying a frequency component in phase and amplitude units, it might be more appropriate to display it as the vector sum of two other components. Each has the same frequency, but amplitudes are different, and phase is 0 degrees for one and 90 degrees for the other (sine and cosine functions resulting in sine and cosine spectra). The relationship of filtering and FFT is important in clinical AER measurement. Digital filtering is often accomplished with FFT technology. First, the FFT of a response, including precise definition of frequency, amplitude, and phase information, is carried out. Then, the frequency response is altered by mathematical manipulation (attenuation or reduction of amplitude) of the sine and cosine properties—for example, reducing or deleting energy at some frequencies. Then, the filtered frequency domain response is returned to the conventional time domain response by means of inverse FFT.

Electrical engineering literature contains numerous papers, monographs, and textbooks on spectral analysis. Briefly, any complex waveform (more than a simple pure tone or sinusoid) consists of a collection of frequencies. Following FFT, the frequency content of a waveform is usually displayed in a graph with frequency (in Hz) on the horizontal axis and some measure of amplitude (μvolt or dB) or power (μvolt^2) on the vertical axis. There are several important considerations and constraints in FFT of a waveform such as the ABR. Vector mathematics produces real and imaginary numbers and both enter into FFT computation. Imaginary values are a concept beyond the comprehension of many clinicians. Fortunately, in FFT of AERs, they are usually set at zero (Marsh, 1988). The smallest difference between frequencies that can be detected with FFT (the frequency resolution) is related to analysis time and the number of sample points used in averaging the response, according to the following equation:

$$\text{Frequency (Hz)} = 1 \, / \, \text{analysis time}$$

Put another way, a given frequency (in Hz) has a specific period (in ms). Frequency resolution is more precise with longer analysis times, and vice versa. For example, with a typical ABR analysis time of 15 ms, the difference between any two frequencies in the FFT plot is 65 Hz, whereas for a 10 ms analysis time the smallest increment of frequency that can be resolved is 100 Hz. Even though the plot of response amplitude as a function of frequency (spectral waveform) may appear continuous, frequency resolution is limited by this relationship. For analysis times typically used in longer latency AERs, frequency resolution for FFT is relatively precise. FFT of an ALR waveform recorded with a 500 ms analysis time, for example, is 2 Hz (according to the formula above).

Another constraint of FFT involves sampling and windowing. The example of frequency analysis used above was based on a continuous signal, or at the least one complete period of the signal. The AER is typically averaged from transient stimulation over a specific analysis time, which is shorter than the period of the response. Technically, the end of the response period (the "end" of the ABR) is difficult to define. One definition of an ABR ending, with rapidly presented stimuli, is where the next ABR begins. For a stimulus rate of 21.1/sec, a new ABR begins 21.1 times per second, or approximately every 47.4 ms (1000 ms / 21.1). Minimally, then, to meet the assumption of periodicity of signal, the FFT should be performed for an ABR recorded over an analysis time of approximately 50 ms, or preferably over multiple repetitions of ABRs over an even longer analysis period (with the same relatively rapid stimulus rate). In any event, the response is really not continuous and is not periodic. That is, it does not go on for an extended time period and does not repeat itself. Instead, the response is quite brief and the waveform is different, or might be different, at each point along the analysis time period.

An obvious problem with performing FFT on an ABR recorded with a typically brief analysis time is the artifactual sharp step between one waveform and the next. This is best visualized by placing two ABRs next to each other. The end of the first waveform is rarely aligned with the beginning of the next waveform. Normally, the baseline would be continuous and this step would be more like a ramp. FFT involves "viewing" this AER waveform through a window. Windowing serves to minimize the negative contribution of the step on the resulting spectrum (introduction of spectral components that are not really in the response). The windowing process, however, can produce errors (leakage and aliasing), evidenced by extra and unwanted spectral components in the resulting frequency domain waveform. It is important to keep in mind that the original response before the FFT process, if recorded with analog filtering, included information that might be altered by the windowing. Also, since AER components often occur at either end of the analysis time, particularly the beginning, the shape of the window might distort (reduce the contribution) of some components and emphasize others. This problem can be reduced by a substantial prestimulus delay (prestimulus baseline period) so that the AER appears more toward the center of the analysis time. More detailed description of FFT principles in evoked response spectral analysis can be found in a number of papers (e.g., de Weerd & Kap, 1981; Marsh, 1988; Norcia, Sato, Shinn, & Mertus, 1986; Reddy & Kirlin, 1979).

SPECTRUM OF ABR. | Beginning within a decade of the discovery of the ABR, dozens of papers have appeared describing investigations of ABR *spectral content* (e.g., Abdala & Folsom, 1995; Beagley, Sayers, & Ross, 1979; Boston, 1981;

Elberling, 1979; Fridman, Zappalla, Bergelson, Greenblatt, Malis, Morrell, & Hoeppner, 1984; Hall, 1986; Kavanagh & Domico, 1986; Kevanishvili & Aphonchenko, 1979; Lang, Jantti, Nyrke, Happonen, 1981; Laukli & Mair, 1981; Malinoff & Spivak, 1990; Sininger, 1995; Suzuki, Sakabe, & Miyashita, 1982; Terkildsen, Osterhammel, & Huis in't Veld, 1975; Wilson & Aghdasi, 2001; Yamamoto, Sakabe, & Kaiho, 1979; Yokoyama, Aoyagi, Suzuki, Kiren, & Koike, 1994). With few exceptions (e.g., Cottrell & Gans, 1995; Hall, 1986; Yokoyama et al., 1994), published information on ABR frequency characteristics is derived from studies of normal children or adult subjects conducted in laboratory settings. FFT analysis confirms that the normal ABR consists of energy in three major frequency regions, as illustrated in Figure 7.7. The greatest amount of energy is in a low-frequency region (below 150 Hz), with prominent energy regions also from about 500 to 600 Hz and 900 to about 1100 Hz. There is little spectral ABR energy above 2000 Hz. The frequency content of specific ABR waves has been inferred on the basis of spectral analysis and offline studies, i.e., ABR waveforms filtered with a digital technique. Some investigators suggest that later waves (IV through VI) consist of energy from the lower two energy regions (about 100 Hz and 500 Hz), wave III is dependent on 100 to 900 Hz energy, and the earliest waves (I and II) consist of relatively higher frequency energy in the range of 400 to 1000 Hz (Kevanishvili & Aphonchenko, 1979; Suzuki, Sakabe, & Miyashita, 1982). Boston (1981) offered a slightly different explanation, finding a correspondence between energy in the 900 to 1100 Hz region and wave I, wave II and wave III; energy around 500 Hz to wave V; and lower frequency energy to the slow wave activity upon which these components are superimposed. The relationship between ABR spectrum and specific components, even in normal subjects, is not yet clear, the topic of some controversy (Elberling, 1979), and clearly requires further investigation.

ABR spectral content is influenced by subject factors and measurement parameters, although systematic study of these interactions is lacking. Reduced consciousness (coma) appears to reduce ABR spectral energy in all frequency regions, especially energy in the high-frequency region, and may seriously alter the normal spectral pattern noted above (Hall, 1986). It is likely that other subject characteristics (age, gender, body temperature, peripheral hearing loss) influence ABR spectrum as well. High-frequency hearing loss that is typically sensorineural in etiology would be expected to diminish high-frequency spectral energy in ABR waveforms. This trend is suggested by data presented in Figure 7.5. Careful documentation of audiologic status is extremely important in basic or clinical investigation of AER spectral content. ABR waveforms recorded from neonates are dominated by lower frequency. Low-frequency ABR spectral content tends to become more prominent as stimulus frequency decreases (from high- to low-frequency tone bursts). As intensity decreases, the overall magnitude of energy decreases, and the proportion of higher frequency energy is diminished (Laukli & Mair, 1981; Suzuki et al., 1982). The magnitude of spectral energy in the ABR is also diminished in pathologies in children and adults affecting the central auditory nervous system, such as head injury (e.g., Hall, 1986, 1992) and developmental disorders (Cottrell & Gans, 1995). Some acquisition parameters, such as filter settings, obviously have a marked effect on ABR spectrum. Others (e.g., electrode site) may also influence ABR spectrum, although data in support of a relationship are not available.

Fsp

A statistical variance ratio measure—Fsp—is a commonly applied algorithm for automatic and statistically confirmed quantification of the ABR signal-to-noise ratio, particularly in newborn hearing screening. The Fsp is based on the magnitude of the response when the stimulus is present (the "signal") divided by the magnitude of the response when the stimulus is not present (the "noise"). In an individual patient and for a given stimulus intensity level, the magnitude of an ABR is remarkably stable assuming the patient is quiet and not moving. The magnitude of the noise, however, varies widely depending on patient-related factors (e.g., muscle activity, EEG unrelated to the response), environmental factors (e.g., electrical artifact), and selected ABR stimulus and acquisition parameters (e.g., number of sweeps, filtering). Ongoing signal averaging reduces the noise and enhances detection of the ABR. As a general rule, noise is lowered as signal averaging is increased and, as a reflection of the larger SNR, the Fsp value increases (e.g., from 1.0 to 3.0). In

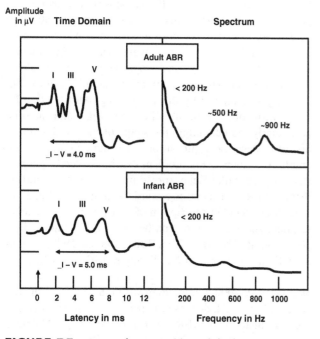

FIGURE 7.7. Spectral composition of the ABR.

patients who do not produce an ABR under adequate measurement conditions (e.g., a stimulus is presented and there are no technical problems), the measured response is approximately the same as the noise, with a resulting signal-to-noise ratio of approximately 1.0. On the other hand, the measured response for patients with who do generate an ABR is larger than the noise, as indicated by a signal-to-noise ratio value greater than 1.0. Generally, an Fsp value of > 2.1 is consistent with the presence of an ABR. For newborn hearing screening with ABR, the Fsp value of > 2.1 would indicate a "Pass" outcome. As first described (Don et al., 1984), the signal-to-noise ratio was evaluated with the F statistic using a value at a single point in the ABR waveform, hence the abbreviation *Fsp*. Statistical calculations of signal-to-noise ratio values in ABR with current evoked response systems are based not on a single data point but, rather, on multiple points. However, the term Fsp continues to be used in reference to the automatic analysis technique. The Fsp analysis technique is incorporated in most newborn hearing screening devices, and now is also applied for objective identification of cortical auditory evoked responses, e.g., the MMN (see Chapter 14).

Miscellaneous Analysis Techniques

The literature contains references to a variety of strategies for automated or quantified analysis of the ABR, although few are ever applied clinically with commercially available evoked response systems (Hall & Rupp, 1997). *Cross-correlation* is among earliest and most commonly reported statistical strategies of ABR analysis (e.g., Arslan, Prosser, & Michielini, 1981 Elberling, 1979) that has been applied clinically in different patient populations for diagnosis of auditory dysfunction (e.g., Barajas, 1985; Maurizi et al., 1985; Paludetti et al., 1985) and newborn hearing screening. Assorted cross-correlation measures, such as the maximum correlation coefficient or the coefficient at a defined latency region, are based on comparison of the ABR recorded from a patient to previously collected templates of normal ABRs from well-defined subjects, e.g., males and females or infants at different ages.

Kidd, Burkard, and Mason (1993) described an interesting analysis in which the neurophysiologic signal, the ABR, was converted to an acoustical signal for auditory detection of the response. Representation of an evoked response as a sound is a common strategy for monitoring facial nerve function intraoperatively (noted in Chapter 15). The authors essentially convert ABR detection from a visual inspection task to an *auditory detection task*. Kidd, Burkard, and Mason (1993) assess the effect of several different techniques of presentation on the accuracy of ABR detection by the listeners, e.g., playing back the response-related sound repetitively, more slowly, at a longer duration, or using a pure tone carrier modulated by the ABR waveform. Listeners were required to simply give a Yes-No response to the acoustic signals (i.e., yes, there is a

response, or no, there's no response). Although ABR analysis with the auditory detection task was feasible, accuracy was higher for the conventional visual inspection approach.

In addition to the just-noted algorithms and functions (e.g., Fsp and cross-correlation), a variety of statistical measures have been applied in the objective detection and analysis of the ABR, developed mostly by groups of biomedical or electrical engineers and hearing scientists and evaluated only with audiologically and neurologically normal adult subjects in the laboratory setting. A sample of many diverse statistical, mathematical, and/or computer-assisted measures reported for detection and analysis of the ABR include the Raleigh test, modified Raleigh test, Watson's U^2 test, Kuiper's test, Hodges-Ajne's, Cochran's Q-test, and Friedman test of the distribution of phase angles in the ABR spectrum (Cebulla, Stürzebecher, & Wernecke, 2000; Stürzebecher & Cebulla, 1997) the magnitude-squared coherence (MSC) test (Dobie & Wilson, 1989); automatic computer-assisted recognition of the pattern for ABR latency/intensity functions (Vannier et al., 2001); zero crossing method (Fridman et al., 1982); matched filtering and band-pass filtering techniques (Boston, 1989; Delgado & Özdamar, 1994; Pratt, Urbach, & Bleich, 1989; Woodworth, Reisman, & Fontaine, 1983); composite probability modeling of increased resolution, or CPMIR; minimal repetition adaptive line enhancement, or MALE (Madhavan, 1992); adaptive signal enhancement (Chan, Lam, Poon, & Qui, 1995); single-trial covariance analysis (Galbraith, 2001); multifilters for attribution automation–based pattern recognition (Grönfors, 1993b); syntactic pattern recognition (Madhavan, de Bruin, Upton, & Jernigan, 1986); neural networks (Callan, Lasky, & Fowler, 1999; Tian, Juhola, & Grönfors, 1997); automatic analysis techniques for peak identification relying on a computerized database of raw responses from large number (> 80) normal subjects (e.g., Sundaramoorthy, Pont, Degg, & Cook, 2000; Vannier, Adam, & Motsch, 2002); and wavelet analysis (Samar, 1999; Samar et al., 1999; Popescu, Papadimitriou, Karamitsos, & Bezerianos, 1999). The paper by Samar, Bopardikar, Rao, and Swartz (1999) is a readable yet detailed explanation of "a growing class of signal processing techniques and transforms that use wavelets and wavelet packets to decompose and manipulate time-varying, nonstationary signals" (p. 7).

The two overall objectives of most of these computer-based and automated analysis techniques are to determine the presence versus absence of an ABR and to differentiate between normal versus abnormal responses. Conventional ABR analysis of latency or amplitude is two-dimensional, involving time (latency) and amplitude calculations of the response. Beginning in the early years of ABR research, and usually with Dr. Billy Martin as a co-author, reports occasionally appeared describing three-dimensional analysis of the ABR, e.g., three-channel Lissajous trajectory (3CLT) analysis (e.g., Gardi, Martin, & Jewett, 1980; Kaminer & Pratt, 1987; Yasuhara & Hori, 2002), isochronic mapping (Thornton, Farrell, Reid, & Peters, 1991) or the three-dimensional dipole tracing (3DT) method (Yoshida et al., 1991). The primary objective of each of these sophisticated multichannel analysis approaches is to localize generators of the ABR, but they have never been regularly applied clinically.

OFFLINE WAVEFORM MANIPULATIONS

Optimally, quality of AER waveforms is improved by altering test parameters or conditions before or during data collection. With this adaptive "think on your feet" approach, the clinician first notices that AER waveform quality is less than optimal and then responds by altering the customary test protocol in an attempt to improve quality. If this is not possible, or the result is inadequate, waveform quality can sometimes be improved after data collection is complete. Any processing of AER data after it has been collected, and stored electronically, is referred to as "offline" versus "online" processing. Three offline processing or manipulation techniques for AER waveforms often employed with commercially available instrumentation are digitally adding and subtracting, smoothing, and filtering of AER waveforms. Each will now be briefly discussed and illustrated with ABR waveforms.

Adding, Subtracting, and Inverting Waveforms

With many clinical evoked-response systems, one waveform can be either digitally added or subtracted from another waveform. These same systems usually feature an option for inverting polarity of an ABR wave form, that is, turning it upside down. Instructions for such functions that are specific to a piece of equipment are described in the manual supplied by the manufacturer. In effect, the voltage recorded (and stored) at each data point (e.g., 256, 512, 1,024 total data points) in one waveform is either added or subtracted from the voltage at the corresponding data point in the other waveform. Therefore, two waveforms that are almost identical will appear unchanged when added. Subtracting one from the other produces what appears to be a flat line because the voltage recorded at each data point is essentially subtracted from itself. Actually, multiple waveforms (more than two), and waveforms from different patients, can be added or subtracted. Adding a series of waveforms from different patients or from the same patient results in a "grand average" for the group. Similarly, reversing polarity of a waveform is accomplished by changing the sign of the voltage at all data points. If the voltage at exactly 5 ms is, for example, +0.37 μv, with inversion of polarity it becomes –0.37 μv. When this process is applied to all data points, the waveform becomes totally inverted. AER peaks that are customarily plotted upward flip downward and vice versa. A clinical application of the inverting feature is cited below in a discussion of mistakes involving electrode placement or usage.

There are several constraints to these processes. First of all, the waveforms must be stored before they can be digitally manipulated. Also, waveforms to be added or subtracted must be recorded with compatible equipment (e.g., the same brand and often same model or version), with equivalent time bases (analysis times), filter settings, and numbers of data points (e.g., 512). Other measurement parameters, however, such as the electrode array used in recording the waveform, stimulus rate, stimulus polarity, and the number of sweeps used in averaging each waveform, make no difference. In fact, as described below, adding waveforms serves to add the number of sweeps (or stimulus repetitions) contributing to the final waveform.

Waveform addition and subtraction have a variety of clinical applications. With addition:

• When two waveforms recorded with different stimulus polarities (one waveform with rarefaction and one with condensation stimuli) are added, stimulus artifact is reduced or eliminated. This is because the artifact occurs in opposite directions (upward- versus downward-going) in each of the waveforms. The result of adding voltages at each data point that are opposite in sign (negative in one and positive in the other) is to approximate zero voltage. The same principle holds for any artifact that is of opposite polarity in the two waveforms. This point is reviewed in the discussion of electrical interference in AER recordings.

• Multiple replicated AER waveforms for certain stimulus and acquisition conditions (e.g., all recorded with click stimuli presented to the same ear, at the same intensity level) when added create a waveform that is actually the result of the combined number of sweeps (stimulus repetitions). That is, if four waveforms averaged from 1,000 stimuli each are added together, the resulting waveform is based on a total of 4,000 sweeps. Digital addition of waveforms can thus be a powerful technique for enhancing the signal-to-noise ratio. Clinically, it is usually a better use of time, and statistically preferable, to first record two or even more waveforms for a given set of measurement parameters with a relatively modest number of sweeps, assess reliability, and then add the waveforms together for latency and amplitude calculation, rather than recording a single waveform for the total number of sweeps. Another advantage of first replicating waveforms and then adding them together is that atypical waveforms (those with an unusually great amount of noise) can be deleted from the grand average (not included in the adding process). With continued averaging over a large number of sweeps, these noisy AER data would of course be included and would serve to contaminate the waveform. Deletion of noisy runs is a simplified version of the highly sophisticated mathematical signal-to-noise enhancement and AER analysis techniques described in Chapter 6.

With subtraction:

• ABR waveforms recorded simultaneously with an ipsilateral and a contralateral electrode array (Fz-Ai and Fz-Ac) can be used to derive a horizontal electrode array. This manipulation was reviewed in Chapter 6. Briefly, vector theory predicts, and clinical study confirms, that subtraction of the contralateral (Fz-Ac) recording from the ipsilateral (Fz-Ai) recording yields a horizontal (Ac-Ai) waveform. The validity of this technique is easily proved by then subtracting derived horizontal waveform from a waveform actually recorded, simultaneously, with an ear-to-ear electrode array. The result is a flat line, indicating that the two horizontal waveforms (actual and digitally derived) were equivalent. One obvious implication of digital subtraction, therefore, is the availability of three-channel AER data from only two-channel recordings.

• By subtracting a no-stimulus waveform (just background activity) from an AER waveform to an adequate stimulus, it is theoretically possible to produce a waveform lacking much of the nonstimulus, or ongoing, EEG noise that typically characterizes AERs. Spectral analysis of the waveform resulting from the subtraction process confirms a reduction of low-frequency background brain activity. Although appealing, this approach is not routinely applied clinically. One problem is that the two waveforms (no stimulus versus stimulus) are not recorded simultaneously and, therefore, arise from somewhat different EEG environments.

Smoothing

Smoothing is a digital process that, as the term implies, removes small irregularities in waveforms and produces a smoother waveform. High-frequency noise (electrical or muscular in origin) causes many tiny spikes that are often superimposed on the major components in an AER waveform. With three-point smoothing, a common method, voltage at an actual data point in the waveform is replaced by the average of voltages for this data point plus the two adjacent (one earlier and one later) data points. Actually, smoothing is a moving average that may include more than three nearby data points. Minor AER waveform "wrinkles" are thus "ironed out." A single waveform can be repeatedly smoothed without producing serious latency distortions. When excessive high-frequency artifact interferes with wave component identification, multiple smoothing may be useful. With repeated smoothing, however, amplitude of small wave components may be reduced because in the smoothing process actual peaks are treated the same as high-frequency noise peaks. Also, although smoothing improves the appearance of waveforms and ease of latency and amplitude analysis, rarely do wave components become apparent after smoothing that could not be detected beforehand.

Filtering

Filtering is an important factor in AER measurement. Off-line digital filtering (after data collection) may be useful in enhancing waveform quality, particularly when electrical activity above or below the frequency range of the response is present in the waveform. Large-amplitude, slow-wave (low-frequency) activity is clearly evident to different extents in the recordings for two electrode arrays (ipsilateral versus contralateral) with a filter setting of 30 to 3000 Hz (left panel of figure). Digital filtering at 150 to 3000 Hz (right panel of figure) essentially removes this low-frequency component and facilitates the identification of an apparent wave V in the waveform. Notice, in the figures, that high-frequency activity is unchanged by this filtering.

Filtering may also produce undesirable effects on ABR waveforms if the low-frequency energy contributes to identification of components. With high-pass cutoff frequencies of 150 Hz and 300 Hz, response amplitude is reduced, especially for wave V. All components in each waveform, however, are still clearly identified. High-pass filtering has a much more serious impact on the ABR waveforms for a newborn infant. With a filter setting of 30 to 3000 Hz, ABR components are clearly visible. As the high-pass filter setting is increased to 150 Hz and then 300 Hz, ABR components become indistinct and are not reliably observed. Filtering can, therefore, serve to enhance waveforms but also deteriorate waveform quality. For ABRs recorded from infants, filtering out low-frequency energy may indeed result in elimination of the entire response, and a serious error in ABR analysis and interpretation.

NONPATHOLOGIC SUBJECT FACTORS INFLUENCING ABR RECORDING

Subject Characteristics

Nonpathologic subject factors are those factors with may influence the outcome of an ABR, or any AER, recording in any subject, even persons with normal peripheral and central auditory system status. They include age and gender, body temperature, state of arousal, attention, and the possible effects of drugs. The influence of each of these factors varies markedly among AERs. Some factors may be totally irrelevant for one type of AER yet profoundly alter another type. Subject attention to the stimulus, for example, has absolutely no effect on ABR recordings yet may determine whether a specific event related potential, such as the P300, is even detected. The importance of some subject characteristics is self-evident. The effect of drugs is a clear concern when recording cortical AERs intraoperatively from an anesthetized patient. Effects of other subject characteristics, or interactions among them and stimulus and acquisition parameters and pathology, are often less clear-cut. To be sure, our knowledge of the effects of all subject characteristics on all AERs remains incomplete. Still, the clinician must always rule out, or at least take into account, the possible influence of these factors in recording and analyzing an AER, before the results of testing are interpreted. Fortunately, effects of subject factors on ABR are rather well appreciated and, for certain factors such as state of arousal, attention, and sedation, negligible.

The effect of one or more of these subject characteristics must be considered whenever the quality of ABR recordings is suboptimal, or at least poorer than expected. By keeping in mind a few general principles of subject characteristic effects, the clinician can often promptly determine whether a specific characteristic should be suspected, or can be safely ruled out, as a cause of poor AER outcome. These generalizations are as follows:

- Age: Young age (in children) affects the ABR, whereas advancing (beyond 50 years) primarily affects later latency (cortical) AERs.
- Gender: Male versus female differences are more important for ABR than any other AERs.
- Body temperature: Hypo- and hyperthermia exert a clear and clinically important effect on the ABR.
- State of arousal: There is no effect on the ABR.
- Muscular artifact: Affects the ABR, along with other responses.
- Hearing sensitivity: High-frequency hearing loss especially affects ABR (and specifically wave I).
- Drugs: Drugs that influence the CNS (e.g., sedatives, anesthetic agents) exert the greatest effect on longer latency, cortically generated AERs and less effect on ABR.

AGE: DEVELOPMENTAL. | The effects of subject age vary considerably among AERs. For example, ABR undergoes changes over the first eighteen months of life, whereas AMLR and ALR, along with P300 response, are apparently not adultlike until age 8 to 10 years, or even later. The general principle relating age and AERs is that shorter latency responses mature at an earlier age than longer latency responses. That is, maturation of AERs tends to proceed from the peripheral to the central auditory system and in a caudal-to-rostral direction within the CNS. This generalization, while helpful in understanding the effect of age on AERs, is actually an oversimplification of a very complex process. As in most discussions of AERs, it's impossible to consider the effect of age, or any other single factor, in isolation. Age interacts importantly, and in a complex fashion, with other subject characteristics (e.g., sensorineural hearing loss, with stimulus parameters (e.g., rate and intensity, and with acquisition parameters (e.g., filter settings). Age-related normative ABR are presented in the appendix.

A classic early ABR paper entitled "Brain Stem Auditory Evoked Responses in Human Infants and Adults" was published by Hecox and Galambos in 1974, within several years after the ABR was discovered. Since then scores of clinical investigators have detailed ABR findings in infants and young children, and the differences between findings in pediatric versus adult populations (e.g., Chiappa, 1997; Eggermont & Salamy, 1988; Fria & Doyle, 1984; Galambos, Hicks, & Wilson, 1984; Gorga et al., 1987a, 1988; Jacobson, 1985; Lauter, Oyler, & Lord-Maes, 1993; Mochizuki, Go, Ohkubo, Tatara, & Motomura, 1982; Morgan, Zimmerman, & Dubno, 1987; Salamy, McKean, & Buda, 1975; Salamy, McKean, Pettett, & Mendelson, 1978; Starr, Amlie, Martin, & Sanders, 1977). At least four overall practical conclusions can be drawn from this substantial research effort. First, although the cochlea may

be fully functional by about 35 weeks conceptional age (e.g., Eggermont et al., 1996), the initial component of the ABR (wave I) is not mature at term birth, as wave I latencies do not reach adult values until about 45 to 50 weeks conceptional age (Eggermont et al., 1996). Second, the ABR waveform is incomplete at birth, and certainly immature for preterm infants (e.g., Amin et al., 1999). Generally, only three major components (waves I, III, and V) are observed. Third, interwave latency values (I–III, III–V, and I–V) are initially prolonged. The ABR wave I–V latency interval, for example, is normally about 5.00 ms at term birth. Finally, during the first eighteen months to two years of life, other wave components emerge and waves III and V progressively shorten in latency. After eighteen months to two years of life, the ABR is essentially adultlike in latency and amplitude (Figure 7.8). Age must be taken into account when interpreting ABR findings in children under the age of 18 months.

ABR can be recorded first at approximately 27 to 28 weeks of conceptional age (Amin et al., 1999; Galambos & Hecox, 1978; Starr, Amlie, Martin, & Sanders, 1977; Stockard & Westmoreland, 1981). At this time (well before the normal termination of pregnancy at 40 weeks), wave I may be relatively more prominent than later waves because, as noted above, the peripheral auditory system matures before the auditory central nervous system (Montandon, Cao, Engel, & Grajew, 1979; Stockard & Stockard, 1983). There is some

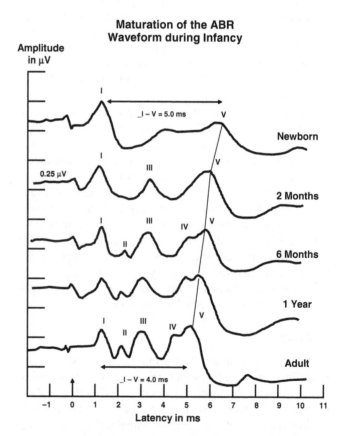

FIGURE 7.8. Changes in ABR waveform as a function of age during infancy.

evidence that wave I amplitude in newborn infants may, in fact, be up to twice as big as in adults (Hecox et al., 1981; Salamy & McKean, 1976; Salamy, McKean, Pettett, & Mendelson, 1978; Starr et al., 1977; Stockard, Stockard, & Sharbrough, 1978). Proximity of the recording electrode to the cochlea, due to relatively small head dimensions, is offered as an explanation for the larger wave I amplitude. Also, some investigators report that newborn wave I latency is prolonged from 0.3 ms (Goldstein et al., 1979; Jacobson, Morehouse, & Johnson, 1982; Morgan et al., 1987; Stockard et al., 1983) to over 1 ms (Cox, Hack, & Metz, 1981), in comparison to adult values. Eggermont et al. (1996) attribute the rather rapid decrease in wave I latency soon after birth to maturation of the first synapse in the afferent auditory pathways. Not all investigators are in agreement on this point, as Schwartz, Pratt, and Schwartz (1989) found wave I latency and amplitude values equivalent for 20 preterm infants and 20 normal adults. The authors of this paper, in reviewing the literature, note two recurring theories to explain the previous finding of wave I alterations in newborn infants. One is the possibility of external and middle ear factors such as collapsing ear canals and middle ear fluid, respectively. Both external and middle ear factors would diminish the effective intensity level of the stimulus. Another possibility is that the peripheral auditory system, in particular the cochlea and eighth nerve, are immature at birth. Schwartz and colleagues (1989) go on to discuss potential sources of differences among studies, including characteristics of the population (age, general health, middle ear status), type of transducer (insert versus supra-aural transducer, stimulus intensity level).

Age, even when marked in hours after birth, is a very pertinent variable affecting the ABR. Maurizi et al. (1986) analyzed ABRs over the first 58 hours of life in 33 full-term newborn infants. By 58 hours, the ABR invariably consisted of three major peaks (I, III, and V), but earlier recordings for two-thirds of the infants lacked a clear and reliable wave I. ABR latency values, including the wave I–V interval, decreased significantly during the first 58 hours. Schwartz et al. (1989) did not specify the time after birth at which their data were collected except for the statement that the infants were recent graduates of the intensive care nursery. There is, therefore, disagreement on absolute ABR latency and amplitude values, and the wave V/I amplitude ratio, in newborn infants. In a study of morphological changes in the ABR within the first week after birth for premature infants (24 to 32 weeks gestational age [GA]), Yamamoto et al. (1990) described marked decreases in the absolute latency for wave I, and the wave I–III interwave latency during the first three weeks after premature birth. Kohelet, Arbel, Goldberg, and Arlasoraff (2000) also found, over the gestational age range of 26 to 43 weeks, significant correlations among ABR latencies, gestational age, postconceptional age, and also a clinical finding, the 5-minute APGAR score. Amin et al. (1999) documented an distinct increase in the frequency of detection of waves (I, III, and V). The most pronounced improvement in the morphology of the ABR waveform was observed for

infants in the 28- to 29-week gestation age group. Along with the morphological changes, the authors noted progressively decreased ABR wave latencies and interwave latencies during the first postnatal week. Although there appear to be rapid changes in the ABR during the first week postpartum for premature infants, Jiang (1995) found no difference between preterm and term infants in the maturational profile as defined by decreases in the ABR wave I–V latency interval and increases in wave V amplitude, even when the babies were followed up to age 6 years. The author concludes that earlier exposure of the preterm infant to a sound environment "extra utero" (after birth) is not likely to have neurophysiological consequences.

There is general consensus that latency values for later ABR waves are very prolonged in neonates when compared to adult values. Consequently, the newborn ABR is characterized by delayed interwave intervals (Figure 7.8). For example, the wave I–V interval in a normal term infant is, on the average, about 5.0 ms versus about 4.0 ms in the mature ABR. Explanations for delayed interwave latencies center on CNS anatomy and physiology, specifically incomplete nerve fiber myelinization, reduced axon diameter, and immature synaptic functioning (Eggermont, 1985b; Eggermont & Salamy, 1988; Fria & Doyle, 1984; Goldstein et al., 1979; Hecox & Burkard, 1982; Jacobson, 1985; Maurizi et al., 1986; Morgan et al., 1987; Salamy et al., 1975; Schwartz et al., 1989; Starr et al., 1977; Weber, 1982). Reported calculations of latency changes (decreases or shortenings) as a function of age in premature infants are approximately 0.15 ms/week for wave I, 0.2 ms/week for wave V, and, variably, 0.45 to as little as 0.1 ms/week for the wave I–V interval (Hecox & Burkard, 1982; Salamy, McKean, & Buda, 1975; Schulman-Galambos & Galambos, 1975; Starr et al., 1977; Stockard et al., 1979; Stockard & Westmoreland, 1981). Age-related changes in ABR latency are not linear. That is, they are not constant across a wide age range. Rather, there are two phases of development. Studies in humans and animals have clearly shown that the rate of latency decrease is greatest in premature infants and then slows from term (40 weeks postconception) to about 18 months (Eggermont, 1983; Fria & Doyle, 1984). Werner, Folsom, and Mancl (1994) provide data of direct relevance to clinical application of the ABR in threshold estimation. Data were reported for a relatively large series of normal-hearing children (96 infants 3 months old and 89 infants 6 months old) and normal-hearing adults (76). The difference in latency for ABR wave V versus wave I (the wave V to wave I latency–intensity intercept difference) was a strong predictor of behavioral threshold for 3-month-old infants, although not for the group of 6-month-old infants or for the adults. Interestingly, the decrease in latency with age in infants and young children occurs despite obvious growth in physical size and, correspondingly, the length of the auditory pathways from the cochlea to and through the brainstem. Moore et al. (1996) estimated developmental changes in the length of the brainstem auditory pathways with a three-dimensional reconstruction of postmortem fetal and infant brainstems. The changes in anatomic dimensions were then analyzed in the context of existing data for ABR latencies (brainstem conduction times) for preterm, term, and older infants. The authors concluded that in premature infants "increasing conduction velocity more than compensates for increasing path length," resulting in decreased ABR latencies.

At this juncture, it is important to keep in mind the difference between conceptional versus gestational estimates of age in newborn infants. Conceptional age is calculated according to calendar dates with obstetric data, from the mother's last menstrual cycle, whereas gestational age is determined from a clinical assessment of physical findings, such as the Ballard examination (Dubowitz, Dubowitz, & Goldberg, 1970). Postconception age is equivalent to gestational age plus chronologic age. There is some imprecision in each approach for estimation of infant age, and up to a two-week margin of error is presumed. This probably accounts for some of the variability in calculated ABR changes with age. As noted by Schwartz, Pratt, and Schwartz (1989), and cited above, differences in measurement conditions among studies also might contribute to the variability. The wave I–V latency interval, for example, appears to vary as a function of stimulus intensity. Wave I–V latency is longer at higher intensity levels, such as 80 dB, and shorter for low intensity levels, such as 30 dB. Normative ABR latency for various stimulus intensity levels can be found in the appendix. In normal adult subjects, changes in ABR interwave latencies as a function of stimulus intensity are less pronounced. Again, ABR waveform morphology also is not adultlike in infancy. Only waves I, III, and V are typically present. Wave III is sometimes not observed and waves II, IV, and VI are rarely observed.

Amin and colleagues (1999) systematically investigated ABR findings for 173 infants at less than 32 weeks gestational age (GA). With the cross-sectional study design, data were collected for infants grouped into four age categories: 24 to 25 weeks up to 30 to 31 weeks. Infants admitted to the NICU were enrolled in the study except for those who had craniofacial anomalies, chromosomal disorders, TORCH infection, and those who were medically unstable. Serial ABR recordings were initially completed at bedside in the NICU within 24 hours after birth, and then for four of the next six days. The stimulus was an alternating polarity click presented at an intensity level of 80 dB nHL and a rate of 39.9/sec. Three test parameters for the otherwise comprehensive clinical study were not consistent with current guidelines for infant ABR assessment. First, the use of a TDH-39 supra-aural earphone "held in place over the infants ear," rather than an insert earphone design, may have affected the inter- and intrasubject precision and consistency of stimulus delivery and stimulus intensity and increased the adverse impact of the high levels of background noise typical of the NICU environment. Second, the high-pass filter setting used in the study (100 Hz) inevitably removed from the ABR waveform much of the low-frequency brain energy that dominates the infant ABR and probably contributed to less than optimal response detection. Finally, the rather high rate of stimulus presenta-

tion (39.9/sec) no doubt contributed to rapid data collection, but the fast stimulation rate also presumably resulted in prolongation of the absolute latencies of ABR components. It is likely that confident identification of ABRs for the infants in this study and the latency values for ABR waves, especially those in the youngest age group, would have been higher with a test protocol that included insert earphones, band-pass filter settings of 30 to 3000 Hz, and a slower rate of stimulation (e.g., in the range of 17 to 21/sec).

The following findings reported by Amin and colleagues (1999) have implications for anyone recording ABRs from premature infants in the NICU setting. The identification of ABR wave I, wave III, and wave V increased for infants from a GA of 24 weeks to 31 weeks. At a GA of 24 to 25 weeks, an ABR wave I was not observed, and wave III and wave V were detected in less than 10 percent of the infants. In contrast, for infants with a GA of 30 to 31 weeks, ABR wave III and wave IV were almost always detected, and wave I was identified in the majority of infants (> 60%). Also, in the oldest group of infants, an ABR was clearly apparent even within the first 24 hours after birth. As one would expect from the well-established gradient of maturation of the auditory system from the peripheral structures to the central nervous system, wave I latency was essentially unchanged from the youngest to the oldest group of infants (24 weeks to 31 weeks GA), whereas the ABR wave I–V latency interval decreased, on the average from 6.86 ms to 5.88 ms during the same time period.

The weakness in the protocol for the study reported by Amin and colleagues (1999) prompts a reiteration of adhering to stimulus and acquisition parameters that will enhance the likelihood of recording an optimal ABR. Three ABR measurement parameters in particular deserve special mention in this discussion of developmental ABR factors— stimulus frequency and rate and recording electrode array. Stimulus frequency appears to be a factor to consider in maturation of the ABR. Even though brainstem maturation, and related changes in ABR interwave latencies are the most prominent dynamic developmental feature in infants, there is recent evidence that cochlear function in the newborn is distinctly different than in older children or adults. Some experimental animals (e.g., chicks) first show responsiveness to low-frequency sounds, even though the base of the cochlea (which in the adult is related to high-frequency hearing) matures before the apex (which in the adult is related to low-frequency hearing). As the animal matures, there are changes in tonotopic organization of the cochlea, with higher frequencies represented in the base and the lower frequency representation shifting toward the apex (Lippe & Rubel, 1983; Rubel & Ryals, 1983). Typically, in the older child or adult, ABR is generated by relatively high-frequency cochlear activity (1000 to 4000 Hz), with little low-frequency contribution. However, greater low-frequency cochlear contribution to ABR would be expected in infants, according to the experimental data of Rubel and colleagues. Several studies of ABR with stimuli of different frequencies suggest that low frequencies are, in fact, more important for ABR generation for newborn infants than adults (Folsom & Wynne, 1987). In a related paper, Eggermont et al. (1996) described a study of the source of age-related changes in latency for the ABR wave I in newborn infants, ranging in age from 30 to 42 weeks conceptional age, and a group of adult subjects. The authors estimated cochlear traveling wave delays by analyzing DPOAE phase delays and derived ABR latencies. No difference in cochlear travel time was found for infants from 34 weeks to 42 weeks conceptional age and young adults. Eggermont et al. (1996) conclude that cochlear functioning is mature at 35 weeks conceptional age.

Increasing stimulus rate produces a more pronounced increase in ABR latency with newborn infants than adults (Hall, 1992; Jiang, Brosi, & Wilkinson, 1998; Parthasarathy, Borgsmiller, & Cohlan, 1998). Among infants, the latency shift increases as gestational age decreases. With very young infants, at a gestational age, for example, of 30 weeks, no ABR may be detected for rapid rates (greater that about 40/sec). ABR repeatability is poor at stimulus rates as low as 21/sec within the first 30 to 58 hours after birth, even in full-term infants (Maurizi et al., 1986). There is conflicting evidence on ABR patterns expected for ipsilateral versus contralateral electrode arrays in infants versus older children. With the ipsilateral array, a conventional electrode configuration, one electrode (noninverting) is located on the forehead (Fz) or vertex (Cz) while the other electrode (inverting) is on the mastoid or earlobe on the side of the stimulus. With the contralateral array, the second (inverting) electrode is on the mastoid or earlobe contralateral to the stimulus. Some investigators recorded a clear ABR with the ipsilateral array, but were unable to detect a response with a contralateral electrode array either within the first 30 hours after birth (Maurizi et al., 1986) or later (Salamy, Eldredge, & Wakely, 1985), while others (e.g., Musiek, Verkest, & Gollegly, 1988) report that a response can be recorded from newborn infants with either electrode array. Given the possibility that an ABR will not be recorded in infants with a contralateral array, this electrode configuration should not be relied upon for clinical purposes, e.g., hearing screening or diagnosis.

AGE: ADVANCING. | The findings of most studies on ABR and age suggest that latency increases within the age range of 25 to at least 55 years, on the order of approximately 0.2 ms. Although the effect of age is not nearly as robust as the gender effect, and was not uniformly demonstrated for both males and females by early investigators (Beagley & Sheldrake, 1978; Rosenhamer, Lindstrom, & Lundberg, 1980; Thomsen, Terkildsen, & Osterhammel, 1978), more recent studies confirm a progressive age-related increase in absolute and interwave latency values (e.g., Lopez-Escamez, Salguero, & Salinero, 1999; Oku & Hasegewa, 1997; Soucek & Mason, 1992; Wharton & Church, 1990). Gender effects on ABR—the characteristically shorter latencies for females than for males—are reviewed in the next section of this

chapter. There are papers describing more pronounced age-related increases in ABR latency for females than for males (Rosenhamer et al., 1981a,b; Wharton & Church, 1990), and vice versa (Kjaer, 1980). The ABR wave I–V interval also appears to increase significantly over the age range of 60 to 86 years, implying brainstem involvement (Allison, Wood, & Goft, 1983; Maurizi, Altissimi, Ottaviani, Paludetti, & Bambini, 1982; Patterson et al., 1981; Rowe, 1978). There is, however, disagreement in the literature on this point, as with absolute latency findings just described above (Rosenhall, Bjorkman, Pedersen, & Kall, 1985). Some investigators have reported a significant decrease in amplitude of all ABR waves, from wave I through VI (Jerger & Hall, 1980, Psatta & Matei, 1988), although this is not a consistent finding (Johannsen & Lehn, 1984).

In considering the effect of aging on the ABR, one must account for interactions among three variables—age, gender, and cochlear (sensory) hearing loss (Hall, 1992; Jerger & Hall, 1980; Jerger & Johnson, 1988; Lightfoot, 1993; Rupa & Dayal, 1993). Jerger and Johnson (1988) reported a comprehensive investigation of the three interrelated factors (age, gender, and sensory hearing loss) and ABR. Gender differences were as described by the many previous investigators. A finding of the Jerger and Johnson (1988) study especially important in clinical interpretation of ABR was that females showed little wave V latency change with increasing hearing loss, whereas wave V latency in male subjects lengthened by approximately 0.1 ms for every decrease of 20 dB in the effective click level of the stimulus (the difference between the click stimulus level and hearing sensitivity at 4000 Hz). Rupa and Dayal (1993) also studied the interaction of age, gender, and sensory hearing loss. Data for 105 ears of 58 persons with otologically normal ears and 177 ears of 64 patients with cochlear hearing loss confirmed an increase in wave V latency with advancing age. The authors developed a mathematical model for predicting the age-related change in wave V latency:

Wave V latency (ms) = $4.892 + 0.007 \times$ age $+ 0.091 \times$ sex

where chronological age is in years, and sex is expressed with a value of 1 for females and 2 for males.

As with gender, reviewed below, there is no ready explanation for these age effects. Brainstem involvement is inferred from increases in ABR interwave latency values (Maurizi et al., 1982). Chen and Ding (1999) also raised the possibility of the role of age-related systemic disorders (e.g., hypertension), in the prolongation of ABR waves. Delayed synaptic transmission associated with age-related loss of neurons and changes in neuron membrane permeability, and contributing to decreased amplitude and increased latency, has been suggested (Johannsen & Lehn, 1984). The observation of unusually poorer waveform morphology in aging prompted Maurizi et al. (1982) to speculate that "biological background activity" was greater in older subjects, leading to a lower signal (ABR)-to-noise ratio. There are numerous papers describing degeneration of auditory CNS structures as a function of age (e.g., Hansen & Reske-Hielsen, 1965).

Age and gender effects appear to contribute substantially to the variability of ABR latency and, especially, amplitude measures (Psatta & Matei, 1988). That is, if each of these measures changes over time and differs between sexes, then both of these sources of variability are included with ABR data for a group of males and females distributed across an age range. According to Psatta and Matei (1988), for example, the standard deviation for amplitude can be reduced to less than 20 percent of the average value by accounting for age-related variation. This compares favorably to the typical magnitude of standard deviation, which is 30 to 40 percent of the mean value. Clearly, inconsistency in measurement parameters, such as stimulus factors (polarity, intensity, rate) and acquisition factors (filter settings), can also contribute importantly to response variability. These observations suggest that clinical interpretation of both ABR latency and amplitude would be more powerful if a patient's findings were compared to normative data matched for gender and age, across the range of childhood to advanced adulthood. (Published normative data are presented in the appendix.)

GENDER. | Distinct ABR differences for female versus male adults have been well appreciated beginning almost with discovery of the response. Since the 1970s, a distinct gender effect on ABR latency and amplitude has been repeatedly reported for *adult* subjects (Beagley & Sheldrake, 1978; Debruyne, Hombergen, & Hoekstra, 1980; Edwards, Squires, Buchwald, & Tanguay, 1983; Elberling & Parbo, 1987; Jerger & Hall, 1980; Kjaer, 1979; Lightfoot, 1993; Lopez-Escamez, Salguero, & Salinero, 1999; McClelland & McCrae, 1979; O'Donovan, Beagley, & Shaw, 1980; Patterson, Michalewski, Thompson, Bowman, & Litzelman, 1981; Robier & Reynaud, 1984; Rosenhall, Bjorkman, Pedersen, & Kall, 1985; Rosenhamer et al., 1980; Rupa & Dayal, 1993; Sand, 1991; Stockard, Stockard, & Sharbrough, 1978; Thomsen et al., 1978; Watson, 1996). Throughout adulthood, females show shorter latency values and larger amplitudes than males for later ABR waves (III, IV, V, and VI). The gender effect is found also in postmenopausal women (Wharton & Church, 1990). Gender-related differences in auditory function occur even in the cochlea. For example, Don et al. (1994) found cochlear response time, as determined from frequency-specific ABRs derived with a high-pass masking technique, was 13 percent shorter in females than males. Because the gender effect is relatively smaller for wave I, and more pronounced for later waves, interwave intervals are significantly shorter for females. Thus, if ABR data are recorded for an unselected group of young normal hearing subjects, absolute wave V latency and the wave III–V and I–V latency intervals are, on the average, from 0.12 to 0.30 ms less for the females. Amplitude is significantly larger for females, although the clinical importance of this finding is generally minimal due to the substantial normal variability of this measure. *A practical implication of these research findings is the importance of balancing the number of male and female subjects when establishing clinical normative data for the ABR.* If normative data in a clinic are gathered mostly from young normal-hearing female subjects (e.g., co-ed college students) there is a high likelihood that a substantial proportion of normal male patients, particularly older ones with some degree of sensory hearing loss, will be classified by ABR analysis as abnormal and, perhaps, considered as at risk for retrocochlear auditory dysfunction.

In contrast to the clear gender difference in adults, the presence of ABR gender differences in *infancy* and *childhood* is open to question. Some early investigators reported no gender differences in newborn infants (e.g., Cox, Hack, & Metz, 1981; Durieux-Smith et al., 1985; Sininger, Cone-Wesson, & Abdala, 1998; Stockard, Stockard, Westmoreland, & Corfits, 1979). Others found shorter latency in female versus male preterm and term infants (Beiser, Himmelfarb, Gold, & Shanon, 1985; Pauwels, Vogeleer, Clement, Rousseeuw, & Kaufman, 1982), but the differences were small and inconsistent in comparison to the striking gender effect for adults. Conditions in the preterm population that may be gender-related, such as risk for neurologic dysfunction, could contribute to such modest ABR differences (Abramovich, Gregory, Slenuck, & Stewart, 1979). Among selected studies, the reported age of onset for the gender differences varied from five years (Mochizuki et al., 1982), to seven years (O'Donovan et al., 1980), and up to fourteen years (McClelland & McCrae, 1979). There are also reports of gender differences in the ABR within adolescence (e.g., Kjaer, 1979; Rosenhall et al., 1985). Subject gender was not even noted in many major and otherwise meticulous investigations of ABR in newborn infants (e.g. Eggermont & Salamy, 1988; Gorga et al., 1987a, 1989; Jacobson, Morehouse, & Johnson, 1982; Stockard, Stockard, & Coen, 1983; Weber, 1982), possibly because it was not considered to be an important variable. Published studies of the role of gender in ABR threshold are also at odds. For example, Cone-Wesson and Ramirez (1997) found lower thresholds in female infants when the ABR was evoked by a 4000 Hz tone burst, but not for a 500 Hz tone-burst stimulus, whereas Sininger et al. (1998) reported lower ABR thresholds for male versus female infants.

Chiarenza, D'Ambrosio, and Cazzullo (1988) initially offered rather compelling evidence of gender differences in the newborn ABR. ABRs were recorded in 80 full-term normal infants (38 males and 42 females). Absolute latencies for positive waves III, IV, and V, and negative troughs following waves II and IV, along with latencies for intervals between positive waves I–IV, II–IV, and negative troughs I–IV, were significantly shorter for females than males. Amplitude was significantly greater for females than males only for wave I and only at one intensity level (70 dB HL). More recently, Stuart and Yang (2001), in an investigation of 202 full-term infants, offered confirmation of clear gender effects for infants for ABRs evoked by air-conduction, but not by bone-conduction, stimulation. For air-conduction stimuli, Wave V latency was, on the average, 0.2 to 0.3 ms shorter for female than male infants, a statistically significant difference (p = .0016). The authors found no difference between male and female infants for thresholds of the ABR evoked by air- and bone-conduction stimulation.

In addition to the rather well defined effects of development on ABRs evoked by air-conduction click stimuli, just reviewed, there are also maturational changes in the ABR for bone-conduction click stimuli and for tone-burst stimuli. The latter are reviewed in Chapter 8.

The mechanism underlying the gender difference is the topic of much investigation and speculation. Two factors, hearing sensitivity and body temperature, must be accounted for at the outset in a consideration of the gender difference. In an unselected group of subjects, females will tend to have better hearing sensitivity in the high-frequency region and higher average body temperature than age-matched male counterparts (e.g., Hall, 1992; Watson, 1996). Each of these variables alone could contribute to shorter latency, but probably not larger amplitude, among female subjects. Assuming that these factors are equivalent across gender, the explanation offered most often for the gender effect is smaller head size and brain dimensions in the females (Allison et al., 1983; Aoyagi et al., 1990; Michalewski et al., 1980; Stockard, Stockard, & Sharbrough, 1978). There is long-standing evidence from gross anatomic study (Parsons & Keene, 1919) and more recent evidence from computerized tomography (Haug, 1977) that females do, indeed, have smaller skull size and less brain volume. The two-part theory here is that interwave latencies (if considered a measure of brainstem conduction time) will be shorter if the distance between the generators for each of the waves is shorter, and amplitude will be larger if the recording electrode is relatively closer to the wave generator. Indeed, other clinical investigations (Conti, Modica, Castrataro, Fileni, & Colosimo, 1988; Dempsey, Censoprano, & Mazor, 1986; Yamaguchi et al., 1991) confirm a strong positive correlation between head size and latency values for ABR wave V and the I–V interval, regardless of the subject's sex. In contrast, Yamaguchi et al. (1991) found a strong negative correlation between head size and ABR amplitude. In other words, in the average person with a big head, ABR latencies are longer and amplitudes are smaller. However, the issue remains cloudy as evidenced by conflicting reports suggesting the absence of a correlation between body height or calculations of head size and the male versus female ABR differences (Edwards et al., 1983; Kjaer, 1979).

Head size and body temperature fail to adequately account for gender differences in the ABR (Costa Neto et al., 1991; Dehan & Jerger, 1990; Hall, 1992). An equally plausible theory is that documented physiologic and biochemical differences between sexes (e.g., Hare, Wood, Manyam, Gerner, Ballenger, & Post, 1982) could, in turn, influence neurotransmission. There are long-standing reports of EEG and ABR changes related to hormonal fluctuations during the menstrual cycle (Creutzfeldt, Arnold, Becker, Langenstein, Tirsch, Wilhelm, & Wuttke, 1976; Doty, Hall, Flickinger, & Sondheimer, 1982; Tasman, Hahn, & Maiste, 1999; Zani, 1989). Elkind-Hirsch and Jerger, with colleagues, conducted several investigations with the overall goal of evaluating the effect of sex hormones on the ABR. In two of the studies (Dehan & Jerger, 1990; Elkind-Hirsch, et al., 1992a, b), wave V and wave I–V latencies were associated with estrogen and estrogen replacement. In a later study, Elkind-Hirsch, Wallace, Malinak, and Jerger (1994) recorded ABRs from men and women (age 23 to 40 years) diagnosed with endocrinologic syndromes (five normal males, nine normally cycling females not receiving hormone therapy, five females "with premature ovarian failure," and five "hyperandrogenized females with polycystic ovarian disease" who were treated with a gonadotropin-releasing hormone agonist). Serum levels for multiple hormones were documented, including estradiol, testosterone, progesterone, prolactic, and two gonadotropics (lutienizing hormone and follicle stimulating hormone). Latency values for ABR wave V were correlated with levels of estrogen or testosterone. Related to these findings of hormone-related changes in the ABR, Tandon, Misra, and Tandon (1990) described in a group of eight young healthy and pregnant women higher ABR thresholds and a significant increase in the wave I–V latency interval in comparison to an age-matched control group of non-pregnant women.

It is clear from accumulated evidence reported in the literature that investigation of gender effects must be conducted with great care, as there may be rather complex interactions among hormonal factors related to gender, stimulus parameters (such as polarity) (Chan, Woo, Hammond, Yiannikas, & McLeod, 1988) and, especially, age and sensorineural hearing loss.

Body Temperature

Body temperature is, obviously, a characteristic feature of every patient. If normothermia (37 degrees centigrade [C] or 98.6 degrees Fahrenheit) is verified at the time of testing, then there is no need to further account for temperature in the interpretation of data for any AER. Temperature exceeding ±1 degree from this value (i.e., below 36 degrees C or above 38 degrees) must be considered as a possible factor in AER outcome. Patients at risk for temperature aberrations include those with infection (high temperature) and those in coma or under the effects of alcohol or anesthesia (low body temperature).

REVIEW OF LITERATURE. | The effect of low body temperature (hypothermia) on the ABR has been extensively investigated for a variety of animal models (see Hall, Bull, & Cronau, 1988, for review). Clinically, most reports of ABR in hypothermia describe changes observed during open heart surgery. Alterations in auditory electrophysiology related to low body temperature are summarized as follows. In vitro depolarization in membrane potentials (a decrease) is recorded in supporting cells (Hensen's) of the organ of Corti (Santos-Sacchi, 1986). Cochlear microphonic (CM) amplitude is reversibly reduced, while CM latency shows little or no change (Butler, Konishi, & Fernandez, 1960; Coats, 1965; deBrey & Eggermont, 1978; Kahana, Rosenblith, & Galambos, 1950). Variable changes during hypothermia are found for the summating potential (Butler, Konishi, & Fernandez, 1960; Manley & Johnstone, 1974). Basilar membrane traveling wave transit time is increased (deBrey & Eggermont, 1978).

Lowered temperature also produces a reversible reduction in eighth nerve compound action potential (ECochG N1 component and ABR wave I) amplitude and a reversible increase of N1 (wave I) latency (Kahana, Rosenblith, & Galambos, 1950). An initial effect of hypothermia may be the selective loss of auditory sensitivity for high-frequency signals, as estimated electrophysiologically (Manley & Johnstone, 1974). Synaptic transmission is delayed and axonal conduction velocity is decreased (Benita & Conde, 1972; deJesus, Hausmanowa-Petrusewicz, & Barchi, 1973). Consequently, ABR latencies are increased, especially for longer versus shorter latency waves. With severe hypothermia (body temperature less than 14 to 20 degrees Centigrade), the ABR disappears (Rosenblum, Ruth, & Gal, 1985).

Less well studied is the effect of *hyper*thermia (increased body temperature) on auditory evoked responses (Hall, Bull, & Cronau, 1988). A handful of experimental studies have shown evidence of decreased latency and amplitude of ECochG N1 component and ABR waves with elevation of body temperature (Barnett, 1980; Gold, Cahani, Sohmer, Horowitz, & Shahar, 1985). Dubois, Coppola, Bucksbaum, and Lees (1981) reported decreased somatosensory evoked response latency as a function of temperature in man. Investigation of ABR and body temperature has been limited to observations in essentially normothermic subjects. Bridger and Graham (1985) recorded ABRs from nine normal subjects while body temperature (measured under the tongue) was raised 1 degree centigrade (C) with a specially constructed heating blanket. Other studies (Geraud et al., 1982; Phillips et al., 1983) were likewise limited to very modest temperature increases (1 degree or less) and conducted in selected patients with neurological disease (multiple sclerosis).

GUIDELINES FOR TEMPERATURE CORRECTION IN ABR RECORDING. | Although body temperature is regularly cited as a factor in ABR measurement (e.g., Hall, 1992; Marshall & Donchin, 1981; Stockard & Westmoreland, 1981), it is probably not necessary to document temperature routinely in ABR assessments for audiological or neurological purposes in generally healthy patients. Documentation of body temperature is required for meaningful and valid interpretation of ABR latency data recorded in seriously ill patients and when monitoring neurological status electrophysiologically.

Examples of patients in this first category are those with infection accompanied by fever or those with hyperthermia caused by certain metabolic diseases, pharmacologic agents, or CNS pathology. Also included in this category are patients with acute illness at risk for hypothermia, including infants of low birth weight (Cox, 1985; Stockard & Westmoreland, 1981) and persons in coma secondary to severe brain injury (Hall & Tucker, 1986). Body temperature must also be taken into account during serial measurements in healthy persons, for example, during sleep studies. Apparent sleep-related alterations in ABR latency and amplitude may actually result from changes in body temperature during various nocturnal sleep stages (e.g., Litscher, 1995).

Temperature is a particularly important parameter to consider in the interpretation of serially recorded ABR data, or sensory evoked responses in general, during CNS monitoring in the operating room, neurointensive care unit, or other acute care setting. The clinical objective of evoked response monitoring is early detection of deleterious changes in neurologic status secondary to dynamic pathophysiology (e.g., brain ischemia). These CNS changes are reflected by increases in the ABR, most often latency. Nonpathologic bases for altered ABR findings, including physiologic factors such as body temperature, must be ruled out before a change in neurological status can be presumed. Guidelines exist for taking hypothermia into account in ABR interpretation (e.g., Britt, Lyons, Pounds, & Prionas, 1983; Stockard et al., 1978). The author recommends a somewhat conservative correction factor for the wave I–V latency of 0.2 ms (200 microseconds) for every degree of body temperature below average normal (37 degrees C). Applying the correction to ABR will sometimes result in wave I–V latency values that initially appear at the upper limit of the normal region, but with the correction are not abnormal bilaterally. There are no published clinical guidelines for correction of ABR latency values in *hyper*thermia. The author, however, has consistently found a ABR wave I–V latency decrease of 0.5 to 0.6 ms throughout the temperature range of 38 through 42 degrees C in young male and female patients (8 to date) with no CNS pathology undergoing hyperthermia therapy. Based on this experience, a correction factor for the wave I–V latency interval of 0.15 ms for each degree of increased body temperature is suggested.

Drugs

Although a wide variety of drugs influence AERs, relatively few affect the ABR. The influence of most drugs is on cortical functioning, rather than brainstem function. Indeed, the anatomic regions important for generation of the ABR are relatively close to other brain centers responsible for vital bodily functions, e.g., heart rate and respiration. The effects of specific CNS-acting drugs on each of the AERs are described in the chapter devoted to the response. As a rule, psychotropic medications, such as antidepressants and sedatives, modify cortical activity and have little or no influence on the ABR. Anesthetics commonly used during pediatric surgery, or for sedation of children, have differential and generally modest effects on the ABR, e.g., latency changes. Potentially ototoxic drugs, on the other hand, by definition can cause peripheral hearing impairment and profoundly alter the ABR.

OTOTOXIC DRUGS. | Ototoxicity is damage to the ear, almost always the cochlear, brought about by a drug. There are many drugs that can cause peripheral hearing impairment. Antibiotics are administered as a treatment of infection. The specific antibiotic used for this purpose depends on many factors, including the type of infecting microorganism, or "bug" (e.g., gram-positive versus gram-negative organisms), the duration and extent of the infection, the clinical diagnosis and part of the body infected (e.g., chronic suppurative otitis media involving the middle ear versus endocarditis involving the heart), age of the patient, allergic reactions, renal functioning, previous antibiotic therapy, and other drugs administered, to name a few. Ototoxic amounts of the drugs are avoided in most cases by carefully selecting the proper dosage (based on age, body weight, and other factors) and monitoring the peak and trough levels of the drug in the blood (the plasma or serum level). The objective is to maintain a serum level that is adequate for killing the microorganism but below the level known to be ototoxic.

There are a number of factors that increase the chance that a potentially ototoxic drug will damage the cochlea and cause a hearing impairment, including: (1) impaired renal function; (2) extended course of treatment (more than 10 days); (3) the concomitant administration of some other drugs, especially loop diuretics, such as furosemide (lasix), or other otoxic antibiotics; (4) previous aminoglycoside therapy; (5) advanced age; (6) and existing sensorineural hearing loss. Since ototoxic drugs are excreted, that is, removed from the blood, mostly by the kidneys, renal function is particularly important as a factor in determining the extent of aminoglycoside ototoxicity. Varied types of patients undergoing AER measurement for audiologic assessment or neurodiagnosis are often treated with potentially ototoxic drugs, such as premature and low birth weight newborn infants at risk for hearing impairment, patients with CNS neoplasms, surgical patients, severely burned patients, and severely head injured patients in the intensive care unit. Audiometric assessment is indicated for patients at risk for ototoxic hearing impairment, before, during, and after medical therapy, and for patients whose serum levels of potentially ototoxic drugs exceed acceptable safe limits.

It is important to emphasize that audiometric testing is not performed to assure safe levels of the drugs but, rather, to document hearing status when ototoxicity is likely or suspected. When indicated, baseline audiometric assessment should be completed either before therapy is started or, at least, within the first 72 hours (3 days) of treatment. Weekly testing during therapy and then follow-up testing after the drug is discontinued is also recommended. Ototoxic effects may occur days, weeks, and even months after a drug is discontinued. For some drugs, such as vancomycin, aspirin, and chloroquine, ototoxicity may be reversible. There is some question about the ototoxicity of vancomycin when not used in combination with other ototoxic drugs. Lasix (furosemide) is noteworthy because of its synergistic effects. That is, lasix in combination with another potentially ototoxic drug (e.g., gentimicin) increases significantly the risk of cochlear damage. Cisplatin, a cytotoxic (antineoplastic) drug now often used as a form of treatment for intracranial neoplasms (brain tumors), causes hearing loss in at least 6 percent of patients, usually within six days after administration begins. The hearing damage is dose related. Chloroquine, a medical treatment for rheumatoid arthritis, appears to produce significant delays in absolute latency values for ABR waves III and V, and abnormal wave I–III and I–V, but not III–V, latency intervals (Bernard, 1980). Vascular side effects are mentioned in an explanation of this finding.

Most ototoxic drugs damage outer hair cells in the cochlea and produce a sensory hearing loss. Damage first occurs in the basal portion of the cochlea, the region important for high-frequency hearing. Therefore, initial evidence of hearing impairment is usually observed for high-frequency sounds (above 8000 Hz). If the hearing deficit progresses, it begins to involve frequencies in the 1000 to 4000 Hz region. This is the frequency region of the cochlea that contributes to ABR generation with click stimuli. AERs, especially ABR, are very useful in initially evaluating and then monitoring auditory status of persons whose age or medical condition precludes conventional behavioral audiometry (an audiogram).

SEDATIVES AND HYPNOTICS (DEPRESSANTS). | These are "controlled drugs" that they can be acquired only with a prescription. Sedatives are the first drugs on a continuum of CNS depressants—drugs that reduce CNS activity. They reduce physical activity and calm the patient. Sedatives and hypnotics cause drowsiness or sleep and, therefore, may be used to quiet patients for AER measurement. Although sedatives and hypnotics facilitate onset and maintenance of sleep, the patient can be easily aroused with stimulation. At the other end of the continuum of CNS depression is anesthesia, which is discussed below. Sedatives commonly used in AER measurement, such as chloral hydrate, are also discussed in Chapter 8. Sedatives are often classified as either long-acting (e.g., diazepam, librium) or short-acting (lorazemam). Controlled drugs are further divided into Schedules, depending on their effect and the penalties for illegal possession. Schedule I drugs (e.g., marijuana, LSD, heroin) are not for clinical use, but only for research purposes. Schedule II controlled drugs can only be obtained with a written prescription (versus given verbally by telephoned) that cannot be refilled. Examples of Schedule II drugs that may be encountered clinically and may influence AERs are pentobarbital, secobarbital, methylphenidate (Ritalin®), synthetic narcotics (meperidine, or Demerol®), and opium narcotics (e.g., morphine). Schedule IV drugs (a prescription must be rewritten after 6 months or five refills) also fall within this general category. Among them are benzodiazepines, such as diazepam (Valium®), lorazepam (Ativan®), chlordiazepoxide (Librium®), and chloral hydrate. The effects of these drugs on the ABR will be described below.

Chloral hydrate is the oldest synthetic "sleeping drug" and, by far, the most popular sedative for quieting children for ABR measurement. It is a halogenated alcohol that undergoes chemical reduction after ingestion and causes CNS depression. Recall that chloral hydrate is a controlled substance and must be stored in a locked area and dispensed only by proper personnel (e.g., physician or registered nurse). The typical pediatric dose is 50 mg per kg of body weight, up to a maximum dose of 1 gram (1000 mg). Chloral hydrate is usually administered in syrup form, but capsules are available (taken with water, juice, or ginger ale). Possible adverse reactions include gastric irritation (upset stomach), nausea, and bad breath. Some children show a paradoxical response and are highly active and excited after the normal dose of chloral hydrate. Serious liver or renal disease are contraindications for use of chloral hydrate.

Accumulated clinical experience and published reports confirm that chloral hydrate does not affect ABR (Mokotoff, Schulman-Galambos, Galambos, 1977; Palaskas, Wilson, & Dobie, 1989; Sohmer & Student, 1978). Cortical auditory evoked responses, including ASSRs evoked by slow modulation frequencies (< 60 Hz), are markedly affected by chloral hydrate, as discussed in Chapters 8 (ASSR), 11 (AMLR), 12 (ALR), 13 (P300), and 14 (MMN response). The reader is referred to Chapter 8 for a more detailed discussion of conscious sedation with chloral hydrate and other drugs and protocols for instituting a sedation policy for diagnostic ABR measurement in infants and other children who cannot be properly assessed in a state of natural sleep.

Phenobarbital and *secobarbital* are also sometimes used as CNS depressants and, therefore, as sedatives for AER measurement. Phenobarbital is a long-acting barbiturate that depresses the CNS. The typical dose for sedation of children is 2 mg/kg/day (by mouth) in four divided doses. Phenobarbital is also used as an anticonvulsant drug. It should not be confused with *pento*barbital, a barbiturate agent sometimes applied in management of severely brain-injured patients. Secobarbital is a short-acting barbiturate drug. Pediatric dosage is the same as for phenobarbital.

Diazepam (Valium), a benzodiazepine, is a frequently prescribed antianxiety drug (minor tranquilizer) that may be used as a sleeping drug. The effect of Valium on ABR is probably minimal (Adams, Watson, & McClelland, 1982; Doring & Daub, 1980), whereas cortical auditory evoked responses are definitely suppressed. Valium is often the drug prescribed by physicians for adult patients whose high-level

anxiety and state of arousal prevent relaxation and preclude valid ABR measurement due to excessive muscle and movement artifact.

Morphine (morphine sulfate), an alkaloid derived from opium, is a narcotic analgesic (pain reliever). The other main types of analgesic (pain reliever) are non-narcotic (e.g., aspirin). In addition to analgesia, morphine produces drowsiness and changes in mood. The suspected site of action is limbic system (hippocampus, amygdala), and it does not affect the major sensory pathways. An IV agent, it is used (in relatively high doses) as a sedative in acute brain-injured patients in the intensive care unit. Morphine does not appear to exert an influence on ABR (Hall, 1988; Samra, Krutak-Krol, Pohorecki, Domino, 1985).

Meperidine is an IV opioid analgesic, like morphine, with no apparent effect on early or late latency AERs, such as ABR (Pfefferbaum, Roth, Tinklenberg, Rosenbloom, & Kopell, 1979).

ANESTHETIC AGENTS. | An appreciation of the effects of anesthetic agents on AERs is essential for those clinicians involved in neuromonitoring during surgery. Anesthesia is defined as loss of sensation (partial or complete), with or without loss of consciousness, that may be drug-induced or due to disease or injury. The following discussion will be limited to general anesthesia affecting the brain and producing loss of sensation and consciousness. Local anesthesia of nerves serving a specific anatomic region may be used in AER measurement. An example would be Phenol (89%), which effectively numbs the transtympanic membrane for transtympanic needle ECochG recordings. The ECochG response and ABR, of course, are not affected.

Depth or stage of general anesthesia may be described according to different schema. According to one description, there are three stages. In stage one, the patient is first excited until voluntary control is lost (hearing is the last of the senses to become nonfunctional). The corneal reflex is still present in the second stage, although loss of voluntary control persists. The third stage is characterized by three criteria: complete relaxation, deep regular breathing, and a sluggish corneal reflex. There are four stages of anesthesia according to another schema, including: (1) analgesia (no feeling), (2) delirium, (3) surgical anesthesia, and (4) medullary depression. From these terms, it is clear that the patient should be maintained in stage 3 during surgery. Stages 1 and 2 represent inadequate anesthesia, while anesthesia is excessive in stage 4.

Before anesthesia, drugs are administered to decrease anxiety, relieve pre- and postoperative pain and provide amnesia for the perioperative period. Examples of these preinduction drugs are benzodiazepines (e.g., Valium), barbiturates, and neuroleptics. There are three major components to anesthesia. The purpose of the first component, induction, is to produce a rapid loss of consciousness. Drugs used to induce anesthesia include benzodiazepines, barbiturates, narcotic analgesics, etomidate, ketamine, and inhalation agents. The second, and longest lasting, component is maintenance of anesthesia. The purpose of this phase, which persists throughout surgery, is to produce a stable state of loss of consciousness and loss of reflexes to painful stimuli. Among the drugs often administered to during maintenance of anesthesia are inhalation agents (gases), narcotic analgesics, ketamine, muscle relaxants, and antiarrhythmic agents. Finally, anesthesia must be reversed so the patient will wake up and return to the preanesthetic state, a process facilitated with opioid antagonists and anticholinesterase agents.

Anesthetic agents are often categorized according to their mode of administration. Some are intravenous (IV) agents, infused directly into the bloodstream via a line inserted into a vein (at the wrist or ankle). Examples of IV agents are barbiturates (thiopental/Sodium Pentothal, methohexital/Brevital, thiamylal), benzodiazepines (diazepam/Valium, midazolam), etomidates (amidate), opioid analgesics (morphine, fentanyl, meperidine), neuroleptics (droperidol + fentanyl), and dissociative anesthetic agents (ketamine). With IV anesthetics, there is fast action and fast recovery. The brain receives one-tenth of the dose within 40 seconds following IV administration. Other anesthetic agents are administered as a gas by inhalation. Inhalation agents, in contrast to those administered intravenously, are slower acting and are measured by partial pressure (tension) in the blood (brain). One commonly used inhalation agent is nitrous oxide, a gaseous anesthetic that is a good analgesic and induction agent, but has low anesthetic potency. Other drugs are called volatile anesthetics (e.g., halothane, isoflurane), which are potent even at low concentrations. Anesthetic agents produce differential effects on AERs. The ABR is not seriously influenced by anesthesia, in comparison to the so-called "extralemniscal" AERs (e.g., AMLR, ALR) that involve multisynaptic nonlemniscal pathways and are sensitive to suppression by anesthetic agents. These responses are also affected to a greater degree by sedatives, such as chloral hydrate.

Propofol is one of the most popular agents for general anesthesia of young children, and it is often used to achieve light anesthesia required for diagnostic auditory assessment with ABR and ASSR. Propofol is a popular pediatric anesthetic because recovery of consciousness is quick when the drug is discontinued, and side effects (e.g., vomiting) are rare (McLeod & Boheimer, 1985; Sanderson & Blades, 1988). In the author's experience in the years following 2000 in performing ABR measurement in the operating room for over 200 children, propofol was by far used most often to maintain anesthesia. Purdie and Cullen (1993) conducted an investigation demonstrating modest effects of propofol anesthesia on 10 children undergoing general surgery that did not involve the ears or brain. Unfortunately, the age of the children was not stated. However, the authors did report performing an ABR while the children were awake, before induction of anesthesia, suggesting that the children were at

least 5 or 6 years old and cooperative. Patients spontaneously breathed through a laryngeal mask a mixture of nitrous oxide in oxygen. Propofol blood plasma concentration was maintained at 4µg ml $^{-1}$ and 8 µg ml $^{-1.}$ Chassard et al. (1989), an a study of the influence of propofol on ABR in adults, also reported modest increases (e.g., 0.15 to 0.5 ms) in absolute and interwave latencies, depending on the dose of the anesthetic up to 8 µg ml $^{-1.}$ Of relevance to clinical measurements of ABR in children, amplitudes do not appear to be adversely affected by propofol. In other words, auditory threshold estimations with ABR are not likely to be elevated secondary to the anesthesia. On the contrary, the absence of myogenic activity with anesthesia markedly enhances the signal-to-noise ratio and, therefore, detection of an ABR wave V at the lowest possible intensity levels.

Halothane and *isoflurane* are potent volatile anesthetics. *Halothane* appears to cause, at most, slight delays in ABR interwave latencies, without altering waveform morphology (Cohen & Britt, 1982; Duncan et al., 1979; Hsu et al., 1992; Stockard et al., 1980). Latency prolongation of approximately 5 percent (e.g., about 0.2 ms for the wave I–V interval) is statistically significant, linear, and dose-related according to some investigators (Thornton, Heneghan, James, & Jones, 1984; Wilson, Wilson, & Cant, 1984). *Isoflurane* may prolong ABR absolute and interwave latencies (Manninen, Lam, & Nicholas, 1984), although some investigators report negligible effects (Stockard et al., 1980).

Fentanyl, a popular narcotic analgesic, is a synthetic opioid that is eighty times as potent as morphine. Fentanyl is used exclusively as an anesthetic, as opposed to morphine which is used as a sedative. At low doses, fentanyl has no apparent effect on ABR interwave latency values (Inoue, Kawasaki, Shiraishi, & Takasaki, 1992; Samra, Lilly, Rush, & Kirsh, 1984). In adults anesthetized with fentanyl, Kileny et al. (1983) observed only slight alterations in AMLR latency and, as with chemical paralysis, noted improved waveform quality as muscle activity subsided.

Sufentanil is a narcotic anesthetic that is ten times more potent than fentanyl, but provides a greater margin of safety (especially in animal research) because it produces less hemodynamic stress than fentanyl.

Enflurane produces increased interwave (wave I–III and wave I–V) latencies of up to 0.85 ms, which are linear and depend on the concentration (Dubois, Sato, Chassy, & Macnamara, 1982; Thornton et al., 1981, 1984).

Small changes in ABR interwave latencies (average of 0.23 ms) are related to anesthesia with *sevoflurane,* at least in children aged 1 month to 15 years (Kitahara, Fukatsu, & Koizumi, 1995).

According to Prosser and Arslan (1985), ABR is not affected by fluorothane.

Methohexital sodium is an IV barbiturate that significantly prolongs wave V latency by as much as 0.4 ms, but latency of waves I and III are unaffected (Kriss, Prasher, & Pratt, 1984).

Althesin and *etomidate* are IV anesthetic agents that have no effect on the ABR.

Thiopental (Sodium Pentothal) is an IV barbiturate that affects ABR minimally, although available information is somewhat confusing. Sanders et al. (1979) found no change in ABR with thiopental (preceded as an anesthetic agent by halothane and nitrous oxide induction). Goff et al. (1977) described an amplitude reduction, but no latency change, when thiopental administration followed diazepam. Drummond, Todd, and Sang (1985) reported the most notable ABR changes. Absolute and interwave latency values for waves I, III, and V were significantly increased (average wave V latency from 6.16 to 6.87 ms), while amplitude was not changed. ABR was never suppressed by thiopental. Effects of thiopental on late AERs were demonstrated by Abrahamian, Allison, Goff, and Rosner (1963).

Pentobarbital is a fast-acting barbiturate that appears to have little serious effect on ABR latency or amplitude (Bobbin, May, & Lemoine, 1979; Cohen & Britt, 1982; Hall, 1985; Marsh, Frewen, Sutton, & Potsic, 1984; Newlon, Greenberg, Enas, & Becker, 1983).

Ketamine (hydrochloride) is a dissociative IV anesthetic that works by altering limbic system activity, but not medullary structures. Afferent neural input probably still reaches the sensory cortex, but activity in association areas may be suppressed. Ketamine does not appear to affect ABR latency or amplitude values (Bobbin, May, & Lemoine, 1979; Cohen & Britt, 1982). In the cat, ketamine produced mixed effects on AERs recorded directly from electrodes placed in inferior colliculus and mesencephalic reticular formation (Dafny & Rigor, 1978). Lower doses of ketamine were associated with reduced amplitude while higher doses appeared to increase amplitude and also latency. Inferior colliculus activity showed greatest sensitivity to ketamine effects.

Nitrous oxide is a gaseous inhalation agent that is a good analgesic. It is used to induce anesthesia, but has low potency (strength) for maintaining anesthesia. ABR is resistant to the effects of nitrous oxide (Sebel, Flynn, & Ingram, 1984). AER components with latency values beyond 50 ms show dose-dependent reduction in amplitude, yet ABR latency is not affected (Lader, 1977).

Lidocaine is used as a lumbar epidural anesthetic in some surgical procedures. *Lidocaine* is also a cardiac drug used in acute treatment of ventricular arrhythmias related to myocardial infarction. Dose-related side effects include tinnitus and speech disturbances, along with serious systemic abnormalities (respiratory depression, heart problems). Interestingly, lidocaine has also been investigated as a possible treatment option for tinnitus. ABR interwave latencies are clearly prolonged by sufficient doses of lidocaine (Javel, Mouney, McGee, & Walsh, 1982; Ruth, Gal, DiFazio, & Moscicki, 1985; Shea & Howell, 1978; Worthington, Brookhouser, Mohiuddin, & Gorga, 1985). However, a single dose of lidocaine and tocainide adequate to relieve tinnitus does not influence ABR latency or amplitude (Wasterstrom, 1985). Kasaba and colleagues (Kasaba et al., 1991; Kasaba, Kosaka, & Itoga, 1991) described latency prolongations for ABR waves III through VII and all interwave latency values after epidural anesthesia with lidocaine (continuous infusion of 60 micrograms/kg/minute after injection of 1.5 mg/kg/1 minute), when data were compared with a control group.

NEUROMUSCULAR BLOCKERS (CHEMICAL PARALYZING AGENTS). | These drugs produce paralysis by interrupting transmission of neural impulses at the skeletal neuromuscular junction. Examples of neuromuscular blockers used in the operating room and intensive care unit are pancuronium (Pavulon), Metocurine, succinylcholine, and curare. All auditory evoked responses can be reliably recorded during chemically induced muscle paralysis with such agents as Pavulon, Metocurine, and succinylcholine (Hall, 1988; Hall, Hargadine, & Allen, 1985; Hall, Mackey-Hargadine, & Kim, 1985; Harker, Hosick, Voots, & Mendel, 1977; Kileny, 1983; Kileny, Dodson, & Gelfand, 1983; Smith & Kraus, 1987). Waveforms are, in fact, often enhanced in paralysis due to the lack of muscle-related noise or artifact.

ANTICONVULSANTS. | Phenytoin, phenobarbital, and carbamazepine (Tegretol®). are anticonvulsants used to limit seizure activity, as in epilepsy (e.g., Dilantin), with or without sedation. ABR interwave latency values are prolonged in phenytoin intoxication, but amplitude is not significantly changed (Chayasirisobhon, Green, Mason, & Berchou, 1984; Faingold & Stittsworth, 1981; Green et al., 1982; Herman & Bignall, 1967). ABR alterations in phenytoin intoxication may be reversible. These studies were primarily carried out in patients with epilepsy.

TRANQUILIZERS AND PSYCHOTHERAPEUTIC AGENTS. | Tranquilizers are referred to as neuroleptic drugs and are thought to block postsynaptic dopaminergic receptors in the mesolimbic region of the brain. Minor tranquilizers are antianxiety and sleeping drugs, such as diazepam and Librium. Major tranquilizers are used as antipsychotic agents. Other psychotherapeutic agents are lithium-based drugs, used treat manic disorders. The mechanism is unknown, but alteration of neuronal and neurotransmitter function is suspected. There is a long list of antipsychotic drugs. All are, by definition, psychotropic and may affect longer latency AERs. Because of this relationship, and because patients for whom late-latency AER testing may be indicated (e.g., schizophrenics) are treated with the drugs, there are literally hundreds of published papers describing changes in ALR, the P300 response, and the contingent negative variation (CNV) response following administration of psychotropic medications. The ABR is not significantly influenced by psychotherapeutic medications.

OTHER DRUGS INFLUENCING AERS. | There is a vast literature on the relationship between *alcohol* and AERs. Dozens of studies conducted before 1980 are thoroughly reviewed in a paper by Porjesz and Begleiter (1981), and many papers have been published since then. The rather pronounced effect of acute alcohol ingestion on cortical auditory evoked responses is reviewed in Chapters 11 through 14. Three overall alcohol-related issues—acute ingestion, chronic abuse, and withdrawal—have generated the most research interest. Acute ingestion of alcohol, without hypothermia, produces decreased amplitude of the ECochG cochlear microphonic (CM). ABR wave latencies (III through VII) are increased but amplitudes are not affected (Chu, Squires, & Starr, 1978; Church & Williams, 1982; Katbamma et al., 1993; Rosenhamer & Silverskiold, 1980; Squires, Chu, & Starr, 1978; Stockard et al., 1976). Substantial prolongations in ABR interwave latencies are also recorded in abstinent alcoholics (Begleiter, Porjesz, & Chou, 1981; Diaz, Cadaveira, & Grau, 1990), a finding correlated with CT evidence of brain atrophy (Chu, Squires, & Starr, 1982). Alcohol intoxication can be associated with lowered body temperature (hypothermia), i.e., body temperature below 37° C. It is important to rule out a temperature effect in study of alcohol effects on AERs. During alcohol withdrawal, ABR latency values (for later waves) may be unusually decreased, a possible reflection of CNS hyperexcitability (Chu et al., 1978). Shortened latencies and increased amplitudes for AERs during withdrawal tend to be more pronounced with longer alcohol exposure. Also, the ABR is more variable in recently detoxified alcoholic subjects (Spitzer & Newman, 1987).

MISCELLANEOUS DRUGS. | There are isolated reports describing effects of miscellaneous drugs on ABR, generally increased latency, including *cholinergics* (Bhargava & McKean, 1977; Bhargava, Salamy, & McKean, 1978), *promethazine, thiamine* (Lonsdale, Nodar, & Orlowski, 1979), and *toluene* (Metrick & Brenner, 1982).

Harkrider, Champlin, and McFadden (2001) published a series of papers on the effects of *nicotine* (an acetylcholinomimetic drug) with the goal of investigating the role of cholinergic mechanisms in the auditory system. Wave I latency was longer, and amplitude smaller, for ten nonsmoker subjects who wore a transdermal nicotine patch (dose of 7 mg/24 hours) than for a control group of ten nonsmoker subjects who wore a placebo patch. All subjects wore the patch for four hours. No other ABR changes with nicotine exposure were reported, suggesting that "afferent transmission through the relay nuclei of the human brainstem is generally normal . . . by the administration of nicotine" (Harkrider, Champlin, & McFadden, 2001, p. 82). The ABR findings of this prospective double-blind controlled study with nicotine exposure are consistent with those reported earlier for chronic smokers (e.g., Kumar & Tandon, 1997).

Pietrowsky, Dentler, Fehm, and Born (1992) studied with a double-blind intrasubject experimental design the effect on ABR of *calcitonin,* a drug that regulates Ca++ and is known to diminish sensitivity to painful stimuli. Subjects were twelve healthy men who received either the salmon calcitonin (sCT) or a placebo. Latency ABR wave V was significantly increased following administration of the sCT, and the extent of latency change was dose-dependent. The authors interpreted the findings as evidence of "a slowing or inhibitory influence of calcitonin on auditory processing."

Synthetic retinoids are used in treatment of severe nodulocystic acne. Nikiforidis et al. (1994) studied in a series of thirty-three patients with this condition the effect of synthetic retinoids on the ABR. Recordings were made before and after administration of oral isotretinoin. Although analysis of group data failed to show changes in the ABR before versus after treatment, there were marked increases in interwave latencies and decreases in amplitudes for 3 of the subjects after versus before therapy.

Mannitol is an osmotic diuretic than increases blood serum osmolality, expands intravascular volume and decreases intracranial (and intraocular and intracochlear) pressures. It is administered intravenously for these purposes. Mannitol is a common medical therapy for increased intracranial pressure in acute brain-injured patients (see Chapter 10). For patients with increased intracranial pressure affecting the ABR (increased wave I latency and interwave latency values), the diuretic-induced reduction intracranial and, secondarily, cochlear pressure is associated with normalization of ABR latencies (e.g., Hall, 1992).

Other Nonpathologic Factors

Sporadic reports appear in the literature on the possible effects of other nonpathologic factors on the ABR. For example, Urbani and Lucertini (1994) examined in six normal-hearing adult subjects the influence of *hypobaric oxygen,* temporary hypobaric hypoxia, on the ABR. With recovery from the induced hypoxia, there was a decrease in the wave I–V latency interval. There is even serious investigation of the possible influence of mobile telephones on the ABR. Kellényi and colleagues in Hungary (Kellényi, Thuroczy, Faludy, & Lnard, 1999) reported significantly increased ABR wave V latency values in a group of ten normal adult subjects on the ear exposed to a "common GSM handy-phone," a finding associated with a 20 dB deficit in hearing sensitivity within the 2000 to 10,000 Hz region on the same side. The authors speculate on the possibility of local thermal effects and ionic membrane shifts within the peripheral auditory system secondary to pulsed radio frequency (RF) exposure, mechanisms similar to those caused by noise exposure.

Litscher (1995) conducted a thorough investigation of the ABR recorded continuously during *nocturnal sleep.* Subjects were nine normal male adults. In addition to the two-channel ABR recordings, detail physiologic measurements were monitored, including EEG, electrocardiography, electrooculography, chin electromyography, respiration, body temperature (rectal), noninvasive blood pressure, and oxygen saturation. Only slight changes in ABR latencies were noted during sleep, but in general they were correlated with body temperature. There were no significant alterations in the absolute amplitude of ABR waves with sleep. Litscher (1995) did, however, describe a significant relation from the awake state to deep sleep for the latencies of waves IV and V and for the wave V/I amplitude ratio.

Mason, Mason, and Gibbon (1995) reported evidence of worsened ABR thresholds in a series of thirteen children (25 "hearing ears") after surgical insertion of grommets (ventilation tubes) into the tympanic membrane. Data suggest the possibility of surgery related *noise induced alteration of auditory function.* The surgical procedure involved a myringotomy, and then the use of suction to remove fluid or glue from the middle ear space. Children who underwent the procedure showed a 15 dB shift (worsening) of ABR threshold, whereas another group of children who did not require suction, either because they had a dry ear or did not have a myringotomy showed no change in ABR thresholds. The finding of a worsening of ABR thresholds is contrary to the expected improvement in air conduction hearing as documented by the ABR following insert of ventilation tubes (e.g., Fria & Sabo, 1980; Hall, 1992; Owen, Morcross-Nechay, & Howie, 1993). Mason, Mason, and Gibbon (1995) attribute the decrease in ABR thresholds in their study to the influence of suction noise on sensory hearing, citing data reported by

Wetmore, Henry, and Konkle (1993) on the high level of sound generated by suction (> 86 dB).

TROUBLESHOOTING IN ABR RECORDING

Some factors that may cause problems in AER measurement or interpretation are easily identified, even before testing begins. The effect on these factors (e.g., age, gender, body temperature, hearing loss) on AER latency, amplitude, or morphology can then be estimated, and perhaps corrected, before response interpretation. Other measurement problems, such as electrical or muscular artifact (see Figure 7.9), produce characteristic deviations in waveform appearance. There are a finite number of such problems. The specific problem must first be analyzed and identified. Then, once recognized, the source of the problem is sought out and, hopefully, the problem is corrected or eliminated. At the very least, deleterious effects on AER waveform are minimized. In some cases, however, these types of problems cannot be minimized, and they preclude valid AER measurement. A final group of measurement problems may have multiple causes. Some are due to operator errors, others mechanical failure, and still others result from a certain characteristic of the subject. Examples of these latter problems are absence of

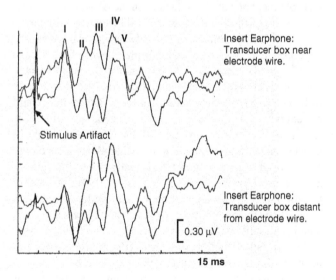

A   **Auditory Brainstem Response**
Stimulus Artifact with Air-Conduction Stimulation

Insert Earphone: Transducer box near electrode wire.

Stimulus Artifact

Insert Earphone: Transducer box distant from electrode wire.

0.30 µV

15 ms

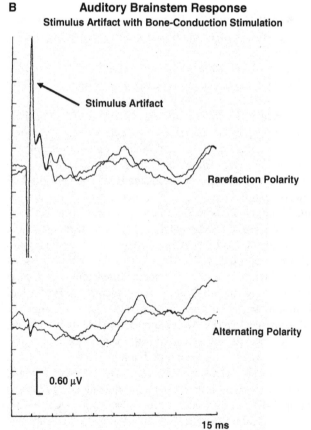

B   **Auditory Brainstem Response**
Stimulus Artifact with Bone-Conduction Stimulation

Stimulus Artifact

Rarefaction Polarity

Alternating Polarity

0.60 µV

15 ms

FIGURE 7.9.   Solving the problem of stimulus-related artifact in the ABR evoked by air-conduction (A) and bone-conduction (B) stimulation.

response components (waves), or even the entire response, or poor waveform morphology.

Troubleshooting is the term used to describe the process of identifying measurement problems, determining their cause, and, whenever possible, finding an adequate and feasible solution. Troubleshooting requires a rational, logical approach to problem solving and is a skill that improves with experience. As a rule, the first time a certain problem is encountered, the clinician may take some time to find a solution. Troubleshooting in these instances may involve a trial-and-error solution method, or even telephone calls or email communications to other more experienced clinicians. The next time this same type of problem interferes with AER measurement, however, the clinician is able to apply prior experiences and more promptly find a solution. The overall objective herein is to help clinicians who are inexperienced with selected AER measures to more quickly and effectively identify and solve problems.

ABR Waveform Analysis

Examples of ABR waveforms produced by various types of errors in technique or measurement are shown in Figure 7.10. The replicated waveform at the top of the figure was re-

corded from a normal-hearing young adult with typical measurement parameters. Stimulus intensity level was 80 dB HL. Waveforms in the figure were generated by altering the test protocol as noted to the right of the waveform. In waveform A there was no stimulus. The earphone was completely unplugged. Many a beginning clinician might imagine a poorly formed component in the waveform at above 7 to 8 ms. Waveform B was recorded during a bone-conduction ABR assessment. Of course, if upon finishing a bone-conduction ABR assessment, a clinician does not unplug the bone vibrator and replace it with the conventional air-conduction earphone, then the next person to use the equipment may very well record nothing but noise, because the bone vibrator is stored somewhere on the evoked response system cart, rather than placed properly on the patient's mastoid bone. The conditions are the same except for the substitution of a bone vibrator for an air-conduction transducer. Waveform B is characterized by absolute latency delay of waves I through V because at 80 dB on the dial, the effective bone conduction intensity is only about 40 dB. The only difference in measurement parameters between the top (normal) waveforms and waveform C is that a 500 Hz tone burst was used as a stimulus, rather than a click. This stimulus has a longer rise time, and the response is associated with cochlear activity arising from a more apical portion of the basilar membrane than the click. Therefore, latency is delayed and wave I is not observed. Again, a clinician might inadvertently record waveform C instead of the top waveforms if equipment was not returned to the "neutral" or customary settings following tone burst stimulation.

The single alteration of measurement parameters for waveform D is inactivation (disenabling) of automatic artifact rejection. Large amplitude movement artifact is allowed to interfere with ABR recording. The result is a waveform with relatively poor morphology and prominent artifact-related peaks that are really muscle activity. Waveform E was recorded with a severely restricted filter setting. Important spectral energy in the ABR is thus filtered out. This waveform was mistakenly recorded because, following an AMLR evaluation, filter settings were not returned to the values appropriate for recording ABR (i.e., 30 to 3000 Hz). Actually, filter settings of 30 to 100 Hz are not even appropriate for AMLR, as explained in Chapter 11. Finally, the results of a similar mistake are seen in waveform F. Here, AMLR measurement preceded the ABR, but upon completion of the AMLR test, analysis time was not shortened from 100 ms back to 15 ms. The entire ABR waveform is compressed into the initial portion of the display. Close inspection of this waveform, at least, that the filter setting was reasonably appropriate, probably about 10 to 1500 Hz. There is good definition of both ABR and AMLR components.

Those who instruct or supervise students or clinicians who are learning how to record, analyze, and interpret ABR may find it useful to develop a similar set of waveforms illustrating the consequences of technical errors for ABR and

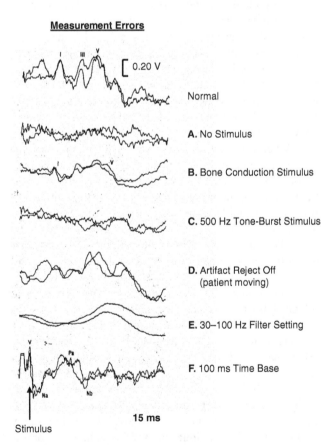

FIGURE 7.10. ABR waveforms recorded with various measurement errors.

other clinically applied AERs (e.g., ECochG, AMLR, ALR, and P300 waveforms). This format lends itself to an interesting and challenging quiz of a student's skills in recognizing symptoms of AER measurement problems and troubleshooting abilities.

Electrode Errors

Figure 7.11 shows selected waveforms recorded from one normal-hearing young adult subject to illustrate the effects of improper electrode placement. Except for electrode locations, all were recorded under the same measurement conditions. The top waveform, recorded with a Fz-ipsilateral earlobe (Ai) electrode array, is normal, with reliable waves I, III and V and possibly waves II and IV. There is also a wave VI. In waveform A, recorded with a horizontal (Ac-Ai) electrode array, wave I, wave II, wave III, and wave IV are prominent, but the wave IV/V complex is diminished and limited to just the wave IV component. In recording waveform B, the conventional (Fz-Ai) electrode array was used, but the ground electrode was totally removed. Under otherwise good measurement conditions, the waveform is almost indistinguishable from the normal replicated waveforms at the top of the figure. The ground electrode is not essential for AER measurement if electrical interference is minimal and impedance between the remaining two electrodes is low and balanced. Waveform quality deteriorates markedly, however, in electrically noisy test environments without a "good ground" electrode (e.g., low impedance and large surface area of contact with the skin).

The inverting electrode (at Ai) was removed prior to recording waveform C, leaving only the Fz noninverting and ground (Fpz) electrodes and, consequently, no "reference" electrode. The result is essentially background activity. This demonstrates the importance of the inverting electrode. As shown by numerous examples of ABRs elsewhere in the book, it is possible and even desirable, in some cases, to record with a noncephalic inverting electrode (located on the body but not on the head). The problem in recording waveform C was that no inverting electrode was used. An electrical potential between two electrodes could not be measured.

Waveform D appears to consist of a very poorly formed response, with only a relatively small and broad component in the expected latency region of wave V. In recording this waveform, electrodes were located at Fz, Ai, and Fpz. Although these are typical electrode sites, waveform C was recorded with reversal of the normal inverting electrode site (Ai) and ground electrode site (Fpz) inputs. Therefore, the noninverting electrode was at Fz, the inverting electrode was at Fpz, and the ground electrode was Ai. ABR activity detected by Fz and Fpz is very similar, since these electrodes are quite close. The Fz and Fpz inputs to the differential amplifier, when subtracted, result in cancellation of most ABR activity. Correct electrode placement and input to the amplifier (at the electrode strip or box) must be verified whenever no response is recorded.

Waveform pattern E lacks a wave I, although other components are observed, and, in fact, there is a distinct wave IV versus V separation. If a two-channel (ipsilateral and contralateral electrode array) recording technique is used, this waveform would be expected in the contralateral channel. The same waveform can be recorded erroneously in two ways. The appearance of this pattern in the ipsilateral channel of the two-channel setup suggests that either the opposite ear is actually being stimulated, unintentionally, or that the two inverting electrode inputs (Ai and Ac) were reversed (plugged in wrong). Once the problem is identified, it is not essential that the electrodes be changed back, since the channels are simply reversed. To avoid confusion and secondary mistakes in data collection, it would usually be wise to reestablish the customary test set up. In some laboratories that routinely employ a dual (ipsilateral versus contralateral) channel recording technique, channel 1 is the Fz-A2 (right earlobe) array, and channel 2 is the Fz-A1 (left earlobe) array. Presumably, this technique follows the audiologic convention of usually testing the right ear first. The author, on the other hand, uses a Fz-A1 (left earlobe) array in the first chan-

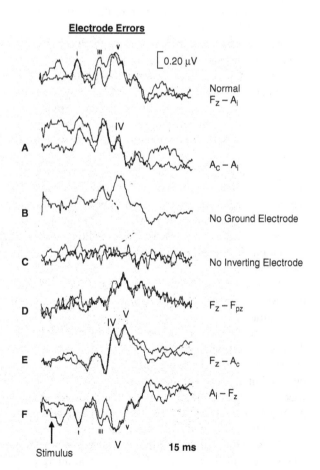

FIGURE 7.11. ABR waveforms recorded with various electrode errors.

nel. Since the left earlobe is "A1" in the 10–20 International Electrode System, it seems more logical to have A1 in channel 1 and A2 in channel 2. Today's software-based evoked response systems can be programmed to automatically plot this information, thus reducing the likelihood of inadvertent reversal of channels during recording. Either way is appropriate as long as it used consistently and understood by all testers in a clinic or laboratory.

The final waveform (F) was recorded by reversing the Fz and Ai electrode inputs. With Ai as noninverting (positive voltage) and Fz as inverting (negative voltage) electrodes, the ABR components are directed downward rather than upward. For most clinicians, this would be unintentional or by mistake. Recall, however, from the discussion on ABR nomenclature in Chapters 1, 3, and 6 that negative-going waves are the convention in Europe and Japan, and also preferred by some investigators in Canada and the United States. Nonetheless, if this upside-down pattern is recorded unintentionally, simply digitally inverting the waveform offline will restore the usual ABR appearance.

Electrical Interference

Since AER measurement involves detection of minute (several μvolts or less) electrical events within the ear, auditory nerve, and brain with electrodes typically located on the surface of the scalp, it is not really surprising that electrical interference can be a major problem. The surface electrodes are just as likely to detect extraneous electrical activity outside of the head as stimulus-related activity within the head. In fact, the unwanted extraneous electrical activity is often far more prominent. Fortunately, if the same electrical artifact (common mode with similar amplitude and phase) is detected by each electrode in a pair, then it will largely be cancelled out (rejected) by the differential amplifier. The process is called common mode rejection. A problem arises, however, when such electrical artifact is mostly detected by just one of the electrodes in the pair.

Another factor contributing to electrical interference in AER measurement is the amount of amplification required in processing the responses. Before the very small electrophysiologic activity (amplitude in millionth of volts, i.e., μvolts) can be processed and analyzed with an evoked response system, it must be amplified by up to 100,000 times. Amplification not only increases the problem with extraneous electrical activity detected by the electrodes, but it also introduces electrical noise to the waveform from the amplifier circuit. Of course, circuitry for various brands of evoked response systems differs in the amount of noise produced during amplification. Finally, transducers that produce acoustic stimuli necessary in generating an AER are electromagnetic devices that themselves can be a source of electrical artifact. Again, the amount of electrical interference varies among transducer types. Major sources and types of electrical interference in AER recordings will now be described and illustrated by actual waveforms. Selected solutions to electrical interference problems in ABR measurement are offered here and also summarized in Table 7.1.

STIMULUS ARTIFACT. | Among electrical interference problems, stimulus artifact is probably the easiest to isolate and solve. This discussion is limited to electrical artifact produced by acoustic stimulus transducers. Acoustic transducers (various types of earphones) produce electromagnetic fields. That is, they generate electrical activity. Very often, the acoustic transducer generating the stimulus for an AER is located close to an electrode that is recording the AER, and stimulus-related artifact would seem to be unavoidable. These undesirable interactions between electrical activity from earphones and recording electrodes can be reduced or eliminated with some common sense precautions (see Figure 7.9).

Early investigators of AERs recommended electromagnetic shielding of earphones with a layer or two of special metal (Coats, 1984; Elberling & Salomon, 1973). The shielding is designed to contain the electromagnetic energy and insulate adjacent electrodes from its effects. Shielding of earphones, which is expensive and may produce unwanted changes in the acoustic properties of the transducer, is not really a practical alternative for most clinicians. Shielding also is not an alternative with bone-conduction transducers (oscillators or vibrators). The best general technique for reducing stimulus artifact is to put as much distance as possible between the transducer (earphone) and cables, and the recording electrodes, as summarized in Table 7.1. For any kind of earphone, the wires leading to the earphone carry an electrical signal and are not completely insulated; therefore, they should be distanced from electrode leads. These two types of wires should not make contact or be draped over one another at any point along their course. One simple method of avoiding such contact is to extend electrode leads in one direction (e.g., up toward the top of the head) and the earphone transducers (for inserts) and cables in another direction (e.g., downward toward the chest), or vice versa. Guidelines for arrangement of electrodes, earphones, and other components of evoked response systems were noted, with illustrations, in Chapter 6. Since electrode leads may function somewhat as antennae in picking up unwanted electrical activity (from the air), shorter leads are desirable. The typical electrode lead, which is 1 meter (about 3 feet), may be adequate in most measurement settings, but specially constructed shorter leads (2 feet or less) are preferable for reducing artifact in especially noisy test environments. A unique combination of electrode and amplifier, the Amplitrode® by Vivosonic, was introduced in Chapter 3. Braiding (intertwining) electrode leads also tends to reduce the likelihood of electrical interference, although in the author's experience braiding electrodes may hamper placement and becomes cumbersome with TIPtrode wires. Tracking a specific electrode from one end to the other if the leads are the same color is particularly difficulty when a group of electrodes are

TABLE 7.1 Selected Auditory Brainstem Response Measurement Problems and Possible Solutions
See text for discussion.

SYMPTOM	POSSIBLE PROBLEMS	POSSIBLE SOLUTIONS
No display	Technical	verify the system power is on
		verify the power cord is plugged in
		verify monitor (screen) power is on
		verify adequate monitor brightness
		verify an evoked program is loaded
		consult the equipment manual
Equipment won't average	Set up error	verify stimulus repetitions are not at "0"
		verify stimulus duration is not "0"
		verify stimulus rate not too fast for the analysis time
		verify all measurement parameters
		restart computer
		consult equipment manual
More than one response in analysis time	Stimulus rate vs. analysis time incompatible	slow stimulus rate so the ISI is longer than the analysis time
		shorten analysis time to less than ISI
		the ISI for a click is analysis time/rate
No response	No stimulus	perform a listening check
		verify the correct transducer is used
		verify the test ear is correct
	Improper electrode site or array	verify correct electrode sites
	Severe hearing loss	obtain an audiogram if feasible
		increase stimulus intensity to maximum
		attempt bone-conduction stimulation
	Inadequate amplification	check gain
Excessive early artifact	Stimulus interference	alternate polarity
		use insert earphones to separate transducer from electrode
		verify electrode wires are not near power cords
		verify electrode wires are not near earphone wires
		reduce stimulus intensity
		use post-stimulus time delay
		stimulus artifact is expected for bone-conduction stimulus
Large, slow artifact	Muscular artifact	attempt to relax patient
		encourage sleep
		sedate patient
		raise high-pass filter cutoff frequency
		sleep status?
		verify artifact rejection is on
Poor waveform morphology	High-frequency loss or retro-cochlear dysfunction?	increase stimulus intensity
		slow stimulus rate
		change stimulus polarity
		increase number of sweeps
		record multiple replicated waveforms
		sum replicated waveforms
		use click versus tone-burst stimuli
		open filter settings
		analyze a prestimulus baseline
		verify that the artifact rejection is on
Excessive noise, spikes, or small fluctuations in waveform	High-frequency electrical interference	rule out electrical devices and lines
		verify good ground
		alter stimulus rate
		lower low-pass filter
		alter electrode array
		increase sweeps
		verify adequate electrode impedance
Small or no wave I	High-frequency hearing loss	increase intensity
		decrease rate
		verify ipsilateral electrode site
		use earlobe versus mastoid electrode

SYMPTOM	POSSIBLE PROBLEMS	POSSIBLE SOLUTIONS
Small or no wave I (continued)		use an ear-canal electrode (e.g., TIPtrode)
		use TM or TT electrode
		change stimulus polarity to rarefaction
		horizontal electrode array
		use click versus a tone burst
		lower high-pass filter
		increase the number of sweeps (averages)
		obtain audiogram
Delayed wave I latency	Conductive hearing loss	Perform an air- versus bone-conduction audiogram
		bone-conduction ABR
		immittance measures
		increase intensity
Bifid wave I	Which peak is used for latency calculations?	decrease intensity
		change polarity
		ECochG electrode
		horizontal electrode array
Small or no wave II or III	High-frequency hearing loss or brainstem dysfunction	obtain audiogram
		increase stimulus intensity
		horizontal or noncephalic electrode array
		change stimulus polarity
		TT or TM electrode
Indistinct wave V	Latency calculation	obtain audiogram
		increase stimulus intensity
		lower high-pass filter setting
		raise low-pass filter setting
		use noncephalic electrode array
		analyze latency–intensity function
		rule out inadvertent ipsilateral masking
		multiple replications
		change polarity
Delayed wave V latency, no wave I	Peripheral or brainstem dysfunction?	obtain audiogram
		increase intensity
		rule out crossover response (masking)
		see wave I enhancement techniques above
		document young age
Prominent wave VI	Really wave V?	lower stimulus intensity
		use contralateral masking
		use horizontal or noncephalic electrode array
Spiked wave V	Really wave IV?	use contralateral and noncephalic electrode arrays
		change stimulus intensity level
		compare with waveform from other ear
Delayed wave I–V latency	Brainstem dysfunction?	rule out hypothermia
		document young age
		calculate interear latency difference
		verify wave V identification (see techniques above)
		use gender-matched normative data
		obtain audiogram
Short wave I–V latency	Brainstem dysfunction?	rule out high-frequency hearing loss
		rule out hyperthermia
		wave I delayed?
		bifid wave I?
		use gender- and age-matched normative data
		verify wave V versus IV identification (above)
Small wave V/I amplitude ratio	Brainstem dysfunction?	verify wave V identification
		verify repeatability of wave V
		is wave V too small or wave I too big or both?
		verify inverting electrode site (smaller V/I amplitude ratio with TIPtrode versus earlobe or mastoid electrode)

braided together. Even if the electrode leads are of different colors, the task when leads are braided is very challenging for a color-deficient tester.

With a conventional supra-aural audiometric earphone (TDH-39 or TDH-49), the earphone is often resting on a mastoid or earlobe electrode. At high intensity levels, stimulus artifact may create a serious problem because stimulus-related waves extend into the time frame of the ABR. There is an additional problem if an automatic display gain option is selected with the evoked response system. The size of waveform displayed on the screen is adjusted on the basis of the largest peaks so that a fixed portion of the screen (e.g., one-third) is filled. If the stimulus artifact is large, the remainder of the waveform (the actual response) may be scaled down excessively, sometimes appearing as a flat line. Some evoked response systems offer a blocking feature in which the portion of the display in the time period of the stimulus (around 0 ms) can be removed from the averaged waveform. Display scaling is therefore determined by the actual response waveform, rather than by stimulus artifact. This technique does not, however, actually solve the artifact problem. The most effective means of reducing stimulus artifact with supra-aural earphones is to rely on alternating polarity stimuli. The artifact produced by each of the two polarities is opposite in direction and when averaged (summed) is mostly cancelled out (the positive plus negative voltages when added approach zero voltage). The obvious limitation of routine use of alternating polarity stimuli is that a single polarity (e.g., rarefaction) may be preferable in most patients. One way around this dilemma is to first record replicate responses with each polarity (rarefaction and condensation) and then, if excessive stimulus artifact is present, to digitally add the waveforms for the two polarities. With some evoked response systems, alternating polarity stimuli are presented, and then waveforms are separately averaged in one channel for rarefaction clicks and another channel for condensation clicks. The process of adding and subtracting waveforms was described above. The effect is a set of waveforms essentially produced by alternating stimuli, so stimulus artifact should be minimal. This approach, of course, is not necessarily time effective nor ideal clinically since averaging a response to both polarities doubles test time and might not have been required. Also, the adding process must be done offline, precluding ongoing data analysis. Figure 7.12 shows the effect of length of time of recording on a ABR in an environment with excessive noise.

Perhaps the most effective method for reducing stimulus artifact is use of insert earphones (tube phones). Clinical advantages of insert earphones were listed in Chapters 3 and 6. Electrical activity is generated from the cable leading from the plug to the box and by the box that houses the transducer. Then, an acoustic signal travels down the plastic tube to the insert cushion. The objective, then, is to keep the earphone cable and box as far away from electrode leads as possible. The plastic tube is not a source of electrical activity

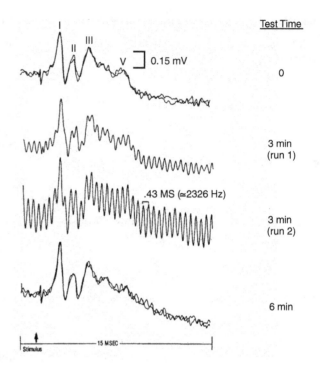

FIGURE 7.12. Effect of time of recording on ABR in an environment with excessive electrical interference.

and will not produce stimulus artifact, even if it is resting on an electrode lead. Insert earphones contribute to reduced stimulus artifact in two ways. The transducer (box) can be positioned away from electrode leads. The greater the separation between the transducer box and electrode wires, the less likely the artifact. Also, the plastic tube produces a time delay between stimulus and onset of the auditory evoked response. The length of tubing produces a delay of 0.8 or 0.9 ms. Therefore, even if stimulus artifact is present, the delay virtually eliminates any interference with identification of early AER components. Other advantages of the insert earphones (e.g., comfort, less acoustic ringing, prevention of collapsing ear canals, increased interaural attenuation), and some associated precautions (e.g., accounting for the time delay in absolute latency calculations) were reviewed in detail in Chapter 3.

ELECTRICAL NOISE. | Electrical power in the United States is supplied with a frequency of 60 Hz; the power line frequency in Europe is 50 Hz. Any electrical outlet or electrical device may produce electrical noise with a frequency of either 60 Hz or of harmonics of this frequency (e.g., 120 Hz), or much higher frequencies that are not multiples of 60 Hz. A few examples of the numerous sources of 60 Hz electrical noise (also referred to as line noise) in a clinical setting are electrical wiring in a test area, fluorescent lights, X-ray viewing boxes, power transformers, copy machines, conveyer belts, escalators, elevators, electrical machinery, patient video monitors, blood pressure transducers, computers and computer monitors, heating blankets and incu-bators, EKG (electrocardiogram) equipment, and operating room microscopes. Even the evoked response system itself, if positioned close to the recording electrodes, can produce excessive electrical artifact in AER measurements. From this partial list of electrical interference suspects, it is clear that some test settings are inevitably quieter electrically than oth-ers. The ideal test environment is a relatively isolated area in which none of the devices listed are on a floor above or below the test area, nor in any nearby room. In addition, the optimal test setting includes new and preferably dedicated wiring (no other equipment or devices are on the same lines) and a radio frequency shielded room for all AER recordings. At the other extreme of the electrical noise continuum is the typical newborn or surgical ICU or OR, which is filled with the above noted electrical devices (many of them life-sup-porting), has electrical wiring that supplies a variety of ma-chines and functions, and is adjacent to other trouble spots (such as an X-ray department).

Electrical interference may be extremely unpredictable, as well as elusive. That is, at one test session there may be so much interference that AER recording is impossible, yet at some other time in the same setting there is electrical si-lence. Serious electrical artifact may appear in one electrode channel but not in another simultaneously recorded channel and then, inexplicably, the artifact problem may appear in the opposite channel. Although this is an extremely frustrat-ing feature of electrical interference, it does suggest that one possible solution is simply to "wait out the storm."

A rather consistent observation regarding electrical interference and electrode arrays deserves mention at this point. In very noisy environments, considerably less elec-trical interference is typically found for a horizontal (ear-to-ear) recording than for electrode arrays consisting of one electrode on the forehead or vertex. This phenomenon is vividly illustrated by Figure 7.13. In these waveforms, each

was recorded with a forehead noninverting electrode char-acterized by excessive high-frequency artifact, although the actual frequency of artifact is different in each case. Yet the horizontal (Ac-Ai) electrode array is remarkably clean. A little personal testimony is in order at this juncture. In the NICU environment, where electrical artifact from multiple essential electric devices creates an extremely hostile place to record an ABR, the author often cannot even begin averag-ing an ABR with the conventional ipsilateral electrode array due to excessive levels of electrical artifact. However, the problems with electrical artifact disappear when the ABR is recorded with a horizontal array. As noted above, if the same electrical interference were present at each of the electrodes in these four pairs, it would be minimized by differential am-plification (cancelled by subtracting the inverting from the noninverting input). Experience and trial by error, however, suggest that the electrical interference is different as detected by the forehead (or vertex) electrode versus ear electrodes. With differential amplification, artifact is, therefore, not re-jected at the amplifier and persists in the Fz-to-ear array. The artifact is apparently common to the two ear electrodes and is largely rejected at the amplifiers. A practical implication of these patterns is that electrical interference in conven-tional electrode arrays (ipsi- or contralateral) that precludes meaningful waveform interpretation might be minimized by digital subtraction of the contralateral waveform from the ipsilateral waveform (as described above). This, in effect, subtracts the activity (including interference) at the forehead (or vertex) site from itself, leaving the ear-to-ear array.

There are two fundamental approaches to dealing with 60 Hz, or any other, electrical artifact. The first, and most effective, is to determine and eliminate the source. The other approach, which is often really a last resort, is to attempt to minimize the effect of the artifact on AER measurement. The following is a general discussion of this topic. Problems are encountered more frequently in specific test environments, such as the newborn ICU, OR, or surgical ICU. Møller (1987) provides a detailed and highly informative discussion on localizing sources of electrical interference and reduc-ing their effects on evoked response recordings. Although his focus is electrical interference in the operating room, the troubleshooting principles presented are equally valuable for any test setting. According to Møller (1987), unwanted elec-trical noise interferes with evoked response equipment and recordings via four pathways: (1) Unshielded electrodes and electrode leads act as antennae in picking up airborne activ-ity from nearby sources, (2) activity may be transmitted to the patient from other electrode leads (not used in evoked re-sponse measurement) connected to other electronic devices (e.g., EKG or heart monitors) and then on to the evoked response equipment, (3) evoked response electrodes pass through magnetic fields and conduct magnetic energy on to the evoked response equipment, and (4) power line electrical activity enters the pre-amplifier or amplifier of the auditory evoked response system and appears in waveforms.

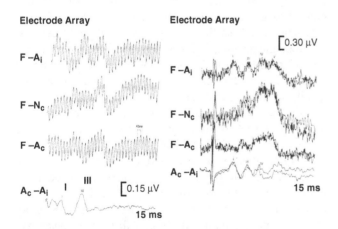

FIGURE 7.13. Two examples of the effect of horizontal electrode array on reduction of airborne electrical artifact in ABR recording.

Table 7.1 lists various sources of electrical interference and some techniques for reducing the effects on evoked responses. Detection of specific sources of unwanted electrical activity in a test area is not always possible, but should be attempted, particularly if the problems are consistently encountered and evoked responses are routinely recorded in the setting. The overall objective in this situation is to systematically and, hopefully, permanently remedy the electrical interference problems rather than spend time during each test session attempting to circumvent the interference. Møller (1987) provided instructions for constructing simple antenna-type devices for detecting sources of electrical and also magnetic interference. A length of wire (for electrical interference) or a wire loop (for magnetic interference) is plugged into one input of the differential amplifier (the positive or negative electrode input) for the evoked response system. The other input is grounded. The amplifier output is sent to an oscilloscope or loudspeaker, rather than the evoked response system. The clinician then places the antennae near suspect sources of electrical interference and notes the presence of electrical activity on the oscilloscope or via the loudspeaker. With this "ghost busting" technique, it is often possible to pinpoint sources of electrical interference and, sometimes, to determine frequency characteristics of the interference. Knowledge of the electrical activity waveform for different electrical devices might be useful in solving future artifact problems.

The alternative to eliminating the source(s) of electrical interference is to manipulate the test protocol so as to minimize the effect on AER recordings. Manipulation of the electrode configuration was noted above. Electrical interference is more likely if the interstimulus interval (the stimulus rate) is even divided into 60 (60 Hz). An odd stimulus rate (e.g., 21.1/sec) reduces the likelihood of an interaction. When 60 Hz noise is present, undulations (waxing and waning) can be created in the appearance of electrical artifact in the waveform by adjusting *stimulus rate*. The extent of electrical artifact may fluctuate also with the number of sweeps. Sometimes, it's possible to manually stop averaging at a point of relatively waveform clarity. Altering filter settings is usually a futile technique for minimizing excessive electrical interference. The use of a notch filter at 60 Hz is rarely helpful because harmonics (higher multiples of 60 Hz) are still passed into the averaging process. As noted above, the frequency of unwanted electrical interference may fall well within the frequency region of the AER being recorded. Furthermore, notch filtering produces undesirable filter ringing and response latency distortion. In short, notch filtering is to be avoided. With electrical interference at 400 Hz, for example, it is impossible to filter out the artifact without eliminating important spectral content of the ABR. Other possible methods of reducing the effects of electrical artifact on AER recordings involve manipulation of the test environment rather that test protocol.

ELECTRICAL SAFETY. | Concern for health and well-being of the patient should always be foremost in the minds of clini-cians carrying out evoked response measurements. Electrical safety is an important consideration in recording AERs, as well as electrically stimulated evoked responses. The unique safety issues in ENoG and electrically evoked auditory evoked responses, such as the importance of stimulus isolation, are discussed in Chapter 15.

Symptoms, Problems, and Solutions

Some measurement problems are common to all AERs, and troubleshooting procedures tend to be fairly consistent among AERs. That is, many of the items in a troubleshooting checklist are the same for all AERs. At the same time, other problems that appear to be quite similar often differ in the extent with which they affect AERs. For example, profound hearing impairment can account for absence of any AER. Certain anesthetic agents, on the other hand, can account for absence of the AMLR or ALR, but not the ECochG or ABR. Also, stimulus artifact occurring within the first millisecond or two after the stimulus can interfere with ECochG and ABR analysis, but it is of no concern with later latency responses. In this section, troubleshooting is discussed separately for each major type of AER using a symptom-oriented format. The symptom-oriented format was chosen because it most closely resembles clinical reality. The clinician with a measurement problem will, armed with the information found in Table 7.1, be able to determine (quickly in some cases) the appropriate solution or solutions, and then go on to successfully complete the AER assessment. This format presumes that the clinician knows, of course, which response is being recorded and, further, recognizes the measurement problem symptom and can locate that symptom among those listed. Because of the common effect of some problems on AERs, there is a certain degree of redundancy in the problems and solutions listed in the series of tables. Selected points are discussed in greater detail within the following text. The beginner at evoked response measurement is advised to purposefully make as many of these mistakes is possible, in a controlled setting, before venturing into clinical AER measurement. The least threatening way to follow through on this recommendation is for the clinician or a good friend, with plenty of time and behind closed doors, to prepare for each type of AER. The first objective is to obtain a high-quality normal response. Then, by systematically altering the measurement parameters or purposefully committing technical errors, such as leaving an electrode unplugged, using an inappropriate filter setting, and so forth, the clinician can view firsthand many of the symptoms that are listed in Table 7.1. A "mistake-making session" can also be valuable laboratory assignment in workshop or a graduate level course on AERs. Of course, clinicians who perform multiple auditory evoked responses on a daily basis will spontaneously and unintentionally participate in many "mistaking making sessions." The threadbare adage "practice makes perfect" certainly applies to ABR recording.

Examples of ABR waveforms produced in a mistake-making auditory evoked response exercise were shown in Figure 7.10. The replicated waveform at the top of the figure was recorded from a normal-hearing young adult with measurement parameters displayed in Table 6.3. Intensity level was 80 dB HL. Each of the subsequent waveforms was generated by altering the test protocol as noted to the right of the waveform.

INTERPRETATION OF ABR IN AUDITORY DYSFUNCTION

Effect of the Degree and Configuration of Hearing Impairment on the ABR

An understanding of the effect of the degree and configuration of hearing impairment on AERs is vital to their application in both neurodiagnosis and assessment of peripheral auditory status. A premise underlying this statement is that pure-tone audiometry should be routinely carried out, whenever possible, prior to AER assessment. Another principle guiding ABR interpretation involves the unpredictable relation between the degree and configuration of hearing loss and the ABR evoked by click stimulation. For the majority of patients with hearing loss, the pattern of ABR findings (e.g., the minimum response level or the shape of the wave V latency–intensity function) provides some information on the type and degree of the hearing loss. For individual patients, however, there may be very marked discrepancies between the ABR and the findings for pure tone audiometry. For example, patients with severe-to-profound sensory hearing loss in high frequencies (greater than about 80 dB nHL for frequencies above 1000 Hz) typically do not yield an ABR, even if hearing sensitivity is normal throughout the region for lower frequencies. Conversely, patients with severe low-frequency sensory hearing loss that may have a serious impact on communication capability will have normal ABR findings if hearing sensitivity is good for the higher frequencies. Balfour, Pillion, and Gaskin (1998) describe a third explanation for major discrepancies between hearing sensitivity and ABR findings. The authors recorded distortion product otoacoustic emissions (DPOAEs) from 5 children with "normal auditory sensitivity for at least one frequency in the 250 to 8000 Hz region" described as "islands of normal sensitivity" using a protocol with six f_2/f_1 ratios per octave (frequency resolution of 1/6 octave). None of the 5 patients had normal DPOAEs at each test frequency. Audiogram configurations were highly variable among the 5 subjects. For each child, an ABR was evoked with click stimuli and with tone bursts of 500, 1000, 2000, and 4000 Hz. Following analysis of their data, the authors stated, "Click-evoked ABR thresholds were ascertained at normal intensity levels for three out of five pediatric ears when a significant communicatively handicapping hearing loss was present. The presence of a click-evoked ABR threshold of < 20 dB nHL is not compatible with the conclusion that hearing is adequate for the development of speech and language skills" (Balfour, Pillion, & Gaskin, 1998, p. 468). The overall conclusion drawn from these 5 case reports underscores the importance of "crosschecking" the results of the click-evoked ABR with frequency-specific (tone-burst) ABR findings and/or DPOAEs, when valid and reliable behavioral audiometry is not possible.

There are at least four clinically pressing questions to consider in a discussion of ABR and cochlear hearing impairment:

- Do various types of peripheral auditory dysfunction differentially affect the ABR? This question is answered affirmatively later in this chapter.
- What is the relation among degree and configuration of hearing loss and the likelihood of observing specific ABR components? For example, how often can the ABR wave I (ECochG AP) be confidently identified in high-frequency sensory hearing impairment using conventional recording techniques? Also, how much sensory hearing impairment can a patient have before the ECochG or ABR cannot be recorded?
- How does ABR wave latency and amplitude change as a function of the degree and configuration of hearing loss?
- Should a clinician correct for ABR latency delay that is presumed to be due to sensory impairment when interpreting the response, in order to more accurately distinguish between sensory versus neural (i.e., cochlear versus retrocochlear) impairment? If so, what correction technique should be used?

Information on the interactions among degree, type, and configuration of hearing impairment on ABR is essential for maximal utilization of ABR in peripheral auditory assessment. Unfortunately, present understanding of these complex interactions remains incomplete.

There are two clinical applications of ABR for which an understanding of hearing impairment is essential. One is neurodiagnosis, in adults or children, and the other is estimation of hearing sensitivity, mostly in children. Thus, in adults, ABR is applied more often for neurodiagnosis than for estimation of auditory sensitivity. An important question is: How does degree and configuration of cochlear (versus retrocochlear) hearing loss affect the ABR? The clinician often has both an audiogram and ABR findings for a patient in hand and must decide whether the ABR findings are consistent with cochlear or retrocochlear hearing impairment. If a distinct wave I is recorded, this decision is relatively straightforward and is based largely on interpretation of the patient's interwave latencies in the context of normative data.

Unfortunately, the ABR for most patients with moderate-to-severe high-frequency sensorineural hearing impairment lacks a clear wave I component. Clinical experience suggests that the most challenging aspect of ABR application in adults is confidently distinguishing between cochlear versus retrocochlear ABR findings in patients with asymmetric sensorineural hearing loss. In a typical hospital audiology or auditory neurophysiology facility, this clinical challenge arises almost daily.

The second routine clinical ABR application that requires an understanding of the effects of degree, type, and configuration of hearing impairment is auditory threshold estimation in children. Currently, click stimuli are most often used in ABR measurement. Thus, an important question is: How are ABR latency and amplitude findings as a function of click stimulus intensity related to the audiogram? Is it possible to estimate confidently the degree and configuration of hearing loss from ABR data for these children? Unfortunately, with current understanding of ABR and peripheral auditory dysfunction (which are reviewed later in this chapter), such estimations, while clinically desirable, are not possible.

In attempting to describe peripheral auditory functioning with ABR, clinicians must always keep in mind two fundamental and related clinical principles: (1) No single auditory measure consistently and adequately evaluates all aspects of hearing, and (2) no diagnostic procedure is infallible. The value of AERs is certain to be enhanced by increased knowledge of neural generators and more sophisticated stimulus and analysis techniques. However, because of their distinctive underlying neuroanatomic and neurophysiologic bases (see Chapter 2), AERs will never be a valid measure of hearing. The clinical implication of this principle is that AER assessment should, whenever possible, be supplemented with other auditory measures, such as aural immittance, pure-tone, and speech audiometry. The intention in the following discussion is to provide the clinician with information that will be useful for meaningful interpretation of ABR in what is presumed to be cochlear impairment. Practical guidelines for dealing with some of the most commonly encountered problems noted in this discussion are summarized in Chapter 9.

Assessment of the Peripheral Auditory System

The peripheral auditory system consists of the external and middle ear, the cochlea (inner ear), and the eighth cranial (auditory) nerve. Sensorineural hearing impairment is due to cochlear and/or eighth-nerve pathology (*sensory* refers to cochlear and *neural* refers to eighth nerve). In assessment of peripheral auditory function, AERs are most valuable clinically in infants and older children who are difficult to test with traditional behavioral audiometry. These include children with serious neurologic and/or emotional problems and newborns (3 months of age or younger). Reasons for hearing impairment, which are numerous and varied, are reviewed in the following sections of this chapter. In these populations, AERs, primarily ABR, provide information on auditory sta-

tus that is not available from other techniques and, therefore, extremely important for effective audiologic and otologic management.

For most adults, peripheral auditory status is evaluated quite effectively and completely with conventional audiometry. AERs are usually not necessary. An appreciation of the relation between degree and type of hearing loss and AER outcome in adults, however, is very helpful for meaningful interpretation of AER findings in persons for whom an audiogram is not available, although this relation remains poorly defined. Knowledge of the anatomy and physiology of the peripheral auditory system, of basic audiometry, and of the types and nature of peripheral hearing impairment is also really necessary to fully utilize this AER application. AERs can contribute importantly and uniquely to assessment of peripheral auditory function in at least five kinds of patients other than very young or difficult-to-test children. Among these are (1) patients with nonorganic hearing impairment (persons feigning a hearing impairment); (2) stuporous, lethargic, or comatose persons who cannot volunteer valid behavioral responses to sounds; (3) patients with severe bilateral conductive hearing loss presenting the masking dilemma; (4) patients undergoing evaluation for Ménière's disease; and (5) those with suspected retrocochlear auditory dysfunction (reviewed in detail in the next chapter). A complete discussion of differential diagnosis of external-, middle-, and inner-ear pathology, as well as audiometric patterns associated with peripheral pathology, is beyond the scope of this chapter and this book. Such information is available from numerous sources, including textbooks cited at the end of Chapter 1. The theme repeatedly emphasized in this chapter is that peripheral auditory system status must always be considered in AER measurement, not only when the objective of testing is estimation of the type and degree of hearing loss, but also when AERs are measured to aid in neurodiagnosis of auditory CNS pathology.

CONDUCTIVE HEARING LOSS (CHL). | An initial step in the interpretation of any abnormal ABR is to verify the middle-ear status. Patients with middle-ear dysfunction may have conductive only or mixed hearing loss, but if middle-ear function is normal, hearing loss is sensorineural. Naturally, verification of middle-ear status is less important if an ABR is recorded with very low stimulus intensity levels that fall within normal limits for hearing sensitivity (20 dB HL or better). Even this ABR outcome (for click stimulation) does not rule out a low-frequency conductive hearing impairment. Middle-ear function is best assessed with aural immittance measurements (e.g., tympanometry). Immittance measurement, in combination with air- versus bone-conduction pure-tone audiometry, are the techniques of choice for defining the extent of the conductive component of hearing impairment for cooperative patients who can be evaluated with traditional audiometry. The effect of the conductive component on ABR latency can then be considered before interpretation for neurodiagnosis. With a young or uncooperative child, at least aural immittance measurement can usually be completed, even though valid pure-tone audiometry may be impossible. When reliable pure-tone audiometry is possible, then ABR assessment is probably unnecessary.

Conductive and sensory hearing-loss components are certainly not mutually exclusive. Interpretation of ABR findings in patients with asymmetric hearing and mixed hearing loss in the poorer ear is clinically challenging, particularly if this interpretation is based on absolute latency of wave V. Failing to take into account the conductive contribution to the loss may lead to an interpretation consistent with retrocochlear dysfunction, perhaps erroneously. Both conductive and retrocochlear hearing impairment typically produce a delay in wave V latency. If wave I is clearly identified, there should be considerably less difficulty in differentiating eighth-nerve or brainstem dysfunction from more peripheral auditory dysfunction. ABR interwave latency values (e.g., I–III, III–V, and I–V) are relatively independent of conductive or sensory hearing impairment. The clinician is obligated first to confirm the presence of a conductive component, then to estimate the degree of impairment in dB, and then, if indicated, to adjust ABR latency values accordingly. Guidelines for taking into account the CHL component are offered later in this chapter.

Effect of the Degree and Configuration of Hearing Loss on the ABR

LOW-FREQUENCY SENSORY HEARING LOSS. | Low-frequency hearing impairment involves audiometric frequencies below approximately 1000 Hz. The configuration of an audiogram characterized by greater hearing impairment in this frequency region and then better hearing for higher frequencies is referred to as "rising." Most low-frequency audiogram patterns reflect conductive hearing loss secondary to middle-ear pathology, or mixed hearing loss due to a disease that may involve both the middle and inner ear, such as otosclerosis. Sensorineural etiologies producing low-frequency hearing loss are less common. Among these are Ménière's disease, genetic and congenital inner-ear anomalies with hearing loss, viral infections, Mondini dysplasia, round window fistula, and, rarely, CPA neoplasms (Laukli & Mair, 1985; Parving, 1984; Soliman, 1987; Vanderbilt University, 1968). Low-frequency hearing impairment is less frequently associated with central auditory nervous system dysfunction (Gravendeel & Plomp, 1960; Soliman, 1987).

Acoustic immittance measurement is extremely useful for differentiating low-frequency sensory hearing impairment from conductive or mixed hearing impairment. Reliance on pure-tone audiometry alone can sometimes lead to errors in interpretation. Invalid high-intensity bone-conduction thresholds, resulting from harmonic bone-conduction distortion or "vibrotactile stimulation" (feeling rather than hearing the sound vibrations), may produce apparent but false and misleading "air-bone gaps" and misinterpretation of the type of hearing loss. With click stimuli, normal-appearing ABR waveforms and latency–intensity functions are typically recorded in low-frequency sensory hearing impairment (e.g., van der Drift, Brocaar, & Van Zanten, 1988a,b; Yamada, Kodera, & Yagi, 1979). The ABR to clicks reflects cochlear activation in the basal turn and is thus largely dependent on hearing status in the 2000 Hz frequency region and above.

One must keep in mind, however, that a normal ABR is not necessarily recorded for low-frequency conductive hearing deficits. In a 1987 study of audiogram configuration and ABR patterns, Keith and Greville showed wave V latencies that were shorter than normal at low intensity levels (below 60 dB HL) for patients with low-frequency sensory hearing loss. Wave I latency, in contrast, was unchanged. The result was a slight decrease in the wave I–V latency interval in comparison to normal hearers or hearing-impaired persons with other audiometric configurations.

Because click-evoked ABRs are often insensitive to low-frequency hearing impairment, alternative techniques are necessary. One option is to elicit the ABR with low-frequency tone-burst stimulation or toned stimuli in notched noise (Stapells, Picton, Durieux-Smith, Edwards, & Moran, 1990). Clinically, this is an attractive option because ABR is not affected by state of arousal or sedation. Normal expectations for tone-burst ABR thresholds can be established for a clinical facility, and ABR findings for tone-burst stimuli can be plotted on audiogram-like graphs. Other possibilities for low-frequency hearing threshold estimation include tone-burst stimulation of the SN10 response, the 40 Hz ERP, and AMLR or ALR (Barajas, Fernandez, & Bernal, 1988; Davis & Hirsh, 1976; Fowler & Swanson, 1989; Galambos et al., 1981; Hawes & Greenburg, 1981; Kavanagh et al., 1984; Kileny & Shea, 1986; Klein, 1983; Sammeth & Barry, 1985; Sturzebecher, Kevanishvili, Werbs, Meyer, & Schmidt, 1985; Suzuki et al., 1977; Szyfter, Dauman, & Charlet de Sauvage, 1984). Unfortunately, each of these responses is influenced to varying degrees by stimulus rate, by subject age and state of arousal, and by the effects of sedation. In addition, evoked-response thresholds may be closely related to behavioral thresholds (Davis & Hirsh, 1976; Fowler & Swanson, 1989; Hawes & Greenberg, 1981; Sturzebecher, Kevanishvili, Werbs, Meyer, & Schmidt, 1985; Suzuki et al., 1977), but they may also exceed behavioral thresholds by as much as 19 dB for AMLR, and by 28 dB for 40 Hz ERP (Barajas, Fernandez, & Bernal, 1988; Szyfter et al., 1984).

EFFECT OF MID- AND HIGH-FREQUENCY HEARING LOSS. | Mid- or high-frequency hearing loss can certainly affect ABR. However, extensive investigation has produced confusing and sometimes contradictory findings (Bauch, Rose, & Harner, 1981; Blegvad, Svane-Knudsen, & Borre, 1984; Borg & Löfqvist, 1982; Chisin, Gafni, & Sohmer, 1983; Coats & Martin, 1977; Gorga, Reiland, & Beauchaine, 1985;

Gorga, Worthington, Reiland, Beauchaine, & Goldgar, 1985; Jerger & Mauldin, 1978; Keith & Greville, 1987; Kileny & Magathan, 1987; Laukli & Mair, 1985a; Lehnhardt, 1981; Møller & Blegvad, 1976; Prosser & Arslan, 1987; Reimer, 1987; Rosenhamer, 1981; Rosenhamer, Lindstrom, & Lundborg, 1981a; Sohmer, Kinarti, & Gafni, 1981; Stürzebecher, Kevanishvili, Werbs, Meyer, & Schmidt, 1985; van der Drift, Brocaar, & van Zanten, 1987, 1988a,b; Yamada, Kodera, & Yagi, 1979). Naturally, there were substantial differences among these studies in stimulus intensity level and subject characteristics (age, gender, degree, and configuration of hearing loss). Many of the studies did not specify each of these factors in the analysis of results. Stimulus intensity is a critical variable in such studies. Group data are misleading because rarely are audiogram configurations equivalent from one subject to the next. Gorga et al. (1985) wisely minimized this problem by analyzing data with the slope of the latency–intensity function as the dependent variable.

A study by Jerger and Johnson (1988) highlighted the complexity of the issue. These investigators found an interactive effect between gender and the degree of hearing loss for wave V latency but not for latency of wave I or III. Study and discussion of ABR in sensory hearing loss should, therefore, incorporate each of these factors. As Jerger and Johnson (1988) point out, "Attempting to control for one possible source of latency variation tends to introduce another source with which the former covaries" (p. 169). In the present discussion, literature regarding the degree and configuration of sensory hearing loss is first briefly reviewed, even though the two features of the audiogram cannot be viewed clinically in isolation, just as sensory deficits cannot always be cleanly separated from conductive deficits.

EFFECT OF DEGREE AND SLOPE OF HEARING LOSS. | Clearly, wave V latency increases as hearing loss at 4000 Hz increases (Coats, 1978; Coats & Martin, 1977; Jerger & Mauldin, 1978; Møller & Blegvad, 1976; Rosenhamer, Lindstrom, & Lundborg, 1981a). The extent of latency increase and the influence of audiogram slope on the increase is less clear. There are numerous accounts of ABR wave V latency changes as a function of sensory hearing loss in the literature. The 1988 study by Jerger and Johnson serves to illustrate some major findings. Latency for ABR wave V in a large series of patients with sensory hearing impairment (for high stimulus-intensity levels of click stimuli) was analyzed as a function of audiometric HTL (hearing threshold level) at 4000 Hz. Latency was stable for hearing loss up to 60 dB HL, and then it increased linearly to a maximum of about 0.4 ms through 90 dB HL. The most pronounced latency change occurred for patients with hearing loss greater than 70 dB HTL.

Some previous studies of ABR and sensory hearing impairment failed to include subjects with hearing loss of this degree. The relation of hearing loss with ABR wave V latency is clearly influenced by age and gender. The latency increase associated with hearing loss is limited to male sub-

jects, both young and old. Female subjects, in contrast, show almost no hearing loss effect. Hyde (1985) showed an effect on ABR wave V latency of high-frequency hearing impairment greater than 40 dB among younger subjects. In contrast, among older subjects, latency values were increased even with mild hearing (20 to 40 dB) impairment, and were further increased with additional hearing impairment latency values.

Earlier investigators suggested that ABR latency increases in sensory hearing impairment were relatively greater for sloping than for flat audiometric configurations (Jerger & Mauldin, 1978; Møller & Blegvad, 1976; Yamada et al., 1979). After showing a statistical relationship between audiogram slope and ABR, Jerger and Mauldin (1978) provided guidelines for taking slope into account in clinical evaluation of ABR. The overall objective was "to predict the likelihood that any observed prolongation of latency can be attributed solely to audiometric configuration" (p. 460), as opposed to retrocochlear pathology. For an ABR stimulus intensity level of 70 to 90 dB HL, one may expect a wave V latency delay of about 0.2 msec for every 30 dB of slope in the audiogram from 1000 to 4000 Hz. Rosenhamer (1981) failed to show a slope effect on wave V latency when hearing loss at 4000 Hz was kept constant. That is, hearing loss at 4000 Hz dominated ABR latency. The study by Jerger and Johnson (1988) also failed to confirm the slope versus latency relation. Latency was comparable for patients with flat and sloping configurations. These findings argue against the wisdom of utilizing an average of HTLs over a high-frequency range, (e.g., from 1000 to 4000 Hz). Over this range, there may be considerable variation in slope and the degree of hearing loss at 4000 Hz.

What about other audiometric frequencies? Coats and Martin (1977) demonstrated a relationship between ABR threshold and audiometric hearing threshold at 8000 Hz. Clinical experience suggests also that auditory sensitivity outside of the 2000 to 4000 Hz region may be a factor in ABR measurement. Even an isolated notch in hearing sensitivity at 6000 Hz or above may alter ABR latency, amplitude, or morphology.

WHAT ABOUT A CORRECTION FOR DEGREE OF SENSORY HEARING LOSS? | One of the more controversial questions in ABR interpretation is whether latency should be adjusted to account for hearing loss. This is especially of interest in neurodiagnosis. Again, ABR threshold is correlated best with audiometric threshold in the 2000 to 4000 Hz region (Coats & Martin, 1977; Møller & Blegvad, 1976). Therefore, if a patient has a severe high-frequency sensorineural loss, should a correction (subtraction) be made on wave V latency *before* this value is compared to group normative data or to latency for the opposite ear? Selected guidelines for correcting for degree of hearing loss are reported by Selters and Brackmann (1977) and by Rosenhamer (1981). Selters and Brackmann (1977) were among the first to apply ABR in identification of eighth-nerve pathology, and, as result, they were among the first to appreciate the problem of ABR interpretation in asymmetric hearing loss. Rosenhamer et al. (1981), recognizing the clinical usefulness of a correction method, tentatively offered their correction method as a "guideline" for ABR interpretation in high-frequency sensory loss, rather than as a firm correction factor. These investigators also suggest that it may be of value to compare ABR findings for equivalent stimulus intensity SLs (sensation levels), rather than HLs (hearing levels) or SPLs (sound pressure levels), in patients with asymmetric hearing impairment. This would, presumably, eliminate the need for correction factors. Jerger and Johnson (1988) revived the concept. Guidelines offered by Jerger and Johnson are summarized in Table 7.2, and endorsed by the present author.

Finally, Prosser and Arslan (1987) described a "diagnostic index" for differentiation of cochlear versus retrocochlear auditory dysfunction, referred to as "Δ (delta) V." It is based on wave V latency for monaural stimulation and incorporates normal wave V latency expectations and the patient's HTL at 2000 and 4000 Hz. According to Prosser and Arslan (1987), a positive Δ V value (greater than Δ 0) is entirely consistent with retrocochlear dysfunction. Approximately 75 percent of patients with confirmed retrocochlear lesions fall within this region. For Δ V values of less than 0, patient data can be plotted and compared to the upper 95 percent confidence level for known cochlear dysfunction. This technique takes advantage of the common observation that at high stimulus intensity levels, there is an approximation of latencies for normal-hearing and cochlear-impaired subjects. The latency approximation for high intensity stimulation occurs on the flattened portion of the latency–intensity function. Latency–intensity functions were introduced in Chapter 6. Obviously, Prosser and Arslan (1987) endorse the general concept of hearing loss correction. However, other researchers who recognize the possibility of interactions among age, gender, and hearing impairment (noted previously) are not in total agreement. For example, Hyde (1985) suggests that different correction criteria be employed for young versus old patients.

TABLE 7.2. Guidelines for Determining Click Stimulus Intensity Level in Neurodiagnostic Auditory Brainstem Response (ABR) Assessment Based on the Degree of Hearing Loss

PURE-TONE AVERAGE (PTA) FOR 1000, 2000, AND 4000 HZ	CLICK INTENSITY LEVEL
0 to 10 dB HL	70 dB nHL
20 to 39 dB HL	80 dB nHL
40 to 59 dB HL	90 dB nHL
60 to 79 dB HL	100 dB nHL

Source: Interactions of age, gender, and sensorineural hearing loss on ABR latency. By Jerger J and Johnson K. 1988. *Ear and Hearing, 9,* 168–176.

A greater interaural latency correction is needed for young versus old patients, assuming comparable audiograms. And, Jerger and Johnson (1988) recommend correction for hearing loss in male, but not female, patients.

What degree of hearing loss obliterates the ABR? Using a 2000 Hz haversine wave stimulus presented at 85 dB HL, Borg and Löfqvist (1982) found an upper cutoff for pure-tone hearing sensitivity of 40 to 50 dB in the 500 Hz region and 80 to 90 dB at 1000 Hz. That is, no ABR for their stimulus conditions was detected from patients with cochlear hearing loss greater than these limits. They emphasized a point made at the beginning of this chapter, namely, absence of an ABR does not necessarily imply total deafness. Other authors have suggested that absence of an ABR is equivocal when hearing loss is greater than 70 dB HL in the 4000 Hz region (Jerger & Jerger, 1988). This finding would be entirely consistent with severe cochlear impairment and, therefore, does not contribute to differentiation of cochlear versus retrocochlear dysfunction.

Patterns for Audiogram and ABR Latency–Intensity Functions

Since the earliest clinical application of ECochG and ABR, investigators have attempted to find a close and predictable relation between the slope of the wave V latency–intensity function and type, degree, and configuration of hearing loss (Eggermont, 1974; Galambos & Hecox, 1978; Hecox, 1983; Keith & Greville, 1987). There are really two separate issues to consider: (1) How can the ABR wave V latency–intensity functions be applied in differentiating conductive versus sensory deficits? (This point is discussed in more detail later in the chapter) and (2) How can the degree and slope of loss be estimated, based on ABR wave V latency–intensity data? The inherent difficulty in such estimations was reorganized as early as 1979 when Yamada, Kodera, and Yagi clearly showed the multiple variations in latency–intensity functions that can be expected in sensory hearing loss.

There are two major clinical limitations to predicting type of loss from the latency–intensity slope. One is the inevitable individual variability among patients with divergent degrees and slopes of impairment, often arising from different etiologies. Second, relatively small intensity increments (less than 10 dB) are necessary to describe fully the slope of the function. The marked slope differences between types of impairment occur within the initial 10 to 15 dB above ABR threshold. Although in normal hearers an ABR is first detectable at 10 to 20 dB SL (above behavioral hearing threshold), the ABR in sensory loss often first appears within 5 dB of hearing threshold (in the 1000 to 4000 Hz region). However, small intensity increments (e.g., 5 dB or less) are not typically used in the clinical application of the ABR for estimation of auditory thresholds. For ABR assessment of infants, constraints in test time usually preclude the use of relatively small increments of stimulus intensity as threshold is approached.

The picture becomes further complicated in steeply sloping high-frequency sensory loss. At low intensity levels, latency is greatly delayed because only more apical (1000 to 2000 Hz) cochlear regions contribute to the response. Higher intensity levels involve the region of 4000 Hz and higher frequencies, and these frequencies are represented at more basal portions of the cochlea, which are activated with less traveling time along the basilar membrane. Therefore, latency decreases sharply. There is some question about whether this ABR latency–intensity slope pattern is unique to high-frequency loss in general. As noted previously, some patients may have serious hearing impairment in the low-frequency region and also in very high-frequency regions, yet reasonably good hearing sensitivity in the 2000 to 4000 Hz region. Typically, the ABR latency–intensity function appears normal with this less common audiometric configuration.

ABR WAVE V LATENCY–INTENSITY FUNCTIONS: CONDUCTIVE VERSUS SENSORY LOSS. | The characteristic finding in conductive loss is a delay in wave I latency and a "horizontal shift" in ABR wave V latency (shown earlier in Figure 7.6) corresponding to the amount of air-bone gap (Borg, Löfqvist, & Rosen, 1981; Fria & Sabo, 1979; Lehnhardt, 1981; McGee & Clemis, 1982; Suzuki & Suzuki, 1977; van der Drift et al., 1988a; Yamada, Yagi, Yamane, & Suzuki, 1975). That is, the ABR latency–intensity function has a normal shape, but it is pushed to the left on the graph by the degree of conductive hearing loss component. van der Drift, Brocaar, and van Zanten (1988a,b) reported data that providing some consistency to the rather confusing literature on this topic. The authors first calculated the average differences in latency–intensity curves (the amount of horizontal shift) for normal hearers versus patients with CHL. Then, they approximated derivative latency–intensity curves by determining the latency difference of wave V for each 10 dB increment in intensity level. The authors draw three main conclusions: First, ABR can*not* be used to distinguish between conductive versus cochlear groups at threshold levels of 35 dB or less (better hearing) because of the overlap among groups. Second, for CHL, wave V latency does not vary as a function of ABR threshold, whereas in cochlear hearing loss, wave V latency decreases as a function of the degree of loss. Third, a combination of the ABR threshold and the amount of horizontal shift—in particular, the derivative horizontal shift—can graphically differentiate patients with conductive versus sensory deficit.

Are steeper-than-normal ABR wave V latency–intensity functions exclusively characteristic of sensory hearing loss? Gorga, Reiland, and Beauchaine (1985) describe an abnormal ABR wave V latency–intensity function for a sleeping 6-year-old boy with high-frequency conductive hearing impairment due to chronic middle-ear disease. Latency of waves I and V was delayed, consistent with CHL. However,

at higher stimulus intensity levels there was a marked shortening of latency values. They cite this as evidence that ABR latency is dependent on an interaction between stimulus intensity and the site of generation along the cochlear partition in general, rather than a reflection of cochlear dysfunction and sensory impairment. That is, the ABR is generated by progressively more apical (low-frequency) portions of the cochlea for both conductive and sensory types of sloping high-frequency loss. Because of the high-frequency deficit, extreme basal portions of the cochlea do not contribute to the response. This is, essentially, an enhancement of expected basal ward shift of cochlear activation associated with a reduction in stimulus intensity (Eggermont, 1976a,b; Eggermont & Don, 1980; Kiang, 1965), described in more detail in Chapter 2.

ABR WAVE V LATENCY–INTENSITY FUNCTIONS: CONFIGURATION OF SENSORY LOSS. | Steeper than normal latency–intensity functions are characteristic of sensory hearing impairment. A fundamental feature of this pattern is the repeatedly described minimal latency increase in wave V at high stimulus intensity levels, despite moderate-to-severe sensory loss (Coats & Martin, 1977; Jerger & Mauldin, 1978; Selters & Brackmann, 1977; Sohmer, Kinarti, & Gafni, 1981). In fact, the ABR wave I–V latency interval is relatively constant in sensory loss, so the minimal latency shift with hearing loss is not due to changes in wave V latency but, rather, to prolongation latency of ABR wave I (ECochG AP) (Aran, 1971; Elberling, 1974; Montandon et al., 1975; Odenthal & Eggermont, 1974; Yoshie & Ohashi, 1969). Two mechanisms (auditory recruitment and cochlear travel time) are offered by various investigators to account for the latency–intensity functions in sensory loss. The concept of travel time along the cochlea's basilar membrane is often cited in explanations of latency–intensity function patterns in normal and sensory-impaired hearing (Borg, 1981a, Coats & Martin, 1977; Don, Eggermont, & Brackmann, 1979; Galambos & Hecox, 1978; Gorga, Worthington, Reiland, Beauchaine, & Goldgar, 1985; Özdamar & Dallos, 1976; Pantev, Lagidze, Pantev, & Kevanishvili, 1985; Sohmer, Kinarti, & Gafni, 1981; Yamada, Kodera, & Yagi, 1979). Understanding this concept is fundamental to meaningful clinical interpretation of ABR.

Briefly, wave V is generated normally by activity along a relatively extended portion of the basilar membrane, whereas wave I is dependent exclusively on activity in the base of the cochlea (the high-frequency region). In general, for normal hearers, high-intensity stimulation, even with a stimulus with maximum energy at 4000 Hz, activates a wider portion of the basilar membrane and approximates the most basal end of the cochlea. High-frequency hearing impairment alters the normal cochlear generator sites for ABR wave I, but not the basilar-membrane sites for wave V. With high-intensity stimulation, which exceeds the degree of hearing loss, wave V continues to be generated in part by basal cochlear activity as well as more apical activity, and latency is reasonably normal. Even a slight shift apically (toward the low frequency end of the cochlea), due to the high-frequency hearing loss, may reduce the neural synchrony required for wave I and limit detection of this component (Goldstein & Kiang, 1958). At lower intensity levels, wave I disappears, and wave V latency increases markedly because *only* more apical regions of the cochlea are activated. For reference, it is estimated that travel time from the 10,000 Hz to the 500 Hz region of the cochlea is approximately 2 ms (Borg, 1981a).

ESTIMATION OF AUDIOMETRIC INFORMATION FROM ABR. | In view of the numerous stimulus and subject variables that may affect ABR outcome, and the limited knowledge about ABR generation in cochlear pathophysiology, it is not surprising that consistently accurate estimation of the audiogram, or even a portion of the audiogram, remains a clinical ideal but not a reality (Brookhauser, Gorga, & Kelly, 1990; Connolly, Stout, Williams, Jorgensen, & Smith, 1990). There is rarely a one-to-one relationship between behavioral and click-stimulus ABR threshold levels, even though agreement within 10 to 15 dB can usually be expected in the 2000 to 4000 Hz region (Bauch & Olsen, 1986; Fjermedal & Laukli, 1989a,b; Kileny & Magathan, 1987; Pratt & Sohmer, 1978; van der Drift, Brocaar, & van Zanten, 1987).

One of the earliest attempts to predict behavioral threshold from ABR threshold was reported by Jerger and Mauldin (1978). This paper provides a thorough discussion of the numerous variables that must be considered in hearing loss prediction from ABR data. These authors proposed a relatively simple predictive equation derived from data collected from 275 ears:

$$PTA^2 = 0.6 \times ABR \text{ threshold}$$

where PTA^2 is calculated as pure-tone-averaged hearing thresholds for 1000, 2000, and 4000 Hz / 3.

The equation is based on statistical analyses (linear regression equations, coefficient of correlation, and standard error of estimate) of various behavioral measures (e.g., PTAs, thresholds for single frequencies, and contour or slope) and ABR threshold. The highest two correlations were between ABR threshold and both 4000 Hz threshold and a high-frequency PTA (1000 to 4000 Hz), as expected. The standard error of estimate, however, was large, due to slope in the frequency region of 500 to 4000 Hz, resulting in inaccuracy on the order of ± 15 dB.

Coats and Martin (1977) found a correlation of .65 between ABR threshold for 4000 and 8000 Hz in 20 patients with cochlear impairment. van der Drift, Brocaar, and van

Zanten (1987) also systematically analyzed correlations between click ABR threshold and high-frequency sensory hearing loss in 209 ears. The correlation coefficient of thresholds for ABR and 2000 to 4000 Hz hearing threshold levels was .93 (versus .48 reported by Jerger & Mauldin, 1978), with a standard error of the estimate of 11 dB (vs. 15 dB reported by Jerger & Mauldin). Findings reported by van der Drift, Brocaar, and van Zanten (1987) provide a clear demonstration of the relationship between hearing at 2000 to 4000 Hz and ABR threshold. Gorga, Worthington, Reiland, Beauchaine, and Goldgar, (1985) also described close agreement between ABR thresholds and hearing thresholds for 2000 to 4000 Hz and independence between ABR and hearing thresholds for 1000 and 8000 Hz.

WAVE I–V LATENCY INTERVAL IN HIGH-FREQUENCY SENSORY LOSS. | There is disagreement as to the effect of high-frequency sensory hearing impairment on the ABR wave I–V latency interval. Some investigators report a significant decrease in the wave I–V latency values for patients with high-frequency sensory hearing impairment (Coats & Martin, 1977; Keith & Greville, 1987; Stürzebecher, Kevanishvili, Werbs, Meyer, & Schmidt, 1985), a finding presumably due to prolongation of latency for the high-frequency–dependent wave I without a corresponding increase in the lower frequency–dependent wave V. Gorga, Reiland, and Beauchaine (1985), however, also reported a similar finding for a patient with high-frequency CHL, not a sensory impairment. The decrease in wave I–V latency is most closely related to the extent of hearing deficit at 4000 Hz. In contrast, some investigators demonstrated no change in wave I–V latency values with high-frequency sensory loss (e.g., Rosenhamer et al., 1981a,b), whereas others associated an *increase* in this latency value with sensory dysfunction (Abramovich & Billings, 1981; Eggermont, Don, & Brackmann, 1980). It is not clear to what extent stimulus parameters (e.g., polarity) and subject factors (e.g., etiology of hearing loss) might contribute to these discrepancies (Coats & Martin, 1977; Ornitz & Walter, 1975). For example, in a comprehensive study of audiogram configurations and ABR latency–intensity functions, Keith and Greville (1987) highlighted various findings that depended on details of both the configuration and the stimulus intensity. The wave I–V latency interval tended to be shorter in sloping high-frequency loss and in rising configurations, unchanged in flat configurations, and prolonged in a notching deficit in the 3000 to 4000 Hz region. Differences in the wave I–V latency–interval were greatest for lower stimulus intensities (below 50 to 60 dB HL), consistent with data reported ten years earlier by Coats and Martin (1977).

Frequency-Specific Auditory Brainstem Response (ABR) and Auditory Steady-State Response (ASSR)

FREQUENCY-SPECIFIC ABR

Research investigations and, to a lesser extent, clinical applications, of frequency-specific measurement of the ABR date back to the 1970s. Indeed, Jewett and Williston in their classic 1971 treatise confirmed the clinical feasibility of eliciting brainstem auditory evoked responses with tonal (tone-burst or tone-pip) signals. Different types of acoustic stimuli used to evoke brainstem responses, including tone-burst stimuli, were reviewed in Chapter 6. The following discussion is focused on the clinical application in infants and young children of tone-burst stimuli for measurement of frequency-specific ABRs and sinusoidal stimuli modulated in amplitude and/or frequency for measurement of the ASSR. The demand for a clinically feasible and reasonably accurate electrophysiological technique for frequency-specific estimation of hearing sensitivity is clearly not met by the click-evoked ABR. As noted elsewhere in this book, the click-evoked ABR may seriously underestimate or overestimate sensory hearing loss, depending on the degree and configuration of the deficit. At the extreme, patients with severe-to-profound high-frequency hearing loss may produce no ABR for click stimulation, even with normal hearing sensitivity in the low-frequency region of the audiogram. An ABR with normal latency values can even be recorded with click stimulation of < 20 dB nHL from patients with severe loss at most audiometric frequencies, so long as there is normal hearing sensitivity somewhere within high-frequency region of the audiogram, including an "island" of normal hearing sensitivity (e.g., Balfour, Pillion, & Gaskin, 1998; Hall, 1992). Conversely, patients with low-frequency hearing loss affecting speech perception and communication often have normal click-evoked ABR findings. Reliance on a click-evoked ABR supplemented with an ABR for a low-frequency tone-burst stimulus (e.g., 500 Hz) does not offer complete assurance that hearing sensitivity is adequate for speech and language acquisition or function. A normal ABR for low-intensity (< 20 dB nHL) click and 500 Hz tone-burst stimuli can clearly be recorded from children

and adults with hearing loss configurations characterized by a mid-frequency notching pattern, although this audiometric pattern is admittedly not common in children (e.g., Hall, 1992; Balfour, Pillion, & Gaskin, 1998).

The overall objective for clinical application of these responses is diagnosis of hearing loss and, specifically, frequency-specific estimation of hearing sensitivity for children whose management includes amplification or cochlear implantation. Strategies reported over the years for recording ABRs with various types of frequency-specific stimuli are first summarized. Then, recent literature on frequency-specific threshold estimation of ABRs with tone-burst stimuli will be reviewed and followed with presentation of a clinical test protocol. A similar review will be offered for the ASSR.

Frequency-Specific ABR Techniques Involving Ipsilateral Masking

The click-evoked ABR is very useful and clinically practical for estimation of auditory functioning in the 1000 to 4000 Hz region. It is adequate for hearing screening purposes. However, information on auditory sensitivity across the audiometric range, especially the speech frequency region of 500 Hz through 3000 to 4000 Hz, is extremely important for rational audiologic management of hearing-impaired patients, such as for the fitting of hearing aids. An estimate of low-frequency hearing status (in the 500 Hz region) is especially desirable. For cooperative adults and most children, this information is best obtained from conventional, behavioral pure-tone audiometry. An auditory electrophysiologic measure that is not seriously influenced by subject state or sedation, such as the ABR, is needed for hearing assessment of very young children and difficult-to-test patients of any age. Because of the pressing clinical need for an electrophysiologic technique to assess auditory sensitivity at different frequencies, especially since the widespread acceptance of universal newborn hearing screening, there is increased clinical interest in frequency-specific ABRs. As noted in Chapter 5, a variation of the technique has also been applied in attempts to record frequency-specific ECochG AP components.

The most obvious approach for generating an ABR reflecting hearing sensitivity at specific audiometric frequencies is to use brief tone stimulation, such as a tone burst, sometimes also referred to as a "tone pip." The tone burst, ideally, has energy at a single pure-tone frequency (e.g., 500 Hz) under all presentation conditions, including high stimulus intensity levels, and contains little or no energy at other frequencies. This ideal stimulus activates the basilar membrane of the cochlea where there are neural units with this characteristic frequency, even for patients with cochlear pathology. There is, however, the well-appreciated trade-off between stimulus duration and frequency specificity. A tone burst with an extremely brief stimulus onset may produce "spectral splatter," that is, acoustic energy at unwanted frequencies. For low-frequency test stimuli, unwanted energy at higher frequencies is most likely to reduce the frequency-specificity of the tone-burst ABR. At higher intensity levels, for acoustic stimuli across the frequency region, this dispersed energy may exceed the threshold levels of higher frequency units and may generate a response due to activation of remote regions of the cochlea.

Over the years, several methods were proposed for recording frequency-specific ABRs:

- Some approaches involved masking of frequency regions that were not intended to be part of the stimulus. With one approach, a click stimulus was presented to the same ear (ipsilateral) as either a high-pass (high-frequency) noise masking signal or noise containing a notch within the region of the desired frequency (band reject masking).
- With another approach, an abrupt pure-tone stimulus was presented with masking at lower and higher frequencies.
- A variant of the stimulus-ipsilateral masking technique utilizes a pure-tone versus noise-masking signal.
- With the derived band method, the ABR to a stimulus at a specific frequency or within a defined frequency region was derived (usually by subtraction) from two other responses. This technique also usually involved a masking paradigm.
- Another more straightforward technique utilized a tonal stimulus (a spectrally constrained stimulus) with carefully selected onset characteristics to enhance frequency specificity. The use of tone-burst stimuli, without ipsilateral masking, is now the most common clinical approach for recording frequency specific ABRs.

The first three general methods are reviewed only briefly here, as they are not regularly applied clinically.

HIGH-FREQUENCY MASKING. | The simplest masking technique for obtaining frequency-specific ABRs involves presentation of high-frequency ("high-pass") masking along with a transient stimulus, i.e., a click or tone burst. This approach uses ipsilateral masking noise, that is, making noise presented though the same earphone as the stimulus. Such masking must be differentiated from *contralateral* masking in ABR measurement, when masking noise is presented to the nonstimulus (nontest) ear to reduce the likelihood of nontest ear participation in generation of the ABR in the event of acoustic crossover from one side of the head to the other. The effect of contralateral masking on the ABR recording was discussed in Chapter 6. With the high-frequency masking method, the stimulus may be a click or a brief tone (usually a tone burst). Use of a transient (rapid onset) stimulus optimizes the likelihood of a clear, well-formed ABR, even at low intensity levels. Some spectral splatter of this transient stimulus is masked by the noise. Because spectral splatter includes unwanted frequencies above the stimulus frequency, high-frequency masking may provide some frequency specificity. Important factors to consider with this technique are the skirt of the masker (the dB/octave roll-off of the filter used in defining the masking), the intensity level of the masker, whether a click or a tone burst is used, and if a tone burst is used, the onset characteristics.

Kileny (1981) and others (Burkard & Hecox, 1983; Conijn, Brocaar, & van Zanten, 1990; Fjermedal & Laukli, 1989b; Jacobson, 1983; McDonald & Shimizu, 1981; Stapells, Picton, Abalo, Read, & Smith, 1985) recorded frequency-specific ABRs using a combination of brief tone stimuli and high-pass masking. Kinarti and Sohmer (1982) similarly evaluated the usefulness of high-pass masking for ABRs generated with low-frequency filtered clicks. Typically, brief-duration tonal stimuli were delivered to the ear in the presence of a high-pass masking noise. For example, the cutoff frequency for noise was 1500 Hz for a 500 Hz brief tone and 2000 Hz for a 1000 Hz brief tone (Kileny, 1981). Latencies were delayed for ABRs to brief tones in the presence of the noise maskers, consistent with a more apical activation site along the basilar membrane than the 2000 to 4000 Hz region activated maximally in normal hearers with a click stimulus. In these early studies, an important factor influencing interpretation of ABR latency for brief-tone stimuli was the reference point from which latency calculations were made. As noted by Kileny (1981), there is variability in this reference point among studies (Coats, Martin, & Kidder, 1979; Elberling, 1976; Klein & Teas, 1978; Mair, Laukli, & Pederson, 1980). For the abrupt unfiltered click, calculation of latency from stimulus onset is straightforward. For brief-tone stimuli, Kileny (1981) recommended latency calculation based on the first rarefaction peak of the waveform, rather than stimulus onset. The stimulus peak is progressively later as stimulus frequency is lowered and stimulus wavelength becomes longer. Failure to appreciate this factor in latency calculations could lead to erroneous inferences regarding generation of the response on the cochlea. That is, ABR latency shifts may be due to a delay in the arrival time of the onset portion of the stimulus that effectively elicits the response, rather than travel time of activation in a basal-ward direction within cochlea.

NOTCHED NOISE. | A similar method involves the use of notched noise or band-reject filtered noise for the masker, along with a transient stimulus. The transient stimulus may be a click or a tone burst. Notched noise is a broad band of noise with a portion of the frequencies removed. When a stimulus is presented along with the notched-noise masker, theoretically only the frequency portion of the stimulus passing through the notch will be involved in generation of the ABR. In concept, this technique is rather straightforward, with the clinical advantage that no more time is required to record frequency-specific ABRs than to record ABRs for a tonal stimulus. The use of notched-noise ABR generation with tone-burst stimulation can be thought of as a two-step process. The general frequency region of interest is selected by use of the appropriate tone-burst frequency (e.g., 500 Hz). Then the notched-noise masker is added to assure both that only this frequency region is activated and that there is no basal-ward (high-frequency) spread of energy and unwanted stimulation by stimulus side-lobe frequencies. Disadvantages of the notched-noise masking techniques include (a) spread of the low-frequency component of the masker into the notch; (b) broad, small amplitude, and sometimes indistinct wave V morphology; (c) extra peaks in the waveform even at high masking levels, which may be misinterpreted as wave V for the stimulus frequency of interest; and (d) overestimation of auditory threshold levels. Furthermore, varying results have been reported with the notched-noise method. For example, Stapells et al. (1985) and van Zanten and Brocaar (1984) found a latency increase of approximately 4 ms as the noise-notch frequency was lowered from 4000 to 500 Hz. ABR estimated auditory thresholds for different notch-noise signals agreed reasonably well to corresponding pure-tone audiometry thresholds. In contrast, studies by Pratt and colleagues (Pratt & Bleich, 1982; Pratt, Yitzhak, & Attias, 1984) showed no latency increase as frequency decreased and found poor agreement between ABR and pure-tone audiometry estimates of hearing threshold levels.

PURE-TONE MASKING. | In the late 1970s and into the 1980s, numerous investigators reported experimental (animal) and clinical findings for a technique for obtaining frequency-specific auditory evoked responses with a pure-tone masking technique, including tuning curves for the AP component of the ECochG (Abbas & Gorga, 1981; Dallos & Cheatham, 1976; Eggermont, 1977; Gorga & Abbas, 1981) and frequency-specific ABRs (Folsom, 1984; Hood & Berlin, 1987; Klein, 1983). An ABR is recorded with a tone-burst or a click stimulus in the presence of a continuous pure-tone (at the frequency of interest), and another ABR is recorded for just the click or the tone-burst stimulus. In theory, the continuous pure tone will mask out the frequency-specific portion of the cochlea. Then, when the ABR for just the click (or tone burst) is subtracted from the ABR waveform for the stimulus plus the pure tone, only the portion of the ABR generated by the pure-tone masker frequency will remain. According to Hood and Berlin (1987), one advantage of this technique versus other frequency-specific ABR recording methods, based on data in guinea pigs, was the apparent consistency of the discrete frequency activation even at high intensity levels. Basal-ward spread of the masker seemed to be minimal. As expected, latency of the ABR components decreased as frequency of the pure tone is increased. It is important to keep in mind, however, that a continuous, high-level, low-frequency stimulus activates fibers in the basal region of the cochlea, as well as in the apical region. The remote activation is not due to spectral splatter; instead, it is due to basilar membrane mechanics (Gorga & Thornton, 1989).

Clinical feasibility and effectiveness of the pure-tone masker derived method was not conclusively documented. One important factor in the effectiveness of the pure-tone derived method was the intensity level of the tone. In early experiments, there was essentially no difference waveform. The subtraction process removed the entire ABR. Possibly the pure-tone intensity level of 10 to 30 dB SL used in these experiments did not provide adequate masking. With a higher pure-tone intensity level, equivalent to or greater than the intensity level of the click, Pantev and Pantev (1982) were able to demonstrate a difference wave. Latency values appropriately increased as frequency decreased. However, at the highest pure-tone masker levels, early latency components were observed. These probably were related to a deleterious high-frequency spread of the pure tone masker. In a follow-up study of 15 normal-hearing subjects, these investigators offered additional evidence that the pure-tone masking method was feasible and valid through the range of 500 to 8000 Hz (Pantev, Lagidze, Pantev, & Kevanishvili, 1985). Pure-tone maskers at intensity levels of 20 to 25 dB were evaluated. The authors especially noted detection of clear responses for low-frequency-region stimuli, providing a thorough argument for the reliability and validity of their technique. An important consideration in this and other derived methods is the electrophysiologic variability and increased noise level that is caused by the subtraction process. That is, the subtraction process has the effect of limiting the noise reduction obtained during signal averaging. Stapells et al. (1985) estimate a noise level 1.4 times larger than the level for unsubtracted ABRs. Sequential ABR waveforms may not have precisely the same latency values. The practical implication of the inherent increase in noise is that averaging with the derived methods must be carried out for twice the usual number of stimuli.

DERIVED RESPONSE METHODS. | The first major study of the use of derived masking methods in generating frequency-specific AERs was that of Teas, Elridge, and Davis (1962), a classic study conducted with ECochG in an animal model.

Other investigators then applied the approach clinically, with both ECochG and ABR (Don, Eggermont, & Brackmann, 1979; Eggermont, 1976b; Eggermont & Don, 1980; Elberling, 1974; Parker & Thornton, 1978). A monograph published in 1979 by Don, Eggermont, and Brackmann was evidence of considerable interest in the technique within the first decade of ABR clinical application. With the derived response methods, an ECochG AP or an ABR is generated by a sound that includes the stimulus plus a second acoustic signal (narrowband noise, high-pass noise, or a pure-tone masker) that has contributions from portions of the cochlea other than those underlying the stimulus. Then, the ABR is generated by the nonstimulus signal (i.e., the noise). The ECochG or ABR waveform for the noise is subtracted from the ABR waveform for the noise-plus-stimulus condition. Theoretically, during the subtraction process, the contribution of the masker to the waveform (and nonstimulus frequency regions of the cochlea) is removed, leaving only the EcochG or ABR for the spectrally constrained stimulus.

One derived masking technique utilizes high-pass noise. In Figure 8.1, adapted from the classic study of the derived response technique by Don, Eggermont, and Brackmann (1979), the high-pass (HP in figure) noise method is illustrated schematically. The letters (A, B, C, D, E, and F) refer to different frequency regions in the cochlea, from higher to lower frequencies, respectively. A click is presumed to include energy in all of these frequency regions (top of figure) and produces the familiar ABR waveform. When the click is presented with a broadband masking noise, assuming an appropriately small signal-to-noise ratio, it is ineffective as a stimulus, and no ABR is generated. This demonstrates the effectiveness of the masker in general. Moving down to the next portion of the figure, a noise band in the 8000 Hz region is presented, along with the click stimulus. This eliminates contribution of the 8000 Hz frequency region (denoted by "A"). Note that the resulting ABR waveform appears to be quite similar to that for the click stimulus. As an aside, if a TDH-39 or TDH-49 earphone were used, however, the stimulus would have limited energy in the 8000 Hz region to begin with.

In Figure 8.1, one of the ABR waveforms was not produced directly by a stimulus but, rather, derived via a subtraction process. The 8000 Hz masked ABR (R2) waveform is subtracted from the click ABR waveform. Because the 8000 Hz masked waveform includes all frequency regions except 8000 Hz, the subtraction process removes all frequency regions but the 8000 Hz region from the click waveform, leaving only the waveform components produced by 8000 Hz (the first derived response shown in the figure as DR1). This is a frequency-specific ABR, theoretically reflecting cochlear activation on the basilar membranes in the 8000 Hz region. A second subtraction process is also shown. An additional frequency region (4000 Hz) is masked, as the high-pass noise cutoff is lowered an octave from 8000 Hz. The resulting ABR (see R3 in the figure), therefore, lacks

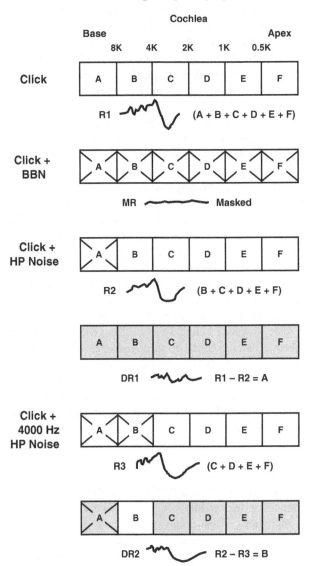

Sequential High-Pass Masking Paradigm for Deriving Frequency-Specific ABRs

FIGURE 8.1. A high-pass noise masking technique used to derive frequency-specific auditory brainstem response (ABR) waveforms.

Adapted with permission from Don, M., Eggermont, J. J., & Brackmann, D. E. (1979). Reconstruction of the audiogram using brainstem responses and high-pass noise masking. *Annals of Otology, Rhinology and Laryngology, Supplement, 57,* 1–20. Copyright © 1979 Annals Publishing Co.

contribution from the frequency region above 4000 Hz, but it contains energy for all other regions. This waveform is subtracted from the waveform (R2) that lacks only the 8000 Hz components. The subtraction process removes the energy for these lower frequency regions (2000 Hz and below) from R2. Energy at 8000 Hz was already gone. What remains (DR2) is the portion of the ABR waveform that was masked by the 4000 Hz high-pass noise. Further subtractions, using already derived responses, are carried out to isolate other frequency regions for a given subject.

In normal hearers, Don, Eggermont, and Brackmann (1979) recorded an ABR with the derived method at intensity levels down to 30 dB SL for cochlear regions above 8000 Hz and 500 Hz and below. Within the 1000 to 4000 Hz region, the derived ABR threshold was observed down to at least 10 dB SL. How well did the derived technique estimate auditory impairment at different frequencies? These authors found very close correspondence between audiometric hearing threshold levels and derived ABR reconstructions of audiograms (usually within 5 to 10 dB) for patients with isolated deficits at 4000 Hz and with low frequency or flat-configuration hearing impairments.

Derived responses were also obtained with *narrowband* (versus high-pass) masking. As usual, ABR waveforms were first recorded with a click stimulus, encompassing a wide frequency region. Then, ABR waveforms were recorded with the click plus a simultaneously presented narrow band of noise centered on the frequency of interest (e.g., 500 or 2000 Hz). The bandwidth of the noise (the range of frequencies from the lower to upper frequency limits) was defined, such as two-thirds of an octave. The band of noise presumably removed the contribution of this frequency region from the ABR waveform. Digital subtraction of the noise-band-masked ABR from the unmasked ABR yielded a difference waveform, with all frequency contributions removed except those in the desired frequency region.

Although the noise-band derived response method appeared to be considerably simpler that the high-pass derived response method, technical and practical problems were subsequently described (Stapells et al., 1985). Noise within the band could spread into other frequency regions, especially to higher frequencies. For example, a 500 Hz noise band could spread into the 1000 Hz to 4000 Hz regions. This complication was greater when the intensity of the masker was increased. A low-intensity masker, however, was not necessarily the solution to this problem because a masker at a low intensity level, relative to the click stimulus, was ineffective. The resulting ABR, therefore, resembled the response to only a click, without frequency specificity, as surmised by the presence of components I, III, and V, along with the shorter latency values for these ABR waves. These ABR features are expected for a click and not for low-frequency stimuli. Stapells and colleagues (1985) observed that if an ABR was generated simultaneously by the low-frequency band (e.g., 500 Hz) and by unwanted activation of higher frequency portions of the cochlea (by spread of masking), the resulting wave V component could have diminished amplitude. This was because the somewhat longer latency positive voltage wave V overlapped in time with the negative voltage trough. Normally the trough (really the SN10 wave) follows wave V, but it occurs earlier when it is due to higher frequencies and generated by more basal portions of the cochlea. Finally, the subtraction process required by the derived methods introduced noise in the ABR recordings.

Interestingly, although the derived band masking strategy is not widely applied clinically for frequency-specific estimation with ABR of auditory thresholds in infants and young children, it is employed in the stacked ABR technique for optimizing the sensitivity of neurodiagnostic ABR measurements in detection of retrocochlear auditory dysfunction. The neurodiagnostic application of stacked ABRs is reviewed in Chapter 10.

SUMMARY. | Although the masking techniques were theoretically appealing, there were serious practical disadvantages to their routine use for frequency-specific ABR measurement. There were two major unknown technical or physiologic variables. First, the actual effectiveness of the masking in limiting the cochlear activation to the portion of the basilar membrane underlying the desired stimulus frequency has not been conclusively defined in the normal or the cochlear-impaired ear. That is, even though hair cells in a portion of the cochlea may be activated by a steady-state (continuous) masking noise, it is conceivable that these or other hair cells in the same region still might be responsive to the transient stimulus. A second unknown concerns the extent and the effect of masking noise spread into the stimulus frequency region, as well as on interactions between masker and stimulus. Complicating the interpretation of ABRs obtained with this method are the steep slopes for the high-frequency side of tuning curves versus the more gradual slopes for the low-frequency side and differences in tuning curve slopes for high-frequency units (sharper slopes) versus low-frequency units (less sharp slopes). In combination, these factors conspired to limit the validity of the techniques, especially for the low-frequency region, which is of greatest clinical concern. Sophisticated ipsilateral masking paradigms have not been incorporated into clinical ABR measurement, as performed with most commercially available evoked response systems.

The preceding physiologic questions regarding the masking techniques, such as spread of masking, effectiveness of masking, the influences of tuning curve shape, apply also to the derived methods. In addition, the high intensity levels required for the masking noise limit the extent of hearing loss for which the methods can be effectively used. The subtracting process introduces progressively greater amounts of noise into the waveforms, which makes response detection more difficult. Perhaps the most limiting factor, at least for routine clinical application of the derived response methods, is the amount of time required to obtain an ABR threshold for even a single frequency. As described in the preceding studies, this technique is simply too time-consuming to be routinely clinically feasible with infants and young children. Don, Eggermont, and Brackmann (1979) point out an additional problem in attempting clinically to correlate an audiogram reconstructed from the derived masking ABR method with traditional pure-tone audiometry. With pure-tone audiometry, the contribution of the basal region of the cochlea is not excluded when lower frequency stimuli (e.g., 250 to 500 Hz) are presented at high intensity levels. Because of the activation of high-frequency auditory fibers by these low-frequency stimuli, a problem described previously, it is not possible validly to assess severe low-frequency hearing impairments. With an effective derived masking technique, then, the ABR would presumably overestimate auditory threshold for low frequencies in comparison to pure-tone audiometry. These authors go on to note that any auditory pathology may disrupt the neural synchrony required to generate a clear, well-formed ABR with a distinct wave V. As a result, the derived technique, or any other frequency-specific method, may appear to be more useful when applied to normal subjects than when applied clinically.

Even in carefully conducted experimental investigations in animals with cochlear pathology, AP thresholds evoked by a specific frequency stimulus and recorded electrophysiologically may be better than threshold for the single unit (fiber) serving the frequency (Pickles, 1988). This implies that the stimulus was not in fact frequency specific and actually activated normal cochlear regions adjacent to the site of lesion. As noted already, intensity level of the stimulus is closely linked to frequency specificity. This is a fundamental principle of auditory electrophysiology. At low stimulus-intensity levels, the AP originates from a discrete site on the cochlea corresponding to the stimulus frequency, but at high levels, the region of response becomes dispersed and corresponds best to the cochlear region with the "best frequency," that is, the most sensitive units.

Tone-Burst Technique for Frequency-Specific ABR Measurement

Although there is an inevitable trade-off between the abruptness of a stimulus needed to produce synchronous firing of neurons in the auditory system reflected by a clear ABR waveform, especially at lower intensity levels, and the spectral constraint of the stimulus, tone-burst ABRs have assumed an important role in pediatric audiologic assessment. There are perhaps three reasons for the persistent interest in this stimulus paradigm for frequency-specific ABR measurement. First, tone-burst stimulation is clinically feasible. The technique is relatively straightforward. Test time is relatively brief, and tone-burst stimuli are already available on all commercial evoked response systems. Second, there is considerable long-standing experimental evidence that at low- to moderate-intensity levels and with proper onset gating, tone bursts can produce frequency-specific early-latency AERs (Abbas & Gorga, 1981; Dallos & Cheatham, 1976; Davis & Hirsh, 1979; Gorga, Kaminski, Beauchaine, & Jesteadt, 1988; Klein & Mills, 1981; Suzuki, Hirai, & Horiuchi, 1977). Early clinical studies of tone-generated ABR demonstrated that behavioral thresholds could be estimated to within 20 dB, although results were not uniformly encouraging and not always audiometrically valid (e.g.,

Coats & Martin, 1977; Fjermedal & Laukli, 1989a,b; Gorga, Kaminski, Beauchaine, & Jesteadt, 1988; Jerger, Hayes, & Jordan, 1980; Jerger & Mauldin, 1978; Møller & Blegvad, 1976; Picton, Ouellette, Hamel, & Smith, 1979; Pratt & Sohmer, 1977; Smith & Simmons, 1982). Third, experimental evidence showed that the spectral splatter associated with tone bursts that have linear onset and offset characteristics—specifically, the amplitude and frequency range of side lobes around the frequency of interest—may be minimized with the use of other nonlinear stimulus-shaping envelopes (e.g., Gorga & Thornton, 1989). Thus, the possibility existed that, with appropriate envelopes, tone bursts offered an optimal stimulus, that is, one that permitted frequency-specific ABR recording simply, quickly, and with relatively inexpensive instrumentation.

As a result of technological advances and careful clinical investigation, the assorted problems with frequency-specific ABR measurement cited in earlier publications have, in general, been solved. Critical review of the literature reveals, in retrospect, a variety of potential methodological weaknesses or even flaws in test protocols used for frequency-specific estimation of hearing sensitivity, particularly in infants and young children. In combination, these factors, and probably others on occasion, conspired to minimize the consistency and the accuracy of tone-burst ABR recordings and, consequently, the impression among some researchers and clinicians that frequency-specific ABR measurement was not clinically feasible or useful in estimating the pure-tone hearing sensitivity of infants and young children. In general, estimation of pure-tone sensitivity with frequency-specific ABR techniques is clinically feasible and reasonably accurate in pediatric populations.

A rather substantial number of publications are devoted to description of tone-burst ABR findings of hundreds of pediatric and adult normal hearers and hearing impaired patients, as summarized in Table 8.1. The following guidelines for a protocol for measurement of frequency-specific ABRs are based on findings from the accumulated published and unpublished thirty-year clinical experience with tone-burst ABR measurement.

A Clinical Protocol for Measurement of Tone-Burst ABR

Adherence to some practical guidelines will lead to reasonably accurate estimation of auditory sensitivity for selected audiometric frequencies in minimal test time. The primary, and most important, is reliance on a proven ABR test protocol. That is, the application of a set of stimulus and acquisition parameters effective in eliciting reliable frequency-specific ABRs from infants. More than thirty years ago, Hecox and Galambos (1974) described the application of ABR in auditory assessment of infants and young children. Since then, accumulated clinical experience with untold millions of children has produced ample evidence in

TABLE 8.1. Published Studies Describing Findings for Auditory Brainstem Response
(ABRs) Elicited with Tone-Burst Stimuli, Arranged Chronologically by Population
Adapted and updated from Stapells (2000).

POPULATION	STUDIES, YEARS
Adult	
Normal hearing	Kodera et al., 1977; Suzuki et al., 1977; Picton et al., 1979; Bauch et al., 1980; Suzuki, Hirai, & Horiuchi, 1981; McDonald & Shimizu, 1981; Klein, 1983; Yamada et al., 1983; Beattie, Moretti, & Warren, 1984; Kavanagh et al., 1984; Klein, 1984; Gorga et al., 1988; Palaskas et al., 1989; Purdy, Houghton, & Keith, 1989; Stapells et al., 1990; Gorga et al., 1993; Werner, Folsom, & Mancl, 1993; Beattie & Torre, 1997; Sininger, Abdala, & Cone-Wesson, 1997; Purdy & Abbas, 1989
Hearing loss	Kodera et al., 1977; Picton et al., 1979; Purdy & Abbas, 1989; Stapells et al., 1990; Conijn, Brocaar, & van Zanten, 1993; Beattie, Garcia, & Johnson, 1996; Nousak & Stapells, 1999; Purdy & Abbas, 2002
Pediatric	
Normal hearing	Hayes & Jerger, 1982; Yamada et al., 1983; Klein, 1984; Werner et al., 1993; Stapells et al., 1995; Sininger et al., 1997; Balfour et al., 1998
Hearing loss	Hayes & Jerger, 1982; Kileny & Magathan, 1987; Stapells et al., 1995; Balfour et al., 1998; Aoyagi et al., 1999

support of specific measurement parameters that are effective for recording tone-burst ABRs. Experience has also clearly demonstrated that the use of improper test parameters will result in inaccurate threshold estimations or, in some cases, a false-negative ABR outcome error, i.e., no detectable ABR in a child for whom an ABR should be present.

An effective protocol for recording frequency-specific ABRs is summarized in Table 8.2 (see page 268). Clinicians are advised to create with their auditory evoked response system a similar protocol for measurement of tone-burst ABRs. The protocol can be appropriately labeled, saved, and then retrieved as needed clinically. Clinicians just beginning to apply tone-burst ABRs in the electrophysiologic frequency-specific estimation of auditory thresholds may wish to have a separate protocol for each test frequency. Experienced clinicians, on the other hand, will probably utilize a generic protocol for recording ABRs with tone-burst stimuli, preferring to change test frequencies and other measurement parameters "on the fly" as the assessment progresses. To assist the reader in creating his or her custom tone-burst ABR protocol, the actual printout of the parameters used in recording ABRs for a case reported in this chapter is displayed in Figure 8.2. A brief discussion of these parameters might be helpful to the reader. Beginning in the top left portion of the parameter display, the electrode locations were Fz (high forehead) for the noninverting electrode and A1 (left earlobe) for the inverting electrode. The "run" mode indicates that averaging was ongoing during data collection. Amplifier sensitivity (i.e., gain) was ± 0.50 µV. The high-pass filter setting (referred to with this system as low-frequency filter or LLF cutoff) was 30 Hz, whereas the low-pass filter setting (high-frequency filter or HFF cutoff) was 1500 Hz. The ter-

minology used in the printout of the protocol for describing filter settings is somewhat confusing. As noted in Chapter 6, manufacturers often use the phrase "low-frequency filter" in reference to the high-pass filter and, conversely, the phrase "high-frequency filter" is used for the low-pass filter. The notch filter option was "off" (i.e., disenabled or not used) to minimize inadvertent removal of low-frequency energy contributing importantly to the infant ABR.

Moving to the next grouping of parameters in Figure 8.2, the maximum number of sweeps per run (stimulus presentations or amount of signal averaging) was preset at 2000. However, this number of stimuli may be exceeded if necessary or, more commonly, signal averaging may be terminated sooner if a clear response is observed. For ABRs evoked with click stimuli and higher frequency tone-burst stimuli, an analysis time of 15 ms is long enough for detection of ABR wave V under all possible conditions. That is, for young infants with ABR latencies delayed due to immaturity, for lower signal intensity levels, and/or for patients who have hearing loss producing longer latency responses. For the 500 Hz tone-burst signal, however, a 20 ms analysis time is needed to encompass ABR wave V under all potential measurement and subject conditions. Lower frequency tone-burst signals activate more apical regions of the cochlea. For lower frequency tone bursts (e.g., 500 Hz), the time required for the traveling wave to reach the more apical portion of the cochlea produces longer latencies for ABR wave. Stimulus rate (the number of stimuli presented per second) was 21.1. An odd number is utilized to minimize measurement interference between stimulus presentation rate and electrical noise at 60 Hz. A somewhat faster rate of stimulation, e.g., 27.3/sec or even higher, would also be appropriate for

UF DEPT. COMMUNICATIVE DISORDERS
SPEECH AND HEARING CLINIC
PO BOX 100174
GAINESVILLE, FL 32610-0174

Gator ABR 1 channel

AMP	Elect	Mode	Sns	Lff	Hff	Notch	Artifact	REM	Remarks
1	Fz-A1	Run	50uV	30	1.5K	Off	90	1	
2	Fz-A1	Run	50uV	30	1.5K	Off	90	2	
3	Fz-A1	Run	50uV	30	1.5K	Off	90	3	
4	Fz-A1	Run	50uV	30	1.5K	Off	90	4	
5	Fz-A1	Run	50uV	30	1.5K	Off	90	5	
6	Fz-A1	Run	50uV	30	1.5K	Off	90	6	
7	Fz-A1	Run	50uV	30	1.5K	Off	90	7	
8	Fz-A1	Run	50uV	30	1.5K	Off	90	8	

ACQ	Comm	Sweep	Time	Delay	Rate	Trigger	Stim	MISC	Type	Ch#	Accept	Reject	Filter	Fsp/SNR	Date	Time	Add	Sub	Inv	Filter	Smooth
1	A	2000	15ms	-1ms	21.1	Inter	Gated	1	Sum	1	677	0	Butter	5.70	06/15/2004	10:08	no	no	no	no	no
2	A	2000	15ms	-1ms	21.1	Inter	Gated	2	Sum	1	648	0	Butter	2.37	06/15/2004	10:08	no	no	no	no	no
3	A	2000	15ms	-1ms	21.1	Inter	Gated	3	Sum	1	696	0	Butter	1.19	06/15/2004	10:09	no	no	no	no	no
4	A	2000	15ms	-1ms	21.1	Inter	Gated	4	Sum	1	611	0	Butter	0.15	06/15/2004	10:10	no	no	no	no	no
5	A	2000	15ms	-1ms	21.1	Inter	Gated	5	Sum	1	305	0	Butter	0.21	06/15/2004	10:10	no	no	no	no	no
6	A	2000	15ms	-1ms	21.1	Inter	Gated	6	Sum	1	245	0	Butter	1.42	06/15/2004	10:11	no	no	no	no	no
7	A	2000	15ms	-1ms	21.1	Inter	Gated	7	Sum	1	611	0	Butter	0.93	06/15/2004	10:11	no	no	no	no	no
8	A	2000	15ms	-1ms	21.1	Inter	Gated	8	Sum	1	570	0	Butter	0.30	06/15/2004	10:11	no	no	no	no	no

STIM	Trans	Type	Pol	Dur	Level	Freq	Pla	Ramp	Env	Noi	NLev	dB	Trans	Type	Pol	Dur	Level	Freq	Pla	Ramp	Env	Noi	NLev	dB
1	Insert	Click	Rar	100us	80					Off		nHL	Insert	Off								Off		nHL
2	Insert	Click	Rar	100us	80					Off		nHL	Insert	Off								Off		nHL
3	Insert	Click	Rar	100us	30					Off		nHL	Insert	Off								Off		nHL
4	Insert	Click	Rar	100us	20					Off		nHL	Insert	Off								Off		nHL
5	Insert	Click	Rar	100us	20					Off		nHL	Insert	Off								Off		nHL
6	Insert	Tone	Alt		100	4KHz	0cy	2	Blk	Off		nHL	Insert	Off								Off		nHL
7	Insert	Tone	Alt		50	4KHz	0cy	2	Blk	Off		nHL	Insert	Off								Off		nHL
8	Insert	Tone	Alt		50	4KHz	0cy	2	Blk	Off		nHL	Insert	Off								Off		nHL

FIGURE 8.2. Test protocol used in performing a frequency-specific auditory brainstem response (ABR) from a young child for assessment of auditory sensitivity. The ABR was recorded in the operating room with the patient lightly anesthetized (anesthetic agent Propofol). Total test time was less than 20 minutes for estimation of auditory thresholds bilaterally for click stimulation, and with three different tone-burst stimuli.

infant ABR measurement. Remember, with faster stimulus rates, assuming the ABR remains well-formed and reliably recorded, test time is shorter and/or more ABR data can be collected within a given amount of time.

In the display of parameters in Figure 8.2, two of the columns describe the number of signal averages accepted (within the sensitivity limits noted above) or rejected (considered artifact because the voltages exceeded the sensitivity limits). Notice that for some runs or averages, there were far fewer than the maximum number of stimulus presentations (sweeps). One of the most important ways to minimize ABR test time is to manually stop signal averaging as soon as a reliable response is detected. Often, at a high intensity level (e.g., 80 dB nHL) a clear and well-formed ABR emerges after only a few hundred stimulus repetitions, whereas up to 2000 stimulus repetitions or more are required to detect a reliable

response as threshold is approached. Naturally, movement artifact was not a problem because the patient was anesthetized. Therefore, there were no "artifact rejections," as documented by the zeros under the "reject" column. The term "Butter" in the column labeled "filter" is an abbreviation for the type of physiologic filter used by the evoked response system (Butterworth filter). The column to the right, labeled "Fsp/SNR," contains statistical calculations of the Fsp (the F-statistic for a single point in the waveform). The Fsp is a statistical measure of the signal-to-noise ratio (SNR) and the presence versus absence of a response. Larger Fsp values correspond to larger SNRs. The Fsp is commonly applied in automated ABR systems used in newborn hearing screening. The test date and time is displayed in the next columns. The reader will note in the figure that stimulus presentation and signal averaging for the case began at 10:08 a.m. (it ended at

10:38 a.m). Although most current auditory evoked response systems have a variety of features for digital manipulation and analysis of waveforms (e.g., adding or subtracting waveforms, and inverting, filtering or smoothing waveforms after data collection), none of these options were used with this case.

In the lower portion of the display of measurement parameters, the reader will note that the transducer was always an insert earphone. There are at least a dozen clinical advantages for the use of insert earphones in ABR measurement in infants and young children (Hall & Mueller, 1997). A rarefaction (negative) polarity (abbreviated "Rar") was used for the click signal, whereas alternating polarity ("Alt") was used for the tone bursts. Although auditory responses can be elicited with single-polarity tone-burst signals, the result for low frequencies often consists of a series of periodic waves, whereas the ABR waveform evoked by an alternating polarity stimulus tends to be more typical in appearance, with a distinct wave V (see Figure 8.3). The conventional duration ("Dur") for a click signal is 100 μsec (or 0.1 ms). Duration of the tone burst signals is shown in several columns to the right. The onset, or "Ramp," consists of 2 cycles of the tone burst (in this example), whereas there is actually no plateau ("Pla"), i.e., 0 cycles for the tone-burst signal frequency ("Freq"), which is 4000 Hz in this example.

The numbers in the column labeled "Level" refer to the intensity level of the signals. A brief explanation of the conventional approach for defining ABR signal intensity is warranted at this point. For click signals, the intensity levels are given in dB nHL, that is, dB above the behavioral threshold for the click signal (or 0 dB nHL) in a group of normal-hearing persons. As a rule, the intensity levels displayed for tone-burst signals on the monitor screen of an auditory evoked system are not referenced to 0 dB nHL but, rather, are equivalent to dB SPL. Thus, before utilizing tone-burst signals in ABR measurement, the clinician should for each signal frequency obtain biologic normative data for a small number of normal-hearing persons. The process of establishing biologic normative data (0 dB nHL or dB normal hearing level) for the tone burst (and also bone-conduction click signals) is simple and rather quick. Using the evoked response system and insert earphones in the typical test settings where ABRs will be recorded from patient populations (e.g., a clinic room, a hospital room, and/or operating room), behavioral thresholds are estimated for each tone-burst signal for a handful of normal-hearing adults. It's not necessary to actually record an ABR in this process. The electrodes can be placed in a cup of water to prevent the equipment from constantly rejecting samples due to artifact, or the artifact reject feature on the evoked response system can be disenabled (turned off) during the normative data collection. Commonly, in a typical quiet but not sound-treated room, and with insert earphones, behavioral thresholds will be obtained at about 35 dB (the intensity level on the screen) for a 500 Hz signal, and about 20 to 25 dB (again, the intensity

number on the screen) for higher signal frequencies. These behavioral threshold values are used as the reference, or as 0 dB nHL. Returning to Figure 8.2, then, the intensity levels for the click signal are already in dB nHL, whereas dB nHL for the 4000 Hz tone-burst signal is actually the value shown (e.g., 100 dB) minus the adjustment for behavioral normative data (e.g., 100 - 25 = 75 dB nHL).

The next column to the right, labeled "Env" (for envelope), indicates the mathematical equation used to shape the onset (ramping, windowing, or envelope) of the tone-burst signals. Blackman ramping or windowing of the onset envelope for tone bursts is often used in clinical measurement of the ABR. Current evoked response systems all offer this and other onset envelope options. Since no masking was used in the ABR recording, the word "off" appears in the Noise ("Noi") column. Indications for masking in ABR measurement were discussed in Chapter 6. With the use of insert earphones, and close analysis of ABR waveforms and the latencies of waves, masking is rarely needed in recording ABRs. For this particular case, a reliable ABR was recorded in the ipsilateral electrode condition (Fz to left earlobe) at a high intensity level (80 dB nHL) for click signals, and with all waves present and at normal latency values. This finding eliminates the possibility that the ABR was generated from crossover of the signal to the nontest (right) ear. Analysis of the initial ABR findings revealed that these criteria were met and immediately confirmed that masking was not necessary. The remaining columns to the right side of the figure are reserved for stimulus parameters for signals presented to the right ear.

The practical application of the measurement parameters displayed in Figure 8.2, and summarized in Table 8.2, is discussed further in the following case report. Key parameters that can make or break successful and accurate ABR are appropriate calibration of stimulus intensity, the inclusion of low-frequency electrophysiological energy with appropriate high-pass filter settings (e.g., 30 Hz), avoidance of the notch filter options, and an adequately long analysis time. When a proven test protocol is used to record a tone-burst ABR from an adequately quiet child, test time is minimal, analysis of the ABR is typically straightforward, and a valid and meaningful test outcome is almost always assured.

RATIONALE FOR A PROTOCOL FOR FREQUENCY-SPECIFIC ABRS. |

A test protocol for eliciting frequency-specific ABRs with tone-burst stimuli is summarized in Table 8.2. As noted above, the selection of parameters used for recording frequency-specific ABRs derives from findings of experimental and clinical investigations during the past thirty years. There are certainly inconsistencies among test protocols for tone-burst ABR measurement published in the literature, cited in textbooks, or included among postings on the Internet. A consortium of audiologists from the United Kingdom (S. Mason, C. Elliott, G. Lightfoot, D. Parker, J. Stevens, G. Sutton, M. Vidler) and from Vancouver, Canada (D. Stapells), have, for example, posted on the Internet recommended guidelines for ABR measurement with air- and bone-conducted click stimuli and for tone-burst stimuli. Relatively minor deviations in parameters for the protocol cited in these guidelines versus the parameters in the protocol displayed in Table 8.2 are noted in the following discussion of stimulus and acquisition parameters. For the most part, similarities among protocols outweigh the differences (e.g., Hall, 1992; Hall & Mueller, 1997; Stapells, 2000; Stapells & Oates, 1997).

The test protocol (Table 8.2) is a logical starting point for the clinical measurement of frequency-specific ABRs from infants and young children. It is not, however, written in stone. A clinician must regularly make changes in stimulus and response parameters as the ABR is recorded from patients in order to elicit a quality and representative response. For any given patient, myriad measurement variables may affect ABR recordings and may require the clinician to modify parameters of the test protocol. Clinical measurement of the ABR is interesting and challenging largely because decisions on test parameters must be made quickly based on information acquired from moment to moment. For consistently successful application of the ABR for diagnostic assessment of infants and young children, the clinician must first understand why certain test parameters are appropriate and under which test circumstances the test parameters should be modified. Then, the clinician must acquire experience in applying this knowledge during ABR measurement clinically with normal-hearing children and children with various types of auditory dysfunction. The rationale for selected parameters in the recommended protocol for measurement of frequency-specific ABRs with tone-burst stimuli is now reviewed briefly.

Stimulus Rate. Data must be collected for a variety of stimulus conditions during a frequency-specific ABR assessment, including different frequencies and multiple intensity levels for each ear. As a result, a full assessment for estimation of hearing sensitivity in a child can require considerably more time than a neurodiagnostic ABR assessment in an adult. Even if each stimuli at each tone-burst test frequency is presented only for three or four stimulus intensity levels, 48 or more waveforms may be recorded during a typical ABR assessment, e.g., 4 frequencies × 3 levels × 2 ears × 2 replications. Although there is no single "correct" or recommended stimulus rate, there are compelling reasons in frequency-specific ABR assessment of infants and young children for employing stimulus rates that are reasonable fast. The general guideline is to elicit an ABR with stimulus rates that are slightly slower than those producing deterioration in response quality and reliability. A stimulus presentation rate somewhere within the range of 27.1/second up to 39.1/second is quite appropriate. In the British/Canadian test protocol, a tone-burst stimulus rate of 37/second is recommended. Slow stimulus presentation rates, e.g., 11.1/sec, unnecessarily prolong test time while providing no benefit

in terms of response detection, reliability, or improved waveform morphology. Obviously, if the quality of an ABR recorded from an infant is equivalent for slow (e.g., 11.1/sec) versus fast (e.g., 39.1/sec) stimulus rates, the faster rate is preferable because test time is one-third as long or, looking at the advantage a different way, three times more ABR data can be collected in the same amount of time. Therefore, even though there is no single recommended stimulus rate, successful and complete measurement of frequency-specific ABRs is greatly enhanced by the use of a relatively high stimulus rate.

Stimulus Polarity. As noted in Chapter 6, rarefaction polarity stimuli are recommended for click-evoked ABRs. There is no clear consensus regarding the optimal polarity for tone-burst stimuli. Some authors suggest the use of alternating polarity tone-burst stimuli (e.g., Hall & Mueller, 1997; Stapells & Oates, 1997), whereas others recommend a single polarity. In most cases, rarefaction polarity tone-burst stimuli are appropriate and effective for generating an ABR, particularly for higher frequency stimuli. Clinically, however, a single polarity stimulus may occasionally produce a highly consistent periodic waveform that does not resemble an ABR. Most common with a high-intensity 500 Hz tone burst, the waveform is distinguished from typical stimulus artifact by a brief period with little or no oscillation immediately following the stimulus, and then prolongation of high amplitude peaks and troughs for many milliseconds after the offset of the stimulus. In such cases, the use of an alternating polarity stimulus appears to eliminate the periodic waveform, revealing a typical ABR wave V. The effect of single (rarefaction) versus alternating stimulus polarity on the ABR elicited with a 500 Hz tone burst is illustrated in Figure 8.3.

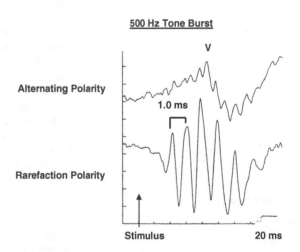

FIGURE 8.3. Auditory brainstem response (ABR) for a 500 Hz tone burst with rarefaction polarity versus alternating polarity showing a distinct difference in waveform morphology. The ABR wave V component is more clearly evident with the alternating polarity stimulus condition.

TABLE 8.2. A Protocol for Measurement of Frequency-Specific Auditory Brainstem Response (ABR)

The conventional ABR protocol for air-conduction click signals must be modified to successfully record ABRs for tone-burst signals. The main differences between protocols for click versus tone-burst ABRs are noted under comments.

PARAMETERS	SUGGESTIONS	COMMENTS
Stimulus Parameters		
Transducer	Insert	Insert earphones offer many advantages in clinical ABR measurement, especially with infants and young children, as delineated in Chapter 3.
Polarity	Alternating	Instead of the usual rarefaction polarity, alternating polarity stimuli can be used to minimize the possibility of a frequency-following-type response.
Ramping	Blackman	Ramping refers to how the rise/fall portions of the tone burst are shaped. Some nonlinear ramping or windowing techniques reduce spectral splatter and increase frequency specificity of tone-burst stimulation. Blackman windowing is the best, and most current AER systems include it in their stimulus package.
Duration	Variable	The rise/fall, and plateau, times for the tone-burst stimuli vary depending on the frequency. As a rule, it's desirable to use longer times for lower frequencies so as to include more cycles to increase the chance that the stimulus sounds like the desired frequency, and not a click. However, as discussed in this section of the chapter, the use of a very brief (0.5 cycles or 2 ms) 250 Hz tone burst will generate a more well-formed and distinct ABR, albeit not quite as frequency specific (an energy band within the frequency range of 100 to 600 Hz). The most common approach for signal duration is to use 2 cycles rise time, 0 cycle plateau, and 2 cycles fall time or, in milliseconds (ms): • 500 Hz: 4 ms rise/fall and 0 ms plateau • 1000 Hz: 2 ms rise/fall and 0 ms plateau • 2000 Hz: 1 ms rise/fall and 0 ms plateau • 4000 Hz: 0.5 ms rise/fall and 0 ms plateau
Intensity	Variable	Keep in mind that the intensity levels on the screen for your ABR system will usually not be defined in dB nHL, as they are for a click. More often, the values are in dB SPL. That is, 95 dB may be selected, but the intensity range for the tone-burst frequency may go as high as 115 dB. Always obtain behavioral threshold data for each tone-burst stimulus to be used for ABR recording (with the earphones specific to the evoked response system and in the room where ABRs will be recorded), and then collect biologic normative data for tone-burst intensity. For example, if the maximum dial setting for a 500 Hz tone burst is 115 dB, but normal subjects have an average threshold of 30 dB for this stimulus, then at 115 dB on the dial the intensity level is really 85 dB nHL (referenced to the normal behavioral threshold for the stimulus). With most evoked response systems, these "correction factors" can be incorporated into the intensities displayed on the screen so that all intensity values are in dB nHL according to clinic normative data. It is then advisable to actually record ABRs for this 500 Hz stimulus from a few of these normal-hearing subjects to estimate the lowest intensity level that produces an observable and reliable ABR wave V.
Acquisition Parameters		
Electrode sites	Fz–Ai	The noninverting (positive) electrode is located in the midline on the high forehead (Fz) and the inverting electrode is located on the earlobe ipsilateral to the stimulus ear (Ai). With an ear clip electrode design, the earlobe electrode is easily applied, impedance is low, and the electrode is removed from the mastoid region. The earlobe electrode records a larger wave I than the mastoid electrode and is associated with less stimulus artifact in bone-conduction ABR recordings. The ground electrode can be located on the low forehead (Fpz) or the contralateral earlobe (limits recordings to a single channel).

TABLE 8.2.   (continued)

PARAMETERS	SUGGESTIONS	COMMENTS
Filter settings	30 to 3000 Hz	A low-frequency cut-off for the high-pass filter (e.g., 30 Hz) is very important because the tone-burst ABR is dominated by low-frequency energy, especially in infants.
Analysis time	15 to 20 ms	For click signals and higher frequency tone-burst signals, an analysis time of 15 ms is adequate to encompass the wave V component even under conditions associated with delayed wave V latency, e.g., low signal intensity level, hearing loss, very young age (immaturity of the auditory pathways). For tone-burst signals of 1000 Hz and below, a 20 ms analysis time is recommended.
Sweeps	Variable	The number of sweeps (stimulus repetitions or number of signal averages for an ABR recording) is dependent on the signal-to-noise ratio. When the signal (ABR amplitude) is larger (e.g., at a high intensity level with a normal-hearing patient) and/or when background noise is low (e.g., the patient is sedated or anesthetized), then relatively fewer stimulus repetitions are needed. On the other hand, when ABR amplitude is smaller (e.g., at lower signal intensity levels and/or in a patient with hearing loss) and noise is greater (a restless unsedated child), more signal averaging (more stimulus repetitions) will be needed. As a rule, fewer stimulus repetitions are required for the second (replication) ABR run when the goal is to simply verify that the response is reliable (and not just artifact).

Stimulus Duration.   When a highly transient (i.e., click) stimulus is used to elicit the ABR, duration is invariably 0.1 ms (100 μsec). For tone-burst stimuli, duration must be selected and specified for the onset, the plateau, and the offset. There are two acceptable, similar, and commonly used options for defining tone-burst duration. Stimulus duration consists of three components (rise-plateau-fall) as shown in Figure 8.4. One option, recommended early on in the history of the ABR by Dr. Hallowell Davis and referred to as the "2-1-2" approach, calls for rise and fall times of 2 cycles with a 1 cycle plateau. The 2-1-2 paradigm for duration of tone-burst stimuli is endorsed by the British/Canadian test protocol. Duration of rise/fall times and the plateau for each stimulus frequency (e.g., 500 Hz up to 4000 Hz) is defined by the same number of cycles. The rationale for this approach is an attempt to assure relative equivalence of acoustic energy among different stimulus frequencies. That is, the absolute times for the rise/fall and plateau components of duration vary among stimuli, but the number of cycles of the stimulus remains constant. The time required for completion of a single cycle of a tone burst is, of course, inversely related to the frequency. Lower stimulus frequencies are characterized by longer times for the completion of a cycle of the waveform, whereas a complete cycle is completed in less time for higher frequencies. Another slightly modified option, now commonly employed clinically, is to define tone-burst duration by 2 cycles for rise/fall time and no plateau, that is,

2-0-2. This approach retains the energy consistency among tone bursts of different frequencies. In addition, there is some evidence that elimination of the stimulus plateau enhances the spectral specificity of the stimulus. In theory, a stimulus

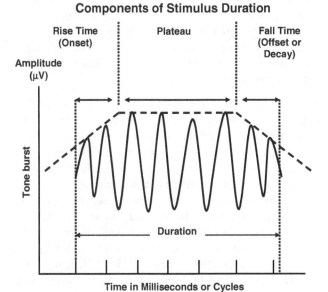

FIGURE 8.4.   Illustration of the components of tone-burst duration.

TABLE 8.3. Duration* of Selected Tone-Burst Stimuli Defined in Cycles versus Time (ms)

Some evoked response systems express duration in units of time, whereas others use cycles.

FREQUENCY (HZ)	CYCLES	TIME (MS)
250	2-0-2	8-0-8
500	2-0-2	4-0-4
1000	2-0-2	2-0-2
2000	2-0-2	1-0-1
4000	2-0-2	0.5-0-0.5

*Duration for tone-burst stimuli in ABR assessment is often indicated using 2 cycles for the onset (rise) portion of the stimulus, 0 cycles for the plateau, and 2 cycles for the offset (fall or decay) portion of the tone burst, i.e., the 2-0-2 paradigm.

plateau is extraneous for evoking an ABR because the response is generated by neurons activated only by stimulus onset. The relationship between stimulus frequency and duration for the rise/fall and plateau for selected tone bursts is displayed in Table 8.3.

Dr. Michael Gorga has described a strategy for evoking with a transient low-frequency tonal stimulus a distinct and easily detected ABR. The stimulus is half a cycle (0.5 cycle) of a 250 Hz tone burst, resulting in an acoustic duration of 2 ms. Predictably, the very brief duration of the stimulus reduces its frequency specificity. The 0.5 cycle 250 Hz tone burst has spectral energy dispersed within a band of frequencies from 100 to 600 Hz. Therefore, a modest loss in frequency specificity is traded for an ABR that is clear, well formed, and relatively easy to record. The transient 250 Hz stimulus still provides information on auditory threshold within the same general low-frequency region targeted by the conventional 500 Hz tone burst. Waveforms elicited with each type of low-frequency tone-burst stimulus are shown in Figure 8.5. Systematic investigation of this strategy for electrophysiologic estimation of auditory sensitivity in infants and young children is underway.

Tone-Burst Envelopes. The envelope of the tone burst refers to how the onset and offset portions of the stimulus are gated or shaped as amplitude for a single stimulus rises from minimum to maximum or falls from maximum to minimum. Different envelopes are associated with different spectral characteristics, especially the extent and amplitude of energy on each side (side lobes) of the center frequency, as shown in Figure 8.6. Most early studies of frequency-specific ECochG and ABR relied on tone-burst stimuli with *linear* stimulus envelopes (Burkard & Hecox, 1983; Davis & Hirsch, 1976a; Gorga & Thornton, 1989; Jacobson, 1983; Kileny, 1981; Mair & Laukli, 1985; McDonald & Shimizu, 1981; Wood, Siltz, & Jacobson, 1979). If low-frequency hearing sensitivity is assessed with brief tone stimuli, the spread of energy to frequency regions where there is better hearing may result

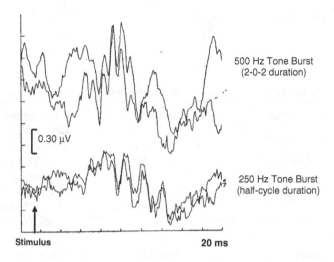

FIGURE 8.5. Auditory brainstem response (ABR) waveforms evoked by a 500 Hz tone burst with the 2-0-2 cycle paradigm for duration versus a very brief duration (half-cycle) 250 Hz stimulus.

in underestimation of audiometric hearing threshold levels. Tonal stimuli with linear gated onsets have distinct theoretical limitations as frequency-specific stimuli. Concerns about the frequency-specificity of linearly gated tone bursts for assessing auditory sensitivity for specific frequency regions led to investigations of nonlinear shaping (ramping, win-

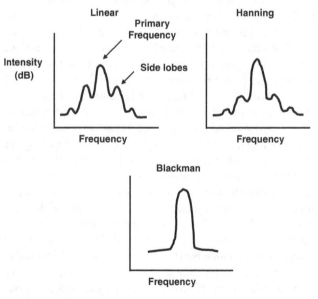

FIGURE 8.6. Spectral characteristics for different types of onset ramps (windowing) available for tone-burst stimuli. Note the greater spectral specificity for Blackman windowing.

dowing, or gating) of tone-burst stimuli (e.g., Gorga et al., 1987; Gorga et al., 1988b; Oates & Stapells, 1997; Stapells, Makeig, & Galamos, 1987).

In theory, nonlinear tonal stimulus gating alternatives are better suited for frequency-specific ABR generation (e.g., Gorga & Thornton, 1989), with optimal stimuli showing maximum side-lobe reduction yet minimal width of the main energy lobe (the test frequency). Blackman windowing or ramping meets this criterion. Citing the work of other authors (e.g., Oates & Stapells, 1997; Stapells et al., 1985), however, Purdy and Abbas (2002) note "frequency-specificity refers to how independent one measure of audiometric threshold is of contributions from surrounding frequencies, whereas cochlear place specificity refers to that portion of the cochlea contributing to the response" (p. 359).

Among window types evaluated by Harris (1978), the cosine^2 (Hanning) and Blackman windows have recently been studied in AER measurement. Gorga and colleagues (Gorga, Kaminski, Beauchaine, & Jesteadt, 1988) recorded ABRs from twenty normal-hearing subjects with tone-burst stimuli gated with cosine^2 functions. Responses were highly reliable within individual subjects. Intersubject variability increased for lower test frequencies. ABR thresholds were higher (worse) than behavioral thresholds, with the differences increasing for the lower test frequencies. In another study, Gorga and colleagues (Gorga, Kaminski, & Beauchaine, 1988) compared behavioral thresholds versus ABR latencies and thresholds in six normal-hearing subjects with brief-duration high-frequency tone bursts (9,000 through 16,000 Hz), gated with Blackman functions. The authors confirmed the clinical feasibility of high-frequency ABR measurement but recommended additional study in hearing-impaired patients before the technique is applied clinically in appropriate populations (e.g., patients receiving potentially ototoxic drugs and therefore at risk for high-frequency auditory deficits). Despite the theoretical advantages of specially shaped tone-burst stimulus-onset envelopes (e.g., Blackman windowing or gating), experimental evidence for greater frequency specificity for ABR recordings in patients with hearing loss is not convincing (e.g., Oates & Purdy, 2001; Oates & Stapells, 1997; Purdy & Abbas, 2002). That is, predictions of pure-tone thresholds with tone bursts having linear versus Blackman onset ramps were equivalent (usually within 10 to 15 dB), at least for adult subjects with sloping high-frequency sensorineural hearing loss. Purdy and Abbas (2002) acknowledge that "There may be more obvious differences between Blackman and linearly gated tone bursts if hearing-impaired listeners with unusually steep hearing losses are investigated. Blackman-gated stimuli may also offer some advantages over linearly gated stimuli for frequencies at or below 1000 Hz, since short rise/fall times can be used to optimize response synchrony, while still maintaining place specificity" (p. 365). Thus, Blackman tone-burst ramping remains an excellent option for estimation with ABR of frequency-specific auditory thresholds.

Stimulus Intensity. Current approaches for verifying the intensity level of click and tone-burst stimuli are certainly less than optimal, particularly for pediatric applications of the ABR. Verification and calibration of stimulus intensity in dB SPL and within the ear canal of a child prior to ABR measurement would be ideal. Designation of click and tone-burst stimulus intensity level in dB SPL, following real ear verification, would contribute to accurate estimation of auditory thresholds in children and would facilitate the inclusion of threshold estimations in prescriptive hearing aid fitting algorithms and programs (e.g., Desired Sensation Level [DSL]) that require data reported in SPL. Of course, technology exists for documentation of stimulus intensity level in the ear canal of patients prior to auditory measurements. Instrumentation for clinical OAE measurement is a good example. Stimulus intensity level is measured with a small microphone located within the probe assembly and then adjusted, taking into account acoustic characteristics of the patient's ear canal in order to match actual stimulus intensity with target intensity level. It is likely that manufacturers of evoked response instrumentation will, before long, design and market devices for clinical documentation in the ear canal of click and tone-burst stimulus intensity. However, lacking this technologic feature with ABR instrumentation currently used in electrophysiologic estimation of auditory thresholds, the clinician is required to rely on biologic calibration of stimulus intensity. Important steps in the process of designating intensity level for click and tone-burst stimuli prior to clinical measurement of ABR in children is summarized in Table 8.4. Although beyond the routine policy of most clinics, it is of course possible with a high-quality sound level meter to verify and calibrate tone-burst stimuli. As with other transient stimuli used to elicit the ABR, intensity is typically designated in dB peak equivalent sound pressure level (peSPL) or peak-to-peak equivalent SPL (ppeSPL). The concept of transient acoustic stimulus calibration in peak equivalent SPL was reviewed in Chapter 6. A selection of data on tone-burst stimulus intensity in ppeSPL corresponding to 0 dB nHL as measured in appropriate couplers at different audiology centers is shown in Table 8.5. Intensity level is defined as the reference equivalent threshold in sound pressure level (RET-SPL), that is, "the difference in decibels, as a function of frequency, between the output from an earphone in a coupler and the audiometer [or evoked response system] dial setting" (Mueller & Hall, 1998, p. 289). Factors that can potentially influence the actual intensity level of tone-burst stimuli in ABR measurement include the rate of stimulus presentation, the type of earphone, and the patient's ear canal acoustics.

Analysis Time. There is consensus in the literature that longer recording epochs or analysis times are required for frequency-specific measurement of the ABR. An analysis time used for recording ABRs evoked by tone bursts in children must be long enough to include the entire wave V component, including the subsequent trough or negative wave,

TABLE 8.4. Steps in the Clinical Implementation of Tone-Burst ABR Measurement for Electrophysiologic Estimation of Frequency-Specific Auditory Thresholds

- Construct tone-burst protocol(s) and save on the evoked response system with clear file names (e.g., 500 Hz TB ABR). See **Table 8.2** for recommended stimulus and acquisition parameters.
- Assemble a small group (N = 5) of normal-hearing young (under 30 years) adult subjects (males and females). Verify normal-hearing status by tympanometry (type A), pure-tone thresholds of 10 dB or better at all audiometric frequencies from 250 Hz through 8000 Hz (including 3000 and 6000 Hz), and amplitudes for otoacoustic emissions within an appropriate normal region.
- Obtain average behavioral thresholds from the group of normal-hearing adults for each tone-burst signal using the evoked response system in the test room(s) to be used for ABR measurement. Simply present tone-burst stimuli one frequency at a time at progressively lower stimulus–intensity levels and request a behavioral response (e.g., hand raising) from each normal-hearing subject to find threshold as done with pure-tone audiometry. Keep the evoked response system as far away as possible from the subject, close the door to the room, and maintain a quiet test setting as done during clinical ABR measurement.
- For each tone-burst stimulus frequency and each set of earphones used with the evoked response system (e.g., insert earphones, TDH earphones, bone-conduction oscillator), calculate the average intensity level on the computer screen (the "dial setting") corresponding to behavioral threshold (e.g., 35 dB for 500 Hz, 20 dB for 1000 Hz, etc). These values are equivalent to 0 dB nHL (normal hearing level).
- Some evoked response systems may indicate intensity for all stimuli (e.g., air-conduction click and tone-burst stimuli, and bone-conduction stimuli) as dB nHL. Verify with several normal-hearing subjects in the clinic test room to be used for ABR measurements that behavioral thresholds are in fact 0 dB nHL for the evoked response system. Make adjustments as needed for stimulus intensity levels, according to the process described above.
- If the evoked response system permits adjustment of stimulus intensity level into dB nHL, enter the "correction factors" obtained from the normative values for 0 dB nHL. For example, for a tone-burst frequency of 500 Hz, the "dial setting" of 35 dB becomes 0 dB HL. See the equipment manual for details on the "clinical biologic calibration" of tone-burst (and bone-conduction) stimuli in dB nHL.
- In the clinic test room, record in practice sessions ABRs for tone-burst signals from several normal-hearing adults and cooperative children (aged 6 to 10 years old). A clear and reliable ABR should be detected for tone-burst

stimulus frequencies of 4000, 2000, and 1000 Hz, and for click stimuli, down to intensity levels of at least 20 dB nHL. An ABR for the 500 Hz tone-burst stimulus should be detected down to at least 30 dB nHL.
- Calculate for the normal ABRs wave V latency values for each stimulus frequency at each intensity level. These values will provide a guideline for expected latencies for patients. For each stimulus frequency, plot an example of ABR waveforms at various intensity levels and keep handy with the evoked response system for reference during clinical tone-burst ABR assessments.
- Prepare and make copies of a data record sheet for tone-burst ABR measurements.
- If possible, perform a tone-burst ABR assessment with a normal-hearing infant no older than 2 months after birth. The "subject" might be the child of a friend or colleague. Obviously, sedation is not required. Modest sleep deprivation (no nap before the ABR session) will increase the likelihood of quiet sleeping during the ABR session. This "dry run" by a clinician under realistic but relaxed clinical conditions will enhance confidence in the test protocol and technique prior to ABR recording from children with unknown auditory status.
- Remember, in performing electrophysiologic estimations of auditory thresholds, that minimal ABR levels, i.e., the lowest intensity level at which a reliable ABR wave V is detected, are not equivalent to pure-tone hearing thresholds. Under adequate clinical conditions (quiet patient and quiet test setting), minimal ABR levels are about 10 dB above (worse than) actual pure-tone thresholds. Therefore, 10 dB should be subtracted from the minimum intensity level producing an ABR to estimate pure-tone hearing threshold.
- During tone-burst ABR measurement, plot estimated auditory thresholds for the click stimulus and for each tone-burst stimulus frequency on "tone burst ABR audiogram" as it is obtained.
- Also during tone-burst ABR measurement, save to computer disk or hard drive and then print out ABR waveforms for all stimulus conditions (click stimulus and tone-burst frequencies at all intensity levels). Typically, replications of ABR waveforms at each intensity level and for each stimulus are superimposed, and waveforms for descending intensity levels are arranged in sequence.
- The "split screen" option can be used to simultaneously plot and print ABRs for two different stimulus conditions, e.g., click ABRs for the left and right ears, or two different stimuli for one ear. Examples of different arrangements for the display of waveforms are shown in figures in this chapter.

---

under conditions that are likely to prolong absolute latency. At least four factors contribute, in combination, to prolongation of latency values for the wave V component of the ABR.

First, latency values increase as stimulus intensity level is decreased toward auditory threshold. Second, latency values are increased by hearing loss and, in particular, conductive or

TABLE 8.5. Tone-Burst Intensity Data in dB Peak-to-Peak Sound Pressure Level (ppeSPL), i.e., Reference Equivalent Threshold in SPL (RETSPL) for Four Different Audiology Centers
Reprinted courtesy of Dr. Steve Mason. The intensity level of a click stimulus delivered with a supra-aural (TDH39) earphone is 33 dB ppeSPL.

CLINIC	REFERENCE	EARPHONE	FREQUENCY IN HZ			
			500	1000	2000	4000
Vancouver	1	TDH39	24.6	23.2	26.1	29.0 dB ppeSPL
Nottingham	2	TDH39	26.5	22.0	29.0	29.5 dB ppeSPL
Los Angeles	3	ER-2 insert	23.2	21.8*	NA**	17.8 dB ppeSPL
Sheffield	4	TDH39	24.1	21.3	24.9	29.0 dB ppeSPL

* data for 1500 Hz

** data not available

1 Stapells, D.R., & Oates, P. (1997). Estimation of the pure-tone audiogram by the auditory brainstem response. *Audiology and Neurotology 2*, 257–280.

2 Mason, S.M. (1999). Calibration of tone pip stimuli. (personal communication)

3 Sininger, Y.S., Abdala, C., & Cone-Wesson, B. (1997). Auditory threshold sensitivity of the human neonate as measured by the auditory brainstem response. *Hearing Research 104*, 27–38.

4 Stevens, J.C. (2001). Calibration of tone pip stimuli. (personal communication)

neural auditory dysfunction. Third, the ABR is immature and latencies longer for children who are less than 18 months old than for older children. Fourth, latency of the ABR wave V component increases progressively as the frequency of tone bursts decreases. Therefore, one can easily develop a worst-case scenario for prolongation of wave V latency for the ABR, i.e., recording an ABR evoked by a 500 Hz tone burst near threshold for a newborn infant with a hearing loss. A 20 ms analysis time will be adequate to encompass the wave V and the following negative trough under such conditions. The British/Canadian ABR protocol includes a recommended "window length" of 20 to 25 ms.

Electrode Array. High-quality ABRs are typically recorded in children with an ipsilateral single channel electrode array, i.e., a noninverting electrode at the Fz location and an inverting electrode on the earlobe ipsilateral to the stimulus (e.g., Ai). The rationale for routine use of these two electrode locations when recording ABRs from children was explained in Chapter 6. Briefly, there are really two options for the noninverting electrode site—Cz and Fz. Although either site is appropriate, the Fz site offers several advantages. With a normal pediatric subject, a well-formed ABR waveform is typically recorded with the Fz site. Also, with the high forehead location, the clinician avoids skin preparation at the child's fontanelle and electrode placement is not complicated by hair. Two options for the inverting electrode site are the earlobe on the side ipsilateral to stimulation (Ai) and the mastoid on the ipsilateral side (Mi). There are three clinical advantages to placement of an inverting electrode on the earlobe, rather than the mastoid: (1) There is less chance of hair sticking to the electrode or the tape used to secure the electrode, (2) the ABR wave I is larger for the earlobe

site, and (3) with bone-conduction stimulation of the ABR at the mastoid, there is greater separation between the electrical energy produced by the oscillator and the recording electrode, i.e., less stimulus artifact. The British/Canadian group ABR test protocol recommends placement for infants of the noninverting electrode high on the forehead as near to Cz as possible, avoiding the fontanelle, and the Cz site for older children, with the inverting electrode on the ipsilateral mastoid or nape.

There are at least three exceptions to this clinical convention of an Fz-Ai electrode array in pediatric ABR measurement. One exception involves the site of the inverting electrode. When the goal of ABR measurement is estimation of auditory threshold rather than a neurodiagnostic application and, specifically, the detection of an ABR wave V at the lowest possible intensity level, a noncephalic (e.g., nape) location is appropriate for the inverting electrode. The nape identified as the bony bump at the base of the neck (see Figure 6.8). The ABR waveform recorded with a noncephalic inverting electrode (a true reference electrode) has greater wave V amplitude than one recorded with an inverting electrode near the ear. This principle of ABR measurement was discussed in Chapter 6. Detection of the presence of a wave V component in the ABR waveform is, of course, enhanced when amplitude is larger, because the result is a high signal-to-noise ratio. The application of a two-channel ABR protocol is the second exception. ABRs can always be recorded simultaneously with both an ipsilateral and contralateral electrode array, although there are no clear benefits in most cases. If a clinician inadvertently selects the wrong inverting electrode—for example, the left earlobe (Ai) site when stimulating the right ear—ABR analysis is not seriously affected, as the correct (ipsilateral) inverting electrode arrangement is available in the opposite channel. With bone conduction ABR measurement, however, a two-channel (ipsilateral and contralateral electrode array) protocol offers a distinct advantage over conventional signal channel (ipsilateral electrode array) measurement. As noted in Chapter 6, the wave I component should be clearly visible in the ipsilateral electrode array, but not in the contralateral electrode array. Comparison of the ABR waveform in the latency region of the wave I component helps to confirm the presence of wave I with bone conduction stimulation, even if amplitude is small. The third exception to the convention of recording an ABR from children with an ipsilateral electrode array (i.e., Fz–Ai) arises in test settings characterized occasionally by excessive electrical interference, such as the neonatal intensive care unit, a CT or MRI suite, or the operating room. When excessive electrical interference precludes the recording of a quality ABR with the ipsilateral electrode array, the solution is often ABR measurement with a horizontal (Ac to Ai) electrode array. That is, the inverting electrode remains on the earlobe ipsilateral to the side of stimulation, and the noninverting electrode is located on the contralateral earlobe. For infants and young children, the normal ABR recorded with a horizontal electrode array consists of wave I, wave III, and wave V. Attempts to record an ABR from infants with a conventional ipsilateral electrode array (Fz–Ai) may be unsuccessful due to excessive artifact related to electrical interference. In contrast to the findings for a horizontal electrode array in infants, when an ABR is recorded with a horizontal electrode array from a normal adult patient, wave IV is present but there is no detectable wave V (see Chapter 6).

Filter Settings. A crucial acquisition parameter to consider in recording frequency-specific ABRs is filter setting. A high-pass (low-frequency cutoff) setting as low as 30 Hz is essential in order to encompass most of the low-frequency portion of the ABR spectrum. Low-frequency energy in the ABR is prominent for infants and, in addition, for low-frequency acoustic stimuli (Hyde, 1985; Picton, Stapells, & Campbell, 1981; Stapells & Picton, 1981; Suzuki, Hirai, & Horiuchi, 1977; Suzuki & Horiuchi, 1977). Raising the cutoff frequency (e.g., to 100 or 150 Hz) results in decreased wave V amplitude, response distortion, elevated response threshold, and a less detectable response. Early negative experiences in recording reliable ABRs with low-frequency stimuli (Davis, 1976a; Davis & Hirsh, 1976; Klein & Teas, 1978) were probably due, in part, to filter settings that, in retrospect, were inappropriately restricted. It is certainly possible to record an ABR from infants with high-pass filter settings higher than 30 Hz (e.g., 150 Hz). Amplitude of wave V will be diminished and, usually, detection of the ABR at stimulus intensity levels near auditory threshold will be affected. The 60 Hz notch filter, available with most evoked response systems, should not be used for infant ABR assessments, as it will remove important energy from the response. For ABR measurement in children, therefore, filter settings of 30 to

either 1500 or 3000 Hz are strongly recommended. This is consistent with the filter parameter recommended in the British/Canadian guidelines, namely, a high-pass filter setting of 20 or 30 Hz, a low-pass filter setting of 1500 or 3000 Hz, and no notch filter.

Number of Stimulus Repetitions. Stimulus repetitions are also described as the number of trials or averages. The number of stimuli that should be presented during the recording of a single ABR waveform is entirely dependent on the signal-to-noise ratio (SNR); that is, the size of the signal (the ABR) and the amount of measurement noise (electrical or myogenic activity) present during the recording. Under some combinations of measurement conditions, such presentation of tone bursts at a high stimulus-intensity level to a sleeping or sedated patient with normal hearing sensitivity in an electrically quiet test setting, a clear ABR can be detected following the presentation of very few stimuli, e.g., less than 200. With a stimulus rate over 20/sec, an ABR waveform can easily be recorded in less than 10 seconds. On the other hand, with another combination of measurement conditions, such as the presentation of tone bursts at a low stimulus-intensity level to a restless patient with a hearing impairment in an electrically noisy setting, multiple thousands of stimulus representations may be needed to achieve an adequate SNR and to confidently identify an ABR wave V. The above suggestions are not entirely consistent with recommendations made in the British/Canadian ABR protocol (i.e., a minimum of 2,000 sweeps), but the protocol does suggest that the number of stimulus presentations be increased to 3,000 or 4,000 "for identification of small responses close to threshold or if the signal baseline is noisy."

ABR Test Protocol: Saving Test Time without Sacrificing Test Quality. With experience, most audiologists develop strategies for cutting corners and saving time when performing clinical procedures. The goal in diagnostic procedures is to obtain all the information needed to completely describe auditory function, without wasting time with the collection of irrelevant or unnecessary information. The following steps are useful for accomplishing this objective with frequency-specific ABR measurement.

- Always continuously monitor ABR activity during recording, performing visual analysis of ABR presence and reliability. Once a recording is complete, e.g., during the replication recording, begin analyzing latency values for wave I (at a high intensity level) and wave V (at all intensity levels) relative to normal expectations. Remember to take into account in ABR latency analysis patient age for children under 18 months.
- Begin with a click-evoked ABR at a high intensity level (80 dB nHL or higher) that is likely to produce a clear and reliable response. If no clear ABR is readily apparent, then immediately move up to the maximum intensity level. There are at least three practical reasons for

beginning the ABR assessment with a click signal: (1) A click signal is most likely to produce a clear and reliable ABR. A click-elicited ABR can serve as a guide in developing a strategy for recording a tone-burst ABR. That is, analysis of the ABR evoked by the click stimulus will facilitate decisions regarding the most appropriate initial tone-burst frequency and the starting intensity level. (2) Latency values are well-defined for click-elicited ABRs, and age-corrected normative data are available. (3) Analysis of click ABR latency values permits within a few minutes of ABR measurement the differentiation between reasonably normal auditory function (latencies for all components and interwave latency values well-within normal limits), a conductive hearing loss (clear wave I but a delay in wave I latency, and subsequent absolute latencies), a sensory hearing loss (little or no wave I and often poorly formed waveform), and neural dysfunction (delayed wave interwave latency values, e.g., wave I–III, wave III–V, wave I–V, or the absence of a detectable wave V). If there is no click ABR at maximum signal intensity levels (usually 95 to 100 dB nHL), then ASSR measurement is indicated. The specific role of ASSR in pediatric auditory assessment is discussed toward the end of this article.

- Discontinue signal averaging (stimulus presentation) as soon as a clear response is detected. Immediately attempt to replicate the response to verify its presence, and stop the averaging as soon as it is clearly repeatable. It is a waste of valuable test time to stubbornly present the preset number of stimulus presentations (e.g., 2000) with no regard to the presence or absence of an ABR, i.e., without considering the signal-to-noise ratio.

- If at a high stimulus intensity level there is a clear ABR with all major components (waves I, III, and V) present at relatively normal latency values, it is reasonable to decrease intensity level by 40 dB or more before recording the next ABR waveform. I often drop stimulus intensity level immediately from 80 dB nHL to 20 or 25 dB nHL under these conditions (see case report below).

- As signal averaging is ongoing, always think ahead to the next step in the ABR measurement process, e.g., your choice for the next stimulus intensity level, stimulus frequency, stimulus mode of presentation (air- versus bone-conduction), and/or test ear. If signal averaging (stimulus presentation) stops and you're still thinking about what step to take next, then precious test time is slipping away.

SUMMARY. | The two major problems inherent in tonal stimulation, without masking, already have been discussed in relation to the masking paradigms. That is, with linear tone-burst gating or windowing approaches, the abrupt onset tone bursts that must be used to produce a reasonably clear and well-formed ABR (at least in the normal ear) are char-

acterized by (1) side lobes (spectral splatter) that limit frequency specificity, and (2) low-frequency stimuli presented at moderate to high intensity levels that can be expected to activate basal, as well as apical, regions. In considering the clinical usefulness of these stimuli for ECochG or ABR measurement, one must bear in mind that the actual frequency specificity of the stimulus, as evaluated by the precision with which it activates a discrete place on the cochlear partition, is influenced by various factors, in addition to the acoustic spectrum of the stimulus at the diaphragm of the transducer. These factors include cochlear status.

ILLUSTRATIVE CASE REPORT

Background. The following case illustrates a typical sequence of steps in the rapid estimation of frequency specific auditory thresholds with ABR. A few minutes is initially devoted to measurement of a click-evoked ABR to immediately differentiate between normal hearing and 3 types of auditory impairment—conductive, sensory, or neural auditory dysfunction. ABR patterns associated with different types of auditory dysfunction were discussed in Chapter 8. The patient presented herein was a 3-year-old boy who was severely delayed in language development. When behavioral audiometry was attempted, the child was very difficult to test (described as non-compliant in the report). He would not accept earphones (supra-aural or insert) for pure-tone or speech audiometry. Behavioral responses were observed to sound-field warble tone signals as follows: 30 dB HL at 1000 Hz, 50 dB HL at 2000 Hz and 4000 Hz. A speech awareness threshold (SAT) was obtained at 40 dB HL in the sound-field condition. Response reliability was judged good.

The author's ABR experience with this child was typical. Both of the children the author assessed with ABR on this test date were at risk for hearing impairment due to severe language delay, yet the ABR findings for both were consistent with normal hearing sensitivity. A review of all ABR assessments conducted for definition of hearing status in infants and young children indicated that the majority (55%) yielded findings consistent with normal hearing. The tone-burst ABR for each child assessed on the test day required less than 20 minutes, including application of electrodes, earphone placement, and impedance verification. Children who require sedation for ABR are most often between the ages of 4 months and 4 years. Administration of sedation is optimally carried out in a medical clinic setting in accordance with institutional guidelines for administration of conscious sedation (e.g., chloral hydrate), or in an operating room with the patient lightly anesthetized with drugs, such as nitrous oxide in combination with propofol or sevoflurane. A review of over 100 sedated ABRs performed by the author under these conditions in the operating room showed that average test time per child was less than 30 minutes. Age is not a factor in ABR test time with sedated children. The ABR protocol used by the author includes threshold estimations for click signals and two or three tone-burst signals (e.g., 500 Hz, 1000 Hz, 4000 Hz) for each ear. More test time (up to but never exceeding one hour) is required when hearing loss is identified and, particularly, with the measurement of bone-conduction and air-conduction ABRs to define the degree of conductive or mixed hearing loss, whereas less time is needed for children with normal ABR findings. This case report is an example of the brief test time characteristic of normal ABRs recorded from an adequately sedated child.

ABR Measurement, Analysis, and Interpretation. Previous behavioral audiologic assessment of this child suggested the possibility of a bilateral hearing loss. This suspicion was confirmed by the documentation of severe speech and language impairment. There is no single correct strategy or step-by-step process for conducting a pediatric ABR assessment. That is, a clinician is not bound by any specific guidelines or convention in deciding how the ABR recording begins (e.g., which ear is stimulated first and at what intensity level) and what steps will be taken next in the ABR assessment of auditory function.

The initial ABR waveforms recorded for the child are shown in Figure 8.7. Test parameters for these recordings were reviewed in Figure 8.2. A well-formed and reliable ABR was recorded for a click signal presented to the left ear at 75 dB nHL. Relatively few signal repetitions were required to obtain these two replicated waves (less than 300 accepted sweeps at 75 dB nHL). Also, test time for recording the two waveforms at 75 dB nHL was less than 1 minute. Inspection of the latency data in Figure 8.7A shows that stimulation with an 75 dB nHL click signal produced an ABR wave I latency of 2.63 ms. This value is outside of normal limits, suggesting a conductive hearing loss. Absolute latencies for later ABR waves, and the interwave latencies (I–III, III–V, I–V), were within normal limits. Age must always be taken into account in interpreting ABR latencies for children less than 18 months old, as the pathways important in generating the ABR are not mature (myelinization is not complete) until that age. Since the patient was 2 years old, we can rule out age as a factor in ABR latencies. However, two other factors must be considered. One is body temperature and the other is the anesthetic agent(s). In this case, body temperature was normal (within ± 1 degree of 37 degrees centigrade) and, therefore, not a factor. Although conscious sedation (e.g., chloral hydrate or Versed) does not affect the ABR, some anesthetic agents may exert an effect (prolongation) on ABR latencies. The anesthetic agents used with this patient, sevoflurane and propofol, fall into this category. For this patient, it is unlikely that the effect of anesthesia increased the interwave latencies. We would expect, for example, a wave I to wave V latency interval of about 4.0 ms versus the 3.82 ms that was recorded. However, any possible effect of anesthetic

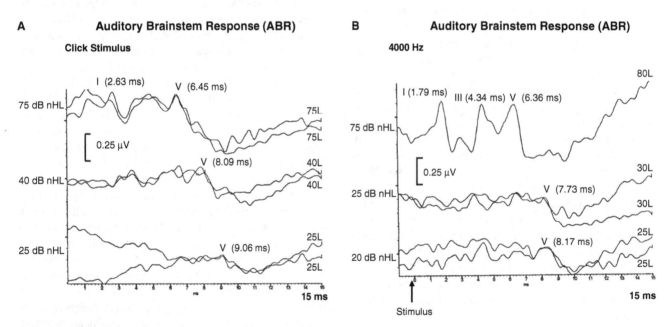

FIGURE 8.7. Auditory brainstem response (ABR) recorded with left ear air-conduction signals from 2-year-old boy under light anesthesia in the operating room, immediately following insertion of ventilation tube. The child had a history of chronic otitis media and conductive hearing loss. Waveforms for a click signal are shown in the left panel (A), and waveforms for a 4000 Hz tone burst are shown in the right panel (B). Measurement parameters were defined in Figure 8.2. The analysis time (x-axis) is 15 ms, including a prestimulus analysis time of –1 ms. Amplitude (y-axis) is displayed with 0.25 µV per division (between sets of short horizontal lines).

agents in this patient was modest and did not alter the ABR interpretation.

Given the normal ABR at 75 dB nHL, the author elected to decrease signal intensity immediately to 40 dB nHL. A reliable ABR wave V was again detected, albeit with a relatively lower amplitude. If the ABR at 75 dB nHL were not normal (e.g., delayed latencies or some waves missing), then the signal intensity level would have been decreased by only 20 to 40 dB initially, to a level of 60 or 40 dB nHL. On the other hand, if at 75 or 80 dB nHL the ABR were absent or only wave V were recorded at a delayed latency, the signal intensity would have been immediately increased to maximum equipment limits (95 or 100 dB nHL). In this case, my decision to decrease the click signal intensity level from 75 dB nHL down to 20 dB nHL paid off by yielding a normal threshold estimation in minimal test time. The cautious reader without clinical ABR experience might, after inspecting the waveforms in Figure 8.7, question the presence of the ABR wave V for both the click and 4000 Hz tone-burst signals at the intensity level of 20 and 25 dB nHL. At least four steps could be taken to confirm the presence of the wave V. First, the display gain could be increased after ABR recording was completed, making the waveform appear larger on the screen. Second, a third replication could be obtained to verify that the deviation in the 8 to 9 ms portion of the waveform was really evoked by the stimulus and was not simply a random variation in voltage. Third, the two

(or three) waveforms could be digitally added to highlight any replicable response (and to cancel out random activity). And, fourth, signal intensity level could be increased to 25 or 30 dB nHL to verify the presence of wave V. With a 5 to 10 dB increase in signal intensity, one would expect the wave V to be slightly shorter in latency and larger in amplitude. Keep in mind that the presence of a reliable ABR wave V at 25 dB nHL for the 4000 Hz tone-burst signal estimates an audiometric threshold (hearing sensitivity) at 4000 Hz no worse than approximately 15 dB HL.

The presence of an ABR wave V down to an intensity level of 20 to 25 dB nHL (displayed in Figure 8.8) confirms that auditory sensitivity in the left ear was within normal limits also for 1000 Hz and 500 Hz. Tone bursts at each frequency produced a repeatable response at a high intensity level (70 and 75 dB nHL), and at 20 dB nHL. Note that the response for the 500 Hz tone burst at 25 dB nHL was repeatable. As expected, the latency for these two lower signal intensity levels was slightly greater than the latency at the higher (70 dB nHL) intensity level. Only 5 minutes of test time were required to confirm by the ABR auditory sensitivity within normal limits in the left ear for the speech frequency region (500 to 4000 Hz). Less than 10 minutes of total test time were needed for ABR assessment of the right ear, including analysis of wave 1 to rule out a conductive component (a wave I latency of 1.70 ms was within normal limits), confirmation that auditory neural function was normal (the wave I to V latency interval of 4.04 ms was within normal

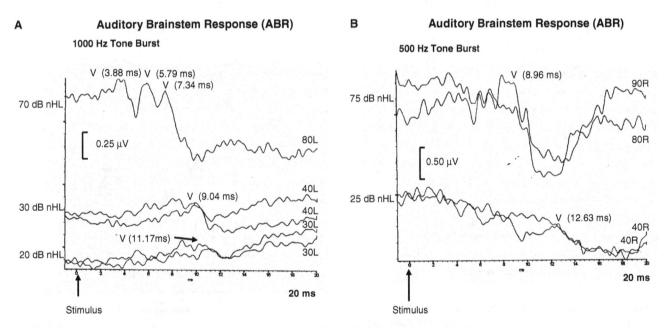

FIGURE 8.8. Auditory brainstem response (ABR) recorded with left ear air-conduction tone-burst stimuli at 1000 Hz (A) and 500 Hz (B) from 2-year-old boy under light anesthesia in the operating room. Not the longer latency for the wave V in comparison to the ABR elicited by click and 4000 Hz tone burst stimuli (see Figure 8.7 A,B). Measurement parameters were defined in Figure 8.2. The analysis time (X-axis) is 20 ms, including a prestimulus analysis time of −1 ms. Amplitude (Y-axis) is displayed with 0.25 µV per division (between sets of short horizontal lines).

limits), and for verification that auditory sensitivity was within normal limits. Also for the right ear (not shown), an apparently replicable wave V at the lowest intensity level (20 dB nHL for the 1000 Hz tone burst and 30 dB nHL for the 500 Hz signal) was confirmed by replicating waveforms at a signal level 5 dB higher. In summary, this typical case illustrates the usefulness of a tone-burst ABR technique for the electrophysiological estimation with reasonable test time of auditory thresholds in infants and young children.

For confident application of tone-burst ABRs in threshold estimation, the clinician must develop the ability to recognize waveform patterns that differ from those evoked by click stimuli. ABR waveforms generated by high-frequency tone bursts often closely resemble click ABRs. For lower frequency tone-burst stimuli, however, the waves have less distinct peaks and appear at longer latencies. Samples of tone-burst ABR waveforms for a child with hearing loss are displayed in Figure 8.9. With sufficient averaging and care

to replicate the waveform, it is possible to consistently identify ABR wave V even at calibrated stimulus intensity levels within 10 to 15 dB of behavioral threshold for tone-burst signals. Once the ABR wave V is detected at minimum stimulus intensity levels (usually in 5 or 10 dB increments), threshold estimations can be plotted on a form resembling an audiogram (Figure 8.10). The author uses a circle to denote ABR threshold for air-conduction stimuli, and a triangle for bone-conduction ABR thresholds. Estimated behavioral thresholds are presumed to be 10 dB better than the lowest tone-burst stimulus intensity level (in dB nHL) generating a repeatable ABR wave V. The estimated behavioral threshold is depicted with a vertical line extending 10 dB on the form and ending in a diagonal mark. The audiogram-like display of frequency-specific behavioral auditory thresholds estimated from ABRs evoked by tone bursts provides a convenient and easy-to-understand summary of the numerous data collected during the assessment and facilitates the inclusion of ABR data into prescriptive hearing aid fitting algorithms, such as the Desired Sensation Level (DSL) or the NAL methods. The pictorial display also permits rapid comparison of ABR findings for different test dates.

A general approach for neurodiagnostic pediatric ABR, and frequency-specific estimation of behavioral thresholds, is illustrated in Figure 8.11. A rather rigid sequence of steps in the ABR assessment can be followed for children with normal auditory function. Myriad permutations of the test

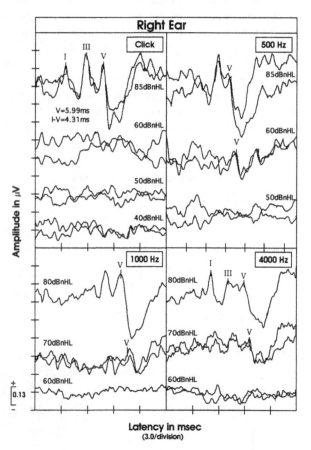

FIGURE 8.9. Auditory brainstem response (ABR) recorded with right ear air-conduction click and with tone-burst stimuli from a 3-year-old boy while he was sedated with chloral hydrate. Speech and language was markedly delayed, and hearing loss was suspected. Measurement parameters were defined in Figure 8.2. The analysis time (x-axis) is 15 ms for all signals except the 500 Hz tone burst (20 ms). Amplitude (y-axis) is displayed with 0.31 μV per division (between sets of short horizontal lines).

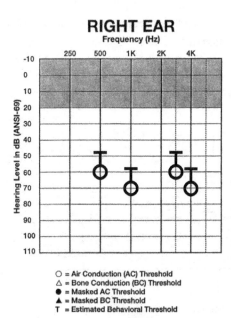

FIGURE 8.10. Auditory thresholds estimated from auditory brainstem responses (ABRs) evoked by air-conduction tone-burst stimuli. Waveforms were shown in Figure 8.9. Minimal ABR levels are depicted by a circle, whereas estimations of behavioral thresholds are depicted by short horizontal lines estimating hearing levels that are 10 dB.

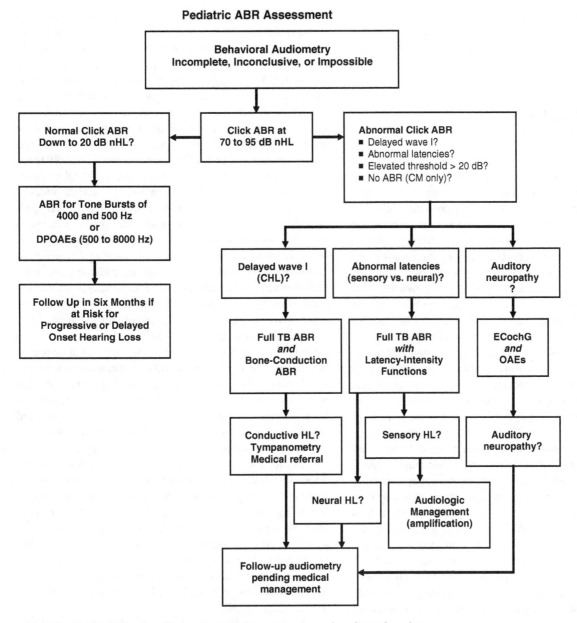

FIGURE 8.11. Flowchart for pediatric ABR assessment of auditory function.

approach arise as evidence of hearing loss emerges. Decisions regarding stimulus-intensity level and frequency, test ear, and mode of stimulus delivery (air versus bone conduction) are made as ABR data are collected and immediately analyzed. When available, background information about the patient, e.g., previous audiologic test results, otologic findings, the diagnosis of a specific syndrome or malformation, will offer the clinician some guidance. The experienced clinician will efficiently proceed from one step to the next, acquiring information on auditory status required for rational and effective management of the patient. The author offers the general guidelines outlined in this section, and summarized in Figure 8.11, based on clinical experience acquired

over the past thirty years. Mistakes will be minimized by adherence to a consistent test protocol and sequence. However, it is certainly appropriate and often necessary to vary from this sequence to obtain as quickly as possible the information on auditory function that is most important for audiologic management of a child. If a child is well sedated and sleeping for an adequate amount of time (i.e., for at least 45 minutes), and if both ears for the child are always accessible (i.e., the child is supine), then the exact sequence of data collection for each ear and each signal condition (click versus tone burst, air conduction versus bone conduction) is not critical. Frequency-specific ABR measurement with tone-burst stimuli is a valuable tool for early identification and confirmation of hearing loss in infants and young children. However, the ASSR also plays a critical role in this communicatively important and clinically challenging diagnostic process.

AUDITORY STEADY-STATE RESPONSE (ASSR)

With the availability of clinical instrumentation (FDA-approved in the United States), the ASSR is quickly assuming a valuable, and unique, position in the current audiologic armamentarium employed by clinicians around the world. The ASSR has a number of clinical advantages, as summarized in Table 8.6. One clinical advantage alone—the capability of estimating electrophysiologically auditory thresholds of up to 120 dB HL in infants and young children—has guaranteed the ASSR a secure place in the pediatric test battery. With the advent of universal newborn hearing screening and the requirement for hearing aid fitting of infants within months after birth, there is a clear clinical demand for objective, e.g., electrophysiologic, estimation of hearing sensitivity as a critical step in prescriptive hearing aid fitting. Recent research on early intervention for childhood hearing impairment has demonstrated the dramatic benefits of providing adequate auditory stimulation within the first six months after birth (Yoshinago-Itano et al., 1998). Traditional behavioral audiologic techniques are insufficient for this purpose. As reviewed in this chapter, it is certainly possible to estimate auditory thresholds for audiometric frequencies with frequency-specific ABR. The threshold estimation information can then be incorporated into prescriptive fitting algorithms, such as desired sensation level (DSL), permitting a reasonably accurate initial hearing aid fitting for hearing-impaired infants. The ABR is evoked most effectively by transient (very brief) acoustic signals, with onset times on the order of a few milliseconds. The ABR consists of bioelectric activity that reflects synchronous firing of thousands of neurons in the auditory (eighth cranial) nerve and auditory system pathways within the brainstem (pons and midbrain). Abrupt, transient signals must be utilized to produce this synchronous firing. The maximum effective intensity level of these signals is limited by their very brief duration. That is, because of their short duration, less energy is delivered to the auditory system. The use of sophisticated equations (e.g., Blackman) for ramping or shaping of the signal onset solves, for the most part, another potential practical problem associated with the very brief duration of the signal, that is, reduction in the frequency-specificity of ABR measurement. As its name implies, the ASSR is generated with steady-state (ongoing sinusoidal rather than transient) acoustic signals. The inherent limitation of maximum intensity associated with the transient signals does not, therefore, apply to ASSR signals.

When a new technique is introduced clinically, audiologists have a tendency to ask whether the technique is better or worse than existing techniques. When, for example, clinical instrumentation for measurement of otoacoustic emissions (OAEs) became commonplace, there was almost immediately ongoing comparison among some audiologists of the merits of OAEs with pure-tone audiometry. I distinctly recall listening at professional meetings to conversations among concerned audiologists who wondered whether OAEs as a technique for hearing assessment would replace pure-tone audiometry and, taking this concern one (illogical) step further—whether automated OAE devices would minimize the need for audiologists! There is now ample clinical evidence that OAEs provide more information on cochlear auditory function, in comparison to pure-tone audiometry. And, although OAEs are a very sensitive and site-specific measure of auditory function at the cochlear (outer hair cell) level, they are most certainly not a measure of "hearing." Hearing, of course, involves a vast array of anatomic pathways and structures throughout the auditory system, especially at the cortical level. Hearing also involves complex auditory functions and processes. Although the cochlea (and of course the outer hair cells), contribute importantly to auditory function, in essence we hear with our brain. During the late 1990s, as audiologists began to use OAEs in their clinical practice, audiometers were not discarded. In fact, before long audiologists realized that pure-tone audiometry would not be supplanted by automated OAE devices. On the contrary, audiologists have discovered that their clinical assessment and management of hearing loss is enhanced by the application of OAE techniques.

Among the criteria that are desirable for auditory evoked responses used in the clinical estimation of auditory thresholds are accuracy, feasibility of measurement from patients in varying states of arousal, the possibility of detection of the response across the age range, recording of the response with stimuli at audiometric frequencies, and frequency-specificity. Reasonable test time is another important criterion for any auditory evoked response to be effective in pediatric threshold estimation (e.g., Hall, 1992; Swanepoel, Schmulian, & Hugo, 2004).

We are now discovering the clinical strengths of ASSRs and, inevitably, some weaknesses of this technique (refer again to Table 8.6). One common misconception is that tone-burst ABR assessment is excessively time-consuming and, also, that the ASSR requires relatively little test time. Fortunately, tone-burst ABR assessments typically require less than one hour. Indeed, with an effective tone-burst protocol, a clear plan of action, an efficient use of test time (as reviewed above), and a quiet child, total test time for a frequency-specific ABR assessment is often less than 30 minutes.

Historical Perspective

As a technique for clinical assessment of auditory function, particularly in the United States, the ASSR is a relative newcomer. Occasional reports of scalp-recorded steady-state responses to auditory stimuli appeared in the 1960s (Geisler,

TABLE 8.6. Clinical Advantages and Disadvantages of Auditory Steady-State Response (ASSR)

Note that brief test time is not listed as a clinical advantage of the ASSR. There is no clear evidence from clinical investigations that ASSR measurement is faster than threshold estimation with tone-burst ABR techniques.

Advantages

- Frequency-specific signals are employed for estimation of auditory sensitivity at audiometric frequencies.
- Frequency-specific auditory information can be obtained with air- or bone-conduction signals.
- Signal intensity levels can be as high as 120 dB HL. The ASSR is, therefore, useful for electrophysiologic assessment of severe-to-profound degree of hearing loss in infants and young children.
- Automated response detection and analysis (i.e., experience in waveform analysis is not necessary).
- Clinical devices are available.

Potential Disadvantages

- ASSR recording requires a very quiet state of arousal. Movement artifact (interference) is likely to produce invalid results or overestimation of actual auditory threshold levels. Sedation is required with infants and young children.
- The influence of deep sedation and anesthesia on the ASSR evoked by high modulation frequencies (e.g., > 60 Hz) requires further investigation. Sedation and anesthesia clearly affect the ASSR for slow modulation frequencies (e.g., < 60 Hz).
- Discrepancies between ASSR thresholds and either behavioral and/or ABR thresholds have been reported in the literature.
- Discrepancies between ASSR thresholds and behavioral thresholds have been reported for patients with conductive hearing loss.
- Estimation of ear-specific thresholds with bone-conduction signals requires the use of masking to the nontest ear.
- Measurement artifact with high-intensity bone-conduction stimulation may be confused with an ASSR, i.e., the device may inaccurately identify a response in a patient with no response.
- Measurement artifact with high-intensity air-conduction stimulation may be confused with an ASSR, i.e., the device may inaccurately identify a response in a patient with behavioral evidence of hearing.
- Since the waveform cannot be analyzed, there is little site-specific information for patients with hearing loss, e.g., identification or differentiation of conductive versus sensory versus neural auditory dysfunction.
- The absence of a response may result from either a profound sensory hearing loss or marked neural dysfunction (e.g., auditory neuropathy).

1960) and the 1970s (Campbell, Atkinson, Francis, & Green, 1977). Ongoing investigation of auditory evoked responses evoked by either frequency and/or amplitude modulation of sinusoidal stimuli, however, began in the early 1980s with the well-known paper by Robert Galambos and colleagues on the "40 Hz response" (e.g., Galambos, Makeig, & Talmachoff, 1981) and follow-up studies of auditory responses evoked with stimulus rates of in the region of 40 Hz as a potential clinical tool (e.g., Griffiths & Chambers, 1991; Levi, Folsom, & Dobie, 1993; Stapells et al., 1984). Since then, papers on the 40 Hz response have appeared consistently in the literature, and many comprehensive articles on the ASSR devote considerable attention to the 40 Hz response (e.g., John, Dimitrijevic, & Picton, 2003a,b). The 40 Hz response is poorly suited as a clinical procedure for auditory assessment, particularly in infants and young children. For this reason, the discussion of the ASSRs in this chapter largely avoids mention of the 40 Hz response.

During the period when the 40 Hz response was generating plenty of interest, a group of researchers in Australia (e.g., Rickards & Clark, 1984) and another group of researchers in Canada (e.g., Stapells, Linden, Suffield, Hamel, & Picton, 1984) confirmed that stimuli modulated in amplitude and/or frequency (i.e., "mixed modulation"), and at a variety of modulation rates as high as 100 Hz, were also effective in eliciting auditory responses. Indeed, further study showed that the combination of frequency modulation with amplitude modulation could enhance ASSRs in comparison to AM alone (e.g., Cohen, Rickards, & Clark, 1991).

Over the years, a variety of terms were used in addition to the 40 Hz response to describe auditory steady-state responses, including amplitude modulation following response (AMFR), the envelope following response (EFR), steady-state evoked response (SSER), and steady-state evoked potential (SSEP). Despite its initial appeal as a clinical procedure for hearing assessment of children, the traditional 40 Hz response was not incorporated into the pediatric audiology test battery due to several practical limitations, namely the pronounced and combined effect of age in young children and sleep (see Hall, 1992, for review). Study of steady-state responses evoked by faster rates of amplitude and frequency modulation, however, has continued up to the present time by researchers within or once part of the groups in both Australia (e.g., Cohen, Rickards, & Clark, 1991; Cone-Wesson, Rickards, Swideski, & Parker, 2002; Rance et al., 1995; Rickards & Clark, 1984) and Canada (e.g., Dimitrijevic et al., 2002; John, Dimitrijevic, & Picton, 2003a,b; Linden, Campbell, Hamel, & Picton, 1985; Perez-Abalo et al., 2001; Picton, John, Dimitrijevic, & Purcell, 2003; Stapells et al., 1984; Stapells, Galambos, Costello, & Makeig, 1988; Valdes et al., 1997). Each of these research groups, and later other authors from other countries, confirmed that steady-state responses (the ASSR) evoked with high rates of stimulus modulation can be applied in the electrophysiologic estimation of auditory thresholds in infants and young children, even in sleep and with sedation.

Two developments contributed to markedly increased interest in and clinical application of the ASSR beginning in about the year 2000. With the expansion of programs for universal newborn hearing screening (UNHS) and early intervention for hearing loss in children, there is greater demand for a technique that permits electrophysiologic estimation of auditory thresholds in infants. Information on auditory thresholds is required for appropriate and timely management with hearing aids and cochlear implants of infant hearing loss. Behavioral techniques are not a feasible or reliable option for hearing assessment within months after birth. The ASSR is particularly valuable for estimation of thresholds in children with severe-to-profound hearing loss, as clinical application of the ABR in pediatric audiologic assessment is constrained by limits in the maximum effective intensity level for transient stimulus. Within the same time period, two manufacturers of evoked response equipment in the United States introduced instrumentation for recording and analyzing ASSRs approved for use in clinical settings. One of these devices (the Audera from Grason Stadler/VIASYS) is based on the ASSR system developed by the Australian group, whereas the other device (the MASTER from Bio-Logic Systems, Corp) is based on instrumentation and algorithms developed by the Canadian group.

For over twenty years, clinical investigations by the Australians, Canadians, and a group in Cuba (some of whom acquired ASSR knowledge and adapted ASSR technology while affiliated with the laboratory in Canada) have documented in infants and young children the feasibility of auditory threshold estimation with the ASSR. More recently, with the availability of clinical ASSR instrumentation, practitioners around the world have further confirmed the diagnostic value of the technique in confirming and defining degree of peripheral hearing loss (e.g., Firzt et al., 2004; Han et al., 2005; Jeng, Brown, Johnson, & Vanderwerff, 2004; Luts et al., 2004; Roberson, O'Rourke, & Stidham, 2003; Stueve & O'Rourke, 2003; Swanepoel, Hugo, & Roode, 2004; Vander Werff, Brown, Gienapp, & Schmidt Clay, 2002). Despite the growing application of ASSR in pediatric hearing assessment, the answers to some rather basic questions will contribute to the clinical value of the technique. Some questions are listed in Table 8.7. The years immediately following the introduction of a technique to clinical practice typically yield new and often unexpected applications in different patient populations. For example, within the first decade after publication of the classic paper on the ABR by Jewett and Williston (1971), curious clinical investigators explored the application of the technique in infants with hearing loss and adults with diverse neuropathologies (e.g., acoustic tumors, brain tumors, multiple sclerosis) and in a variety of test settings (audiology clinics, well-baby and intensive-care nurseries, neurointensive care units, and operating rooms). A by-product of the accumulated clinical experience with

ABR was not only an appreciation of its strengths and clinical advantages but, in addition, recognition of its limitations. Limitations of the ABR as a clinical tool are reviewed in Chapters 9 and 10.

Continued clinical experience and experimentation with the ASSR will also probably lead to new and unexpected applications in a variety of patient populations. And, distinct limitations of the ASSR as a clinical tool will be documented and recognized. In short, as its strengths and weaknesses are appreciated, the ASSR will assume a valued and well-defined role in the audiologic test battery, complementing but not supplanting other time-tested procedures, such as the ABR.

The literature on ASSR is rather substantial, even though the technique is just being incorporated into the audiologic test battery. The reader who is interested in supplementing the following review with more information on the ASSR, particularly technical details on stimulus and analysis options, is directed to the 42-page review paper by Picton, John, Dimitrijevic, and Purcell (2003), as well as dozens of other published articles cited herein. Copies of publications on the ASSR can be readily obtained in PDF format from several websites maintained by major research groups, such as the Rotman Research Institute in Toronto directed by Dr. Terence Picton, the Human Auditory Physiology Laboratory at the University of British Columbia directed by Dr. David Stapells, and the School of Audiology affiliated with the Department of Otolaryngology at the University of Melbourne in Australia. Of course, an Internet search will reveal various other sources of information about the ASSR.

Principles of ASSR Measurement

In many respects, the ASSR as evoked with rapidly modulated stimuli is a variation of the ABR. David Stapells and colleagues (2005) have noted, "It is quite likely that the 80 Hz ASSRs are actually ABR waves V to rapidly presented stimuli. Referring to these 80 Hz ASSRs as 'brainstem ASSRs,' then, is both technically correct as well as useful clinically" (p. 2). Indeed, the same general instrumentation is typically used to record both the ABR and ASSR. Although different software for stimulus generation and response analysis is required for the ABR versus ASSR, stimuli are delivered with the same earphones, and the response is detected with the same electrodes. The clinician who understands ABR measurement, analysis, and interpretation is off to a good start in learning how to apply ASSR clinically. There are two major distinctions between the ABR and the ASSR, one involving the stimulus and the other response analysis. The ABR is evoked with transient stimuli separated by periods of silence, whereas the ASSR is evoked with essentially constant sinusoidal (pure-tone) stimuli modulated rapidly in amplitude and/or frequency. The clear advantage of the ongoing steady-state stimulus used to elicit the ASSR—higher effective intensity levels—will be reviewed in more detail

TABLE 8.7. Questions about the ASSR as a Clinical Technique for Auditory Assessment in Children and Adults

Evidenced-based answers to the questions will contribute to the clinical value of the ASSR.

- Where are the anatomic generators of the ASSR recorded with different stimulus characteristics (slow versus fast modulation rate), i.e., the regions of the auditory system and, specifically, types of neurons?
- Can the ASSR be reliably recorded from children during natural sleep, or is sedation is required?
- What effect does auditory nervous system maturation have on the ASSR, and for the ASSR evoked by slow and fast rates of stimulus modulation?
- Does deep sedation and anesthesia affect the ASSR evoked by high modulation frequencies (e.g., > 80 Hz)? Sedation and anesthesia clearly affect the ASSR for slow modulation frequencies.
- How closely can auditory thresholds be estimated with the ASSR, and with what level of confidence can estimations be made?
- How closely do ABR thresholds agree with ASSR thresholds when test protocols are optimized for each technique?
- Does the accuracy of estimation of auditory thresholds with ASSR vary as a function of common subject factors, e.g., age, normal hearing versus type of hearing loss (conductive, sensory, mixed, neural), and degree of hearing loss from normal hearing through severe-to-profound?
- What factors contribute to discrepancies between ASSR thresholds and either behavioral and/or ABR thresholds that have been reported in the literature?
- What is the explanation(s) for discrepancies between ASSR thresholds and behavioral thresholds reported for patients with conductive hearing loss?

- Are different commercially available devices marketed for measurement of the ASSR, and the ASSRs recorded actually equivalent, including instrumentation utilizing stimuli that are essentially rapidly presented abrupt onset tone bursts versus equipment utilizing amplitude and frequency modulated sinusoidal stimuli?
- Are adequate experimental data available in support of algorithms for stimulation and analysis of the ASSR with various, particularly new, clinical instrumentation?
- Are there equipment-specific differences in ASSR findings for normal hearers and patients with varying types of auditory dysfunction related to algorithms employed in analysis of the response?
- Does measurement artifact with relatively high-intensity bone-conduction stimulation preclude use of the ASSR in defining sensory hearing level in conductive hearing loss?
- What sources of measurement artifact with high-intensity air-conduction stimulation contribute to spurious detection of an ASSR in patients with no behavioral evidence of hearing?
- Even though the waveform cannot be analyzed, does the ASSR provide any site-specific information for patients with hearing loss, e.g., identification or differentiation of conductive versus sensory versus neural auditory dysfunction?
- Can the ASSR be used to document benefit from amplification or cochlear implant use in infants and young children?
- Does the ASSR have neurodiagnostic value in the identification of central auditory nervous system dysfunction in specific patient populations, e.g., acoustic tumors, multiple sclerosis, dyslexia?

---

later in this chapter. The rate of stimulus modulation affects the site of ASSR generation within the auditory system, i.e., at the level of the brainstem versus cerebral cortex. Anatomic principles important for clinical application and interpretation of the ASSR were reviewed in Chapter 2.

The strategy for response analysis is distinctly different for the ABR versus ASSR. For the former, the clinician typically inspects visually a characteristic relatively invariant waveform and manually calculates response parameters, such as the latency and amplitude of specific waves or components. With ASSR measurement, in contrast, a complex waveform is recorded containing EEG activity and, if there is an ASSR, increased brain activity within the spectral region of the amplitude modulation frequency. The ASSR within the complex waveform cannot be detected visually. Rather, it is detected by either automated spectral analysis of stimulus-related brain energy in the frequency domain (*Fast Fourier Transform, FFT*) or by automated analysis of the phase of the response relative to stimulus phase, i.e., the similarity

of the response (replicability of the response) with repeated stimulation or *phase coherence*. In either case, the presence of a response versus only background noise is verified statistically (e.g., a t or T^2 test for phase coherence or F test for signal in noise determination). ASSR analysis approaches are reviewed briefly below. ASSR analysis is automated and, in fact, the sequence for stimulus presentation can even be controlled automatically. Even so, clinical experience and judgment is important for determining how the ASSR should be applied with individual patients, whether ASSR findings are reliable and valid, and how ASSR findings should be interpreted within the context of the overall pattern of audiologic test findings. These points are developed further later in this chapter.

STIMULATION OF THE ASSR. | The ASSR is elicited with sinusoidal (pure-tone and steady-state) stimuli (carrier tones) that are modulated in amplitude and, sometimes, frequency. Thus, the nature of the steady-state stimulus for eliciting the

ASSR differs in theory from the highly transient stimulus used to evoke the ABR. A typical stimulus is a 1000 Hz carrier tone with 100 percent amplitude modulation at a rate of 100 Hz. That is, for any given intensity level, the amplitude of the tone is decreased from maximum to minimum 100 times per second. The stimulus activates the cochlea at the 1000 Hz region with rather high frequency specificity. In addition, energy is generated within the auditory regions of the brain at the frequency of the modulation (100 Hz in this example). To increase its effectiveness in eliciting an ASSR, a sinusoidal stimulus may be modulated in amplitude (e.g., 100% modulation) and frequency (e.g., 10% modulation). The inclusion of frequency modulation (FM), in addition to amplitude modulation (AM), referred to as mixed modulation (MM) may increase ASSR amplitude but, of course, it also broadens the spectra of the stimulus, resulting in a less frequency-specific ASSR. Other terms used to describe types of modulation reported in ASSR measurement include AM^2 (exponentially modulated) and independent amplitude and frequency modulation (IAFM). In the words of Dimitrijevic, John, and Picton (2004), "An IAFM stimulus consists of a carrier that is modulated in amplitude and frequency, with different rates of modulation for the AM and FM" (p. 69). With the ASSR, hearing sensitivity of the peripheral auditory system is estimated at the frequency of the carrier tone, but the response within the brain is detected at the modulation frequency. The ASSR can be evoked with a modulated sinusoidal stimulus at one frequency (e.g., 1000 Hz) presented to one ear, with threshold estimated by repeated measurements as intensity is manipulated. The test approach is very similar to that typically taken in performing behavioral pure-tone audiometry. It is also possible to simultaneously record multiple ASSRs evoked by more than one stimulus frequency (e.g., John, Lins, Boucher, & Picton, 1998; Lins et al., 1995; Lins et al., 1996; Picton et al., 1987). With fast stimulus modulation rates (e.g., 70 to 110 Hz), amplitude is comparable for ASSRs evoked by single versus multiple carrier frequencies, as long as the carrier frequencies are separated by at least one octave. Indeed, the term used for one ASSR instrument—the MASTER system—is an acronym for **m**ultiple **a**uditory **ste**ady-state **r**esponse. ASSRs with the MASTER device can be measured with up to eight stimuli presented at the same time, i.e., four stimuli at different frequencies presented simultaneously to both ears. The modulations rates are distinctive for each of the eight stimuli. Analysis of the ASSR, therefore, involves detection of brain activity elicited by each of the modulation rates. Strategies and techniques available for ASSR measurement with clinical instrumentation are discussed further in the next section of this chapter. At high rates of modulation, and with rapid onset times (abrupt transitions from minimum to maximum amplitude), the stimuli used to elicit the ASSR approximate rapidly presented tone bursts and, therefore, the ASSR is very similar, if not the same as, an ABR. Whether there are inherent anatomic or audiologic differences between ASSRs evoked with sinusoidal stimuli that are modulated rapidly in amplitude and frequency versus ABRs evoked with rapidly presented tone bursts is not yet clear. Such distinctions in stimulus paradigms, however, are found among clinical devices that, collectively, are marketed for measurement of the ASSR.

ANALYSIS OF THE ASSR. | Complex brain activity (i.e., a complex waveform) is detected with electrodes during ASSR measurement. If a response is present, ASSR energy elicited by the modulation of the stimulus is embedded within the spectrum of the EEG recorded during stimulation. Several variations of analysis strategies and techniques are used to detect the presence of stimulus-related brain activity during ASSR measurement and to verify that the presumed response is statistically different than background electrical activity (noise). Methods for detection of the ASSR, and measurement of response magnitude or amplitude, commonly involve analysis of brain activity within the frequency domain—Fast Fourier Transform (FFT)—and/or calculation of the variability or, conversely, coherence of the phase of the response. Analysis of the ASSR in the frequency domain involves calculation of amplitude of brain activity (average power) at the modulation frequency(ies) and also activity (average power) for bins at a certain number of adjacent frequencies (e.g., 120) above and below the MF (e.g., 60 on either side of the MF). Then, the energy at the MF is statistically compared to the nonresponse energy (noise) in the same frequency region using the F-ratio to determine the probability (e.g., $p < .05$) that a response is really present versus simply background noise. With both the FFT and the phase coherence analysis approaches, probability of the presence of a response versus nonresponse (noise) within ongoing EEG is determined statistically. As reviewed below, the many publications by Drs. Picton, Stapells, Dimitrijevic, John, Herdman, and other authors among the Canadian group are a good source of information on the FFT approach for ASSR analysis, whereas details on the ASSR analysis technique that relies on calculation of phase coherence can be found in the publications of the Australian research group, e.g., papers authored by Drs. Rance, Rickards, Clark, Cohen, Cone-Wesson, and others. Picton, Dimitrijevic, John, & Van Roon (2001) provide evidence that detection of ASSR is enhanced by combined analysis of phase and spectral calculation of response amplitude in noise.

ASSR Test Protocol

There are as of yet no clear conventions for ASSR measurement or accepted test protocols and clearly no standards for equipment. In fact, stimulus and acquisition parameters and analysis algorithms vary widely among laboratory instrumentation and among devices marketed by different manufacturers for clinical measurement of the ASSR. A problem that has for some time plagued OAE instrumentation is now apparent also with ASSR equipment—namely, the evolution of test parameters, test protocols, and even analysis algorithms motivated by good intentions (e.g., reducing test time or more rapid estimations of auditory threshold) or laboratory experiences in normal hearers, rather than peer-reviewed published research evidence and findings in clinical populations. General test parameters are displayed in Table 8.8. There are substantial differences among manufacturers for selected parameters, such as mode of stimulation (monaural versus binaural), for the number of sweeps accumulated within an averaged waveform, analysis strategies and algorithms, and even basic parameters, such as electrode locations. Some of the more common variations in test parameters are noted in the discussion below.

TABLE 8.8. General ASSR Measurement Parameters Used by Manufacturers of Clinical Devices

Specific stimulus and acquisition options vary for each manufacturer. Consult with equipment manual for details.

PARAMETER	SELECTION
Stimulus Parameters	
Transducer	Insert earphone
Type	Sinusoid
Frequencies	500, 1000, 2000, 4000 Hz*
Modulation depth	Amplitude (100%)
	Frequency (20%)
Modulation rate	82 to 106 Hz
Duration	Variable
Polarity	Alternating
Intensity	0 to 100 dB SPL
Repetitions	Variable
Masking	Available for use as indicated.
Mode	Monaural or binaural (dichotic)*
Acquisition Parameters	
Electrodes	
Noninverting	Cz or Fz
Inverting	Nape, inion, or ipsilateral mastoid
Ground	Shoulder, contralateral mastoid, or low forehead
Filters	
HP	1 Hz or 10 Hz
LP	300 Hz or 500 Hz
Slope	6 dB/octave
Notch	None
Amplification	×10,000
Artifact rejection	On
Analysis time (epoch)	1 second
Number of epochs	16
Sweeps (# stimuli)	Variable
Averaging time	40 seconds to 15 minutes
Analysis algorithm	FFT with F-test or phase coherence

*Four stimuli may be presented to each ear simultaneously.

STIMULUS PARAMETERS. | The ASSR is evoked with sinusoidal stimuli—pure tones—that are modulated in amplitude and, sometimes, frequency. The practice of modulating a stimulus in either the amplitude and/or frequency dimension is not unique to ASSR measurement. For over fifty years, modulation of frequency (FM) or amplitude (AM) of stimuli has been used in psychoacoustic studies of auditory perception, including detection of very small or rapid changes in each acoustic property in normal-hearing subjects (e.g., Viemeister, 1979; Zwicker, 1955) and persons with auditory dysfunction (e.g., Bacon & Viemeister, 1985; Formby, 1987). The possible relevance of these psychoacoustic investigations to potential clinical applications of the ASSR will be noted in a subsequent section of the chapter. A typical stimulus is illustrated in Figure 8.12. The carrier frequency, sometimes abbreviated "f_c," can be amplitude and/or frequency modulated at varying depths. Maximum amplitude modulation, often employed in clinical studies, is 100 percent. At the other extreme, 0 percent AM of a carrier tone results in a simple sinusoid or pure tone. The depth of frequency modulation is usually no more than 20 percent to preserve reasonable spectral selectivity. AM and FM can also be described in terms of phase. The cochlea is certainly stimulated by the carrier frequency, but energy also activates the cochlea at the carrier frequency plus or minus the modulation frequency—that is, somewhat higher and lower frequencies. Although there is no energy in the stimulus at the modulation frequency, nonlinear distortion or "distortion products or combination tones" within the cochlear are produced at various frequencies related to the three stimulus frequencies (carrier frequency plus the two other modulation-related frequencies). Mathematically, it is possible to predict that one distortion product will occur at the modulation frequency. Undesirable, and complicated, interactions adversely impact on effective stimulation of the ASSR when multiple amplitude modulated sinusoidal stimuli each generating a series of distortion products, are presented within an octave. Increasing the intensity levels of multiple simultaneously presented modulated stimuli also increases the likelihood of interaction among stimuli and the cochlear distortion they generate.

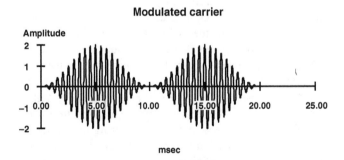

Modulated carrier

FIGURE 8.12. Sinusoidal stimulus (a 2000 Hz tone) modulated in amplitude at a rate of 100 Hz used to evoke the auditory steady-state response (ASSR).

There is, therefore, an upper limit to the intensity level that will produce ASSRs without concerns that undesirable interactions among stimuli affect the accuracy of analysis and interpretation of the response. The interactions among multiple modulated sinusoidal stimuli (presented to the same ear), absolute frequency and intensity of the stimuli, and distortion products are extremely complicated even in normal-hearing subjects and simply cannot be predicted in patients with cochlear dysfunction. Perhaps most concerning for clinical ASSR measurement is the attenuation of lower frequency carrier stimuli by energy produced by higher frequency carrier tones (e.g., John et al., 1998). Two other potential clinical issues raised in discussions of multiple amplitude and frequency-modulated sinusoids are temporary threshold shift secondary to ongoing stimulation of the cochlea and adaptation of the auditory system to continuous stimulation (e.g., John et al., 1998).

Although the concept of stimulation of the ASSR with pure tones that are modulated in either amplitude or frequency is rather straightforward, there are in fact a number of stimulus variables that interactively influence the ASSR. The major variables—stimulus frequency, modulation rate and method (e.g., amplitude, exponential amplitude, frequency, mixed modulation), and the mode of presentation (monaural or binaural, i.e., dichotic)—are reviewed herein. The ASSR can also be evoked with stimuli other than modulated sinusoids, including broadband noise, narrowband noise, and very rapidly presented click and tone-burst stimuli.

The ability to generate an auditory evoked response with sinusoidal versus a series of transient stimuli offers two apparent clinical advantages. First, the maximum intensity level for sinusoidal stimuli can be as high as 120 dB HL, perhaps even higher with special earphones. With transient stimuli—clicks or very short-duration tone bursts—used clinically to elicit the ABR, maximum intensity level is generally limited to about 80 to 85 dB nHL. The reader will note in the previous statement that intensity level for the sinusoidal stimulus used to evoke the ASSR was defined in dB HL, not dB nHL. Like the pure-tone stimuli used in behavioral threshold estimation, intensity level of the sinusoidal stimuli used to evoke the ASSR can be measured and calibrated with a sound level meter in dB SPL, and then converted to and designated in dB HL. Despite the correspondence of stimulus intensity level for the ASSR and pure-tone audiometry, an ASSR is typically not detected at audiometric zero (i.e., 0 dB HL). This point is discussed below in relation to the clinical application of the ASSR. Nonetheless, with maximum stimulus-intensity levels of 120 dB HL, and perhaps higher, it's possible with the ASSR to estimate auditory thresholds in patients with severe-to-profound hearing loss, a region beyond the intensity limits for stimuli that evoke an ABR. The other advantage of sinusoidal stimuli used to evoke the ASSR, at least in theory, is a high degree of frequency specificity. Most of the spectral energy in the stimulus is centered on the carrier-tone frequency, although even with amplitude

modulation of the carrier tone there are also spectral "side lobes" above and below the carrier frequency related to the modulation frequency (see Figure 8.13). In the preceding discussion of frequency specificity of auditory threshold estimations with ABRs elicited by tone bursts, a distinction was made between the acoustic frequency specificity of stimuli ("cochlear place specificity") and the frequency precision of the actual responses ("neuronal specificity"). The same concept applies to the ASSR evoked by AM or FM sinusoidal stimuli. The distinctions among acoustic specificity, place specificity, and neuronal specificity in ASSR measurement of normal hearers and persons with sensory hearing loss are discussed in detail by Stapells et al. (1994), Herdman, Picton, and Stapells (2002), and particularly Picton et al. (2003). Naturally, a reduction in any of the three types of specificity, or any combination of the three, will adversely affect the accuracy of frequency-specific threshold estimation with the ASSR. Citing evidence from earlier studies (Herdman, Lins, et al., 2002; Herdman, Picton, & Stapells, 2002) of frequency specificity for the ASSR evoked with 80 Hz stimulus modulation in persons with precipitous sloping hearing loss and with high-pass masking noise, Stapells et al. (2005) state, "ASSR frequency specificity was not as good as would be expected from the acoustic specificity of the AM stimuli. Further, ASSR frequency specificity was very similar to that previously shown for the tone-evoked ABR . . ." (p. 5). As noted in Chapter 2, an ASSR evoked by rapid (80 to 100 Hz) modulations in amplitude and frequency is generated mostly at the brainstem, rather than cortical, level in the auditory system. Unlike the 40 Hz response, therefore, ASSRs for high rates of AM or FM are not significantly influenced by sedation or sleep, even in infants and young children.

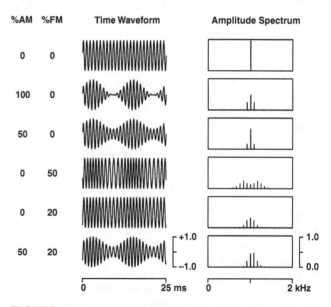

FIGURE 8.13. Frequency specificity of modulated tonal stimuli used to evoke the auditory steady-state response (ASSR).

The simplest stimulus used to evoke the ASSR is a sinusoidal carrier frequency modulated in amplitude at a depth of 100 percent, usually at a high modulation rate (> 80 Hz). Combining frequency modulation (at a depth of 20 to 25%) with amplitude modulation—a mixed modulation technique—enhances ASSR amplitude or gain on the average 1.35 versus AM alone (Cohen, Rickards, & Clark, 1991; John & Picton, 2000). Adding frequency modulation of 10 percent to the 100 percent AM, however, produces only a slight increase in ASSR amplitude. Even with only amplitude modulation there is some reduction in frequency specificity of sinusoidal stimulation. Most of the stimulus energy is, of course, at the carrier frequency at two side lobes or bands at frequencies lower and higher than the carrier frequency (abbreviated f_c) as determined by the modulation frequency (abbreviated MF or f_m). For example, with a carrier frequency of 1000 Hz modulated at 80 Hz, the cochlea is stimulated at 1000 Hz and a spectral width of 160 Hz (920 to 1080 Hz). Including frequency modulation further expands the spectrum of the stimulus and reduces frequency-specificity (Figure 8.14). Larger ASSR amplitudes are also produced with modifications in the stimulus modulation technique, such as exponential modulation (abbreviated AM^2). Other more complex stimuli, including nonsinusoidal carriers (e.g., narrow- and broadband noise) are effective in evoking ASSRs with larger amplitudes, but the inevitable tradeoff is even less spectral specificity (John, Dimitrijevic, & Picton, 2003). Different modulation frequencies (MFs) or rates are typically used with different stimulus frequencies to evoke the ASSR, e.g., an MF of 74 Hz at 500 Hz; an MF of 81 Hz at 1000 Hz; an MF of 88 Hz at 2000 Hz; and an MF of 95 Hz at 4000 Hz.

Experimentation with various stimulus paradigms soon confirmed that more than one ASSR could be recorded at the same time, with presentation of different stimuli simultaneously to each ear and also with up to at least eight separate modulation frequencies (Dolphin, 1997; Lins & Picton, 1995). The term "dichotic" paradigm is used when a different acoustic stimulus is presented simultaneously to each ear. John, Lins, Boucher, & Picton (1998) coined the term *multiple auditory steady-state response* (MASTER) for the technique. Frequency specificity appears to be comparable for multiple frequencies presented simultaneously versus a single-carrier frequency and modulation rate. An important constraint with the MASTER technique is the separation of stimulus frequencies presented to an ear by at least an octave to eliminate interactions. In theory, simultaneous measurement of the ASSR for multiple frequencies in both ears would reduce test time. Although this possibility is supported by studies (e.g., Herdman & Stapells, 2001, 2003; John, Purcell, Dimitrijevic, & Picton, 2002) utilizing one type of equipment (the MASTER device), direct comparison of test time in clinical settings and populations with different devices is lacking. The reduction in ASSR test time resulting from recordings evoked by the presentation of multiple stimuli to both ears will be affected by clinical factors, such as the degree and configuration of hearing loss, whether the patient is sedated with little measurement noise versus awake, and the magnitude of the ASSR at different frequencies. The practical implications of single- versus multiple-frequency ASSR techniques, including test time, are discussed further in the section on clinical applications.

Dimitrijevic, John, Van Roon, and Picton (2001) conducted a study of "independent amplitude and frequency modulation," abbreviated IAFM. That is, the authors recorded two ASSRs each evoked by a single carrier frequency with AM at one rate and FM at another rate. This approach is in contrast to the conventional modulation of amplitude and frequency at the same rate for a single carrier tone, i.e., mixed modulation, described above. Dimitrijevic et al. (2001) were able to clearly distinguish independent ASSRs for each type of modulation. Amplitude of the ASSRs was only slightly (14%) less than the amplitude for ASSRs recorded separately for either AM or FM alone. Furthermore, the authors reported in 21 young normal-hearing adults a significant correlation between amplitudes of the ASSRs elicited with the IAFM stimulus paradigm and word recognition performance.

Using the MASTER technique, John, Dimitrijevic, and Picton (2003a,b) systematically investigated in 12 adult normal-hearing subjects with four experiments the efficiency of various stimuli in eliciting the ASSR. Stimuli included pure-tone stimuli of 500, 1000, 2000, and 4000 Hz modulated

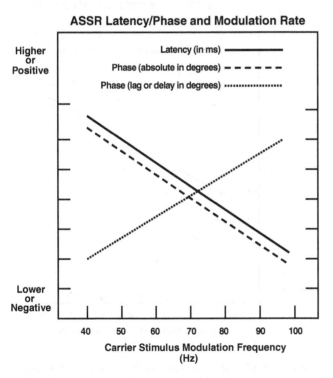

FIGURE 8.14. Relations among modulation frequency, absolute phase, phase lag, and latency of the ASSR.

in amplitude (AM), exponential amplitude (AM^2), or with mixed modulation at rates of 80 to 95 Hz, narrowband and broadband noise stimuli modulated at rates of 80 to 87 Hz, and rapidly presented clicks and tone bursts. Efficiency was operationally defined by the magnitude of the ASSR and the amount of measurement time needed to identify confidently (statistically significant) the presence of a response. Frequency–specificity is important for accurate estimation of auditory thresholds. The size of an ASSR, however, contributes to rapid detection of the response, a distinct asset for hearing screening. Confirming the findings for an earlier study (John et al., 1998), the authors found larger amplitudes for ASSRs for noise stimuli than conventional modulated sinusoidal stimuli.

Stürzbecher, Cebulla, and Pschirrer (2001), in a paper with nearly the same title as the one just noted by John et al. (2003b), also examined in normal-hearing adult subjects the efficiency stimuli used to evoked the ASSR. The stimuli were multiple simultaneously presented sinusoidal carriers (500, 1000, 2000, and 4000 Hz) all modulated at the same rate. As the authors point out, the multiple-carrier stimulus (AM3MF2) increased the signal-to-noise ratio (SNR) to 1.6, an enhancement that "is notable if one takes into consideration the fact that by doubling the number of averaged epochs (doubling the examination time), the SNR is improved only by a theoretical factor of 1.4" (p. 67). Higher SNRs for evoked responses typically are associated with increased response detection near threshold and, therefore, more accurate results for hearing screening and with estimation of hearing threshold with the response. Further investigation with the types of stimuli used in the study by Stürzbecher, Cebulla, and Pschirrer (2001) is warranted with infants and other patients with different types of hearing loss.

As with any AER, manipulation of *stimulus intensity* affects the amplitude and latency (or phase) of the ASSR (Dimitrijevic et al., 2002; Small & Stapells, 2005). As the intensity of typical carrier stimulus frequencies (e.g., audiometric frequencies of 500 to 4000 Hz) is increased, there is a significant increase in response amplitude (in μvolt) and a decrease in the phase delay of the ASSR (in milliseconds and degrees). John and Picton (2000) reported an average decrease in latency of the ASSR of 2.4 ms with a change in intensity from 35 to 75 dB SPL. A basal-ward change or shift in activation of the cochlea as stimulus intensity is increased is offered as the physiologic explanation for the intensity–latency relation with ASSR, even for the sinusoidal stimuli used to evoke the response (e.g., John & Picton, 2000). Latency of the ASSR also decreases by about one-half as the modulation frequency of the sinusoidal stimuli is doubled (Cohen et al., 1991; John & Picton, 2000; Rickards & Clark, 1984). Latency of the ASSR also, predictably, decreases as the carrier frequency is increased. John and Picton (2000) reported a latency decrease of 5.5 to 6.0 ms across the frequency range of 500 to 6000 Hz. The intensity dependence

of ASSR amplitude and phase is apparent for both air- and bone conduction stimulation (Small & Stapells, 2005). Relations among modulation frequency, absolute phase, phase lag, and latency of the ASSR are illustrated in Figure 8.15.

Insert earphones are now used almost exclusively to present stimuli in ASSR measurement. The multiple and varied advantages of insert earphones in clinical auditory evoked response measurement were reviewed in Chapter 3, and again with reference to specific responses in other chapters. One advantage of insert earphones versus supra-aural earphones that appears to be unique for stimulation of the ASSR is reducing the likelihood of inadvertently generating with very high intensity (> 100 dB HL) and very low frequency (< 500 Hz) stimuli a somatosensory evoked response, rather than an auditory response (e.g., Rance et al., 1998).

An apparent clinical advantage of the ASSR in the possibility of evoking a response with frequency-specific *bone-conduction stimuli,* and perhaps at higher intensity levels than are feasible with highly transient clicks or tone bursts. Several papers describe ASSR findings for bone-conduction stimulation in normal-hearing subjects (Dimitrijevic et al., 2002; Jeng et al., 2004; Lins et al., 1996; Small & Stapells, 2004, 2005), or with normal subjects with simulated conductive hearing loss (Jeng et al., 2004). In most studies, subjects were normal hearers with conductive hearing loss simulated by plugging insert earphone tubing and sensory hearing loss

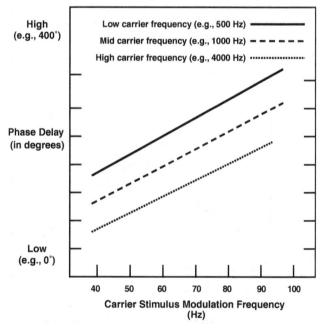

FIGURE 8.15. Relations between modulation frequency and phase delay for different categories of carrier tone frequency.

simulated by masking noise. Measurement methodology varied among the studies, particularly the site of bone-conduction stimulation (forehead versus mastoid). Two consistent themes among the studies were the feasibility of eliciting an ASSR with bone-conduction stimulation and, unfortunately, the likelihood of producing an artifactual ASSR at relatively modest bone-conduction stimulus intensity levels. Lins et al. (1996) described ASSR findings with bone-conduction stimulation (RadioEar B-71 forehead oscillator placement) for 8 normal-hearing young adult subjects with sensory hearing impairment simulated by masking noise. The authors reported reasonably close agreement (5 dB ± 5 dB) between behavioral and ASSR estimations of hearing levels for air-conduction stimulation. However, thresholds estimated by the ASSR with bone-conduction stimulation were consistently and significantly higher than those measured with conventional bone-conduction pure-tone audiometry for normal-hearing subjects (26 to 33 dB higher) and for simulated sensory hearing impairment (9 to 14 dB higher). In a similar study, Dimitrijevic et al. (2002) described ASSRs evoked with bone-conduction stimulation with a Radioear B-71 vibrator at the forehead from 10 normal hearing subjects with simulated conductive hearing loss. At equivalent intensity levels, the amplitude of ASSRs was greater for bone-conduction versus air-conduction stimulation, raising the possibility of bone conduction stimulus artifact.

Jeng and colleagues (2004) at the University of Iowa recorded the ASSR with air- and bone-conduction stimuli from a group of 10 normal-hearing adult subjects with simulated conductive hearing impairment and 5 adult subjects with profound bilateral sensory hearing loss (cochlear implant users). The authors' stated goal was to further define the accuracy and reproducibility of the ASSR in estimating air-bone gap in conductive hearing loss and the upper intensity limits for bone-conduction stimulation. ASSR measurement was conducted with the MASTER system. In simulated conductive hearing loss, Jeng et al. (2004) found a strong correlation (r = 0.81) for the air-bone gap determined with pure-tone audiometry versus the air-bone gap estimated with the ASSR. Presumably, bone-conduction measurements were made with forehead placement for both behavioral audiometry and the ASSR. Nonetheless, there was a trend toward overestimation of the magnitude of the air-bone gap with ASSR. Thresholds for the ASSR with bone-conduction stimulation were quite consistent (3 to 0 dB across the frequency region of 500 to 4000 Hz) for two types of simulated conductive hearing loss (occluding insert earphone tubes with epoxy versus lamb's wool). These values for bone-conduction ASSR thresholds were comparable to reported test–retest accuracy for bone-conduction pure-tone thresholds. Perhaps the most discouraging finding reported by Jeng et al. (2004) was incorrect identification of an ASSR in patients with profound hearing loss with bone-conduction stimulation within the intensity range of 53 to 54 dB (for carrier frequencies of 500, 2000, and 4000 Hz) and as low as 36 dB HL for a carrier frequency

stimulus of 1000 Hz. It appears that rather low intensity levels must be used with bone-conduction stimulation of the ASSR to avoid the possibility of recording an apparent response that is really an artifact.

Small and Stapells (2005) recorded the ASSR with bone-conduction stimulation from 10 normal-hearing young adults using a higher than typical A/D rate in an attempt to minimize stimulus artifact. Bone-conduction stimuli were presented to the mastoid with a RadioEar B-71 oscillator located close to the pinna (within 2 cm) and held in place with 450 to 550 g of force with an elastic headband. As the authors point out, "A significant problem with bone-conduction stimulus artifact in the EEG is that this energy can alias to exactly the same frequency of the ASSR modulation rate of the stimulus, and be interpreted as a response" (Small & Stapells, 2005, p. 174). One useful step in reducing the possibility of bone conduction stimulus artifact is to alternate the polarity of the stimulus, a well-appreciated and effective strategy for minimizing stimulus artifact with bone conduction ABR. As documented by Small and Stapells (2004, 2005), careful selection of A/D rates, and reliance on a low pass (300 Hz) electrophysiologic filter with a steep slope are also effective strategies for minimizing the chance of a spurious (false) ASSR produced by aliasing. The authors found thresholds for ASSRs evoked by bone-conduction stimulation (500 to 4000 Hz) in the range of 18 to 26 dB HL. Alternating bone-conduction stimulus polarity did not affect the amplitude or phase of the ASSR and, therefore, offers a potential option for minimizing reducing the likelihood of spurious responses. Regarding clinical application of bone-conduction ASSRs, Small and Stapells (2005) conclude with the cautionary statement, ". . . there are no normative threshold data for infants and no threshold data from any subjects with impaired hearing (infants or adults). Bone conduction ASSRs are, therefore, not yet ready for clinical use" (p. 183). Formal investigation in various clinical populations of bone-conduction stimulation in ASSR measurement with instrumentation produced by different manufacturers is also needed.

Cone-Wesson et al. (2002) applied the sensorineural acuity level (SAL) technique in estimation of the air-bone gap with the ASSR. The SAL technique in behavioral audiometry dates back to clinical studies in the 1950s (see Hall, 2004, for review). With the SAL technique, masking noise is delivered to both ears via bone conduction, with the bone oscillator located on the forehead. Thresholds for tonal stimuli are measured in the unmasked and then the masked condition. Using the SAL technique, Cone-Wesson et al. (2002) recorded the ASSR from 39 infants. Although the infants were at risk for hearing loss, the majority apparently had reasonably normal hearing sensitivity as estimated by click-evoked ABR, with cochlear integrity verified by DPOAE and middle ear status defined by tympanometry. Nine of the infants yielded elevated ABR minimum response levels. ASSR threshold was first determined with air-conduction sinusoidal stimuli (100% amplitude modulation and 15% frequency modulation). Narrowband noise was delivered via a RadioEar B-70 bone-conduction oscillator placed in a superior and posterior position relative to the mastoid bone (Stuart et al., 1990). The bone oscillator was held in place with a custom-made headband made of elastic and Velcro, maintaining a pressure of 325 ± 25 grams. Noise was increased from 0 dB nHL in 10 dB increments until no ASSR was detected (e.g., a "random" outcome), and then the intensity level at the masking level was documented. As anticipated, the amount of bone-conduction narrowband masking needed to affect ASSR threshold measures was markedly higher for children with presumed sensorineural hearing loss than for normal-hearing infants and those with conductive hearing loss. A sensory hearing loss was inferred when bone-conducted narrowband noise of > 20 dB nHL was required to mask the ASSR. Approximately 4 to 5 minutes of test time was required to estimate auditory threshold for a single frequency. Cone-Wesson et al. (2002) concluded "it was possible to estimate AC and BC masking thresholds infants at risk for hearing loss. . . . The SAL method adapted for ASSR was able to separate infants with hearing loss into conductive and sensorineural hearing loss groups" (pp. 274, 275).

Investigation of the ASSR for bone-conduction stimuli in infants suggests the likelihood that results differ as a function of stimulus frequency and in comparison to adult findings (Small, Hatton, & Stapells, 2004). Experimental and clinical evidence with the ABR evoked with bone-conduction stimulation has, for some time, revealed a comparable pattern of findings, that is, differences in thresholds for low versus high frequencies and for infants versus adults. There is, in summary, limited research on the measurement of the ASSR with bone-conduction stimuli. At the least, one can safely conclude that application of clinical experience and normative data from adult subjects in ASSR measurement of infants is inadvisable. One clinically important advantage to recording the ABR versus ASSR with bone-conduction stimulation is the possibility of verifying that the response is ear-specific, even without masking of the contralateral ear. As detailed in Chapter 6, detection of a reliable wave I component in the ipsilateral ABR waveform evoked by bone-conduction stimulation, but not in the ABR recorded with a contralateral electrode array, confirms that the response is due to activation of the stimulus ear and auditory nerve. It is not to visually identify in the ASSR waveform individual components associated with neural generators and, therefore, to ascribe a response to one ear or the other unless an appropriate amount of masking is delivered to the nontest ear.

ACQUISITION PARAMETERS. | An oft-cited potential weakness in pediatric application of ASSR for estimation of hearing threshold is inadequate signal averaging (e.g., Luts & Wouters, 2004; Picton et al., 2003; Stapells et al., 2005).

As noted in the general overview of AER measurement in Chapter 2, and for specific responses in other chapters, the ultimate goal in AER recording is to achieve an adequate signal-to-noise (SNR) ratio. After steps are taken to minimize environmental and physiologic noise, the next best step in enhancing the SNR at low stimulus intensity levels (when the signal (AER) is small) is to continue signal averaging until the noise level approximates the minimal level. With ABR measurement, signal averaging may continue for thousands of stimulus presentations, whereas at high intensity levels with a normal-hearing quiet subject only relatively few (200 or less) sweeps are required. The same principle, of course, applies to ASSR measurement. Under certain conditions—high noise and/or small response—more signal averaging is necessary. Unfortunately, the measurement algorithms and strategies employed by ASSR devices vary considerably in terms of signal averaging stopping criterion and time. Assuming that noise, stimulus intensity level, and hearing threshold status is equivalent among subjects, there is a direct relation between test time and the extent of signal averaging. Shorter averaging time is only a good thing if the resultant SNR permits confident and statistically proven identification of an ASSR. As a rule, more signal averaging and test time is indicated when the SNR fails to meet minimal criteria for detection of a response, a point made clear by John, Brown, Muir, and Picton (2004), who stated, "Since the background electrical noise in the recording decreases with averaging, distinguishing a response from the background noise becomes more reliable as the testing duration is increased" (p. 540).

Inconsistencies in stimulus parameters among studies and for different ASSR devices are detailed throughout this chapter and in review articles (e.g., Picton et al., 2003). Acquisition parameters also vary considerably among published studies. As an example, a variety of electrode locations are described in published studies and equipment manuals, especially for the inverting electrode and the ground (common) electrode. The noninverting electrode site is invariably the vertex (Cz) or high forehead (Fz). Reported inverting electrode sites, however, are diverse, including the mastoid, earlobe, a midline occipital location (Oz), the inion, the right side of the neck, a site midline and low on the posterior surface of the neck (at the hairline), and the nape of the neck. A variety of ground (common) electrode locations are also employed in ASSR measurement, such as the mastoid, low forehead (Fpz), midline parietal scalp (Pz), right or left clavicle (collarbone), cheek, and shoulder. Surprisingly, some authors followed manufacturer-recommended default parameters, but did not specify the location of recording electrodes (e.g., Stueve & O'Rourke, 2003). There are no published investigations of the influence of electrode location on the ASSR.

ASSR TEST PROTOCOL. | At the outset, it is important to stress that subject state is a critical variable for successful

ASSR measurement. Reliable ASSR findings, and accurate estimation of hearing thresholds with the ASSR, are highly dependent on a very quiet EEG, that is, with the patient sleeping, sedated, or lightly anesthetized. Although an ASSR can often be recorded from an awake subject who is resting comfortably and very quiet, threshold estimations (when the response amplitude is smallest) are best made in the natural or sedated sleep state when noise is minimal. As implied in the preceding discussion, agreement is lacking regarding test parameters for recording the ASSR. Given the divergent measurement strategies and analysis algorithms used with ASSR instrumentation, it's not possible to present a consistent test protocol acceptable to clinicians with different devices.

Some authors report average test times of up to 3 hours for estimation of frequency specific auditory thresholds in both ears with the ABR in combination with ASSR (e.g., Stueve & O'Rourke, 2003). However, for the ASSR alone or the ASSR in combination with click ABR measurement, total test times of 1 hour or less for clinical estimation of auditory thresholds with ASSR for each ear at audiometric frequencies of 500 to 4000 Hz are more typical. Luts and colleagues (2005) in Belgium, for example, reported a total test time of 58 minutes for estimation of thresholds for four frequencies in both ears. Overall test time for ASSR measurement, as with tone-burst ABR recordings, is dependent on experience of the clinician and factors essentially beyond control of the clinician, e.g., subject state of arousal, auditory status, and electrical interference. In the author's experience, estimation of auditory thresholds bilaterally for a click stimulus and tone bursts of 500, 1000, and 4000 Hz can, in very quiet normal-hearing children, be completed in less than 20 minutes with maximum use of test time. Strategies for minimizing test time were reviewed earlier in this chapter. On the other hand, there are reports (e.g., Luts & Wonters, 2005) of ABR test times of up to 45 minutes for threshold estimation with only click stimuli. One might expect test time to be shorted by simultaneous presentation of multiple stimulus frequencies to each ear, in comparison to ASSR measurement with one stimulus frequency at a time presented to one ear at a time. Times savings for the simultaneous multi-frequency and two-ear (i.e., MASTER) strategy may be realized for persons with equivalent hearing levels across the range of stimulus frequencies, e.g., from 500 to 4000 or 8000 Hz. However, ASSR test times are less noticeable for the MASTER versus single-frequency and single-ear approach with patients who have rising or sloping audiometric configurations. There are substantial differences in such cases in the sensation level of stimulus intensities among test frequencies. For example, if the starting stimulus intensity level is 70 dB HL and hearing sensitivity is 0 dB at 1000 Hz and 70 dB at 4000 Hz, then the statistical criterion for detection of the ASSR will be readily met in the audiometric region where hearing sensitivity is normal (1000 Hz in this example). In contrast, signal averaging may continue for 15 minutes or more at the frequency with severe hearing loss (4000 Hz in this example), as stimulus intensity is very close to actual behavioral auditory threshold. Similarly, differences in hearing levels between ears may result in highly divergent ASSR detection outcomes among frequencies and ears.

When stimulus frequency and intensity, as well as the test ear, is under manual control by an experienced clinician, as it is with pure-tone audiometry, logical decisions on starting stimulus intensity levels and the size of decrements or increments in intensity for individual frequencies (and for each ear) can be made as indicated. That is, the steps taken to estimate auditory thresholds with the ASSR are determined based on already acquired data, or expectations on the degree and configuration of hearing loss derived from other audiometric measures (e.g., click or tone-burst ABR, acoustic reflexes, or OAEs). The end result can be increased efficiency in ASSR assessment, even though data are not collected simultaneously for two ears or multiple stimulus frequencies. A formal study comparing test performance and time for an ASSR device using each of these general strategies is reviewed in the next section.

Critical stimulus parameters in ASSR measurement can be varied along rather wide ranges. For example, stimulus carrier frequencies cover the audiometric region from 250 to 8000 Hz, stimulus intensity may be as low as −10 dB and as high as 130 dB HL (usually in either 10 or 5 dB increments), and modulation frequency with most clinical evoked response systems can be varied from 10 to 20 Hz up to 200 Hz or more. Similarly, the depth of modulation of the sinusoidal stimulus may be decreased from 0 percent (a typical pure tone) to 100 percent, and frequency modulation changed from 0 to 20 percent or more. The concept of amplitude modulation (from full amplitude to total decrease in amplitude) is rather straightforward, but frequency modulation requires a brief explanation, as it is a function of the absolute frequency and the percentage of modulation. As example, for a carrier frequency of 2000 Hz, frequency modulation of 10 percent produces a deviation in stimulus frequency of 200 Hz, but a change (or swing) in frequency of 400 Hz (i.e., ± 200 Hz or from 1800 to 2200 Hz). Or, for a carrier frequency of 500 Hz, frequency modulation of 10 percent produces a deviation in stimulus frequency of 50 Hz, and a change (or swing) in frequency of 100 Hz (i.e., ± 100 Hz or from 400 to 600 Hz). The relative AM/FM phase angle may also be manipulated, although changes in the latter from manufacturer default values should only be made based on experimental and statistically confirmed evidence. Clearly, myriad permutations of stimulus variables are possible in for ASSR measurement when one considers combinations of stimulus carrier frequency, intensity of the stimulus (in dB SPL or dB HL), modulation frequency, and the depth of amplitude and frequency modulation. In estimating hearing threshold levels with the ASSR, it is very important to utilize only test parameters either recommended by the manufacturer or demonstrated by formal investigation to be effective and appropriate for the clinical purpose and population. As an aside, automated stimulus presentation is an option with clinical ASSR systems whereby the sequence begins at an established initial intensity level, and then stimulus intensity is decreased with user determined increments (e.g., 5 or 10 dB) under computer control until a response is confirmed at a lower limit for stimulus intensity or threshold is estimated.

Given the seriousness of the consequences, a warning stated in review of test protocols for the ECochG and ABR is repeated here: Never turn the power of any component of the ASSR system on or off with the patient connected via electrodes to the system. Always turn the power on before connecting the patient to the device via electrodes and, at the conclusion of the ASSR assessment, first either unplug the electrodes from the ASSR device or remove the electrodes from the patient before powering off.

ASSR ANALYSIS. | In a departure from other AERs that are analyzed almost exclusively in the time domain, analysis of the ASSR is in the frequency domain. That is, there is no attempt to inspect or process information in a temporal waveform arising after stimulus presentation. The ABR, for example, is characterized by a series of distinct wave components occurring at different latencies after the stimulus. The ASSR, in contrast, appears as a repeating sequence of waves with constant amplitude and frequency (phase) characteristics over time. There are several related approaches for analysis of ASSR activity in the frequency domain. One general analysis approach for detection and confirmation of the ASSR relies on a Fourier analysis or fast Fourier transformation (FFT) of brain activity during acoustic stimulation. Confirmation of ASSR activity with the FFT technique is illustrated in Figure 8.16. Brain activity at the frequency of interest is mathematically processed (multiplied by the sine and cosine of the stimulus frequency) to derive the amplitude and the phase of the response. The FFT, computed digitally and including both real and imaginary values, yields estimations of amplitude and phase simultaneously over a range of frequencies. Brain activity is sampled and signal averaged during repeated sweeps. Brain energy is acquired and quantified for a spectral band defined by the high-pass and low-pass filters. Special attention is focused on the region of the modulation frequency or, for multiple stimuli, at the frequency region for each of the modulation frequencies. Amplitude and phase at the modulation frequency(ies) is determined relative to background electrical activity (noise), generally over a duration of about 1.5 ms. The ASSR activity can also be displayed in a polar plot, where amplitude of activity is depicted by the amplitude of a vector and phase of the vector is shown in relation to the x-axis, i.e., the reference for phase of the stimulus. The vector plot method for displaying the results of ASSR analysis is shown in Figure 8.17. Although there are different techniques available for

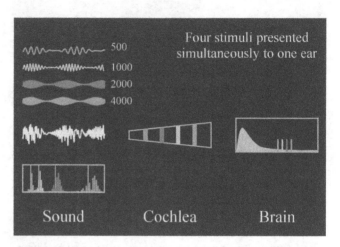

FIGURE 8.16. An example of a method for displaying and analyzing the auditory steady-state response (ASSR) that is based on spectral analysis of brain activity at modulation frequencies. Note the presence of EEG activity in the low-frequency region. Multiple stimuli with different carrier frequencies and different modulation frequencies were presented simultaneously to both ears. Presence of a response (versus only noise) is verified statistically with the F statistic.

calculation of phase of the ASSR, a common approach is to quantify phase delay (or lag) between the onset phase of the stimulus and the onset phase of the response. The result of the phase calculation is typically diagrammed in a polar plot with vector lines projecting from the center. Amplitude or size of brain activity, perhaps including a response, is designated by the length of the vector in μV or power (square of the amplitude), whereas phase (in degrees) is indicated by the angle between the vector lines and a 0^0 phase line (usually the X-axis). There are three possible outcomes with the vector plot or view approach for analysis of the ASSR:

- Phase Locked: A response is present, as defined by a coherent relation between the stimulus and the phase of the ASSR.
- Random: Under adequate measurement conditions (low noise), no coherent relation is detected between the stimulus and the phase of the ASSR.
- Excessive Noise: The level of ambient electrical, EEG, or myogenic noise is excessively high precluding confident detection of an ASSR.

As ASSR is sampled, the coherence of response phase is assessed statistically. According to John and Picton (2000), phase delay (in degrees) can be converted to latency (in seconds) by dividing by 360f, where f is the stimulus modulation frequency (in Hz).

ASSR activity always occurs within background activity (noise) arising from physiologic sources (the brain and muscles in the region of the head and neck) and electrical

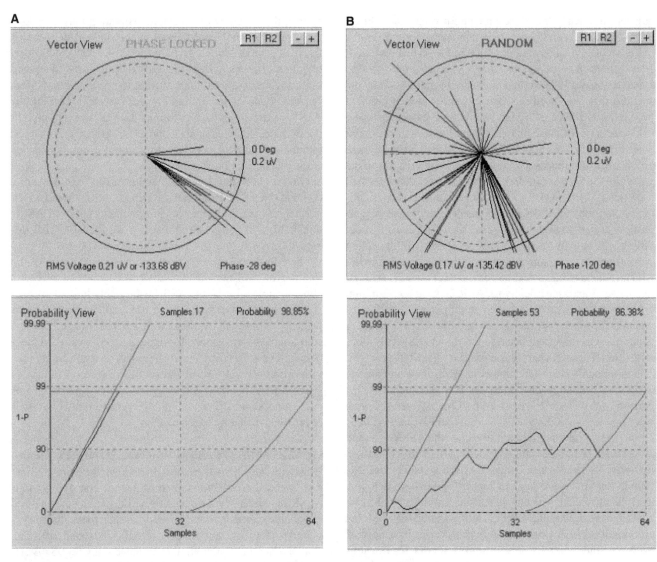

FIGURE 8.17. An example of a method for displaying and analyzing ASSR phase and amplitude used by one equipment manufacturer. A. Phase coherence (phase locking) is shown in the top portion of the figure, with vectors clumped together and related consistently to phase of the stimulus (horizontal line). Probability of the presence of a response (versus only noise) meets criterion of 98.85 percent (top right portion of bottom figure). B. Lack of phase coherence (random activity) is shown in the top portion of the figure, with vectors projecting in different directions and not related to phase of the stimulus (horizontal line). Probability of the presence of a response (versus only noise) fails to meet criterion of 98.85 percent after a period of stimulus presentation (bottom portion).

sources (the evoked response instrument and transducers, plus electrical devices in the vicinity of the test setting). As reviewed in Chapter 3 for AER measurement in general, two important strategies for enhancing detection of desired brain activity by minimizing background noise are filtering out unwanted spectral activity and signal averaging during repeated stimulation. Artifact rejection of noise that is clearly not stimulus-related, e.g., due to bodily movement, is also an important step in confident detection of the ASSR. The primary

goal, therefore, is ongoing detection of the signal (the ASSR) within the noise (non-ASSR activity), with statistical proof that the signal is different from the noise. In ASSR measurement, a variety of techniques, with differing mathematical assumptions, equations, and statistical tests, have been applied to achieve this essential goal. As noted above, the F-test is most commonly applied to verify that the activity in the brain spectrum related to the stimulus (power at the signal frequency) is statistically different from the average power in adjacent frequency bins. The literature reveals many different mathematical and conceptual approaches for each of the major steps in the measurement of ASSRs, as just reviewed. It is important to appreciate that ASSR findings reported since the early 1980s were, without doubt, influenced by the specific strategies used for such fundamental measurement processes as filtering, signal averaging, measurement and calculation of response phase and amplitude, and statistical determination of the signal within noise. Even today, there are distinct differences among devices on the market in the ways the ASSR is recorded, processed, and distinguished statistically from background noise. Even some fundamental assumptions of ASSR measurement affecting instrument design vary among manufacturers. One of the most distinct differences among ASSR devices has to do with the extent of, or time spent on, signal averaging. The direct relation between signal averaging and response detection was reviewed in Chapter 3 and, specifically for ABR, in Chapter 5. At high intensity levels, especially when hearing sensitivity is normal at the frequency of the carrier stimulus, signal averaging is not quite as important because the signal (ASSR) is more robust relative to background noise (i.e., the SNR is large). The time required for detection of an ASSR does not appear to differ significantly among devices. For example, in a comparison of the MASTER device (Bio Logic Systems, Corp.) with the Audera (GSI/VIASYS), Luts and Wouters (2005) reported that the time required to record the ASSR from ten normal hearing adults and ten adults with sensory hearing loss was, on the average, equivalent for the two devices. Although test time was 6 minutes longer for the MASTER system, the difference was not statistically significant. The two devices were differentiated by the time required for ASSR recording in subjects with normal-hearing versus hearing loss. With the Audera device, test time was shorter for hearing-impaired subjects, in comparison to normal hearers, but just the opposite pattern emerged for the MASTER device. Schmulian, Swanepoel, and Hugo (2005) in a group of 25 cooperative young adult hearing-impaired subjects found no significant difference in the time required for completing a multiple-frequency ASSR protocol (28 minutes; standard deviation 11 minutes) versus a ABR protocol for click and tone burst (500 Hz only) stimuli (24 minutes; standard deviation 9 minutes).

As the stimulus intensity level approaches auditory threshold, or at low intensity levels in normal-hearing subjects, amplitude of the ASSR is smaller and more signal averaging is typically required to achieve an adequate SNR. Under such measurement conditions, signal averaging should continue until it is clear that further averaging will not substantially lower the SNR and improve signal detection. If a device includes stopping rules for signal averaging based on a time limit (e.g., 100 seconds) or a limit in the number of sweeps (e.g., 16, 32, or 64), the ASSR will not be consistently detected close to auditory threshold, particularly when there is considerable measurement noise. Of course, the accuracy of threshold estimation may vary as a function of a number of factors, including carrier stimulus frequency, modulation rate (amplitude of ASSR), definition of stimulus intensity level (e.g., dB HL versus dB SPL), and both physiologic and nonphysiologic noise levels. Unfortunately, consistency among clinical devices is lacking for ASSR parameters and algorithms at virtually every step in the measurement and analysis process. Perhaps due to these factors, accuracy of behavioral threshold estimation varies among devices in normal-hearing subjects and persons with hearing impairment. Luts and Wouters (2005), in the direct comparison of two devices described above, found in 10 normal-hearing subjects closer agreement between ASSR thresholds and behavioral thresholds for the MASTER device, whereas accuracy was equivalent for the two devices in the hearing-impaired group. However, generalization of the findings of the Luts and Wouters (2005) study to everyday clinical application of the ASSR is probably limited, as data were collected from cooperative adult subjects in a double-walled sound booth outfitted with a Faraday cage. Clearly, additional data are needed for larger and more varied subject populations before firm conclusions can be made on interdevice differences in the clinical setting. The reader, again, is referred for more details to original articles describing specific devices and strategies for ASSR measurement, as well as review papers on the topic.

STIMULUS ARTIFACTS AND ARTIFACTUAL RESPONSES. | Problems with ASSR measurement include stimulus-related artifacts and the possibility of mistakenly identifying as an ASSR in persons with no hearing activity from some source (physiologic or electromagnetic) other than the auditory system. Artifacts are most likely for ASSRs evoked with air-conduction stimuli at high intensity levels, e.g., > 95 dB HL (Gorga et al., 2004; Picton & John, 2004; Small & Stapells, 2004) and with bone-conduction stimuli at moderate intensity levels, e.g., 40 dB HL and higher (Dimitrijevic et al., 2002; Small & Stapells, 2005). The phenomenon of *aliasing* in ASSR measurement is a common explanation for spurious findings due to artifact. Indeed, distortion of evoked electrophysiologic activity, or even the misidentification of measurement artifact as evoked electrophysiologic activity, by aliasing is not only a problem with the ASSR. Rather, aliasing can contaminate any auditory evoked response recording. As described in Chapter 3 and articulated by Picton and John (2004), "aliasing occurs when a signal is sampled at a rate lower than twice its frequency. The signal is then seen at a frequency equal to the absolute difference between its frequency and the closest integer multiple of the sampling rate" (p. 542). An AER waveform is not, of course, a display of continuous ongoing brain activity. Rather, it consists of a series of sampling points of voltage distributed over the analysis time. On first-generation evoked response systems, the oscilloscope display revealed a series of dots or data points, each representing a sampling (measure) of the voltage of electrical activity at a specific latency after the stimulus. AER waveforms recorded with current instruments for evoked responses appear as a solid display of brain activity, but manual operation of the cursor along the waveform reveals the discrete rather than continuous reflection of voltages at different latency points within the analysis time. That is, the cursor jumps from one frequency to another, with temporal resolution (interval from one latency point to the next) equivalent to the analysis time divided by the number of data points (e.g., 15 ms/1024 = 0.015 ms). With higher sampling rates, there are more data points within the analysis time and, of course, a higher degree of temporal resolution.

The concepts of analog-to-digital (A/D) conversion, the Nyquist frequency (N_f) for determining minimal sampling rate, and signal averaging—each fundamental to AER measurement in general—were reviewed in Chapter 3. The primary objective in analysis of the ASSR is detection within a restricted spectral band surrounding the stimulus modulate rate (or frequency) of stimulus-related brain activity that is statistically higher in amplitude that background brain activity (EEG) in the same frequency region. Since even the faster stimulus modulation rates used in ASSR measurement are less than about 110 per second (an MF of < 110 Hz), relatively slow sampling rates of 1000 Hz (1K) or even 500 Hz (0.5 K) would appear to be adequate, as they are at least five to ten times the rate of stimulation. However, the carrier frequency—the frequency of the sinusoid that is modulated—is much higher (e.g., 500 Hz up to at least 4000 Hz) than the modulation frequency. Transducers used to evoke AERs invariably generate an electromagnetic field (see Chapter 3). The strength of the electromagnetic field is directly related to the proximity of the transducer to the recording electrodes and is influenced also by the orientation of electrode array with respect to the field and the type of transducer (greatest for a oscillator, less for supra-aural earphones, and least for insert earphones). An apparent ASSR, i.e., energy within the region of the modulation frequency, can be detected when the electromagnetic field produced by stimuli presented at high-intensity levels is sampled at an inadequately low rate. That is, the sampling rate is too slow to faithfully reflect the relatively high frequency of the signal. Instead, a lower frequency waveform is generated as some of the data points of the high-frequency waveform are sampled, whereas the rest are not. The resulting lower frequency signal is an incomplete and misleading measurement of the actual waveform. The stimulus artifact at a higher frequency, due to aliasing, appears as spectral energy near the modulation frequency. The alias frequency can be determined with a formula (National Instruments LabVIEW Measurement Manual, 2000; Small & Stapells, 2004):

Alias frequency = Sampling frequency – input frequency

Let's assume the carrier frequency in an ASSR assessment is a 500 Hz sinusoid modulated at a rate (frequency) of 80 Hz. As noted above, stimulus energy would be found at 500 Hz and at spectral lobes 80 Hz below and above 500 Hz (e.g., 420 and 580 Hz). A common sampling (A/D conversion) rate is 500 Hz. If each of these values is inserted into calculations with the equation (e.g., 500 Hz – 420 Hz = 80 Hz), one of the products is precisely the modulation frequency (80 Hz). Reduction of the likelihood of aliasing affecting ASSR measurement, including the possibility of incorrect detection of artifactual ASSRs, can be accomplished by increasing the sampling and A/D conversion rate. For example, if a sampling A/D conversion rate is selected at an appropriate Nyquist frequency (at least two times the signal frequency) relative to the carrier frequency (not the modulation frequency), then any possible aliasing artifact will appear within a frequency region well away from the modulation frequency. The reader is referred for more details on this important topic to reviews presented within published papers describing formal investigations of artifacts in ASSR measurement with air- and bone-conduction stimulation (e.g., Gorga et al., 2004; Picton & John, 2004, Small & Stapells, 2004).

Picton and John (2004) and Small and Stapells (2004) have verified experimentally the validity of this solution to the problem of aliasing in ASSR measurement with a research version of the MASTER system. In the study reported by Picton and John (2004), stimulus artifacts were intentionally created with 12 normal-hearing young adult subjects by presenting carrier tones by bone conduction at 50 dB HL and also via air conduction at intensity levels of 115 dB above hearing threshold with earphones on the neck. Picton and John (2004) investigated potential artifacts with an A/D conversion rate of 500 Hz and four different types of stimuli: a basic amplitude modulated (100%) sinusoid (SAM), the SAM stimulus inverted in polarity, an alternating polarity SAM stimulus, and "the fourth stimulus was composed of two tones separated by the required envelope frequency to form beats" (p. 544). The ASSR evoked by air-conduction stimuli was recorded in two conditions. In one condition, without ipsilateral masking, the subjects could hear the stimulus, and the response recorded was a combination of stimulus artifact and actual stimulus-evoked physiologic activity. In the other condition, only artifact was recorded because a masking noise of 50 dB was presented via insert earphones so the subjects could not hear the stimulus. The authors clearly demonstrated artifacts secondary to aliasing that affected measurement of ASSRs evoked by air-conduction stimulation at 90 dB HL and greater and bone-conduction stimulation at 30 dB HL and greater. There were examples of artifacts contaminating the recording of actual physiologic responses, that is, an ASSR was present but it was recorded in combination with (vector added to) artifact, and also apparent ASSR activity that was entirely due to artifact. Strategies employed to eliminate the possibility of artifacts included the use of anti-aliasing filters with steep slopes to process the electrical signal before A/D conversion, manipulating the A/D rate to avoid submultiples of the carrier frequencies and vice versa (changing the carrier frequencies so that they are not multiples of the rate of A/D conversion), minimizing current leakage and "cross talk" between the digital-to-analog and analog-to-digital circuits after amplification.

Small and Stapells (2004) examined the potential for artifacts affecting ASSR measurement in 17 adult subjects with severe-to-profound hearing loss who could not hear the air-conduction stimuli presented at 120 dB HL or the bone-conduction stimuli presented at 60 dB HL used to evoke the ASSR. In concurrence with John and Picton (2004) and others (Gorga et al., 2004; Jeng et al., 2004), Small and Stapells (2004) showed conclusively that high-intensity air- and bone-conduction stimuli can be associated with detection of activity that is inappropriately identified as ASSR—spurious ASSRs—in persons with hearing impairment who do not respond behaviorally to the stimuli. The authors found that alternating stimulus polarity by 180 degrees reduces markedly the likelihood of artifactual responses, and proper A/D sampling rates and EEG filter slopes and low-pass settings generally solved measurement problems related to aliasing. Interestingly, with a 500 Hz carrier stimulus frequency these steps failed to entirely eliminate "spurious ASSR." Small and Stapells (2004) speculate that the responses were indeed physiologic, but were generated from the vestibular versus the auditory system. One example of nonauditory responses elicited by high-intensity sounds—vestibular evoked myogenic potentials (VEMPs)— is reviewed in Chapter 15.

Gorga and colleagues (2004) at the Boys Town National Research Hospital also studied the issue of artifactual responses with the goal of determining the maximum stimulus intensity level for reliable measurement of the ASSR. Subjects were 10 adults (age 30 to 77 years) with profound hearing loss managed with cochlear implants. Cochlear implants were turned off, and none of the subjects had a behavioral response for the ASSR stimuli or for pure-tone stimuli. ASSR recordings were conducted with the MASTER system. In calibrating the stimulus intensity levels for the equipment with a specially built impedance network, the authors discovered that "ASSRs" were detected even when the electrodes were not connected to a subject. Background noise with the impedance network is, of course, much lower than that encountered in ASSR recordings from patients, enhancing the chances that a spurious ASSR would be detected. The authors conducted further investigation with human subjects to better assess the possibility of artifactual ASSR in clinical settings. Gorga et al. (2004), " . . . under conditions that presumably are the same as those used in the clinic" (p. 306), found apparent ASSRs for stimuli at 100 dB HL and higher intensities in subjects with no behavioral response to the same stimuli, concluding that the responses were due to measurement artifact.

In each of the published investigations of artifacts in ASSR measurement just reviewed, data were collected with the MASTER device, either a research version or the clinical instrumentation available from a manufacturer (Bio-Logic System Corp., Inc). The manufacturer has since modified the ASSR software to minimize the problem of artifacts in ASSR measurement. The next step in the process of assessing the validity of ASSR recordings evoked at high intensity levels for air- and bone-conduction stimulation is to verify the absence of artifactual responses in clinical populations (e.g., profound hearing loss) with the latest version of the equipment. There are no published reports of problems with artifact at high intensity levels for other ASSR devices. The author has applied one of the devices (the GSI Audera device) in assessment of hearing in children and adults with profound hearing loss, including patients subsequently undergoing cochlear implantation. The ASSR was regularly measured with AM and FM sinusoidal stimuli at frequencies from 500 to 8000 Hz, and occasionally also 250 and 8000 Hz, presented at intensity levels up to 120 dB HL. In no case were there examples of statistically verified responses, that is, phase coherent vector plots that met probability criteria (99.85%) for "phase locking."

Nonpathologic Factors

AGE: DEVELOPMENT IN CHILDREN. | The following review focuses on maturational changes in the ASSR. Estimation of auditory thresholds with the ASSR in infants and young children is reviewed in the next section of this chapter. Given the well-known time course for maturation of the central auditory nervous system from birth through at least the early teenage years, the caudal to rostral maturational gradient, and developmental effects on other auditory evoked responses, one would anticipate pronounced maturational changes with the ASSR, with complex and important interactions between age and stimulus parameters. Indeed, factors playing a role in developmental effects on the ASSR include, in addition to chronological age and intersubject variability, the intensity level and the mode of stimulation (air- versus bone-conduction), stimulus frequency, and the type of stimulus modulation (AM, FM, MM, and AM^2, or IAFM). Much of the published information on age and the ASSR is limited to the 40 Hz response and will not be reviewed here. The ASSR for fast stimulus modulation rates (e.g., around 80 Hz) used clinically in infants for hearing assessment is certainly present from birth (e.g., Lins et al., 1996; Rickards et al., 1994), but not yet adult-like. From the neonatal period to adulthood, amplitude of the ASSR for fast stimulus modulation frequencies more than doubles. For most carrier stimulus frequencies, phase of the ASSR remains relatively constant throughout childhood. There is some evidence that the low-frequency (e.g., 500 Hz) stimuli may be associated with a slightly earlier onset phase (approximately 90 degrees) although, once again, data are limited and small age-related changes in ASSR phase could easily be obscured by intersubject variability in ASSR measurements (e.g., Lins et al., 1996; Picton et al., 2003). However, the time schedule for development of the fast MF ASSR and the age at which it reaches maturation is not precisely known.

Cone-Wesson, Parker, Swiderski, and Rickards (2002) investigated detection of the ASSR in premature and full-term infants, all of whom passed hearing screening with ABR and otoacoustic emissions (TEOAE and DPOAE). Using stimulus intensity levels (e.g., approximately 50 to 60 dB SPL) adequate for detecting mild hearing loss, or greater, pass rates for an ASSR elicited with amplitude-modulated carrier tones were higher for full-term versus premature infants, and for a 2000 Hz versus 500 Hz stimulus.

John et al. (2004) described ASSRs evoked by these various types of stimulus modulations for a group of 70 normal hearing full-term infants. ASSRs were recorded within 74 hours after birth for 50 infants at gestational ages between 37 and 42 weeks and another group of 20 infants born at 36 to 42 weeks gestational age but undergoing ASSR measurement between 3 and 15 weeks after birth. As expected from investigations with adult subjects, ASSR amplitude was larger when evoked with MM (13% for the younger infants and 22% for the older infants) and AM^2 (16% for the younger group and 13% for the older group) sinusoidal stimuli in comparison to ASSRs evoked by AM stimuli. The authors acknowledge the slightly wider spectra of the MM and AM^2 stimuli, although frequency-specificity remained adequate for estimation of auditory thresholds. Importantly, however, the larger ASSR amplitudes and correspondingly larger SNRs with the more complex stimuli should contribute to shorter test time and, in theory, increased accuracy of threshold estimations. The study confirmed a clear age effect, even within the first few months after birth. As John et al. (2004) state, "The incidence of significant responses rose substantially when the infants were tested at the age of 1 to 3 months rather than within 3 days of birth. There were no differences in the EEG noise levels of the recordings of these two groups, but the responses became significantly larger in the older infants" (p. 549).

Stapells and colleagues (Small, Hatton, & Stapells, 2004) described clear differences in *bone-conduction* evoked ASSRs for infants versus adults, specifically lower (better) thresholds infants for low-frequency stimuli and lower thresholds for adults for high-frequency stimuli. Systematic investigation of development effects on the ASSR is clearly needed, particularly with instrumentation used already clinically.

AGE: ADVANCING AGE IN ADULTS. | Advancing age does not appear to have a major influence on ASSR phase or amplitude (e.g., Picton et al., 2003), even for the 40 Hz response. As Picton et al. (2003) note, however, considerable intersubject variability could make it difficult to detect modest age effects in various ASSR parameters.

GENDER. | John and Picton (2000) reported a subtle trend toward shorter ASSR latency (0.78 ms) for female (N = 16)

than male (N = 18) subjects, but a high degree of intersubject variability may have obscured clear differences.

ATTENTION, STATE OF AROUSAL, AND SLEEP. | The pronounced effect of sleep on the 40 Hz ASSR, is one of the main reasons why the response never gained widespread pediatric use as a clinical measure of auditory function. Attention and state of arousal may also influence the 40 Hz ASSR. Sleep is certainly a factor in ASSR measurement for other relatively slow stimulus modulation frequencies (< 70 Hz), and especially for rates lower than 50 Hz. Recall from Chapter 3 that the ASSR for slower modulation rates is generated mostly in cortical auditory regions. Sleep has a minimal effect on the ASSR elicited with fast stimulus modulation rates (> 70 Hz) in children and adults (e.g., Cohen et al., 1991; Levi et al., 1993; Lins & Picton, 1995), although even in adults there appear to be intersubject differences in the effect of sleep on the fast MF ASSR (Purcell, John, Schneider, & Picton, 2004). There are no formal investigations of the possible effects of attention and state of arousal on the ASSR for fast stimulus modulation rates.

Clinical Applications and Populations

The leap from auditory evoked recordings in the predictable laboratory setting with unequivocally normal and cooperative subjects to the clinical environment with patients presenting with diverse, and often undiagnosed, peripheral and central auditory dysfunction is large and fraught will unknown variables and sources of measurement error. Clinical experience has shown that correlations among pure-tone thresholds, estimations of auditory thresholds with the tone-burst ABR technique, and ASSR estimations of auditory thresholds are reasonably close on the average, but rather poor for occasional individual patients. Picton et al. (2004) raise the important issue of terminology used in discussion of the relations among findings for behavioral and electrophysiologic auditory measures. In their words,

> We suggest "physiologic thresholds" to describe the lowest intensity at which an auditory steady-state response is recognized, and "predicted behavioral thresholds" if one is predicting behavioral thresholds from physiologic thresholds. Predicted behavioral thresholds would have to be further qualified, since the prediction could derive from a regression equation or from a simple subtraction of the mean difference between physiologic and behavioral thresholds" (Picton et al., 2003, p. 206)

Perhaps most disconcerting is recent evidence of false (artifact-related) ASSRs for air-conduction stimuli in persons with no behavioral response to sound (e.g., Gorga et al., 2004; Picton & John, 2004; Small & Stapells, 2004) and for bone-conducted stimuli at moderate (e.g., 50 dB HL) intensity levels (Jeng et al., 2004; Small & Stapells, 2005). As reviewed in Chapter 15, a vestibular evoked myogenic potential (VEMP) can be recorded from the sterno-cleido-mastoid muscle with very high intensity acoustic stimulation. After modifying the technique for stimulation and analysis of the ASSR to minimize the likelihood of recording artifacts rather than true responses, Small and Stapells (2004) still detected in some persons with profound hearing loss ASSRs evoked by high-intensity, low-frequency (500 and 1000 Hz) sinusoidal stimuli. These authors considered the possibility that the apparent ASSR was, in reality, a true physiologic response generated by the vestibular system, rather than the auditory system.

Therefore, despite the already substantial and still growing clinical literature on the ASSR, particularly on the topic of estimating auditory thresholds in children, much remains unknown. Stapells and colleagues (2005) state this point concisely: "Having gone through the literature on ASSR thresholds to air-conduction stimuli, one must conclude that the clinical database is very small and therefore *preliminary* [author's italics]" (p. 13).

AUDITORY THRESHOLD ESTIMATION: ADULTS. | The most obvious clinical application of the ASSR is estimation of auditory thresholds in infants and young children, when behavioral audiometry cannot provide valid and/or reliable information on hearing. However, as evidenced by the number of publications in the literature, many initial experiences with ASSR as an objective measure of auditory sensitivity in clinical practice and in research laboratories were acquired in adult populations (N of 10 up to 60), including normal hearers (e.g., Aoyagi et al., 1994; Dimitrijevic et al., 2002; Herdman & Stapells, 2001; Lins et al., 1996; Perez-Abalo et al., 2001; Picton et al., 1998) and adults with hearing impairment (e.g., Dimitrijevic et al., 2002; Herdman & Stapells, 2003; Picton et al., 1998; Rance et al., 1998; Rance et al., 1995; Schmulian, Swanepoel, & Hugo, 2005; Vander Werff & Brown, 2005). Stimuli among studies include stimuli with amplitude modulation or mixed modulation (amplitude and frequency). The published studies include some reporting ASSR analysis based primarily on phase coherence and others that relied on an F-test of the ASSR spectra.

One explanation for the early exploration of ASSRs in adults is readily apparent. Adult patients are generally capable of performing behavioral audiometry and, therefore, offer the opportunity for comparison of ASSR estimations of auditory sensitivity with valid pure-tone thresholds. The results of behavioral hearing assessments are, of course, not always reliable or accurate in adults. Definition of the degree of hearing loss at audiometric frequencies is a common challenge among patients who have some type of nonorganic hearing impairment, e.g., malingering, pseudohypacusis, and psychogenic or functional hearing loss.

A substantial number of papers (listed above) describe encouraging findings on the accuracy of ASSR estimations of hearing threshold in adults. Picton et al. (2003) and Herdman and Stapells (2003) have published comprehensive reviews of the literature. For adults with sensory hearing loss,

the agreement between pure-tone thresholds, as defined by statistical correlation, is approximately 0.8 to 0.9 for higher frequency stimuli (1000 to 4000 Hz) and slightly poorer (0.7 to 0.8) for a 500 Hz stimulus. The slope of high-frequency sensory hearing loss is approximated with the ASSR, with correlations between ASSR and behavioral thresholds holding up even for varying audiometric configurations, including steeply sloping patterns (e.g., Herdman & Stapells, 2003; Vander Werff & Brown, 2005). Furthermore, these studies provide evidence that the average discrepancy between ASSR and behavioral thresholds (again for sensory hearing loss) is reasonably close, i.e., 6 to 7 dB for frequencies of 1000 to 4000 Hz and about 10 dB for 500 Hz. However, among other studies comparing behavioral versus ASSR estimated thresholds in adults with hearing loss, the mean difference for the physiologic minus behavioral threshold estimation ranges from a minimum of 3 dB to over 25 dB, and the value for one standard deviation is on the order of 9 to 13 dB. Configuration of sensory hearing loss in adults does not influence accuracy of hearing threshold estimation with ASSR (e.g., Schmulian, Swanepoel, & Hugo, 2005). As a rule, particularly among the earlier studies, the estimations of behavioral thresholds with ASSR were more accurate for hearing-impaired subjects than normal hearers, with accuracy increasing as a function of the degree of hearing loss. Indeed, least accurate estimations of auditory thresholds with ASSR are reported for normal-hearing subjects and, especially, for a 500 Hz carrier frequency (Cone-Wesson et al., 2002; Lins et al., 1996; Perez-Abalo et al., 2001; Picton et al., 2001; Rance & Rickards, 2002; Rance et al., 1995; Swanepoel, Schmulian, & Hugo, 2004; Schmulian, Swanepoel, & Hugo, 2005; Vander Werff & Brown, 2005). In general, ABR recordings near auditory threshold are the product of signal averaging for 2000 or more stimuli, whereas less signal averaging is employed in ASSR measurement. It is reasonable, therefore, to speculate on the possibility of improved accuracy for ASSR estimation of auditory thresholds with markedly more signal averaging. Accuracy in the estimation of normal auditory thresholds with the ASSR seems to increase directly with recording time (e.g., Herdman & Stapells, 2001; Perez-Abalo et al., 2001; Swanepoel, Schmulian, & Hugo, 2004), probably reflecting the effect of continued averaging on the signal-to-noise ratio and detection of the ASSR. Unfortunately, for clinical application of the ASSR in unselected patient populations, behavioral threshold even in cooperative normal-hearing adults appears to be regularly overestimated on the average by 20 to 30 dB at 500 Hz, 15 to 20 dB for 1000 Hz, and 10 to 15 dB for higher frequencies, even when ASSR data are recorded in a sound-treated booth. Errors in agreement between behavioral thresholds and detection levels for the ASSR tend to be skewed to overestimation of hearing loss (e.g., Vander Werff & Brown, 2005). Since standard deviations for the difference between behavioral and ASSR thresholds are on the order of 10 dB, normal-hearing subjects not infrequently yield ASSRs at stimulus intensity levels no better than 45 dB HL. Put another way, and from the clinician's perspective, the ASSR does not consistently permit differentiation of children with mild hearing loss that may require amplification versus those with perfectly normal hearing sensitivity. In a tertiary audiology setting, especially when auditory electrophysiologic techniques are used to confirm and define hearing loss in infants failing hearing screenings, normal hearing status is ultimately confirmed for the majority of patients. An inability to consistently differentiate with ASSR between normal hearing and mild hearing sensitivity loss would preclude prompt and confident decisions regarding audiologic management for infants.

The relation between ABR and ASSR thresholds is close, with mean differences of less than 5 dB, according to most studies. As noted above, the ASSR offers a clear clinical advantage over ABR in patients with suspected severe-to-profound hearing loss, namely, the possibility for stimulus intensity levels well above the upper limit for transient stimulus intensity level (80 to 90 dB nHL). However, as cited elsewhere in the chapter, concerns were raised recently about the possibility in patients with profound sensory hearing loss of apparent ASSRs that were really measurement artifacts at high air- and bone-conduction stimulus intensity levels. Another lingering question is whether the ASSR is as accurate in predicting auditory thresholds in conductive hearing loss as in sensory hearing loss. The author discovered with early experience in recording the ASSR from adult graduate students (Hall, 2003) a tendency for the ASSR to overestimate thresholds in simulated conductive loss (e.g., produced by occluding insert earphone tubing with cotton). This observation is supported by published experimental evidence, albeit rather limited (Dimitrijevic et al., 2002; Jeng et al., 2004). Data are lacking for series of patients with conductive hearing loss secondary to middle ear disorders, and further formal investigation is warranted. However, anecdotal case reports reveal an apparent discrepancy between estimations of auditory thresholds with the ASSR versus behavioral audiometry, with the former overestimating the latter. Systematic investigation with multiple clinical devices is required to better define accuracy of the ASSR technique in estimating auditory threshold in patients with middle ear disease and associated conductive hearing loss.

Dimitrijevic, John, and Picton (2004) investigated the ASSR in young normal-hearing subjects and 20 older subjects (age 57 to 86 years) with hearing ranging from normal (average hearing levels for 500, 1000, and 2000 Hz less than 25 dB HL) to varying degrees of sensorineural hearing impairment. The main purpose of the study was to assess the relation between the ASSR elicited by independent amplitude and frequency modulated (IAFM) sinusoidal stimuli and word recognition scores (WRS). The sinusoidal IAFM stimuli were manipulated in an attempt to approximate human speech, specifically consonant-vowel (CV) signals, vowel-vowel signals, and fricative phonemes. Properties

of speech were modeled by overall stimulus intensity, carrier frequencies within the speech spectrum, intensity levels among the different frequencies, depth of frequency and amplitude modulation, and the modulation frequencies. Details of the stimuli used in the study are provided in an appendix to the article. In the words of the authors, "The general idea behind using multiple IAFM to predict WRS is that speech contains acoustic information that varies rapidly in intensity and frequency" (Dimitrijevic, John, & Picton, 2004, p. 80). Word recognition in quiet was assessed with W-22 and NU-6 50-word lists presented via two free-field sound speakers at 70 dB SPL. Hearing in the nontest ear was eliminated with the use of earplugs. The authors also described effects of amplification on the ASSR for a subgroup of the hearing-impaired subjects. Consistent with their previous reports (e.g., Dimitrijevic et al., 2001; Picton et al., 2003), the authors found a significant relation between the ASSR for an 80 Hz MF and word recognition scores for normal hearers (correlation coefficient of 0.73) and the hearing-impaired group (correlation coefficient of 0.65). The correlation between word recognition score and the ASSR evoked with 40 Hz IAFM stimuli was slightly lower. However, assessment of the ASSRs for stimulus modulation frequencies of 40 Hz and 80 Hz in combination yielded the highest correlation with word recognition scores, perhaps according to the authors because the resulting ASSRs reflected function of auditory system at levels of the brainstem and cortex.

Using the Audera™ device in a study of a small number (N = 10) of adults with hearing impairment, Johnson and Brown (2001) confirmed agreement between ABR and ASSR thresholds, and also the advantage of the ASSR in estimating auditory thresholds within the severe-to-profound range of loss. In addition to examining the accuracy of estimations of behavioral auditory thresholds with the ASSR, Vander Werff and Brown (2005) investigated in a small group of adult subjects with varying degrees of hearing loss the potential clinical usefulness of intensity-amplitude growth functions for the ASSR. There were three categories of hearing status with 10 subjects in each: normal hearing (thresholds of < 15 dB HL), flat hearing loss (moderate-to-severe with no more than 15 dB HL difference among frequencies), and sloping hearing loss of 40 to 75 dB in high frequencies with at least a 25 dB/octave decrease between 1000 and 2000 Hz. Citing the lengthy test time required for actual threshold estimation with multiple-stimulus frequencies presented simultaneously, the authors reasoned that it might be possible to predict auditory threshold more efficiently by predicting ASSR threshold from more robust responses evoked at higher (supra) threshold levels. However, Vander Werff and Brown (2005) concluded that "the form of the ASSR amplitude growth function did not distinguish between the two configurations of hearing loss, and attempts to predict behavioral thresholds from the amplitude growth function were unsuccessful. . . ." (p. 319).

AUDITORY THRESHOLD ESTIMATION: CHILDREN. | As an electrophysiologic measure like the ABR, the ASSR offers an opportunity for estimation of auditory thresholds in infants and young children who cannot be properly assessed with behavioral audiometry techniques. The ASSR provides a distinct edge over behavioral audiometry, and in several respects even the ABR, in this clinically challenging patient population. One strong feature of the ASSR, in comparison to the ABR, that must be reiterated is the capacity for defining severe-to-profound hearing loss—that is, estimating hearing thresholds within the range of 80 to 120 dB. The limitation of ABR in defining the degree of severe-to-profound hearing loss (> 90 dB HL) is well appreciated by clinicians and well documented in the literature. As noted by Brookhauser, Gorga, and Kelly (1990), "The absence of a click-evoked ABR does not indicate that benefit cannot be obtained from the use of conventional amplification" (p. 807) and, furthermore, "As a consequence, the clinician confronted with a severely to profoundly deaf young child must often make an initial determination regarding the most appropriate rehabilitative strategy with less-than-complete information" (p. 809). Unfortunately, differences in stimulation and analysis approaches and algorithms among clinical ASSR instruments influence auditory threshold estimations and perhaps other response parameters. Other important measurement factors also probably affected the accuracy of hearing threshold estimations, among them the level of acoustic noise in the test setting and the age of subjects. Consequently, a clear picture of the clinical value and role of ASSR in pediatric audiology has not yet formed.

A handful of published papers describe estimation of auditory thresholds with ABR and ASSR in infants and young children including those with normal hearing and those with hearing impairment (Aoyagi et al., 1999; Cone-Wesson et al., 2002; Firszt et al., 2004; Han et al., 2005; Levi et al., 1993; Lins et al., 1996; Luts et al., 2004; Perez-Abalo et al., 2001; Rance & Briggs, 2002; Rance et al., 1998; Rance & Rickards, 2002; Rance et al., 2005; Rance et al., 1995; Rickards et al., 1994; Roberson, O'Rourke, & Stidham, 2003; Stueve & O'Rourke, 2003; Swanepoel, Hugo, & Roode, 2004; Vander Werff et al., 2002). Among some published studies, ASSR thresholds for tonal stimuli, or an average of ASSR thresholds for more than one tonal stimulus, are compared to the ABR elicited with non-frequency-specific click stimuli. Evidence generally supports good agreement in detection thresholds for ABR and ASSR. For example, in a study of 32 children (ranging in age from 2 months to 3 years) with undefined behavioral hearing thresholds, Vander Werff et al. (2002) reported a correlation between ASSR and tone-burst ABR thresholds of 0.86 at a 500 Hz stimulus frequency, and up to 0.97 for frequencies within the 2000 and 4000 Hz region. Stueve and O'Rourke (2003) reported for 144 ears among children with sensory hearing impairment a correlation coefficient of 0.79 for a 500 Hz tone-burst ABR and an ASSR evoked also by a 500 Hz signal. Other authors

confirm the relatively close relation between ASSR and ABR thresholds in pediatric populations (e.g., Dimitrijevic et al., 2002; Perez-Abalo et al., 2001). Another rather consistent finding is the possibility of recording a statistically confirmed ASSR from patients lacking a detectable ABR. The proportion of children with hearing impairment with an ASSR, yet no ABR at intensity limits for click or tone-burst stimuli, was reported as 77 percent by Stueve & O'Rourke (2003) and over 90 percent by Swanepoel and Hugo (2004). There are no published examples of the opposite pattern in sensory hearing loss, that is, the presence of an ABR for patients with no ASSR.

Fewer authors describe the relation between the ASSR and behavioral thresholds (Cone-Wesson et al., 2002; Firszt et al., 2004; Luts et al., 2004; Rance & Briggs, 2002; Rance & Rickards, 2002; Rance et al., 2005; Stueve & O'Rourke, 2003; Swanepoel, Hugo, & Roode, 2004; Vander Werff et al., 2002). Rance and Rickard (2002) studied the relation between behavioral and ASSR estimations of auditory thresholds for 211 infants aged 1 to 8 months. None of the subjects had middle ear dysfunction. Correlations between behavioral thresholds and the ASSR were high (Pearson product-moment correlation values of 0.96 to 0.98). Errors in prediction of behavioral hearing thresholds with ASSR were largest for normal-hearing subjects. Stueve and O'Rourke (2003) report correlations of 0.82 to 0.90 between ASSR minimum response levels and behavioral thresholds for frequencies of 500 to 4000 Hz. According to the authors, ASSR thresholds were within ± 20 dB of behavioral thresholds for at least 72 percent of the subjects (with closer agreement for higher frequencies). Swanepoel, Hugo, and Roode (2004) report smaller average differences between behavioral hearing thresholds and ASSR (6 dB for 500 Hz and 4 dB for 1000, 2000, and 4000 Hz, but correlations between ASSR and behavioral auditory thresholds are lower (in the range of 0.58 to 0.74) than those in the study by Stueve and O'Rourke (2003). Consistent with findings summarized above for adult subjects, the discrepancies between behavioral thresholds and threshold estimations with the ASSR are most pronounced for normal-hearing infants, particularly for ASSRs evoked with a carrier frequency of 500 Hz (e.g., Rance & Rickards, 2002). Of course, one could also take the "cup is half empty" perspective and conclude that discrepancies exceeding 20 dB in the estimation of behavioral thresholds with ASSR exist for about 25 percent of the subjects. Clinicians attempting to apply the ASSR in fitting hearing aids on infants might not be comforted by the likelihood of serious over- or underamplification in one out of four children. Most data, however, were obtained from children with normal hearing or severe-to-profound hearing loss, as few subjects had hearing loss within the 30 to 80 dB range. Consensus is clearly lacking on the relationship between ASSR and actual hearing thresholds due to limited data and serious inconsistencies among studies in methodology. Some methodological weaknesses are understandable—that is, the difficulty of establishing a "behavioral gold-standard" for frequency-specific hearing thresholds in samples of infants who are too young to volunteer valid and reliable behavioral responses or comparison of ASSR findings with those obtained for behavioral audiometry weeks or even months later. Other discrepancies among studies include small sample sizes (e.g., as few as 10 subjects), different statistical measures of calculating correlation (e.g., parametric versus nonparametric), reliance on ABR thresholds estimated only with broad spectrum (not frequency-specific) clicks or clicks plus 500 Hz tone-bursts at limited maximum intensity levels, the use of questionable measurement parameters for tone-burst stimulation of the ABR in infants, differences is the approach taken for dealing with cases with no response at stimulus intensity limits (e.g., eliminating the cases from analysis or assigning an arbitrary threshold), and very few subjects in certain hearing loss groups (e.g., mild and moderate).

Rance et al. (1995, 1998) were among the first investigators to point out the value of ASSR in estimating auditory thresholds for severely hearing impaired patients with no detectable ABR at maximum transient stimulus intensity levels. Indeed, correlations between ASSR and behavioral thresholds generally increase directly with the degree of hearing loss, while differences between behavioral and electrophysiologic thresholds decrease to as little as 3 dB (e.g., Rance et al., 1995; Swanepoel & Hugo, 2004). Stimulus intensity level is limited to about 90 dB nHL for clicks and tone bursts used to evoked the ABR (Hall, 1992). Since the ASSR is elicited by steady-state (sinusoid) signals with maximum intensity levels of 120 dB HL or higher, it is the technique of choice for obtaining vital information on auditory sensitivity required for definition of candidacy for cochlear implantation. Rance et al. (1998) analyzed retrospectively ASSR data for 108 infants and young children (aged 1 to 49 months) with sensorineural hearing impairment as documented by behavioral audiometry. The ASSR was elicited with sinusoids of 500, 1000, 2000, and 4000 Hz, each amplitude-modulated at 90 Hz and delivered via supra-aural earphones. None of the subjects yielded an ABR at maximum intensity levels (100 dB nHL) for a click stimulus. Rance et al. (1998) also noted a relationship between ASSR findings and aided behavioral auditory thresholds. That is, the likelihood of a behavioral hearing threshold of < 60 dB SPL was predicted by the detection of an ASSR, whereas children who yielded no ASSR at equipment stimulus intensity limits rarely showed benefit from amplification.

Cone-Wesson et al. (2002) examined the relation between auditory thresholds estimated behaviorally with ABR elicited with clicks and ASSR elicited with 90 Hz modulated carrier frequencies for 16 children with normal hearing or mild hearing loss (< 40 dB HL), 18 with moderate hearing loss (45 to 75 dB HL), and 17 with severe-to-profound hearing loss (> 75 dB HL) with an average age of 16 months (mean age of 9 months). The authors reported that 31 children had sensorineural hearing loss and 10 with conductive

hearing loss, with the remaining subjects with mixed hearing loss or normal hearing. The correlation between behavioral thresholds and auditory evoked responses was comparable for the click-evoked ABR and ASSR elicited by 1000, 2000, and 4000 Hz, whereas the relation was slightly closer for the behavioral threshold and ASSR threshold at 500 Hz.

Swanepoel and Hugo (2004) also emphasize the critical role of the ASSR in defining for infants and young children hearing sensitivity in the severe-to-profound range. Using sinusoidal stimuli at intensity levels of 120 dB HL (500 Hz) up to 128 dB HL (1000 Hz), the authors report that an ASSR was present in 63 percent of the subjects at 500 Hz, 80 percent at 1000 Hz, 83 percent at 2000 Hz, and 70 percent at 4000 Hz. Fully 90 percent of the patients yielded ASSRs for stimulus intensity levels exceeding 90 dB HL, that is, outside of the intensity range for recording an ABR. Looking at these figures from another perspective, between about one-fourth and one-third of the children had no detectable ASSR even at maximum stimulus intensity levels.

There is at this time no established normative database for ASSR thresholds appropriate for use with various clinical devices. In fact, as John, Brown, Muir, and Picton (2004) report in a comprehensive paper on ASSR in infants, which includes a review of the literature, threshold levels in normal subjects vary widely among published studies and among stimulus frequencies. For examples, among studies thresholds for a 2000 Hz stimulus range from a minimum of 17 dB HL up to 51 dB HL, and for a 500 Hz stimulus ASSR thresholds range from 33 dB HL to 57 dB HL. The standard deviation for thresholds estimated with ABR and ASSR, for example, is often on the order of 15 dB or greater, revealing considerable intersubject variability and inaccuracy in findings. Unfortunately, if the possibility of the magnitude of error in threshold estimation in a normal infant is as high as 60 dB or greater, then it is not possible to make confident decisions on whether amplification is even indicated. Once a hearing loss is identified, decisions on the implementation of amplification must be made within months after birth. Delaying intervention beyond six months because estimations of auditory thresholds are uncertain has a very serious adverse impact on the child's communicative outcome. On the other hand, providing amplification within a specific frequency when hearing is really normal poses the risk of iatrogenic hearing loss, i.e., noise induced by management with amplification, and may, ironically, interfere with normal speech and language acquisition. Clearly, the possibility of errors as large as 60 dB in estimating behavioral threshold severely limits the usefulness of ASSR in providing the data on threshold estimation required for accurate prescriptive hearing aid fittings. As Stapells et al. (2005) point out, "mean and median normative thresholds are of interest, but they do not directly establish the criterion for 'normal' for clinical testing. Whereas the mean threshold is closer to the level were 50% of normal infants demonstrate a response, to establish criterion levels for 'normal' at least 90–95% of infants should show a response at that level" (p. 11). With these guidelines and based on available published normative data, even under good recording conditions (low ambient acoustic noise in a quiet patient), criteria for normal are as high as 60 dB HL for low-frequency stimuli (e.g., 500 Hz) and 50 dB HL for higher stimulus frequencies. Thus, confident differentiation of patients with normal hearing versus mild and even moderate degrees of hearing loss would appear to be problematic.

Luts et al. (2004) were able to define auditory thresholds at 1000, 2000, and 4000 Hz for 95 percent of both ears for a small group of infants (N = 10) between the ages of 3 and 14 months. In contrast, thresholds could be estimated with ABR for only 60 percent of the ears. Even at an average of five months later, behavioral audiometry yielded frequency-specific threshold estimations for barely half (51%) of the children. As noted by Swanepoel, Hugo, and Roode (2004), "Because the ASSR allows for better hearing aid fittings, resulting in true hearing aid trials, and absent ASSR thresholds predict poor hearing aid benefit, the ASSR is uniquely suited, above the ABR, to assist in the assessment of young children for cochlear implantation" (p. 534).

In a study of 200 children with moderate-to-profound sensorineural hearing loss, Rance and Briggs (2002) found a strong relation (Pearson r correlations of 0.81 to 0.93) between behavioral and ASSR thresholds. Then, expanding the number of subjects, Rance and Australian colleagues (Rance et al., 2005) conducted a retrospective multi-site investigation of ASSR estimation of hearing thresholds for a large infant population (N = 575 subjects and 1091 ears). Subjects included 285 with normal hearing, 271 with sensorineural hearing loss, and 19 with audiologic findings consistent with auditory neuropathy. ASSR findings obtained during infancy (within the first three months after birth) with the GSI Audera device were related to reliable behavioral hearing thresholds acquired with visual reinforcement audiometry from children between the ages of 6 to 23 months (average of 9.8 months). Stimuli for behavioral audiometry were warbled tones at octave frequencies of 500 to 4000 Hz presented for intensity levels up to 120 dB HL. Rance et al. (2005) confirmed with their sizable patient population the following four general findings reported also by others in clinical studies with modest numbers of infants. First, correlations between behavioral hearing thresholds and ASSR threshold estimations were consistently high (Pearson product moment correlations of 0.96 to 0.98) for stimulus frequencies of 500 to 4000 Hz. Second, the relation between hearing thresholds and ASSR was markedly poorer for children with the diagnosis of auditory neuropathy (Pearson product moment correlations of 0.46 to 0.55). Third, for normal-hearing infants (conditioned hearing thresholds < 15 dB HL), estimations of threshold with the ASSR (ranging from 24.3 to 32.5 dB HL) were usually higher than actual hearing thresholds, i.e., the ASSR overestimated hearing levels. Finally, accuracy of hearing threshold estimation with the ASSR improved with

the degree of hearing loss. Rance et al. (2005) point out that "the ASSR thresholds for the normal hearing cohort in this [their] investigation were significantly higher than those reported for the tone-burst auditory brainstem response (TB-ABR) technique" (p. 298). Furthermore, based on the data reported in the paper, the ASSR "cannot reliably differentiate between normal ears and those with mildly elevated hearing levels" (p. 298).

SENSORINEURAL HEARING LOSS. | In an examination of ASSR amplitude in adult subjects as a function of stimulus intensity in dB sensation level (SL), Dimitrijevic et al. (2002) found larger amplitudes for subjects with sensorineural hearing loss than normal hearers. Some of these authors (Dimitrijevic, John, & Picton, 2004) also described the effects of sensorineural hearing loss on the ASSR for a modest number of elderly subjects. Amplitude of the ASSR elicited by fast stimulus modulation rates (e.g., 80 Hz) was smaller in elderly hearing-impaired subjects than in normal-hearing young or elderly subjects. According to the authors, "This is probably related to decreased frequency resolution associated with hearing loss" (Dimitrijevic, John, & Picton, 2004, p. 79). The possible influence of age as a factor in these findings could not be assessed as there were no young hearing impaired subjects enrolled in the study.

In one of the conditions in the study on the ASSR and word recognition scores by Dimitrijevic, John, and Picton (2004), the ASSR was recorded from hearing-impaired elderly subjects with "spectrally shaped speech noise" presented at 70 dB SPL to the same ear as the IAFM stimulus. Elderly subjects with hearing loss showed poorer word recognition scores than elderly subjects with essentially normal hearing and young normal hearers. However, the effect of ipsilateral masking noise on the ASSR for IAFM stimuli was equivalent for young and old subjects, including older subjects with hearing loss.

AUDITORY NEUROPATHY. | The ASSR is not useful for estimating auditory thresholds in patients meeting criteria for the diagnosis of auditory neuropathy. In many cases of auditory neuropathy, no ASSR is detected under any stimulus or measurement conditions. Based on the findings of formal investigation of 20 infants and young children with repeatable cochlear microphonic (CM) and absent click-evoked ABRs, Rance et al. (1999) conclude, "the high rate SSEP [ASSR] appears to have little or no predictive value for hearing levels in children with AN [auditory neuropathy]" (p. 248). It appears that the disruption of neural synchrony in auditory neuropathy that adversely affects generation of the ABR also interferes with the capacity of auditory neurons to consistently lock into the phase of the amplitude and frequency modulated sinusoidal stimulus. Overall accuracy of the estimation of auditory thresholds with the ASSR as a function of the degree of hearing threshold level, and in

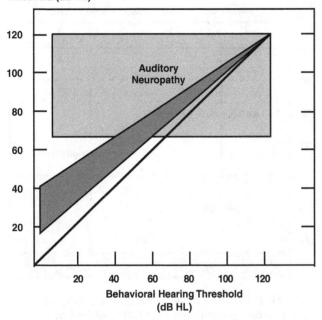

General Relation of Thresholds for ASSR and Behavioral Audiometry in Infancy

FIGURE 8.18. Estimation of auditory thresholds with the auditory steady-state response (ASSR) for patients with sensory hearing loss versus auditory neuropathy. Accuracy of threshold prediction increases directly with the degree of sensory hearing loss. Hearing thresholds cannot be predicted for auditory neuropathy.

auditory neuropathy, is shown schematically in Figure 8.18. In normal hearers, the ASSR has a tendency to overestimate hearing threshold. Accuracy of the ASSR in predicting hearing threshold as defined by pure-tone audiometry increases directly with the degree of sensory hearing loss. For patients with auditory neuropathy, however, the relation between ASSR and pure-tone threshold is unpredictable. No published data exist on the estimation of pure-tone thresholds by ASSR in conductive hearing loss. Anecdotal case reports, however, suggest the possibility of marked overestimation errors for the ASSR in conductive hearing loss.

HEARING AIDS. | One promising application of the ASSR evoked by stimuli presented in the sound field via speakers is objective confirmation of hearing aid gain (Picton et al., 1998). Earlier attempts to apply electrophysiologic auditory measures, e.g., the ABR, in objective estimation of the acoustic benefit of amplification were largely unsuccessful because of limitations of hearing aids in processing with a high degree of fidelity the transient stimuli required to evoke the response. Dimitrijevic, John, and Picton (2004) reported for their group of 10 hearing-impaired elderly subjects that

number of significant ASSRs evoked by IAFM stimuli at an intensity level of 70 dB SPL increased with amplification. Also, amplitude for ASSRs evoked with the 80 Hz modulation-frequency stimulus were larger, especially for lower frequency carrier frequencies. The authors note that "At the present time the presence or absence of a response seems to be a more reliable indicator of the benefits of amplification than response amplitudes" (Dimitrijevic, John, & Picton, 2004, p. 80).

COCHLEAR IMPLANTS. | For infants and young children, information from audiologic assessment with the ASSR can facilitate and speed up decisions regarding cochlear implantation (Firszt et al., 2004; Rance et al., 1998; Roberson, O'Rourke, & Stidham, 2003), as well as amplification. For children with no ABR at maximum stimulus limits (> 80 dB nHL), the ASSR differentiates among those with residual hearing who might benefit from hearing aids versus those with no response to tonal stimuli up to 120 dB HL or higher. Most of the latter cases are best managed as soon as feasible with cochlear implants. In the author's experience, the availability of ASSR permits the early identification of infants and young children who are likely to be candidates for cochlear implants. Confirmation of potential candidacy for cochlear implantation in infancy is well appreciated by parents and others entrusted with management of the child's aural habilitation, including audiologists and otolaryngologists.

AUDITORY PROCESSING. | Although the focus of clinical interest and investigation to date, the objective estimation of auditory thresholds is, of course, not the only clinical application of the ASSR. As noted above, manipulation of acoustic stimuli with AM or FM has been applied in psychoacoustic investigations of auditory perception. The ASSR has promise as a suprathreshold measure auditory processing of temporal and spectral features of sound. Test paradigms include calculation of ASSR amplitude elicited by stimuli at a fixed suprathreshold intensity level, yet at varying rates of amplitude or frequency modulation, or with systematic decreases in the amount of modulation until the difference limen or "just noticeable difference" for detection of the modulation is evidenced by a change in the ASSR (e.g., John, Dimitrijevic, Van Roon, & Picton, 2001). Or, as suggested by Dimitrijevic, John, Van Roon, and Picton (2001), "another approach would be to present a set of stimuli with multiple modulations in amplitude and frequency and to determine how many of these modulations are detected by the auditory system. This could provide a measurement of how much information is available to be used for speech perception" (p. 101). As an electrophysiologic measure of temporal and spectral auditory processing, the ASSR offers the additional advantage of feasibility in very young children and others whose ability to volunteer valid behavioral responses is compromised.

Complementary Roles of ABR and ASSR in Clinical Audiology Today

The ABR and ASSR each contribute importantly to the pediatric audiologic test battery. In discussing the ABR and the ASSR, Cone-Wesson et al. (2002) pose a question perhaps asked by many clinicians: "Can we determine which is the 'better' technique?" (p. 185). In defining the most effective role of ASSRs in the audiologic test battery, we would probably be better guided not by the question, "Which procedure is better—ABR or ASSR?" but, instead, "How can I best exploit both ABR and ASSR clinically in the electrophysiologic assessment of auditory function?" In other words, the relationship between the two techniques is not competitive but, rather, complementary. The clinical strengths and weakness of the ABR and ASSR techniques for assessment of different types of hearing loss are summarized in Table 8.9. Clinical experience with these techniques in pediatric assessment suggests that the ABR is most useful in the differentiation of types of auditory dysfunction, whereas the ASSR is uniquely valuable in estimating auditory thresholds in infants and young children with moderate to profound sensory hearing loss. This latter advantage is perhaps the most important for ASSR in comparison to the ABR. As shown in Figure 8.19, the upper limit for intensity of transient click and tone-burst stimuli used to evoke the ABR is approximately 80 dB nHL. In contrast, the ASSR is evoked by amplitude or frequency-modulated sinusoidal stimuli with maximum intensity levels of up to 120 dB HL or higher. This observation forms the basis for the approach to incorporating the ASSR technique into the audiologic assessment of infants that is illustrated in Figure 8.20. The diagnostic audiologic follow-up to an infant hearing screening failure begins with a simple click ABR. If the findings are entirely normal (i.e., a reliable wave V at 20 dB nHL and a normal wave I to V latency interval), then either tone-burst ABR or OAEs can be used to confirm normal peripheral auditory function. A

Stimulus Intensity Limits of ABR versus ASSR in Estimating Auditory Thresholds

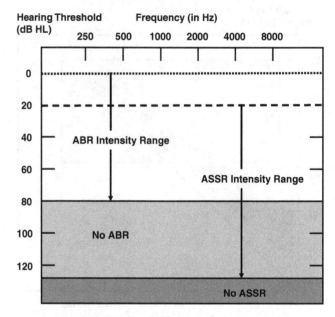

FIGURE 8.19. The range of stimulus intensity for the auditory brainstem response (ABR) elicited by transient (click and tone-burst) stimuli and for the ASSR with sinusoidal stimuli modulated in amplitude and/or frequency.

finding of delayed ABR wave I latency with a click signal suggests the likelihood of a conductive hearing loss and ABR measurement with bone-conduction stimulation can be used to confirm the conductive hearing loss, and to estimate the air-bone gap. I should point out that the ASSR technique could also be used for either of these diagnostic applications following the click ABR—that is, estimating normal auditory function within the speech frequency region

TABLE 8.9. Relative Contributions of Auditory Brainstem Response (ABR) and Auditory Steady-State Response (ASSR) in Pediatric Audiologic Test Battery for Assessment of Different Types of Auditory Dysfunction

AUDITORY DYSFUNCTION	ABR	ASSR
Normal hearing	Accurate estimation of thresholds.	Tends to overestimate thresholds.
Conductive HL	Ear-specific bone-conduction threshold estimation of hearing thresholds is possible without the need for masking.	Frequency-specific bone-conduction threshold estimation is possible, but masking is required.
Sensory HL	Accurate in estimating mild-to-moderate hearing loss (HL), but not greater HL.	Accurate threshold estimation for patients with moderate-to-profound HL (120 dB HL).
Neural / Auditory Neuropathy	Neural dysfunction can identified with analysis of interwave latencies and peripheral components (e.g., wave I and cochlear microphonic).	Cannot distinguish between profound sensory HL and auditory neuropathy.

Role of ASSR in Frequency-Specific Estimation of Hearing Thresholds in Infants

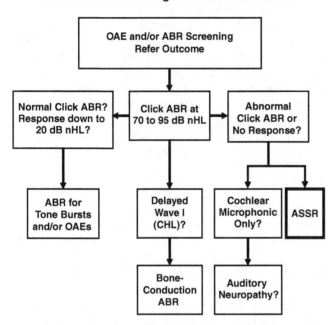

FIGURE 8.20. An approach for incorporating the auditory steady-state response (ASSR) into the pediatric test battery (see lower right portion of figure), along with otoacoustic emissions (OAEs) and the click- and tone-burst-evoked ABR.

or estimating the air-bone gap. However, as noted above, the ABR technique has the advantage of more closely estimating normal hearing and the advantage of providing ear-specific bone-conduction information without masking. The ASSR is most useful for estimation of auditory thresholds for patients with no evidence of auditory neuropathy by the click ABR, ECochG, and OAEs, and who have an ABR only at high click intensity levels, or no ABR at maximum signal levels.

One of the distinct clinical advantages of beginning the auditory electrophysiologic assessment of infants and young children with a click ABR is identification of auditory neuropathy. With reliance only on the ASSR for electrophysiologic estimation of auditory status, profound sensory hearing loss cannot be distinguished from auditory neuropathy. Each type of auditory dysfunction is usually characterized by an absent ASSR. Of course, the same is true for brainstem components of the ABR, i.e., waves III and V, and often ABR wave I, are not recorded in auditory neuropathy. Rance et al. (1999) found that when the ASSR was present in auditory neuropathy, there was a "weak relationship" with behavioral thresholds, i.e., the ASSR grossly overestimated pure-tone thresholds (by up to 90 dB HL). ABR measurement in auditory neuropathy, however, yields a waveform analyzed with visual inspection, permitting the detection of the cochlear microphonic (CM). The value of the CM in detection and

diagnosis of auditory neuropathy was discussed in detail in Chapter 5. As documented by Rance et al. (1998) and subsequently others, beginning a pediatric electrophysiologic assessment with the ABR evoked by click stimuli will permit more valid measurement and accurate interpretation of the ASSR, particularly for patients with auditory neuropathy. In addition to contributing to early detection of auditory neuropathy, click-evoked ABR measurement also leads quickly to differentiation among normal auditory function and all major types of auditory dysfunction—conductive, sensory, mixed, and neural. Therefore, the few minutes required for completion of click-evoked ABR measurement yield information that guides the strategy for subsequent auditory electrophysiologic recordings, including the ASSR.

Conclusions

The ABR and ASSR each can contribute importantly, and rather uniquely, to the diagnostic auditory assessment of children. It is very important, however, to realize and consistently remember clinically that neither the ABR nor the ASSR are tests of hearing. Each technique must be applied within an appropriate test battery, such as that recommended by the Joint Committee on Infant Hearing (see Table 8.10). As noted earlier in the chapter, audiologic assessment of children should be guided by the cross-check principle (Jerger & Hayes, 1976). The author's clinical experience with simultaneous measurement of ABR and ASSR indicates that test time is equivalent for the two techniques. Audiologists who are involved in the auditory assessment of infant and young children will discover that the modest time and effort they expend to acquire skills in the measurement of tone-burst ABRs will yield valuable diagnostic dividends and will contribute to the timely and effective audiologic management

TABLE 8.10. Summary of the Pediatric Test Battery Recommended by the Joint Committee on Infant Hearing (2000) for Audiologic Assessment of Infants in the Age Range of Birth to 6 Months

---

- Child and family history
- Auditory brainstem response (ABR) during initial evaluation to confirm type, degree, and configuration of hearing loss (may include auditory steady-state response, ASSR)
- Acoustic immittance measures (including acoustic reflexes)
- Behavioral response audiometry *(if feasible)*
- Otoacoustic emissions (OAEs)
- Visual reinforcement audiometry *or* conditioned play audiometry
- Speech detection and recognition
- Parental report of auditory and visual behaviors
- Screening of infant's communication milestones

---

of this clinically challenging patient population. Based on review of the literature, and clinical experience, the author concurs with Dr. David Stapells (Stapells et al., 2005) who advises, "The ASSR . . . is appropriate if it used *in conjunction with* [author's italics] the tone-evoked ABR" (p. 13).

SEDATION AND ANESTHESIA IN ABR AND ASSR ASSESSMENT

A complete frequency-specific ABR or ASSR assessment usually requires up to 45 minutes and, with the inclusion of bone-conduction recordings or in complicated cases, as long as one hour. Very young infants (e.g., up to 2 or 3 months of age) may sleep naturally for most of the time required to complete the ABR or ASSR recording, especially if the child is sleep deprived and then fed before the recording begins. Sedation or light anesthesia is almost always required for older infants and children up to age 4 or 5 years. Confident identification and analysis of an ABR or ASSR is dependent on detecting the signal (response) within background noise (e.g., nonresponse electrical signals). Accurate estimation of ABR or ASSR thresholds is particularly influenced by measurement noise, as the "signal" is smallest for very low stimulus-intensity levels. Muscle artifact and movement interference is, of course, the most troublesome source of noise in recording auditory evoked responses. The effect of myogenic (muscle) artifact in ABR recording, and options for solving the problem, were discussed in Chapter 7. A quiet and sleeping child is essential when the ABR or the ASSR is applied for estimation of auditory thresholds. Patient restlessness and movement will contribute to overestimation of hearing thresholds and, if the assessment cannot be completed, inconclusive test results. With the exception of young infants, conscious sedation or light anesthesia is often required to induce an adequate patient state for pediatric applications of ABR and/or ASSR.

The American Academy of Pediatrics (AAP) has developed clear guidelines for conscious sedation (see Table 8.11). Guidelines for sedation can be found in several publications (e.g., Guidelines for Monitoring and Management of Pediatric Patients During and After Sedation for Diagnostic and Therapeutic Procedures, *Pediatrics 89,* 1992, pp. 1110–1115, and Guidelines for Monitoring and Management of Pediatric Patients During and After Sedation for Diagnostic and Therapeutic Procedures: Addendum, *Pediatrics 110,* 2002, pp. 836–838). Sedation guidelines are also available at the AAP website (www.aap.org/policy). Other organizations (e.g., Anesthesiology Society of America and American Dental Association) also have formulated detailed protocols for conscious sedation that can be accessed on and downloaded from websites. These resources include definition of terms important in the discussion of sedation. In addition, conscious sedation in various clinical units at most hospitals (e.g., EEG lab, radiology service) is conducted according to institutional policies and procedures developed by a conscious sedation committee. The following section summarizes information on common sedatives and anesthetic agents used with children undergoing assessment of auditory evoked responses. The reader is strongly encouraged to review documents available from professional organizations (e.g., the American Academy of Pediatrics) and local hospitals for more details on sedation policies and procedures. Results of a survey reported by Reich and Wiatrak (1996) suggest that, despite the available of published guidelines, there is a lack of "uniformity" in the type of sedation administered, at least in the United States.

Sedation

CHLORAL HYDRATE. | Chloral hydrate is a commonly prescribed sedative. It is the drug used most often for inducing sleep or at least a drowsy state in infants and young children undergoing AER assessment (e.g., Hall, 1992; Reich & Wiatrak, 1996). Categorized as a hypnotic or "sleeping" drug, it is a halogenated aliphatic alcohol that depresses the CNS, specifically the cerebral cortex. The half-life of chloral hydrate is 8 hours. Chloral hydrate is classified as a "conscious sedative" (e.g., Guidelines for Elective Use of Conscious Sedation, Deep Sedation, and General Anesthesia in Pediatric Patients, Committee on Drugs, Section on Anesthesia, American Academy of Pediatrics, *Pediatrics 76,* 1985, pp. 317–321). That is, consciousness is minimally depressed, the patient breathes independently (maintains an open airway), and can be aroused by physical or verbal stimulation. The gag reflex, a protective reflex, may be sluggish but is present (not suppressed). An example of physical stimulation is pinching the skin (e.g., earlobe) lightly. Loss of consciousness with such a sedative is extremely unlikely. With the typical protocol for clinical use of chloral hydrate, medical personnel (e.g., nurse or physician) administer the sedation and monitor vital signs, skin color, and O_2 (oxygen) saturation, while the audiologist performs the auditory electrophysiologic procedure(s).

Side Effects. Adverse reactions to chloral hydrate include, occasionally, nausea and gastric irritation and, rarely, excitement, delirium, disorientation, and erythematous (edema) and urticarial (rash) allergic reactions. Severe itching is associated with these reactions. With infants and young children, vomiting is probably the most common adverse reaction. It is extremely important in these cases to prevent aspiration, one of the few serious complications of this sedation approach. The second most common problem is a paradoxical reaction to the drug, that is, arousal, excitement, and a high level of activity as opposed to quieting and sleep. Even without a paradoxical reaction, some children become light-headed or disoriented after chloral hydrate is ingested. During induction of sedation and also during emergence from sedation, it is very important for the clinician to assure that the patient is closely supervised and protected from physical injury (e.g.,

TABLE 8.11. Personnel, Procedures, and Terminology Involved in Conscious Sedation of Patients for Pediatric ABR Assessment

Detailed information on conscious sedation of children is available from the American Academy of Pediatrics (www.aap.org/policy), and websites for other professional organizations (e.g., American Dental Association, American Society of Anesthesiology).

Personnel

- The physician responsible for the patient or supervising the procedure should be present at the procedure or within the procedure area during the entire sedation period.
- A registered or licensed practical nurse or other appropriately qualified professional must be present to monitor and document the patient's physiologic parameters and assist in any supportive or resuscitative measures.
- Sedative and anxiolytic medications should only be administered by or in the presence of individuals skilled in airway management and cardiopulmonary resuscitation.

Sedation Procedures

- Obtain informed consent for conscious sedation, as well as the procedure (e.g., ABR) as indicated.
- Patient must undergo a documented presedation medical evaluation, including a focused airway examination on the same day, or within recent days, to include:
  - Age and weight
  - Medical history, including drug allergies, current medications, relevant diseases, adverse drug reactions (e.g., paradoxical reaction to the planned sedative), and any relevant family history.
  - Review of systems, especially any airway or respiratory problems.
  - History of specific drug, dosage, and time of any medications taken on the day of the procedure.
  - History of food or fluid intake within 8 hours before sedation.
  - Vital signs, including heart rate, blood pressure, respiratory rate, level of consciousness, and temperature.
- There should be an appropriate interval of fasting before sedation.
- Conscious sedation orders for patients must be written. Prescriptions or orders from areas outside the area where conscious sedation is administered are not acceptable.
- An individual must be specifically assigned to monitor the patient's cardiorespiratory status during and after the procedure; for deeply sedated patients, that individual should have no other responsibilities and should record vital signs at least every 5 minutes.

- A physician or nurse administers all medication.
- Children should *not* receive sedative or anxiolytic medications without supervision by skilled medical personnel (i.e., medication should not be administered at home or by a technician without medical supervision). Age- and size-appropriate equipment and appropriate medications to sustain life should be checked before sedation and be immediately available.
- Physicians or their designee will maintain a time-based record including the name, route, site, time, dosage, and patient effects of any drugs administered during the procedure.
- The patient's vital signs and oxygen saturation will be monitored by the physician or nursing staff during the procedure and documented in the record at intervals.
- All patients sedated for a procedure must be continuously monitored with pulse oximetry.

Postsedation Procedures

- After the procedure, the patient must be observed in a facility appropriately staffed and equipped.
- Specific discharge criteria must be used.
- If a patient is discharged following completion of the procedure, the physician or designee will identify a person responsible for the patient and provide verbal and written instructions and information about limitations of activity, anticipated changes in behavior, etc., to this person.
- Discharge criteria must be met and documented prior to discharging a patient following sedation.
  - Vital signs are stable and within the pre-procedure range.
  - The patient has returned to his or her presedation level of consciousness.
  - The patient has written instructions for post-procedure care.

Selected Terminology

Analgesia: The elimination or diminution of pain.
Anxiolysis: The elimination or diminution of anxiety.
Conscious sedation: A minimally depressed level of consciousness. The patient retains the ability to independently maintain an adequate airway and will respond to verbal command or physical stimulation.

falling). The patient should, for example, not be allowed to walk unassisted or lie in a bed without guardrails. As an aside, before going ahead with chloral hydrate as the seda-

tive of choice, it is useful to question the child's parents or physician about these types of adverse reactions to previous attempts at sedation with chloral hydrate).

Contraindications. Contraindications, or reasons not to use chloral hydrate, are marked hepatic and renal impairment. The drug should be used only with extreme caution in children with a history of active respiratory disorders or seizure activity. Precautions include pregnancy, gastritis, and severe cardiac disease. Chloral hydrate may produce an abnormal response in persons with Crigler-Najjar syndrome (a rare congenital disease producing jaundice or yellow-appearing skin). There is reported drug interaction between chloral hydrate and furosemide (lasix), causing flushing, sweating, and blood pressure variations. Lasix is a commonly used and potentially ototoxic loop diuretic. Chloral hydrate in combination with alcohol may inhibit the metabolism of both drugs and lead to prolonged CNS depression and also produce vasodilation and hypotension.

Administration. Chloral hydrate is available in three forms: syrup, capsule, and suppository. Clinical experience suggests that, for infants and young children (4 to 5 months and older), administration of the syrup PO (by mouth) is the most consistently successful approach. Suppositories were often used for ABR assessments in the early years of (e.g., Jerger, Hayes, & Jordan, 1980), but are definitely not preferred by the author, whose aversion to the approach is based on the rather unpleasant experience of searching for potentially expelled suppositories by the patients in the study reported by Jerger et al. (1980). With oral administration, the proper dose of syrup is poured into an oral syringe or cup. A oral syringe is better suited to very young children. The syrup is squirted into a back corner of the mouth while the child is encouraged to swallow. Water can be available as a chaser. The syrup, which is sweet, sticky, and not very tasty, can also be mixed with water, juice, or ginger ale. While this technique may facilitate compliance with administration, unless all the liquid is consumed, it is difficult to document the amount of sedation ingested. PR (per rectum) administration via suppository is also appropriate and sometimes effective with young children. Capsules are used with older children or adults (e.g., the mentally retarded) who require light sedation.

Initial Dosage. Dosages to induce sleep range from 500 milligrams (mg) to 2 grams (gm), which is 2000 milligrams. For light sedation the dosages are halved. A typical pediatric dose is 50 mg of chloral hydrate per kilogram (kg) of body weight, that is, 50 mg/kg (Reich & Wiatrak, 1996). One kg is equal to 2.2 pounds. Clinical experience suggests that some physicians, pediatricians in particular, prefer to initially administer one-half this dose (25 mg/kg). Then, if the child does not fall asleep within a defined period of time (e.g., 45 minutes) a second half dose (12 mg/kg) may be administered. In contrast, an acceptable clinical policy, with experienced medical personnel (nurses and physicians) on hand, is to administer an initial dose of 75 mg/kg, after verifying that the drug is not medically contraindicated. The maximum amount of chloral hydrate administered on a day is 1000 mg (1 gram). Baranak, Marsh, and Potsic (1984) described an equivalent policy for sedation with chloral hydrate.

The author's recommendation to begin with 75 mg/kg, rather than the traditional 25 or 50 mg/kg, was made after reviewing the success rate with the standard dose with over 50 children during a period of three years, and also after consultation with physicians on the pharmacokinetics of chloral hydrate. With a dose of 50 mg/kg, we encountered a sizable proportion of infants who initially became more, rather than less, active after administration. Physical stimulation, such as scrubbing the skin during electrode placement, immediately aroused the child, and if sedation did occur the duration was often inadequate to complete testing. With our initial policy, the standard 50 mg/kg, we often found it necessary to readminister a half dose. This did not seem to be consistently effective, led to questions about the amount of sedation that the child actually ingested, added considerably to test time, frustrated the tester and parent alike, and ultimately was not effective in sedating an unacceptable proportion of children.

Second Dosage. Guidelines are necessary for managing the patient who either does not fall asleep with sedation or who awakes before sufficient AER data are recorded. With the 50 mg/kg initial dose, if the patient is still awake after 45 minutes has elapsed, a repeat dosage (also 50 mg/kg) or a half dosage (25 mg/kg) is often administered. With an initial dose of 75 mg/kg, additional sedative may be administered after 45 minutes, but the total dose should not exceed 100 mg/kg. The decision to resedate is, to a large extent, a matter of clinician judgment and medical policy. It is reasonable to defer resedating a child for up to 1 hour (assuming total ingestion of a 75 mg/kg initial dose). If the child is comfortable and soothed by a parent in a quiet, darkened room, experience suggests that a sleep state adequate for ABR testing is likely. Naturally, with any pediatric AER assessment, but particularly after sedation, the clinician should have all equipment and supplies ready, have a test strategy planned out, and be prepared to immediately and quickly perform an efficient AER assessment. With adequate preparation and optimal test conditions, it is often possible to obtain vital AER data on auditory status from an adequately sedated patient in 15 minutes or less.

If the preceding dosage(s) of chloral hydrate are not effective in sedating a patient, the AER assessment must be postponed to another day. The decision at this point is whether to attempt sedation again with chloral hydrate or to take a different approach. A second attempt with chloral hydrate is reasonable if the patient became drowsy and, in the clinician's judgment, would fall asleep under similar circumstances with the aid of sleep deprivation. On the other hand, if the ineffective sedation was already a second attempt or the patient's response was clearly paradoxical (increased activity rather than sleep), then an alternative to chloral hydrate is indicated. The usual alternative is light anesthesia in a day surgery setting.

Although accumulated clinical experience and published reports confirm that chloral hydrate does not affect ABR (Mokotoff, Schulman-Galambos, Galambos, 1977; Palaskas, Wilson, & Dobie, 1989; Sohmer & Student, 1978), amplitude of the Pa component of the AMLR is decreased and latency may be increased (Okitsu, 1984; Osterhammel, Shallop, & & Terkildsen, 1985; Palaskas et al., 1989). Changes in the AMLR with chloral hydrate sedation are more pronounced when the stimulation rate is increased (from 4 stimuli per second to 10 stimuli per second). This experimental finding has obvious clinical implications for AMLR evaluation of children. Chloral hydrate sedation (2 grams) also reduces the amplitude and increases the latency of the auditory 40 Hz response (Palaskas et al., 1989). In addition, the threshold level of response detection is increased by 9 to 12 dB HL in the sedated state. Presumably, chloral hydrate will have a similar effect on an ASSR evoked by slow rates of modulation (e.g., < 60 Hz), but not for faster stimulus modulation rates. Other sedatives (e.g., Versed) are also useful for achieving a restful state adequate for measurement of ABR and ASSR in young children.

Diazepam (Valium), a benzodiazepine, is an anti-anxiety drug (minor tranquilizer) that may be used to relax adult patients undergoing auditory evoked response assessment. The effect of Valium on ABR is probably minimal (Adams et al., 1982; Doring & Daub, 1980). ALR N1, P2, and N2 component amplitude is reduced by benzodiazepines, but latency is not usually affected (Lader, 1977).

Anesthetic Agents

Light anesthesia to assure that the patient is sleeping during ABR or ASSR measurement is an option to the reliance on conscious sedation, or it may be used when a conscious sedative (e.g., chloral hydrate) is ineffective. Propofol is an example of an anesthetic agent commonly used to achieve light anesthesia required for an ABR or ASSR. An appreciation of the effects of anesthetic agents on the ABR is essential for any clinician involved in the electrophysiologic assessment of infants and young children or in neurophysiologic intraoperative monitoring during surgery. Anesthesia is defined as loss of sensation (partial or complete), with or without loss of consciousness, that may be drug-induced or due to disease or injury. The following discussion will be limited to general anesthesia that affects the brain and produces loss of sensation and consciousness. Depth or stage of general anesthesia may be described according to different schema. According to one description, there are three stages. In stage one, the patient is first excited until voluntary control is lost (hearing is the last of the senses to become nonfunctional). The corneal reflex is still present in the second stage of anesthesia, although loss of voluntary control persists. The third stage of anesthesia is defined as complete relaxation, deep

regular breathing, and a sluggish corneal reflex. There are four stages of anesthesia according to another schema, including: (1) analgesia (no feeling), (2) delirium, (3) surgical anesthesia, and (4) medullary depression. From these terms, it is clear that the patient should be maintained in stage 3 during surgery. Stages 1 and 2 represent inadequate anesthesia, while anesthesia is excessive in stage 4. Only light anesthesia is required during pediatric applications of the ABR and ASSR, as the goal is simply to induce restful sleep and a motionless state.

Before anesthesia, drugs are administered to decrease anxiety, relieve pre- and postoperative pain and provide amnesia for the perioperative period. Examples of these drugs are benzodiazepines (e.g., Valium), conscious sedatives (e.g., Versed), barbiturates, and neuroleptics. There are three major components to anesthesia. The purpose of the first component, induction, is to produce a rapid loss of consciousness. Drugs used to induce anesthesia include benzodiazepines, barbiturates, narcotic analgesics, etomidate, ketamine, and inhalation agents. The second, and longest lasting, component is maintenance of anesthesia. The purpose of this phase, which persists throughout surgery, is to produce a stable state of loss of consciousness and loss of reflexes to painful stimuli. Among the drugs often administered to during maintenance of anesthesia are inhalational agents (gases), narcotic analgesics, ketamine, muscle relaxants, and anti-arrythmic agents. Finally, anesthesia must be reversed so the patient will wake up and return to the preanesthetic state. This is achieved with opioid antagonists and anticholinesterase agents.

Anesthetic agents are often categorized according to their mode of administration. Some are intravenous (IV) agents, infused directly into the bloodstream via a line inserted into a vein (at the wrist or ankle). Examples of IV agents are barbiturates (thiopental/Sodium Pentothal, methohexital/Brevital, thiamylal), benzodiazepines (diazepam/Valium, midazolam), etomidates (amidate), opioid analgesics (morphine, fentanyl, meperidine), neuroleptics (droperidol + fentanyl), and dissociative anesthetic agents (ketamine). With IV anesthetics, there is fast action and fast recovery. The brain receives one-tenth of the dose within 40 seconds following IV administration. Other anesthetic agents are administered as a gas by inhalation. Inhalational agents, in contrast to those administered IV, are slower acting and are measured by partial pressure (tension) in the blood (brain). One commonly used inhalational agent is nitrous oxide, a gaseous anesthetic that is a good analgesic and induction agent, but it has low anesthetic potency. Others are called volatile anesthetics (e.g., halothane, isoflurane), which are potent even at low concentrations.

Anesthesia and Auditory Evoked Responses

Anesthetic agents produce differential effects on AERs. Most anesthetic agents have minimal effect on the ABR. A good example is *propofol,* perhaps the anesthetic agent used most often with children undergoing an ABR and/or ASSR procedure. Propofol at anesthetic levels generally produces a very modest delay in ABR interwave latencies, as detailed below. Other drugs (e.g., enflurane and halothane) also prolong ABR latency. *Halothane* appears to cause, at most, slight delays in ABR interwave latencies, without altering waveform morphology (Cohen & Britt, 1982; Duncan et al., 1979; Stockard et al., 1980; Wilson et al., 1984). Latency prolongation is statistically significant, linear, and dose related, according to some investigators (Thornton, Heneghan, James, & Jones, 1984; Wilson, Wilson, & Cant, 1984). *Isoflurane* may prolong ABR absolute and interwave latencies (Manninen, Nicholas, & Lam, 1984), although some investigators report negligible effects (Stockard et al., 1980). In contrast, so-called "extralemniscal" AERs (e.g., AMLR, ALR), involving multi-synaptic nonlemniscal pathways, are highly sensitive to the effects of anesthetic agents on the central nervous system. Cortical responses are also affected to a greater degree by sedatives, such as chloral hydrate.

Fentanyl is a popular narcotic analgesic. It is a synthetic opioid that is eighty times as potent as morphine. Fentanyl is used exclusively as an anesthetic, as opposed to morphine, which is used as a sedative. Fentanyl has no apparent effect on ABR (Samra, Lilly, Rush, & Kirsh, 1984). In adults anesthetized with fentanyl, Kileny et al. (1983) observed only slight alterations in AMLR latency and, as with chemical paralysis, noted improved waveform quality as muscle activity subsided. *Sufentanil* is a narcotic anesthetic that is ten times more potent than fentanyl, but provides a greater margin of safety (especially in animal research) because is produces less hemodynamic stress than fentanyl. *Enflurane* produces increase interwave (wave I–III and I–V) latencies of up to 0.85 ms, which are linear and depend on the concentration (Dubois, Sato, Chassy, & Macnamara, 1982; Thornton et al., 1981; Thornton et al., 1984). *Methohexital sodium* is an IV barbiturate that significantly prolongs wave V latency by as much as 0.4 ms, but latency of waves I and III are unaffected (Kriss, Prasher, & Pratt, 1984). *Etomidate* is an IV anesthetic agent that has no effect on the ABR.

Sodium Pentothal (thiopental) is an IV barbiturate that affects ABR minimally, although available information is somewhat confusing. Sanders et al. (1979) found no change in ABR with thiopental (preceding as an anesthetic agent by halothane and nitrous oxide induction). An amplitude reduction, but Goff et al. (1977) reported no latency change when thiopental administration followed diazepam. Drummond, Todd, and Sang (1985) reported the most notable ABR changes. Absolute and interwave latency values for waves I, III, and V were significantly increased (average wave V latency from 6.16 to 6.87 ms), while wave V amplitude was not changed. ABR was never suppressed by thiopental. Effects of thiopental on late AERs were demonstrated by Abrahamian, Allison, Goff, and Rosner (1963). *Pentobarbital* is

a fast-acting barbiturate that appears to have little serious effect on ABR latency or amplitude (Bobbin, May, & Lemoine, 1979; Cohen & Britt, 1982; Hall, 1985; Marsh, Frewen, Sutton, & Potsic, 1984, Newlon, Greenberg, Enas, & Becker, 1983).

Ketamine (hydrochloride) is a dissociative IV anesthetic that works by altering limbic system activity, but not medullary structures. Afferent neural input probably still reaches the sensory cortex, but activity in association areas may be suppressed. Ketamine does not appear to affect ABR latency or amplitude values (Bobbin, May, & Lemoine, 1979; Cohen & Britt, 1982; Sasaki, 1991). In contrast, ketamine has pronounced effects on the ASSR elicited by slow modulation rates (< 80 Hz), but ASSRs for faster modulation rates ASSR (Kuwada, Batra, & Maher et al., 2002). *Nitrous oxide* is a gaseous inhalation agent that is a good analgesic. It is used to induce anesthesia, but has low potency (strength) for maintaining anesthesia. ABR interwave latencies are not affected by nitrous oxide. The drug (a gas) can fill the middle ear space via the Eustachian tube producing positive middle ear pressure and temporary conductive hearing impairment. The conductive hearing loss component may result in delays in the absolute latencies of the ABR, e.g., a delay in wave I and in subsequent waves.

Propofol is an anesthetic agent commonly used with children undergoing auditory evoked response recordings for assessment of hearing sensitivity. Propofol produces in children slight but clinically significant prolongations in interwave latencies of the ABR (e.g., Purdie & Cullen, 1993). Masui (1995) studied the effect of *sevoflurane* and *nitrous oxide* anesthesia on auditory brainstem responses in children. Both agents are popular for anesthesia with children during clinical assessment with ABR and ASSR. Subjects were 70 infants and children ranging in age between 1 month and 15 years. Nitrous oxide (60%) and sevoflurane (2.5%) increased the latency of wave V and the I–V interwave interval significantly. The changes were small for nitrous oxide (mean of 0.26 ms with standard deviation of 0.16 ms) and for sevoflurane (mean of 0.23 ms with a standard deviation of 0.19 ms). Although a clear ABR is recorded with children anesthetized with nitrous oxide and sevoflurane, latency increases under anesthesia could lead to misinterpretation of ABR abnormalities in some patients, particularly when the effects were combined with those associated with other factors (e.g., age or body temperature).

Neuromuscular Blockers (Chemical Paralyzing Agents)

These drugs produce paralysis by interrupting transmission of neural impulses at the skeletal neuromuscular junction. Examples of neuromuscular blockers used in the operating room and intensive care unit are pancuronium (Pavulon), Metocurine, succinylcholine, and curare. All AERs can be reliably recorded during chemically induced muscle paralysis with such agents as Pavulon, Metocurine, and succinylcholine (Hall, 1988; Hall, Hargadine, & Allen, 1985; Hall, Mackey-Hargadine, & Kim, 1985; Harker, Hosick, Voots, & Mendel, 1977; Kileny, 1983; Kileny, Dodon, & Gelfand, 1983; Smith & Kraus, 1987). Waveforms are, in fact, often enhanced in patients under the influence of chemical paralysis due to the lack of muscle-related noise or artifact. Children who are lightly anesthetized for auditory evoked response recordings in hearing assessment do not usually require chemical paralysis.

SEDATION GUIDELINES FOR ABR OR ASSR MEASUREMENT

General Guidelines and Protocols

PRESEDATION PROTOCOL. | Important features of the policy followed before and after sedation with chloral hydrate are summarized as a checklist in Table 8.11. Beforehand, it is important to provide clear information in writing to the parents regarding the sedation. The following items might be noted:

- Reason(s) for sedation: Parents are more likely to comply with the requests for sedation if they understand the reason for both sedation and AER assessment.
- Prescription (dosage): Generally, a prescription for a specific dosage of a specific sedative is requested of the patient's physician. The testing clinician's or clinic's telephone number should be provide in writing so that the referring physician can call with questions or concerns.
- Eating: Some food (a light breakfast or lunch) one or two hours before testing reduces the likelihood of gastric irritation, which, as noted above, is one possible side effect of chloral hydrate. This recommendation also is not universally endorsed.
- Sedative administration: The written instructions should make it clear that the patient is NOT to be given sedation by the parents or caregiver before arrival at the clinic or hospital. Trained medical personnel should administer all of the sedative (the entire dose) with close attention to the precautions described above (under administration and monitoring/documentation). There are several potential medical problems associated with administration by others. The actual amount administered and ingested is not known, the time of ingestion may be unclear, there is no medical support to manage emergencies, such as aspiration or respiratory arrest, and the patient may not be closely supervised after sedation. A result of this latter item may be serious accidental injury (e.g., head injury secondary to fall). Furthermore, with sedation for an unpredictable time before arrival at the clinic, the patient is more apt to sleep in transit and awake before or during testing.

With the patient in the clinic, but before sedation is administered, medical personnel should take a history, determine medical contraindications to sedations (e.g., congestion, respiratory problems), document any pertinent physical conditions (e.g., congenital heart problems, seizure disorders) and other medications (e.g., anticonvulsant drugs). A recent physical examination, especially including the airway, is advised. The patient must be weighed, with weight converted to kilograms. Then, the proper dose of sedation is drawn and administered (as described above).

MONITORING STATUS DURING SEDATION. | Emergency equipment, including an emergency ("crash") cart must be easily accessible in the test area in the unlikely event of complications. Respiration is monitoring visually or with a stethoscope. If the tester is outside of a test booth, a family member or assistant should remain in the room with the patient. Respiration can be monitored acoustically with a talk-back system microphone placed near the patient's head. The clinician, with this arrangement, must have quick and easy access to the test room. Medical personnel are alerted if respiration slows markedly or becomes shallow or labored. If the child is on a surface off the floor (e.g., a bed or table), care is taken to prevent the patient from striking his or her head against hard or sharp objects or falling to the floor.

POSTSEDATION PROTOCOL. | Supervision must be as close after as during sedation. The patient, although arousable, is generally "floppy" and has poor motor control. The patient should not be allowed to sit or stand unassisted in the first few hours after awaking from sedation. Climbing on chairs or tables is prohibited. Family members or guardians must be given explicit instructions about the need for close supervision. The patient may take a long nap. Until he or she is completely awake and alert, playing with other children, returning to school or daycare, or other usual activities are not appropriate. Other drugs with alcohol (e.g., cough medicine) should be avoided during this period. Fluids are encouraged to reduce stomach irritation, but young children should not lie flat if drinking from a bottle or if feeding. The gag reflex may be sluggish, and aspiration of the liquid is possible. A patient must not leave the clinical area until he or she is awake. Medical personnel (physician or nurse) document in medical records patient status and the instructions given to family members or guardians during the postsedation period before discharge. A telephone number for emergency consultation is provided. The prescription receipt or a copy of the prescription form is attached to medical records.

ALTERNATIVES TO SEDATION. | A common nonmedical alternative to chloral hydrate sedation, i.e., sleep deprivation, was noted above. In the nursery setting, nonsedative substances may help a child sleep naturally. One example is "SweetEase," a glucose substance. Commercially available over-the-counter drugs that induce drowsiness or sleep, such as

Benadryl, are also an option. Approval of the patient's primary care physician (PCP) is suggested for young children or patients who have any health problems, who are treated with other medications, or for whom there is a risk of a complication. The typical sequence for sedation begins with chloral hydrate, unless previous attempts to sedate with chloral hydrate were clearly unsuccessful. The next alternative is light anesthesia in an operating room setting, often an ambulatory surgery facility. Describing medication experiences with a series of 167 children, Jerger, Hayes, and Jordan (1980) found that for only 6 was sedation not effective, and only 1 patient was tested under general anesthesia. Similarly, Baranak, Marsh, and Potsic (1984) reported that with adequate sleep deprivation and chloral hydrate dosage (60 to 80 mg/kg as described above), 80 percent of children who weighed less than 15 kg (33 pounds) were sufficiently sedated for ABR with the first dose, and only 1 of 40 children was given a third dose. These authors do not administer a third dose because of disruptions of eating and sleeping habits for up to two days. They note that 50 percent of the sedative (the active metabolite) is still on board 12 hours later. Chloral hydrate is least likely to be effective in very large children or adults, where the mg/kg dosage exceeds 1 gram (1000 kg). Often, these patients are mentally retarded and have long defied behavioral testing and routine sedation. With these patients, the author recommends questioning the referring physician about the possibility of general anesthesia in the future. If sedation was needed for AER assessment, and was not effective, there is a good chance that other diagnostic or therapeutic procedures (e.g., CT scanning or dental work) were also precluded by the patient's uncooperativeness or high level of activity. AER assessment can then be put on the list of procedures to be carried out under general anesthesia. This approach is usually agreeable to all involved and provides an optimal setting for valid AER measurement.

Conscious Sedation: Safety and Risk Issues

Extensive clinical experience accumulated during the past thirty years by hundreds of clinicians strongly supports the argument that chloral hydrate is a safe sedative. The risk of chloral hydrate sedation in children is minimized by strict adherence to accepted policies and protocols for its administration. Cote and colleagues at Northwestern University (Cote et al., 2000) confirmed this point in a paper entitled "Adverse Sedation Events in Pediatrics: Analysis of Medications Used for Sedation" and published in the journal *Pediatrics*. The authors analyzed clinical findings for 95 case reports of adverse sedation events. Among the series of patients, the outcome for 60 of the patients was death or permanent neurologic injury. The authors found no relation between outcome and drug class (e.g., sedatives vs. opioids) or route of administration (e.g., oral, rectal, IV, inhalation). Negative outcomes were invariably associated with drug overdoses, drug interactions, and drug combinations (espe-

cially three or more sedating medications). That is, problems with chloral hydrate usage were due to failure to follow established and accepted clinical protocols for its administration in children.

Sedation versus Anesthesia

Whether infants and young children undergo auditory evoked response assessment with conscious sedation in a clinic setting or with light anesthesia in the operating room may depend on institutional policy, medical status of the child, or clinician preference. There are distinct advantages and disadvantages associated with each approach, as summarized in Table 8.12. The author's experience with pediatric ABR assessment in a medical center setting reflects a clear shift toward more rigorous protocols for administration of sedation and a parallel trend away from conscious sedation and toward light anesthesia. Colleagues in anesthesiology argue strongly for light anesthesia (e.g., propofol or sevofluorane) in the operating room, rather than chloral hydrate in a clinic environment. Selected advantages for light anesthesia in the operating room cited in Table 8.12 are weighted heavily by anesthesiologists, particularly the ability to respond promptly to complications involving vital functions (e.g., breathing), however unlikely, and the relatively short time required for return to the awake state. The latter advantage is, of course, welcome to all involved in pediatric measurement of the ABR.

TABLE 8.12. Advantages and Disadvantages Associated with Conscious Sedation in a Clinic Setting versus Light Anesthesia in an Operating Room Setting for Children Undergoing ABR and/or ASSR Assessment for Estimation of Hearing Sensitivity

SETTING	ADVANTAGES	DISADVANTAGES
Clinic	Less expensive	Limited sedation options
	Near or in audiology clinic	Limited medical support
	Scheduling ease	Increased liability
		Uncertain success (child never is sedated)
		Potentially greater test time
Operating room	Medical (ENT) support	More expensive
	Ideal patient state	Remote location (away from audiology clinic)
	Controlled sedation	Noisier environment
	Limited liability for audiologist	Complicated scheduling and delay in test date

9 CHAPTER

ABR
Pediatric Clinical Applications and Populations

This chapter consists of a review of the literature on major applications of the ABR in children, with a summary of findings, and guidelines for ABR measurement in selected patient populations. Chapter 8 is devoted to one of the most important pediatric applications of the ABR—estimation of auditory threshold in infants and young children. Information within this chapter on diseases and disorders and pediatric applications of ABR is grouped within general categories as follows:

- Newborn hearing screening
- Risk factors for infant hearing loss
- ABR in primarily peripheral auditory disorders and pathologies
- ABR in primarily CNS disorders and pathologies

Since the first reports of clinical application of the ABR in children appeared over thirty years ago (e.g., Hecox & Galambos, 1974), a vast amount of information on ABR findings, patterns, and applications has been disseminated in many thousands of publications. A comprehensive review of the literature on this topic is far beyond the scope of this chapter. Even a passing reference to each published article or book chapter describing the application of ABR in myriad pediatric populations would require an entire book. Decisions on what material would be included in the following review were based mostly on the practical value of the information for clinicians faced with the daily task of diagnosing auditory dysfunction with ABR. Large chunks of the literature are condensed in the form of tables and, regrettably, many good studies are not cited. The reader encountering a patient with a specific diagnosis and requiring more information for proper interpretation of ABR findings or patient management is strongly encouraged to conduct a formal search of literature on the particular clinical entity. In this age of computers, everyone has essentially immediate access to diverse and limitless sources of information. Reliance on a well-established search engine, such as Medline, is a good starting point. To access all of the scientific and medical articles available in the National Library of Medicine in the United States, just access the website: www.nlm. nih.gov, and then the link to Medline Plus. With a few carefully selected keywords, the curious student, clinician, or researcher can within minutes locate primary resources on a topic, including review articles and abstracts, of virtually every publication that includes the keywords within its abstract or text. Many readers around the world have access to, and familiarity with, other search engines and databases. A more generic search of the Internet is likely to uncover nonpublished but still useful sources of information on the ABR in various pediatric populations. Websites of major medical schools with active research programs in audiology, hearing science, otolaryngology, neurology, and related disciplines, and auditory evoked responses in particular, are a handy additional source of information.

NEWBORN HEARING SCREENING

Newborn auditory screening is a routine clinical application of ABR. The overall goal is to identify as early as possible hearing impairment that will affect the normal acquisition of speech and language. Although concerns about the efficacy and rationale for newborn hearing screening and other related issues (e.g., parental anxiety) are periodically raised (e.g., Bess & Paradise, 1994; Thompson et al., 2000), there is now unequivocal scientific evidence that early intervention results in remarkable benefits for language acquisition (e.g., Yoshinago-Itano et al., 1998). Attempts to screen hearing of newborn infants began in the late 1960s (Downs & Sterritt, 1967; Froding, 1960). Behavioral techniques for hearing screening of neonates were less than satisfactory and not widely applied. Moderate-to-high intensity sounds are required to elicit a behavioral response from newborn infants, even those with normal auditory function. In addition, criteria for the presence or absence of a response are often unclear and highly subjective (Ling, Ling, &

Doehring, 1970). Behavioral assessment should be carried out in a sound-treated environment, but in hospital settings newborn infants at risk for hearing impairment are typically too ill or unstable medically to be transported to an audiology test facility. Behavioral audiometry in neonates, therefore, is not accurate for estimating auditory sensitivity and is not clinically feasible in most cases. In fact, in early position statements, the Joint Committee on Infant Screening discouraged the use of behavioral screening methods.

During the 1970s, nonbehavioral techniques for diagnostic auditory assessment in general, and infant screening in particular, were introduced. Most popular among these techniques were the Crib-O-Gram type devices (Bennett, 1980; Durieux-Smith et al., 1985; Simmons & Russ, 1974) and auditory brainstem response (ABR). With the Crib-O-Gram or Linco-Bennett techniques, the infant lies in a special crib designed to detect movement. Under computer control, a sound (a band of noise in the 3000 Hz region) is presented via a speaker toward the infant's head at an intensity level of 92 dB SPL. A response is determined automatically when the infant moves within a brief interval after the stimulus presentation. The physiologic response may be as subtle as a change in respiration pattern.

Early identification of infant hearing impairment was altered dramatically by the discovery in 1971 of the auditory brainstem response (ABR) by Jewett and Williston and a subsequent paper by Hecox and Galambos in 1974 describing the clinical application of ABR in auditory assessment of infants and young children. The evolution of ABR as a newborn hearing screening technique, and other major developments in newborn hearing screening over time, are depicted in Figure 9.1. Only a few years after his classic article introducing the ABR as a tool for audiologic assessment of children, Dr. Robert Galambos published a series of papers documenting the clinical feasibility of ABR as a technique for screening infants at bedside in the nursery setting, even premature infants confined to the neonatal intensive care unit (NICU). Within the next decade, dozens of articles describing ABR experiences with newborn hearing screening of at-risk infants were published by well-known audiologists, pediatricians, neurologists, and others at hospitals and medical centers across the United States (see Hall, 1992 for review). Failure rates were rather high (e.g., over 20%) in some of these early studies. However, as clinical experience accumulated for screening personnel and screening equipment, earphones, protocols, techniques, and strategies were modified for this new ABR application, the reported failure

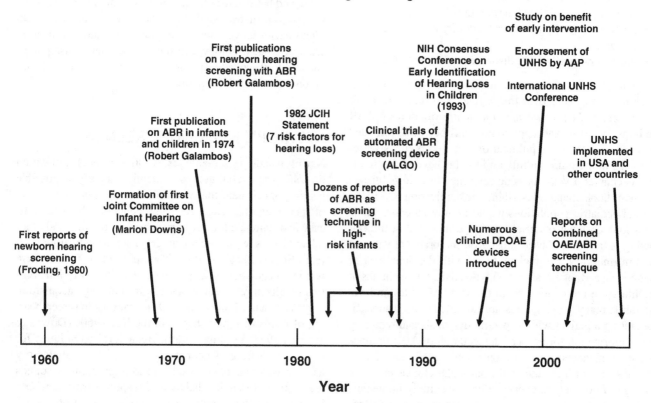

Evolution of Newborn Hearing Screening with ABR

FIGURE 9.1. Timeline of major developments in the application of the auditory brainstem response (ABR) as a technique for newborn hearing screening, including universal newborn hearing screening (UNHS).

rates decreased to under 10 percent, an impressive figure for infants at high risk for hearing loss. The Joint Committee on Infant Hearing, a multidisciplinary group with an interest in early identification of hearing loss initially inspired by Dr. Marion Downs, published in 1971 the first set of risk indicators. In 1982, ABR was endorsed as a screening technique of choice by multiple disciplines (e.g., JCIH, 1982). Hearing screening efforts in this era were focused almost exclusively on infants at risk for hearing loss; screening was performed, and results interpreted, by skilled audiologic personnel manually operating what were essentially large and rather sophisticated diagnostic evoked response systems. Most of the infants identified as at risk for hearing impairment were found in the NICU. Risk factors or indicators for an infant, established by the JCIH, were identified by a medical chart review. Risk indicators for neonatal hearing loss, including delayed onset and progressive hearing loss, and central auditory nervous system dysfunction are discussed later in this chapter.

The risk criteria approach to determining which children were screened was an efficient means of identifying approximately 50 percent of children born with permanent hearing loss, even though only about 1 out of 10 children are born with a risk factor. The serious limitation of the risk criteria approach, well-appreciated even in the early 1980s (e.g., Stein, Clark, & Kraus, 1983), was the impossibility of detecting early hearing loss in the other 50 percent of infants—those who were born healthy in a well-baby nursery, with no obvious risk factors. Among the healthy well-baby population, an estimated 1 to 3 infants per 1000 have permanent hearing loss sufficient to interfere with normal speech and language acquisition (American Academy of Pediatrics, 1999). At the time, however, the idea of routinely screening the other 90 percent of infants born in well-baby nurseries (over 3,600,000 babies in the United States alone) was more than a daunting task—it was simply out of the question for many reasons. Even if every audiologist devoted all of his or her time to newborn hearing screening with the existing diagnostic evoked response systems, personnel were lacking. The majority of well babies were born in hospitals that did not employ audiologists. And, importantly, mass hearing screening by audiologists and sophisticated equipment was not cost efficient.

During the same time period—the mid-1980s—clinical devices for automated ABR were designed, evaluated with clinical trials, and then introduced to the market (Hall, Kileny, & Ruth, 1987; Kileny, 1987; Stewart et al., 2000). The availability of automated ABR instrumentation was a major breakthrough as it permitted cost-efficient and accurate hearing screening of large numbers of babies by nonaudiologic personnel (e.g., nurses, technicians). Within a decade, the JCIH and other well-respected groups also identified otoacoustic emissions as an acceptable technique for newborn hearing screening. Over a period of about five years—from the mid-1990s to year 2000—universal newborn hearing

screening (UNHS) expanded remarkably throughout the United States and other countries in the world. The rapid expansion of UNHS was really a product of three converging variables—technology, research, and policy. The four main reasons for the introduction and expansion of UNHS are development of automated technology, research evidence of benefit from early intervention, widespread multidisciplinary professional support, and public policy endorsement. Detailed information on the historical evolution of UNHS and widely accepted protocols and procedures for newborn hearing with ABR is available from multiple and easily accessible sources. The reader is referred to formal position statements endorsed by multiple disciplines with an interest in infant hearing and published by the Joint Committee on Infant Hearing (JCIH). Indeed, the latest JCIH statement is mandatory reading for anyone involved in some aspect of early hearing detection and intervention, now known as EHDI. The JCIH statements can be found in publications and on the websites for the professional organizations participating on the Committee, including the American Academy of Audiology (www.audiology.org), the American Speech-Language-Hearing Association (www.asha.org), the American Academy of Otolaryngology-Head & Neck Surgery (www.aaohns.org), and the American Academy of Pediatrics (www.aap.org). The published statements include a wealth of information on risk factors for infant hearing loss (including progressive and delayed onset hearing loss), detailed guidelines for establishing an early intervention program, recommendations for screening techniques, benchmarks or goals for each aspect of a program for early identification of hearing loss in children, and a comprehensive roadmap for timely and appropriate intervention. For quick and easy access, the above-noted websites, and other sources of information on newborn hearing screening, are summarized in Table 9.1.

TABLE 9.1. Selected Sources of Information on Early Identification and Intervention for Hearing Loss in Infants and Young Children

- American Academy of Audiology (www.audiology.org)
- American Speech-Language-Hearing Association (www.asha.org)
- American Academy of Otolaryngology-Head & Neck Surgery (www.aaohns.org)
- American Academy of Pediatrics (www.aap.org)
- Centers for Disease Control, U.S. Department of Health. Early Hearing Detection Intervention Program, National Center for Birth Defects and Developmental Disabilities (www.cdc.gov/ncbddd/ehdi)
- National Center for Hearing Assessment and Management (NCHAM) (www.infanthearing.org)
- Alexander Graham Bell Association for the Deaf and Hard of Hearing (www.agbell.org)
- International Working Group on Childhood Hearing (IGCH) (www.childhearinggroup.isib.cnr.it)

Given the volume of published information on UNHS, and the worldwide endorsement, acceptance, and implementation of UNHS, little would be gained by providing herein a historical overview of or a treatise on the rationale for screening hearing in newborn infants or a regurgitation of the information already easily accessible in its original form from many sources. The literature on ABR in newborn hearing screening has, likewise, been summarized in detail within numerous other publications. The reader utilizing a specific technique for newborn hearing screening, e.g., automated ABR or otoacoustic emissions (TEOAE or DPOAE), should review published information on the technique, including original papers describing clinical trials, test performance, and cost analysis.

Test Protocol for Infant Screening with ABR

Automated techniques, either ABR and/or OAE, are now relied upon for screening almost all infants born healthy and not at risk for hearing loss. The multiple benefits of automated ABR (AABR) as a screening technique will be discussed in the next section, to be followed by a review of the most effective strategy—combined automated OAE/AER—for hearing screening of all newborn infants, well baby or at risk. Even in the current era of UNHS, the demand exists for a conventional ABR assessment at bedside in the intensive care nursery (i.e., NICU) setting performed by a skilled clinician. Most weeks, the author conducts one or two complete ABR measurements in the NICU to document auditory status of infants at risk for hearing loss. In most cases, the infants either yielded a "Refer" outcome on AABR or automated OAE or are diagnosed with a syndrome strongly associated with hearing loss, such as Cornelia de Lange, Goldenhar's, or CHARGE syndrome. These and other high-risk indicators for infant hearing loss are reviewed in a subsequent section on pediatric auditory disorders. A diagnostic ABR at bedside before hospital discharge, with the option for manipulating stimulus and acquisition parameters as indicated, generally permits documentation of the type and degree of hearing loss even under adverse measurement conditions (e.g., considerable electrical and myogenic artifact). The availability of air- and bone-conduction stimulation, the opportunity for close visual analysis of waveform replicability, and calculation of absolute and interwave latencies for all ABR components permit verification that an ABR is present and allow for differentiation of conductive, sensory, mixed, and neural auditory dysfunction, including auditory neuropathy.

Accumulated experience over the past thirty years with ABR as a diagnostic procedure, and as a screening technique, has led to the development of a proven test protocol. The many lessons about ABR measurement in infants learned (sometimes the hard way) and reported collectively in the literature by dozens of clinical researchers during the 1970s and 1980s (reviewed above) are now integrated into ABR instrumentation and test protocols. That is, the ABR protocol

and equipment used for neurodiagnostic assessment, mostly of adults, was modified and adapted to permit successful ABR measurement with infants. Changes in the protocol involved an assortment of stimulus and acquisition parameters. Alterations in the equipment included, for example, the use of insert earphones and miniature lightweight probe assemblies and probe tips to couple the earphone properly to the tiny infant ear. Equipment adaptations also included the development and manufacture of small, highly adhesive, disposable electrodes for single use with an infant.

Concepts important in ABR measurement of infants will now be discussed briefly. Key components of a protocol for newborn hearing screening with ABR, and the reason for their use in infants, are summarized in Table 9.2. Close review of the information in the table is recommended as a starting point for clinicians who apply the ABR as a screening tool in infants. The recommendations for a test protocol summarized in the table and below are supplemented by a detailed review of ABR stimulus and acquisition parameters in Chapters 3 and 6. To prepare for application of the ABR in hearing screening and diagnosis of auditory function in neonates and young children, the clinician is also advised to study carefully the information presented in Chapters 3 and 6. For confident and consistently successful ABR measurement in this challenging patient population, one must be capable of making rapid and on-the-spot decisions about changes in the protocol based on a variety of interrelated variables, e.g., test and subject conditions, and ongoing analysis of ABR data. The foundation for this capacity to appropriately "think on one's feet" is a thorough understanding of the principles of ABR measurement, and the "hows and whys" of the test protocol.

STIMULUS PARAMETERS. | The first step in successful infant screening with ABR is the use of insert earphones with a probe assembly and miniature probe tips, or some other earphone arrangement, designed specifically for use with newborn infants. Examples of several such earphone and cushion or probe tip designs are illustrated in Figure 9.2. The many benefits of insert earphones in ABR measurement are cited in Chapter 3. The selection of other stimulus parameters cited in Table 9.2 is rather straightforward. Although the exact stimulus rate is not important, minimizing test time is an obvious advantage to using a relatively fast rate of stimulation for newborn hearing screening. Years of clinical experience confirm that stimulus rates within the region of 25 to 35 clicks per second permit rapid signal averaging without adversely affecting the quality or reliability of an infant ABR. Minor manipulations in stimulus rate during infant ABR recordings can be useful in minimizing undesirable electrical artifact that deteriorates waveform morphology and confounds identification of wave V. The NICU is an electrically hostile environment, with multiple potential sources of electrical activity (e.g., monitoring devices, fluorescent lights, pumps) close to the baby and the auditory evoked response instrumentation

TABLE 9.2. Guidelines for an ABR Test Protocol for Auditory Screening of Infants and Young Children

Stimulus and acquisition parameters for measurement of auditory evoked responses, including the ABR, are reviewed thoroughly in Chapter 3. Literature pertaining to the test protocol for ABR is reviewed in Chapter 6.

PARAMETER	SELECTION	RATIONALE/COMMENT
Stimulus Parameters		
Transducer	Insert earphone	Insert earphones are essential for infant ABR assessment with probe tips and coupler designed for use with very small external ear canals.
Type	Click	Click stimuli are typically used for infant hearing screening. Tone-burst stimuli may also be used, especially for higher frequencies (e.g., 2000 or 4000 Hz).
Duration	0.1 ms (100 μs)	Although the electrical signal for a click is 0.1 ms, the acoustical signal is longer in duration. Tone-burst duration is 2–0–2 cycles.
Polarity	Rarefaction	ABR wave V may have larger amplitude and shorter latency for a rarefaction polarity stimulus than for condensation or alternating polarity; however, immediately change to another polarity if the waveform is suboptimal.
Rate	> 20/sec, e.g., 27.3 or 31.7	A faster rate saves time without affecting quality of ABR. An odd number (21.1 or 27.3) for stimulus rate (versus an even integer, e.g., 20) reduces the chance of an interaction during signal averaging between the usual electrical frequency (50 or 60 Hz depending on the country). Changing the rate slightly may minimize any interaction with electrical interference, indicated by an undulating artifact affecting the waveform.
Intensity	35 dB nHL or lower	A conventional screening stimulus intensity level of 35 dB nHL is adequate for detecting hearing loss of > 25 dB HL. Detection of a reliable ABR wave V at 20 dB nHL for a click stimulus, however, confirms normal hearing sensitivity (< 15 dB HL) somewhere within the high range of audiometric frequencies (e.g., 1000 to 8000 Hz). The term "dB nHL" and its derivation is reviewed in Chapter 3.
Repetitions	Variable	The appropriate number of stimulus repetitions (or sweeps) is determined by how many or few are needed during signal averaging to produced an adequate signal-to-noise ratio (SNR) for confident detection of wave V either visually or with a statistical algorithm. For a click stimulus-intensity level of 35 dB nHL, between 1000 to 4000 sweeps is adequate. The amount of noise encountered during ABR screening is a major factor affecting the SNR and, therefore, the minimum acceptable number of stimulus presentations.
Masking (nontest ear)	Unnecessary	The stimulus intensity level in a screening ABR (e.g., 35 dB nHL) is far below the minimal level for acoustic crossover, i.e., interaural attenuation is adequate.
Mode	Monaural	The stimulus must be presented to only the test ear.
Acquisition Parameters		
Electrodes		
Noninverting	Fz	In infants, a high forehead site (Fz) is preferable to a vertex site. A noninverting site on the contralateral ear (a horizontal electrode array, or Ac-Ai) is helpful for recording an ABR when there is excessive electrical artifact with the typical ipsilateral (Fz-Ai) electrode array.
Inverting	Ai or nape of neck	Nape of neck (noncephalic) electrode yields the largest wave V, thus permitting more confident detection of wave V at low stimulus intensity levels.
Ground (common)	Fpz	A low forehead site is convenient for the common electrode, but the ground electrode can really be located anywhere on the body.

(continued)

TABLE 9.2.   (continued)

PARAMETER	SELECTION	RATIONALE/COMMENT
Filters		
High pass	30 to 75 Hz	Low frequencies are important and essential for recording maximum amplitude of wave V for an infant ABR. High-pass filter settings of 100 Hz or higher should be avoided.
Low pass	1500 or 3000 Hz	Either low-pass filter setting is appropriate for ABR screening.
Notch	None	Use of the notch filter is not advised because it removes low-frequency energy that contributes importantly to the infant ABR spectrum. With the notch filter "enabled," amplitude of the infant ABR wave V is diminished, making confident identification more difficult.
Amplification	× 100,000	Amplification of × 100,000 is equivalent to sensitivity of ± 25 mV and is adequate for ABR screening of infants.
Analysis time	15 ms	An averaging epoch of 15 ms encompasses the entire ABR waveform, including wave V and the following trough, which is evoked by click stimuli in infants, even at low intensity levels and for premature babies. Remember, the ABR is not mature in newborn infants and the wave V latency is normally delayed in comparison to values for older children and adults.
Pre-stimulus time	−1 ms	Inspection of a baseline waveform before stimulus presentation provides information on recording conditions and response quality and influences analysis of the infant ABR.
Sweeps (# stimuli)	Variable	Whatever number is needed to produce a good SNR (a clear and reliably recorded ABR wave V with relatively low background electrical activity, or noise).
Runs (replications)	≥ 2	Confirmation that an ABR wave V is present is enhanced greatly by verification that the response is reliable, i.e., the wave V is observed in the same latency region in two or more separately averaged waveforms. Remember . . . *If the waveform doesn't replicate, then you must investigate.*

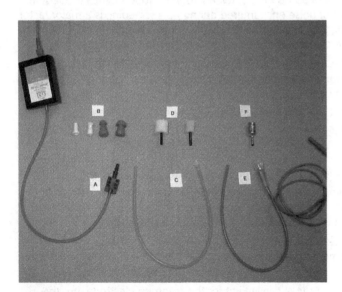

FIGURE 9.2.   Earphones and couplers for transducers and ear cushions specifically designed for use with infants and young children.

(electrodes and wires and physiologic amplifier and cable). In some cases, there is an interaction during signal averaging between the rate of stimulation and electrical interference. The source of the electrical interference is rarely apparent. The interaction is detected during averaging by large amplitude and highly periodic peaks and troughs in the ongoing display, artifactual activity that obscures any evidence of an ABR. A very slight change in the stimulus rate, e.g., from 27.1 to 29.7/sec, often reduces the undesirable contamination of electrical artifact and results in an adequate signal (ABR) to noise (extraneous electrical activity) ratio and confident identification of the wave V component. On occasion, it's necessary during an ABR screening or assessment in the NICU or other electrically active settings to repeatedly alter the stimulus rate (always to another odd number) to elude the mysterious electrical interference.

ACQUISITION PARAMETERS. | Proper selection of certain acquisition parameters listed in Table 9.2 is crucial to recording and confidently detecting an ABR in an infant or young child. Indeed, for some of the acquisition parameters an unwise choice can lead to a false-positive error in waveform analysis, e.g., the conclusion that no response is present when, in fact, the child has normal hearing. An example of such a mistake in measurement of an ABR in infant is the use of a contralateral electrode array, rather than an ipsilateral array. Rarely is an ABR recorded from a newborn infant with the inverting electrode located near the ear contralateral to the side of stimulation. With an older child or adult, in contrast, if an ABR is present in the ipsilateral array, then a reliable response is invariably recorded with a contralateral electrode array, lacking the wave I component but with clear waves III and V. The influence of electrode array on ABR waveforms for newborn infants versus older children and adults is illustrated in Figure 9.3. The precise explanation for the characteristic absence of a contralateral ABR in newborn infants is not clear, but contributing factors might include the plane of the electrode array relative to the generators of ABR components, small head size, and perhaps immaturity of the nervous system. In any event, an infant who yields a clear and reliable ABR with a noninverting electrode on the forehead and an inverting electrode on the ear ipsilateral to the stimulus will typically show no response when the inverting electrode is on the other ear. Actually, it's quite easy to mistakenly depend on a contralateral electrode array in recording an infant from a child. During hasty and/

or hectic preparation for an ABR procedure in a busy clinical setting, the inverting electrode from one ear can be inadvertently plugged into the receptacle for the opposite ear. Or, the electrode that was intended for the right ear may be placed by mistake on the left ear. About 10 percent of males (the author is among them) have a genetically determined "red/green color deficiency," often referred to incorrectly as "color blindness." Mixing up electrode wires with colors that are not primary and distinct is not difficult when one cannot distinguish among the colors.

How can simple mistakes be minimized in ABR measurement of infants and young children? As noted in Chapter 3, the author has a long-standing policy of consistently using an obviously different color for each electrode lead, i.e., yellow or white for the noninverting (forehead) electrode lead, a red lead for the right ear (one inverting) electrode, and a blue lead for the left ear electrode, and then a gray or black color for the ground (common) electrode. If sets of new electrodes are not available for purchase in specific colors, each wire can be identified with a removable tag labeled appropriately (e.g., Fz, RE, LE, Gnd). Consistency in test protocols and practices, even for little steps like electrode placement, helps to minimize operator error in ABR measurement.

Returning to ways an ABR can be perhaps unknowingly recorded with the contralateral electrode array, this mistake will occur if the clinician delivers the stimulus to the incorrect ear. Even if the electrodes are placed properly, a contralateral ABR will be recorded if the earphones are reversed. To minimize the likelihood of this mistake with insert earphones, the clinician should always verify that the red insert tube is connected to the right insert earphone transducer box, and vice versa. Then, just before the command is given to begin signal averaging, the clinician should make a final inspection of the location of each electrode and each earphone. Taking a few seconds to double-check the equipment setup before recording an ABR will save many minutes of precious test time, and considerable consternation, during an ABR recording. There's one more flaw in ABR measurement that can consistently result in incorrect contralateral recordings, particularly if newborn hearing screenings are performed by volunteer or inexperienced personnel. Electrodes are each placed on the appropriate sites, including each inverting electrode on the correct ear. The earphones are also situated on the correct ear. The appropriateness of the electrode and earphone placement is double-checked by the tester, according to protocol. The baby is lying on one side, so a decision is made to first screen hearing of the uppermost ear, using an electrode array with the inverting electrode on that ear (the noninverting electrode is always on the forehead). Then, perhaps in haste to complete the screening while the baby remains sleeping, the tester turns the baby over and immediately begins to deliver stimuli to the other ear, without switching to the inverting electrode on the new test ear. Speaking from experience, it's not hard to make this mistake. If the error goes unrecognized or is committed often by an

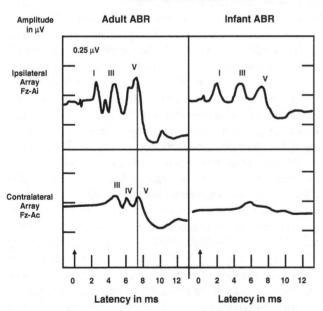

FIGURE 9.3. Effect of electrode array on the auditory brainstem response (ABR) waveform in infants versus older children and adults. A horizontal electrode array is a viable option for recording infant ABRs, especially in electrically noisy environments. The contralateral electrode array, in contrast, is not a good choice, as most infants have no detectable ABR with this recording arrangement.

inexperienced tester, the newborn hearing screening program will be fraught with a very high proportion of unilateral ABR "Refer" outcomes. Most infants will yield a "Pass" outcome with the ipsilateral ABR and most will yield a "Refer" outcome for the ABR recorded, inadvertently, with the contralateral electrode array.

A proper high-pass filter setting is also essential for consistently successful ABR hearing screening results. As discussed in Chapters 3 and 6, the spectrum of the infant ABR is dominated by low-frequency energy that is included in, and contributes to, the magnitude of the response only if the high-pass filter setting is adequately low. Since much of the infant ABR spectrum is below 100 Hz, a high-pass filter cutoff of 30 Hz is recommended in the hearing screening protocol, rather than higher filter cutoff values (e.g., 100 or 150 Hz). The same rationale applied to the recommendation for avoiding the notch filter during ABR measurement from infants. In modifying a template test protocol for ABR applications in adults for infant hearing screening, a default "enabled" or "on" setting for notch filter could easily be overlooked and not changed. The typically analog (rather than digital) notch filter removes a rather broad chunk of frequencies from the EEG of the brain before the ABR is averaged. Although the purpose of the notch filter is to eliminate electrical activity at the 60 Hz frequency, assumed to be electrical artifact, a broader band of energy in energy above and below 60 Hz is also filtered out. Use of the notch filter in a infant hearing screening protocol invariably has the undesirable effect of removing substantial energy from the ABR and rarely produces the desired effect—elimination of electrical artifact.

Another acquisition parameter that can easily be set improperly is analysis time. An analysis time of 10 ms is often employed with neurodiagnostic application of the ABR in adults because for a high stimulus intensity level the entire ABR waveform, including wave V and the following trough, appears within the first 7 to 8 ms after stimulus onset. If a 10 ms analysis time is used to record an ABR from an infant, however, especially at a low stimulus–intensity level, there's a good possibility that the ABR will not be detected. An example clearly makes this point. For a normal-hearing infant at a gestational age of 33 to 34 weeks, the average latency of the wave V component for a click stimulus at an intensity level of 25 dB nHL is 10.35 ms (van Riper & Kileny, 2002), with the subsequent negative wave following over an additional 1 to 2 ms. Clearly, the entire ABR for a normal-hearing infant would fall outside an inappropriately brief analysis time of 10 ms, resulting in a serious error in analysis—the assumption of a screening failure ("Refer" outcome) when in fact the infant has normal hearing. A variety of commonly encountered measurement and subject factors—e.g., hearing loss, prematurity, raster stimulus presentation rate, etc.— actually prolong the infant ABR wave V latency far beyond 10 ms, enhancing the likelihood of an error in ABR screening outcome with an inappropriate analysis time. The simple solution to this serious problem with recording and analysis

in infant screening with the ABR is the consistent use of an analysis time of 15 ms or more.

Two other acquisition parameters warrant a brief comment. Decisions about the number of stimulus presentations, or sweeps, required in infant ABR screening must be based on the size of the response in comparison to background activity—the signal-to-noise ratio—not on a predetermined and fixed number of stimuli (e.g., 1500 or 2000). The number of stimuli required during infant ABR screening is entirely dependent on subject factors (e.g., hearing status and state of arousal) and measurement conditions (e.g., electrical noise in the test setting). For a normal-hearing infant who is sleeping soundly in an electrically quiet test setting, an ABR might be easily detected with only 500 to 1000 sweeps. On the other hand, under adverse measurement conditions, more than 4000 sweeps may be necessary to either confirm the presence of a wave V component (a "Pass" outcome) or to verify with confidence that no response is present (a "Refer" outcome). Finally, it is good clinical policy to always confirm the presence of an ABR at the screening intensity level (e.g., 35 dB nHL) by recording a second ABR and then superimposing the two waveforms for analysis of replicability of the wave V and the negative trough after wave V, (i.e., to verify that the ABR wave V is repeatable within the same general latency region. Strategies contributing to efficient and successful ABR measurement in infants and young children are summarized in Table 9.3.

INFECTION CONTROL. | Precautions to prevent the spread of infection are important with any clinical service and with any population. Extra precautions are appropriate, however, with newborn infants and young children, especially in the hospital setting where nosocomial infections (spread from human to human) are a serious problem, and a patient's resistance to infection may be compromised by poor health status. Immediately following an ABR screening or assessment, and particularly just before a screening or assessment begins, clean and disinfect the earphones, probe assemblies, electrode cables, preamplifier boxes, and other components of the evoked response system that may come into contact with the patient. Reusable components that make contact with infants (e.g., probe tips and tubing) can be properly disinfected with hospital-approved substances (e.g., Cidex). Commercially available germicidal disposable cloths (e.g., SaniCloth Plus®) work very well for this purpose. An Internet search will uncover many options for disinfecting clinical equipment. Also, representatives from the infectious disease prevention office in a medical center can provide specific recommendations on disinfecting practices that are effective, recommended by the institution, and pose no risk to the patient.

Automated ABR (AABR) Technique

Substantial literature has accumulated on the application of ABR in newborn hearing screening since Robert Galambos

TABLE 9.3. Summary of Some General Techniques and Strategies for Clinical Application of the ABR in Estimating Auditory Threshold, Usually in Children

General Strategy

- For young children (under age 2 years), verify and record chronological age in months (gestational age for neonates).
- Ready equipment, instruct and prepare patient. Encourage restful state, with sleeping if possible.
- Administer sedation if appropriate. Document dose and patient status (see Chapter 8). Wait for patient to fall asleep. To facilitate patient sleep and make best use of time, it is often advisable for the clinician to leave the test room, periodically returning to check the patient's status.
- Apply electrodes, verify impedance (reapply any electrode with absolute impedance exceeding 5000 ohms or impedance that is 2000 ohms or more than other electrodes), place transducers, and dim test room lighting. Electrode application, or at least preparation of electrode sites, may precede sedation.
- Obtain two ABR waveforms with an air-conduction click stimulus at a moderate to high intensity level (e.g., 60 to 80 dB HL) in one ear. The starting intensity level is determined by the patient's sleep state and prior information on hearing status. A lower intensity level at the start of the ABR assessment is appropriate for the possibility of normal-hearing infants who are sleeping naturally. The higher level is appropriate for children who are lightly anesthetized (they won't be awoken by the loud sound) and/or children with moderate hearing loss or greater. Only continue signal averaging (presenting stimuli) until an ABR is detected and ongoing averaging has minimal effect on morphology and ease of detection. As soon as a clear ABR is detected, manually stop the averaging process and immediately begin averaging the second ABR to assure that the response is replicable. *At high stimulus intensity levels in quiet normal-hearing children, no more than 250 to 500 sweeps (stimulus presentations) are required to yield a well-formed and replicable ABR waveform.*

If . . .

- Replicated wave I, wave III, and wave V are present at normal latencies, go to a screening intensity level (e.g., 30 or even as low as 20 dB HL) and complete two runs. Then, if a replicated wave V is present, decrease intensity level in 10 dB steps to the minimal level at which a wave V is present. If a replicated response is not present at the screening intensity level, increase the intensity level in 10 dB steps as just described to find minimal response level.
- Replicated waves III and V, or only V, are present, go to 40 dB nHL. Depending on whether a replicable response is or is not present, decrease or increase intensity level in 10 dB steps to find minimal response level.
- No replicated wave V is present at 40 dB nHL, go to 80 or 90 dB HL. It's not inappropriate to apply 50 dB HL masking (white noise) to nontest ear, although masking is not always necessary if insert earphones are used (higher interaural attenuation). Depending on whether a replicable response is or is not present, de-

crease or increase intensity level in 10 dB steps to find minimal response level.
- If no response at highest stimulus intensity level, verify that the stimulus is present and check earphone placement.
- If patient remains quiet (sleeping or not restless), then:
  - Beginning at minimal response level determined first in 10 dB steps (above), redetermine minimal response level in 5 dB steps for each ear.
  - At high intensity level (e.g., 80 to 95 dB), attempt to record clear waves I, III, and V for each ear. Calculate absolute and interwave latencies. Compare values to age-matched normative data.
- If wave I latency is abnormally delayed, and/or wave V latency–intensity function is consistently delayed versus age-matched normative data, consider bone-conduction stimulation at the mastoid.
  - Begin at 40 dB HL (usually 80 to 85 dB dial reading) with a two-channel ipsi- versus contralateral electrode array with stimulation of the ear showing greater air conduction latency delay. Follow guidelines for enhancing wave I (Table 7.1, Chapter 7). Apply 50 dB masking to contralateral ear. An important objective is to first identify wave I in ipsilateral channel. Wave I in ipsilateral channel assures response from test ear (versus crossover response). Then, decrease intensity level in 20 dB or 10 dB increments to determine minimal wave V response level. Plot air-conduction and bone-conduction wave V latency values on a latency–intensity function sheet.
  - Repeat the same process for other ear. If there is a difference for air- versus bone-conduction ABR wave V latency, attempt to carry out immittance audiometry (especially tympanometry) while patient remains asleep.
- If air-conduction click ABR minimal level exceeds 60 dB and ABR pattern is not conductive (as described above), consider tone-burst stimulation to define frequency-specific hearing sensitivity.
  - For auditory threshold estimation in a cooperative adult (e.g., suspected malingerer), use ASSR or ABR with tone-burst stimulation at frequencies of 500, 1000, 2000, and 4000 Hz.
  - For threshold estimation in a child, follow steps above, for each ear first for 500 Hz tone burst and then for 1000 Hz.
- Assure the reliability of responses and plot wave V latency–intensity functions for air- and bone-conduction click stimulation at each intensity level and for each ear as responses are identified. Do not wait until test is completed to plot these data. Information plotted on latency–intensity functions is useful in developing ongoing test strategy.
- Verify that sedated patient can be aroused. Obtain medical clearance to dismiss sedated patient, if necessary.
- Plot out replicated waveforms with appropriate labels for ear, stimulus level, and location of peaks. Prepare a chart note and/or report.

and colleagues first demonstrated the feasibility of ABR screening over thirty years ago (Schulman-Galambos & Galambos, 1975). Clinical reports of ABR in newborn screening regularly provided practical information that contributed to modifications of the test protocol, instrumentation, and techniques and, in turn, improved test performance and efficiency. Information presented within the protocol in Table 9.2 is a compendium of dividends derived from dozens of clinical studies during the 1980s (see Hall, 1992, for review), most of them conducted following the publication by the JCIH of an updated list of risk indicators for hearing loss (Joint Committee on Infant Hearing, 1982). The most obvious benefit of the collective clinical experience and knowledge was a sharp decrease in ABR screening failure rate and test time. By the mid-1980s, failure rates of less than 10 percent were commonly reported for ABR screening, even for the at-risk population where actual hearing loss can be documented in about 5 to 6 percent of the infants. The first automated devices designed specifically for newborn hearing screening also were introduced during the mid–1980s. Hall, Ruth, and Kileny (Hall, Kileny, & Ruth, 1987; Kileny, 1987) reported clinical trials of an automated ABR device—the ALGO-1—that compared the ABR waveform from an individual infant to a template derived from the composite ABRs from a series of infants with confirmed normal hearing sensitivity. The template, heavily weighted for detection of wave V and the negative trough following ABR wave V, shifted in time over a range of ±1.5 ms so that infants with minor differences in wave V latency due to maturation or inconsequential middle ear dysfunction would not be classified as (false) "Refer" outcomes. The clinical trials involved screening infants in the nursery setting with the ALGO-1 while simultaneously recording ongoing EEG during stimulation. Then, for each of a series of infants, screening results for the ALGO-1 device were validated against a "gold standard" ABR screening outcome. The gold standard was an ABR averaged in the laboratory from the recorded EEG data collected in the nursery, and then interpreted by a skilled and experience audiologist who was unaware of the screening outcome. In NICU populations from each of three different university hospital research sites, Hall, Ruth, and Kileny reported failure rates well under 10 percent. Importantly, these investigators found no examples of false-negative screening errors, as determined by performing a separate "no stimulus" hearing screening with the earphone cushion of the ALGO-1 device affixed to the surface of the bed several feet away from the baby's ear. Within a few years, test performance of the ALGO-1 was further defined by other clinical trials (e.g., Herrmann, Thornton, & Joseph, 1995; Jacobson, Jacobson, & Spahr, 1990).

Over course of the next twenty years, published studies of the automated ABR (AABR) newborn hearing screening technique regularly appeared in the peer-reviewed literature, confirming the findings of the initial small-scale clinical trial of the ALGO-1 device. Selected studies are summarized in Table 9.4. Failure rates as low as 4 percent or less are commonly achievable with AABR screening in the well-baby population, even when screening is conducted within 24 hours after birth. After a brief setup period of 3 to 4 minutes for electrode application and earphone placement, reported AABR test time is typically less about 5 to 6 minutes, and just over a minute (71 seconds) with more advanced technology (e.g., Murray et al., 2004), with screening for both ears sometimes requiring only 30 seconds. Data from a multisite study of over 11,000 infants, reported by Stewart et al. (2000), will be described to illustrate the application of automated ABR in infant hearing screening. As summarized in Table 9.5, the automated ABR technique in the well-baby population produced failure rates of 2 percent or less, even when screening was performed within the first 36 hours after birth. In fact, there were with the AABR technique no differences in failure rates as a function of time after birth beginning within five hours after delivery. Median screening time was consistently less than 6 minutes. There was also evidence of a false-positive rate of less than 2 percent for infant hearing screening with automated ABR. Each of these values meets benchmarks set by the American Academy of Pediatrics (1999) of < 4 percent for "Refer" rate and < 2 percent for false-positive rate. Variations in failure rates among the five sites in the study were closely analyzed in an attempt to ascertain factors contributing to the differences. Data analysis confirmed that the type of hearing screening personnel (e.g., audiologist, nurse, technician, volunteer) was unrelated to screening test performance. Rather, the experience of screening personnel was most important factor determining test performance. Other investigators have confirmed that test performance with AABR is acceptable even with entirely volunteer-based or nurse-based UNHS programs (e.g., Messner et al., 2001; Meurer et al., 2000). "Refer" rates reported by Stewart et al. (2000) were indirectly correlated with tester experience—the more babies a person screened, the lower the average "Refer" rate. Consistent with data reported in other studies on the AABR technique (e.g., Lemons et al., 2002), the learning curve was relatively short (several weeks) for the AABR device used in the multi-site study. That is, minimal and stable "Refer" rates were obtained within a few weeks after screening personnel were trained and gained a modest amount of experience with the AABR screening technique in the nursery setting.

There are now many options for commercially available instrumentation designed expressly for hearing screening of infants and young children. Devices designed specifically for newborn hearing screening include the following features: (1) transducers and probe tips or ear couplers permitting precise stimulus delivery into the very small infant ear canals and attenuation of ambient noise reaching the ear canal, (2) small size and light weight for portability and ease of use at the bedside in a nursery setting, (3) the option for battery operation, (4) a selection of test protocols appropriate for different test conditions (e.g., quiet versus

TABLE 9.4. Published Reports of Automated Auditory Brainstem Response (AABR) in Newborn Hearing Screening (arranged chronologically)

STUDY (YEAR)	N	POPULATION	DEVICE	REFER RATE	COMMENT
Hall, Kileny, & Ruth (1987)	600	HR*	ALGO-1	<10%	Clinical trial of early automated ABR device
Jacobson & Jacobson (1994)	119	HR/WB	ALGO-1	3.8%	TEOAE refer rate was 38.4%
Chen et al. (1996)	260	HR	ALGO-1	15%	Prevalence of SNHL was 3.1%
Oudesluys-Murphy & Harlaar (1997)	277	WB*	ALGO-1	3.5%	Screening in infant's home in Netherlands
Doyle, Sininger, & Starr (1998)	116	WB	ALGO-2	8%	Refer rate of 43% for TEOAE
Mason & Hermann (1998)	10372	WB	ALGO-2	4%	Incidence of bilateral hearing loss of 1.4/1000
Hahn et al. (1999)	388	WB	ALGO-2	9%	Total average screening time was 8.26 minutes
Meyer et al. (1999)	777	HR	ALGO-1 Plus	5%	Bilateral refer rate was 2%
van Strääten et al. (1996)	250	HR	ALGO-1 Plus	2%	No false negatives were discovered
van Strääten (1999)	review article				Summary of AABR technique and rationale
Iley & Addis (2000)	44	WB	ALGO-2	4.5%	Screening time of 5 minutes
Sininger et al. (2000)	4831	HR	custom (Fsp)	<10%	Excellent review of AABR screening technique
	2348	WB	custom (Fsp)	14%	
Stewart et al. (2000)	11711	HR/WB	ALGO-2	<2%	Screening personnel not factor in refer rate
Messner et al. (2001)	5771	WB	ALGO-2	5%	Only volunteers used for screening
van Strääten et al (2001)	90	HR	ALGO-1 E	0%	Pass/refer rate decreased with gestational age
Vohr et al. (2001)	12081	WB	ALGO-2	3.21%	TEOAE refer rate was 6.49%
Meier, Narabayashi, Probst, & Schmuziger (2004)	150	WB	ALGO-3	2%	TEOAE and DPOAE refer rate was 3%
Murray et al. (2004)	194	WB	ALGO 3	5.7%	Average screening time was 70.8 seconds

* HR = high risk; WB = well babies with no risk factors; ALGO device by Natus, Inc.

noisy), (5) algorithms for automated response detection and noise reduction that are based on and validated with data collected during clinical trials with large number of babies with different age and health characteristics (term versus premature infants) and in different settings (e.g., well-baby nursery versus intensive care nursery), and (6) data for each test protocol derived from clinical trials on test performance (e.g., sensitivity and specificity) in identification of children with normal hearing and children with varying types and degrees of hearing impairment. Other features available with selected AABR devices (e.g., ALGO-3 by Natus Medical, Inc.) include simultaneous bilateral stimulation to increase speed of data acquisition, rapid and efficient detection and rejection of myogenic noise and sweeps contaminated by ambient acoustic noise, and methods for automatic detection of human errors in equipment setup and operation.

All AABR devices determine the presence or absence of the ABR using a "machine scoring" method, without the need for visual inspection by a skilled operator. Data collected are processed with an algorithm for statistical

TABLE 9.5. Summary of Selected Findings for a Multi-Site Study of Automated ABR in Newborn Hearing Screening

SITE OF SCREENING	REFER RATE	SCREEN TIME Minimum (secs)	SCREEN TIME Median (mins:secs)	SCREENING PERSONNEL	FALSE POSITIVE RATE	LOST TO FOLLOW-UP RATE
Boulder	2%	31	5.57	volunteers	2.0 %	19%
Louisville	<1%	30	5:34	nurses	0.35%	45%
Memphis	3%	31	5:35	technicians	2.5 %	13%
Huntsville	1%	32	3:31	audiologists	0.05%	21%
Nashville (ICN)	6%	32	4:40	varied *	2.0 %	32%

*Audiologists, nurses, graduate audiology students
From Stewart et al., 2000.

verification of the outcome ("Pass" or "Refer"). As noted in the review of the study by Hall, Ruth, and Kileny, one AABR screening instrument (the ALGO device marketed by Natus Medical, Inc.) determines the presence of an ABR by matching the measurement to a template representing a normal response. Most other ABR screening devices verify the presence of the response at a low click stimulus intensity level (e.g., 35 dB nHL) by assessing whether the measured ABR signal-to-noise ratio exceeds a specified criterion.

Other techniques for "machine detection and scoring" of ABR waveforms that take into account latency and amplitude response parameters are reported in the literature (e.g., Mason, Davis, Wood, & Farnsworth, 1998). The algorithm employed most often for calculating the ABR signal-to-noise ratio is based on the magnitude of the response when the stimulus is present, i.e., the signal, divided by the magnitude of the response when the stimulus is not present, i.e., the noise (e.g., Hall, Smith, & Popelka, 2004; Sininger et al., 2000). The measured response for infants who have an ABR is larger than the noise, with a signal-to-noise ratio greater than 1.0. In contrast, for babies who do not have an ABR, the measured response is no greater than the noise, producing a signal-to-noise ratio of approximately 1.0. As originally described, the signal-to-noise ratio was evaluated with the F statistic using a value at a single point in the ABR waveform and therefore was labeled Fsp (Don et al., 1984). In modern automated ABR screening devices, signal-to-noise ratio values are based on multiple points rather than a single point. The term Fsp, however, is still commonly used in reference to the algorithm. As noted in Chapter 7, the magnitude of an ABR is quite stable in an individual for stimuli at a fixed level. On the other hand, the magnitude of the noise varies greatly depending on factors involving the patient (e.g., ongoing EEG and muscle activity), environmental factors (e.g., electrical artifact from lights and other equipment) and, importantly, measurement parameters (e.g., stimulus intensity level and the number of stimulus presentations or sweeps. Signal averaging, a parameter directly related to the number of stimulus presentations or sweeps, reduces the noise and, therefore, enhances detection of the ABR. As the amount of signal averaging increases the level of noise decreases, and the value of the Fsp grows larger. Fsp was used for automated ABR in a large NIH sponsored multi-center study of over 7000 newborns (Norton et al., 2000). The results of the study confirmed that a criterion Fsp value of 3.1 effectively separates normal-hearing infants (a "Pass") from infants who must be referred for a follow-up hearing screening or a diagnostic assessment (a "Refer" outcome).

Factors other than test performance (e.g., sensitivity and specificity) influence decisions regarding the costs and benefits of UNHS. Numerous clinical investigators have calculated he cost per infant of AABR screening, and the accumulated costs associated with identification of each child with bilateral hearing loss. Some of the papers summarized in Table 9.4 include such financial data. As a rule, the cost for screening an infant with AABR is in the range of $15 to $35 USD, whereas the cost to identify an infant with true bilateral hearing loss is on the order of $17,000 to $20,000 USD (e.g., Boshuizen et al., 2001; Gorga et al., 2001; Iley & Addis, 2000; Lemons et al., 2002; Mason & Hermann, 1998; van Strääten, 1999). Statistics on the comparative costs of hearing screening with AABR versus OAEs, and other performance parameters for the two techniques, are cited in the next section.

Experience confirms that an adequately low "Refer" rate for hearing screening with AABR (< 4%) can be achieved and maintained by adherence to some rather simple guidelines and techniques:

- Quiet baby: Conduct AABR screening soon after the baby is fed, during usual sleeping time.
- Earphone placement: Assure that the earphone is coupled snugly to the baby's ears and remains secure throughout the screening.
- Electrode placement: Properly prepare the skin before electrode placement to obtain adequately low and balanced interelectrode impedance.
- Screening time after birth: For infants born prematurely, delay hearing screening until close to discharge to allow for infant development and maturity.

- Follow manufacturer recommendations for test protocol and technique.

Combined ABR/OAE Screening Technique

One of the most recent and promising technological advances in newborn hearing screening is the integration of OAE and AABR into a single device. Since their discovery by David Kemp in 1978, otoacoustic emissions have assumed an important role as a hearing screening tool and a valuable procedure in the diagnostic audiology test battery. The reader is referred to a textbook by Hall (2000a) for a comprehensive review of OAE principles, protocols, and clinical applications. The OAE and AABR software share a common lightweight portable computer-based instrument, and one probe is used to deliver stimuli for OAE and AABR measurement. The availability of both screening technologies in one commercially available piece of equipment facilitates the application of combined OAE and AABR screening. There are really three options for combining the techniques in newborn hearing screening. One option, recommended in the NIH 1993 Consensus Conference Report (National Institutes of Health, 1993) and now commonly used in the well-baby population, is a two-step screening strategy that relies on OAEs as the primary technique and AABR as a secondary technique (e.g., Boshuizen et al., 2001; Kaldestad, Wingaard, & Hansen, 2002; Kennedy, 1999; Morlet et al., 1998; Vohr et al., 2001; Watkin & Baldwin, 1999). Most babies (90% or more) are expected to yield a "Pass" outcome with OAE and, assuming no risk factor for progressive or delayed onset hearing loss, the child is released from the screening program. Babies who yield a "Refer" outcome for OAE screening undergo a second screening with the AABR technique before hospital discharge. The advantages of this two-step combination screening strategy are short screening time for the majority of infants, yet a very low overall failure rate for the program. Another option for combining the techniques, clearly feasible and advisable for the NICU population, is to rely on AABR as the primary screening technique, with OAEs as the secondary technique (e.g., Morlet et al., 1998; Valkama et al., 2000; Wood et al., 1998). As detailed in the subsequent review of risk factors for infant hearing loss, children with neurologic risk indicators and associated retrocochlear and central auditory nervous system dysfunction, including children ultimately diagnosed with auditory neuropathy, are likely to be found in the NICU. With this approach, infants who yield a "Refer" outcome for AABR undergo a secondary screening with OAEs before hospital discharge. The third option is, of course, to complete both OAE and AABR hearing screening before hospital discharge for a subset of infants.

A study reported by Hall, Smith, and Popelka (2004) highlights the clinical benefits of a combined OAE/AABR screening strategy. Data were collected with a combined ABR and OAE screening technique for a sample of 600 ears and 300 neonates (161 females and 139 males). ABRs were recorded 13 to 42 hours after birth in the well-baby nursery with battery-operated handheld hearing screener (AUDIOscreener, Everest Biomedical and GSI). Distortion product OAEs at $2f_1$-f_2 were stimulated with four f_2 signal frequencies (2000, 3000, 4000, and 5000 Hz), with an f_1 intensity level (L_1) set at 65 dB SPL and an f_2 intensity level (L_2) set at 55 dB SPL ($L2 - L1 = -10$ dB). A "Pass" outcome for DPOAE screening was defined by a minimum signal-to-noise level difference ($L_{dp} - L_{nf}$) of 6 dB, an minimum L_{dp} values of -7 dB SPL for 2000 Hz, -8 dB SPL for 3000 Hz, -5 dB SPL for 4000 Hz, and -7 dB SPL for 5000 Hz. ABRs for the AUDIOscreener were recorded from scalp electrodes placed at Fz (noninverting) and the ipsilateral masoid (Mi) in response to click signals presented through a probe assembly coupled to the ear. The same probe was used for DPOAE and ABR measurements. The device was configured to present rarefaction clicks at 35 dB nHL at a rate of 37.1/sec. A unique feature of this device is that the level of the stimulus is determined in the actual ear being measured instead of relying on a coupler calibration, as is typically done. The real ear ABR stimuli are determined automatically using a microphone built into the probe. The ABR was collected with a high-pass filter setting of 100 Hz and a low-pass filter setting of 1500 Hz. Maximum electrode impedance was 12 K ohms, while the maximum electrode impedance mismatch was 5 K ohms.

Response presence or absence was determined with the Fsp statistic. The criterion for a "Pass" outcome was an Fsp value of 3.2 or greater. In the analysis of ABR screening data, OAEs provided an independent indication of peripheral auditory status. OAEs were present at four frequencies at levels that exceeded normative values in all ears that received an ABR "Pass" outcome. Therefore, we presume that all of the ears that received an ABR "Pass" result had normal peripheral auditory status. No further testing was performed on these babies. Each ear that yielded an ABR Fsp value of less than 3.2 was categorized as a "Refer" result. All babies who received a "Refer" result in one or both ears also received a full diagnostic evaluation on an outpatient basis within several weeks after the initial screening. Based on an analysis of initial hearing screening findings and follow-up diagnostic audiologic findings, the combination screening strategy was associated by high sensitivity and acceptable specificity. In addition, for babies with a "Refer" outcome with the combination hearing screening approach, differentiation of type of possible auditory disorder was inferred by the pattern of findings for the ABR versus OAE technique (see Table 9.6).

The benefits of the combination ABR/OAE approach for newborn hearing screening, as revealed by the study conducted by Hall, Smith, and Popelka (2004) and others (e.g., Norton et al., 2000), are summarized as follows:

- OAE technology permits for individual patients in-ear calibration of signal intensity for ABR, as well for OAE signals.

TABLE 9.6. Patterns of Findings for a Combined Auditory Brainstem Response and Otoacoustic Emissions Screening Strategy in Relation to Type of Auditory Dysfunction

	SCREENING PROCEDURE	
TYPE OF DISORDER	**ABR**	**OAE**
Normal hearing	normal	normal
Conductive disorder*	normal	abnormal
Sensory disorder	abnormal	abnormal
Neural disorder (e.g., auditory neuropathy)	abnormal	normal

* Mild conductive disorder or occlusion of the external ear canal with vernix

From Hall, Smith, & Popelka, 2004.

- Screening efficiency is enhanced by a combined OAE and ABR strategy. That is, most babies can be rapidly screened with automated OAEs, and then OAE "Refer" outcomes can be immediately screened secondarily by AABR.
- With the combination of OAE and ABR technologies, newborn hearing screening can yield a refer rate of < 2 percent and a false-positive rate of < 0.2 percent.
- A low "Refer" rate results in minimal parental anxiety in the interim between newborn screening in the hospital and the secondary screening, or the diagnostic assessment.
- Follow-up rates for infants who do not pass hearing screening are often far below the 95 percent target set by the American Academy of Pediatrics. With low "Refer" rates, fewer hearing-impaired infants are lost to follow-up.
- Also, the low "Refer" rates characteristic of combined OAE/ABR screening result in the need for fewer diagnostic follow-up assessments and markedly lower costs associated with the identification of each hearing-impaired child.
- The combined use of OAEs and ABR in newborn hearing screening permits differentiation of conductive versus sensory versus neural auditory dysfunction, before hospital discharge. For example, the combination of an OAE "Refer" with AABR "Pass" suggests a peripheral explanation, such as vernix casseosus in the external ear canal or subtle middle ear dysfunction. This possibility can then be confirmed with another technique, e.g., tympanometry. Immediate differentiation among major types of auditory dysfunction, in turn, permits quicker and more appropriate management.
- Finally, the combined application of OAE and ABR in newborn hearing screening leads to early identification of auditory neuropathy in the well-baby population, as well as in the intensive care nursery. A "Pass" outcome

for OAE screening, coupled with a "Refer" AABR outcome, raises the question of auditory neuropathy and certainly warrants follow-up diagnostic audiometry.

Given the availability now of both OAE and AABR techniques, it's reasonable to ask how they compare with regard to test performance and economic considerations. A remarkable number of investigators have evaluated these characteristics for hearing screening with OAE and AABR. Space does not permit an exhaustive review of the literature on the topic of the application of both OAE and AABR techniques in hearing screening of newborn infants. In general, infant hearing screening failure rates and associated screening costs are lower for the AABR technique than for OAEs. A study reported by Lemons and colleagues (2002) offers a representative example of the findings of the papers listed in Table 9.4. Data were collected from 1500 newborn infants with a transient OAE (TEOAE) technique and an AABR technique. OAE screening was conducted by licensed audiologists, whereas AABR screening was performed by neonatal nurses. Average age at the time of screening was 29 hours for the TEOAE technique and 9.5 hours for AABR. Within the first 24 hours after birth, screening was successfully completed with AABR for 84 percent of the infants, whereas during the same time period only 35 percent of the infants could be screened by TEOAE. Throughout the duration of the study, referral rate remained at 15 percent for the TEOAE screening procedure. In contrast, for the AABR technique the referral rate was initially 8 percent, then decreased to 4 percent by the end of the study. Lemons and colleagues (2002) also performed detailed cost analysis of newborn hearing screening with the two techniques. Total predischarge costs for initiating and implementing the newborn hearing screening program were $49,316 USD for TEOAEs and $47,553 USD for AABR, while the cost of screening each infant was $32.23 for TEOAEs and $33.68 for the AABR technique. Finally, costs were calculated for postdischarge hearing screenings and follow-up diagnostic audiologic assessments. The average total costs of procedures performed after hospital discharge will, of course, be influenced by the referral rate—that is, the proportion of babies who fail the initial screening in the hospital and require follow-up assessments. Postdischarge costs for screening and diagnostic hearing procedures were $58.07 USD for the TEOAE procedure and $48.85 USD. Lemons et al. (2002) conclude that "AABR appears to be the preferred method for universal newborn hearing screening. AABR was associated with the lowest costs, achieved the lowest referral rates at hospital discharge, and had the quickest learning curve to achieve those rates" (p. 120).

PEDIATRIC DIAGNOSTIC AUDITORY ASSESSMENT

Although a complete discussion of pediatric AER applications could certainly be the topic of an entire book, the majority of AER principles applied in assessment of peripheral or central auditory function in children are equally appropriate and useful in assessment of adults. For example, an appreciation of the effects of age on AERs is extremely important for interpretation of findings in young children, but also in older adult patients. Also, sedation is often required in pediatric ABR measurement, but sedatives may be a factor to consider in the response interpretation of adults as well, particularly for certain kinds of patients, such as mentally retarded adults, or in certain test settings, such as the ICU. There are some unique pediatric AER measurement considerations. Perhaps the most important of these is the relationship between AER findings and behavioral measures of auditory function. A major motive for AER assessment in children is either to supplement or to confirm information from behavioral audiometry. That is, because of the patient's young age, nonauditory handicap (emotional or neurological), or lack of cooperation, adequate behavioral testing cannot be completed, or for those same reasons, the validity of existing behavioral information on hearing is questioned. Not unexpectedly, then, many of the published papers on pediatric auditory assessment with AERs have focused on their relationship with behavioral findings.

Although a valuable tool for the diagnostic assessment of auditory, otologic, and neurologic disorders in children, the ABR is not a test of hearing. This important qualification was emphasized in Chapter 3. ABR findings should, whenever possible, be analyzed and interpreted in the context of a test battery including other independent electrophysiologic, and also behavioral, measures of auditory function. Recommendations of the JCIH for the diagnostic approach for assessment of hearing of infants, summarized in Table 9.7, offer an excellent example of the importance of a diverse test battery. The importance of the test battery approach for

diagnostic assessment of hearing in children was also emphasized in Chapter 8.

Application of a comprehensive test battery approach for pediatric audiologic assessment offers valuable dividends for accurate diagnosis and appropriate management. One advantage is confidence in the validity of the diagnostic outcome. Over thirty years ago, Jerger and Hayes stressed the importance of the test battery approach in children in their classic paper on the "cross-check principle." An excerpt from the classic paper highlights the main point:

> In summary, we believe that the unique limitations of conventional behavioral audiometry dictate the need for a "test battery" approach. The key concept governing our assessment strategy is the cross-check principle. The basic operation of this principle is that no result be accepted until it is confirmed by an independent measure. . . . We believe that the application of the cross-check principle to our clinical population has had an appreciable effect on the accuracy with which we can identify and quantify hearing loss during the critical years for language learning. (Jerger & Hayes, 1976, p. 65)

The cross-check principle remains relevant for pediatric audiology today. The ABR is an essential component of the test battery, because it provides information about auditory function that is not available from other audiologic procedures. But the ABR should not be applied at the exclusion of other procedures, with test results interpreted in isolation. The diagnostic power of well-selected audiologic procedures incorporated within a test battery greatly exceeds the value of any single procedure within the test battery.

PERIPHERAL AUDITORY DISORDERS

Risk Factors for Infant Hearing Loss

Careful documentation of and close attention to risk indicators for infant hearing loss remains very important, even in the current era of universal newborn hearing screening (UNHS). In the past, the early identification of infants with hearing loss depended almost entirely on risk indicators documented by chart review or parental history. With the advent of UNHS, however, it is reasonable to question the rationale for ongoing efforts to document risk indicators. In other words, if all babies undergo hearing screening at birth, won't all infants with hearing impairment be identified at a very early age? The answer to this question is unequivocally "no," for at least two important reasons. First, UNHS is really not yet universal worldwide. Infant hearing screening programs are scarce in a number of countries and nonexistent in most developing countries. Although interest in and efforts to implement programs for early identification in developing countries is increasing (e.g., Swanepoel, Delport, & Swart, 2004), major national financial, educational, and healthcare challenges must be addressed. In addition, countries or remote regions within countries lacking newborn hearing screening programs also typically have no human,

TABLE 9.7. Summary of the Pediatric Test Battery Recommended by the Joint Committee on Infant Hearing (2000) for Audiologic Assessment of Infants in the Age Range of Birth to 6 Months

---

- Child and family history
- Auditory brainstem response (ABR) during initial evaluation to confirm type, degree, and configuration of hearing loss (may include auditory steady-state response, ASSR)
- Acoustic immittance measures (including acoustic reflexes)
- Behavioral response audiometry (if feasible)
- Otoacoustic emissions (OAEs)
- Visual reinforcement audiometry or conditioned play audiometry
- Speech detection and recognition
- Parental report of auditory and visual behaviors
- Screening of infant's communication milestones

---

technological, or financial resources required to create an infrastructure for intervention for hearing impairment, including providers of hearing care (e.g., audiologists and otolaryngologists) and devices used in management of hearing loss (e.g., hearing aids and cochlear implants). In countries and other geographical regions where such resources are very limited, a focused effort to identify infants at greatest risk for hearing loss is a logical, and possibly feasible, first step toward an ultimate goal of UNHS.

Also, risk indicators remain an essential feature of early identification of hearing loss because a proportion of children with serious and communicatively important hearing loss are born with normal hearing sensitivity. UNHS in the immediate postnatal period is not effective for early identification of children with hearing loss that progresses after birth or is delayed in onset. Progressive and delayed onset hearing loss is associated with specific risk indicators, to be discussed momentarily. The onset of progressive hearing loss may, in some cases, begin at birth. However, it may be so subtle that it escapes detection with current hearing screening techniques. Or, the progressive hearing loss may, at least initially, affect cochlear function for frequencies outside of the range of current hearing screening techniques, e.g., frequencies below 1000 Hz or above 8000 Hz. As the term implies, children with delayed onset hearing loss have normal auditory function at birth and will, of course, pass even the most sensitive hearing screening measure.

Beginning in 1973, the JCIH has recommended hearing screening of infants with one or more risk indicators. Over the years, the list expanded from five risk indicators, as new causes for infant hearing loss were identified through clinical research, to the list of risk indicators noted in the 2000 statement of the JCIH. Space does not permit a detailed explanation of the risk indicators. For a review of the research evidence in support of the selection of the risk indicators, the reader is referred to the most recent JCIH statement, the bibliography cited at the end of the statement, and the rather substantial published literature on risk factors and etiologies for childhood hearing impairment. Two points warrant emphasis at this juncture. First, several of the most commonly encountered risk indicators for hearing impairment are among those least likely to be related to hearing loss. Second, an infant with a risk factor does not necessarily have a hearing impairment. In fact, the majority of infants at risk for hearing impairment do not and will not have hearing impairment. Accumulated clinical experience dating back to the early 1980s confirms that the risk for hearing impairment increases for infants with two or more risk indicators, and some risk indicators are more strongly related to hearing impairment than others.

RISK INDICATORS FOR NEONATAL HEARING LOSS (BIRTH TO 28 DAYS). | Risk indicators recommended by the Joint Committee on Infant Hearing (2000a,b,c) for neonatal hearing loss, e.g., for babies from birth up to 28 days after birth) are

summarized in Table 9.8. Any infant with one or more of the risk factors listed requires hearing screening within the first month after birth. Of course, in most countries infants undergo hearing screening within days after birth and before discharge from the hospital nursery. Screening equipment and personnel are most often available in the hospital setting. In addition, the probability that a child will be located or available to undergo hearing screening drops dramatically after discharge. Differences in the occurrence of risk factors in an infant population, and the likelihood of risk individual risk factors to hearing loss, are summarized in Table 9.9. Although the risk indicator most often identified by chart review, ototoxic medications, is not strongly associated with neonatal hearing loss, it is a risk indicator for progressive hearing loss. Three other risk indicators found relatively infrequently by chart review—congenital infections, bacterial meningitis, and family history—are among those more likely to be found among children with confirmed, permanent, and severe hearing loss. Of considerable concern in a newborn hearing screening program are those risk factors, e.g., severe asphyxia and mechanical ventilation, that are near the top of both lists—frequency of occurrence and association with hearing loss. Professionals involved with early identification of hearing loss in infants must be very familiar with the risk factors listed in Table 9.8 and make every attempt to document the risk factors from chart review and reported medical and family history. Although risk indicators are most often found in the medical charts of children in the NICU, a small proportion of children in the well-baby nursery will also be classified as at risk for hearing loss. Family history of hearing loss is the most prevalent risk indicator among healthy babies.

Although any of the risk indicators may occur in isolation, some of them are features of syndromes or are found among collections of multiple congenital anomalies and disorders detected immediately at birth. More than a hundred syndromes may be associated with conductive, sensory, or mixed hearing loss. An example is aural atresia, a severe malformation in the development of the ear, usually involving the middle ear and external ear, that produces moderate or severe conductive hearing loss. Aural atresia may occur in isolation, in combination with less obvious otologic anomalies (e.g., pre-auricular pits or tags), or as part of a syndrome, such as Treacher-Collins syndrome. Children with Treacher-Collins syndrome typically have, in addition to aural atresia, heart, kidney, genital, and skeletal defects. Preauricular pits and tags often occur in isolation, without any other obvious otologic or craniofacial abnormalities. Kugelman et al. (1997) reported the presence of preauricular pits and tags in 5.7 infants per 1000 births. The authors reported the presence of associated congenital anomalies in 19 percent of the infants with preauricular pits and tags. Either conductive and sensorineural hearing loss was confirmed in approximately one out of four infants with preauricular pits and tags. Two collections of serious physical anomalies of disorders that include ear abnormalities and hea-

TABLE 9.8. Risk Factors (Indicators) for Infant Hearing Loss (Peripheral), Central Nervous System (Auditory Dysfunction), and Delayed Onset Hearing Loss, Arranged Alphabetically

The risk factors also referral indicators for infant hearing screening. The association of risk factors to subsequent documentation of hearing loss for infants ages 29 days through 2 years, including progressive hearing loss, is discussed in the text and summarized in Table 9.10.

Hearing Loss	Neurological Deficits*

• Bacterial meningitis
• Birth weight < 1500 grams
• Congenital infections
  • Cytomegalovirus (CMV)
  • Syphilis
  • Herpes
  • Toxoplasmosis
  • Rubella
• Craniofacial anomalies (CFA)
  • Microcrotia
  • Aural atresia
  • Preauricular pits or tags
  • Stigmata
  • Syndromes associated with hearing loss
• ECMO (extracorporeal membrane oxygenation)
• Family history of hearing loss (permanent congenital or delayed onset hearing loss)
• Hyperbilirubinemia requiring transfusion or as defined by specific blood levels
• Mechanical ventilation for > 5 days
  • Pulmonary hypertension in newborn infant
  • Bronchopulmonary dysplasia
• Ototoxic medications > 3 treatment days or with loop diuretics, e.g.,
  • gentamicin
  • furosemide (lasix)
• Physician and/or parent concern
• Severe respiratory depression at birth (severe asphyxia)
  • Apgar score of 0 at 1 minute
  • Apgar score of 0 to 6 at 5 minutes
	• Hyperbilirubinemia
	• Asphyxia
	• Meningitis
	• CMV
	• Intracranial hemorrhage (IVH)
	• Other cranial or CNS pathology
	  • Encephalopathy
	  • Ventriculomegaly
	  • Hydrocephalus
	• Known risk for neurological handicaps
	• Seizure activity
	• Abnormal findings on clinical neurological examination
	
	**Delayed Onset Hearing Loss ** (1/56 children with permanent hearing loss at 1 year)
	
	• Low birth weight
	• Respiratory distress syndrome
	• Bronchiopulmonary dysplasia
	• Mechanical ventilation for > 36 days

* The 2000 JCIH also recommends as a risk factor for auditory neuropathy infants with a compromised neonatal course who receive intensive neonatal care.

** Children who pass OAE or ABR screening at birth and show evidence of severe hearing loss at 1 year of age by reliable behavioral audiometry. Cone-Wesson et al. (2000) estimate that hearing loss has a delayed onset for 1/56 children with permanent hearing loss at 1 year of age.

From Joint Committee on Infant Hearing, 2000a,b,c; Van Riper & Kileny, 1999.

ing loss, or risk factors for hearing loss, are referred to by the acronyms CHARGE and TORCH. The letters in CHARGE are labels for the following defects: coloboma of the eye, head anomaly, atresia (stenosis) of choana in the nose, retardation of growth and/or development, genital hypoplasia, and ear anomalies and/or hearing impairment. The acronym TORCH refers to toxoplasmosis, other (including syphilis), rubella, cytomegalovirus (CMV), and herpes simplex. The majority of infants with the CHARGE disorders have some degree of hearing loss (Edwards, Kileny, & van Riper, 2002; Thelin & Fussner, 2005).

Also listed in Table 9.8 are risk indicators for neurologic dysfunction and possible retrocochlear or central auditory nervous system dysfunction. In the general newborn population, cochlear hearing impairment is by far more common than central auditory dysfunction. The incidence of neurologic insults and risk factors is considerably higher in the NICU population. Also, it's important to recognize that selected risk factors, such as hyperbilirubinema, asphyxia, meningitis, and CMV, are associated with both cochlear and retrocochlear auditory dysfunction. The possibility of central auditory dysfunction—hearing impairment that can adversely

TABLE 9.9. Relation of Risk Factors and Subsequently Diagnosed Hearing Loss for a Series of 2,103 Infants According to the Frequency of Occurrence Ranked from Most Likely (top) to Least Likely (bottom)

FREQUENCY OF OCCURRENCE (% OF TOTAL)

Risk Factor	Hearing Loss
Ototoxic medications (>70%)	Craniofacial anomalies (>50%)
Severe asphyxia (>50%)	Severe asphyxia (>15%)
Mechanical ventilation >5 days (>25%)	Congenital infections (>15%)
Low birth weight (<1500 grams (>20%)	Family history (>15%)
Parental/physician concern (>15%)	Mechanical ventilation (>10%)
ECMO (>10%)	Bacterial meningitis (>10%)
Hyperbilirubinemia*	Low birth weight*
Craniofacial anomalies*	Hyperbilirubinemia*
Family history*	Ototoxic medications*
Congenital infections*	ECMO*
Bacterial meningitis*	Substance abuse (maternal)*
Substance abuse (maternal)**	Parent/physician concern**
Neurodegenerative disorders**	Neurodegenerative disorders**

* Frequency of occurrence as risk factor or hearing loss < 10%

** Negligible frequency of occurrence

From Cone-Wesson et al., 2000; Van Riper & Kileny, 2002.

impact the acquisition of speech, language, and communication function—in children with neurologic risk indicators has two very fundamental implications for the strategy used to identify and diagnosis newborn hearing screening. In the NICU, where most of the infants with neurologic risk factors are found, ABR must be the primary screening technique. Otoacoustic emissions are inadequate as the sole screening technique in the NICU because children with even marked retrocochlear or central auditory nervous system abnormalities will go undetected. As discussed in a previous section of this chapter, a combination of the ABR and OAE techniques has merit in both the NICU and well-baby nursery. Given the higher proportion of infants with neurologic dysfunction in the NICU, the ABR should be used there as the primary hearing screening technique, with a secondary screening by OAEs for infants who yield a "Fail" ABR screening outcome to differentiate retrocochlear versus cochlear auditory dysfunction. Neurologic risk indicators also have implications for early detection and timely diagnosis of auditory neuropathy. Most children who eventually meet criteria for the diagnosis of auditory neuropathy are identified by the neurologic risk indicators listed in Table 9.8, along with selected risk indicators for progressive hearing loss to be discussed next.

RISK INDICATORS FOR DELAYED ONSET HEARING LOSS. | Some children with communicatively important hearing loss at 1 year of age or later will have normal hearing at birth and will, therefore, yield a "Pass" outcome with any newborn hearing screening technique. The design of a hearing screening program must take into account the probability of either

a progressive or delayed onset hearing loss and mandate follow-up screening for any child meeting an appropriate risk indicator. The four risk indicators associated with delayed onset hearing loss, listed at the bottom of Table 9.8, are initially documented by medical chart review immediately after the child's birth. Then, each child with one or more of these risk indicators undergoes follow-up hearing screenings at six-month intervals until the child is either 3 years old and until there is no evidence of hearing impairment or there is a "Refer" outcome for a hearing screening. A child with a risk indicator for delayed hearing loss and a "Refer" outcome for a follow-up hearing screening requires diagnostic audiologic assessment to confirm and define the extent of the hearing impairment, with audiologic management and medical consultation to follow promptly as indicated. A strategy for hearing screening in the nursery setting and follow-up hearing screening or diagnostic assessment is illustrated in Figure 9.4.

RISK INDICATORS FOR PROGRESSIVE HEARING LOSS AND INFANT HEARING LOSS (29 DAYS TO 2 YEARS). | Even after discharge from the nursery, the onset of infant hearing loss can be associated with a variety of factors. Table 9.10 contains the rather lengthy list of risk indicators for infant hearing loss after the neonatal period. Professionals involved in pediatric health care, including pediatricians, family physicians, audiologists, public health nurses, and other early intervention specialists and personnel (e.g., in the United States persons working in Early Head Start programs), must be well aware of and consistently attempt to identify risk indicators

Infant Hearing Screening and Follow-Up Diagnostic Assessment

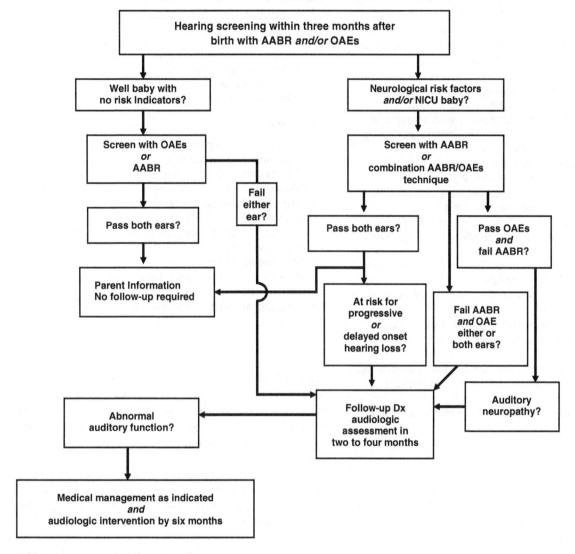

FIGURE 9.4. Flowchart for infant hearing screening and follow-up diagnostic assessment.

for hearing loss in children within the age range of 29 days to 2 years. First on the list is parent or caregiver concern about a child's hearing. The concern often is triggered by either apparent unresponsiveness to sound (e.g., speech or environmental sounds) or perceived delay in the acquisition of speech and language. Put in simple terms, the proper response by a physician or other pediatric health care provider to a parent's expressed concern about a child's hearing is an immediate referral for hearing assessment by an audiologist. Clearly, in a discussion of newborn hearing screening it's superfluous to make the point that no child is too young to undergo a hearing evaluation. In addition, intervention can be implemented at any age for a child diagnosed with hearing impairment.

Careful review of the indicators in Table 9.10 reveals at least two that are often associated with the subsequent diagnosis of auditory neuropathy, including hyperbilirubinemia and a variety of neurodegenerative disorders. Also, as noted in the review of auditory neuropathy in Chapter 5, there are reports of auditory neuropathy among persons with genetically determined disorders. In contrast to the neonatal risk indicators that are, with only one exception (congenital anomalies), associated with permanent sensorineural hearing loss (cited previously in Tables 9.8 and 9.9), several risk indicators in Table 9.10 pertain to conductive hearing loss (e.g., stigmata of selected syndromes and recurrent or persistent otitis media). Note also that one of the risk indicators—head trauma—is unrelated to a disease or pathology but, rather,

TABLE 9.10. Joint Committee on Infant Hearing Risk Indicators for Infants from Age 29 Days through 2 Years, Including Infants at Risk for *Progressive* or *Delayed Onset* Sensorineural Hearing Loss and/or *Conductive Hearing Loss*

JCIH recommends children with these risk indicators who pass newborn hearing screening undergoing regular audiologic monitoring every six months until age 3 years.

- Parental or caregiver concern regarding hearing
- Speech, language, and/or developmental delay
- Stigmata or other findings associated with a syndrome known to include a sensorineural or conductive hearing loss or Eustachian tube dysfunction
- Postnatal infections associated with sensorineural hearing loss, including bacterial meningitis
- In-utero infections such as cytomegalovirus (CMV), herpes, rubella, syphilis, and toxoplasmosis
- Neonatal (birth to 28 days) indicators—specifically hyperbilirubinemia at a serum level requiring exchange transfusion
- Persistent pulmonary hypertension of the newborn associated with mechanical ventilation
- Conditions requiring the use of extracorporeal membrane oxygenation (ECMO)
- Syndromes associated with progressive hearing loss, such as neurofibromatosis, osteopetrosis, and Usher's syndrome
- Neurodegenerative disorders, such as Hunter syndrome, or sensory motor neuropathies, such as Friedreich's
- Head trauma
- Recurrent or persistent otitis media with effusion for at least three months

TABLE 9.11. Summary of Selected Otologic Pathologies Involving the External and the Middle Ear That Are Associated with Conductive Hearing Impairment

External ear

- Cerumen (earwax) impaction
- External ear canal stenosis
- Otitis externa (acute)
- Otitis externa (chronic)

Middle ear

- Aural atresia (congenital)
- Cholesteatoma (acquired)
- Cholesteatoma (congenital)
- Discontinuity of ossicular chain
- Eustachian tube dysfunction
- Fixation of the ossicular chain
- Glomus jugulare tumor (carotid body tumor, chemodectoma)
- Otitis media without effusion
- Otitis media with effusion (serous or purulent)
- Otosclerosis
- Tympanic membrane perforation

secondary to some type of injury or accident. Finally, progressive hearing loss is associated with disorders categorized within one of the risk indicators in infants after the neonatal period, specifically neurofibromatosis, osteopetrosis, and Usher's syndrome.

External and Middle Ear Pathology

Diseases of the external and middle ear associated with CHL are listed in Table 9.11. The literature on AERs in adults with these pathologies is somewhat sparse, because conventional clinical procedures, such as aural immittance (impedance) and pure-tone audiometry, are usually adequate to evaluate external and middle ear functioning in most patients. Measurement of AERs in children with external and/or middle ear pathology is a common clinical practice. For example, among infants failing hearing screening, over 10 percent may have middle ear dysfunction and CHL. Also, otitis media is the most common heath problem among children in general. Young children suspected to have hearing impairment on the basis of delayed speech and language development must be considered at risk for recurrent middle ear pathology. Furthermore, middle ear pathology is a

frequent finding among certain types of patients who require AER assessment because they cannot be evaluated adequately with behavioral audiometry, such as mentally retarded children. Investigations of AERs findings, primarily ABR, in middle ear pathology are reviewed later in the chapter.

It is very important to keep in mind that even though AER measurement in many patients is carried out for neurodiagnosis, the external and middle ear are always the first link in the auditory system for air-conduction stimulation. AER measures used for identification of eighth-nerve or auditory CNS dysfunction, such as interaural latency difference (ILD) for wave V, can be strongly influenced by peripheral auditory deficits. Unsuspected or unrecognized CHL (e.g., which may be due to otitis media or even simple impacted cerumen) can lead to the erroneous interpretation of retrocochlear pathology. Therefore, while evaluation of external/middle ear function may not be the *reason* for AER evaluation, peripheral pathology must always be *ruled out* when interpreting AERs in neurodiagnosis.

Three general principles should be remembered during ABR assessment of patients with suspected or documented middle ear dysfunction resulting in CHL:

- CHL essentially attenuates the level of sound reaching the cochlea.
- Many middle ear pathologies produce relatively greater low-frequency than high-frequency hearing loss.
- Air- versus bone-conduction measures are needed for complete description of CHL.

The effective stimulus intensity level activating the AER is reduced by the amount of CHL component that has been caused by the attenuation of sound intensity reaching the cochlea. Simply put, ABR latency values at a given stimulus intensity level are prolonged in conductive loss, and these values are consistent with latencies expected for the intensity level actually reaching the cochlea. This ABR pattern was illustrated in Figure 7.5. The attenuation of air-conduction stimulus intensity caused by the CHL corresponds roughly to a "shift" or prolongation in latency. Within several years after the ABR was introduced clinically, there were suggestions that the latency–intensity function could be used in differentiating conductive versus sensorineural hearing impairment (Hecox & Galambos, 1974; Yamada, Yagi, Yamane, & Suzuki, 1975; Yamada, et al., 1979).

In accounting for the effect of CHL component on AER latency, one must consider the stimulus intensity level, the amount of the CHL component, the configuration of the CHL, and any concomitant sensorineural hearing loss component. Although early reports suggested that the latency shift caused by a CHL (the air-bone gap in hearing thresholds) could not be predicted (Clemis & McGee, 1979), there are now data mathematically relating CHL component and the observed pattern of latency–intensity function (Borg, Lofqvist, & Rosen, 1981; van der Drift, Brocaar, & van Zanten, 1988a,b). The second general principle is that many middle-ear pathologies produce a relatively greater degree of CHL for low frequencies (1000 Hz and below) than for higher frequencies. Thus, the click-evoked ABR, which is generated primarily by cochlear activity in the frequency region above 1000 Hz, may underestimate HTL (hearing threshold level) in CHL. The complex relation between AER outcome and audiometric configuration is explored at the end of this chapter.

Finally, complete description of CHL, by conventional audiometry or AERs, requires a comparison of findings for air- versus bone-conduction stimulation. Bone-conduction ABR measurement is clinically feasible, as indicated in Chapter 6, but it requires an appreciation of the substantial differences in bone- versus air-conduction transducer and stimulus characteristics.

Marked prolongation of absolute latencies for ABR wave I and later waves, a finding that is characteristic of CHL, can also result from other nonconductive causes. These causes, including collapsed ear canals, imprecise earphone placement, and movement in earphone location during testing, must also be ruled out prior to meaningful interpretation of ABR waveforms.

OTITIS MEDIA. | *Otitis media* is commonly referred to in lay terms as an "ear infection." The site of the disease is the middle ear space, behind the eardrum. Normally this space is filled with air and ventilated regularly by the eustachian tube, which connects the middle ear to the *nasopharynx* (back of the throat). When the eustachian tube becomes blocked,

such as during an upper respiratory infection, the middle ear space is not adequately ventilated. *Negative pressure* develops within the space (pressure within the middle ear is less than atmospheric pressure), and fluid seeps into the middle ear from the mucous membrane that lines the cavity. This is called "otitis media with effusion" (or "nonsuppurative otitis media") and is actually *not* an "ear infection." The eardrum may appear retracted, and bubbles or a fluid level may be seen through the eardrum. Middle ear fluid can cause a mild, usually low-frequency, hearing impairment. Several other forms of otitis media also affect hearing:

- *Chronic serious (secretory) otitis media,* also known as "glue ear," causes greater hearing deficit. The eardrum appears bluish grey or yellowish.
- In *acute bacterial (or viral) otitis media,* the eardrum appears red and sometimes bulging. The patient complains of ear pain. Over time, without treatment, the eardrum can rupture spontaneously, and pus will flow out. This perforation of the eardrum usually heals spontaneously as the disease resolves.
- *Chronic purulent otitis media* ("chronic ear") is an ear infection that does not resolve. There is persistent, sometimes foul-smelling, drainage from the perforation, which is often quite large. A mild-to-moderate CHL is usually present.
- *Acute serous otitis media* ("middle ear infection") occasionally affects the majority of otherwise healthy children. The overall incidence is as high as 60 to 70 percent, and it tends to be higher in males than females. There is extensive literature on its detection, diagnosis, and treatment.

Also, considerable controversy surrounds several otitis media issues, particularly the effectiveness of different treatment modalities (e.g., decongestant/antihistamine medications, ventilation tubes) and the long-term impact of otitis media on speech and language development.

ABR FINDINGS. | Even the earliest clinical reports on ABR (Hecox & Galambos, 1974) implied that responses could be useful in differentiating conductive versus sensorineural hearing impairment. Since then, studies of ABR in otitis media have addressed several issues. There are reports describing (1) latency, (2) amplitude, and (3) morphology as a function of CHL, with the goal of accurately estimating the degree of loss (Borg, Löfqvist, & Rosen, 1981; Conijn, van der Drift, Brocaar, & van Zanten, 1989; Fria & Sabo, 1980; McGee & Clemis, 1982; Mendelson, Salamy, Lenoir, & McKean, 1979). Some of these investigators considered CHL in general but did not specifically describe results for patients with otitis media (e.g., Borg, Löfqvist, & Rosen, 1981). Their findings are incorporated into the preceding discussion on the effects of type and configuration of hearing loss on AERs. Others have attempted to relate brainstem auditory functioning, as measured with ABR, to chronic otitis media in children (Anteby, Hafner, Pratt, & Uri, 1986; Chambers, Rowan, Matthies, & Novak, 1989; Folsom, Weber, & Thompson, 1983).

In a relatively early paper on clinical applications of ABR, Yamada et al. (1975) presented latency–intensity data for 11 subjects with simulated CHL (produced artificially) and 12 patients with unspecified middle ear disease and CHL. The authors described displacement of the latency–intensity function to the right (i.e., toward increased intensity levels) as a function of the degree of CHL. Amount of CHL was predicted by calculating the increase in stimulus intensity level necessary to produce ABR wave V latency value equivalent to normal expectations (i.e., to shift the value back into the normal region). This technique is still widely used clinically. Not unexpectedly, with a click stimulus, Yamada et al. (1975) found the best correlation between ABR latency values and hearing sensitivity above 1000 Hz. The discrepancy between the degree of hearing loss estimated by ABR and the actual CHL at 4000 Hz was less than 15 dB for more than 80 percent of the subjects.

Mendelson et al. (1979) evaluated the usefulness of ABR wave I and wave V latency prolongations in identification of conductive hearing deficits in 40 children with clinical evidence of otitis media and 23 normal children. Normal ABR latency values correctly predicted that there was no otitis media with effusion (OME) in approximately 90 percent of the ears. Wave I was abnormally prolonged (greater than 1 standard deviation above the mean), however, for 81 percent of the children with suppurative otitis media. These investigators also reported a decrease in ABR latency after treatment of the disease.

Fria and Sabo (1980) published one of the first systematic studies of ABR in OME. Their subjects were 14 infants and young children (10 male and 4 female, ages 4 to 39 months) and 12 school-aged children (six of each gender, ages 6 to 12 years). In contrast to earlier investigators, they carefully defined the population by including only patients with OME that was validated by surgery. That is, the OME was confirmed upon *myringotomy* (cutting an opening in the eardrum and draining the fluid) versus OME presumed by *otoscopy* (viewing the eardrum with an otoscope). This study led to two main conclusions, each of which is clinically useful: (1) ABR latency is a sensitive indicator of OME, and (2) ABR data can be used to estimate the amount of conductive hearing component. The *sensitivity* of abnormal latency for wave I versus V in detecting OME was 82 percent versus 100 percent. *Specificity* of normal ABR latency for wave I versus V in correctly predicting no OME was 100 percent versus 25 percent. Therefore, wave I was slightly less sensitive, but overall a better indicator of the presence of OME. Wave V tended to be abnormally delayed even in children without OME. In 5 of 28 ears (18%), wave I was not detected. Age-related variability in wave V versus I is cited as an explanation for this finding. The possible confounding effect of auditory brainstem dysfunction in younger patients

with concomitant otitis media could also argue against clinical reliance on wave V.

Fria and Sabo's second conclusion was that the amount of CHL component can be estimated. Using the simple Yamada et al. (1975) approach for predicting the degree of CHL component, Fria and Sabo (1980) found a difference between actual CHL and ABR estimation of the loss to be less than 15 dB in 70 percent of subjects and less than 20 dB in 90 percent. These authors also applied another relatively simple, and clinically feasible, prediction technique. They assumed a 0.3 ms latency increase above normal values in latency for wave I (1.5 ms) and wave V (5.5 ms) for every 10 dB of CHL component at a stimulus intensity level of 60 dB nHL. For example, a CHL component of 30 dB was predicted by a latency delay (in comparison to normal) of 0.9 ms. the difference between actual and predicted CHL component did not exceed 20 dB among this small group of subjects. Fria and Sabo (1980) presented linear regression equations for predicting the extent of CHL from ABR latency delays at a 60 dB nHL stimulus level. In a 1989 critical review of ABR in assessment of conductive hearing impairment, Stapells and colleagues (Stapells, 1989; Stapells & Ruben, 1989) discussed the advantages and disadvantages of this clinical technique.

CONGENITAL AURAL ATRESIA. | Congenital aural stenosis, microtia, or atresia are malformations of the external and/or middle ear. It may occur as part of a syndrome (e.g., Treacher Collins syndrome) or in isolation. *Congenital aural stenosis* is an excessive narrowing of the external auditory canal so that the canal actually ends before reaching the TM (tympanic membrane) or the middle ear space. In place of the TM, there may be a relatively thick wall of soft tissue. The external ear may appear normal. This type of malformation usually produces a conductive hearing loss of 35 to 40 dB and may not be detected for a number of years during childhood. Associated with the stenosis may be preauricular pits.

There are varying grades of external ear malformation, ranging from slightly abnormal appearance, such as a low-set or posteriorly rotated ear, a total absence of the pinna, or just a small tag in the normal location of the external ear. In addition to the external ear malformation, there may be a bony plate separating the external and middle ear sites, as well as various kinds of ossicular malformations. Occasionally, a sensorineural component may accompany the severe conductive hearing loss, even though these two regions of auditory anatomy have different embryologic origins. Patients with aural atresia, especially very young children or patients of any age with bilateral malformations, present an apparently insolvable audiometric problem—the "masking dilemma." That is, noise adequate to mask the nontest ear during pure-tone or speech audiometry exceeds interaural attenuation levels and crosses over to influence perception of the test signal. Put simply, enough masking is too much masking. With infants or young children, it may be impossible to use earphones or bone oscillators in behavioral assessment of auditory sensitivity.

According to prevailing opinion, ABR by air conduction and bone conduction is similarly limited by masking problems. Crossover levels of 50 to 75 dB have been reported for click stimuli (Humes & Ochs, 1982; Reid & Thornton, 1983). Bone-conduction ABR is, additionally, constrained by maximum stimulus output levels of 50 to 55 dB nHL. There are, as reviewed in this chapter, numerous clinical reports of ABR used in defining conductive hearing loss. However, the clinical emphasis in the past was on applying ABR in accordance with the principles, and inherent limitations, of behavioral audiometry, rather than on utilizing the distinctive advantages of ABR "as with any audiometric procedure, a masking noise must be administered to the non-test ear when the poorer ear is being evaluated" and "because a bone-conducted signal reaches each cochlea with about the same intensity, masking the nontest ear is essential if information about individual ears is desired" (Weber, 1983b, p. 348). Other authors (e.g., Finitzo-Hieber, Hecox, & Kone, 1979) reiterate a similar theme.

A major objective in audiometry is to obtain results that are specific to the test ear, without contribution from the nontest ear. In fact, with ABR, the masking dilemma can be successfully circumvented; masking is *not* always necessary and ear-specific information on auditory sensitivity (conductive and sensorineural status) can be routinely obtained from most patients with atresia-related conductive impairment, regardless of age. In fact, ABR is the best available technique for evaluating auditory function in congenital aural atresia. Jahrsdoerfer, Hall, and Gray (1988) point out that: "As hearing is recognized as the most important parameter that needs to be measured early in the life of the individual [with congenital aural atresia], the advent of ABR testing has been of inestimable help" (p. 59). Next, an ABR protocol specifically for audiologic assessment of aural atresia is presented, followed by an evidence-based discussion of the distinctive advantages of ABR in this population.

A general test protocol for bone conduction ABR was presented in Chapter 6. Key concepts and components of the test protocol for recording quality ABR waveforms in patients with aural atresia are summarized in Table 9.12. *The first and foremost principle in assessment of hearing status in patients of all ages with aural atresia—estimation of auditory thresholds for both ears and for air and bone conduction—cannot be overemphasized.* For patients presenting for the first time in the clinic with medical evidence of middle ear disease, and at considerable risk for conductive hearing loss, it would be almost inconceivable, and certainly inconsistent with minimum standard of care, to only assess hearing for one ear or to only assess hearing with bone-conduction stimulation and not air-conduction stimulation. There is simply no rationale for assuming normal sensory and/or conductive auditory status for either ear. A thorough ear-specific evaluation of overall (air-conduction) hearing status and purely sensory (bone-conduction) hearing status is obligatory. *Standard of care should not be compromised for patients with aural atresia.* ABR assessment of patients with aural atresia should always consist of careful estimation of hearing sensitivity of each ear by air conduction and bone conduction. As an electrophysiologic auditory measure, the ABR of course permits definition and air- and bone-conduction hearing status at any age, including infancy within days after birth. There's absolutely no reason to delay audiologic assessment of children with aural atresia. In fact, there are some compelling reasons for immediately defining with an ABR assessment auditory status of infants who have aural atresia. Clearly, aural atresia does not resolve spontaneously over time. The initial ABR findings will remain a valid representation of the patient's hearing throughout childhood. There's another very practical advantage to early audiologic assessment. Within the first few months after birth, the ABR can be recorded without the need for sedation. Also within the first few months, the temporal bones have not yet fused with other cranial bones. Thus, it's possible to record with air- and bone-conduction stimulation ABRs that are ear-specific, without masking the nontest ear and without concerns about acoustic stimulus crossover to the nontest ear.

The author has encountered audiologists who, for reasons that remain unclear, perform for patients with bilateral aural atresia ABR measurement with only bone-conduction stimulation, and sometimes only for one side, and also clinicians who, for patients with unilateral aural atresia, only perform ABR measurement for the involved ear. Two faulty assumptions presumably underlie these unacceptable audiologic practices. Exclusive bone-conduction ABR measurement of bilateral aural atresia presumes, incorrectly, that it is not possible to present stimuli via air conduction and/or valid air conduction ABR recordings are impossible. This is simply not the case. Unequivocally, ear-specific ABR findings can be obtained by presenting via supra-aural earphones air-conduction click stimuli to the temporal bone (in the normal location of the external ear). The overall degree of conductive hearing loss can then be rather accurately estimated for each ear. Depending on the anatomic features of the otologic malformation (e.g., soft tissue mass versus bony plate), the degree of hearing loss may vary considerably among patients with aural atresia or microtia. The degree of hearing loss can only be determined by systematic ABR assessment with air-conduction stimulation.

Literature. Hall and colleagues (Hall, Brown, & Mackey-Hargadine, 1985; Hall, Morgan, Mackey-Hargadine, Aguilar, & Jahrsdoerfer, 1984; Hayes, 1994; Jahrsdoerfer & Hall, 1986; Jahrsdoerfer, Yeakley, Hall, Robbins, & Gray, 1985) have systematically applied air-conduction versus bone-conduction ABR in ear-specific assessment of a series of patients with congenital aural atresia. These investigators assert that success in obtaining ear-specific information is highest for infants and young children, but such measurement can be enhanced in all patients by adhering to the guidelines and implementing the test protocol summarized in Table 9.12.

TABLE 9.12. Concepts and Techniques Important for Audiologic Assessment with ABR of Patients with Aural Atresia

The same general principles apply to ABR assessment for other etiologies of conductive hearing loss. Details on application of the bone-conduction ABR technique are presented in Chapter 6. A protocol for ABR measurement in infants and young children is summarized in Table 9.2.

Concepts

- Always record an ABR with stimulation of each ear by air conduction and bone conduction. Do not simply perform an ABR assessment with stimulation of the obviously involved ear (for apparently unilateral aural atresia) or with only bone-conduction stimulation.

- Whenever possible, perform an air- and bone-conduction ABR within several months after birth to minimize parental concern about hearing status, to permit early intervention with appropriate audiologic management, and to avoid the need for sedation during ABR measurement. Diagnostic ABR measurement with air- and bone-conduction stimulation after birth in the nursery before hospital discharge is feasible and advisable.

- Rely on the presence of a repeatable wave I in the ipsilateral electrode array (see details below and in Chapter 6) for verification that the ABR is ear-specific (i.e., evoked by stimulation of the test ear).

Techniques

- Use earlobe electrode placement (as opposed to mastoid placement) to augment wave I by as much as 30 percent. If the patient does not have an earlobe, affix the electrode to an auricular tag of skin if present.

- For air-conduction ABR measurement, place supra-aural (e.g., TDH) cushions on the head in the normal region of the external ear, using auricular tags or skin remnants as a guide.

- For bone-conduction ABR measurement, place the oscillator (e.g., Radioear B70A) on the temporal bone posterior to the normal region of the external ear, using auricular tags or skin remnants as a guide.

- A high-pass filter setting of 30 Hz (rather than a higher cutoff, such as 150 or 300 Hz) is important to encompass the relatively low-frequency energy in the ABR, especially for bone-conduction stimuli.

- The ABR should be evoked with relatively slow click presentation rate (e.g., 11.1) to enhance amplitude of the wave I component.

- A very quiet patient state (soundly sleeping naturally, sedated, or lightly anesthetized) is essential for confident detection of possibly small-amplitude wave I components with bone-conduction stimulation. Measurement noise or interference during ABR measurement hampers the clear identification of the wave I component.

- The ABR should be recorded with a simultaneous two-channel electrode technique (ipsilateral and contralateral electrode arrays) for both air- and bone-conduction stimulation (see Chapter 6 for details). The ABR wave I component, generated by the distal portion of the eighth cranial (auditory) nerve, should be apparent only in the response evoked by stimulation of the test ear and detected with the ipsilateral electrode array.

CRANIOFACIAL ANOMALIES (CFA). | Children with various craniofacial anomalies, such as external ear anomalies, dysmorphic features, aural atresia, and cleft lip and/or palate are at very high risk for hearing impairment, particularly conductive hearing loss. Among risk factors for neonatal hearing loss, CFA ranks as one most often associated with a subsequent confirmation of hearing loss by diagnostic audiometry. ABR findings in aural atresia were just reviewed. Hayes (1994) reported "significant hearing loss is commonly prevalent in infants with CFA . . . even at a very young age" (p. 43). The author documented ABR abnormalities in almost 50 percent of a series of 145 infants with craniofacial anomalies. Among them, children with normal hearing were identified only among those with external ear anomalies (N = 24, or 82%) and dysmorphic features (N = 5, or 55.6%). All other children had some degree of hearing loss, usually bilaterally.

OTOSCLEROSIS. | *Otosclerosis* is a genetic disease of the bone around the cochlea. It is a process of bone resorption and reformation, often known as "otospongiosis." The stapes footplate, which is the junction between the middle and inner ear, is often involved in the disease. Bony structural abnormalities of the cochlea (the labyrinthine capsule) in otosclerosis can produce sensorineural hearing deficit, and stapes footplate (ossicular chain) fixation often produces a conductive hearing deficit. There may be either a pure sensorineural hearing loss or a pure CHL, but often, both components occur together, and the resulting hearing loss is mixed. An apparent mixed loss may be due to depression of bone-conduction hearing associated with abnormal middle-ear mechanics in otosclerosis. In these cases, bone-conduction thresholds often improve with effective medical or surgical therapy (e.g., Ghorayeb, Yeakley, Hall, & Jones, 1991).

Otosclerosis affects between 0.5 and 1.0 percent of the population, and it is more likely in women than in men. It tends to be bilateral, first appearing in the first three or four decades of life. The effects of otosclerosis on hearing are more pronounced during pregnancy. An otoscopic finding in some otosclerotic patients is *Schwartze's sign,* a pinkish blush seen through the TM, due to *hyperemia* (extra blood collection) at the promontory. This indicates an active disease process. Otosclerosis can be treated with medical and surgical therapy. Medical therapy usually consists of sodium fluoride treatment, sometimes supplemented with vitamin D and calcium carbonate. This therapy is presumed to affect the overall disease process (middle ear and cochlear components). The surgical treatment is *stapedectomy,* in which various surgical techniques and prostheses are used to recreate a flexible and functional connection between the TM and the oval window. The objective of surgery is to correct the reduction in sound transmission to the inner ear, which was caused by stapes footplate fixation.

Because otosclerosis is a disease that almost always affects otherwise healthy adults who can cooperate for traditional audiometry, including air- and bone-conduction pure-tone threshold measurement, AERs are infrequently indicated for auditory assessment. Theoretically, air- versus bone-conduction ABR might be useful in persons with severe CHL secondary to otosclerosis, when the masking dilemma precludes meaningful interpretation of behavioral pure-tone audiometry. However, bone-conduction ABR in these patients is typically of little value because the likelihood of a response is diminished by the sensorineural deficit (or at least the decreased bone-conduction sensitivity) that is often a component of the disease.

Relatively few investigations of AERs have included patients with otosclerosis (McGee & Clemis, 1982). McGee and Clemis (1982) analyzed ABR data for a diverse group of patients with CHL, including 6 patients (7 ears) with otosclerosis. Importantly, among the 32 ears tested, no wave I could be detected in 17. ABR findings in otosclerosis (ossicular chain fixation) were described as comparable to those with ossicular chain discontinuity. A characteristically conductive increase in wave V latency was reported, but the increase was greater than anticipated from the pure-tone air- versus bone-conduction gap in the 1000 to 4000 Hz region.

DISCONTINUITY OF THE OSSICULAR CHAIN. | There are various causes for discontinuity or interruption of the ossicular chain. A key example is head trauma. The blow to the head dislodges the tiny ossicles, usually at the joint between the incus and the stapes, although other regions (the stapes crura) can also be damaged. Chronic middle ear disease can also eventually erode or cause necrosis of one or more of the ossicles and can produce a complete break in the chain. The audiometric pattern in complete ossicular chain disruption is distinctive. It consists of a highly compliant tympanogram, absent acoustic reflexes, and a moderate or severe (typically 40 dB or more) CHL component that is even greater for the higher frequencies (above 1000 Hz).

There are few published references to AERs in ossicular chain discontinuity. In the study by McGee and Clemis (1982), just noted in the discussion of otosclerosis, there were 4 subjects (5 ears) with confirmed ossicular chain discontinuity. The authors did not provide detailed description of ABR findings among these patients, but they did cite greater wave V latency increases than were expected, based on the amount of air-bone gap. A comparable observation was made for otosclerotic patients. In contrast, 11 patients with otitis media (15 ears) showed ABR wave V latency increase consistent with the reduction of effective stimulus intensity due to air-bone gap. Another point made by McGee and Clemis (1982) was that in patients with mixed hearing loss (conductive plus neural), ABR changes due to CHL in some patients obscured identification of abnormal latency increases resulting from confirmed retrocochlear dysfunction.

As with ossicular chain fixation in otosclerosis, there is generally little value in applying AERs in the assessment of hearing sensitivity in ossicular chain disruption because this can be done better with traditional audiometry. An exception to this rule, of course, is the comatose, severely head-injured patient undergoing AER assessment for neurodiagnosis or for neuromonitoring. It is important for the clinician to determine from medical colleagues or from chart review whether the patient has a temporal bone fracture, and, if so, whether ossicular chain disruption is suspected. An abnormal or absent ABR by air conduction (but not by bone conduction) would be expected in this patient. Among middle ear pathologies producing CHL, however, ossicular chain disruption would be expected to have greater impact on ABR findings than most. This is because, for the majority of middle ear pathologies (such as otitis media), hearing loss is greater for lower frequencies and less for higher frequencies. ABR (with a click stimulus) tends to underestimate the degree of low-frequency hearing impairment. In contrast, the high-frequency deficit in ossicular chain disruption occurs in the frequency region most important for ABR generation.

COCHLEAR PATHOLOGY

ABR findings in cochlear pathology are distinctively different than those just described for CHL. The ABR in all but severe sensory (cochlear) impairment is remarkably robust, although a wave I component may be indistinct or not detectable. The ABR is virtually independent of low-frequency hearing loss. A normal-appearing ABR may be recorded in sensory-impaired patients with only "islands" of residual good hearing sensitivity in the 2000 to 4000 Hz region. Even sensory hearing loss within the ABR frequency region of 1000 to 4000 Hz typically does not influence appreciably the response appreciably the response latency or amplitude for high stimulus–intensity levels (e.g., 80 dB HL or above) until it reaches at least 50 to 60 dB HTL. Again, wave I is often not present. No ABR is typically observed with severe-to-profound high-frequency loss, despite better HTLs for low frequencies.

With moderate high-frequency sensory hearing loss, the ABR wave V latency–intensity function is steeper than normal. No ABR wave V is recorded for low intensity levels. A response first appears as click stimulus intensity level approaches HTLs in the 1000 to 4000 Hz region. Actually, the appearance of the ABR for somewhat lower stimulus intensity levels suggests the contribution of audiometric frequencies below 1000 Hz to the response. Latency of the response at these intensities is abnormally prolonged because at these intensities it is generated by a more apical portion of the cochlea and requires somewhat greater travel time along the basilar membrane. Then, as stimulus intensity level exceeds HL (hearing level) in the region of 1000 to 4000 Hz, latency of wave V decreases rapidly and eventually falls within the normal region.

The relationship between sensory hearing impairment and ABR as just outlined is oversimplified and not always encountered clinically. In fact, there is a complex and poorly understood interaction among ABR findings and (a) degree, slope, and overall configuration of sensory hearing impairment; (b) subject age and gender; (c) stimulus parameters; and (d) acoustic characteristics of the transducer. The relationship is further complicated by apparent differences in the effects of various etiologies of sensory hearing impairment on ABR. Additionally, even patients with apparently equivalent audiograms produce ABRs with divergent and sometimes unexplainable latency–intensity functions. ABR findings reported for etiologies of sensory impairment are now reviewed. Some common pathologies and disorders associated with sensory and neural hearing impairment of children, and adults, are summarized in Table 9.13.

TABLE 9.13. Listing of Some Types of Cochlea or Eighth Nerve Pathology That Are Associated with Sensorineural Hearing Impairment in Children and Adults

Cochlea

- Basilar skull fracture
- Endolymphatic hydrops
- Genetic syndromes (over 70)
- Head trauma
- Kernicterus
- Labyrinthine fistula
- Ménière's disease
- Meningitis (*Hemophilus influenza,* meningococcal)
- Otosclerosis
- Ototoxic drugs, e.g., aminoglycosides, loop diuretics, cis-platin, carbo-platin)
- Presbycusis (hearing loss in aging)
- Rubella
- Temporal bone fracture

Eighth nerve

- Meningioma
- Presbycusis
- Temporal bone fracture
- Schwannoma (neuroma, neurinoma, "acoustic tumor")
- Vascular loop
- von Recklinghausen's disease (neurofibromatosis)

OTOTOXICITY. | Ototoxicity was reviewed earlier in the discussion of risk factors for infant hearing loss. A brief period of exposure (< 5 days) to most ototoxic drugs, particularly aminoglycosides, does not typically result in cochlear auditory dysfunction and sensory hearing impairment. Many infants receive antibiotics in as a prophylactic measure while laboratory tests are conducted to confirm or rule out infection (e.g., sepsis). The risk of auditory dysfunction is substantially increased, however, by prolonged administration of the drug, by drug serum (blood) levels exceeding the accepted therapeutic range (e.g., in an inadvertent overdose), by the synergistic effects caused by the simultaneous administration of more than one drug (e.g., an aminoglycoside plus a loop diuretic) or previous exposure to an ototoxic drug, and by other systemic health problems (e.g., impaired renal function). Some of the many drugs used therapeutically in children that are potentially ototoxic are listed in Table 9.14.

Chayasirisobhon et al. (1996) reported abnormal ABRs for 7 of 21 neonates (33.3%) treated for > 10 days with gentamicin, but only 4.5 percent of a group of 15 infants who received the drug for ≤ 7 days. ABR latency–intensity functions were recorded from 80 dB nHL down to 30 dB nHL. These findings are consistent with another report of ABR abnormalities associated with gentamicin (Kohelet et al., 1990). Interpretation of studies of ABR and potentially ototoxic drugs in newborn infants requiring intensive care is complicated by the presence in the same population of multiple risk factors for hearing impairment, e.g., asphyxia, severe infection, etc.

CONNEXIN 26 MUTATIONS. | The rapid growth in sophisticated molecular genetic research in recent years has led to the

TABLE 9.14. Selected Potentially Ototoxic Therapeutic Drugs Used with Children

- Aminoglycoside antibiotics
  - gentamicin
  - tobramycin
  - amikacin
  - gentamicin
  - kanamycin
  - neomycin
  - netimicin
  - streptomycin
- Other antibiotics (e.g., vancomycin)
- Anti-neoplastic (chemotherapeutic) drugs (e.g., cis-platin, carbo-platin)
- Diuretics, including loop diuretics (e.g., furosemide, or lasix)
- Salicylates (aspirin)
- Quinine drugs (e.g., Larium)
- Environmental chemicals (e.g., solvents)

discovery of well over 30 genes involved in nonsyndromic hearing loss. A computer-assisted literature search will uncover hundreds of publications summarizing advances in our understanding of hereditary hearing loss, as well as websites and homepages devoted to the topic. Mutations of the gap junction protein connexin 26 (designated at locus GJB2) affect the cochlea in humans. Beginning in the mid–1990s, a number of investigators from around the world documented nonsyndromic hearing loss as an expression of connexin 26 mutations (see Cohn et al., 1999, for review). The ABR is useful for confirming the presence and type of hearing loss in very young children at risk for or suspected of having connexin 26 mutations, including infants who cannot yet be properly evaluated with behavioral audiometry. Results of an ABR assessment in infancy can lead to early intervention for serious hearing impairment, and may also contribute to genetic counseling.

The ABR is now often included in the audiologic test battery utilized by researchers who are investigating the genotype-phenotype relations of connexin 26 mutations, particularly the type, configuration, degree, onset, and clinical course of hearing loss (e.g., Cohn et al., 1999; Sobe et al., 2000). The ABR can be applied clinically in children with connexin 26 mutations for documentation and diagnosis of auditory dysfunction as it is with other etiologies associated with hearing loss.

PRIMARILY CNS AUDITORY DISORDERS

AER findings reported for children with a wide variety of diseases involving the peripheral and/or central nervous system are reviewed briefly in this section of the chapter. Table 9.15 includes ABR findings for the selected diseases and disorders. Figures illustrating ABR waveform patterns associated with CNS neuropathologies were shown in Chapter 7. The following information is offered as a resource for the clinician preparing for neurodiagnostic application of AER, that is, to facilitate ready access to information that will be of value in planning ABR test strategy and interpreting ABR findings for patients encountered in the clinical setting. Additional, and more detailed, information is available from textbooks devoted to the medical disciplines of neurology, otology, neurosurgery, neuropathology, and pediatrics, and, of course, the Internet. A host of neurologic conditions are not here, mainly because systematic study of ABRs in affected patients is lacking.

Auditory Neuropathy

ABR findings in pathologies associated with auditory neuropathy, such as Charcot-Marie-Tooth syndrome and Guillain-Barre syndrome, are reviewed elsewhere in this chapter. Auditory neuropathy is reviewed in detail in Chapter 5.

Neoplasms and Tumors

NEUROFIBROMATOSIS TYPE I AND II. | The two types of neurofibromatoses are genetically distinct autosomal dominant inherited multisystem progressive disorders. Auditory abnormalities include tumors involving the auditory nerve bilaterally. ABR findings in NF2, particularly in adults, have been reported for many years. Pikus (1995) reported ABR data for a series of 43 children with NF1 and for 13 children with NF2. ABR abnormalities confirmed involvement of retrocochlear pathways. Pastores, Michels, and Jack (1991) described normal ABR findings in two asymptomatic children (age 7 and 11) in a family at risk for NF2. The small tumors were confirmed with gadolinium-enhanced MRI scans.

Acoustic tumors not associated with NF are very unusual in children. Sells and Hurley (1994) report a case study of 15-year-old male with an acoustic neuroma (vestibular schwannoma) confirmed surgically. Suspicion of a unilateral hearing loss first arose by a failed school hearing screening. Diagnostic audiologic assessment showed unilateral sensorineural hearing loss, absent acoustic reflexes, and an abnormal ABR on the involved ear.

BRAINSTEM GLIOMAS. | *Brainstem gliomas* are tumors arising from glial cells. Gliomas are often not found in the pure form but, rather, may include mixtures among the types. Brainstem gliomas are mostly seen in children or adolescents and account for approximately three-fourths of brainstem tumors in children. Although the tumors tend to grow slowly, most are highly invasive, infiltrating the brainstem so that total surgical removal is often not possible and recurrence is often likely. Central nervous system tumors afflicting children, including gliomas, are listed in Table 9.16.

By virtue of the anatomy of ABR and the availability of CT and MRI scanning, it is not surprising that since the mid-1970s numerous investigators have described findings for children with radiologically (or surgically) confirmed brainstem neoplasms varied as to type and location within the brainstem (Fischer, Mauguiere, Echallier, & Courjon, 1982; Hashimoto, Ishiyama, & Tozuka, 1979; Kjaer, 1980; Musiek & Geurkink, 1982; Nodar, Hahn, & Levine, 1980; Starr & Achor, 1975; Starr & Hamilton, 1976; Stockard & Rossiter, 1977; Stockard, Sharbrough, & Stockard, 1977; Stockard, Stockard, & Sharbrough, 1986; Yagi & Kaga, 1979). Considerable accumulated clinical experience confirms that ABR is a valuable neurodiagnostic procedure, especially when diagnosis via neuroradiology or clinical findings is not conclusive. ABR is particularly useful, of course, when auditory pathways are primarily involved. It is pertinent to note, in this regard, that early generation CT scanners utilized during the late 1970s and even into the early 1980s were relatively poor at resolving brainstem anatomy. Bony artifact problems were not uncommon in CT scans of the brainstem. MRI has to a large extent overcome this limitation for neuroradiologic examination of the brainstem and, perhaps, reduced the clinical

TABLE 9.15. Summary of Auditory Brainstem Response (ABR) Findings in Selected Pediatric Patient Populations, Arranged Alphabetically

ABR findings in infants with risk factors (e.g., asphyxia, hyperbilirubinemia, meningitis, etc.), are also reviewed in the text and summarized in Tables 9.8, 9.9, and 9.10. N = normal; A = abnormal; V = variable; NS = not specified.

| | | ABR FINDINGS | | | |
CLINICAL ENTITY	STUDY(S)	N	I	I–V	COMMENTS
Acute facial palsy	Hatanaka, Takedatsu, Yashuhara, & Kobayashi, 1992	2	N	A	ABR contributes to diagnosis
Agyria-Pachygyria	Liang et al., 2002	10	N	N	Normal ABR; abnormal SSER* and VER findings
AIDS	Frank, Vishnubhakat, & Pahwa, 1992	16	V	A	More ABR abnormalities at faster stimulus rates
Anemia	Li, Wang, & Wang, 1994	48	A	N	Peripheral impairment; reversible with treatment
	Shankar et al., 2000	19	N	A	Abnormal findings associated with iron deficiency
Angelman syndrome	Sugimoto et al., 1992	3	A	N	ABR confirmed sensory hearing loss
Anoxia (near drowning)	Kaga et al., 1996	16	N	A	5 of 16 with abnormal ABR (no wave V)
Brain death	Ushio, Kaga, & Sakata, 2001	1	N	A	ABR useful for definition of brain death in infants
Carbohydrate-deficient-glycoprotein (CDG)	Veniselli, Bianchieri, Rocco, & Tortorelli, 1998	1	A	N	ABR confirmed sensorineural hearing loss
CHARGE syndrome	Edwards, Kileny, & Van Riper, 2002	22	A	A	81% with hearing loss; early ID with ABR
Chiari malformation type I	Kamuro, Inagaki, & Tomita, 1992	8	N	A	Rostral ABR abnormalities (III–V latency delay)
	Saito et al., 1997	1	A	A	Delay in wave I and I–III latency; normal III–V
Chromosome 10	Kinoshita et al., 1992	1	A	A	Deletion of short arm of chromosome 10p14
Connexin 26	Sobe et al., 2000	75	A	N	ABR useful in confirming sensorineural hearing loss
Craniofacial anomalies**	Hayes, 1994	145	A	N	50% of infants with abnormal ABR findings
DIDMOAD syndrome	Higashi, 1991	2	N	N	Also known as Wolfram syndrome; normal ABRs
ECMO***					
Encephalopathy (anoxic)	Kaga, Shindo, Gotoh, & Tamura, 1990	2	N	A	
	Anand, Gupta, & Raj, 1991	24	N	A	Perinatal asphyxia; 22% with abnormal ABR
Epilepsy	Zgorzalewicz & Galas-Zgorzalewicz, 2000	100	N	A	Abnormal latencies with CBZ and VGB therapy
Fetal alcohol syndrome	Church & Kaltenbach, 1997	—	N	A	Review article
Gaucher's disease	Kaga et al., 1990	1	N	A	
Hydrocephalus	Sood & Mahapatra, 1991	1	N	A	Improved ABR findings with shunt procedure

CLINICAL ENTITY	STUDY(S)	N	ABR FINDINGS I	ABR FINDINGS I–V	COMMENTS
Hyperbilirubinemia	Agrawal et al., 1998	30	V	A	Serial ABR abnormalities correlate with bilirubin
	Rhee, Park, & Jang, 1999	11	V	A	OAE limited for screening in hyper-bilirubinemia
	Yilmaz et al., 2001	22	N	A	ABR not useful in prognosis of neu-rologic disorders
	Hosono et al., 2002	58	V	A	Albumin priming associated with improved ABR
Intestinal aganglionosis	Shimotake & Iwai, 1994	1	A	A	A rare genetic neural crest migra-tion disorder
Intra-cranial hemorrhage	Negishi et al., 1993	41	A	A	Wave V/I amplitude ratio has prog-nostic value
Kawasaki disease	Sundel et al., 1992	23	A	N	ABR documents sensory hearing loss in infants
Lead exposure	Osman et al., 1999	155	A	A	Delayed wave I latency in high blood lead levels
Learning disorders (spe-cific)	von Deuster & Axmann, 1995	10	A	A	Absent ABR in 7 children; possible desynchrony
Meningitis	Bao & Wong, 1998	101	A	A	Included bacterial, virus, and aseptic meningitis
Meningitis (purulent)	Charuvanji, Visudhiphan, Chiemchanya, & Tawin, 1990	18	A	A	ABR most effective method for hearing assessment
Multiply handicapped	Cottrell & Gans, 1995	20	N	A	Poor morphology; less spectral energy
Noise exposure	Chen & Chen, 1993	228	N	N	Airport/aircraft noise affects hear-ing, but not ABR
Ondine's syndrome	Litscher et al., 1996	1	N	A	Also central alveolar hyperventila-tion syndrome
Ototoxicity	Chayasirisobhon et al., 1996	200	V	V	ABR abnormalities rare in gentamicin
Pelizaeus-Merzbacher	Kaga et al., 1990	3	N	A	Abnormal ABR findings are not uncommon
Pneumonia (neonatal)	Wu, Zhang, & Lu, 1993	433	V	N	About 7% of infants had elevated ABR thresholds
Renal disease (end stage)	Suppeij et al, 1992	14	A	A	ABR abnormalities associated with anemia
Rhett syndrome	Stach et al., 1994	36	N	N	No ABR abnormality, consistent with literature
Syphilis (congenital)	Gleich, Urbina, & Pincus, 1994	75	N	N	Normal ABRs with Apgar >9 at 5 minutes
Temperament	Woodward et al., 2001	56	N	A	Larger wave V in highly reactive children
Toxoplasmosis (congenital)	McGee et al., 1992	30	A	A	Conductive hearing loss, but not sensorineural

* SSER = somatosensory evoked responses; VER = visual evoked responses

** aural atresia, cleft lip/palate, external ear anomalies, dysmorphic features

*** ECMO = extracorporeal membrane oxygenation

TABLE 9.16. Proportion of Primary Intracranial Tumors Found among Children versus Persons of All Ages*

TUMOR TYPE	CHILDREN	ALL AGES
Glioma	>75%	45–50%
Astrocytoma	>50%	>75%
Cerebellar	30%	Malignant 50 to 60%
Brainstem	10%	Benign 25 to 30%
Oligodendroglioma	<2%	5%
Ependymoma	8%	5%
Medulloblastoma	25%	6%
Schwannoma	rare	6%
Meningioma	rare	15%
Hemangioblastoma	rare	1–2%
Sarcoma	rare	1–2%
Lymphoma	0%	<1%
Germ cell tumor	2–4%	1–2%
Dermoid, epidermoid	1–2%	<1%
Craniopharyngioma	5–10%	3%
Pituitary adenoma	rare	5%
	100%	100%

*15 to 20% of all intracranial tumors occur in childhood. Approximately 70% of intracranial tumors in children are located in infratentorial regions. In contrast, in adults, approximately 70% are located supratentorially.

Adapted from Okazaki, 1983.

value of the ABR in some patient populations. Always keep in mind, however, that conventional neuroradiology provides information on structure, whereas as an electrophysiological measure, the ABR assesses function. What follows is a brief review of selected papers describing ABR findings in a sample of CNS disorders affecting children. Nodar, Hahn, and Levine (1980) described ABRs for 7 children (aged 2.5 to 13 years) with diagnosed *brainstem neoplasms,* including one with astroependymoma, one with medulloblastoma, one with intraparenchymal ependymoma, and two with glioma. No tumor type was specified for the other two patients. All children showed abnormalities for at least two of seven response parameters. The seven were absolute wave latency, wave latency difference between ears, wave I–V latency interval, response stability, amplitude, morphology, and presence of waves.

Weston, Manson, and Abbott (1986) recorded ABRs from 14 children with clinical and radiological evidence of *brainstem glioma* and found that all with pontine involvement (13 of the 14) had abnormalities of wave V (delayed latency, reduced amplitude or absent). According to these authors, there were at that time (1986) a total of 52 cases of brainstem glioma reported in the literature (Guthkelch, Sclabassi, Vries, 1982; Hashimoto, Ishiyama, & Tozuka, 1979; Hecox, Cone, & Blaw, 1981; Kjaer, 1980; Nodar, Hahn, & Levine, 1980; Starr & Achor, 1975; Starr & Hamilton, 1976; Stockard & Rossiter, 1977; Stockard, Sharbrough, & Stock-

ard, 1977; Yagi, Kaga, & Baba, 1980) and in no case were normal ABR reported when the lesion involved the pons. ABR abnormalities for subjects in the Weston et al. (1986) study were consistently found for the stimulus ear ipsilateral to the tumor, but were not invariably related to tumor size.

In a comprehensive clinical study, Rotteveel et al. (1985) described ABR and somatosensory evoked response (SSER) findings for 26 children (aged 1 to 19 years, mean 9.9) with *infra- and supratentorial tumors.* The fourteen infratentorial tumors included six medulloblastomas (all but one in the fourth ventricle), four gliomas, two arachnoid sarcomas, two astrocytomas, and a ganglioneuroblastoma. The twelve supratentorial tumors were three craniopharyngeomas, three astrocytomas (grade I, II and III) in different regions, an optic nerve astrocytoma, a lipoma, an ependymoma, a chromophobe adenoma, a germinoma, and an unspecified tumor in the left thalamus. Occasional ABR abnormalities in the supratentorial group were associated with brainstem dysfunction secondary to intracranial pressure effects (e.g., compression of inferior colliculus). The majority of children in the infratentorial group had ABR abnormalities, including delayed interwave latencies and total absence of waves. Abnormalities were not uncommon for ABRs elicited with stimulation of the ear contralateral to the tumor (pressure effect). Tumors near the eighth nerve typically produced asymmetric findings, whereas symmetric findings were related to tumors in the midline fourth ventricle region. Serial ABRs had clinical value in documenting the progression of pathophysiologic changes, including development of hydrocephalus. The authors emphasize the clinical importance of ABR by stating that large tumors are easy to detect but removal surgically is difficult or impossible. With ABR, it may be possible to detect small tumors in some cases, which permits effective surgical therapy.

Fischer, Mauguiere, Echallier, and Courjon (1982) summarized ABR findings for a group of 66 patients with various CNS tumors, including meningiomas (8), two fourth ventricle ependymomas, five cerebellar tumors, two third ventricle colloid cysts, a craniopharyngeoma, a cyst, a pinealoma, an astrocytoma, a germinoma, and over 40 with unspecified tumors involving the brainstem. The effect of posterior fossa meningiomas and cerebellar tumors on the ABR depended on the size of the tumor and its location relative to auditory structures. CT information was generally more useful than ABR in characterizing location and size. The authors stated that useful, and sometimes unique, diagnostic information was obtained from ABR for 36 patients, including evidence of a tumor by ABR before CT scanning.

Brainstem Encephalitis

In a report of ABR findings in children with *brainstem encephalitis,* Rosenblatt and Majnemer (1984) also describe the ABR pattern for two 6-year-old children with brainstem gliomas (and one with an extra-axial tumor, Burkitt's lymphoma). Clinical symptoms and signs were diplopia (double vision), neck pain, ataxia, dysarthria, dysphagia (swallowing difficulty), cranial nerve palsies (nerves VI, VII, IX and X), horizontal nystagmus, and hyperreflexia. Each child died. One of the children with brainstem glioma showed a markedly prolonged wave III–V interval on the left and prolongation of all latencies on the right. The other had an abnormal delay for the wave III–V and wave I–V latencies bilaterally and reduced wave V amplitude. The child with Burkitt's lymphoma had normal ABR findings.

Epilepsy

Studies of children, and adults, show prolonged latencies for wave III and wave V, and interwave latencies, in a proportion of patients with epilepsy (Yuksul et al., 1995; Zgorzalewicz, Galas-Zgorzalewicz, & Steinborn, 1995). Zgorzalewicz and Galas-Zgorzalewicz (2000) further relate ABR interwave latency abnormalities to subclinical toxicity induced by long-term therapy with carbamazepine (CBZ) and valproate acid (VPA).

Demyelinating Diseases

This is a group of diseases that affect the myelin sheath of neurons, sparing the axons of CNS and peripheral nervous system neurons. Two categories are demyelinating diseases (disease process affects normal myelin sheath) and dysmyelinating diseases (defective myelin metabolism). The following diseases fall into the CNS demyelinating category: acute disseminated encephalomyelitis (ADEM), acute hemorrhagic leukoencephalitis, multiple sclerosis, and Schilder's disease. Guillian-Barre syndrome demyelination affects the peripheral nervous system. Dysmyelinating diseases encompass leukodystrophies, such as metachromatic leukodystrophy, globoid cell leukodystrophy, sudanophilic (orthochromatic) leukodystrophy, adrenoleukodystrophy, Pelizaeus-Merzbacher disease, and Alexander's disease.

MULTIPLE SCLEROSIS (MS). | MS is the most common type of demyelinating disease and a major cause of neurologic impairment in adults except the elderly. Young adults are usually affected (about 50 to 70% of patients have onset between age 20 and 40 years). MS in children is extremely rare.

SCHILDER'S DISEASE. | This is a progressive childhood disease with usually bilateral, large, and continuous patches of demyelination and associated severe axonal damage. It is sometimes referred to as "diffuse cerebral sclerosis." Brainstem tracts may show demyelination. Some authors consider Schilder's disease a childhood variant of MS. Schilder's disease may be misdiagnosed as subacute sclerosing panencephalitis or adrenoleukodystrophy. Diagnosis is made by CT and MRI scanning (showing bilateral white matter hypodensity) and CSF examination (with elevation of gam-

malobulin or IgG fractions). Symptoms include an unreversible, progressive loss of intellectual functions, cortical blindness, bilateral spastic paresis, and deafness, leading to death in one to five years. Effectiveness of the typical treatment of corticosteroids or ACTH has not been demonstrated conclusively.

LEUKODYSTROPHIES. | These are rare familial abnormalities of myelination formation that are found in infants and children and affect white matter (gray matter is spared). There is widespread and often symmetrically bilateral failure or degeneration in the formation of myelination in the CNS with some degree of axonal degeneration. Diagnosis is suggested by neuroradiologic scanning, which shows extensive white matter hypodensity. Metachromatic leukodystrophy is inherited as an autosomal recessive trait and has its onset around 12 to 18 months of age with progressive leg weakness and ataxia and then upper limb involvement, progressive dementia, and speech/language deficits. There are six different types of metachromatic leukodystrophy. Death occurs by age 7 in most cases. Adrenoleukodystrophy is a childhood disease affecting boys only with an onset at approximately 7 years. Long-chain fatty acids are elevated in the CNS. Neurologic and mental deterioration progressively develop secondary to diffuse cerebral sclerosis. There may also be spinal cord or peripheral nerve demyelination. Death occurs within one to four years. Krabbe's leukodystrophy (globoid cell leukodystrophy) has three forms: infantile, juvenile, and adult. Infantile is most common and recognized by failure to thrive, myoclonic seizures, spasticity, macrocrania, loss of acquired skills, and early death. Pathology is characterized by multinucleated giant cells in the white matter. There are three leukodystrophies with no known biochemical markers. Pelizaeus-Merzbacher disease is inherited and usually sex linked, affects only males, and has an onset as early as the first months of life. Symptoms include head trembling, roving eye movements, ataxia, slow motor and mental development, which worsen during adolescence. The disease has an extended course, with death occurring in early adulthood. Alexander's leukodystrophy begins in infancy. Symptoms are deterioration of psychomotor functioning, seizures, and spasticity. During the second year, macrocephaly becomes apparent with death by age 6 years. Canavan's sclerosis begins also in infancy. Symptoms are hypotonia, optic atrophy, seizures, spasticity, megalencephaly, and failure to thrive. Another form of this disease begins at age 5 and develops at a slower rate. Along with a variety of diseases, leukodystrophies produce neurologic degeneration.

ABR abnormalities are typically found in this white matter disease and are useful in distinguishing white versus gray matter involvement. Prolonged ABR interwave (I–V) latencies characterize adrenoleukodystrophy and a related disease adrenomyeloneuropathy (Garg, Markland, DeMyer, & Warren, 1983; Grimes, Elles, Grunberger, & Pikus, 1983; Markand, DeMyer, Worth, & Warren, 1982; Tobimatsu et al.,

1985; Vercruyssen, Martin, & Mercelis, 1983). The abnormal ABR findings are associated with increased central conduction times for somatosensory evoked responses (SSERs) and visual evoked responses (VERs). Absence of ABR waves III or V, or all components after wave I and II, are not uncommon (Markand et al., 1982; Yagi, Kaga, & Baba, 1980). Wave I is usually present, but the ABR is rarely normal, and then only in patients with a mild form of the disease. Eighth-nerve pathology has been reported (Igarashi et al., 1976). Isolated unilateral absence of wave VI has also been given diagnostic significance in adrenoleukodystrophy (Black, Fariello, & Chun, 1979).

Similarly markedly abnormal ABRs are recorded in most patients with Pelizaeus-Merzbacher disease and both infantile and juvenile onset metachromatic leukodystrophy (Brown et al., 1981; Carlin et al., 1983; Davis, Aminoff, & Berg, 1985; Hecox, Cone, & Blaw, 1981; Markand et al., 1982; Nuwer et al., 1982). In patients with metachromatic leukodystrophy, there may be, in addition, a delayed latency wave I (Carlin et al., 1983; Hecox, Cone, & Blaw, 1981; Markand et al., 1982; Ochs, Markand, & DeMyer, 1979). These types of ABR were normal in carriers of Pelizaeus-Merzbacher disease who were unaffected. ABR aberrations in leukodystrophies are correlated with demyelination and are again useful clinically in differentiating white matter versus gray matter disease.

Varied ABR findings were reported in other demyelinating diseases. Jacobson, Means, and Dhib-Jalbut (1986) described eighth-nerve involvement evidenced by increased wave I latency and slight high-frequency pure-tone hearing threshold deficit for a 30-year-old male patient with acute inflammatory demyelinating disease. Twelve patients with inflammatory acute transverse myelopathy had normal ABRs. This disease involves neural tracts on both sides of the spinal cord. In West syndrome, absence of waves after I was reported by Yagi, Kaga, and Baba (1980).

METABOLIC DISEASES

This group of diseases includes those resulting from inherent abnormalities in CNS metabolism, as opposed to metabolic abnormalities secondary to specific etiolologies such as trauma, vascular pathology and infection, and from the effects of an exogenous toxin or poison.

Storage Diseases

BACKGROUND. | These entities are related to abnormalities in lipid metabolism (Tay-Sachs disease, Gaucher's disease, metachromatic leukodystrophy, Krabbe's disease, Austin's disease, Fabry's disease, Niemann-Pick disease, Refsum's disease), mucopolysaccharide metabolism (Hurler's disease, Hunter's disease, Sanfilippo's disease), carbohydrate metabolism (glycogen storage disease), galactosemia, Leigh's disease (a subacute necrotizing encephalopathy that can af-

fect the brainstem tegmentum), Lafora's disease, amino acid metabolism, metal metabolism (Wilson's disease, iron and calcium metabolism disorders), and pigment metabolism. Clinical signs and symptoms are varied.

As a rule, children with three of the mucopolysaccharidoses (Hurler, Hunter, and Sanfilippo diseases) are severely mentally retarded. For Hunter's syndrome, signs and symptoms include mental and skeletal abnormalities (with dwarfing), vertebral defects, atypical flexion posture, distinct facial features, and mental abnormalities. Hearing loss, often mixed (conductive and sensorineural components), is a frequent feature of Hunter's syndrome. Peck (1984) reviewed auditory manifestations of Hunter's syndrome. Gaucher's disease was among the first of the lipidoses storage diseases described. An early feature is hepatosplenomegaly. There are two main types of Gaucher's disease, one involving the viscera and the other the CNS. With this latter type, young children are affected and there is rapid neurologic deterioration. Various diseases afflicting children or adults have as a major feature CNS degeneration. These are also discussed above in the sections on demyelinating diseases, degenerative diseases, and perinatal neuropathologies.

TAY-SACHS DISEASE. | This is inherited as an autosomal recessive trait and is the most common lipid storage disease in children. It's also known as infantile gangliosidosis. Actually, there are two types of Tay-Sachs disease, with the infantile type more common. At approximately 6 months of age, the child becomes less active, more lethargic, weak, spastic, and begins to lose developmental milestones. Blindness may also be a feature of the disease. Neurologic deficits progress (including seizures, myoclonus, and spastic quadriplegia) and death usually follows within two years of onset. Onset of a second type, juvenile Tay-Sachs disease, is at 3 to 4 years and is characterized by seizures, spasticity, and dementia. The carrier rate for Tay-Sachs disease is especially high in Jewish families originating from Poland and Lithuania. The cause is an enzyme deficiency that results in excessive accumulation of a certain type of ganglioside (GM2) in CNS neurons. This enzyme abnormality can be detected in amniotic fluid within the first trimester of pregnancy, permitting genetic counseling and abortion if indicated therapeutically.

MAROTEAUX-LAMY SYNDROME. | Maroteaux-Lamy syndrome is a mucopolysaccharidosis VI (MPS VI) disorder. Shigematsu et al. (1991) published a case report of a 13-month-old Japanese boy with a respiratory infection who was subsequently diagnosed with mucopolysaccharidosis type VI based on urinary glycosaminoglycan analysis and low activity of arylsulfatase B in peripheral leukocytes. Although the authors report that MPS VI is usually characterized by normal hearing, the child's ABR findings confirmed a moderate hearing impairment.

GAUCHER'S DISEASE (CEREBROSIDE LIPIDOSIS). | This is a rare lipid storage disease that, like Tay-Sach's disease, is caused by an enzyme deficiency (a different enzyme) and the accumulation of ganglioside (cerebroside) in the nervous system, as well as the viscera (liver, spleen, lungs). The result is diffuse neuronal damage and progressive and marked CNS dysfunction (e.g., muscle paralysis), usually beginning at 6 months, with death by 1 year. The phenotype of this rare autosomal recessive disorder, particularly neurologic involvement, is variable. There is a non-CNS form of Gaucher's disease with a much longer survival time.

ABR FINDINGS. | Grossly abnormal ABRs are found in Gaucher's syndrome (e.g., Campbell, Harris, Sirimanna, & Vellodi, 2003; Campbell, Harris, & Vellodi, 2004; Kaga, Marsh, & Fukuyama, 1982; Kaga et al., 1998; Lacey & Terplan, 1984). Kaga et al. (1982) recorded serial ABRs from an infant with Gaucher's disease. Onset of the disease was at 3 months. Symptoms were first stridor, strabismus, failure to thrive, and inguinal hernia, and then muscular rigidity, ocular palsies, and respiratory failure. The initial ABR showed delayed wave I–III latency and no later waves. On subsequent ABRs, this latency became further prolonged, then wave components disappeared as neurologic status deteriorated. Notably, an autopsy showed no structural damage in the auditory brainstem, suggesting to the authors that metabolic and electrophysiologic changes precede histopathologic changes. In a case report of infantile Gaucher's disease, Lacey and Terplan (1984) described similar markedly abnormal ABR findings (only wave I and II consistently, with an unreliable wave III). The authors cite experience with two other infants with this ABR pattern. However, they did correlate these ABR abnormalities with bilateral absence of cochlear nucleus neurons and changes in the superior olivary complex. In a later study, the authors (Kaga et al., 1998) correlated abnormal ABR findings (only wave I and wave II were recorded) with neuropathology. In summary, autopsy findings showed Gaucher's cells in the cerebrum and thalamus, dorsal brainstem gliosis, and pathologic cells in the superior olivary complex with marked gliosis in the cochlear nucleus.

Campbell, Harris, and Vellodi (2004) studied specifically the ABR in 8 children with type 3 Gaucher's disease. Patients were treated for Gaucher's disease with exogenous enzyme replacement therapy (ERT), a management option that generally increases life expectancy and quality of life. Peripheral auditory findings (pure-tone audiometry, tympanometry, and otoacoustic emissions) were normal for all of the subjects. A diverse collection of ABR abnormalities were reported, including absence of all waves except wave I (a common pattern) and delays in later waves (III and V). Campbell, Harris, and Vellodi (2004) conclude that "ERT does not prevent ABR deterioration in GD3 children" (p. 386), and "it seems most likely that the progressive deterioration in ABRs reflects underlying subclinical brainstem deterioration. . . ." (p. 387).

FABRY'S DISEASE. | Fabry's disease is a lipid storage disease, again caused by an enzyme deficiency. It is inherited (X-linked) and can affect the peripheral and central nervous system, along with other major organ systems (kidney, skin, eye, and heart). Pain in the extremities is often an early symptom. Evidence of cerebral ischemia usually develops first in adolescence, secondary to glycolipid storage in the muscles lining arteries and subsequent vascular occlusion. There is no cure.

REFSUM'S DISEASE. | A recessively inherited lipid storage disorder first described in 1946, Refsum's disease is caused by a phytanic acid enzyme deficiency that results in excessive accumulation of phytanic acid in many bodily tissues. Refsum's disease is also known as "heredopathia atactica polyneuritiformis." In the nervous system, this process leads to severe demyelinating peripheral neuropathy, ataxia, visual deficits (pigmentary retinopathy), and hearing impairment. Refsum's disease can be managed by dietary modifications.

Progressive sensory hearing loss is a common characteristic of Refsum's disease, affecting up to 80 percent of patients (Bergsmark & Djupesland, 1968), a finding verified by histopathologic evidence of cochlear and saccular degeneration, collapse of Reissner's membrane, and atrophy of the organ of Corti and spiral ganglion. Oysu and Turkish colleagues (Oysu, Aslan, Basaran, & Baserer, 2001) report a case study of a 6-year-old boy with the diagnosis of Refsum's disease. Although the audiogram initially showed essentially normal hearing and DPOAEs were normal, no ABR was detected bilaterally. Unfortunately, the boy did not follow a prescribed specialized diet, and he returned at age 11 years with a severe-to-profound sensorineural hearing loss, yet normal DPOAEs. The authors concluded from the absence of the ABR and normal DPOAEs that "the boy might have an auditory neuropathy" (p. 130). Auditory neuropathy is discussed in detail in Chapter 5.

Other Metabolic Disorders

MAPLE SYRUP URINE DISEASE. | Blood chemistry abnormalities result in urine that smells like maple syrup. The pathology resembles phenylketonuria (PKU), but is more severe. Clinical signs include ocular muscle abnormalities, epilepsy, spasticity, hypoglycemia, and mental retardation. The disease can be managed with proper dietary adjustments, but most children have residual intellectual deficits.

Marked delay in ABR interwave latencies are common in children with Maple Syrup Urine disease (Hall, 1992), with improvement in ABR findings following appropriate medical therapy.

PHENYLKETONURIA (PKU). | PKU is an inborn error of amino acid metabolism first identified in 1934. It can cause severe mental retardation if not treated. Because PKU causes no other signs or symptoms in the infant but can be detected by analysis of amino acids in blood and urine, newborn screening is routinely done. PKU is an autosomal recessive disorder occurring in 1 of 10,000 to 12,000 births in the United States. Without treatment, the infant develops vomiting within the first two months and signs of delayed intellectual development within the first six months. CNS pathology may be widespread and include defective myelination, diminished brain growth, and focal neurologic abnormalities. PKU can be effectively treated with a special diet.

HURLER'S SYNDROME. | This is one of the more severe types of a group of about eight rare inherited disorders of acid mucopolysaccharide metabolism that are related to enzyme deficiencies. Clinical signs include mental retardation, facial abnormalities, congenital heart disease, severe skeletal abnormalities, dwarfism, and eye defects. Hurler's syndrome has its onset in infancy and clinical progressively worsens with death usually occurring at approximately age 10 years.

FETAL ALCOHOL SYNDROME. | Fetal alcohol syndrome (FAS) consists of a pattern of malformations (e.g., craniofacial anomalies, reduced growth, CNS deficits, malformations of the skeletal system and internal organs) in children following prenatal exposure to maternal alcohol abuse.

A modest number of studies show abnormally prolonged latencies for ABRs in children with FAS, in comparison to age-matched normal children (Church, Eldis, Blakley, & Bawle, 1997; Church & Kaltenbach, 1997; Pettigrew & Hutchinson, 1985; Rintelmann et al., 1995; Rössig, Wässer, & Oppermann, 1994). There are, however, no large-scale and longitudinal investigations documenting long-term and permanent ABR abnormalities.

FRAGILE X SYNDROME. | Children with fragile X syndrome, the most common hereditary type of mental retardation, may demonstrate behavior disorders (autistic-type disorder), attention-deficit disorder, and speech-language impairment.

Longer latencies for ABR components, including interwave latencies, have been reported in children with fragile X syndrome (Arinami et al., 1988; Gillberg et al., 1986; Wisniewski et al., 1991). Miezejeski et al. (1997) conducted a study of 13 children with fragile X syndrome mental retardation, a group of 18 control subjects with other mental retardation, and 44 "nondisabled" control subjects. There were no ABR abnormalities in the subjects with fragile X syndrome when latency data were compared to control subjects without retardation. Interestingly, however, mentally retarded subjects in both groups had longer ABR latencies under sedation than comparable subjects who underwent ABR assessment without sedation. The authors speculate that the apparent effect of sedation on the ABR for mentally retarded children might explain the discrepancy in reported findings for fragile X syndrome.

WOLF-HIRSCHHORN SYNDROME. | Wolf-Hirschhorn syndrome arises from a chromosomal abnormality (partial deletion of chromosome arm 4p) that is characterized by craniofacial anomalies (e.g., a broad beaked nose, epicanthal folds, slanting palpebral fissures, short philtrum, preauricular pits), cleft lip and/or palate, genitourinary abnormalities). Peripheral hearing loss may also be a feature of Wolf-Hirschhorn syndrome.

Lesperance, Grundfast, and Rosenbaum (1998) report ABR data for five patients with Wolf-Hirschhorn syndrome. Peripheral hearing loss was confirmed with ABR for the children, ranging in severity from mild, unilateral conductive impairment to severe-to-profound bilateral sensorineural hearing loss. Otitis media was found in three children with cleft anomalies. One of the patients had abnormal ABR interwave latencies consistent with retrocochlear auditory dysfunction. The authors conclude, "Comprehensive audiologic and otologic evaluation of children with Wolf-Hirschhorn syndrome should be performed as early as possible. Even difficult-to-test, mentally retarded children can be tested with BAER [ABR] . . ." (Lesperance, Grundfast, & Rosenbaum, 1998, p. 195).

DIDMOAD SYNDROME (WOLFRAM SYNDROME). | The acronym DIDMOAD refers to collection of multisystem abnormalities (Diabetes insipidus [DI], diabetes mellitus [DM], optic atrophy [OA], and deafness [D]). Although the expression of the abnormalities in the rare DIDMOAD syndrome varies considerably, deafness is documented in the majority of patients (Dreyer et al., 1982; Gunn & Belmonte, 1977).

Higashi (1991) reported two cases (10- and 12-year-old brothers) with DIDMOAD syndrome. Each of the children had clinical features including polyuria and polydipsia, diabetes mellitus, optic atrophy, and only a moderate hearing loss at 8000 Hz. ABR findings were normal.

PROGERIA. | First described in 1880, progeria is a rare syndrome, estimated at 1 case per 250,000 births, characterized by the unusual appearance of premature aging or senility. The term is actually misleading because patients with progeria do not have the physical or biochemical findings associated with old age. Although most children with progeria appear normal at birth, the characteristic features develop rapidly in early childhood. In one of the only case reports of progeria studied with a comprehensive audiologic test battery, Hall and Denneny (1993) found in a 5-year-old girl a mild-to-moderate conductive hearing loss bilaterally and a pattern of findings consistent with fixation of the ossicular chain, confirmed surgically. ABR thresholds were elevated, and the ABR wave I to V interval was prolonged in comparison to normative data.

MOEBIUS SYNDROME. | Hamaguchi et al. (1993) described markedly abnormal ABR findings for three children with Moebius syndrome. ABR abnormalities included reduced amplitude for waves, delayed interwave latencies, and absence of the wave V.

INFANTILE OPSOCLONUS-POLYMYOCLONIA SYNDROME. |
Horikawa et al. (1993) collected serial ABR data over a period from 15 to 39 months of age from a child with infantile opsoclonus-polymyoclonia syndrome. Interestingly, ABR interwave latency values showed no change over time measurement period. The ABR findings were, therefore, initially normal but as the child matured, ABR latencies were progressively prolonged in comparison to age-appropriate normative data. The ABR remained abnormal, even though one of the primary symptoms (opsoclonus) resolved.

INFANTILE NEUROAXONAL DYSTROPHY. |
Itoh et al. (1992) report ABR findings for children diagnosed with infantile neuroaxonal dystrophy, a disorder characterized by poor vision, marked hypotonia in the legs, and regression of neurocognitive status. Neurologic degeneration was confirmed by MRI evidence of atrophy of the brainstem and cerbellar vermis. The ABR deteriorated over time until no response could be detected by the age of 2.5 years.

INTESTINAL AGANGLIOSIS. |
Total intestinal aganglionosis is a hereditary disease that is associated with cells derived embryologically from neural crest cells. Ganglion cells are often found within the intestinal tract, including the stomach.

Shimotake and Iwai (1994) recorded the ABR from three children with total or near total intestinal aganglionosis. Each had undergone surgery as newborn infants for "severe gut motility disorders." One of the three children (a 2-year-old) had normal ABR findings. The other two children had elevated ABR thresholds bilaterally. One child (a 5-month-old infant) showed delays in absolute latencies for waves I, III, and V, but interwave latency values were within normal limits. According to the authors, the ABR findings were consistent with inner ear pathology due to common embryologic origin of the cochlea and the intestinal ganglionosis (neural crest derived cells).

MITOCHONDRIAL ENCEPHALOMYOPATHIES. |
Mitochondrial disorders are a varied collection of progressive diseases that have in common morphological, biochemical, and/or genetic abnormalities of mitochondria. Features include accumulation of mitochondria and metabolic disorders. Examples of mitochondrial disorders include Kearns-Sayre syndrome, MELAS syndrome (mitochondrial encephalomyopathy, lactic acidosis, stroke-like episodes), MERRF syndrome (myoclonic epilepsia with red ragged fibers), and Leigh syndrome. Hearing loss is a common feature (about 50 to 70%) of Kearns-Sayre, MELAS, and MERRF syndromes. As noted by Zwirner and Wilichowski (2001), "Because of the unique significance of ATP as a fuel source for all cells, mitochondrial cytopathies may be evident as multisystem diseases affecting particularly, tissues with the highest energy demand, such as the nervous system, muscle, retina, ear, kidney, and liver" (p. 515).

Zwirner and Wilichowski (2001) report abnormal ABRs consistent with sensorineural hearing loss in 10 children with mitochondrial encephalomyopathy. Absence of an ABR due to the severity of hearing loss was a common finding.

Kaga, Naitoh, and Nihei (1987) and Yoshinaga, Ogino, and Ohtahara, et al. (1993) reported hearing loss and markedly abnormal ABR findings in patients with Leigh's syndrome, including prolongation of inter-wave latencies, even in early stages of the disease. Sakai et al. (2004) present two case reports of two sisters (age 4 and 11 years) with Leigh's syndrome with a T8993G point mutation of mitochondrial DNA. Clinical medical findings included low density areas in the basal ganglia and posterior limb of the internal capsule by CT, high levels of lactate and pyruvate in the spinal fluid, muscle weakness, ataxia, retinitis pigmentosa, epileptic seizures, and mental retardation. The children were referred to the authors because they responded poorly to sounds. The older sister yielded essentially normal ABR findings. Hearing sensitivity, however, progressively worsened in the younger sister, a finding associated with delayed ABR latencies and elevations of the ABR threshold to >70 dB.

Yoshinaga et al. (1993) reported a case study of a 7-month-old girl with Leigh's syndrome diagnosed with neurophysiologic, radiologic, enzymatic, biochemical, and molecular studies. Over time the patient developed additional clinical symptoms of brainstem dysfunction (irregular respiration and dysphagia), hypotonia, and then seizures and tonic spasms. Blood analysis showed elevated levels of lactate and pyruvate and a mitochondrial DNA point mutation at 8993 from the patient and the mother. ABR abnormalities were among the first clinical signs found in this patient.

ENZYME DEFICIENCY. |
ABR abnormalities are found in children with peroxisomal enzyme deficiency (Akaboshi et al., 1997; Barth et al., 1990). Akaboshi et al. (1997) describe abnormal ABR findings in a 21-month-old girl with peroxisomal bifunctional enzyme deficiency, a disorder characterized by the loss of a single peroxisomal enzyme beginning in the perinatal period. Initially, at the age of 3 months, wave I was observed with normal latency, but the wave I–V latency was abnormally prolonged. Amplitude of wave III and wave V decreased by 11 months, and the ABR was not detectable at 15 months of age. The ABR abnormalities were attributed to disruption in the role of peroxisomal bifunctional enzyme in neuronal maturation, i.e., to dysmyelination.

DIABETES MELLITUS |
Neurologic complications of diabetes mellitus, as well as peripheral hearing loss, occur in adults and children. For example, Reske-Nielsen reported in long-term diabetic children a pattern of diffuse degenerative changes in the brain, probably secondary to severe and far-reaching vascular disease and angiopathy (Reske-Nielsen et al., 1968).

Sieger et al. (1983) found no ABR wave I–V latency delays among diabetic children in comparison to normative data taken from the literature. In another pediatric study, Sabo, Nozza, and Finegold (1987) examined ABR data for 7 patients with newly diagnosed diabetes and 8 with established diabetes plus acute ketoacidosis. No ABR abnormalities were found in either group. However, a more recent larger scale investigation showed evidence of ABR abnormalities in diabetic children. Niedzielska and Katska (1998) analyzed basic audiometric findings (e.g., pure-tone audiometry and aural immittance measures) and ABR data for a series of 37 insulin-treated children ranging in age from 6 to 18 years. All of the patients enrolled in the study had normal hearing sensitivity (< 15 dB HL) bilaterally and normal middle ear function. Prolongation of wave I latency was observed in 4 ears, but the most common ABR abnormalities were latency delays in wave III and wave V and an abnormally prolonged wave I to V latency interval (23 ears). Furthermore, children with abnormal ABR findings were more likely to have unstable diabetes, with HbA–1c and fructosamine levels that fluctuated widely. Duration of the disease, however, was not related to ABR changes. The authors point out that their findings are in agreement with a previous report (Grosse-Aldenhovel, Gallenkamp, & Sulemana, 1991) of retrocochlear auditory dysfunction in diabetes mellitus.

END STAGE RENAL DISEASE (ESRD). | Peripheral and central neuropathy is a feature in some patients with ESRD and anemia. Recombinant human erythroprotein is applied as a treatment for children adults with ESRD, in addition to dialysis. There are reports of abnormal ABR findings in patients with chronic renal failure (e.g., Pratt et al., 1986; Rossini et al., 1984), and ESRD in adult patients (Di Paolo et al., 1988). Suppiej et al. (1992) recorded ABRs from 14 children with ESRD who were maintained with dialysis. Wave I latency was delayed for the group with ESRD in comparison to a control group. Before anemia correction, 6 of the 14 patients had abnormalities of ABR wave I, 2 of the children with ESRD had abnormal latency prolongations for wave III and wave V and interwave latency abnormalities. Abnormal brainstem findings by ABR were reversed with anemia correction (by recombinant human erythroprotein treatment).

HYPERORNITHINEMIA. | Hyperornithinemia is an inborn disorder of amino acid metabolism caused by mutations in the enzyme ornithine aminotransferase, commonly with peripheral nervous system dysfunction including gyrate atrophy (GA) of the choroids and retina and vision deficits and type II muscle fiber atrophy.

Peltola et al. (2002) recorded ABRs from 40 patients with GA ranging in age from 5 to 74 years (mean age of 32 years). Five of the patients had no detectable ABR, and others had variable ABR abnormalities.

NONKETOTIC HYPERGLYCINEMIA (NKH). | NKH is an inherited metabolic abnormality caused by deficiency of the glycine cleavage enzyme in the liver and brain. The result is a deficit in serine (an amino acid) conversion and increased glycine levels in blood plasma (2 to 4 times the normal amount) and in the cerebral spinal fluid (15 to 30 times the normal amount). Neuropathology is characterized by decreased myelin, especially in the nerve fiber tracts that myelinate postnatally, and spongy CNS tissue degeneration. Usually, symptoms first appear shortly after birth. Some children die because of severe brainstem dysfunction, and survivors have serious neurologic deficits including seizures, muscular hypotonia, lethargy, and mental retardation. Therapy generally consists of medication to correct the biochemical imbalances and dietary reduction of glycine, but these measures are not usually effective. Strychnine, which is an antagonist of glycine, has also been administered, with varied success.

In a paper on evoked responses in NKH, Markand, Garg, and Brandt (1982), reported that in all four children studied ABRs were consistently recorded and well-formed, but the wave I–V latency was abnormally prolonged (greater than 3 standard deviations above normal in 3 and greater than 2 standard deviations in the other patient). In two patients, the ABR wave I–III interval was abnormal, and in the other two there was a delay in the overall I–V interval. Grossly abnormal EEGs and VERs were also described.

Chu and Yang (1987) studied ABRs in 69 patients with various hepatic (liver) diseases, among them 16 with chronic active viral hepatitis, 16 with liver cirrhosis after viral hepatitis, 17 with alcoholic liver disease, and 20 with Wilson's disease. Abnormal ABR interwave latencies (wave I–III, III–V, and/or I–V) were found in liver cirrhosis, alcoholic liver disease, and especially Wilson's disease, whereas these latency values were within normal limits in viral hepatitis.

RICKETS (HYPOPHOSPHATEMIC OSTEOMALACIA). | X-linked hypophosphatemic rickets is a disorder of renal proximal tubular function characterized by decreased reabsorption and subsequent loss of phosphorus. Hypophosphatemic results in osteomalacia and, in growing patients, rickets. This disorder, the most common form of a familial hypophosphatemic rickets, has been mapped to the xp21.2 site of the distal short arm of the x-chromosome. Treatment is comprised of phosphorus supplementation and administration of calcitriol, which promotes both healing of rickets and restoration of linear bone growth, although biopsy evidence of osteomalacia may persist despite therapy.

Sensorineural hearing deficits are associated with X-linked hypophosphatemic rickets (Davies, Kane, & Valentine, 1984; Meister, Johnson, Popelka, Kim, & Whyte, 1986; O'Malley, Ramsden, Latif, Kane, & Davies, 1985; Weir, 1977). Auditory data for these studies were, collectively, obtained from fewer than 50 patients, three-fourths of whom were adults. Hearing assessment consisted mainly of pure-tone audiometry, although Davies et al. (1984) and Meister et al. (1986) also measured word recognition, acoustic immittance (tympanometry and stapedial reflexes), and tone decay. In a follow-up study, Davies et al. (1984) also evaluated cochlear function with transtympanic ECochG for 13 of their original 25 patients.

On the basis of these findings, it appears that cochlear auditory impairment may be a component of both recessive and X-linked forms of hypophosphatemic osteomalacia (rickets), at least in older adults. However, varied audiogram configurations were described, including hearing impairment affecting frequencies below 1000 Hz (O'Malley et al., 1985), primarily the mid-frequency region or high-frequency threshold (Weir, 1977). Hearing deficits are not an invariant feature of this disorder, as Meister et al. (1986) failed to detect any auditory abnormality in a series of 19 patients ranging in age from 1 to 58 years. The pathophysiologic basis for auditory deficits in rickets is also unclear. Davies and colleagues (Davies, Kane, & Valentine, 1984; O'Malley et al., 1985) speculated that rickets-related bony abnormalities of the cochlea contribute to hydrops and hair cell atrophy and, therefore, a low-frequency hearing impairment similar to the audiometric configuration of Ménière's disease. In contrast, Weir (1977) presumed an eighth nerve site of lesion, because of his observation of high-frequency hearing impairment and radiologic evidence of internal auditory canal narrowing. Although the foregoing studies are intriguing, the information they provide on auditory function in rickets is incomplete and somewhat contradictory. Data were reported for predominantly adult population. There is no systematic study of hearing in children with this disease. Also, none of the studies analyzed data for patients versus and age- and gender-matched control groups.

Hall and Jonas (1988) studied auditory function in 15 children with diagnosed rickets (8 male and 7 female) ranging in age from 5 through 16 years (mean 9.7) and a control group of 15 unrelated children (8 male and 7 female) ranging in age from 4 through 15 years (mean 9.3). Diagnosis was based on family history, physical examination, X-ray evidence of rickets, blood chemistries, and low tubular reabsorption of phosphorus without evidence of other disturbance of renal tubular function. The test battery consisted of immittance, pure-tone, speech, and ABR audiometry. Tympanometry and static immittance measures were within clinically normal limits for all subjects. There were no statistically significant (0.05 level of confidence) differences between groups for acoustic reflex threshold measures, pure-tone audiometry (for traditional and high frequencies), and speech audiometry procedures.

ABR data were separated for gender in recognition of established differences for males versus females (see Chapter 7). Absolute latency for wave I was equivalent between groups. Interwave latency values were similar for females in the rickets in comparison to the control groups, but wave I–III and I–V latencies in males were distinctly prolonged compared to the controls. Prolongation of ABR latency in males with rickets appeared to be related to age and was clustered within one family.

TOXINS AND POISONS

Toxins and poisons include anesthetics and hypnotics, carbon monoxide, heavy metals (inorganic and organic lead and mercury), and industrial agents. Before dementia is apparent, toxins typically produce other more clinically notable signs and symptoms. Lead poisoning in children, for example, results in convulsions, lethargy, irritability, papilledema, and projectile vomiting. In adults, chronic lead poisoning is very rare. Chronic paint or toluene sniffing causes toxic neuropathology, including optic nerve lesions, acute muscle weakness, dementia, cerebellar dysfunction, and varied peripheral neuropathies.

Lead Poisoning

Lead poisoning is a risk factor for auditory abnormalities. Although some studies fail to demonstrate abnormal ABR findings with exposure to lead (e.g., Counter, Buchanan, Ortega, & Laurell, 1997; Grandjean et al., 2001; Wong, Ng, & Yeung, 1991; Yokoyama et al., 2002), others found variable audiologic findings (e.g., Musiek & Hanlon, 1999), including a rather complex relation between blood lead level and ABR response parameters (Robinson et al., 1985). In a more comprehensive follow-up investigation to a previous study (Rothenberg, Poblano, & Garza-Morales, 1994), Rothenberg, Poblano, and Schnaas (2000) collected ABR data from 100 children aged 5 to 7 years who were exposed during the prenatal period to maternal blood lead. ABR interwave latency values were associated with blood lead content. Rothenberg, Poblano, and Schnaas (2000) "hypothesize that the simultaneous effects of lead on brainstem length and myelogenesis and/or synaptic transmission cause the BAER [ABR] conduction interval to decrease up to 8 -µg/dl blood lead level, and then to increase thereafter" (p. 508).

Osman and colleagues (1999) performed ABR recordings in 155 children exposed to lead who were living in an industrial region in Poland. Hearing sensitivity, as measured with pure-tone audiometry, was impaired with increasing blood lead levels. Associated with this finding were delays in ABR wave I latency in the children with the highest blood lead levels (P-Bb > 100 µg/L, 0.48 µmol/L). The authors acknowledge that "the BAEP [ABR] methodology chosen might have been too crude in detecting possible lead-induced alterations . . ." (p. 7).

Methylmercury (MeHg)

ABR has also been applied in the study of children exposed to methylmercury (MeHg), a contaminant of seafood and freshwater fish throughout the world (e.g., Hamada et al., 1982; Inayoshi, Okajima, Sannomiya, & Tsuda, 1993;

Murata et al., 2004; Murata, Weihe, Renzoni, 1999). Methylmercury ingestion can lead to nervous system dysfunction and disruption of brain development for infants born of mothers exposed during pregnancy to dietary methylmercury. The presence and quantity of MeHg exposure is determined from analysis of hair samples. Damage to the developing nervous system is, if detected early, potentially reversible. In a very thorough investigation of 149 children, Murata et al. (2004) correlated delayed latencies of wave III and V, and interwave latencies, with intrauterine MeHg exposure biomarkers. Abnormalities were most pronounced for the wave I–III and wave III–V intervals. In contrast the evidence of auditory brainstem dysfunction, hearing sensitivity was generally within normal limits.

INFECTIONS AND INFLAMMATORY DISEASES

Brain Abscess

BACKGROUND. | Approximately 60 percent of brain abscesses result from spread of infections from the middle ear and mastoid or from the paranasal cavities or nasal cavity. In these cases, the abscess is located in the adjacent inferior temporal lobe or cerebellar hemisphere or frontal or anterior temporal lobes. Other sources are metastatic infection, congenital anomalies, trauma, and postsurgical development. Abscesses begin with an infection and inflammation (*S. aureus,* streptococci, gram-negative bacilli, or anaerobes in 80 percent of cases) that destroy brain tissue, forming a cystic mass. The mass becomes surrounded by a thin layer of compressed brain tissue. Abscesses are found most often in deep cerebral white matter (versus cortical gray matter) and are distributed in certain sites with the brain. Neurologic symptoms and signs are headache, fever, systemic illness, nausea, reduced alertness, and seizures. Diagnosis is based on these clinical findings and CT scanning. In contrast to meningitis, lumbar puncture (LP) in suspected abscess is contraindicated because of the possibility of herniation of brain tissue from the supratentorial compartment due to mass effect and increased intracranial pressure (ICP). The overall mortality for brain abscess is approximately 45 percent. Without surgical intervention, virtually all patients die. With early diagnosis (e.g., by CT scanning), antibiotic therapy is often successful in effecting a cure. There is a male:female ratio of occurrence of 3:1.

ABR FINDINGS. | Goitein, Fainmesser, and Sohmer (1983) describe the relation among ABR findings, clinical findings (neurologic status), physiologic parameters (e.g. mean arterial blood pressure, intracranial pressure, cerebral perfusion pressure), and outcome for a group of children with varied brain pathologies. Within this group are eleven children with meningitis, five with encephalitis, and one with a brain abscess. A potential pathophysiologic process in each of these pathologies, including brain abscess, is increased intracranial pressure that can lead to brain ischemia. Absence of waves IV and V were noted in the child with a brain abscess, presumably because of the effect of supratentorial pressure (due to the mass of the abscess) on upper brainstem functioning.

Kawasaki Disease

BACKGROUND. | Kawasaki disease is an acute, idiopathic, vasculitis affecting infants and children that is related to systemic inflammation and serious alterations in immunoregulation. The disease involves mostly medium-size arteries serving extraparenchymal muscles. Involvement of the coronary arteries occurs in about one out of five patients and is a factor in morbidity in Kawasaki disease. The coronary artery abnormalities, e.g., inflammation, aneurysms, immunoregulatory changes, can be treated successfully with medical therapy (high-dose intravenous gamma globulin, or IVGG).

ABR FINDINGS. | Sensorineural hearing loss may accompany Kawasaki disease (Dreyer et al., 1982). Sundel et al. (1992) included ABR in an audiologic test battery in a study of the prevalence and type of hearing loss in a series of 40 children with Kawasaki disease. The average subject age was 3.2 years. Sensorineural hearing loss was found in 7 of 23 patients who yielded valid audiologic results. The ABR is useful for documenting the type and degree of hearing loss in infants and young children with Kawasaki disease. The authors question the possible role of aspirin ototoxicity as a factor in the development of sensory hearing loss in children with Kawasaki disease.

Meningitis

BACKGROUND. | The typical routes of entry for bacterial infection of the CNS in meningitis are the cardiopulmonary system, the nasopharynx and sinuses, the middle ear, and along the nerves and skull fractures secondary to trauma. The term *meningitis* is not entirely accurate, as the bacterial infection and inflammation may involve, in addition to the meninges, the subarachnoid CSF and ventricles and brain parenchyma. Intracranial complications include brain swelling and increased intracranial pressure, which can produce diffuse encephalopathy, stupor, and coma. Convulsive seizures may occur as well. Cranial nerve abnormalities and hydrocephalus (from inflammatory exudate blocking the foramina of Luschka and Magendie or the reabsorptive apparatus at the arachnoid villi).

Meningitis occurs most often in the very young and the very old (70% of cases in children under 5 years and 20% in patients over age 70 years). Approximately 70 percent of meningitis cases are caused by *Streptococcus pneumoniae, Haemophilus influenzae* (H. flu), and *Neisseria meningitidis,* whereas the causative organisms for most of the other 30 percent are *Staphylococcus aureus* and species of *Streptococcus, Proteus, Pseudomonas,* and *Escherichia (E) coli.* Between age 3 months to 4 years, *H. flu* is the major pathogen. Neonates are resistant to *H. flu* for immunologic reasons. Preterm neonates are susceptible to gram-negative organisms (*Proteus, Pseudomonas,* and *E. coli*), and full-term neonates are affected by gram-positive organisms (*Staphylococcus*). Diagnosis is made by clinical symptoms (fever, irritability, headache, lethargy, disorientation), analysis of CSF, blood culture, and biochemical testing.

ABR FINDINGS. | Peripheral auditory deficits in meningitis are a common cause for pediatric hearing loss. For example, Özdamar and colleagues reported peripheral deficits in 35 percent of a series of 60 patients. Among these, about 20 percent had evidence of only sensorineural loss and another 15 percent had conductive loss (Özdamar, Kraus, & Stein, 1983; Özdamar & Kraus, 1983; Stein & Kraus, 1988). In addition, auditory CNS dysfunction may be a component of bacterial meningitis (Guerit, 1991; Özdamar et al., 1983; Özdamar & Kraus, 1983) as reflected by increased ABR wave I–III latencies. Among 60 patients recovering from meningitis, Özdamar, Kraus, and Stein (1983) found six (10%) with ABR interwave latencies exceeding 3 standard deviations of age-matched average normal values, indicating neurologic dysfunction. ABR abnormalities were more commonly found in children with seizures, cranial nerve palsies (other than the auditory or 8th nerve), hydrocephalus, and extended duration of pretreatment symptoms (longer than three days). CNS dysfunction in acute meningitis was clearly demonstrated with ABR findings in the study by Goitein, Fainmesser, and Sohmer (1983), noted above. Among the eleven children with acute meningitis, five showed normal ABRs, but two had abnormal prolongations of interwave latency values and another four had no detectable response. The underlying pathophysiology in the ABR abnormalities was brainstem ischemia associated with increased intracranial pressure and reduced cerebral perfusion pressure. ABR findings were related to survival, as all children with some evidence of an ABR survived the acute meningitis and all those with no response died.

Bao and Wong (1998) recorded the ABR from 101 children with meningitis including bacterial (N = 52), viral (N = 6), and aseptic (N = 43). Abnormalities in the ABR were found for 27.7 percent of the patients, including patterns consistent with unilateral and bilateral, and conductive and sensorineural, hearing loss. ABR abnormalities were observed more often for bacterial meningitis (34.6%, and mostly for *H. flu* bacteria) than for aseptic meningitis (20.9%). Only one child with viral meningitis (coxackie virus) had what was described as "mild impairment" of the ABR. Interestingly, with antibiotic treatment ten children with normal ABRs showed no change, and four out of ten children who initially had abnormal ABR findings showed a return to normal.

Kapoor et al. (1997) conducted a study of the ABR in 50 children with tuberculosis meningitis and 50 control subjects. One-half of the meningitis subjects showed ABR ab-

normalities. Prolonged absolute and interwave latencies were the most common finding, but 4 percent of the subjects had no detectable ABR either unilaterally or bilaterally. ABR abnormalities were correlated with some clinical findings, including elevated intracranial pressure (ICP), Glasgow Coma Scale (GCS), but were not related to age, gender, duration of meningitis, neurologic deficits, or CSF findings. Serial recordings in seven patients documented complete reversal of ABR abnormalities.

Cherian, Singh, Chacko, and Abraham (2002) investigated ABR in 32 children (aged 1 month to 12 years) with acute bacterial meningitis. Among the group, 28 percent had sensorineural hearing loss (bilateral in 22% and unilateral in 6%) as confirmed by ABR and, when feasible, behavioral audiometry. Clinical findings (e.g., vomiting, seizures, aminoglycoside usage) was not related to the likelihood of hearing loss. ABR measurement contributed to early identification and intervention of hearing loss in meningitis.

Mycotic (Fungal) Infections

BACKGROUND. | Meningitis and CNS abscesses are more common now because of increased reliance on immunosuppressive medical therapy in management of cancer and other various diseases (collagen vascular diseases, myasthenia gravis, and multiple sclerosis) and in organ transplant recipients. These medical therapies have also contributed to an increase in problems with other opportunistic infections, including viruses such as Herpes simplex and zoster. Clinically, fungal infections present similarly to chronic meningitis or brain abscess. The most common fungal CNS infection is cryptococcal meningitis. Other fungi that produce CNS infection in immunocompromised hosts include *Norcardia, Aspergillus,* and, most commonly, *Candida.* Mycotic infections are diagnosed by sophisticated CSF analysis. Treatment for mycotic infections is difficult, but often involves the antibiotic amphotericin B (a potentially ototoxic drug).

Viral Infections

BACKGROUND. | Viral diseases involving the nervous system are varied and include herpes zoster (Ramsay-Hunt syndrome), herpes simplex encephalitis, congenital cytomegalovirus (CMV), meningoencephalitis, meningitis, poliomyelitis, rabies, and slow virus infections (Jakob-Creutzfeldt disease), progressive multifocal leukoencephalopathy, subacute slerosing panencephalitis, Progressive rubella panencephalitis, and human immune virus (HIV) or acquired immune deficiency syndrome (AIDS). Congenital and perinatal viruses may affect the nervous system in many ways, producing chromosomal damage, encephalitis, congenital defects, mental retardation, and fetal death. To a large extent, the amount of damage caused by the virus is related to the embryonic time of exposure. In childhood, encephalitis may result from different viral diseases, among them measles, rubella, varicella, and mumps. Herpes zoster infections have been appreciated since 1831. They are now known to result from a virus infection that affects peripheral or cranial nerves, although which anatomic structures are necessarily involved is still debated. The disease more commonly affects persons over age 45 years and males versus females. Patients with the Ramsay-Hunt syndrome from herpes zoster can present with skin eruptions on areas of the head and neurotologic pathology including external ear lesions, facial nerve paralysis, eighth nerve lesions, and inner ear (cochlea) abnormalities, along with related sensorineural hearing impairment. Neurotologic findings are usually unilateral.

ENCEPHALITIS. | Rosenblatt and Majnemer (1984) illustrated the effect of brainstem encephalitis on ABR with two case reports (a 10-month-old boy and an 11.5-month-old girl). Typical clinical symptoms in the disease include reduced level of consciousness (lethargy), dysarthria, dysphagia (swallowing problems), cranial nerve deficits, and ataxia. Among proposed etiologies for selected cases are herpes simplex infection and influenza inoculation. Serial ABRs for each patient initially showed an abnormal delay for interwave latencies. Over time (eight months for case 1 and three months for case 2), the ABR improved substantially. Other abnormalities reported were poor morphology, decreased wave V/I amplitude ratio, and absence of wave components. There was evidence of peripheral auditory deficit for each patient. The authors point out that initial ABR findings in these two patients with brainstem encephalitis were indistinguishable from those of children with brainstem glioma (also discussed in the paper), but that over time the ABRs for brainstem encephalitis improved, whereas those for the neoplasm did not, or even worsened.

Jain and Maheshwari (1984) recorded ABRs from fifteen patients (aged 13 to 51 years) comatose (mean Glasgow Coma Scale score of 8.2) secondary to meningoencephalitis (see Chapter 16 for definition of Glasgow Coma Scale). Etiology was unknown for four patients and included pyogenic meningitis, tubercular meningitis, enteric encephalopathy, and fungal meningoencephalitis for the remainder. Five patients in the group had normal ABRs bilaterally, in comparison to control group data. The other ten showed abnormalities (reported only for the most involved ear) that consisted of either delayed interwave latencies (eight patients) or missing wave components (two patients). This proportion of comatose patients with abnormal ABRs is far greater than would be expected for coma due to head injury.

REYE SYNDROME. | Among possible viral-related diseases in childhood, Reye syndrome is a common cause of death, with mortality estimated a from 60 to 80 percent. Encephalopathy, reflecting brain edema, is a major component. The exact etiology is not well defined, but most children have a prior viral illness. Abdominal organs (e.g., liver), in addition to the brain, may be involved. Reye syndrome is associated by some with aspirin use, but the exact relationship is unclear.

LUES (SYPHILIS). | This is a chronic infection caused by the microorganism *Treponema palidum* (a spirochete). It may be congenital or acquired. Congenital syphilis is due to infection of the fetus during pregnancy. The traditional clinical findings of neurosyphilis (paresis or tabes dorsalis, with delusions, poor judgment, motor and language dysfunction, pains in trunk region, primary optic atrophy, Argyll Robertson pupils) are now very uncommon. Congenital syphilis with onset of symptoms in infancy is more severe and may result in death. Diagnosis is more secure when based on the fluorescent treponema antibody (FTA) test rather than on VDRL (Venereal Disease Research Laboratory) test. Treatment of choice is benzathine penicillin. Auditory deficits in patients with congenital syphilis are usually progressive and occur in from 20 to 40 percent of patients, more often males than females. Hearing impairment may begin in childhood or be delayed until some point in adulthood. Hearing loss associated with acquired syphilis is a less serious clinical problem because of antibiotic medical therapy. Vascular syphilis of the brain is less common today than in the past. Neurologic symptoms are also less apparent.

ACQUIRED IMMUNE DEFICIENCY SYNDROME (HUMAN IMMUNODEFICIENCY VIRUS). | HIV (AIDS) is among the major health problems in the United States, and a devastating health concern in some regions of the world, e.g., Africa. Central nervous system infection is often a component of AIDS (in over three-fourths of patients as determined by autopsy), and neurotologic complications may also be a feature (Koenig et al.,1986). Subacute encephalitis is common, with cortical atrophy, abnormal histopathologic findings, myelination degeneration, and both white and gray matter involvement. There are cases of central auditory nervous system lesions by autopsy (Hart, Cokely, Schupbach, Dal Canto, & Coppleston, 1989). CNS-related disorders include dementia and depression. AIDS is a terminal disease. Death is often due to unrelated infection, such as pneumonia.

PRECOCIOUS PUBERTY. | Theodore et al. (1983) studied ABR, along with EEG and VERs, in nineteen children with precocious puberty ranging in age from 2 years 9 months to 8 years. All had normal ABR and VER findings. The authors indicate that these data do not support the theory of widespread neurologic pathology or dysfunction in persons with precocious puberty.

RETT SYNDROME. | Rett syndrome is a pediatric neurologic disorder affecting only girls and characterized by dementia, seizures, spasticity, hyperreflexia, autistic behavior, microcephaly, spontaneous hyperventilation, and certain stereotypical behaviors (e.g., rocking, grinding teeth). Etiology is unknown, although it is thought to be a disease involving the CNS gray matter.

Verma, Nigro, and Hart (1987) found no evidence of auditory, somatosensory, or visual evoked response abnormality but did report abnormal EEGs in nine girls with diagnosed Rett syndrome, confirming the concept that the disease affects gray matter and does not involve white matter. Stach, Stoner, Smith, and Jerger (1994) also reported normal ABR findings, and in a study of thirty-six subjects, mostly children, a finding in agreement with findings of previous and subsequent studies of auditory function in Rett syndrome (e.g., Hagberg, Aicardi, Dias, & Ramos, 1983; Lenn, Olsho, & Turk, 1986; Pillion & Naidu, 2000; Zoghbi et al., 1985). In contrast, some investigators describe abnormalities in the ABR (Pelson & Budden, 1987; Wu et al., 1988). In addition, Pillion, Rawool, and Naidu (2000) correlated abnormally prolonged latencies for all ABR waves in about 20 percent of a group of thirty-four female children with Rett's syndrome, with an especially high rate of abnormalities for wave III in children with moderate and severe hyperventilation. The authors state that "ABR abnormalities in RS can be expected, considering the finding of a decrease in volume of gray and white matter in RS" (p. 83).

TOURETTE'S SYNDROME. | Gilles de la Tourette's syndrome is an involuntary movement disorder with onset in childhood. Clinical manifestations are varied, but include motor tics, myoclonic or choreiform movements; it may also be associated with hyperactivity or learning disabilities. The cause appears to be organic, although different etiologies are likely. There may be a family history of tic disorders.

Krumholz et al. (1983) described normal ABR findings (latency and amplitude values for all major components) for seventeen patients (children and adults) with Tourette's syndrome. SSERs and VERs for the patient group also did not differ from those of control subjects.

COCKAYNE SYNDROME. | Cockayne syndrome is a rare autosomal recessive disease, first described in 1936, characterized by progressive neurologic dysfunction, microcephaly, growth retardation, and severe developmental delay. Signs and symptoms are highly variable and may include sensorineural hearing loss. Consanguinity is reported in some patient series.

In an investigation of twenty-five patients with Cockayne syndrome, Özdirim, Topey, Ozon, and Cila (1996) found sensorineural hearing loss by pure-tone audiometry in ten of fourteen patients who could be evaluated. The authors reported ABR abnormalities in three of eleven patients. Details on the ABR findings were, unfortunately, not described, but they were apparently consistent with sensorineural hearing loss.

GUILLAIN-BARRE SYNDROME AND MILLER FISHER SYNDROME. | Guillain-Barre syndrome is an acute, but uncommon, type of progressive peripheral neuropathy that often follows a viral infection. The exact cause is not known. Symptoms include first a sensation of tingling and then numbness, proceeding to weakness, areflexia, and sometimes

paralysis spreading from hands and feet to other regions of the body. Breathing may be affected in severe degrees of paralysis. These symptoms, and the disease, may be only temporary.

Miller Fisher syndrome, sometimes also referred to as simply Fisher's syndrome, was first described in 1956. Similar to, and considered a variant of, Guillain-Barre syndrome, *Miller Fisher syndrome* is characterized by a rapid onset of symptoms (as described above), general areflexia, and then resolution of symptoms (i.e., a good prognosis). Unlike Guillain-Barre syndrome, there is no limb weakness or early ataxia in Miller Fisher syndrome. Peripheral neuropathy in Guillain-Barre syndrome is associated with the diagnosis of auditory neuropathy, along with other demyelinating neuropathies, e.g., Charcot-Marie-Tooth disease.

Five of six patients with Guillain-Barre syndrome (without Miller Fisher variant) reported by Schiff, Cracco, and Cracco (1985) showed ABR abnormalities, mainly in the I-III latency interval. Ropper and Chiappa (1986) also noted abnormal ABR findings in three out of twenty-one patients. Wong (1997) described varied combinations of abnormal ABR findings in two children with Miller Fisher syndrome, including in one child or the other absence of waves (wave I unilaterally, wave III, and wave V), but then a resolution of the ABR abnormalities in one child. The author reported normal ABR recordings for two children with Guillain-Barre syndrome.

Minoda et al. (1999) describe audiologic and vestibular findings in fourteen patients with Fisher's syndrome, including several children age 11 years and older. Modest ABR abnormalities were found in four patients (e.g., delayed absolute and interwave latencies), but there was no consistent pattern for the abnormalities. The authors do not specify whether the abnormal ABR findings were in pediatric or adult subjects.

CEREBROVASCULAR DISEASES. | Cerebrovascular disease is largely a problem in adults. Rupture of an aneurysm under the age of 15 years is unusual, while 90 percent rupture between ages 30 and 70 years.

Minami, Kurokawa, Inoue, Takaki, and Goya (1984) described a correlation between ABR findings and clinical status in a 13-year-old child with primary brainstem hemorrhage. Often related to systemic hypertension (high blood pressure), primary brainstem hemorrhage usually features abrupt onset of coma and severe neurologic damage. Peak incidence is in the 40- to 50-year age region. Death often occurs due to respiratory arrest. These investigators found that the ABR interwave latencies were initially prolonged, but the abnormalities reversed as CT scanning showed resolution of the lesion and as the patient's clinical status improved.

MOYAMOYA DISEASE. | Moyamoya disease (MMD) is a rare and progressive cerebrovascular disorder characterized by bilateral occlusion of the carotid artery system, particularly the circle of Willis, the internal carotid arteries, and the anterior and middle cerebral arteries. Although rare, MMD mostly affects children, females more than males, sometimes in isolation, but often as a feature of another condition, e.g., Fanconi's anemia, congenital heart disease, Down syndrome, Noonan syndrome, neurofibromatosis, and other diseases.

Setzen and colleagues (1999) conducted a very comprehensive diagnostic audiologic assessment of two Caucasian children with MMD, a 3-year-old male Caucasian child and a 15-month-old male. For the older child, speech and language development was significantly delayed, prompting audiologic assessment with a battery of auditory procedures, including behavioral audiometry, aural immittance measures, TEOAEs, DPOAEs with input/output functions, ABR, and multiple-channel cortical auditory evoked responses (AMLR and ALR). The children also underwent neuroradiologic studies (CTMRI, and magnetic resonance angiography, or MRA), EEG. Peripheral auditory function was intact, and ABR findings were entirely normal. Cortical auditory dysfunction was, however, confirmed by the absence of the AMLR and ALR, a finding consistent with an abnormal behavioral response to sound.

DEGENERATIVE DISEASES

Charcot-Marie-Tooth Disease

BACKGROUND. | This is an inherited disease that involves degeneration of the myelin sheaths and axons of distal portions of peripheral nerves. Charcot-Marie-Tooth disease is strongly associated with the diagnosis of auditory neuropathy, as discussed in Chapter 5.

ABR FINDINGS. | By definition, the ABR is absent or grossly abnormal in auditory neuropathy secondary to Charcot-Marie-Tooth disease (see Chapter 5). Cassandro et al. (1986) and Campanella et al. (1984) reported grossly normal ABR and ALR findings in five patients with Charcot-Marie-Tooth disease. ABR abnormalities in a family with this disease were described by Satya-Murti, Cacace, and Hanson (1979). Yet, ABRs were essentially normal in five patients presented by Campanella et al. (1984).

Familial (Hereditary) Spastic Paraplegia

BACKGROUND. | This is one of the hereditary spinocerebellar degenerative diseases affecting corticospinal tracts and posterior columns.

AER FINDINGS. | An 11-year-old patient with familial spastic paraplegia reported by Campanella et al. (1984) and Cassandro et al. (1986) had a normal ABR.

Friedreich's Ataxia

BACKGROUND. | Friedreich's ataxia is classified as one of the spinocerebellar degenerative diseases. It has many clinical variants. Degeneration is found in dorsal root ganglia, dorsal roots, dorsal columns, spinocerebellar tracts, pyramidal tracts, and brainstem nuclei and tracts. Degeneration in the spiral ganglion (in the cochlea) causes auditory impairment. Signs and symptoms include gait disturbances, dysarthria, reflex abnormalities (areflexia), and sensation deficits. The diagnosis of Friedrich's ataxia is ultimately made is some children with auditory neuropathy, characterized by the absence of an ABR.

ABR FINDINGS. | Among the spinocerebellar degenerative diseases, ABRs and auditory function in general have been studied most extensively for Friedreich's ataxia. Satya-Murti, Cacace, and Hanson (1980) administered a comprehensive audiometric test battery (pure-tone audiometry, aural immittance measurements, simple and complex [synthetic sentence identification] speech audiometry) and ABR measurements to four patients with early onset progressive ataxia and two patients with late onset ataxia. Auditory deficits included bilateral sensorineural pure-tone hearing deficits, pronounced "rollover" on performance intensity functions for single syllable words, bilaterally depressed scores for synthetic sentence identification with an ipsilateral competing message (SSI-ICM), and markedly abnormal ABRs. There was no recognizable ABR in the four patients with early onset of disease, whereas the two patients with late onset ataxia both had unequivocally normal ABRs. The pattern of findings strongly suggested peripheral (eighth nerve) auditory dysfunction, presumably at the level of the spiral ganglion.

Hereditary Motor Sensory Neuropathy (Dejerine-Sottas Disease)

BACKGROUND. | This disease, identified by French physicians in 1893, is classified as a hereditary motor sensory neuropathy HMSN type III. Cranial nerves are involved. It is related pathophysiologically to olivopontocerebellar degeneration. Involvement of subcortical auditory pathways would not be predicted in this neuropathology. Hereditary motor sensory neuropathy is a disease closely associated with auditory neuropathy (see Chapter 5).

ABR FINDINGS. | Italian neurologists Baiocco, Testa, d'Angelo, and Cocchini (1984) presented ABR, pure-tone and speech audiometry for two patients with Dejerine-Sottas disease. The diagnosis was confirmed with nerve biopsies. Pure-tone and complex speech auditory measures were consistent with retrocochlear dysfunction. The ABR was markedly abnormal with wave I–V latency values of greater than 5.5 msec and absence of wave III. Rossini and Cracco (1987) studied the ABR in three patients with HMSN type I, three with HMSN type II, and one patient with HSMN type III.

Only one of the patients with HMSN type III had abnormal ABR findings (markedly increased wave I–V latencies). Likewise, Satya-Murti et al. (1979) found ABR abnormalities, including prolongation of the wave I–III latency interval and poor morphology or absence of wave V, in two patients with hereditary motor sensory neuropathy type II. Behavioral audiometry confirmed normal peripheral auditory status, however, for meaningful clinical interpretation of ABR, it is important to keep in mind that eighth-nerve involvement and related serious hearing deficit may be a feature of this disease. Stockard, Stockard, and Sharbrough (1986) provide further evidence of ABR wave I–V latency prolongations in HMSN. In some cases, the delay was between wave I and II, indicating eighth-nerve dysfunction and consistent with polyneuropathy (multiple peripheral nerve lesions), that is, auditory neuropathy. Intrinsic brainstem dysfunction as evidenced by wave III to V latency increases was documented in other cases. Also, Garg, Markand, and Bustion (1982) found prolongation of the ABR wave I–III latency interval (greater than 3 standard deviations above normal mean value) in three patients with hereditary motor sensory neuropathy type I. This latency prolongation was largely due to an increase in the interval between wave I and II. Later latency intervals were normal. These findings imply eighth-nerve dysfunction, perhaps related to deficient Schwann cell myelin.

Sclerosing Panencephalitis

BACKGROUND. | Subacute sclerosing panencephalitis is a progressive neurological disease caused by a persistent measle virus infection that is characterized by long asymptomatic periods. Eventually, when it reaches the acute stage, subacute sclerosing panencephalitis leads to death, usually within one year. CNS structures affected include the cerebral hemispheres and subcortical regions (brainstem, cerebellum, spinal cord).

ABR FINDINGS. | Inagaki and Japanese colleagues (1999) made a total of 98 ABR recordings from 17 children with subacute sclerosing panencephalitis. The children were exposed to measles early (average age of 1.8 years), with the onset of disease occurring on the average at 8.8 years. Consistent with other investigators (e.g., Hecox, Cone, & Blaw, 1981; Miyao et al., 1983), Inagaki and colleagues (1999) found multiple ABR abnormalities, including elevation in the thresholds for wave V, delayed absolute latencies for waves I, III, and V, and delays also in the wave I–V latency interval. ABR abnormalities were detected within one to two years after the onset of the disease and steadily worsened in a rostral-to-caudal direction as the disease progressed in stages.

NEURODEVELOPMENTAL DISORDERS

Perinatal diseases are associated with some of the well-established risk factors for auditory impairment (e.g., hyper-bilirubenia, asphyxia, perinatal infections, meningitis). Most of the risk factors for infant hearing loss were reviewed earlier in the discussion of newborn hearing screening. Congenital CNS malformations are abnormally formed organs present from birth that are produced by an inborn (genetic) error in morphogenesis or environmental problems during the formation of the structure. They include dysraphism or neural tube defects (anencephaly, cranium bifidum, spina bifida with meningocele, meningomyelocele, myelocystocele), aqueductal malformations, failure of cleavage (Arnold-Chiari malformations, Dandy-Walker syndrome), disorders of size (megalencephaly, microencephaly), disorders of commiseration, anoxic-ischemic lesions, and hydrocephalus.

Diseases that usually affect children after the perinatal period (generally after the chronologic age of 3 months) and may also affect adults, such as tumors, leukodystrophies, and trauma, are described in other sections of this chapter. Storage diseases affecting children (e.g., Tay-Sachs, Gaucher's, Fabry's, Refsum's, and Hurler's diseases) are discussed elsewhere in the section (see section on "Metabolic Diseases").

Hydrocephalus

BACKGROUND. | Hydrocephalus is by definition an excessive amount of cerebrospinal fluid (CSF) in the ventricular system. Congenital hydrocephalus has an incidence of approximately 1:1000 live births, and is the main pathophysiology in these infants. These may be secondary to a malformation syndrome (e.g., Arnold-Chiari or Dandy-Walker malformation) or, less often, an intracranial tumor. In older patients, the hydrocephalus is usually a feature of another disease (e.g., alcoholic cerebral atrophy, posttrauma). The major mechanisms leading to hydrocephalus are (1) blockage of CSF circulation in the ventricles and subarachnoid space (occurring at various sites, including foramina of Monro, the third ventricle, the aqueduct of Sylvius, the fourth ventricle), (2) excessive production of CSF (an uncommon cause due to choroid plexus papilloma), and (3) hemodynamic disruption of the venous pulse wave (in which the normal pulsating increase in arterial pressure is not damped by the venous system and is, instead, transmitted to the ventricular system with subsequent ventricular enlargement over time). Mortality of hydrocephalus can be as high as 50 percent without treatment. A shunt operative procedure is the treatment of choice. CSF is routed from the ventricular system to another bodily space, such as the peritoneal space.

ABR FINDINGS. | Since 1980, clinical reports have occasionally appeared describing ABR findings in pediatric hydrocephalus (Edwards, Durieux-Smith, & Picton, 1985; Hall, 1992; Hall, Tucker, Fletcher, & Habersang, 1988; Kraus et al., 1984; Venkataramana, Satishchandra, Hegde, Reddy, & Das, 1988). Intracranial pressure increases associated with hydrocephalus clearly can disrupt rostral brainstem function and prolong latencies of ABR wave V, and sometimes III. In severe cases of hydrocephalus, the ABR may be absent (Hall, 1992). Reversal of ABR abnormalities, however, can follow treatment of hydrocephalus with a CSF shunt (Hall, 1992).

Kraus et al. (1984) recorded ABRs from forty patients (80 ears) with medically confirmed hydrocephalus. All but two of the patients were children, and twenty-nine were less than 3 years of age. Among the group, 88 percent showed some evidence of ABR abnormalities. The percentages of abnormal findings were distributed as follows: wave I–V latency delay, 38 percent; decreased wave V/I amplitude ratio, 33 percent; wave III latency delay, 27 percent; wave V latency delay, 53 percent. Wave I latency was normal for all of the patients. Important clinical findings were absence of any detectable response for 25 percent of the series and evidence of a peripheral auditory sensitivity deficit (ABR threshold greater than 20 dB HL) for 70 percent. The proportion of wave I–V abnormality in hydrocephalus (33%) was higher than the figure reported by these authors for 100 multiply handicapped children (23%) or 60 with meningitis (10%). Evidence of peripheral auditory deficits was also more commonly found in hydrocephalus. This is supported by audiometric data for forty-seven hydrocephalic children (multiple etiologies) recently reported by Lopponen, Sorri, Serlo, and von Wendt (1989). A high-frequency sensorineural loss was found in 38 percent (18/47) of the children. The loss did not differ among etiologic groups. Kraus et al. (1984) present a thoughtful discussion of the pathophysiology of hydrocephalus in relation to the reported ABR patterns. ABR is a valuable technique for estimating peripheral hearing status in hydrocephalus, since these children are often too ill or too young to be tested behaviorally. This raises an important clinical point. Estimation of peripheral function with ABR wave V data in hydrocephalus must be done very cautiously, since CNS pathology may also produce marked ABR abnormalities.

Sood and Mahapatra (1991) reported abnormal baseline (pretreatment) ABR findings (delayed interwave latencies) for the majority of patients (N = 30) with hydrocephalus secondary to brain tumors, including abnormalities in 80 percent with cerebellar tumor, 70 percent with third ventricle tumor, and 100 percent of patients with brainstem tumor. Following a CSF shunt procedure, the ABR was improved in 70 percent of the patients with brainstem tumor and 40 percent of ventricular tumor group. In several patients, only an ABR wave I was present before the shunt procedure, whereas a normal ABR appeared post-shunt procedure. However, deterioration of the ABR was found for a smaller proportion of the cerebellar and brainstem tumor group following the shunt procedure, and the ABR was unchanged after the shunt procedure for all of the patients with cerebellar tumors.

Myelomeningocele and Arnold-Chiari Malformation

BACKGROUND. | Myelomeningocele is a complex neuropathy that presumably has multiple etiologies. Approximately

1 in 1,000 infants are born with myelomeningocele. There are probably genetic factors that increase risk. The role of dietary and environment factors (e.g., maternal medications) in affecting the risk of myelomeningocele has also received attention. The embryologic basis of the disease appears to involve both incomplete closure of the neural tube and rupture of an already closed neural tube. In myelomeningocele, the anatomic deformity is a sac on the infant's back that encloses cerebral spinal fluid and misplaced neural tissue and spaces, including spinal cord, arachnoid space, dorsal and ventral nerve roots, dura mater, epidural space. There are numerous texts providing details on the surgical management of myelomeningocele (to close the dysraphic defect). Possible sequelae of myelomeningocele are hydrocephalus, mental retardation (usually secondary to CNS infection), learning disabilities, problems with bladder and bowel control, and difficulties ambulating (moving about).

Arnold-Chiari malformation type II is a common feature of myelomeningocele. It develops within the first three months after birth in about two-thirds of patients, but may also appear in childhood or adolescence. In Arnold-Chiari malformation type II, there is a displacement of the caudal brainstem and cerebellum through the foramen magnum and an elongation of the fourth ventricle into the cervical canal. Some cranial nerves are stretched and deformed as the brainstem moves downward. Other anatomic defects, such as aqueductal stenosis, "beaking" of the quadrigeminal plate, cervicomedullary kinking, extension of cerebellar tissue over the cervical spinal cord, arachnoid bands in the superior cervical region, and abnormal brainstem nuclei (including specifically pons and collicular regions), are also found in the majority of patients. There is no consensus on the preferred surgical management of Arnold-Chiari malformation type II.

ABR FINDINGS. | There are a handful of papers specifically describing ABR findings in Arnold-Chiari malformation (Hall, Browns, Mackey-Hargadine, 1985a; Holliday, Pillsbury, Kelly, & Dillard, 1985; Lutschg, Meyer, Jeanneret-Iseli, & Kaiser, 1985; Mori, Uchida, Nishimura, & Eghwrudjakpor, 1988). Lutschg et al. (1985) described ABR findings for twenty-seven children (aged 4 to 15 years) with myelomeningocele and Arnold-Chiari malformation type II. Clinical symptoms included cranial nerve deficits (stridor, fasciculation of the tongue, paretic strabism), and cerebellar signs. Among this series was a group of seventeen children with hydrocephalus that had been managed with a shunt procedure and ten children with no clinical signs of increased ICP who were, therefore, not shunted. ABR wave I latency was equivalent among normal subjects and patient groups. There were statistically significant increases in wave V latency and the wave I–V latency interval between the following pairs of groups: normal subjects versus the entire myelomeningocele group; myelomeningocele patients without versus with hydrocephalus; myelomeningocele without versus with cranial nerve deficits. ABR interwave latency values were greatest for the patient group with hydrocephalus and cranial nerve deficits, and shortest for the group with myelomeningocele but neither hydrocephalus nor cranial nerve deficits. The authors propose several hypotheses for the increased interwave ABR latencies. In addition to compression of brainstem structures as they are displaced into the foramen magnum the possible effect on auditory function, it is plausible that elongation of the brainstem (which is a component of this mechanism) of approximately 0.5 cm would increase the auditory pathways and produce a delay in the ABR wave I–V interval by 1 to 2 ms.

Holliday, Pillsbury, Kelly, and Dillard (1985) described ABR findings for a series of twelve infants with myelomeningocele and eight with Arnold Chiari malformation type II and present in detail a case report. ABRs were abnormal (interwave latency delay) in eight patients and normal in four. All four infants with myelomeningocele but without Arnold-Chiari malformation showed the age-corrected normal ABRs. Myelomeningoceles in these patients were located in the lumbar or lumbosacral region (below the thoracic level). Two were shunted and two were not. Five children with Arnold-Chiari malformation II but with no clinical symptoms (of posterior fossa or cervical spinal cord neurologic dysfunction) had abnormal ABRs. For all but one, the dysraphic defect affected the spinal cord in the thoracic region. Three infants with symptomatic Arnold-Chiari II malformation showed abnormal ABRs. Interestingly, one had the defect only in the lumbosacral region. These authors also presented group data and a case report confirming that initially abnormal interwave latencies could be reversed and brought within a clinically normal range (age-matched mean plus 2.5 standard deviations) by surgical decompression of bony and fibrous material. Ear differences were noted, emphasizing the importance of separate stimulation if each ear in clinical recordings.

Autism

BACKGROUND. | Autism is a neurodevelopmental disorder affecting verbal and nonverbal communication and a child's inability to develop normal relationships with other persons, even parents. This characteristic feature of autism may be present from birth, or the ability to develop social relationships may regress within the first few years of life. In addition, traits of autistic children include stereotyped behavior (e.g., rituals involving objects or repetitive movements), severe impairment of speech acquisition and communication, absence of smiling and facial expression, inappropriate reactions to different situations and events, unpredictable behavior (ranging from violence to motionlessness), unawareness of dangers, strange postures and mannerisms, and abnormal responses to sensory stimulation. The estimated prevalence of autism is 2 to 5 children per 10,000, with a boy:girl ratio of about 4:1. The precise etiology of autism remains a mys-

tery, but neurochemical, neurobiologic, and genetic factors are all suspected. Autism may occur or co-exist with other neurodevelopmental disorders, such as fragile X syndrome, seizure disorders, phenylketonuria, neurofibromatosis, and tuberous sclerosis. AER assessment may be indicated because hearing impairment is suspected due to unresponsiveness to sounds and heightened responsiveness or attention to light sources. Toilet training and feeding are difficult. The literature on autism spectrum disorders is rapidly increasing, including auditory evoked responses studies of potential neurobiological markers. The ABR is an important diagnostic tool in autism because behavioral audiometry is often not feasible for young children or those who do not cooperate due to their abnormal behavioral traits.

ABR FINDINGS. | Dating back to the early years of ABR clinical application, a number of investigators have described ABR findings in autism (Courchesne, Lincoln, Kilman, & Galambos, 1985; Coutinho, Rocha, & Santos, 2002; Gillberg, Rosenhall, & Johansson, 1983; Grillon, Courchesne, & Akshoomoff, 1989; Harris, Broms, & Mollerstrom, 1981; Klin, 1993; McClelland et al., 1992; Rosenhall, Nordin, Brantberg, & Gillberg, 2003; Skoff, Mirksy, & Turner, 1980; Sohmer & Student, 1978; Tanguay et al., 1982; Taylor, Rosenblatt, & Linschoten, 1982; Thivierge, Bedard, Cote, & Maziade, 1990; Wong & Wong, 1991). Collectively, the literature on ABR and autism is confusing, with some investigators reporting consistently normal ABR findings, or even shorter than normal latencies (e.g., Courchesne et al., 1985; Rumsey et al., 1984), but the majority of authors describing various types of ABR abnormality in at least some autistic children. A variety of factors probably contribute to the inconsistencies among studies, including differences in ABR test protocols, peripheral hearing status, the possibility of other co-existing disorders, inadequate numbers of subjects (often case reports), and analysis of ABR data without data from an age- and gender-matched control group. Sohmer and Student (1978) described ABR findings for thirteen children (aged 4 to 12 years) with the diagnosis of autism. There was no detectable ABR at maximum stimulus intensity levels for four children with autistic traits, which the authors presumed was due to profound cochlear loss. The remaining nine autistic children showed normal ABR threshold levels, but increased interwave latency values were reported for an unspecified portion of these children. The authors acknowledged considerable overlap among normal and patient groups in ABR findings. However, they conclude that the ABR abnormalities in some of the autistic children are evidence of functional (and perhaps structural) deficits in this population.

Harris, Broms, and Mollerstrom (1981) recorded ABRs from two subjects with autism as well as a larger group of mentally retarded children, but did delineate their findings. Tanguay et al. (1982) found a high proportion of ABR abnormalities in sixteen children (ranging in age from 33 to 169 months) with the diagnosis of early infantile autism, based on criteria recommended by the American Psychiatric Association (1980) published *Diagnostic and Statistical Manual of Mental Disorders (DSM III)*. All of the infants reportedly passes an audiometric screening. It is important to point out that testing was carried out with the patients aware or sleeping naturally (no sedation was used) and the authors indicated that 29 percent of the subjects were moving during the test and more than one test session was necessary in a number of cases. Three showed marked prolongations of wave I latency (presumable indicating a peripheral deficit) and in eight ABR interwave latency values were greater than 3 standard deviations above the mean for a control group. Group data comparison (with gender matched), however, revealed no statistically significant difference in ABR interwave latency parameters. In general, alterations in stimulus latency and rate failed to produce any ABR differences for autistic as compared to control groups. Harris, Broms, and Mollerstrom (1981) conclude that some autistic children show increased "brainstem transmission time," that abnormal ABR findings are not necessarily symmetrical but may be unilateral, and that wave I latency delay in autistic children signifies a peripheral auditory processing deficit. They do not explain how this latter finding can occur in children who have passed an auditory screening. This paper presents a rather detailed discussion of the nature of autism and speculation on possible mechanisms for the ABR results.

Taylor, Rosenblatt, and Linschoten (1982) recorded ABRs from thirty-two children with autism, as defined by criteria recommended in 1977 by the National Society for Autistic Children. Sedation was used for ABR assessment because the authors indicated that without sedation, the children were uncooperative, and excessive muscular artifact precluded reliable recordings. Eleven of the thirty-two children had abnormally elevated ABR threshold levels consistent with a moderate (40 to 60 dB HL) hearing impairment (three unilateral and eight bilateral), while another three subjects showed evidence of a severe-to-profound hearing impairment (thresholds of 70 dB HL or greater). Among autistic subjects with a detectable wave I, there were significant prolongations in the interwave latency values (wave I–III and I–V, but not wave III–V) when compared to data from the control group. Children were subdivided into those with accompanying neurologic pathologies (e.g., perinatal encephalopathy, microcrania) versus those without secondary pathology. ABR findings were comparable for the two groups. The authors conclude that 44 percent of this population had a significant peripheral hearing impairment, at least unilaterally.

Courchesne, Lincoln, Kilman, and Galambos (1985) conducted a systematic study of ABR in fourteen autistic subjects. There were several remarkable methodologic strengths of the study. Data for autistic patients were compared to those for an age- and gender-matched control group. Subjects were carefully selected to exclude those with "sec-

ondary and tertiary" pathologies (e.g., mental retardation or other handicaps) but include only those who were sufficiently cooperative to participate in measurement of ABR and also later latency ERPs. Only high-functioning autistic subjects were enrolled in the study. Finally, body temperature of subjects was taken into account as an important factor in AER interpretation. All autistic subjects in the study by Courchesne et al. (1985) had normal-appearing ABRs when data were analyzed in relation to the control group, even with manipulation of measurement parameters (rate of stimulation, stimulus intensity, and click polarity). There were no statistically significant latency differences between groups nor clinically abnormal ABR latency values for any of the individual subjects. The authors conclude that the etiology of autism does not include dysfunction in the part of the auditory brainstem underlying the ABR. Other possible sites of dysfunction elsewhere in the brainstem, or certainly the CNS, cannot be ruled out by the findings of this study. In reconciling these normal findings with previously reported ABR abnormalities (Gillberg et al., 1983; Sohmer & Student, 1978; Tanguay et al., 1982; Taylor et al., 1982), the authors cite the possible influence of secondary pathologies or lesions in anatomic regions near the ABR generators (e.g., in extralemniscal pathways), which, in some patients, extend into the generators. Also, the present study was limited to high-functioning subjects, whereas different ABR findings might be more characteristic of lower functioning autistic children.

Grillon, Courchesne, and Akshoomoff (1989) published in the *Journal of Autism and Development Disorders* a study of ABR and AMLR in eight nonretarded subjects with infantile autism (average age 23 years), eight subjects with receptive developmental language disorder (mean age 16 years), and a normal control group. No differences were found between groups for ABR or AMLR. Other studies of ABR in autism were reported by Gillberg et al. (1983) and Skoff et al. (1980). Differences among ABR studies of autism are probably due, in part at least, to variable definitions of autism and subject characteristics (e.g., age, gender), the rather limited numbers of subjects, and inadequate subject cooperation.

In the most comprehensive investigation of the ABR in autism, Rosenhall and colleagues (2003) collected data over a twelve-year period from a series of 101 children and adolescents selected from among 153 on the basis of normal hearing sensitivity. The diagnosis of autism was agreed upon by two experts according to DSM-III-R criteria. ABR data for the children with autism were compared to data for an age-matched control group. Analysis of group data confirmed significant prolongation of absolute latencies for wave I and V, and the wave III to V interwave latency, in the autistic children in comparison to the control group. ABR latency and amplitude parameters were not correlated with mental development (IQ scores). Among 101 patients, 58.4 percent had some type of ABR abnormality, with prolongations of absolute latencies (waves I, III, and V) in one-half of the group (50.5%), and abnormal interwave latency values (typically wave I–V) in just over one-third of the subjects (36.6%). Rosenhall et al. (2003) conclude that "ABR abnormalities are common in young people with autism" (p. 211). The authors also provide a thoughtful discussion of the possible relationship between the ABR findings and current theories on risk factors, neuroanatomic anomalies, and neurobiological impairment in autism.

Cornelia de Lange Syndrome

BACKGROUND. | Of unknown etiology, Cornelia de Lange syndrome is named after the physician who first described several cases of patients whom she had evaluated with the following characteristics: distinctive facial features (excessive hair and long curly eyelashes), characteristic appearance of the hands and feet (e.g., syndactyly), cleft palate, and severe mental retardation.

ABR FINDINGS. | Kaga, Tami, Kitazumi, and Kodama (1995) described in detail audiologic findings, including ABR results, for ten children with Cornelia de Lange syndrome. Severe bilateral hearing loss was confirmed by ABR for four of the ten patients, and some degree of hearing impairment was documented in eight of the ten (80%). Two patients had a unilateral hearing loss, and another two patients had a mild bilateral hearing loss. Importantly, ABR findings were essential for accurate definition of hearing status as behavioral audiometry was consistent with severe hearing impairment for all of the children.

Mental Retardation (MR)

BACKGROUND. | Mental retardation is found in about 780,000 children of school age. In persons with mental retardation, general intellectual functioning is significantly below average. Classification ranges from mild (Wechsler IQ score of 55 to 69) to profound (Wechsler IQ score of 24 or less). Mild mental retardation is the most common form. It is apparently not a result of catastrophic problems during pregnancy or during birth but, rather, to social and environmental factors. It is associated with a variety of such factors, including lifestyle of the mother, cigarette smoking, alcohol and drug abuse, and poor nutrition during pregnancy. These maternal characteristics are also related to premature birth and reduced intrauterine growth. In contrast to mild or moderate mental retardation, severe mental retardation usually has a distinct etiology (genetic, biochemical, viral, or developmental causes) but, like mild retardation, is usually not due to medical problems occurring at birth. It is associated with physical handicaps and multiple neurologic signs. Even though approximately 3 percent of children born are mentally retarded, 90 percent of these are only mildly impaired. Some of the prenatal causes of mental retardation are inherited, such as malformation of the CNS, chromosomal abnormali-

ties, and familial retardation. Some prenatal causes are metabolic, including phenylketonuria, cretinism, and cystinuria. Some are acquired, such as maternal disease and intrauterine exposure to infection or drugs. Perinatal etiologies include prematurity, hypoxic-ischemic events during delivery, intracranial hemorrhage, metabolic encephalopathy, and toxemia of pregnancy. In as many as 40 percent of mentally retarded persons, there is no clear etiology. Neuroanatomic correlates of mental retardation include whole brain weight that is 76 percent of normal and brainstem/cerebellum weight 66 percent of normal.

Hearing deficits detected by behavioral and impedance audiometry are not uncommon in children with mental retardation. Exact figures on the proportion of MR children with serious hearing loss vary considerably among studies, in part because of difficulties in consistently obtaining valid behavioral audiometric data in this population and in part because of differences in hearing status of institutionalized versus noninstitutionalized children (Balkany, Downs, Jafek, & Krajicek, 1979; Fulton & Lloyd, 1968; Lloyd & Reid, 1967; Schwartz & Schwartz, 1978; Squires, Ollo, & Jordan, 1986). The greatest proportion (from about 20 to 40%) of hearing deficits, in Down syndrome children at least, are conductive (often secondary to otitis media), but high-frequency sensorineural hearing loss is a characteristic finding (occurring in from 10 to 20% of MR children). Hearing loss is generally more common among the institutionalized mentally retarded. Squires, Ollo, and Jordan (1986) reported that the incidence of serious hearing deficit was 73 percent in young adults with Down syndrome as opposed to only 22 percent in non-Down retarded young adults. The differential effect of Down versus non-Down syndrome mental retardation sensorineural hearing deficits on ABR outcome is reviewed below.

ABR FINDINGS. | Sohmer and Student (1978), in a study of ABR in ten children (ages 2 to 8 years) with "psychomotor retardation," found interwave latency values that were, on the average, statistically greater than those for a control group. For some patients, there was no apparent wave V component, which the authors present as evidence of structural CNS damage. The study also included children with autism and children with minimal brain damage. This latter group showed the most abnormal ABRs.

Harris, Broms, and Mollerstrom (1981) recorded ABRs from eleven institutional mentally retarded subjects ranging in age from 3 to 23 years. Subjects were described as "psychomotorically" retarded, and hearing loss was suspected in all. Testing was done under general anesthesia. Notably, in five patients with suspected or questionable hearing impairment on the basis of behavioral testing, the ABR was interpreted by the authors as consistent with normal peripheral auditory function and hearing aid use was discontinued. ECochG was employed in selected cases. In at least one patient with no detectable ABR, an ECochG response was observed.

Folsom, Widen, and Wilson (1983) recorded ABRs from thirty-eight infants with Down syndrome at the age of 3, 6, and 12 months and compared the findings to data for a group of thirty-five normally developing age-matched infants. Morphology was comparable for all subjects. The main observation was a decrease in wave III and V latencies, especially at higher intensity levels, and a steeper latency–intensity function in older subjects (12 months of age) in the group with Down syndrome. The authors concluded that latency–intensity curves derived from normally developing infants are inadequate as normative data for clinical interpretation of ABR findings in Down syndrome patients. Because of the unusually short latency values in the older Down syndrome children, the authors suggest that ABR might underestimate hearing impairment and lead to false-negative interpretation (presuming less hearing impairment than the child actually has). They further suggested that these ABR latency differences between normal and Down syndrome children might be a reflection of high-frequency sensorineural hearing loss, citing previously reported evidence of abnormally rapid decrease in latency for ABR wave with increased stimulus intensity in high-frequency cochlear impairment (Coats, 1978; Yamada, Kodera, & Yagi, 1979).

Maurizi, Ottavani, Paludetti, and Lungarotti (1985) studied twenty-nine children (aged 1 month through 16 years) with Down syndrome with ABR. Pure-tone audiometry, impedance (immittance) audiometry, and otologic examination were also carried out whenever possible. Middle ear pathology was a common finding. Electrophysiologic assessment techniques were extremely useful, as fewer than 30 percent of the children yielded reliable behavioral audiometric findings. ABR thresholds and morphology were described as normal in sixteen of the twenty-nine patients (55%). The authors concluded that ABR is the assessment technique of choice in the uncooperative child, although they acknowledge the difficulty in differentiating normal hearing sensitivity versus mild (low-frequency) conductive hearing impairment.

Kaga and Marsh (1986) used ABR to assess auditory function of thirty-seven Japanese infants and children with Down syndrome who were suspected of having hearing deficits. Behavioral audiometry was also done. Twelve children showed no response by behavioral testing and ABR. ABR findings were varied, including wave I latency prolongation (thirteen patients), wave V latency prolongation (five patients), shorter wave I latency value (two patients), and shorter wave V latency value (seven patients). Notably, there were no cases of prolonged wave I to V latency intervals. This population of children with Down syndrome showed a high incidence of middle and inner ear dysfunction.

In a study of twenty-four institutionalized severe-to-profoundly mentally retarded persons, Sikorski and Ruth (1982) found that for one-half of the group there was a serious discrepancy between conventional (behavioral and immittance) audiometry and ABR. In some cases, ABR findings suggested better hearing function than the conventional testing, but in other cases the ABR estimated greater hearing impairment. The authors cite their findings as evidence that ABR should be a part of the audiometric test battery in mentally retarded populations.

A total of 122 profoundly retarded and institutionalized children ranging in age from 7 months to 18 years were studied by Stein, Kraus, Özdamar, Cartee, Jabaley, Jeantet, and Reed (1987). Approximately one-third (32%) of this series of patients showed ABR evidence of hearing impairment and, among these, sensory deficits were more frequent than conductive deficits (20% versus 12% respectively). An additional 11 percent of the children had ABR patterns consistent with neurologic deficit. Notably, only three children in this institutionalized group had Down syndrome. One had a conductive hearing loss and none showed unusually short ABR wave I–V latencies.

Kavanagh, Gould, McCormick, and Franks (1989) reported ABR and AMLR data for forty-eight subjects with "mental handicaps," among them seven with Down syndrome. The average age of subjects was 8.5 years, with a range of 8 months to 32 years. Sedation was required for all subjects, regardless of age, because of mental handicap and, presumably, uncooperative behavior. The main purpose of the study was to compare detectability of ABR versus AMLR for low-intensity stimuli. Data were not analyzed separately for patients with Down syndrome. The authors concluded that ABR had lower test-retest variability and is, in most cases, more identifiable near threshold than AMLR. Still, among twenty-five patients with hearing loss, there were four who showed reliable AMLRs in the absence of ABRs. Recording ABR with wide filter settings was strongly recommended to increase identifiability and threshold detection with ABR.

Landau and Kleffner Syndrome

BACKGROUND. | First described in 1957, Landau and Kleffner syndrome is an acquired aphasia, a rare form of epilepsy, with an onset usually between the ages of 3 and 8 years. Normal-functioning children with Landau and Kleffner syndrome show a progressive decline in neurocognitive development. Communication disorder is one of the most common and noticeable features, especially very poor auditory comprehension (speech understanding).

ABR FINDINGS. | Koeda and Kohno (1992) describe a case report of Landau and Kleffner syndrome. The patient was an 8-year-old girl who had nonverbal agnosis, convulsions, and diffuse EEG abnormalities. ABR findings were reported as normal. Wioland, Rudolf, and Metz-Lutz (2001) conducted thorough auditory evoked response recordings in five children with Landau and Kleffner syndrome. The ABR and AMLR were normal in each of the subjects, whereas some abnormalities were found for the N1c component of the ALR.

Cerebral Palsy (CP)

BACKGROUND. | Cerebral palsy is associated with prematurity, retarded growth, and asphyxia (e.g., an Apgar score of less than 3 at 10 to 15 minutes) at birth. The most common specific causes of cerebral palsy are cerebral anoxic–hypoxic events occurring in the perinatal period, either in utero, at delivery, or immediately following birth. It is important to realize, however, that most children with these risk factors do not have subsequent evidence of cerebral palsy, and, conversely, over three-fourths of children with cerebral palsy have had none of the risk factors. Therefore, in children with cerebral palsy, as well as mental retardation, a distinct etiology often cannot be documented. Other causes are viral infections in utero and neonatal meningitis. Cerebral palsy is characterized by nonprogressive but varied neurologic deficits, including cerebellar ataxia, athetosis and spasticity (di- or hemiplegia), and sometimes associated neurologic disorders (epilepsy and mental retardation). Incidence of cerebral palsy is estimated at 0.5 percent, of which approximately one out of ten is severely handicapped. Speech disorders are found in the majority (about 60%) of persons with cerebral palsy and approximately 30 percent have seizure disorders.

ABR FINDINGS. | Since cerebral palsy is a motor disease, normal findings would be expected for sensory responses, such as AERs. Nonetheless, AERs may be requested for children with cerebral palsy because of the high incidence of speech problems in the population. Conversely, children identified as infants with auditory neuropathy upon referral for neurodevelopmental assessment sometimes are diagnosed with CP. AERs can be useful in ruling out peripheral hearing deficit. Movement and related muscle artifact may make AER assessment in cerebral palsy somewhat difficult.

Auditory Processing Disorders (APD) and Learning Disorders (Disabilities)

BACKGROUND. | A learning disability by definition (e.g., according to Public Law 94–142) is not mental retardation or limited intellectual capacity. Characteristics of children with learning disabilities are varied and may include developmental dyslexia (the most common), writing disorders, and/or problems with arithmetic calculations. Mild (sometimes referred to as "soft") neurologic signs may also be observed in children with learning disabilities. Often, poor academic performance in grade school is the first indication of a learning disability. The largest proportion of learning-disabled children (accounting for from 40 to 60% of such children) are school-age children with language difficulties, including language comprehension and expression, word-finding deficits, and impaired speech discrimination. Failure to properly recognize a learning disability may lead to the erroneous assumption that a child is mildly mentally retarded or emotionally disturbed. Learning disabilities are thought by many to be secondary to CNS dysfunction. Consequently, a collection of terms is sometimes used to describe children with learning disabilities, such as agnosia, apraxia, childhood or developmental aphasia, minimal brain dysfunction, or injury. There is, in turn, considerable confusion among educational and medical professionals in evaluating and describing children with learning disabilities.

ABR FINDINGS. | Mason and Mellor (1984) compared AER findings for eight children with severe language disorders and six with severe motor speech disorders. Data were also collected for an age-matched normal control group. ABR latency was equivalent among groups, although amplitude was smaller for all wave components. AMLR and ALR latency values were also comparable among groups.

In the study of autistic persons noted above, Grillon, Courchesne, and Akshoomoff (1989) also recorded ABR and AMLR from eight subjects (mean age of 16 years) with "receptive developmental language disorder" (RDLD). There was no significant difference between an RDLD group and an age-matched control group for ABR or AMLR. Previously, Courchesne, Grillon and colleagues (Courchesne et al., 1989) reported endogenous ERP findings in these same RDLD patients, as well as an autistic group. The P3b component was unusually large in the RDLD group and smaller than normal in the autistic group. On a similar theme, Kraus, Smith, Reed, Stein, and Cartee (1985) likewise found no difference in the detectability of AMLR Na and Pa components among groups of normal, learning-disabled, and mentally handicapped patients.

For over twenty-five years, auditory evoked responses have been applied in children for objective evaluation of *auditory processing disorders (APDs)* (Jerger & Jerger, 1985; Musiek, Gollegly, Kibbe, & Verkest, 1988). Auditory evoked response assessment, particularly of AMLR, ALR, and the P300 response, is now being applied in evaluation of this poorly defined population. Preliminary evidence suggests that AER findings, including computed evoked response topography, may complement diagnostic speech audiometry and other central auditory procedures in evaluation of APD (Jerger, 1987; Jerger, Jerger, & Loiselle, 1989).

Among the auditory evoked responses, the ABR is most likely to be normal in children with APD. Hall (1992) described case reports of children with APD and normal ABR findings. Hall & Mueller (1997) report findings for the ABR, AMLR, and P300 in a series of over 200 children evaluated for APD at a diagnostic audiology center. Fewer than 10 percent showed ABR abnormalities, whereas the majority of the children had abnormal findings for the cortical auditory evoked responses (AMLR and P300). Abnormal ABR findings consisted of modest delays in interwave latencies.

Attention-Deficit/Hyperactivity Disorder (ADHD)

BACKGROUND. | There is a large and rapidly growing literature on attention-deficit/hyperactivity disorder (ADHD).

Three types of ADHD are recognized: (a) attention deficit with hyperactivity, (b) an inattentive type of attention deficit (without hyperactivity), and (c) a mixed type consisting of features of the other two types. One criterion for the diagnosis of ADHD is the onset of symptoms before the age of 8 years. There is a strong male predominance for ADHD. Core features of ADHD include developmentally inappropriate levels of attention (i.e., attention is not as expected for the child's age), concentration, activity, distractability, and impulsivity. ADHD often co-exists with other disorders, such as auditory processing disorder (APD), conduct disorder, and other behavioral conditions. Treatment includes behavioral modification and medication with CNS stimulant drugs (e.g., Ritalin, Concerta, Adderall).

ABR FINDINGS. | Puente and Mexican colleagues (2002) recorded the ABR, and the auditory late response, in eighteen children, sixteen boys and one girl aged 6 to 10 years (mean age of 9 years) diagnosed with ADD and a control group of twenty subjects (college-age young adults), 10 male and 10 female, with a mean age of 22 years. Latencies for ABR wave III and wave V, and for the wave I–III and I–V latency intervals, were significantly delayed for the group of children with ADD when compared with the control group. Latency of the P300 response was also delayed for the children with ADD. Close inspection of the data for this study revealed average ABR latency values for the children with ADD that were consistent with normal expectations. For example, the average wave V latency was 5.70 ms (standard deviation of 0.19 ms), and the I to wave V latency interval was 4.14 ms (standard deviation of 0.13 ms). Even ADD subjects at 2 standard deviations from the mean value for the group had a wave I to V latency interval (4.40 ms) well within clinical normal limits (see normative ABR data in the appendix). The explanation for the statistically significant prolongation of ABR latencies in the ADD group may be related to gender. Males and females were equally distributed in the normal group, and the average age was 22 years, whereas sixteen out of seventeen of the children with ADD were male and the average age for the children was 9 years. Confidence in the interpretation of the ABR data for the ADD group would be enhanced by the inclusion of a control group matched with the ADD group for age and gender.

Congenital Neonatal Hypotonia

BACKGROUND. | The etiology of congenital hypotonia, accompanied by horizontal pendular nystagmus, but not following perinatal accidents, is presumably in the brainstem. Kaga et al. (1986) evaluated with ABR five male Japanese infants with this clinical status. All showed only waves I and II. Curiously, four of the five infants responded to environmental sounds and voices. The authors suspect a nonprogressive inborn disorder in myelination. Polizzi, Mauceri, and Ruggieri (1999) presented a case report of a child (a 5-year-old Italian boy) with a history of failure to thrive, hypotonia, truncal ataxia, psychomotor retardation, and congenital horizontal pendular nystagmus. ABR findings also were markedly abnormal, with only waves I and II recorded.

Infantile Spasms

BACKGROUND. | The symptoms of infantile spasms are sudden, brief jerking movements (flexions or extensions) of the head, arms, and legs that occur in a series and then are followed by no movement. The disease usually appears first in the first year of life and spontaneously disappears by age 4 to 5 years, however, mild-to-severe mental retardation develops by this time in up to nine out of ten children. Neuropathologic findings associated with the disease include lesions in both white and gray matter of the brainstem and cerebrum. Cytomegalovirus (CMV) infection has also been documented in some cases.

ABR FINDINGS. | Kaga, Tanaka, and Fukuyama (1981) and later Kaga, Marsh, and Fukuyama (1982) reported ABR wave I–V latency delays in 30 percent of thirty patients with infantile spasms. One of these patients also had a serious peripheral auditory deficit by ABR (no response). An important implication for audiometric evaluation was that behavioral hearing testing (conditioned orientation response procedure) was consistent with elevated pure-tone thresholds for 86 percent of the series, even though ABR did not confirm peripheral hearing deficit. Cortical dysfunction is cited in an explanation of this pattern of auditory findings.

Hypotonia

ABR FINDINGS. | Kaga, Yokochi, Kodama, Kitazumi, and Marsh (1986) report ABR findings for five male infants (ranging in age from 3 to 13 months at initial examination) with a previously undescribed syndrome consisting of congenital horizontal pendular nystagmus and general hypotonia of head and limbs. Absence of all ABR components after waves I and II was considered a feature of this syndrome. Follow-up of the infants showed no progression of the disease. Interestingly, behavioral response to sounds, including speech stimuli, was normal among the infants.

Ondine's Syndrome (Curse)

BACKGROUND. | This is a rare congenital or acquired disorder usually first appearing in infants soon after birth. Also referred to as central alveolar hypoventilation syndrome, it is characterized by depressed central ventilatory drive, slow and shallow breathing, and hypercapnic (increased carbon dioxide) and hypoxic (decreased oxygen) responses during quiet sleep. The initial clinical signs are cyanosis and respiratory acidosis, often accompanied by generalized hypotonia and hyporeflexia, and sometimes cranial nerve abnormalities. Neuropathologic studies generally fail to demonstrate obvious structural causes of these clinical problems. The pathophysiological basis of Ondine's syndrome may be dysfunction of chemoreceptor neurons in the CNS respiratory centers (located in medullary brainstem near nuclei of cranial nerves VIII, IX, and X).

ABR FINDINGS. | There are just a few reports of ABR in this disease (Beckerman et al., 1986; Litscher, Schwarz, & Reimann, 1996; Long & Allen, 1984). Beckerman et al. (1986) recorded ABRs from 4 infants with severe congenital central alveolar hypoventilation syndrome who ranged in age from 6 weeks to 15 months. All patients had well-formed responses of appropriate amplitudes. The patients differed from age- and gender-matched control infants by showing a statistically significant delay in the wave I–III interval, which did not produce a significant prolongation of the wave I–V latency. The ABR abnormalities were consistently observed on repeated assessments and were not correlated with ventilatory status (hypoxia or hypercapnia) nor chloral hydrate sedation. Litscher, Schwarz, and Reimann (1996) confirmed in a case report of a 3-year-old girl with the diagnosis of central alveolar hypoventilation syndrome delays in ABR interwave latencies and also absence of the ABR wave III.

Sudden Infant Death Syndrome (SIDS)

BACKGROUND. | The term "crib death" is also used to describe the sudden, unpredictable, and apparently unexplained death of a previously healthy infant while sleeping. SIDS usually occurs within the age range of three weeks to six months after birth. Although there is some evidence that the overall risk of SIDS is greater in winter and in infants with CNS-related respiratory problems (neurologic immaturity of brainstem respiratory regions), the cause of SIDS is not known. Histopathologic examination of the brainstems of SIDS victims shows evidence of gliosis in respiratory centers, but the same histopathologic pattern of findings also characterizes infants with other serious neurologic deficits (e.g., respiratory distress syndrome). When an infant has extended periods of sleep apnea characterized by hypoxemia (reduced oxygen in the blood reaching the brain) and associated cyanosis and flaccidity, is successfully resuscitated (revived), and again begins breathing independently, it is sometimes referred to as a "near-miss sudden infant death" episode. There is less likelihood of SIDS when an infant sleeps in the supine position (on his or her back).

ABR FINDINGS. | In part because neuroanatomy of ABR and respiration are relatively close within the brainstem, several investigators have studied ABR in infants potentially at risk for SIDS, that is, near-miss SIDS. Based on findings reported in the first, and most controversial, studies by Nodar and colleagues (e.g., Nodar, Lonsdale, & Orlowski, 1980), ABR appeared to be consistently abnormal in near-miss SIDS infants. These authors concluded that ABR might be useful in predicting which infants were at risk for SIDS as the response provided evidence of brainstem dysfunction in the region of respiratory centers. Prompted by these initial data, Stockard and Hecox (1981) retrospectively analyzed ABR findings in a series of twenty-eight near-miss SIDS infants and found abnormalities in only three. In the same year, Gupta, Guilleminault, and Dorfman (1981) reported than none of their series of nine near-miss SIDS infants showed evidence of ABR abnormalities. During the early 1980s, the relationship between ABR and SIDS generated considerable interest and debate among the authors just cited and others. Central to the debate were the rather atypical criteria for normality utilized by Nodar and colleagues of the Cleveland Clinic.

The issue of ABR in near-miss SIDS infants was thoroughly reviewed, and reinvestigated, by Stockard (1982). The subjects were six near-miss SIDS infants, tested by ABR within the first two weeks after the incident. Stockard (1982) also reported ABR data for one infant before and after a near-miss SIDS incident (the only incident this infant had). Two weeks after the near miss, this subject died of SIDS. The initial ABR, which was performed as part of routine auditory screening, was normal by age-matched criteria. In addition, ABR latency (interwave) data for each of the near-miss SIDS infants were within age-matched normative limits. Group ABR data recorded between 2.5 and 3.5 months of age, however, showed a statistically significant prolongation in the wave I–V latency for near-miss SIDS infants (4.91 ms) versus an age-matched control group (4.66 ms). The author was unable to demonstrate any individual subject abnormalities even by using various techniques that sometimes increase ABR sensitivity to CNS dysfunction (e.g., increased stimulus rate). The overall conclusion from this study was that ABR results have no value in predicting SIDS. ABR data are helpful in documenting brainstem integrity of infants who have experienced hypoxic and ischemic insults, and longitudinal ABR data are perhaps useful in documenting trends in neurological status.

Craniopagus (Conjoined Twins)

BACKGROUND. | Conjoined twins are extremely rare (less than one in 2.5 million births). They are typically conjoined in the parietal occipital regions, and they share some cerebral blood supply.

ABR FINDINGS. | Hughes and Fino (1984) studied serial EEG, VERs, and ABRs in premature conjoined twins. Brains were separate but venous vasculature was shared. There were differences between each of the twins in ABR latency, suggesting that brainstem maturity may progress at variable rates in conjoined twins.

Pediatric Head Injury

BACKGROUND.   Trauma is the leading cause of injury and death in children aged 1 to 14 (Bruce et al., 1978; Raimondi

& Hirschauer, 1984; Walker, Mayer, Storrs, & Hylton, 1985; Wegman, 1982). Head injury is usually a component of life-threatening trauma. Each year head injury kills five times as many children as the second ranking lethal disease—leukemia—and kills or causes permanent disability in more children than all other neurologic diseases combined. Head injury is the most common CNS pathologic entity in many pediatric ICUs. The mode of injury for the majority of children is generally a motor vehicle or auto-pedestrian or auto-bicyclist accident. Other causes of injury are falls, child abuse, and gunshot wounds.

ABR FINDINGS. | ABR abnormalities following severe closed head injury in children are well documented (Hall, Hargadine, & Allen, 1985; Hall & Tucker, 1985, 1986). The reader is referred to Hall (1992) for a thorough review of the literature on ABR in pediatric head injury. ABR can be applied in multiple ways following head injury in children. ABR offers a tool for early and objective assessment of peripheral auditory function in children at risk for trauma-related hearing loss secondary temporal bone fracture or medical therapy that includes potentially ototoxic medications. Neurodiagnostic ABR assessment can document or rule out brainstem auditory dysfunction. Serial ABR measurements during the acute phase following head injury provide a means of monitoring pathophysiologic status in comatose children and providing information useful for making important decisions regarding medical and surgical management. The ABR can also be applied in the definition of brain death (see Hall, 1992, for review).

Neonatal Brain Injury

BACKGROUND. | Risk factors for infant hearing impairment include diseases and disorders that can affect the CNS, including auditory pathways and centers. The general topic of risk factors in newborn infants was reviewed earlier in the chapter. In addition to the many publications on principles, procedures, and clinical findings in ABR-based screening of neonatal auditory sensitivity, there also reports describing systematic ABR assessment of CNS status in this population (Cevette, 1984; Hecox & Cone, 1981; Minoli & Moro, 1985; Stockard et al., 1983; Watanabe et al., 1984). A variety of diseases encountered in the neonatal ICU can result in auditory CNS dysfunction, as well as peripheral hearing loss. Among these diseases are CNS infections (e.g., cytomegalovirus [CMV], rubella, toxoplasmosis, herpes), hyperbilirubinemia, hypoxic-ischemic encephalopathy secondary to respiratory distress, asphyxia and apnea, intraventricular hemorrhage (IVH) and hydrocephalus (Guthkelch, Sclabassi, & Vries, 1982; Hecox & Cone, 1981; Kraus et al., 1984; McPherson, Amlie, & Foltz, 1985; McSherry, Walter, & Horber, 1982; Sklar et al., 1979; Watanabe et al., 1984). The discussion above on pathophysiology in brain injury is in general applicable to the neonate, although cerebral

metabolic needs and normal cerebrovascular characteristics may vary significantly. There are, however, differences between the pediatric population and newborns in the distribution of etiologies and, importantly, in procedures for assessment of CNS dysfunction and neurological and intellectual outcome (Raimondi & Hirschauer, 1984; Walker et al., 1985). Clearly, neurologic grading scales standardized with adults and older children, such as the GCS, are inappropriate for infants who are neurologically immature. This immaturity ranges from incomplete reflex development to virtually no speech and language development and, therefore, confounds grading CNS status from the brainstem to the cortex. The clinical neurologic examination, likewise, is relatively imprecise in the evaluation of neonatal CNS functioning. Furthermore, the long-term neurologic and cognitive effects of certain diseases, such as hydrocephalus, meningitis, and traumatic head injury, appear to be more pronounced for infants than older children and adults (Raimondi & Hirschauer, 1984; Walker et al., 1985). For these reasons, ABR can play an important role as a neurophysiologic index of CNS integrity in the neonatal ICU setting.

HYDROCEPHALUS. | From antiquity to the present, hydrocephalus has been recognized as a distinct neurologic disease. Rational management strategies, however, were not introduced until the early 1900s, following classic laboratory experiments by Walter Dandy on the pathophysiology of hydrocephalus. Current surgical shunt techniques for treating hydrocephalus can be traced to the early 1950s (Milhorat, 1984). Hydrocephalus is more difficult to diagnose in infants than in adults. Clearcut neurologic symptoms may be delayed because ICP increases are dissipated by cranial enlargement. In time, ICP increases will exceed the capacity of the skull to expand, but even then typical symptoms of neurologic dysfunction, such as headaches, cannot be described by the infant. Symptoms are vomiting, lethargy, and irritability. Subsequent clinical signs of infantile hydrocephalus include separation of the cranial sutures, engorgement of the superficial scalp veins, enlargement of the fontanels and ocular abnormalities (bilateral gaze deficits). The diagnosis is confirmed with computerized tomography and ultrasonography.

In determining whether neonates with dilated ventricles by CT or ultrasound require surgical intervention (shunt procedure), it is extremely useful to have direct information on the functional effects of increased ICP. The ABR may, in many cases, provide this information. Studies of hydrocephalic children have shown that ABR abnormalities may contribute to the decision to surgically intervene, and serial postoperative ABRs can assess the effect of surgery on brain function (Cevette, 1984; Hall, Brown, & Mackey-Hargadine, 1985; Hall & Tucker, 1986; Kraus et al., 1984). ABR wave I–V latency intervals exceeding age-matched normal limits are unequivocal evidence of brainstem compression secondary to hydrocephalus. Postoperative decreases in this brainstem transmission time index reflect reduction in ICP, whereas a persistence or worsening of auditory brainstem abnormalities suggests the need for a shunt revision. It is important to point out that the ABR may, in fact, be a less-sensitive indicator of CNS dysfunction in hydrocephalus than other sensory evoked responses, such as the visual evoked response (Guthkelch et al., 1982; Hall & Tucker, 1986; Sklar, Ehle, & Clark, 1979). Therefore, a normal ABR does not necessarily infer that a shunt procedure is inappropriate, particularly if there is evidence of visual evoked response (VER) abnormalities. On the other hand, a prolonged ABR wave I–V interval is rather conclusive evidence of significant CNS dysfunction. The degree of pre- versus postshunt ABR changes is influenced by the presence of other intracranial pathology (e.g., IVH), the mechanism of hydrocephalus (e.g., congenital obstruction) leading to noncommunicating hydrocephalus versus cerebrospinal fluid (CSF) oversecretion and the extent of CNS structural damage, as evidenced by CT.

Severe Burns

Critical care management of severely burned children is extremely challenging because this population is subject to numerous serious medical problems in the acute post-burn period. One of these medical problems is sepsis, which usually is treated with potentially ototoxic drugs. The ototoxicity of aminoglycosides (e.g., gentamicin, amikacin, tobramycin), other antibiotics (vancomycin, erythromycin, amphotericin B), and loop diretics (e.g., furosemide [Lasix]) is well established. There is also evidence of complex pharmacokinetic interactions among drugs—that is, potentiation of the ototoxicity of one drug by another. It is clear that cochlear auditory impairment may be an unfortunate consequence of medical therapies commonly used in severely burned children. The auditory deficits are first observed in the high-frequency region and are due mainly to outer hair cell alterations.

It would be desirable to have a clinically feasible means of predicting the ototoxic effects of a drug, or combination of drugs, for an individual patient. Predictive information might contribute to both acute medical therapy and long-term rehabilitation plans. Unfortunately, prediction of ototoxicity on the basis of medical data or patient characteristics is very difficult. Numerous factors must be considered in the determining the likelihood of ototoxicity. Among these factors are duration and magnitude of drug dosage, differences in perilymph penetration among drugs, synergism among drugs, liver and renal function, body temperature, familial predisposition, individual susceptibility, and, perhaps, noise exposure during hospitalization (Bess, Peek, & Chapman, 1979; Bock & Saunders, 1977; Moore, Smith, & Lietman, 1984; Quick, 1980). Further complicating the picture is evi-

dence that cochlear damage may, in rare cases, be reversible and conversely, in perhaps many cases, delayed. These latter patients are especially troublesome since auditory deficits may first appear weeks or even months after the ototoxic therapy has been discontinued.

Traditional audiometry is not feasible in the acute severely burned child. Transportation to a sound-treated test chamber is medically contraindicated and, in addition, most patients are stuporous and unable to volunteer valid behavioral responses. For the infant with burns, behavioral assessment would be of limited value regardless of test site or mental state. In our experience, ABR offers a clinical means of detecting auditory deficits in children, including infants, in the acute period after a severe burn. This ABR application is the topic of papers (Hall, Winkler, Herndon, & Gary, 1986) and is reviewed also by Hall (1992).

Auditory Neuropathy

ABR assessment at this stage may be relatively straightforward, as in the initial newborn hearing screening. The application of ABR in diagnosis of auditory neuropathy is reviewed in detail in Chapter 7. If the ABR abnormality is characterized by elevation of threshold (minimum response) levels, and all components are reliably observed and interwave latency values are within normal limits, the pathology may be limited to inner hair cells. Although the term "auditory neuropathy" has been used to describe this pattern of findings (Harrison, 1998), it is anatomically speaking an uncommon form of cochlear (sensory) hearing impairment (Prieve, Gorga, & Neely, 1991). Possible explanations can include a genetically based inner hair cell disorder (Deol, 1981; Schrott, Stephan, & Spoendlin, 1989), certain etiologies that can affect inner hair cells, such as measles or mumps (Prieve, Gorga, & Neely, 1991), or ototoxicity due to carboplatin (discussed below). OAEs are normal, or at least detectable, because all or some outer hair cells are functionally intact. The ABR, including wave I, is dependent on synchronous firing of afferent eighth-nerve fibers in the region of the spiral ganglion secondary to synaptic activation by the inner hair cells. Inner hair cell dysfunction will, to some extent, elevate ABR thresholds. Normal interwave latencies reflect intact retrocochlear pathways. Audiologic follow-up assessments with the inner hair cell pattern should be scheduled often until behavioral thresholds and speech audiometry findings are available. An otologic and genetic consultation would also be indicated. If a hearing loss by pure-tone audiometry is confirmed, it would be appropriate to proceed cautiously with hearing aid selection and fitting. If, on the other hand, ABR interwave latencies are abnormally delayed, relative to age-appropriate normative data, or wave I or other ABR components are not reliably observed, then more extensive electrophysiologic assessment is warranted.

10

CHAPTER

ABR
Adult Diseases and Disorders and Clinical Applications

PERIPHERAL AUDITORY DISORDERS

Conductive Hearing Loss (Middle Ear Disorders)

OTOSCLEROSIS. | Otosclerosis is a genetic disease of the bone around the cochlea. It is a process of bone resorption and reformation, often known as "otospongiosis." The stapes footplate, which is the junction between the middle and inner ear, is often involved in the disease. Bony structural abnormalities of the cochlea (the labyrinthine capsule) in otosclerosis can produce sensorineural hearing deficit, and stapes footplate (ossicular chain) fixation often produces a conductive hearing deficit. There may be either a pure sensorineural hearing loss or a pure CHL, but often, both components occur together, and the resulting hearing loss is mixed. An apparent mixed loss may be due to depression of bone-conduction hearing associated with abnormal middle ear mechanics in otosclerosis. In these cases, bone-conduction thresholds often improve with effective medical or surgical therapy.

Otosclerosis affects between 0.5 and 1.0 percent of the population, and it is more likely in women than in men. It tends to be bilateral, first appearing in the first three or four decades of life. The effects of otosclerosis on hearing are more pronounced during pregnancy. An otoscopic finding in some otosclerotic patients is Schwartze's sign, a pinkish blush seen through the TM, due to hyperemia (extra blood collection) at the promontory. This indicates an active disease process. Otosclerosis can be treated with medical and surgical therapy. Medical therapy usually consists of sodium fluoride treatment, sometimes supplemented with vitamin D and calcium carbonate. This therapy is presumed to affect the overall disease process (middle ear and cochlear components). The surgical treatment is stapedectomy, in which various surgical techniques and prostheses are used to recreate a flexible and functional connection between the TM and the oval window. The objective of surgery is to correct the reduction in sound transmission to the inner ear, which was caused by stapes footplate fixation.

Because otosclerosis is a disease that almost always affects otherwise healthy adults who can cooperate for traditional audiometry, including air- and bone-conduction pure-tone threshold measurement, auditory evoked responses are infrequently indicated for auditory assessment. Theoretically, air- versus bone-conduction ABR might be useful in persons with severe CHL secondary to otosclerosis, when the masking dilemma precludes meaningful interpretation of behavioral pure-tone audiometry. However, bone-conduction ABR in these patients is typically of little value because the likelihood of a response is diminished by the sensorineural deficit (or at least the decreased bone-conduction sensitivity) that is often a component of the disease. Relatively few investigations of ABR have included patients with otosclerosis (McGee & Clemis, 1982). McGee and Clemis (1982) analyzed ABR data for a diverse group of patients with CHL, including six patients (seven ears) with otosclerosis. Importantly, among the thirty-two ears tested, no wave I could be detected in seventeen. ABR findings in otosclerosis (ossicular chain fixation) were described as comparable to those with ossicular chain discontinuity. A characteristically conductive increase in wave V latency was reported, but the increase was greater than anticipated from the pure-tone air-versus bone-conduction gap in the 1000 to 4000 Hz region.

DISCONTINUITY OF THE OSSICULAR CHAIN. | There are various causes for discontinuity or interruption of the ossicular chain. A key example is head trauma. The blow to the head dislodges the tiny ossicles, usually at the joint between the incus and the stapes, although other regions (the stapes crura) can also be damaged. Chronic middle ear disease can also eventually erode or cause necrosis of one or more of the ossicles and can produce a complete break in the chain. The audiometric pattern in complete ossicular chain disruption is distinctive. It consists of a highly compliant tympanogram, absent acoustic reflexes, and a moderate or severe (typically 40 dB or more) CHL component that is even greater for the higher frequencies (above 1000 Hz).

There are few published references to AERs in ossicular chain discontinuity. In the study by McGee and Clemis (1982), just noted in the discussion of otosclerosis, there were four subjects (five ears) with confirmed ossicular chain discontinuity. The authors did not provide a detailed description of ABR findings among these patients, but they did cite greater wave V latency increases than were expected, based on the amount of air-bone gap. A comparable observation was made for otosclerotic patients. In contrast, eleven patients with otitis media (fifteen ears) showed ABR wave V latency increase consistent with the reduction of effective stimulus intensity due to air-bone gap. Another point made by McGee and Clemis (1982) was that in patients with mixed hearing loss (conductive plus neural), ABR changes due to CHL in some patients obscured identification of abnormal latency increases resulting from confirmed retrocochlear dysfunction. There is generally little value in applying auditory evoked responses in the assessment of hearing sensitivity in ossicular chain disruption because this can be done better with traditional audiometry. An exception to this rule, of course, is the comatose, severely head-injured patient undergoing AER assessment for neurodiagnosis or for neuromonitoring, reviewed later in this chapter. It is important for the clinician to determine from medical colleagues or from chart review whether the patient has a temporal bone fracture, and, if so, whether ossicular chain disruption is suspected. An abnormal or absent ABR by air conduction (but not by bone conduction) would be expected in this patient. Among middle ear pathologies producing CHL, however, ossicular chain disruption would be expected to have greater impact on ABR findings than most. This is because, for the majority of middle ear pathologies (such as otitis media), hearing loss is greater for lower frequencies and less for higher frequencies. ABR (with a click stimulus) tends to underestimate the degree of low-frequency hearing impairment. In contrast, the high-frequency deficit in ossicular chain disruption occurs in the frequency region most important for ABR generation.

Sensory Hearing Loss (Cochlear Disorders)

ABR findings in cochlear pathology are distinctively different than those just described for CHL. Some common etiologies for sensory and neural hearing loss are listed in Table 10.1. The ABR in all but severe sensory (cochlear) impairment is remarkably robust, although a wave I component may be indistinct or not detectable. The ABR is virtually independent of low-frequency hearing loss. The relation of ABR findings to degree and configuration of sensorineural hearing loss was reviewed in Chapter 7. A normal-appearing ABR may be recorded in sensory-impaired patients with only "islands" of residual good hearing sensitivity in the 2000 to 4000 Hz region. Even sensory hearing loss within the ABR frequency region of 1000 to 4000 Hz typically does not influence appreciably the response latency or amplitude for high stimulus-intensity levels (e.g., 80 dB HL or above) until it reaches

TABLE 10.1. Selected Pathologies Affecting the Cochlea and Eighth Cranial (acoustic) Nerve Associated with Sensory and Neural Hearing Impairment (arranged alphabetically)

Cochlea
- Basilar
- Endolymphatic hydrops
- Genetic syndromes (there are over 50 affecting children)
- Head trauma
- Kernicterus
- Labyrinthine fistula
- Ménière's disease
- Meningitis
- Otosclerosis
- Ototoxic drugs
- Prebycusis
- Rubella
- Temporal bone fracture

Eighth Cranial Nerve
- Meningioma
- Presbycusis
- Temporal bone fracture
- Vestibular schwannoma (i.e., acoustic tumor, acoustic neuroma)
- Vascular loop
- Von Recklinghausen's disease (Neurofibromatosis II)

at least 50 to 60 dB HTL. Again, wave I is often not present. No ABR is typically observed with severe-to-profound high-frequency loss, despite better HTLs for low frequencies. In patients with moderate high-frequency sensory hearing loss, the ABR wave V latency–intensity function is steeper than normal. No ABR wave V is recorded for low intensity levels. A response first appears as click-stimulus intensity level approaches HTLs in the 1000 to 4000 Hz region. Actually, the appearance of the ABR for somewhat lower stimulus intensity levels suggests the contribution of audiometric frequencies below 1000 Hz to the response. Latency of the response at these intensities is abnormally prolonged because it is generated by a more apical portion of the cochlea and requires somewhat greater travel time along the basilar membrane. Then, as stimulus intensity level exceeds HL (hearing level) in the 1000 to 4000 Hz region, latency of wave V decreases rapid and eventually falls within the normal region.

The relationship between sensory hearing impairment and ABR as just outlined is oversimplified and not always encountered clinically. In fact, there is a complex and poorly understood interaction among ABR findings and (a) degree, slope, and overall configuration of sensory hearing impairment; (b) subject age and gender; (c) stimulus parameters; and (d) acoustic characteristics of the transducer. The relationship is further complicated by apparent differences in the effects of various etiologies of sensory hearing impairment on ABR. Additionally, as noted at the outset of this chapter, even patients with apparently equivalent audiograms produce ABRs with divergent and sometimes unexplainable latency–intensity functions. ABR findings reported for etiologies of sensory impairment are now reviewed.

MÉNIÈRE'S DISEASE. | Electrocochleography is, of course, the auditory evoked response most useful for electrophysiological confirmation of Ménière's disease, and endolymphatic hydrops in general. The topic of ECochG in Ménière's disease is reviewed with considerable detail in Chapter 5. With two exceptions, the ABR as typically recorded has limited clinical value in the diagnosis or management of Ménière's disease. For patients with unilateral or asymmetric sensorineural hearing undergoing work-up for possible Ménière's disease, the ABR certainly contributes to the differentiation of sensory versus neural auditory dysfunction. Immediately prior to measurement of the ECochG, a neurodiagnostic ABR assessment helps to rule out retrocochlear auditory dysfunction (e.g., an acoustic tumor) and to focus the diagnostic process on differentiation among types of cochlear auditory disorders. The ABR is also applied intraoperatively as a neurophysiologic monitoring technique for patients with Ménière's disease who are undergoing surgical management, e.g., an endolymphatic sac decompression procedure or a vestibular nerve section operation. The topic of intraoperative monitoring with the ABR is discussed later in this chapter.

There is one possible direct application of ABR in the diagnosis of patients with suspected endolymphatic hydrops. Don and colleagues at the House Ear Institute have reported at scientific meetings preliminary, but promising, evidence of patterns of abnormalities for the stacked ABR technique in Ménière's disease. As noted in Chapter 9, the stacked ABR technique isolates auditory function for five specific frequency regions. Stacked ABR is more useful than conventional click-evoked ABR in the evaluation of patients with suspected small acoustic tumors because "it represents a measure that assesses the activity of essentially all the eighth nerve fibers, not just a subset" (Don et al., 2005, p. 275). For the stacked ABR technique to assess separately nerve fibers representing each of five different frequency regions, it must of course activate separately portions of the basilar membrane also representing the five different frequency regions. Velocity of traveling waves along the basilar membrane from the basal to apical extremes is influenced by biomechanical disruptions with the cochlea related to Ménière's disease. In theory, wave V latencies for different frequency regions of the cochlea, as determined with the stacked ABR technique, will be affected by the disruption in traveling wave velocity in Ménière's disease.

PRESBYCUSIS. | The term *presbycusis* is often used in reference to sensorineural hearing loss accompanying the aging process. The root word *presby* is derived from the Greek word for "old," and the word *kousis,* also from Greek, means "hearing." Aging is associated with anatomic and physiologic changes in the cochlea, the eighth cranial nerve, and central auditory nervous system. Age-related sensory hearing loss, due to cochlear changes, is encountered most often clinically. In fact, presbycusis is the most common etiology of sensorineural hearing loss for persons over the age of 60 years. An understanding of the effect of presbycusis on the ABR is, therefore, not esoteric but, rather, practical information that will prove useful in the analysis and interpretation of ABR findings for many older patients undergoing neurodiagnostic assessment. In recording a neurodiagnostic ABR from older patients with sensorineural hearing loss, it's important to differentiate the effect of age-related sensory or neural auditory dysfunction from other explanations for an abnormal ABR, such as those associated with neoplasms (tumors) and other retrocochlear or CNS pathologies. Comprehensive audiologic assessment is also very helpful in delineating the contribution of age-related auditory dysfunction to ABR findings. For example, presbycusis is usually bilaterally symmetrical, whereas most neuropathology involving the eighth cranial nerve is unilateral. The pattern of findings for other audiologic procedures, e.g., word recognition and acoustic reflexes, also contribute to the differentiation of sensory versus neural auditory dysfunction. In addition, the form of presbycusis related to age-related changes in the central auditory nervous system must be considered in the analysis and interpretation of ABR findings. The ABR changes associated with normal aging tend to be relatively minor (e.g., Jerger & Hall, 1980; Rosenhamer et al., 1980), bilaterally symmetrical, and distributed over the entire wave I to wave V latency interval, rather than within a specific latency region (e.g., wave I to III or wave III to V). The effect of retrocochlear auditory pathology on the ABR, in contrast, is typically pronounced, unilateral, and often greatest for the latency interval between wave I and wave III.

ABR investigations in adult patient populations often include older subjects with apparent presbycusis. As noted in the chapters devoted to cortical auditory evoked responses, there are plenty of examples in the literature of indiscriminant inclusion in studies of specific of patient populations (e.g., Alzheimer's dementia), older patients with apparent age-related hearing loss, apparently without concerns about the possible influence of presbycusis. In one of the few reports of a specific and systematic investigation of the ABR in presbycusis, Rosenhall et al. (1985) recorded responses from 373 subjects divided into two groups: young (50 years or less, with a mean age of 38 years) and older (60 years or older, with a mean age of 70 years). The investigators ruled out conductive, retrocochlear, and neurologic disorders for all subjects. Data were analyzed separately for male and female subjects. Severe high-frequency sensorineural hearing loss, presumably presbycusis, produced a delay of 0.3 to 0.6 ms in the absolute latency of ABR wave V, a delay that was greater for males than females with the same degree of hearing loss. Relevant to clinical application of the ABR in older patient populations, the authors concluded that the correction of ABR latency according to hearing loss was not appropriate for females and, for males, was not consistently accurate. Also, the ABR wave I to V latency interval increased as a function of age, but mostly for the more central wave III to wave V portion. The results of this study (Rosenhall et al., 1985) confirm that presbycusis must be carefully documented, or ruled out, for meaningful interpretation of ABR findings in elderly patient or subject populations.

NOISE-INDUCED SENSORINEURAL HEARING LOSS. | Exposure to high-intensity sounds has long been recognized as a common cause of hearing impairment. A review of the vast literature on noise-induced hearing loss, including the pathophysiology, therapeutic protective mechanisms, and prevention with hearing conservation, is far beyond the scope of this discussion. Hearing loss resulting from noise exposure reflects damage or dysfunction of the cochlea, especially in the region of frequencies from about 3000 to 6000 Hz. A characteristic pattern for pure-tone audiometry in patients with chronic noise exposure or an incident of acoustic trauma (e.g., an abrupt and very high intensity noise) is a "notch" in the audiogram in the region of 4000 Hz. Noise-induced hearing loss may, of course, be present in patients undergoing neurodiagnostic ABR assessment, particularly adult males.

There are several practical implications of noise-induced hearing loss for the technique used in ABR assessment and for analysis of ABR findings. Because of the high-frequency nature of noise-induced sensorineural hearing loss, wave I may not be clearly observed unless the ABR is recorded with an ECochG-type electrode (e.g., TIPtrode or tympanic membrane electrode). During a neurodiagnostic ABR assessment, every attempt should be made to reliably record a wave I component so neural transmission times can be calculated from interwave latencies (e.g., wave I to wave III, wave I to wave V).

Noise-induced sensorineural hearing loss can pose another problem in the analysis of neurodiagnostic ABR findings. Although often bilaterally symmetrical, the effects of excessive noise exposure on hearing can be greater for one ear than the other. Etiologies for asymmetric noise-induced hearing loss include exposure to a blast or sudden high-intensity sound (e.g., a firecracker) or chronic exposure to higher intensity levels of sound on one side. For example, a right-handed person who shoots rifles may develop greater hearing loss for the less-protected left ear.

Almadori et al. (1988) conducted a study of ABR findings in fifty-four subjects (108 ears) with permanent noise-induced hearing impairment. Other etiologies were ruled out by history, otologic examination, and neuroradiology. All subjects were males exposed to occupational noise, and age ranged from 25 to 51 years. Audiograms consistently showed a sensorineural hearing loss with the 4000 Hz notching configuration. The ABR evoked with a click stimulus presented

at an intensity level of 70 dB and at a rate of 21/sec, and recorded with an inverting electrode on the mastoid, lacked a clear wave I component for 11 percent of the ears, even when the degree of hearing loss was less than 40 dB HL. With a faster rate (51/sec), wave I was not detected for 37 percent of the subjects. ABR interwave latencies were within normal limits, when they could be calculated (i.e., when wave I was present). The findings of this study highlight at least 3 practical guidelines for neurodiagnostic ABR measurement in adult patients with noise-induced hearing loss and, particularly, for enhancing the likelihood of recording a wave I component:

1. If necessary, increase stimulus intensity to the maximum level (e.g., 95 dB nHL) in an attempt to generate a clear and reliable wave I component, and then calculate interwave latency values.
2. Use a relatively slow rate of stimulation for neurodiagnostic ABR applications (e.g., 21 stimuli per second or slower.
3. Always rely on an ECochG-type electrode when recording a neurodiagnostic ABR from a patient with high-frequency sensorineural hearing loss.

OTOTOXICITY. | A variety of therapeutic drugs are potentially ototoxic, typically interfering with normal metabolism within the cochlea and damaging outer and eventually inner hair cells. The application of the ABR in documenting ototoxicity in children was discussed in Chapter 9, and some of the more common potentially ototoxic medications were summarized. Adults are exposed to potentially ototoxic medications during treatment for chronic and potentially life threatening diseases (e.g., cystic fibrosis and cancers), with nonsurgical management of brain neoplasms, and during intensive care following surgery or traumatic injury. In most adults, conventional behavioral audiologic procedures (e.g., pure-tone and speech audiometry) are adequate for monitoring auditory function and documenting hearing loss. Persons with acute brain injury or other serious medical conditions are the exception to this statement. Antibiotics are commonly administered in such patients for treatment of infections, and other potentially ototoxic medications (e.g., loop diuretics) may also be indicated for maintenance of systemic or cerebral homeostasis. The topic of ABR neurophysiologic monitoring of adults in the neurointensive care unit is reviewed toward the end of this chapter.

Hotz and colleagues (1990) documented with serial ABR recordings changes in absolute latencies for wave I and wave V in a series of twenty patients confined to the intensive care unit and treated medically with two aminoglycoside antibiotics—netilicin and tobramycin. The authors reported peripheral and central effects of the drugs on the ABR.

BAROTRAUMA. | Rapid changes in atmospheric pressure, such as compression and decompression experienced by divers and in hyperbaric environments, can affect different portions of the auditory system, including the middle ear and inner ear. Divers exposed to very high levels of atmospheric pressures show symptoms of high-pressure nervous syndrome, including brainstem findings (e.g., vertigo, tremors).

With four experienced and normal-hearing divers serving as subjects, Wang, Jiang, Gong, Zheng (1994) experimentally simulated in a hyperbaric chamber compression with helium-oxygen to 350 m. ABR recordings were normal immediately after the subjects exited the chamber. The authors attributed transient changes in ABR latency and morphology within the hyperbaric chamber to pressure-related alterations in stimulus intensity and the presence of background noise. Lorenz et al. (1995) exposed four divers to an experimental deep helium–oxygen saturation dive equivalent to 450 meters of seawater and reported findings in apparent contradiction to those reported by Wang et al. (1994). Serial ABR recordings during the simulated dive were characterized by decreased absolute latency for wave I and prolongation of the wave I to III and wave I to V latency intervals. The magnitude of changes in the ABR with compression varied among the four subjects. The authors offered explanations for the ABR findings, suggesting the shortened wave I latency might have been related to enhanced sound transmission and a high-frequency shift in middle ear resonance in dense helium. Explanations for the ABR interwave latency prolongations included pressure-induced reduction in the velocity of nerve conduction, synaptic delays, and inhibitory effects on auditory brainstem pathways.

NONORGANIC HEARING IMPAIRMENT. | The term *nonorganic hearing impairment* refers to apparent hearing loss with no clear anatomic or physiologic explanation. Falling into this general category are hearing conditions described with a variety of other terms, including *malingering* (willful feigning of a hearing loss or exaggeration of an existing hearing loss), *functional hearing loss,* and *pseudohypacusis.* The motive for malingering may be monetary compensation, personal gain, or avoidance of something perceived by the patient as unpleasant or undesirable (e.g., school, work, or military service), or even to gain attention from others. Nonorganic hearing loss is distinguished from *psychogenic hearing impairment,* an apparent hearing loss that is the physical manifestation of a psychological disorder, e.g., "conversion hysteria." Different management strategies are taken for these two general categories of nonorganic hearing impairment.

Auditory evoked responses offer an electrophysiologic approach for identifying and confirming actual hearing level in nonorganic hearing impairment. Although the ABR was recommended as the technique of choice for clinical documentation of nonorganic hearing loss (e.g., Hall, 1992), the ASSR in conjunction with otoacoustic emissions is now a viable option for frequency-specific estimation of auditory sensitivity with the added advantage of objective computer-based analysis of findings.

RETROCOCHLEAR (EIGHTH CRANIAL NERVE) DISORDERS

Background

In addition to neurons (excitable cells), the nervous system consists of a variety of nonexcitable support cells, referred to as neuroglia. Up to 45 percent of intracranial tumors arise from neuroglia. Most neuroglia cells are smaller than neurons. They do not have axons and do not synapse with other cells. Neuroglial cells outnumber neurons by five to ten times and make up about one-half of the volume of the nervous system (Snell, 1987). There are four major types of neuroglial cells:

- *Astrocytes* (star-shaped cells) support nerve cells, function as electrical insulators, and provide a barrier at synapses to contain neurotransmitters.
- *Oligodendrocytes* are active in the formation of myelin sheaths for nerve fibers, including Schwann cells.
- *Microglia* are, as the name implies, small glial cells. They are activated in the presence of inflammation and degenerative process in the nervous system, at which time microglia also have a phagocytic function (i.e., they ingest and remove neural residue).
- *Ependymal* cells line cavities of the brain, such as the ventricles. Some ependymal cells are ciliated and facilitate CSF (cerebrospinal fluid) circulation in the ventricular system. Others actually produce CSF.

The estimated annual incidence of intracranial tumors in the United States is between 4.5 and 12 persons per 100,000 in the general population (Davis & Robertson 1991; Okazaki, 1983). Approximately 1 percent of hospital admissions are for management of brain tumor. Brain tumor is a general term that refers to a variety of intracranial lesions, including neoplasms and mass lesions of the brain parenchyma and meninges and also tumors from structures near the brain that can affect indirectly brain tissue and function, such as pituitary adenomas and chordomas. Consequently, the term "intracranial tumors" is probably more anatomically accurate than "brain tumor." As displayed in Table 10.2, there is a difference in the distribution of intracranial tumors in children versus adults. The most common childhood brain tumors are medulloblastoma, cerebellar and cerebral astrocytoma, craniopharyngiomas, ependymomas, optic path glioma, pinealomas, and brainstem gliomas (Davis & Robertson, 1991).

Intracranial tumors can be described as follows:

- Medulloblastomas are very invasive and highly malignant. They appear mostly in infants or children younger than 5 years of age and more often in boys. Anatomic structures that may be involved include the fourth ventricle, cerebral hemispheres (subarachnoid spaces), brainstem, and spinal cord.
- Astrocytomas are found most often in the cerebellum, especially in children ages 5 to 8 years. Cerebral astro-

TABLE 10.2. Proportion of Primary Intracranial Tumors Found among Children versus Persons of All Ages*

TUMOR TYPE	CHILDREN	ALL AGES
Glioma	>75%	45–50%
Astrocytoma	>50%	>75%
Cerebellar	30%	Malignant 50 to 60%
Brainstem	10%	Benign 25 to 30%
Oligodendroglioma	<2%	5%
Ependymoma	8%	5%
Medulloblastoma	25%	6%
Schwannoma	rare	6%
Meningioma	rare	15%
Hemangioblastoma	rare	1–2%
Sarcoma	rare	1–2%
Lymphoma	0%	<1%
Germ cell tumor	2–4%	1–2%
Dermoid, epidermoid	1–2%	<1%
Craniopharyngioma	5–10%	3%
Pituitary adenoma	rare	5%
	100%	100%

*15 to 20% of all intracranial tumors occur in childhood. Approximately 70% of intracranial tumors in children are located in infratentorial regions. In contrast, in adults, approximately 70% are located supratentorially.

Adapted from Okazaki, 1983.

cytomas are not as common in children, but they are highly malignant. The frontal lobe is frequently involved.

• Craniopharyngiomas are congenital and develop quickly in children.

• Ependymomas are found in infants and young children, most often in the posterior fossa. When in the cerebral regions (often frontal or parietal lobes), they become rather large.

• Pinealomas usually occur in adolescent boys.

• Gliomas (e.g., optic path or brainstem gliomas) are more common in children, whereas other tumor types, such as acoustic neuromas, pituitary adenomas, and meningiomas, are rare in children.

• Meningiomas have their origin in the meninges (an outer covering of the brain). They invade the skull and dura, but usually not actual brain tissue. Because they become very vascular, CNS dysfunction can result from compression and displacement of brain tissue, which varies depending on the location.

An important distinction for understanding clinical findings associated with brain tumors has to do with their general location. In adults, approximately 70 percent are found in the supratentorial compartment of the brain (above the tentorium posterior fossa), whereas children, 70 percent are infratentorial. Some brain tumors show a different distribution for males versus females. For example, astrocytomas, glio-

bastomas, ependymomas, medulloblastomas, and pinealomas are more often found in males. Meningiomas, in contrast, are seen more in females. As with any classification system, the categories shown in Table 10.2 divide a spectrum of biologic findings into arbitrary units. For example, the implication of terms such as benign and malignant is not always clear-cut. A large benign tumor (e.g., an acoustic tumor, or properly, a vestibular schwannoma) pressing against vital brainstem structures can lead to serious medical problems, even death. On the other hand, a small malignant tumor (e.g., and astrocytoma), although highly invasive, initially may not interfere with neuron function and temporarily may escape detection. The actual impact of tumor type on brain function is dependent on many factors, such as invasiveness, size, location, and rate of growth. Also, tumors may evolve from benign to malignant. In assessment of auditory function, it is important to keep in mind the patients with brain tumors rarely have subjective auditory complaints. Clinical evidence of auditory abnormality generally is increasingly subtle as the level of the tumor is more rostral (toward the cerebral cortex). For most auditory tests, depressed performance is found for the ear contralateral to the side of the lesion. General clinical signs of cerebral tumors affecting the auditory regions (temporal cortex) include hemiparesis, personality abnormalities, memory impairment, auditory hallucinations, and seizures (a frequent finding). Tumors in the brainstem may produce clinical signs, such as abnormal corneal reflex, nystagmus, dizziness, cranial nerve deficits (e.g., facial paralysis), ataxia, diminished gag and cough reflexes, movement abnormalities, and hemiparesis. In this chapter, detailed information is presented mostly for those intracranial neoplasms that have been reported in the ABR literature.

Types of Retrocochlear Tumors

Supporting neuroglia tissue covers the bundle of fibers making up the eighth nerve near the CNS, specifically the pons in the brainstem. Distal to the pia mater (away from the brainstem), in the vicinity of the porus acusticus, Schwann cells replace the neuroglia and surround the nerve until it reaches the cochlea. The three major types of tumors involving the eighth cranial nerve are schwannomas, neurofibromas, and meningiomas. Other pathologies are also found in the region of the CP angle, including dermoid tumors, arteriorvenous malformations, vascular loops, and others (e.g., Hirsch et al., 1996; Schwaber & Hall, 1992).

VESTIBULAR SCHWANNOMAS. | Vestibular schwannomas are most often found on the eighth cranial nerve, and less often on the fifth, seventh, or twelfth cranial nerves. The estimated incidence of symptomatic vestibular schwannomas in the general population is 1:100,000. Interestingly, however, the prevalence of vestibular schwannomas as documented at autopsy may be as high as 900 in 100,000, or about 9 per 1000 persons (e.g., NIH Consensus Panel, 1993). The terms *acous-*

tic neuroma, acoustic neurinoma, and *acoustic neurilemoma,* frequently used interchangeably with vestibular schwannoma involving the eighth cranial nerve, are in fact inaccurate in two ways. The tumor usually arises from Schwann cells on one of the vestibular portions of the eighth nerve (superior or inferior), not the nerve ("neur-" or "neuro-") fibers of the auditory ("acoustic") portion, as the vernacular would imply. The relation of the superior and inferior vestibular nerves to the auditory and facial nerves within the internal auditory canal is shown schematically in Figure 10.1. About 70 to 80 percent of CPA (cerebellopontine angle) neoplasms are vestibular schwannomas. These constitute approximately 5 to 10 percent of intracranial neoplasms and are the third-ranking type of intracranial tumor. Gliomas and meningiomas rank first and second, respectively. Almost always unilateral (95 percent of cases), vestibular schwannomas are found most often in middle age (the highest proportion between ages 35 and 60 years) and are twice as common in females as in males. The schwannoma of the eighth nerve is considered benign. It usually arises from a focal point within the nerve trunk of the peripheral portion of one of the two vestibular branches of the nerve (superior or inferior), either within the internal auditory canal (intracanalicular) or outside it. The tumor is an encapsulated, homogeneous mass projecting from the side of the nerve as depicted in Figure 10.1. The vestibular schwannoma typically grows to displace, deform, and/or stretch the normal auditory nerve fibers, which may eventually be compressed into a thin ribbon. A vestibular schwannoma can erode the walls of the internal ear canal and increase the size of the canal lumen. The easiest route for expansion is toward the CP angle. Once in the CP angle, the tumor can grow to rather large proportions. At this stage, the tumor consists of a stalk (within the canal) attached to a mass (in the CP angle). Eighth-nerve tumors grow slowly and sometimes stop growing spontaneously. However, in some patients, the tumor may over the course of years become sizable (greater than 4 to 5 cm in diameter). At the extreme, the tumor may compress and distort other cranial nerves (e.g., the seventh [facial] and/or fifth [trigeminal]), may produce a contralateral shift of the brainstem, and may even compress the fourth ventricle. Compression of the fourth ventricle results in elevation of intracranial pressure and may produce hydrocephalus.

In addition to compressive effects of the eighth-nerve tumor, symptoms may be due to compromise of the blood supply to the nerve or inner ear or to interruption of cochlear fluid flow. Clinical symptoms first occur after progressive growth of the tumor, when the tumor is 1 to 4 cm in size. Interestingly, symptoms described in the early literature on eighth-nerve tumors were more pronounced (ataxia, headache, papilledema) because the tumors tended to be detected later when they were larger. According to some reports (Hart & Davenport, 1981; Hart, Gardner, & Howieson, 1983; Portmann, Dauman, Duriez, Portmann, & Dhillon, 1989), the approximate distribution of initial symptoms in patients with eighth nerve tumors is as follows: hearing loss in 53 to 85 percent; headache in 0 to 20 percent; imbalance/dizziness in 4 to 7 percent; unsteady gait in 0 to 8 percent; tinnitus in 0 to 18 percent; and facial paresthesia in 0 to 2 percent. Tinnitus usually accompanies hearing loss, but it may initially be the only symptom. A frequently mentioned first complaint is difficulty hearing over the telephone. Although a vestibular portion of eighth nerve is the origin of these tumors, balance problems are not among the earliest or most pronounced symptoms at diagnosis is somewhat different. On the other hand, there are almost always hearing complaints (97 to 100 percent of patients) and some unsteadiness is typical.

NEUROFIBROMAS. | In the otolaryngology literature, neurofibromatosis was at one time referred to as simply von Recklinghausen's disease. In 1882, a German physician, Friedrich von Recklinghausen, first described in five patients a specific collection of signs and symptoms, among them café au lait spots (a skin blemish having, literally, the color of coffee with milk), cutaneous neurofibromas, tumors within the CNS, mental retardation, and skeletal abnormalities. The disease is now referred to as either neurofibromatosis (NF) 1, peripheral form, or as NF2, a central form. An important point for the present discussion is that bilateral eighth-nerve

Internal Auditory Canal

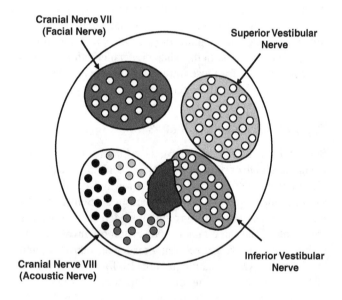

FIGURE 10.1. Major neural structures within the internal auditory canal (IAC), including the superior and inferior vestibular nerves that give rise to vestibular schwannomas, i.e., "acoustic tumors." A vestibular schwannoma is shown arising from the inferior vestibular nerve and impinging on the auditory nerve.

pathology may be a feature of both of these clinical entities, although it is far more likely with NF2.

Both types of neurofibromatosis are genetically transferred and autosomal dominant. However, the gene for NF1 is on chromosome 17, and the gene for NF2 is on chromosome 22 (Lanser, Sussman, & Frazer, 1992). NF1 is, however, much more common than NF2. A prevalence estimate, for example, is 60 out of 100,000 for NF1 and only 0.1 per 1000,000 for NF2. For NF1, the age of onset is often within the first decade after birth, whereas the NF2 type of disease does not appear until the second or third decade. More than one café au lait spot is found in 94 percent of patients with NF1 and less than one-half this portion (42%) in patients with NF2. Moreover, three-fourths of patients with NF1 will have more than six café au lait spots, as opposed to no patients (0 percent) with NF2. Importantly, eighth-nerve tumors are found in only 5 percent of NF1 patients but in over 95 percent of those with NF2. Therefore, although bilateral tumors are often considered a characteristic feature of what was formerly called von Recklinghausen disease (now properly categorized as peripheral neurofibromatosis or NF1), they are in fact commonly associated with the central type of neurofibromatosis (NF2). Both types of neurofibromatosis affecting the eighth cranial nerve arise from Schwann cells. The development of unilateral tumors in NF1 is similar to that of the eighth-nerve schwannomas described previously. Bilateral tumors, in contrast, develop as a multilobulated mass, with the auditory (eighth) and facial (seventh) cranial nerves coursing through, rather than around, the tumor. That is, unilateral tumors displace the nerves (Baldwin & LeMaster 1989). Also, bilateral tumors, unlike schwannomas, are not encapsulated, although they are usually well defined.

In general, hearing impairment is found in over 90 percent of patients with neurofibromatosis, and it may be the initial complaint in 50 percent. The degree of hearing impairment associated with neurofibromas is typically less a function of tumor size than is impairment with unilateral schwannomas, probably because of a different relation between the tumor and the nerve. Also, hearing deficits may be due to lesions within either the peripheral auditory system (eighth-nerve pathology) or the central auditory nervous system. Thus, normal air-conduction hearing thresholds and good word-recognition scores in conditions of quiet (implying peripheral integrity) do not necessarily rule out auditory system involvement. Patients with bilateral eighth-nerve tumors present some rather unusual diagnostic and rehabilitation challenges. Because the tumor infiltrates, rather then compresses, the eighth nerve, there may be less pronounced retrocochlear auditory findings initially when the tumor is small. This feature of the tumor also seriously limits the possibility for hearing preservation during surgical removal of tumors, and it increases the importance of intraoperative monitoring with ECochG and ABR (discussed in Chapter 5 and later in this chapter). Detection of bilateral neurofibromas by comparing ABR latency values between ears, such as the interear latency difference (ILD)

for wave V or for the wave I–V interval, is not necessarily a sensitive strategy for detection of the tumors. In fact, ABR abnormalities are likely to be bilateral. Because neurofibromatosis has its onset in young adulthood (usually in the productive period of life), it can produce a precipitous, profound, and often devastating communication disorder. Auditory assessment, including otoacoustic emissions and the ABR, can contribute not only to early identification and description of the neuropathology, but also lead to the audiologic rehabilitation process that these patients unfortunately often require. Neurofibromatosis often takes a progressive, disabling, and disfiguring course, with subsequent emotional consequences in addition to the auditory and neurological features.

MENINGIOMAS. | Meningiomas are found in various intracranial regions, although certain sites are more common. Meningiomas are more common in females than males, and usually appear later in life. The tumors originate from meningothelial arachnoid cells, and are often attached to the dura. Typically, they have a rubbery consistency, are distinct from the brain, and are slow growing. Tumor size at discovery is related to location. That is, very large tumors may develop in regions of the brain that do not readily produce clinical symptoms. The meningioma's relationship to the dura leads to one of the following classifications: sessile (broad attachment to dura), pedunculated (flat), and no dural attachment (often located within the lateral ventricles). Over 90 percent of meningiomas are found in the supratentorial compartment, and more than 67 percent are in the anterior half of the cranium. Among posterior fossa meningiomas, more than half are found either within the cerebellum or within the CP angle. Meningiomas involving the eighth nerve are sometimes difficult to distinguish from schwannomas. Meningiomas are almost always (98 to 99 percent of the time) found singly. Because they may originate and grow exclusively within the CP angle (as opposed to within the internal auditory canal), meningiomas may produce relatively subtle audiometric signs. In the author's experience, for example, patients may have symmetrical audiograms and may evidence abnormality only with diagnostic screening procedures, such as acoustic reflex decay or word-recognition rollover. With involvement of the auditory system, however, ABR findings are unequivocally abnormal.

ABR Findings in Retrocochlear Tumors

Soon after the discovery of the ABR, in the mid-to-late 1970s, numerous investigators reported clinical data and experience with ABR in identification of eighth-nerve and/or CP-angle tumors. The earliest clinical investigations of ABR in retrocochlear pathology were cited in Chapter 1. Neuroradiologic techniques at the time were quite limited and certainly not sensitive to abnormal growths of tissue and mass lesions. CT scans were not yet a clinical option, and MRI was not yet discovered. As measurement of the ABR became available clinically, usually in major medical centers and university settings, its diagnostic value in the early detection of retrocochlear pathology was readily apparent. Publications describing neurodiagnostic ABR findings soon followed. Although the titles of the papers in the early literature often describe the pathology as "acoustic tumor" or "CP angle tumor," rarely are data reported only for a single type of tumor. Indeed, not all tumors originating from the eighth nerve expand into the CP angle; conversely, not all tumors in the CP angle arise from the eighth nerve. The most common eighth-nerve and CP-angle mass is the vestibular schwannoma, accounting for anywhere from 75 to 90 percent of the tumors in this anatomic region. The second-ranking tumor type, the meningioma, is found in 2 to 10 percent of patients. In a typical unselected series of twenty-five to thirty patients with retrocochlear neoplasms, therefore, perhaps twenty or twenty-one will have vestibular nerve schwannomas, and the remainder will have meningiomas, neurofibromas, or infrequently, miscellaneous tumor types such as lymphomas, gliomas, hemangioblastomas, chordomas, and dermoid tumors.

ABR developed a well-deserved reputation as a sensitive measure of retrocochlear function, that is, one capable of detecting a huge proportion of cases, yielding few false-negative findings. Over 90 percent of surgically confirmed eighth-nerve or CP-angle tumors were identified on the basis of ABR abnormalities, and often reported "hit rates" were as high as 96 to 100 percent. The strength of ABR within the diagnostic audiology test battery in the pre-CT era was clearly evident when findings for patients with retrocochlear versus cochlear auditory dysfunction were compared with those for other more conventional "site-of-lesion" procedures, as seen in Table 10.3. In retrospect, the early claims of apparently high sensitivity of the ABR in the detection of retrocochlear

pathology were somewhat misleading. Because neuroradiologic technology available in the 1970s was rather crude, it is likely that few of the patients with confirmed retrocochlear pathology had small tumors. The high proportion of abnormal ABR findings in patients with retrocochlear pathology was probably a function of the size of tumors, and not the sensitivity of the procedure. As reviewed later in this section, as MRI became the "gold standard" for acoustic tumors, the hit rate for ABR in retrocochlear pathology dropped rather sharply. Also, clinical researchers became more aware of concerns about the false-positive rate for ABR in retrocochlear pathology, reported as anywhere from 10 to 33 percent (see Legatt, Pedley, Emerson, Stein, & Abramson, 1988 for review). A false-positive ABR outcome, in this context, is an abnormal ABR that is suggestive of retrocochlear pathology. Instead, the patient may have some other auditory dysfunction, such as a sensory (cochlear) hearing impairment. False-positive errors are troublesome because most patients with sensorineural hearing loss undergoing neurodiagnostic actually have sensory, rather than neural, auditory dysfunction. Even a modest false-positive rate in the differentiation of cochlear versus neural auditory dysfunction, therefore, affects a large number of patients, with corresponding increases in medical costs and patient anxiety.

Many studies evaluate ABR criteria for differentiation of cochlear versus eighth-nerve lesions and factors influencing ABR findings in retrocochlear pathology. Some investigators attempt to correlate ABR findings to tumor size or to radiologic findings, such as CT (computerized tomography) or MRI (magnetic resonance imaging). Often in the literature, the diagnostic power of ABR is compared with that of ECochG or other audiometric procedures (acoustic reflex and traditional

TABLE 10.3. Meta-analysis of Early Published Data Showing the Relation between Traditional Diagnostic Audiology "Site-of-Lesion" Procedures and the Auditory Brainstem Response (ABR) in Detection of Eighth Cranial Nerve (Acoustic) Tumors

Data were collected and analyzed by the author.

PROCEDURE	EIGHTH-NERVE DISORDER		COCHLEAR DISORDER	
	N	%	N	%
Short increment sensitivity index (SISI)	720	64	696	92
Tone decay*	737	64	2069	91
Alternate binaural loudness balance (ABLB)	620	68	1067	90
Phonetically balance word recognition**	737	69	250	60
Supra-threshold adaptation test (STAT)	20	70	75	83
Békèsy threshold tracing test	44	84	327	96
Békèsy comfortable loudness (BCL) test	16	80	101	97
Acoustic reflex measures***	126	85	218	84
Auditory brainstem response (wave V IAD)	*292*	*96*	*793*	*88*

* Tone decay data were combined for Carhart, Rosenberg, and Olsen/Noffsinger procedures.

** Abnormal findings for either maximum score (PBmax) or rollover.

*** Abnormal findings for acoustic reflex threshold and/or decay.

From Hall & Mueller, 1997.

diagnostic audiometry test procedures). Much research attention has been directed to the relative sensitivity (i.e., ability to detect a specific disorder and to avoid false-negative findings) and specificity (i.e., ability of avoid false-positive findings) of these various auditory measures. The influence of subject characteristics—such as age, gender, and degree of hearing loss—on ABR interpretation is also emphasized in the literature.

INDICATIONS FOR A NEURODIAGNOSTIC ABR. | A fundamental question to ask at the outset of a discussion of ABR in retrocochlear pathology is: What audiologic or medical signs, symptoms, or factors prompt a referral for neurodiagnostic ABR? Symptoms typically cited as "red flags" for possible retrocochlear pathology are:

- Unilateral or unexplained asymmetrical tinnitus
- Asymmetrical (unequal) audiometric findings, including:
  - Hearing thresholds by pure-tone audiometry
  - Maximum word recognition scores or rollover in performance
  - Acoustic reflex thresholds or decay
- Vertigo or unilateral vestibular findings (e.g., by ENG)
- Certain neurological findings, particularly involving cranial nerve function (e.g., facial nerve paresis)

There are no official or widely accepted guidelines as to exactly what constitutes "unequal hearing thresholds," in terms of both the degree of difference in hearing between ears and the number of test frequencies that must be involved in the asymmetry. Some evidence exists, however, for hearing threshold differences that should prompt a referral for neurodiagnostic assessment. Mangham (1991) addressed the issue of how much difference in pure-tone thresholds between ears puts a patient at risk for an acoustic tumor. Subjects were 210 patients with surgically confirmed unilateral acoustic tumors and a control group of 112 patients. Asymmetry was calculated by subtracting the hearing thresholds of the "non-suspect ear" from those of the "suspect ear." Effectiveness of pure-tone hearing threshold asymmetry varied among test frequencies. The rank order of effectiveness of threshold difference in referral for diagnostic assessment as a function of test frequency was 2000 Hz, 4000 Hz, 1000 Hz, 8000 Hz, 500 Hz, and 250 Hz. The authors describe as the most effective strategy for referral for neurodiagnostic assessment (MRI in this study) an average threshold difference of ≥ 20 dB for the 1000 to 8000 Hz region of the audiogram. The pure-tone threshold criterion warranting a referral for an ABR was an average threshold of 5 to 20 dB. Magdziarz, Wiet, Dinces, and Adamiec (2000) also examined audiologic findings in patients with confirmed acoustic tumors. Data for pure-tone and speech audiometry were reported for 369 patients. The authors conclude "a high level of suspicion appears warranted in any case involving unexplained unilateral audiovestibular symptoms . . ." (Magdziarz et al., 2000, p. 157).

The literature suggests that sudden onset of unilateral sensorineural hearing loss also should be considered a risk indicator for retrocochlear auditory pathology and, therefore, justification for a neurodiagnostic ABR (e.g., Chaimoff et al., 1999). In making a decision about the need for an ABR from audiologic test results, the author's long-standing motto and recommendation to beginning clinicians is simply: "When in doubt, refer out!" Strategies for recording the ABR from patients with suspected retrocochlear auditory pathology are summarized in Table 10.4. The sensitivity of ABR

TABLE 10.4. Summary of Techniques and Strategies for Assessment of Retrocochlear Auditory Function with a Neurodiagnostic ABR

The goal is differentiation of sensory versus neural auditory dysfunction in a patient with an asymmetric hearing loss.

- Obtain and analyze audiogram and aural immittance results to rule out middle ear dysfunction and conductive hearing loss component for either ear. Determine suspect ear, if possible. Determine the appropriate inverting electrode design for detection of the ABR wave I component (e.g., TIPtrode with mild hearing loss or tympanic electrode with a moderate hearing loss).
- Ready equipment, instruct and prepare patient.
- Apply ECochG and ABR electrodes, verify impedance (reapply electrodes as indicated above).
- Place transducers (insert earphones) and verify that electrodes and earphones are on the correct side.
- Record an ABR with high-intensity (70 to 90 dB nHL) click stimuli presented at a rate of approximately 21.1/sec. Identify waves I, II, III, and V. Calculate absolute and interwave latency values, analysis symmetry, and compare to normative data.
  - If hearing sensitivity in the 1000 to 4000 Hz region is asymmetric (greater than 10 dB difference between ears), record ABR for several stimulus intensity levels over a 20 to 30 dB range for the better hearing ear or for both ears. Compare interear latency values at equivalent sensation levels (SLs) according to guidelines displayed in Table 7.2 (Jerger & Johnson, 1988).
  - If waves I, II, III and V are not clearly identified, follow guidelines for waveform enhancement described in Chapter 7 on troubleshooting.
- Record replicated ABR as above but at a very rapid stimulus rate (91.1/sec). Identify and calculate latency for wave V. Compare absolute and interaural wave V latency values to normative data.
- Before the data collection is completed and the patient is disconnected, verify that the ABR waveforms are replicable and major wave components are confidently identified.
- Calculate interwave latency values and compare to normative data.
- Calculate interaural latency values and compare to normative data.
- Plot out replicated waveforms with appropriate labels for ear, stimulus level, and location of peaks. Prepare a chart note and/or report.

to retrocochlear pathology and the likelihood of detecting a clear waveform for confident analysis will be enhanced by adherence to these simple guidelines. The next sections of the chapter offer a review of common approaches for analysis of the ABR in retrocochlear pathology.

ABR LATENCY CRITERIA IN RETROCOCHLEAR PATHOLOGY. | Retrocochlear pathology almost always alters ABR waveforms. Regardless of the analysis criteria employed, early studies showed that ABR was abnormal in over 95 percent of a typical series of patients with eighth-nerve and/or CP-angle pathology (specifically tumors). As CT and later MRI technology was introduced clinically, the "hit-rate" of the ABR in retrocochlear pathology declined. Possible ABR findings in retrocochlear pathology range for an entirely normal response to no detected response, even at maximum stimulus intensity levels. Absence of a response is not directly related to degree of hearing impairment, and it may occur in patients with eighth-nerve pathology causing little or no deficit in hearing sensitivity. Therefore, absence of an ABR in combination with normal hearing, or at most a mild or moderate sensorineural hearing impairment, is pathogomonic of eighth-nerve (neural) auditory dysfunction and not consistent with cochlear (sensory) dysfunction. Interestingly, acoustic tumors may present in patients with sudden onset of hearing loss. Chaimoff et al. (1999) reported that nineteen of forty patients (47.5 percent) evaluated for sudden sensorineural hearing loss had a tumor in the CP angle. The ABR is noncontributory to the diagnosis of retrocochlear pathology for patients with severe-to-profound hearing loss, as even sensory hearing loss of that degree will preclude the detection of an ABR. The finding of an absent ABR is highly variable, and in unselected groups of patients with eighth-nerve tumors, it may occur in as few as 15 percent of patients and up to as many as 75 percent (Barrs, Brackmann, Olson, & House, 1985; Cashman & Rossman, 1983; Clemis & McGee, 1979; Kusakari et al., 1981; Musiek, Josey, & Glasscock, 1986; Olsen & Harner, 1983; Prosser, Arslan, & Pastore 1984; Rosenhall, 1981a,b; Terkildsen, Osterhammel, & Thomsen, 1981). Lack of detectable ABR however, commonly occurs in patients with large tumors.

Before interpreting an absent response as consistent with eighth-nerve pathology, one must exclude the possibility of a conductive component to the hearing impairment—that is, a mixed hearing loss (conductive and sensory hearing loss in combination). A conductive hearing component is ruled out with an otologic examination, aural immittance measurements, and pure-tone (air- vs. bone-conduction) audiometry. Also, a valid finding of an absent response presumes that there were no technical or measurement errors. Naturally, absence of an ABR precludes analysis of latency or amplitude parameters. Differentiation of a normal versus an abnormal ABR is based most often on analysis of the latency of major waves. Examples of ABR abnormalities in retrocochlear pathology are illustrated in Figure 10.2. Traditionally,

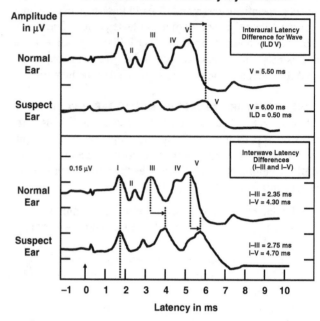

Techniques and Criteria for Analysis of ABR in Retrocochlear Auditory Dysfunction

FIGURE 10.2. ABR waveforms in retrocochlear auditory dysfunction illustrating major techniques for latency analysis, including the interaural latency difference (ILD) and the wave I–V latency interval.

four latency criteria for retrocochlear pathology were employed (Clemis & McGee, 1979; Clemis & Mitchell; 1977; Daly, et al., 1977; Rosenhamer, 1977; Selters & Brackmann, 1977; Sohmer, Feinmesser, & Szabo, 1974; Terkildsen, Huis in't Veld, & Osterhammel, 1977; Thomsen, Terkildsen, & Osterhammel, 1978). These include:

- Absolute latency of wave V exceeds some clinical definition for normal limits, such as 2.5 standard deviations above normal mean latency for a laboratory, or it is greater than a fixed absolute normal latency value, such as 6.2 ms.
- There is an abnormal ILD (interear or interaural latency difference) for wave V. That is, wave V latency is greater when the suspected side (ear) of pathology is stimulated than on the opposite ear. The definition for an abnormal ILD is usually a value of greater than 0.40 ms, but some authors recommend values of greater than 0.30 or 0.20 ms. Lower values for criteria for an abnormal ILD, e.g., 0.20 ms instead of 0.40 ms, will result in higher ABR sensitivity to retrocochlear auditory dysfunction. The trade-off, however, is a distinct increase in false-positive outcomes, that is, reduced specifity (apparent retrocochlear finding in a patient with cochlear auditory dysfunction). Analysis of the ILD may be made with or without a correction of wave V latency for hearing sensitivity loss. As a rule, correction factors are not advisable as there is the possibility an

abnormal ABR will be overcorrected and interpreted as normal.

- The wave I–V latency value is abnormally prolonged, relative to clinical normative data. Sometimes, the wave I–III latency intervals are also analyzed.
- There is an abnormal ILD for the I–V latency interval (and perhaps for wave I–III and wave III–V intervals.

These criteria involve either a comparison of ABR latency for the patient versus group normative data, or an intrasubject comparison of interwave latencies from one ear versus the other ear.

Each latency criterion is clinically useful, but each also has clinical limitations. One weakness shared by all of these criteria, and rarely noted in the literature, is the assumption that wave components recorded from patients with eighth-nerve pathology can be consistently identified correctly and confidently and, furthermore, that latency values for each ABR wave can be precisely calculated. This assumption is not supported by clinical experience. Eighth-nerve tumors often markedly distort waveform morphology, rendering confident identification and individual wave components very difficult and accurate calculation of latency sometimes impossible (Musiek, Josey, & Glasscock (1986). For example, Musiek, Josey, & Glasscock (1986) noted that eighteen of sixty-one patients with eighth-nerve or CP angle tumors had no reliable waves, and the ABR for another twenty-seven (44 percent of total group) was characterized by presence of only one or two major waves.

Poor ABR morphology may also confound identification of wave components for pure cochlear pathology (Bauch & Olsen, 1986, 1989; Bauch, Rose, & Harner, 1982), especially when the hearing loss in the 3000 or 4000 Hz region approaches or exceeds 75 dB HL. There is no doubt in these cases that the ABR is grossly abnormal. However, it is misleading and really inappropriate to proceed with a formal analysis of latency and amplitude parameters, followed by rigid adherence to certain latency criteria for interpretation. The first step toward accurate interpretation of any AER waveform is manipulation of measurement parameters during data collection in order to optimize the quality of the response. The next step is to ensure response reliability (replicability) before analysis (see Chapter 7 for a discussion of ABR analysis techniques).

ABR WAVE V ILD. | The difficulties associated with analyzing either absolute or interwave latency values for a patient in the context of group normative data were recognized in early clinical investigations of ABR in eighth-nerve pathology. Recognition of the limitations led to the practice of comparing latency differences between ears for a patient. A scattergram for the distribution of interwave latency differences for ABR wave V is illustrated in Figure 10.3. Using the patient essentially as her or his own control obviously eliminates the possible influence of certain subject factors, such as age, gen-

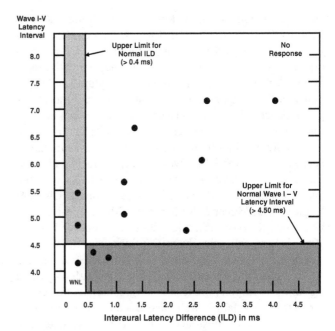

FIGURE 10.3. Scattergram distribution of ABR interaural latency difference (ILDs) intervals for wave V and wave I–V latency intervals in a series of patients with confirmed acoustic tumors.
Adapted from Eggermont, J. J., Don, M., & Brackmann, D. E. (1980). Electrocochleography and auditory brainstem responses in patients with pontine angle tumors. *Annals of Otology, Rhinology & Laryngology, 89,* 1–19. Copyright © 1980 Annals Publishing Company.

der, and body temperature. Still, normative data, or expectations, are required to evaluate the significance of interear differences. ABR latency values for equivalent right- and left-ear stimulation are typically rather symmetrical, but it is necessary to define the normal limits for an ear difference.

The difference for absolute latency of wave V with stimulation of the ear on the involved side (with suspected retrocochlear pathology) versus the uninvolved side—the ILD for wave V—was the ABR criterion used most often by early investigators of ABR, and clinicians apply ABR in neurodiagnosis. This index is also referred to as "interaural time for wave V," or "IT." In one of the earliest papers on ABR in detection of eighth-nerve pathology, Selters and Brackmann (1977) noted that for a group of twenty normal hearers, the ILD for wave V latency was between 0 and 0.20 ms for the two remaining subjects. (Note: This original article actually contains a critical error in this passage [on p. 182], stating that the interear difference was 2.0 ms for these two subjects. The authors' subsequent reference to these data indicates that they meant to state 0.2 ms).

Many other researchers cited in clinical reports a wave V ILD criterion of either 0.30 ms or 0.40 ms (e.g., Bauch & Olsen, 1989; Cashman & Rossman, 1983; Clemis & McGee, 1979; Eggermont, Don, & Brackmann, 1980; Hyde & Blair,

1981; Josey, Glasscock, & Musiek, 1988; Telian, Kileny, Niparko, Kemink, & Graham, 1989; Terkildsen, Osterhammel, & Thomsen, 1981; Thomsen, Terklidsen, & Osterhammel, 1978). In generating interaural latency normative data, it is important to ensure interaural equality in stimulus parameters (intensity, rate, polarity, duration) and transducer performance. The same transducer (earphone) can be used for testing each ear to further optimize equivalent interaural test conditions. In a high proportion of cases with eighth-nerve tumors (over 90%), wave V latency for the affected ear exceeds the latency value of the opposite ear by more than 0.3 or 0.4 msec (Bauch & Olsen, 1989; Bauch, Olsen, & Harner, 1983; Møller & Møller, 1983; Musiek, 1982; Musiek, Josey, & Glasscock, 1986; Prosser, Arslan, & Pastore, 1984; Selters & Brackmann, 1977; Stürzebecher, Werbs, & Kevanishvili, 1985; Terkildsen, Osterhammel, & Thomsen, 1981). Actually, for the majority of patients with confirmed eighth-nerve tumors, the ILD is far greater than this cutoff for abnormality, falling well beyond a commonly used cutoff of 0.40 ms, as illustrated in Figure 10.3. An interaural prolongation of the wave V latency for the involved ear of over 1.0 ms, or even total absence of the wave V component, is not uncommon in patients with eighth nerve tumors. In their pioneering article about neurodiagnostic ABR in retrocochlear pathology, Selters and Brackmann (1977) reported that a wave V could not be detected in 43 percent of a series of 46 patients with CP-angle tumors. This observation is supported by data reported by Bauch and Olsen (1989). These authors evaluated ABR findings for 88 patients with confirmed eighth-nerve tumors, but only 36 (41 percent) had repeatable wave V components bilaterally. Other investigators report that well over half of tumor patients characteristically have no apparent wave V (Eggermont, Don, & Brackmann, 1980; Rosenhall, 1981a, b). One very important factor contributing the likelihood of wave V presence versus absence is, of course, the degree of hearing sensitivity deficit in the 1000 to 4000 Hz region. This factor is discussed later in this chapter. In general, however, the wave V ILD (IT) is a very sensitive measure of eighth-nerve pathology. This is because the definition of abnormality is made on the basis of an intrasubject, as opposed to intersubject, comparison. Again, the patient is used as his or her own control, eliminating the possible influence of subject characteristics (e.g., age, gender, and body temperature) as sources of variability in ABR data.

There are, however, other problems associated with reliance on only the interaural wave V latency difference. That is, not all test variables are accounted for by the interaural latency comparison approach. Concomitant unilateral middle ear or cochlear dysfunction, unrelated to eighth-nerve pathology, can confound analysis of interaural latency differences. Patients with sensorineural hearing loss and suspected retocochlear pathology may, in fact, have diverse etiologies. According to data for 229 nontumor patients reported by Bauch, Rose, and Harner (1982), most common diagnoses include sensorineural loss of undetermined etiology (39%), Ménière's disease (14%), cochlear otosclerosis (6%), and labyrinthitis (3%), although nine other causes were also listed. The distribution of etiologies will naturally vary among ABR test facilities.

Different types of otopathology are not mutually exclusive. If unrelated auditory dysfunction is on the suspected side (the ear ipsilateral to the suspected eighth-nerve lesion), the ILD will be spuriously enhanced. On the other hand, when ABR of delayed latency due to eighth-nerve pathology is compared to the opposite ear, which has unrelated auditory dysfunction, the ILD may be minimal and within normal expectations. Lack of an ILD may also be a function of the size of a tumor, as discussed in some detail later in this chapter. Briefly, very large tumors may produce ABR abnormalities with stimulation of the contralateral ear, as well as the ipsilateral ear (e.g., Deans, Birchall, & Mendelow, 1990; Hall, 1992), a combination of abnormalities may actually result in a deceptively reduced (more normal) ILD. This complicating effect of a large tumor on interaural comparisons applies to both the absolute wave V latency and the wave I–V latency interval.

The main problem with relying on the absolute latency of wave V is the possible confounding influence of middle ear or cochlear pathology on interpretation of the ABR. An auditory abnormality distal (peripheral) to the eighth-nerve may produce an absolute latency delay that is incorrectly attributed to the suspected eighth-nerve pathology. Clinically, it is not uncommon to apply ABR for identification of retrocochlear pathology in patients with one or more multiple unrelated otologic pathologies (and hearing deficits), such a presbycusis or hearing impairment that is noise or drug induced (Musiek, 1982). Prolonged ABR latency values are a typical finding in conductive hearing impairment. Thus, an abnormal ABR wave V ILD may be due to a relatively common disease entity, such as otitis media or otosclerosis, in addition to retrocochlear pathology. The potential influence of cochlear pathology on interpretation of absolute wave V latency is not always as obvious and straightforward. A severe high-frequency sensorineural hearing impairment that involves a cochlea (e.g., due to presbycusis) can also produce wave V latency delay. In the case of presbycusis, however, the hearing impairment is bilateral. However, one form of presbycusis involves neural dysfunction that is age-related, and not secondary to a neoplasm. Thus, a delay in wave V for one ear cannot confidently and consistently be attributed to an eighth-nerve tumor until conductive and severe sensory auditory dysfunction is first ruled out.

Comparison of an absolute latency value (or an interwave latency value) for a patient versus for group normative data is a common analysis technique, but it too can be problematic. All group data are statistically variable. The upper limit for normal latency values must be defined. Usually, the definition is based on simple statistics, such as latency value that is 2.5 or 3.0 standard deviations above the average value, or above the 95th percentile, for a group of audiologically and neurologically normal adults. As noted in Chapter 7, these normative data are gathered by most clinical facilities for a relatively small number of subjects, with the equipment and usual test protocol for the facility. However, reliance on any group normative data for ABR latency interpretation in retrocochlear pathology is complicated by the influence of a variety of subject related factors (especially gender), as noted earlier, and hearing loss unrelated to the pathology. It is perhaps appropriate to begin analyzing ABRs with reference to large-scale published normative databases, that is, normative standards collected with carefully defined test protocols from samples of hundreds of even thousands of subjects.

ABR INTERWAVE LATENCIES. | Coats (1978) was among the first to point out that some of the problems inherent to absolute ABR latency analysis appear to be resolved by the us of interwave latency values. Interwave latency intervals are sometimes abbreviated as "IWIs." The practice of interwave latency analysis is based on the assumption that replicable waves I and V, and also perhaps III, are recorded and identified clearly in the ABR waveform. However, with typical ABR recording techniques, not all patients with retrocochlear pathology meet this minimal requirement. For example, Musiek, Josey, and Glasscock (1986) reported that only sixteen of sixty-one patients (26%) showed wave I, wave III, and wave V in two ABR averages under the same stimulus conditions. Cashman and Rossman (1983) found only five of thirty-five tumor patients (14 percent) met those interwave criteria. Note that these studies were reported more than twenty years ago. The likelihood of detecting reliable waves I and V is considerably higher when an ABR is recorded with current electrode designs (e.g., a TIPtrode or tympanic membrane electrode) with a maximum stimulus intensity level of 95 to 100 dB nHL.

The I–V latency interval is often referred to as a reflection of "brainstem transmission time" or "central conduction time" (e.g., Brackmann, 1984; Fabiani, Sohmer, Tait, Gafni, & Kinarti, 1979; Sohmer, Kinarti, & Gafni, 1981) implying that it, unlike absolute latency measures, is not subject to influences of middle ear and cochlear pathology. Certainly, the wave I–V interval is less affected by these disorders and more consistently related to brainstem function than is the absolute latency for wave V. In this respect, it is preferable for identification of eighth-nerve pathology. In particular, an interaural comparison of the wave I–V latency value can reduce the likelihood of false-positive interpretation error (Zöllner & Eibach, 1981a,b). Figure 10.3 depicted a scattergram for the distribution of ABR wave I –V (interwave) latencies in patients with acoustic tumors. The ABR wave I–V latency interval, however, is not a pure measure

of brainstem transmission time. Alterations in the wave I–V latency value clearly can be associated with conductive or cochlear auditory dysfunction. For example, high-frequency hearing impairment may produce a delay in wave I latency without a corresponding prolongation of wave V. This results in a slightly shortened wave I–V latency interval. The term "brainstem transmission time" is, therefore, misleading and not entirely accurate. False-negative findings, although exceptionally rare for this ABR application, are attributed to reliance on the wave I–V latency normative criterion (Feblot & Uziel, 1982). Failure to recognize the possible influence of auditory sensitivity status on the wave I–V interval is likely to increase the chance of errors in interpretation in some patients.

Another clinical limitation is shared by each of the traditional latency criteria. The wave V and wave I–V latency measures are both dependent on brainstem integrity, at least at the level of the pons and probably also to more rostral brainstem regions (the lateral lemniscus and perhaps the level of the inferior colliculus). By analysis of wave V or the wave I–V latency interval, eighth-nerve pathology cannot be consistently distinguished from other types of pathology involving brainstem auditory structures, such as vascular disease, MS (multiple sclerosis), or intra-axial brainstem neoplasms. Robinson and Rudge (1983) conducted a thorough study with ABR, AMLR, and CT of ninety-two patients who were suspected of having a CP-angle tumor on initial presentation. Ultimately, sixty-four patients actually had tumors confirmed. For forty of these patients, the tumor was an eighth-nerve schwannoma. In the study by Robinson and Rudge (1983), auditory findings for patients with vascular lesions closely resembled those for the tumor group. ABR, in particular, was abnormal on the affected side for all vascular lesion patients. ABR findings in these patients were indistinguishable from findings for patients with eighth-nerve tumors. (Note: AER findings in brainstem and cerebral neuropathology are reviewed later in the next chapter.) One probable solution to this limitation of the overall I–V latency parameter is close analysis of more discrete latency intervals, such as wave I–III, wave III–V, or even the wave I–II latency interval. This technique is discussed next.

Perhaps the most reliable precise ABR criterion for identification of eighth-nerve pathology is the wave I–III latency interval (Antonelli, Bellotto, & Grandori, 1987; Eggermont, Don, & Brackmann, 1980; Feblot & Uziel, 1982; Maurer, Strumpel, & Wende, 1982; Møller & Møller, 1983, 1985; Musiek, Josey, & Glasscock, 1986). The anatomic presumption for relying on the wave I to II or the wave I to III latency interval is that wave I arises from the distal end of the nerve (at the cochlea), and wave II arises from the proximal end (near the brainstem). Maurer, Strumpel, and Wende (1982) found a prolongation of the wave I to II latency interval (and subsequent I–V interwave latency value) for seven out of thirty-seven patients with confirmed eighth-nerve pathology. Among those patients with an identifiable wave (N = 24), the wave I to II latency delay, therefore, occurred in 29 percent. On the basis of this finding, these investigators logically conclude that the lesion is intracanalicular (confined to within the internal auditory canal) and localized directly to the eighth nerve. Møller and Møller (1983) provide further evidence that wave I–II interval prolongation is the ABR signature of eighth-nerve tumors. Among a series of twenty-seven patients with surgically confirmed tumors, twenty-four (92%) showed a latency delay for wave II.

Later, Antonelli, Bellotto, and Grandori (1987) analyzed directly the accuracy of the wave I–II and I–III latency intervals in identification of eighth-nerve tumors. For all patients with detectable waves I and II, or waves I and III, the latency intervals were abnormally prolonged. The overall wave I–V latency interval was abnormally prolonged for 90 percent of the group of fifteen patients. Perhaps equally important, the wave I–II interval was also the most specific latency criterion for differentiating eighth-nerve versus pontine brainstem dysfunction. That is, the wave I–II interval was normal in 87.5 percent of patients with brainstem lesions, yet no eighth-nerve tumor. In comparison, the proportion of normal findings (true negative outcome for eighth-nerve tumors) in lower pons pathology was 0 percent for the wave I–V latency interval, 83 percent for the wave III–V latency interval, and 14.3 percent for the wave I–III latency interval. Unfortunately, with conventional recording techniques, wave II is often not clear even with audiologically and neurologically normal subjects. Methods that can be used to enhance ABR wave I and wave II are described in detail in Chapter 7. Furthermore, aside from these reports, few investigators appear to have specifically analyzed the effect of pathology on wave II.

The wave I–III and III–V latency intervals, in contrast, are now regularly scrutinized in ABR interpretation. Møller and Møller (1983) reported that twenty-three of their twenty-seven patients (85 percent) had abnormally prolonged III–V latencies, and for two patients there was an abnormal ILD for wave III and wave V (greater than 0.30 ms). Overall, then twenty-six out of twenty-seven patients (96 percent) with tumors, and measurable hearing, yielded an ABR consistent with pathology in the CP angle. Musiek, Josey, and Glasscock (1986) found that fourteen of sixteen patients (88 percent) showed an abnormal wave I–III latency interval (greater than 2 standard deviations above mean and normal value). This was compared to an abnormal rate of 43.8 percent for the wave III–V latency interval, and a 100 percent abnormal rate for an ILD for wave V of more than 0.30 ms. Importantly, only twelve of the sixteen patients had prolonged latency for the I–V interval, suggesting that the most sensitive criteria for abnormality is an interaural wave V asymmetry (>0.30 ms) and/or a prolongation of either the wave I–III or the wave III–V latency measure. It is possible

to record a delay for only one of these interwave measures (I–III or III–V), with even a correspondingly shorter value for the other, resulting in a normal wave I–V latency value.

Calculation of ABR interwave latencies is, of course, dependent on confident identification of the wave I component. Strategies for enhancing wave I amplitude, and the likelihood of wave I detection are emphasized in Chapters 4, 6, and 7. With reliance on a few simple techniques, including inverting electrodes within the ear canal (e.g., TIPtrode) or even more proximal to the cochlea, a reliable wave I can be recorded in the majority of patients undergoing neurodiagnostic ABR assessment for detection of retrocochlear auditory pathology (e.g., Bauch & Olsen, 1990; Brantberg, 1996; Hall, 1992).

ABR AMPLITUDE CRITERIA IN RETROCOCHLEAR PATHOLOGY. |

ABR amplitude criteria are relied on less often than latency criteria for identification of eighth-nerve pathology, mainly because amplitude is considerably more variable. The variability in ABR amplitude characterizes repeated measurements in a single subject and between subjects, even in audiologically and neurologically normal subjects. A relative amplitude measure, the ratio of amplitude for wave V to wave I for a given subject (the wave V/I ratio), is more consistent and has some clinical value (Chiappa, Gladstone, & Young, 1979; Hecox & Cone, 1981; Musiek, Kibbe, Rackliffe, & Weider, 1984; Rosenhall, Hadner, & Bjorkman, 1981; Stockard & Rossiter, 1977). For normal subjects, wave V is larger than wave I, resulting in a wave V/I ratio of more than 1.00. Because variability of even this relative amplitude measure is substantial, the criterion for abnormality is usually a ratio of less than 0.50. That is, the ABR is described as abnormal only when the amplitude for wave V is less than one-half of the amplitude for wave I. The type of inverting electrode used in recording an ABR affects the wave V to wave I relation. The expectation of a wave V/ I ratio of about 1.00 is derived from calculations with an inverting electrode on the earlobe or the mastoid. If an inverting electrode is placed in the ear canal (e.g., TIPtrode) or closer to the cochlea (e.g., tympanic membrane or a transtympanic electrode on the promontory), then wave I is much larger whereas the wave V amplitude is unchanged. The result is a smaller wave V to wave I amplitude ratio in normal hearing. General concepts and techniques for ABR analysis, including amplitude analysis, are reviewed in Chapter 7.

Experience with various kinds of neuropathologies suggests that this rule for the relative amplitude of ABR wave V to wave I should be qualified to include a requirement that wave I amplitude not exceed normal expectations. Exceptionally large wave I amplitude, in combination with a normally sized wave V component, has been reported for patients with eighth-nerve and auditory CNS pathology (see Hall, 1992). Although this pattern is by definition not normal, it cannot be equated with the usual reduction of the wave V/I amplitude due to diminished wave V. One study specifically addressing the V/I amplitude ratio in eighth-nerve pathology was reported by Musiek, Kibbe, Rackliffe, and Weider (1984). The ABR wave V/I amplitude measure was compared for twenty-five normal ears, twenty-five with cochlear hearing impairment, and twenty-five with retrocochlear hearing impairment. The retrocochlear group consisted of patients with either eighth-nerve or brainstem pathology, including seven patients with tumors. Amplitude for wave V was significantly greater than for wave I in the normal and cochlear group, but not the retrocochlear group. Also, absolute amplitudes for both wave I and wave V were reduced below 1.00 for 8 percent of normal ears, none of the cochlear ears, and 44 percent of the retrocochlear ears. In comparison, 84 percent of the retrocochlear ears had latency abnormalities. Arguing for the inclusion of the wave V to wave I ratio as a response parameter in neurodiagnostic ABR assessment, Musiek, Kibbe, Rackliffe, and Weider (1984) found for four of the retrocochlear ears that a reduced amplitude ratio was the only abnormal ABR parameter. Therefore, even though the ABR wave V/I amplitude ratio is not a highly sensitive ABR measure for identification of retrocochlear pathology, an abnormally reduced ratio must be considered suspicious because it is infrequently associated with normal retrocochlear function or with cochlear dysfunction. If either an increased ABR wave V latency or a decreased wave V/I amplitude ratio is viewed as an abnormal sign, then most patients will be correctly identified as at risk for retrocochlear pathology.

DEFINITION OF ABR WAVE I IN RETROCOCHLEAR PATHOLOGY. | The clinically valuable ABR wave I–V latency interval cannot, of course be calculated without confident and accurate identification of wave I. Given the anatomic site of tumors, a clear and easily identified wave I would be expected in most patients with posterior fossa lesions (Shanon, Gold, & Himmelfarb, 1981a). Wave I is generated by the distal (cochlear end) of the eighth nerve (see Chapter 2 for a detailed discussion of ABR anatomy). The tumor is usually located considerably medial to this site, near the proximal (brainstem end) of the eighth nerve. Yet among patients undergoing ABR assessment to rule out eighth-nerve pathology, wave I component is not reliably observed for anywhere from 15 to 80 percent, at least when recorded with the conventional mastoid or earlobe inverting-electrode location (Antonelli, Bellotto, & Grandori, 1987; Elberling & Parbo, 1987; Kusakari et al., 1981; Maurer, Strumpel, & Wende, 1982; Musiek, Josey, & Glasscock, 1986; Rosenhall, 1981a,b). When wave I is identified, it may have normal latency, but reduced amplitude, and often poor morphology and repeatability. Prolongation of latency relative to normal values is also not uncommon, even with little or no hearing sensitivity deficit (Kusakari et al., 1981; Rosenhall, 1981a, b; Shanon, Gold, Himelfarb, 1981a). Conversely, as just noted,

there is evidence of an unusually large-amplitude wave I component in some patients with eighth-nerve or CP-angle tumors.

Given these anatomic points, why is wave I undetectable so often in patients with retrocochlear pathology? There are several possible explanations. First of all, even some normal-hearing persons without pathology inexplicably show no ABR wave I (Worthington & Peters, 1980), particularly at reduced effective intensity levels. Second, a characteristic effect of high-frequency hearing loss on the ABR is poor wave I morphology or absence of wave I (Bauch, Rose, & Harner, 1982). For example, Hyde and Blair (1981) reported observing a definite wave I component for only 42 percent of a group of 400 patients with unspecified cochlear hearing impairment (mostly with noise-induced etiology). Pathophysiologic explanations for the absence of wave I in eighth-nerve tumors must also be considered (described in a following section of this chapter). These would include tumor-related retrograde (toward the cochlea) neural degeneration, interference with blood supply to more distal portions of the nerve and the cochlea, or, rarely, an extremely distal site of lesion. Perhaps the most straightforward and accurate explanation for an absent ABR wave I in about one-third of patients with confirmed eighth-nerve tumors is a deficient recording technique.

The mastoid site for an inverting electrode is inadequate in neurodiagnostic applications of ABR. With an external ear canal electrode design, e.g., the TIPtrode, the majority of patients undergoing ABR assessment for detection of retrocochlear pathology have a clear wave I (e.g., Bauch & Olsen, 1990; Brantberg, 1996; Hall, 1992). And the likelihood of recording a clear wave I is markedly higher with a transtympanic ECochG recording technique. For example, Gerhardt, Wagner, and Werbs (1985) found an ABR wave I (ECochG AP component) with a promontory inverting-electrode placement in twenty-four of twenty-five patients who had no distinct wave I with the conventional mastoid placement for the inverting electrode. Similarly, Antonelli et al. (1987) reported that only three of fifteen (20%) patients with acoustic schwannomas yielded an ABR wave I at maximum stimulus intensity level with mastoid electrode placement, but fourteen of the fifteen (93.3%) had a wave I with TT (transtympanic) measurement. Schwaber and Hall (1990) also consistently observed a clear wave I with a TT electrode from patients with confirmed eighth-nerve tumors, whereas an ear canal (TIPtrode) electrode produced a wave I in less than 20 percent. Many investigators have confirmed markedly improved rates of detect ability of wave I with ear canal, TM, or especially, TT promontory placement of the inverting electrode (see Hall, 1992 for review). This point is highlighted in the discussion of electrodes in ECochG measurement (Chapter 4).

As expected, latency values are generally equivalent for the ECochG AP and ABR wave I components, although in selected cases, differences of up to 0.5 ms may be observed (Elberling & Parbo, 1987). The discrepancy is attributed to vague definition of the ABR wave I peak, mostly in patients with serious hearing impairment. Recording ECochG and ABR simultaneously requires minimally a two-channel measurement protocol with minor alteration of the usual ABR stimulus and acquisition parameters. This is certainly not novel and as a general clinical technique has been advocated often in the past (Coats, 1974; Elberling, 1978; Kusakari et al., 1981; Lambert & Ruth, 1988; Okitsu, Kusakari, Ito, & Tomioka, 1980). Difficulty in identification of wave I in differentiation of cochlear versus retrocochlear lesions with ABR is a common, but solvable, clinical measurement problem. Ear canal, TM, or TT electrode placement in ABR evaluation of suspected eighth-nerve pathology is clinically warranted and valuable whenever the wave I component is not reliably recorded with conventional techniques. Other strategies for enhancing the amplitude of the ABR wave I are identified in the section on troubleshooting in Chapter 7. Reiterating an important point, stressed in the discussion on intraoperative monitoring with ECochG (in Chapter 5) and with ABR (later in this chapter), it is certainly possible to record a clear and reliable ABR wave I (ECochG AP component) in patients with no later ABR waves and no response to pure-tone or speech stimuli at maximum intensity levels (e.g., Hall, 1992; Kaga et al., 1997).

INFLUENCE OF AGE, GENDER, AND HEARING LOSS. | In the analysis and interpretation of ABR findings for a patient with suspected retrocochlear pathology, some response parameter (e.g., a latency value) is compared to expectations for a population without this pathology—a reference data set. The typical reference data are descriptive statistics for ABR latency, and sometimes amplitude, gathered from a small group of young normal-hearing subjects by clinicians in a particular facility (see Chapter 7). At the very least, subject characteristics such as age, gender, and body temperature, which have reasonably well-defined effects on the ABR (Allison, Wood, & Goff, 1983; Beagley & Sheldrake, 1978; Hall, Bull, & Cronau, 1988; Jerger & Hall, 1980; Kjaer, 1979; Rosenhall, Bjorkman, Pedersen, & Kall, 1985), must be considered in clinical analysis of the response in any patient, including those with suspected eighth-nerve pathology. Both age and gender factors may influence absolute and interwave ABR latency values (see Chapter 7).

The importance of these subject characteristics is readily apparent in a simple, yet not really hypothetical, example. The shortest ABR latency values are typically found in young females. When data are analyzed for subjects without high-frequency hearing loss, latency is relatively longer for males and for older versus younger adult subjects. The usual effect of high-frequency hearing loss is to shorten the wave I–V interval (Coats & Martin, 1977; Keith & Greville, 1987; Otto & McCandless, 1982; Stürzebecher, Kevanishvili, Werbs,

Meyers, & Schmidt, 1985). In some subjects with hearing loss, this effect probably offsets the wave I–V prolongation due to age (Elberling & Parbo, 1987). In any event, if normative ABR data for a clinical facility are collected from young females, then some older male patients will invariably yield statistically abnormal latency findings. Rarely, in attempts at identification of eighth-nerve tumor are ABR findings interpreted according to gender, that is, with different sets of normative reference data for males and females. Thomsen, Terkildsen, and Osterhammel (1978) plotted wave V latency data for stimulation of tumor and nontumor ears as a function of age and gender. These researchers were among the first to show the expected effects of these two factors. These authors did not specifically comment on the need to consider gender in the interpretation of ABR data. The implication was, of course, that ILDs are independent of gender effects. However, Stürzebecher, Werbs, and Kevanishvili (1985) applied separate criteria for abnormality in male versus female patients. These investigators recorded ABRs from 84 normal-hearing subjects and 372 patients with sensorineural hearing loss. Analysis showed shorter wave I–V latency values for females than for males. The authors suggested different analysis criteria as a function of gender, specifically an interaural wave I–V difference of > 0.25 ms for females and > 0.30 ms for males as criteria for retrocochlear findings. As stressed in Chapter 7, the effect of gender on the ABR interacts with the effect of advancing age.

To maximize the sensitivity and specificity of ABR to eighth-nerve pathology, it is useful to include within the reference database findings for patients with sensory hearing loss. As mentioned previously, a test with high sensitivity identifies most or all patients with the target disorder (i.e., there are few or no false-negative findings). A test with high specificity rarely or never indicates that the target disorder is present in a patient who, in fact, does not have the disorder (i.e., there are no false-positive findings). Including patients with sensory auditory pathology in a normative database is not common, but quite logical. The rationale for the practice is straightforward. Hearing impairment can affect absolute and also interwave ABR latencies, and can contribute to variability of the response within group of subjects. In attempting to differentiate cochlear from retrocochlear auditory dysfunction with ABR, it makes sense to compare the ABR latency and amplitude for a patient with suspected retrocochlear pathology with data for patients with cochlear dysfunction, not a group of normal hearers. There is also logic in matching, whenever feasible, the data for the group of subjects with cochlear (i.e., nonretrocochlear) auditory dysfunction on the basis of age and gender. The main objective in developing the optimal reference database for differential diagnosis, then, is to include a heterogeneous group of subjects (or patients) who, by definition, show unequivocally normal ABRs. These patients can have varied otologic pathology—such as Ménière's disease, presbycusis, noise-induced hearing deficits, vestibular complaints—and can actually include patients for whom retrocochlear pathology was initially suspected. The only difference between reference data subjects and the patient, in this case, is that none of the reference data subjects have the pathology of interest, in this case eighth-nerve pathology. The reference database subjects are neurologically, but not necessarily audiologically, normal (Elberling & Parbo, 1987; Joseph, West, Thornton, & Hermann, 1987). This approach is justified clinically because combined cochlear and retrocochlear deficits are found in one-third to about one-half of patients with this pathology, because of the pathophysiologic characteristics of eighth-nerve tumors (Djupesland, Flottorp, Modalsli, Tevete, & Sortland, 1981; Hirsh & Anderson, 1980; Rosenhammer, 1977; Terkildsen et al., 1981). Joseph, West, Thornton, and Hermann (1987) offered a reference database for a large group of patients with cochlear auditory dysfunction that is well suited for analysis of ABR findings in patients with suspected retrocochlear pathology (see the appendix).

The rather large number of tumor patients showing no ABR wave V for click stimuli, due in part to the degree of high-frequency hearing sensitivity deficit, can apparently be reduced by use of tone-burst stimuli. This is potentially an important clinical finding. The ABR pattern characterized by absence of a wave V component, while still showing a clear wave I, is a distinctive and strong retrocochlear sign. However, the total absence of an ABR including wave I in a patient with severe high-frequency sensorineural hearing impairment is an equivocal finding. That is, because this finding can occur with a severe sensory (cochlear) hearing impairment, it cannot be considered a retrocochlear finding. The probability of not observing an ABR increases systematically as a function of high-frequency hearing impairment. One possible solution to this interpretation problem is stimulation of the ABR with lower frequency tone bursts, in the frequency region where hearing sensitivity is relatively good or at least is bilaterally symmetrical. Clemis and McGee (1979) provided early evidence suggesting the clinical value of this approach. They found that wave V for tone-burst stimuli was present for approximately 85 percent of their series of patients, whereas with click stimuli, the ABR was entirely absent for more than one-half. Telian and Kileny (1989) also successfully applied this technique in identification of eighth-nerve tumors. According to Desaulty, Lansiaux, Moreau, and Vandorpe (1992), ABR sensitivity to retrocochlear pathology is enhanced when the response is evoked by a 4000 Hz tone-burst stimulus.

Bauch and colleagues (Bauch & Olsen, 1989; Bauch, Olsen, & Harner, 1983; Bauch, Rose, & Harner, 1982) addressed the issue of hearing loss and ABR outcome. In the 1983 study, ABR data were analyzed for thirty patients with surgically confirmed CP-angle tumors and thirty patients with cochlear hearing impairments. Each of the patients in

this second group was carefully selected on the basis of degree and configuration of hearing loss to resemble a patient in the tumor group. The ABR findings for the tumor group were consistent with expectations. That is, twenty-nine of thirty (97 percent) had an abnormal ABR. Among these twenty-nine, 52 percent showed no detectable response, 45 percent yielded an abnormally large ILD for wave V (> 0.2 ms after correction for hearing loss using the Selters and Brackmann (1977) technique, and one patient (3 percent) had an abnormally delayed absolute wave V latency value. As an aside, the single tumor patient with normal ABR results had no acoustic reflexes, a strong retrocochlear audiometric sign. In the Bauch, Olsen, and Harner (1983) study, 23 percent of the nontumor patients had abnormal results (false-positive findings), including three patients with no ABR. The authors described very precipitous, steeply sloping configurations for the sensorineural hearing impairments of these patients. For example, HTLs (hearing threshold levels) were in the mid-to-moderate range (40 to 50 dB HL) in the 500 Hz and even the 1000 Hz region, then dropped to 80 dB or greater for higher frequencies. An absent or abnormal ABR was not an invariant finding among nontumor patients with these audiometric configurations, as five showed completely normal ABR. The diagnosis of cochlear otosclerosis appeared to be a factor among those patients with an abnormal ABR yet no tumor.

Bauch, in a follow-up study (Bauch & Olsen, 1989), provided clinically valuable data on the effect of asymmetric sensory hearing impairment on the ABR wave V ILD. Impairment was described for the better hearing ear and the poorer hearing ear by a three-frequency (2000, 3000, and 4000 Hz) PTA (pure-tone average) taken from the patients' audiogram. Patients with evidence of conductive or mixed hearing impairment were excluded from analysis. For subjects with better-ear hearing within the normal region, there was a definite increase in false-positive ILD findings (ILD > 0.40 ms) as a function of hearing impairment in the poorer ear. For example, with normal hearing in one ear and a high-frequency sensory hearing impairment of greater than 60 dB in the poorer ear, 83 percent of subjects had an ILD exceeding the normal cutoff of 0.40 ms. When hearing in the better ear was decreased, then the proportion of false-positive findings increased for an even smaller ILD in the high frequencies. Jerger and Johnson (1988) report the most recent comprehensive study of the effects of age, gender, and hearing loss on evaluation of ABR findings in differentiation of cochlear versus retrocochlear pathology that is summarized in Chapter 7.

Is the degree of hearing loss in retrocochlear pathology, as assessed with traditional pure-tone audiometry, consistent with electrophysiologic estimates of hearing sensitivity? The basis of this question is actually more physiologic than procedural. Group data for tumor patients generally support a direct relationship between hearing loss and ABR threshold elevation, with the likelihood of an absent ABR increasing with the degree of threshold deficit. This is by no means an invariable relationship, however. As noted at the outset of this discussion, even patients with retrocochlear pathology who have normal hearing sensitivity or just a mild sensitivity deficit may have no detectable ABR, including absence of a wave I component. There is some evidence from studies of patients with retrocochlear pathology that subjective HTLs (from the pure-tone audiogram) are usually equivalent to estimations of auditory threshold based on ECochG. In the study by Eggermont, Don, and Brackmann (1980), several ears showed an AP threshold worse than the subjective HTL for the corresponding stimulus. This pattern of findings was attributed to the greater dependency of the AP on synchronously firing nerve fibers. Any transmission of neural information along the eighth nerve, even with a limited number of functional neurons, can possibly be perceived subjectively, but an AP will be produced only with time-locked firing of many nerve fibers. A few other ears showed just the reverse pattern. Subjective threshold was poorer than ECochG threshold. This suggested to the authors that there was in these cases an additional retrocochlear (more central) component to auditory deficit, presumably caused by tumor effects on the brainstem. The limited cases with discrepancies between behavioral and electrophysiologic thresholds were viewed as exceptions, especially patients with acoustic tumors (vestibular schwannomas). Meningiomas, with more central origins, produced such discrepancies more often.

Recent experiences with ECochG and ABR monitoring of eighth-nerve function before, during, and after surgical removal of tumors confirm the possibility of marked differences between electrophysiologic and behavioral estimations of auditory threshold. At the extreme, a normal-appearing ECochG AP (ABR wave I) component can be recorded from patients showing a profound hearing impairment by pure-tone audiometry—that is, no behavioral response to pure-tone stimuli at maximum intensity levels. Sabin, Prasher, Bentivoglio, and Symon (1987) presented a case report demonstrating cochlear potentials and the ECochG AP and N2 components but no measurable hearing by audiometry after surgery to remove an eighth-nerve tumor. Fifteen months later, only the CM (cochler microphonic) and SP (summating potential) remained. There was neither an ECochG AP component and ABR nor behavioral response to sound. Shanon, Gold, and Himmelfarb (1981a) also reported preservation of the CM in severe hearing loss by pure-tone audiometry. Now, with the recognition of the entity referred to as "auditory neuropathy," the possibility of a CM component in severe hearing loss is not unexpected. Auditory neuropathy is reviewed in detail in Chapter 5 and noted also later in this chapter.

The CM and SP are clearly cochlear in origin. It has been proposed that ECochG AP may arise from afferent fibers exiting the basal portion of the cochlea, while N2 is from corresponding afferent fibers leaving the apical regions (Eggermont, 1976a, b). Later components of the ABR, after wave I, clearly reflect activation of more central structures (proximal eighth nerve and brainstem). The physiologic basis of the preceding set of findings would appear to be preserved cochlear integrity, which implies adequate blood supply, in combination with total eighth-nerve dysfunction. The eighth-nerve abnormality is due perhaps to serve mechanical compression by the tumor on the auditory portion of the eighth nerve or to surgical section of the eighth nerve. Ruben, Hudson, and Chiong (1963) years ago described comparable sparing of ECochG AP in eighth-nerve section during experiments with the cat. Clinically, this ABR pattern is somewhat disconcerting, particularly when intra- or postoperative recordings of wave I are reviewed for evidence of hearing preservation.

HEARING LOSS CORRECTION FACTOR IN ABR INTERPRETATION. | In view of the known effects of high-frequency hearing impairment on ABR soon after the response was discovered, correction techniques were introduced to account for the contribution of conductive or cochlear impairment to latency prolongation (Hyde & Blair, 1981; Jerger & Johnson, 1988; Jerger & Mauldin, 1978; Prosser, Arslan, & Pastore, 1984; Selters & Brackmann, 1977). Briefly, the correction method proposed by Selters and Brackmann (1977) required subtraction of 0.1 ms from the wave V latency for every 10 dB of hearing loss above 50 dB at the audiometric frequency of 4000 Hz. Hearing loss exceeding 75 dB at both 2000 and 4000 Hz precludes valid application of ABR in identification of retrocochlear pathology, according to these authors. There is evidence, however, that this approach is not appropriate for all configurations of hearing impairment, leading to too much correction for flat configurations and, perhaps, too little correction for very precipitous, steeply sloping high-frequency hearing loss configurations (Jerger & Mauldin, 1978). Hyde and Blair (1981) noted that a limitation of the original Selters and Brackmann (1977) method in their clinical population was an unacceptably high false-positive rate of 14 percent. That is, the correction failed to account adequately for cochlear loss and too often led to the incorrect interpretation of an eighth-nerve finding (i.e., an ILD for wave V exceeding 0.30 in a cochlear ear). These authors modified the correction by subtracting 0.1 ms for every 5 dB of hearing loss above 55 dB at 4000 Hz. Cashman et al. (1993) evaluated ABR test performance (sensitivity and specificity) with and without the application of the Selters and Brackmann correction factors in a series of 1,539 consecutive patients with sensorineural hearing loss. False-positive rates (ABR pattern consistent with retrocochlear pathology in patients with sensory hearing loss) decreased from 25 percent to 12.5 percent with application of the correction factors, but false-negative errors (missed retrocochlear pathology) increased from 2.9 percent to 5.8 percent. In other words, the findings for this rather comprehensive investigation confirmed the inevitable trade-off between sensitivity and specificity. That is, when one parameter of test performance is increased (a good thing), the other is reduced. Each clinician needs to determine which of the two parameters of test performance should be optimized in the neurodiagnostic application of ABR.

In fact, correction for cochlear hearing impairments is probably not necessary for most patients. When ABR data are analyzed as a function of patients with diagnosed unilateral purely cochlear hearing impairment (e.g., Ménière's disease), the ILD for wave V is less than 0.30 ms across a wide range of hearing loss (Terkildsen, Osterhammel, & Thomsen, 1981; Thomsen, Terkildsen, & Osterhammel, 1978). Even with a unilateral cochlear deficit of greater than 60 dB HL, the ILD for wave V rarely is asymmetric. Rosenhall (1981a,b) found little correlation between degree of hearing loss and ABR morphology. Jerger and Johnson (1988) suggest an adjustment of the click stimulus SL for the better hearing versus the poorer hearing ear in neurodiagnostic application of ABR in patients with asymmetric sensorineural hearing impairment. Their guidelines are displayed in Table 7.2 and explained in Chapter 7. Correction for a conductive component to hearing loss is very important. The average conductive component in dB for 1000, 2000, and 4000 Hz is determined by air- and bone-conduction pure-tone audiometry. Then, the expected latency shift (increase) for this amount of conductive loss is calculated and subtracted from the wave V latency. Another alternative to circumventing the effect of conductive hearing impairment is to present the ABR stimulus via bone conduction or, if the conductive impairment is limited to lower frequencies, to use a high-frequency air-conduction tone-burst stimulus.

RELATION OF ABR FINDINGS WITH TUMOR SIZE AND LOCATION. | A close and predictable correlation between tumor size and the extent of ABR abnormality would obviously provide extremely valuable information for identification and medical management of eighth-nerve pathology. For this reason, numerous investigators have specifically analyzed the relationship between tumor size and ABR, as well as other neurodiagnostic procedures (Bergenius, Borg, & Hirsch, 1983; Djupesland et al., 1981; Feblot & Uziel, 1982; Musiek, Josey, & Glasscock, 1986; Prosser, Arslan, & Pastore, 1984; Rosenhall, 1981a, b; Selters & Brackmann, 1977; Shanon, Gold, & Himmelfarb, 1981a; Thomsen, Terkildsen, & Osterhammel, 1978; Zappalla, Greenblatt, & Karmel, 1982; and others).

Patterns of ABR findings do in part depend on the size and location of the lesion. There is general agreement that a greater proportion of patients with large tumors than small tumors have no detectable ABR. Also, a tumor of a given size is more likely to be associated with ABR abnormali-

ties if it is located within the internal auditory canal. However, within categories of ABR findings, there may be a wide range of tumor sizes. For example, Musiek, Josey, and Glasscock (1986) reported a comparable intergroup distribution of tumor size between those patients showing all ABR wave components (1.0 to 4.5 cm) and those with missing components (0.5 to 5.0 cm). Methods for measuring size of tumors, and definitions of large, vary. As a rule, tumors larger than 1.5 to 2 cm in diameter are referred to as "large," and there is no question that tumors in the 3 to 5 cm range are considered "large." Among reported series of patients, there is a diversity in the proportions of patients with both large tumors (arbitrarily defined as larger than 1.5 to 1.7 cm) and detectable ABR (among total patient groups), such as seven out of ten (Bergenius, Borg, & Hirsch, 1983) and eleven out of twenty-eight (Eggermont, Don, & Brackmann, 1980). Absence of an ABR is certainly less likely in patients with small tumors (arbitrarily defined as smaller than 1.5 to 1.7 cm), but it does occur. In fact, two out of twelve patients with small tumors reported by Bergenius et al. (1983), and four out of forty-three reported by Eggermont, Don, and Brackmann (1980) showed no ABR. Conversely, normal ABRs in patients with confirmed tumors (false-negative findings) are most likely when the tumors are small (Legatt et al., 1988).

Thus, it is not possible to predict tumor size from a specific ABR parameter, such as the I–V latency interval, for a given patient. Although group data have occasionally produced statistically significant correlations between tumor size and the wave I–V latency interval (Feblot & Uziel, 1982), the relationship is typically weak (Musiek, Josey, & Glasscock, 1986). Most investigators do suggest that ABRs, as interpreted by all the traditional latency criteria, are more likely to be abnormal for larger tumors (Clemis & McGee, 1979; Eggermont, Don, & Brackmann, 1980; Selters & Brackmann, 1977), but even this general claim is not universally supported (Rosenhall, 1981; Rosenhammer, 1977). There does not seem to be a tendency for the wave I–V latency interval increase systematically as a function of tumor size.

The lack of a close correlation between tumor size and ABR abnormality is not unexpected because factors other than tumor size—principally the location, the consistency of the tumor (soft versus firm), and the status of the blood supply-also exert important influences on auditory pathophysiology (Eggermont, Don, & Brackmann, 1980). Small tumors within the confines of the internal auditory canal can produce marked ipsilateral ABR abnormalities either by direct compression of the nerve or by interrupting blood flowing to the cochlea and nerve. However, tumor effects on the brainstem in the CP-angle region are unlikely. In contrast, considerably larger tumors within the more spacious CP angle may have relatively subtle effects on selected ABR wave components and perhaps no detectable effect on some audiologic tests (e.g., audiogram, simple speech-recognition tasks). Rate of tumor growth probably is a factor in the degree of ABR abnormality as well.

Contralateral effects of CP-angle tumors on ABR are often noted in the literature (Deka, Kacker, & Tandon, 1987; Eggermont, Don, & Brackmann, 1980; Møller & Møller, 1983; Musiek, 1982; Musiek & Kibbe, 1986; Musiek, Weider, & Mueller, 1983; Musiek, Josey, & Glasscock, 1986; Rosenhall, 198aa, b; Rosenhammer, 1977; Selters & Brackmann, 1977; Shanon, Gold, & Himmelfarb, 1981a; Wieland & Kemp, 1979; Zappalla, Greenblatt, & Karmel, 1982). Tumors limited to the internal auditory canal or smaller-to-moderate-sized tumors (less than 2 cm diameter) within the CP angle in the posterior fossa produce ABR abnormalities only with the stimulus ipsilateral to the lesion. ABR abnormalities found with stimulation of the ear contralateral the side of the lesion, as well as ipsilaterally, are a strong indication of a large (greater than 2 or 3 cm) posterior fossa mass. Contralateral findings vary. Patients may demonstrate normal wave I–III latency values by a prolonged wave III–V latency, abnormal wave I–III and normal wave III–V, delayed latency for both of these latency interval, or no detectable wave V with either normal or an abnormal wave I–III latency interval (Deka et al., 1987; Møller & Møller, 1983; Musiek & Kibbe, 1986; Zappalla, Greenblatt, & Karmel, 1982).

In general, contralateral ABR abnormalities appear to be relatively evenly distributed among these three categories, although a common denominator is contralateral wave I–V prolongation. Tumor size is probably a factor in the pattern of latency abnormality observed, and it may account to some extent for the divergent conclusions of various authors. For example, Zappalla, Greenblatt, and Karmel (1982) found a significant correlation between increasing tumor size for the contralateral wave III–V latency interval, but not for the other latency parameters. There are, however, reports of abnormalities limited to wave V (Musiek & Kibbe, 1986; Wieland & Kemp, 1979). The reported proportions of all eighth-nerve tumor patients showing contralateral ABR abnormalities, of any type, are usually on the order of 20 to 35 percent (Maurer, Strumpel, & Wende, 1982; Møller & Møller, 1983), but for very large tumors (greater than 3 cm diameter), it may exceed 70 percent (Musiek & Kibbe, 1986).

An appreciation of these contralateral effects of eighth-nerve tumors is clinically important for two reasons. First, in ABR, interpretation of contralateral effects must be differentiated from abnormalities actually due either to bilateral tumors or, if wave I or wave III are not clearly recorded, to other serious hearing impairment. Second, ABR recordings from the contralateral ear may provide diagnostically useful information on tumor size and functional effects, even though the degree of hearing deficit on the involved ear precludes meaningful ABR recording. Postoperative reversal of

contralateral ABR abnormalities is possible (Deka, Kacker, & Tandon, 1987), and this is probably due to decompression of the involved auditory regions secondary to removal of the mass. Strictly speaking, the only ABR latency finding that exclusively and consistently localizes eighth-nerve pathology is prolonged I–II interval, as well as—perhaps—a prolonged I–III interval. All other latency abnormalities, such as wave V latency or the I–V interval, whether analyzed with respect to the contralateral ear or to group reference data, simply reflect general auditory brainstem dysfunction. These criteria do not effectively distinguish among various etiologies, such as brainstem tumors, MS, or brainstem vascular diseases. This, of course, is not a unique clinical limitation. Rarely can neurodiagnosis be made solely on the basis of AER findings.

Three consistent findings emerge from the literature on ABR and tumor characteristics. First, the relation between tumor size and ABR outcome is clear only for very small or large tumors. Sensitivity of the ABR is lowest (< 80 percent) for acoustic tumors that are less than 1 cm in size and essentially 100 percent for acoustic tumors > 2.5 cm. Within the extremes for tumor size, ABR findings are highly variable and dependent instead on other factors. A second, and related, finding has to do with the location of the tumor. There is ample evidence that sensitivity of the ABR is considerably higher for tumors extending into the CP angle (extracanalicular) versus tumors confined to the internal auditory canal (intracanalicular). Of course, smaller tumors tend be limited to the IAC, whereas tumors originating within the IAC with growth expand into the CP angle, so the location of the tumor is often related to size. And, finally, experience with intraoperative monitoring during surgical removal of acoustic tumors shows that hearing preservation is more likely for patients with acoustic tumors (really vestibular schwannomas) arising from the superior vestibular nerve than from the inferior vestibular nerve. It's possible that ABR sensitivity is lower for retrocochlear tumors arising from the superior vestibular nerve than the inferior vestibular nerve, although clear clinical evidence of this supposition is lacking.

Chandrasekhar, Brackmann, and Devgan (1995) reported data for 197 patients (98 male and 99 female, ranging in age from 13 to 78 years) with acoustic neuromas who underwent diagnostic assessment with gadolinium-enhanced MRI and ABR. An ILD for wave V of 0.2 ms and an assessment of morphology were used as ABR indices for a retrocochlear response. Analysis of the ABR with the ILD index yielded a general sensitivity of 92.3 percent, whereas with the morphology index sensitivity was 81.6 percent. Sensitivity of the ABR was dependent on tumor size. ABR sensitivity for the ILD measure was 100 percent for tumors > 3.0 cm, and then decreased to 83.1 percent for tumors ≤ 1.0 cm. ABR sensitivity for the morphology measure was 100 percent for tumors > 2.0 cm, and diminished to 76.5 percent for tumors ≤ 1.0 cm.

RELATION OF ABR WITH TUMOR TYPE AND PATHOPHYSI-OLOGY. | There are two main ways in which a tumor can interfere with generation of the ECochG and ABR. Perhaps the most commonly cited mechanism is either compression or stretching of the eighth-nerve fibers by the expanding tumor mass, with resulting increases in nerve-conduction velocity (Selters & Brackmann, 1977) or, even more likely, tumor-related desynchronization of eighth-nerve fibers. The second mechanism of tumor interference is a compromised blood supply to the eighth nerve and to the cochlea. To understand the first mechanism, recall that the ECochG or ABR with click stimulation is, as noted in Chapters 3 and 4, mainly dependent on hearing sensitivity in the 1000 to 4000 Hz frequency region. A proportion of the high-frequency fibers, those tonotopically coded for high-frequency sounds and originating in the basal region of the cochlea, are located on the outer portion of the eighth nerve (see Chapter 2). These fibers, then, are the first to be affected by a vestibular schwannoma (not a meningioma or neurofibroma). Wave I latency is not slowed because, as noted previously, it arises from the source of the afferents near the cochlea, at the peripheral end of the internal auditory canal. Waves II and maybe III, generated by the central end of the eighth nerve and probably by the cochlear nucleus, respectively, are directly affected.

As mentioned, the second mechanism is compromise of blood supply to the eighth nerve and the cochlea. In some cases, this mechanism interacts with compression of the nerve, and in other cases it may be the primary cause of pathophysiology. Vasculature of the auditory system, including the eighth nerve, was also noted in Chapter 2. The eighth nerve gets its blood supply via the internal auditory artery, which usually originates directly from the AICA (anterior inferior cerebellar artery), and ultimately from the vertebral basilar artery system serving the brainstem. The internal auditory artery runs through the internal auditory canal, next to the eighth nerve. Therefore, a tumor involving the eighth nerve may concomitantly interrupt blood flow through the internal auditory artery, which, in turn, can result in ischemia of the nerve peripheral to the tumor (retrograde degeneration) and also to the cochlea. The reported rapid deterioration of audiologic measures, including ABR findings, in a relatively short time in some patients with eighth-nerve tumors (Eggermont, Don, & Brackmann, 1980) is not reflecting a fast-growing mass. Eighth-nerve tumors, as noted, are typically slow growing. Rather, these dynamic auditory findings occur when the tumor has reached a critical mass, and with further expansion, it compresses blood vessels and/or nerve fibers. Different types of tumors, or different neurotologic pathologies in general, do not each produce predictable and unique alterations in the ABR abnormality. Invariably, the most pronounced ABR abnormalities in eighth-nerve tumors are observed with stimulation of the ear ipsilateral to the site of lesion. In a patient with suspected tumor, a less

pronounced ABR abnormality with stimulation of the unaffected (presumably nontumor) side may be associated with a very large tumor (greater than 3 cm). It also may reflect an intrinsic (intra-axial) tumor, originating from within the brainstem, rather than a lesion growing from a site on the eighth nerve. Symmetrically abnormal ABR findings (i.e., an equivalent pattern of latency prolongation and/or amplitude reduction for stimulation of each ear) suggest either bilateral eighth-nerve tumors (neurofibromatosis) or, in the presence of normal hearing sensitivity, perhaps MS. As noted, ABR abnormalities observed with stimulation of the ear contralateral to the side tumors are found in 20 to 35 percent of most patient series. An obvious pathophysiologic explanation for contralateral ABR abnormalities, and one typically cited, is brainstem compression and probably distortion, which affects auditory pathways, such as the lateral lemniscus, on the side opposite a large tumor (Deka, Kacker, & Tandon, 1987). Zappalla, Møller, and Møller (1983) offer a specific theory for the latency delays of early wave components (the wave I–III prolongation): The cerebellum is a major neuroanatomic structure in the posterior fossa, forming one boundary of the CP angle. The flocculus of the cerebellum is attached to the eighth nerve. A large tumor in the CP angle can displace the cerebellum and lead to traction on the contralateral eighth nerve.

The basis of contralateral ABR abnormalities is debated. Those investigators who attribute them to brainstem shift and contralateral compression of auditory structures presume that the ABR is dependent on stimulus-ipsilateral brainstem pathways. For example, a large tumor in the right CP angle would produce marked ABR abnormalities with right-ear stimulation due to a direct effect on the right eighth nerve. This large tumor would also shift the brainstem from the right to left side, producing an indirect compression of the left brainstem auditory regions. With stimulation of the left ear, contralateral to the tumor, ABR abnormalities would be observed because the pathways leading from the left eighth nerve up to the left side of the brainstem eventually course through the compressed (involved) regions (probably in the upper pons or midbrain). There are several rather detailed discussions of the pathophysiologic basis of the contralateral effects of tumors on ABRs. Robinson and Rudge (1983) observed ABR abnormalities for stimuli presented to the ear that was contralateral to the side of eighth-nerve schwannomas, but the finding was not invariably associated with tumor size. Furthermore, even very large CP-angle meningiomas causing an equivalent amount of brainstem shift did not produce contralateral ABR abnormalities. These investigators maintain that the pathways underlying the ABR are contralateral to the stimulus ear, at least for the generation of wave III and later waves. With progressive expansion in the CP angle, a tumor originating on the eighth nerve will eventually press on the ipsilateral brainstem and in this manner involve the auditory regions that generate the ABR in response to stimulation of the contralateral ear. Meningiomas and other CP-angle tumors, rarely arising from the eighth nerve, would be less likely to expand in the vicinity of these vital auditory structures.

Musiek and Kibbe (1986) also speculate on possible reasons for their finding of contralateral abnormalities for the wave IV/V complex, yet not for earlier waves. Wave I and wave II are, of course, not involved because they arise from within the internal ear canal contralateral to the tumor and are thus completely isolated from any effects of the mass. Assuming that wave III is generated from the cochlear nucleus region, it too would be little influenced by a contralateral posterior fossa tumor by virtue of the relatively distant location of its generator in relation to the tumor, as well as the compliance offered by the CP-angle cistern adjacent to the cochlear nucleus. The explanation for the primary effect of the tumor on wave V is based largely on the presumption that this component originates in the vicinity of the nucleus of the lateral lemniscus ipsilateral to the tumor, after crossover (decussation) of most auditory fibers from the contralateral cochlear nucleus. Compression of the ipsilateral nucleus of the lateral lemniscus leads to desynchronization of neural impulses contributing to wave V. Even the otherwise intact fibers running up the brainstem contralateral to the tumor are, according to Musiek and Kibbe (1986), susceptible to the desynchronization by mediation via decussating fibers at the lower (caudal) pontine level.

In any event, the contralateral compression effect of large tumors may, at the extreme, cause obstruction of the ventricular (aqueduct) system and may compromise CSF flow, leading to transtentorial herniation. The pathophysiologic process would almost certainly be reflected by marked rostral-to-caudal deterioration of the ABR (Hall, Mackey-Hargadine, & Kim, 1985) and would be associated with severe clinical neurologic impairment. With modern neurodiagnostic technology and surgical therapy, this devastating progression of neurologic events is, fortunately, rarely allowed to occur. Without adequate techniques for surgical intervention, until the early 1900s, this deterioration was commonplace. This difference of opinion on the pathophysiologic effects of eighth-nerve tumors illustrates an important principle that can be generalized to all neurodiagnostic applications of AERs. That is, a firm understanding of AER anatomy in humans, such as laterality of the ABR, is essential for maximum utilization and meaningful interpretation of clinical findings.

RELATION OF ABR WITH CT AND MRI. | CT with a contrast medium is one of two radiologic imaging techniques used for detection and localization of eighth-nerve tumors. In the era before CT, conventional polytomography of the temporal bone was regularly used to detect bony destruction and enlargement of the internal auditory canal. Unfortunately, one out of ten patients with eighth-nerve tumors may have

symmetrical internal auditory canals, as visualized by convention tomography. Conventional polytomography is an unacceptable imaging technique for this purpose (Bonafe et al., 1985). The typical CT appearance of an eighth-nerve tumor is an isodense or hyperdense mass with homogenous contrast enhancement. Internal auditory-canal erosion and expansion is characteristic of a vestibular schwannoma, whereas a meningioma typically shows a broader tumor base and perhaps calcification. Some tumor types uncommonly found in the CP angle, such as lymphomas, may resemble vestibular schwannomas in CT appearance, while others (epidermoids, arachnoid cysts, and glomus tumors) have a more distinctive appearance.

Following a review of 303 eighth-nerve neuroma cases, Barrs, Brackmann, Olson, and House (1985) concluded that the combination of ABR plus enhanced CT identified 99 percent of the neuromas. The CT scanner used in this study was a relatively high-resolution machine (General Electric 8800). Previous reports of tumor identification with earlier scanners, with poorer resolution, showed a miss rate of about 30 percent. One of the significant findings of the study by Barrs and colleagues (1985) was the effect of tumor size on the success of CT. With intravenous (iophendylate dye)-enhanced CT, 97 percent of the tumors of 1.5 cm or smaller were not detected. Of the entire series of patients, these smaller tumors were found in only 12 percent. Tumor size was determined at the time of surgery and included the dimension of the tumor within the internal auditory canal and any portion extending into the CP-angle cistern. To put this relationship into perspective, tumors larger than 1.5 cm in diameter usually extended into the CP angle more than 5 mm (0.5 cm). Of the 229 patients in the study who underwent ABR assessment, only 5 (2%) showed normal (i.e., false-negative) findings. Three of these patients had tumors of 1 cm or less, while tumors were in the 2 to 2.5 cm range for the other two. A direct comparison of ABR versus CT results was quite informative. There were thirty-one patients with abnormal ABR findings and a normal CT. An additional six patients showed no ABR (no response) and still had a normal CT. Conversely, there were only two patients in the series with abnormal CT yet normal ABR findings. The authors point out that two patients with neurofibromatosis had no otologic symptoms, including normal ABRs. Wong and Brackmann (1981) reported a similar theme with an earlier generation of CT scanner. CT did not produce false-positive findings, and it detected 95 percent of relatively large tumors (greater than 2.5 cm), but small tumors (less than 1.5 cm) were detected at a rate of only 5 percent.

During the 1980s, CT with gas (oxygen) cisternography was recommended for definitive and most accurate CT diagnosis of tumors in patients showing no evidence of pathology on normal enhanced CT studies (Bockenheimer, Schmidt, & Zöllner, 1984; Maurer, Strümpel, & Wende, 1982). Although gas cisternography facilitated detection of small lesions within the internal auditory canal (less than 5 mm protrusion into the CP angle), which are not revealed by enhanced CT, it was associated with the possibility of a false-negative rate of over 20 percent for tumors extending less than 5 mm into the CP angle and as high as 50 percent for smaller tumors, protruding less than 2 mm into the CP angle (Barrs, Luxford, Becker, & Brackmann, 1984). A problem with a false-positive conventional CT outcome was also reported (Robinson & Rudge, 1982). These investigators reviewed diagnostic findings for ninety patients with clinical evidence leading to the suspicion of a CP-angle tumor. Of the remaining group, eleven had normal ABRs, and for three of them, the CT reportedly showed a tumor. After prolonged clinical follow-up and continued neuroradiologic evaluation, no tumor was demonstrated. The diagnostic significance of this finding is apparent. If CT were used as the final definition for the presence of a tumor, and the normal ABR was discounted, the three patients might have undergone surgery for no reason.

During the 1980s, the relative roles of ABR and CT in early identification of eighth-nerve pathology were debated in the literature. Diagnostic efficiency of different combinations of auditory, clinical, and neuroradiologic tests in detection of eighth-nerve tumors traditionally generated considerable research interest. Clusters of papers on this topic appeared periodically as new diagnostic procedures were introduced (Antonelli et al., 1987; Cohn, LeLiever, Hokanson, & Quinn 1986; Harner & Laws, 1981; Hart & Davenport, 1981; Jerger & Jerger, 1983; Portmann et al., 1989; Robinson & Rudge, 1983; Thomsen, Nyboe, Borum, Tos, & Barfoed, 1981; Turner & Nielson, 1984). A variety of diagnostic models or test sequence algorithms, some relying on human decision making and others on computer-based expert systems, were also proposed for detection of eighth-nerve tumors. Most of these models, reviewed by Cohn et al. (1986), incorporated both ABR and CT. The over all objective in developing diagnostic models for eighth-nerve tumor detection was to find an approach that has the highest sensitivity and specificity at the lowest cost.

Proponents of CT as the procedure of choice argued that it was the definitive study for detecting, localizing, and estimating the size of lesions. The main disadvantage of this approach was substantially increased health cost. Considerable health care costs are also associated with reliance on MRI as a screening technique, as noted below. The case for ABR as the first-line method for identification of eighth-nerve dysfunction was actually presented throughout this chapter. In summary, ABR is a readily available, relatively inexpensive, noninvasive, office procedure with a proven high sensitivity in detecting eighth-nerve auditory dysfunction. ABR abnormalities reflected lesions that were rather small and not always visible on CT with scanning devices available during the 1980s (Musiek, 1982).

One recommended diagnostic approach was to consider ABR as a screening tool to be applied with patients at risk for eighth-nerve pathology, as determined by clinical symptoms and audiometric signs (Bonafe et al., 1985; Jerger & Jerger, 1983; Maurer, Strumpel, & Wende, 1982). The symptoms and signs include, but are not limited to, unilateral sensorineural hearing impairment, retrocochlear findings by acoustic-reflex measurement (acoustic-reflex decay), speech audiometry findings (inordinately poor maximum performance or rollover on performance intensity functions), as well as several clinical findings, such as tinnitus, ataxia, and cranial nerve deficits. ABR abnormality consistent with retrocochlear pathology indicated the need for carbon dioxide-enhanced CT scanning or MRI (magnetic resonance imaging). The reader is referred to the aforementioned review articles for detailed discussion of the advantages and disadvantages of various clinical approaches to diagnosis of eighth-nerve tumors.

ABR can also be applied as a cross-check to reduce false-negative and false-positive errors associated with neuroradiologic techniques (Josey, Glasscock, Musiek 1988). The cross-check principle is one of the foundations of diagnostic audiology. Josey, Glasscock, and Musiek (1988) analyzed ABR and CT data for a series of 100 patients with surgically confirmed eighth-nerve tumors. Among the tumors, ninety-one were described as "acoustic neurilemmomas," four as meningiomas, and five as neurofibromas. ABR findings were consistent with eighth-nerve pathology for ninety of the ninety-three patients (96.7%) with interpretable waveforms (hearing loss was excessively severe in the other seven patients). However, initial neuroradiology studies (enhanced CT or MRI) showed evidence of eighth-nerve pathology for only 69 percent of the 100 patients. These authors conclude that ABR is a valuable technique not only for early identification of eighth-nerve pathology, but it also offers a method for cross-checking neuroradiology studies in the neurodiagnosis. If ABR is abnormal in the presence of normal neuroradiologic studies, then air-contrast CT or MRI can be considered, or the neuroradiologic study can be repeated in six to twelve months. An abnormal ABR, in the presence of normal CT or MRI, should not be dismissed as a false-positive finding. Conversely, a normal ABR in combination with positive (abnormal) neuroradiologic findings suggests the need for further diagnostic workup and may argue against immediate surgical therapy.

MRI, also sometimes called nuclear magnetic resonance (NMR) or simply magnetic resonance (MR), has rapidly assumed an important role in clinical neuroradiology. Numerous investigators have assessed the usefulness of MRI in detection of suspected eighth-nerve pathology within the internal auditory canal and the CP angle (Cohn et al., 1986; Daniels et al., 1987; Haberman & Kramer, 1989; Jackler, Shapiro, Dillon, Pitts, & Lanser, 1990; Maslan, Latack, Kemink, & Graham, 1986; Portmann et al., 1989; Valvassori, 1986; Young, Bydder, & Hall, 1983). The reported advantages of MRI versus CT include elimination of bone artifact in the brainstem and temporal bone region and earlier and more accurate detection of small soft-tissue masses, particularly those accompanied by edema. This first advantage is also a disadvantage because bone changes are a characteristic feature of some otologic lesions, and bony landmarks are useful in determining the exact location of the lesion. Naturally, a major objective of research is to describe the value of MRI in detection of smaller sized (less than 1.5 cm) tumors. Experience to date supports this effectiveness. MRI, especially gadolinium DTPA enhanced MRI, is an effective neuroradiologic technique for diagnosis of CP-angle tumors, especially eighth-nerve Schwannomas (Jackler et al., 1990; Portmann et al., 1989; Valvassori, 1986). The eighth nerve can be visualized as it leaves the brainstem. Small tumors produce a thickened appearance of the nerve and obscure the normally seen perineural plane separating the vestibular from the auditory portions. Small vestibular schwannomas (< 0.5 cm) may be asymptomatic. A large tumor is seen as a mass having a different appearance than the brainstem tissue and surrounding CSF.

Technical limitations for MRI did emerge in the early 1990s with the scanning machines and computer software available then. There is at least one published example of technical problems leading to a false-negative MRI outcome in a patient with confirmed tumor (Barkovich, Wippold, & Brammer, 1986), as well as other apparently valid interpretations of false-negative MRI findings (Josey, Glasscock, & Musiek, 1988; Telian & Kileny, 1988). There is certainly the possibility of a false-positive MRI outcome in patients with other abnormalities, such as Paget's disease or a vascular loop (Crain & Dolan, 1990; Haberman & Kramer, 1989; Loftus & Wazen, 1990). Von Glass and colleagues (1991), for example, described two case reports of patients with greater-than-normal arachnoidal tissue in arachnoidititis who were mistakenly identified with vestibular schwannomas. Saito, Handa, and Kitahara (1993) report a case study of a patient with an intracanalicular mass on MRI. Symptoms included a unilateral tinnitus, a severe unilateral hearing loss and absence of an ABR on the involved ear. An acoustic tumor was presumed from Gd-MRI scanning. At surgery, however, no tumor could be found. The eighth cranial nerve appeared swollen and discolored. Histopathology revealed a lesion consisting of edematous nerve fiber and inflammatory cells, described by the authors as eighth cranial neuritis.

Clinical trade-off for the high sensitivity of MRI to retrocochlear pathology may be detection of anatomic structures that are mistakenly considered tumors and, based on this radiologic evidence, inappropriate intracranial surgery is performed. Although the cost of MRI is generally greater than the cost of ABR, and availability is more restricted, screening MRI techniques have been reported. Linker, Ruckenstein, Acker, and Gardener (1997) described the application of a T2-weighted fast-spin echo MRI as a screening tool for retrocochlear lesions in a series of 155 patients. According to the authors, "this imaging technique is rapidly performed and provides superb visualization of the relevant anatomic structures at a global cost of $475" (Linker et al., 1997, p. 1525).

Robinette, Bauch, Olsen, and Cevette (2000) at the Mayo Clinic in Rochester, Minnesota, conducted a very thorough examination of the costs and benefits of the identification of acoustic tumors with gadolinium-enhanced MRI alone and when MRI was combined with ABR. Financial data were calculated for seventy-five patients with surgically confirmed acoustic neuromas defined by size ranging from small (< 1.0 cm) to large (> 2.0 cm). Using hypothetical costs associated with identifying the tumors in a large intermediate-risk patient population (N = 900), Robinette et al. (2000) estimated a total cost of $1.35 million USD for screening with Gd-MRI and a cost of $486,000 for a combined Gd-MRI and ABR screening approach. The latter was associated, however, with four missed acoustic tumors. For a low-risk patient population (N = 1600), the cost of the Gd-MRI screening strategy was estimated at $2.4 million USD, whereas the ABR plus MRI screening approach was associated with a cost of $787,500. The authors conclude that combining MRI and ABR in screening for acoustic tumors "allows considerable savings when patients are in the intermediate- or low-risk groups" (Robinette et al., 2000, p. 963).

Most of the literature on the relative costs for MRI and ABR is based on studies in countries with highly developed health care systems. Recognizing the rarity of acoustic tumors and costs borne by health care systems for "more commonly encountered diseases," Murphy and Selesnick (2002) performed a meta-analysis of data reported in the English language literature from 1966 to 2001 on detection and diagnosis of retrocochlear pathology. Despite its clear sensitivity to acoustic tumors, MRI with gadolinium is cost prohibitive within the health care systems of some countries. The authors make an interesting point in concluding, "Which modality to use in acoustic neuroma diagnosis is just as much a philosophical and macroeconomic question as a technological one. . . . The cost of a timely diagnosis of acoustic neuromas must be weighed against using resources for other, more pressing, health concerns" (Murphy & Selesnick, 2002, p. 253).

RELATION OF ABR WITH MRI FINDINGS. | The diagnostic value of the ABR was initially challenged in the 1980s, as CT scanning, particularly with contrast enhancement techniques, became commonplace in medical facilities (e.g., Barrs et al., 1985; Hart, Gardner, & Howieson, 1983; Josey, Glasscock, & Musiek, 1988; Portmann et al., 1989; Telian & Kileny, 1988). The role of the ABR in the identification of retrocochlear pathology during the 1980s evolved from a primary to a complementary or supportive role, with CT serving

TABLE 10.5. Selected Studies Published since 1990 of Auditory Brainstem Response (ABR) Test Performance in the Diagnosis of Retrocochlear Auditory Dysfunction Secondary to Eighth Cranial Nerve (Acoustic) Tumors
Studies are limited to those including MRI (usually with gadolinium enhancement) and are listed chronologically.

STUDY (YEAR)	N	ABR MEASURE	FINDINGS
Chandrasekhar et al. (1995)	197	Wave V IAD*	ILD sensitivity of 100% for large tumors (>3 cm)
		Morphology	Sensitivity of 83.1% for small tumors (≤1.0 cm)
Gordon & Cohen (1995)	105	Wave I–V ILD	Sensitivity of 87.6% overall, and 69% for tumors <10 mm
Gosepath, Maurer, & Mann (1995)	17	???	Sensitivity of 76.5% for intracanalicular tumors
Ferguson et al. (1996)	237	???	False negative CT in a patient with a small intracanalicular tumor
Zappia et al. (1996)	111	Wave V ILD*	Sensitivity of 95% overall, and 89% for tumors ≤1 cm
Godey et al. (1998)	89	Wave V ILD	Sensitivity of 94% for extracanalicular tumors; 77% for intracanalicular
El-Kashlan et al. (2000)	25	???	Sensitivity of 92% for small tumors (<1 cm)
Haapaniemi et al. (2000)	41	???	Sensitivity of 98% in all tumors (extra- and intracanalicular)
Don et al. (2005)	54	Stacked ABR	Sensitivity of 95% to small tumors (≤1 cm)

* IAD = interaural difference; MRI = magnetic resonance imaging; PTA = pure-tone audiometry; WR = word recognition; ART = acoustic reflex threshold; ARD = acoustic reflex decay; ILD = interaural latency difference.

as the frontline procedure. In the mid-1990s, as MRI technology became routinely applied in medical facilities, more questions arose regarding the test performance and place of ABR in the identification of retrocochlear pathology. The title of a paper by Dr. Karen Doyle in 1999 expresses succinctly the emerging concern of many neuro-otologists: "Is there still a role for auditory brainstem response audiometry in the diagnosis of acoustic neuroma?" Some of the many papers addressing the topic of ABR versus MRI in the detection and diagnosis of acoustic neuromas are summarized in Table 10.5. Skepticism about the diagnostic power of ABR in early detection of retrocochlear pathology is evident from some publications, most of which appear in the otolaryngology literature (e.g., Burkey et al., 1996; Cueva, 2004; Gordon & Cohen, 1995; Levine, Antonelli, Li, & Haines, 1991; Marangos, Maier, Merz, & Laszig, 2001; Naessens, Gordts, Clement, & Buissert, 1996; Ruckenstein, Cueva, Morrison, Sataloff, & Press, 1996; Schmidt et al., 2001; Wilson et al., 1992; Zappia, O'Connor, Wieta, & Pinces, 1997). The most common weakness cited for ABR is, of course, the problem of false-negative ABR findings (misses) in patients with small acoustic tumors (< 0.5 cm). Marangos et al. (2001) conducted an investigation of ABR in the detection of neuroradiologically confirmed retrocochlear pathology in 309 patients that took into account several important variables, including tumor histology (e.g., vestibular schwannoma versus meningioma), tumor size (small tumors < 15 mm to very

large tumors > 40 mm). The authors' conclusions are representative of other opinions expressed in the literature: "ABR is not sufficient for early detection of small CPA tumors" (Marangos et al., 2001, p. 95). Cueva (2004) also evaluated in 312 patients with asymmetrical hearing loss the use of ABR versus MRI for detecting in thirty-one patients a variety of retrocochlear abnormalities, among them patients with vestibular schwannomas, glomus jugulare tumors, ecstatic basilar arteries with brainstem compression, and petrous apex cholesterol granulomas. Citing an overall ABR false-negative rate of 29 percent for vestibular schwannomas coupled with a high false-positive rate (76.84%), corresponding to sensitivity of 71 percent and specificity of 74 percent, Cueva (2004) "recommends abandoning ABR as a screening test for symmetric SNHL and adoption of a focused MRI protocol as the screening test of choice (within certain guidelines)" (p. 1686).

Even as CT scans were referred to as the "gold standard" for acoustic tumors, clinical reports documented the possibility of false-negative and false-positive outcomes. The former would result in a missed tumor. Since the tumor remained undetected by the "definitive" measure of the day, diagnosis and management was markedly delayed, with potentially increased morbidity and mortality and reduced likelihood of medical management with hearing preservation. False-positive errors for the CT scans were also associated with serious problems, namely, a craniotomy and very risky (and expensive) otologic and/or neurosurgical procedure for a patient who in fact had no tumor.

No diagnostic procedure is infallible, with 100 percent sensitivity and 100 percent specificity. The MRI is no exception to this principle of test performance. The false-negative rate for detection of acoustic tumors with ABR has clearly increased directly with advances in the sophistication of neuroradiology technology, specifically CT, enhanced CT, MRI, and then MRI with gadolinium (Gd). As sensitivity of neuroradiogic studies increases, however, there is an inevitable increase in the possibility, albeit small, of false-positive diagnostic errors, that is, a neuroradiologic finding consistent with a tumor when no tumor exists. Jacobson, Newman, Monsell, and Wharton (1993) illustrated with two case studies "the complex issues raised by the detection of small asymptomatic VS [vestibular schwannoma] by Gd MRI that were missed by ABR. The role of ABR testing in the diagnosis and management of VS remains well established and will continue to evolve" (p. 355). The authors clarify a distinction "between the clinical *diagnosis* and clinical *detection* of VS. Whereas the clinical *diagnosis* of VS is made histologically, the clinical *detection* of VS is currently made through the use of gadolinium-DTPA MRI (Gd MRI), which serves as the "gold standard" (Jacobson et al., 1993, pp. 356–357). One of the cases reported in this paper reveals three potential clinical disadvantages associated with reliance on ABR for early detection of retrocochlear pathology, specifically what are later confirmed as false-negative errors. First, hearing may deteriorate following the normal ABR finding. Second, surgical approaches used for tumor removal with hearing preservation may not be appropriate. Finally, the likelihood is increased of tumor involvement with neural structures outside of the auditory system, e.g., the seventh cranial (facial) nerve (Jacobson et al., 1993).

ABR AND THE DIAGNOSTIC AUDIOLOGY TEST BATTERY. | There are numerous articles describing the relative diagnostic value of different traditional audiologic procedures, such as alternate binaural loudness balance (ABLB), speech audiometry, tone-decay tests, and, more recently, acoustic reflexes (Antonelli, Bellotto, & Grandori, 1987; Hall, 1991; Hirsh & Anderson, 1980; Jerger & Jerger, 1983; and others). The interesting history of diagnostic audiometry is not covered here, but it is reviewed in published papers (e.g., Hall, 1991; Jerger, 1987). The cross-check principle, described initially by Jerger and Hayes (1976), remains important in the identification of eighth-nerve tumors: No single test is invariably accurate. A test battery approach optimized correct identification in cochlear loss. However, as the data presented next on sensitivity and specificity dramatically demonstrate, ABR was by far the single best audiometric procedure for this purpose.

The relative sensitivity of the ABR in identifying retrocochlear pathology, in comparison to the traditional site-of-lesion procedures, is clearly evident in Table 10.3. The most important component of the audiologic test battery for rational interpretation of ABR data is the simple pure-tone audiogram. Normal hearing sensitivity is not incompatible with a markedly abnormal or even an absent ABR and confirmed retrocochlear pathology, as supported by evidence from formal investigation (e.g., Marangos, Schipper, & Richter, 1999; Valente, Peterin, Goebel, & Neely, 1995) and emphasized at the outset of the chapter. In fact, the absence of an ABR in a patient with normal hearing sensitivity is a very strong audiometric sign of eighth-nerve pathology. The same ABR finding in a patient with severe sensorineural impairment is less significant (Musiek, Josey, & Glasscock, 1986). Also, information from immittance measurement is very useful in interpreting ABR findings. Immittance testing is the most sensitive measure of middle-ear status, and it is invaluable for ruling out conductive hearing impairment. Further, the acoustic reflex has an accuracy rate of about 85 percent in identifying eighth-nerve pathology (Hall, 1985) and thus is useful not only for corroborating ABR findings, but also as a first-line screening test to determine which patients should undergo ABR assessment. Finally, speech audiometry performance, or at least single-syllable word recognition, has traditionally been included in the diagnostic test battery for differentiating cochlear versus retrocochlear audiotory pathology (Hall, 1991). Speech-recognition findings (maximum scores) tend to be rather variable and, importantly, not correlated statistically with ABR patterns (Musiek, Josey, & Glasscock, 1986). In fact, word-recognition rollover provides increased sensitivity to retrocochlear pathology.

TEST PERFORMANCE OF ABR IN RETROCOCHLEAR PATHOLOGY. | In the era before MRI, there was widespread agreement that ABR had a remarkably high hit rate for identification of eighth-nerve pathology. In most reported series of patients with surgically confirmed pathology, between 96 percent and 100 percent were correctly identified. Usually, the tumors missed by analysis of ABR were extremely small (Legatt et al., 1988). This accuracy, viewed also as a minimal rate for false-negative findings (i.e., for missing tumors), is unquestionably a unique clinical advantage and a major reason for the rapid inclusion of ABR as a neurodiagnostic procedure. Even among the earlier studies, however, there was some acknowledgment that ABR recordings could produce false-positive findings in 8 to 30 percent or more of nontumor patients (Bauch, Olsen, & Harner, 1983; Clemis & McGee, 1979; Selters & Brackmann, 1977), a problem cited also in later studies, e.g., Gstoettner et al. (1992) and Cueva, (2004). That is, if ABRs were recorded from 100 tumor patients, the findings would be consistent with eighth-nerve pathology for about ninety-six of them (tumors for approximately four patients would be missed). However, if ABRs were recorded during the same period from 1,000 nontumor patients, findings for up 30 percent for more (or as many as 300 or more patients) would also incorrectly suggest eighth-nerve pathology where it did not exist. The incorrect suggestion of eighth-nerve pathology in patients with no lesion is a false-positive error. As the preceding example clearly implies, the problem of false-positive errors in assessment of suspected eighth-nerve pathology is potentially a clinical concern because the diagnostic errors lead to overreferral and unnecessary medical costs for large numbers of patients.

The invariably related concepts of test sensitivity, specificity, and receiver operating characteristics (ROC) curves have been applied in an assessment of ABR clinical effectiveness (Antonelli, Bellotto, & Grandori, 1987; Turner & Nielsen, 1984; Turner, Shepard, & Frazer, 1984). These concepts are most often used in defining the efficiency of ABR in differentiating cochlear versus retrocochlear dysfunction, but they are also appropriate for defining the efficiency of differentiating any two general sites of lesions (e.g., eighth-nerve vs. lower brainstem dysfunction). Sensitivity and specificity values may however differ substantially for other sites of lesions, such as the brainstem. The operating characteristics of a test are often described with a 2×2 contingency table or an ROC curve. Schwartz (1987) plotted the relative characteristic of different audiologic and radiologic procedures, as reported by Turner, Shepard, and Frazer (1984). ABR was clearly the most sensitive measure, but it was slightly less specific than another audiometric test (Békèsy Comfortable Loudness). Radiologic procedures were among the most specific, yet with the exception of gas cisternography, they were not as sensitive as ABR.

An important factor in evaluating the sensitivity and specificity of tests is predictive value, i.e., the probability of a disease (e.g., eighth-nerve tumor) being present (positive predictive value). Predictive value is directly linked to the prevalence of the disease, and it decreases systematically as prevalence decreases. This point is especially relevant in a discussion of ABR for identification of eighth-nerve pathology because the prevalence of the disease of interest is very low. The vast majority of patients suspected of eighth-nerve pathology will, in fact, have none. Therefore, incorrect prediction of this pathology in a nontumor patient is more likely than the failure to identify true pathology. From a practical policy standpoint, it is probably a wise clinical policy to first set stringent criteria for an abnormal ABR finding, and then to be sure to follow up borderline abnormal findings with a repeat ABR in six to nine months, to correctly identify small and slowly growing eighth-nerve tumors. When this is done, the reduced sensitivity at the time of the test is balanced by the increased specificity and by the continued sensitivity and specificity when following the patient over time.

Callan, Lasky, and Fowler (1999) applied neural networks in an evaluation of the test performance of five au-

diologic procedures in the identification of retrocochlear pathology. The article begins with a detailed review of the literature on MRI in retrocochlear pathology, on test battery theory and clinical decision making, and on neural networks, particularly learning vector quantization self-organizing map (LVQ-SOM). Subjects included twenty-one patients with confirmed acoustic tumors and forty-eight patients in a "tumor absent" group. Curiously, despite this thorough review, no details were provided on the features of the patients with retrocochlear pathology, such as the specific pathology, size, or location of the tumors, nor other pertinent subject characteristics (e.g., age and gender). The five audiologic procedures were the ABR (interaural latency difference and wave I–V latency interval), contralateral and ipsilateral acoustic reflexes (at 2000 Hz), tone decay, and word recognition score. The audiologic procedures were evaluated on six measures of test performance: (1) number of hits (accurate detection of tumors), (2) number of correct rejections (number of cases a nontumor patient was correctly identified), (3) hit rate (sensitivity, or proportion of hits among all patients with tumors), (4) correct rejection rate (specificity, or proportion of patients without tumors who were correctly identified), (5) A″, a single test performance measure that includes sensitivity and specifity, and (6) efficiency, an overall measure of correct results. In summarizing their results, Callan, Lasky, and Fowler (1999) concluded, "Of the audiological tests evaluated in the present analysis, the superiority of the auditory brainstem evoked response in predicting retrocochlear disease was again demonstrated. However, the results also demonstrated that identification accuracy could be improved by combining the ABR with other tests" (p. 287). The benefits of combining other audiologic tests (e.g., rollover for word recognition performance–intensity functions and acoustic reflex measures) cited by Callan, Lasky, and Fowler (1999) were not, however, consistent with finding reported by other investigators (e.g., Kotlarz, Eby, & Borton, 1992).

Can ABR test performance in retrocochlear pathology be improved with some manipulation of the measurement technique? Several investigators provide evidence in the affirmative. Lightfoot (1992) investigated in thirty-one patients with confirmed acoustic neuroma the value of increasing the rate of stimulus presentation (11.1/sec to 88.8/sec) to increase ABR sensitivity to retrocochlear auditory dysfunction. Sensitivity and specificity of the ABR in patients with sensorineural hearing loss, including those with acoustic tumors, increased when a "dual interpretive criterion" was used for ABR analysis, i.e., a greater than normal rate-induced latency shift (RLS) in the ABR wave V, or the loss of wave V at the high stimulus presentation rate.

AN ARGUMENT FOR ABR IN NEURODIAGNOSIS OF RETROCOCHLEAR AUDITORY DYSFUNCTION. | In the era of MRI, should the ABR still play a role—leading or supporting—in

the diagnosis of auditory dysfunction? There is no doubt that MRI is the technique of choice for the documentation of the site and size of retrocochlear tumors in the IAC and/or CP angle that potentially affect the auditory pathways. The results of MRI are essential for final medical management decisions regarding patients with retrocochlear pathology. Questions usually answered by MRI include: Does the patient have a tumor? How large is the tumor? Where is the tumor located? What is the best management option, such as surgical removal, another intervention approach (e.g., gamma [photon] knife), or close monitoring? Nonetheless, the concept of applying the ABR as a screening test for retrocochlear pathology, much as it is used for hearing screening of infants at risk for hearing loss, can be applied in the cost-effective detection of acoustic tumors. Based on evidence of a sensitivity rate of 92 percent in patients with small (< 1.0 cm) acoustic neuromas (AN), El-Kashlan, Eisenmann, and Kileny (2000) conclude that "With strict adherence to optimal technique and evaluation criteria, the ABR remains a viable option for AN screening, especially in elderly patients or when there is a low index of suspicion" (p. 257). Scherler and Bohmer (1995) compared MRI and ABR for detecting acoustic tumors in a series of 391 patients. Less than 5 percent of the patients with acoustic neuromas (AN) had normal ABR findings. The authors conclude "Patients with high suspicion for AN from history, PTA, and caloric responses should be sent directly for MRI. . . . Patients with low suspicion for AN from screening tests should have BERA [ABR] performed to exclude a retrolabyrinthine lesion" (Scherler & Bohmer, 1995, p. 487). Ferguson et al. (1996) conducted a prospective investigation of the efficacy of ABR, MRI, and other procedures, in detection of CP angle tumors. The authors conclude based on their study "There is no effective screening procedure for CPA tumours, as MRI scanning with gadolinium enhancement will identify virtually all tumours. Where MRI is available but waiting lists are long, the described strategy using ABR to select priority referrals for MRI scanning is recommended" (Ferguson et al., 1996, p. 159). Other researchers also have reported positive clinical experiences with ABR in early detection of retrocochlear pathology, when validated against MRI (e.g., Kochanek et al., 1998).

In comparison to assessment of auditory function in infants and young children, neurodiagnostic ABR measurement with cooperative adult patients is straightforward and not time consuming. Total duration for completion of a pediatric ABR for estimation of auditory thresholds may exceed an hour when the time is totaled up for administration of sedation, for achieving an adequate sleep, and for recording and analyzing dozens of ABR waveforms bilaterally that are evoked by various permutations of stimulus conditions (e.g., clicks, three or four tone bursts, and multiple intensities levels down to threshold). In contrast, a skilled and experienced clinician can perform a neurodiagnostic ABR

assessment bilaterally in less than 30 minutes, including the time required to prepare the patient (electrode application, earphone placement), and to record replicable waveforms at one or two high stimulus intensity levels, and for slower and faster rates of stimulation. ABR is available as a clinical procedure in most audiology and neuro-otology facilities were patients with suspected retrocochlear pathology are likely to undergo diagnostic assessment. The combination of availability and brief test time, coupled with sensitivity to auditory dysfunction and a reasonable charge for the service, renders the ABR attractive as a screening procedure for retrocochlear pathology. The natural history of acoustic tumors is another variable that should be considered in evaluating the role of ABR in detection and neurodiagnosis of acoustic tumors. As noted elsewhere in this chapter, acoustic tumors are typically slow growing. Rosenberg (2000) conducted a retrospective chart review study of 129 patients with acoustic tumors who underwent either conservative treatment by serial neuroradiologic imaging or subtotal surgical resection. The growth rate for tumors in the nonsurgical group of patients was, on the average, 0.91 mm per year. And, 42 percent of the tumors in this group either did not grow, or they actually regressed in size. Furthermore, the overall postoperative growth rate of tumors in patients who underwent incomplete surgical resection was 0.35 mm per year, with 68.5 percent of the tumors either not growing or regressing in size. Rosenberg (2000) concludes, "The vast majority of patients older than 65 years with acoustic neuromas do not require intervention" (p. 497).

The issue of MRI and ABR in retrocochlear pathology is often inappropriately cast as an either/or decision, or stated with the question "Which diagnostic technique is better for detection of retrocochlear pathology—MRI or ABR?" This approach is inappropriate because it is based on the faulty assumption that MRI and ABR theoretically provide the same type of information about retrocochlear pathology. To use a simplistic and overworked analogy, comparing MRI to ABR in retrocochlear pathology is like comparing apples to oranges. Conventional MRI is a measure of structure, whereas ABR is a measure of function. Clinical experience with auditory neuropathy provides unequivocal evidence of the sensitivity of ABR to non-neoplastic retrocochlear dysfunction and also the insensitivity of CT and MRI to the same retrocochlear dysfunction. At least four types of factors—accessibility, financial, legal, and test performance—can be included in a decision regarding a protocol or strategy for applying MRI and/or ABR in the detection of retrocochlear auditory pathology. Although formal data are lacking regarding the availability of ABR versus MRI in primary or secondary medical facilities (e.g., physician's offices and general hospitals), it is reasonable to presume that equipment and personnel for ABR measurement are more accessible than scanners to perform MRIs and neuroradiologists to interpret the results. From the financial perspective, the charge (fee), or cost to the patient, in most facilities is probably less for a screening ABR than for a screening MRI scan. MRI clearly is superior to ABR in terms of limiting legal liability or risk, specifically for failure to diagnose a serious health problem. A blanket statement about superior test performance for either procedure would be ill advised. Without question, MRI is far superior to ABR for confirmation of small mass lesions in the retrocochlear region of the head. That is, MRI has a clear edge in test performance for tumors. This statement, however, must be qualified on two counts. First, only ABR, and not MRI, will detect non-neoplastic auditory dysfunction secondary, for example, to infections, metabolic abnormalities, and degenerative pathophysiologies. Also, the overwhelming majority of patients considered at risk for acoustic tumors, according the indicators cited at the beginning of the discussion of ABR in retrocochlear pathology, will have cochlear or non-tumor auditory dysfunction, rather than a tumor. Put another way, a tumor will be confirmed for only a small percentage of patients undergoing an MRI scan. ABR can also play an ongoing role in medical decisions regarding management of small tumors that are not associated with abnormalities in the neurologic examination or audiologic assessment. In such patients, surgical removal of the tumor is not invariably indicated. Rather, the decision on management "is best determined by the patient and physician together taking into account a number of factors. They include the size, location, and growth rate of the tumor; the presence of brainstem compression; the results of balance function testing; the progression of symptoms; age and general health; the prospects for preservation of usuable hearing; and the general wishes of the patient" (Jacobson et al., 1993, p. 359).

Depending on how one prefers to weight the above-noted factors—that is, which are more important in the decision-making process—multiple strategies exist for applying either MRI, ABR, or both techniques in neurodiagnosis of retrocochlear pathology. If minimizing liability and legal risk is a top priority, then MRI should be the front-line procedure, and, if a tumor is detected, an ABR need not be performed. If cost containment is a top priority, if accessibility to MRI is limited, and/or if a patient has claustrophobia or marked intolerance to loud sounds, then ABR should be the primary procedure, with MRI to follow only if the ABR findings are consistent with retrocochlear auditory function or are non-contributory due to the severity of hearing loss. Another option for combining the two technologies is to document the presence of a tumor with MRI. If the tumor is small or for another medical reason the decision is made to monitor the patient, rather than intervene surgically, the ABR is a viable tool for periodic follow-up assessment of the patient's status. Underlying this strategy is the assumption that with growth the tumor will affect eighth cranial nerve function, and the abnormality in function will be detected by the ABR. Finally, test performance for detection of retrocochlear pa-

thology can be maximized by routinely combining MRI with ABR for all patients meeting risk criteria (reviewed at the beginning of this section).

STACKED ABR. | A contemporary review of ABR as a tool for screening for acoustic tumors would not be complete without mention of the stacked ABR technique. Principles underlying measurement and analysis of the ABR with this technique can be traced back to the late 1970s. Dr. Manny Don and colleagues at the House Ear Institute then developed a technique for deriving with sequential high-pass masking manipulations the ABR for different frequency regions (Don & Eggermont, 1978; Don et al., 1997). The stacked ABR technique was described in Chapter 6. Failure of the conventional ABR to consistently detect small acoustic tumors, as reviewed in the foregoing sections, was the primary motivation for resurrection and clinical adaption of the derived high-pass masking technique in the form of the stacked ABR (Don, 2002; Don & Kwong, 2002). Sensitivity of the conventional ABR to retrocochlear pathology is certainly reduced in small tumors and lesions not directly impinging on auditory nerve fibers. However, with respect to the failure of conventional ABR to detect small tumors, Don et al. (2005) suspect that "the key problem is that small tumors often do not affect a sufficient number of the subset of eighth nerve fibers whose activity dominates the generation of the peak latency of the wave V to click stimuli" (p. 275). In other words, if the auditory nerve fibers carrying information from the high-frequency region of the cochlea are not sufficiently affected by a small tumor, then the click-evoked ABR appears normal, even if other populations of auditory nerve fibers are compromised by the tumor. If an ABR were recorded that was dependent on each frequency region (rather than just one), it would probably be abnormal when the contribution of one or more frequency regions was limited or eliminated by the compressive effects of a small tumor.

Don et al. (2005) recorded stacked ABRs from a series of fifty-four patients with small acoustic tumors (SAT) and a control group of seventy-eight normal-hearing nontumor subjects. Tumor size as documented by gadolinium-enhanced MRI ranged from 1.5 cm down to 0.2 cm. The ABR was evoked with click stimuli delivered to supra-aural earphones at an intensity level of 93 dB peSPL. Derived band ABRs were extracted with pink noise presented to the same ear as the click stimulus under six high-pass stimulus conditions, with filter cutoffs at 8000, 4000, 2000, 1000, and 500 Hz. The process used to derive an ABR for different frequency regions was illustrated in Figure 8.1 (on page 261). Test performance of the stacked ABR technique exceeded that of more conventional analysis measures of interaural latency difference (ILD) for wave V and the wave I to wave V latency interval. For example, sensitivity of the ILD in the SAT population was 45 percent, whereas for the wave I to wave V latency interval sensitivity was 38 percent. In contrast, Don et al. (2005) report sensitivity of 95 percent and specificity of 88 percent for the stacked ABR technique. Furthermore, if specificity were held at 50 percent (a high level of false positive screening errors), then 100 percent of the SATs were detected with stacked ABR. The authors conclude "the stacked ABR can be a sensitive, widely available, cost-effective, and comfortable tool for screening SATs" (Don et al., 2005, p. 288).

Philbert et al. (2003) compared the effectiveness of the stacked ABR technique with the derived band method versus an ABR technique that utilized tone-burst stimuli within the same six general regions of frequencies (cited above). Subjects were six patients with unilateral retrocochlear pathology (vestibular schwannoma). Size of the tumors was not specified. The two methods yielded similar values for ABR wave V latency, wave V amplitude, and waveform reproducibility. The results suggest that the tone-burst technique has promise as an alternative to the stacked ABR technique, but results are preliminary. Furthermore, test performance of the tone-burst technique in detection of SATs was not examined.

OTHER TYPES OF TUMORS. | Wang, Tien, and Hsu (2001) present a case report of a woman with a lipoma in the internal auditory canal. The patient had multiple lipomas on her trunk and limbs. CT confirmed a tumor in the IAC on the left side, confirmed as a lipoma. Audiometry showed an asymmetric left-side hearing loss and ABR findings consistent with retrocochlear auditory dysfunction.

AUDITORY CENTRAL NERVOUS SYSTEM (CNS) DISORDERS

Many papers describe ABR findings for patients with a wide array of diseases involving the CNS, primarily the brainstem. Table 10.6 lists a selection of publications including ABR results in adults with CNS diseases and disorders. The following information is limited to neuropathology in adult patient populations. The strategy for recording the ABR from patients with CNS diseases and disorders is similar to the strategy used for retrocochlear disorders, as is the approach taken for analysis and interpretation. The effectiveness of ABR measurement in CNS pathology can be increased with some modifications in the technique, as summarized in Table 10.7. The techniques are appropriate also for pediatric neurodiagnostic ABR applications. Principles of ABR measurement, reviewed in Chapters 6 and 7, are of course important for this clinical application of the response.

Tumors

Islam et al. (2002) report a case study of an 18-year-old male with MRI confirmation of a multicystic tumor extending into the fourth ventricle, diagnosed as a pineal region germinoma.

The tumor and associated bilateral dilatation of the ventricles compressed the inferior brachium. Apparent mixed hearing loss was caused by two different mechanisms. The conductive component was due to increased intracochlear fluid pressure and increased impedance at the stapes footplate, secondary to hydrocephalus and fluid transmission through the cochlear aqueduct. The neural component of the hearing loss was a result of compression of brainstem auditory structures. With right ear stimulation, ABR interwave latencies were abnormally delayed. There was detectable ABR with left-ear stimulation at 60 dB nHL.

A series of fifty-three patients with varied midbrain or infratentorial lesions reported by Hashimoto, Ishiyama, and Tozuka (1979) included three patients with pontine gliomas, two with medulloblastomas, one with a choroid plexus papilloma, eight with pineal tumors (midbrain), and four with cerebellar astrocytomas. ABR abnormalities were consistently recorded. Only wave I was normal, while latencies of III and V were increased and amplitudes of these components was reduced.

Musiek and Geurkink (1982) analyzed findings for a battery of behavioral tests (competing sentences, rapidly alternating speech perception, binaural fusion, staggered spondaic words, dichotic digits, frequency pattern recognition, low-pass filtered speech) and ABR obtained in a series of ten subjects with confirmed brainstem lesions. ABR latency abnormalities were noted for more subjects than were abnormalities for any single behavioral procedure. However, the pattern of findings for the entire test battery, ABR included, showed greatest sensitivity in confirmation of brainstem pathology. Interestingly, in patients with unilateral brainstem lesions, ABR abnormalities tended to be observed either with stimulation ipsilateral to the lesion or for both ears (lesion was unilateral but latency prolongation was bilateral).

Musiek and Lee (1995) recorded the ABR in a series of thirty-two patients with brainstem lesions, including fourteen subjects with intrinsic or extrinsic tumors, among them gliomas, meningiomas, cerebellar tumors, and a patient with a fifth cranial nerve neuroma. ABR findings were not specified for each type of pathology, but based on an analysis of ROC curves for the ABR, the authors conclude, "the ABR may not be as powerful a clinical tool for detecting brainstem disorders as some early reports suggest" (p. 635). Sensitivity of the ABR to brainstem lesions was enhanced by the use of multiple response indices, e.g., absolute latency of wave V and the three main interwave latency calculations (wave I–III, wave III–V, and wave I–V). In a companion case report, Baran, Catherwood, and Musiek (1995) describe the failure of ABR to detect in an 18-year-old woman a large mass in the low brainstem that, by CT, did not involve the auditory pathways. The case was presented to illustrate the specificity of ABR in patients with brainstem pathology that does not compromise pathways and nuclei in the central auditory nervous system.

TABLE 10.6. Summary of Selected Studies of the Auditory Brainstem Response (ABR) in Adult Patients with Various Diseases and Neuropathologies
Findings for other published studies are described in the text.

STUDY (YEAR)	N	DISEASE/ PATHOLOGY	COMMENTS
Tumors			
Naito et al. (1999)	1	T-cell lymphoma in brainstem	Prolonged wave I–V latency initially, and then loss of ABR.
Cerebrovascular Disorders			
Suzaki et al., 2002	45	Cardiopulmonary arrest	Abnormal interwave latencies for some patients.
Miscellaneous Disorders			
Stach, Westerberg, & Roberson (1998)	1	CNS milary tuberculosis	Only wave I was recorded in 28-year-old female.
Sood, Mahapatra, & Bhatia (1992)	22	Congenital craniovertebral anomaly	Abnormal ABR in basilar invagination.
Yoshikawa & Takamori, 2001	1	Benign segmental myoclonus	Normal ABR findings.
Xu, Cai, & Yang (1997)	65	Hepatolenticular degeneration	Abnormal interwave latencies in untreated patients.
Kondo et al. (1990)	13	Machado-Joseph disease	Abnormal ABR in 8 patients; only wave I in 5 patients.
Tandon, Bhatia, & Goel (1996)	23	Primary hypertension	Absolute and interwave latency delays in type III patients.
Horner, Riski, Weber, & Nashold (1993)	8	Spasmodic torticollis	ABR consistently normal.
Middleton et al. (1997)	14	Spasmodic dysphonia	ABR consistently normal.
Nakano et al. (1997)	17	Chronic respiratory insufficiency	Normal ABR in all subjects.
Souliere, Kava, Barrs, & Bell (1991)	2	Neurosarcoidosis	CPA granuloma with abnormal ABR with normal hearing.
Schmidt et al. (2001)	8	X-linked adrenoleukodystrophy	Abnormal interwave latencies in all patients.
Karp & Laureno (1993)	14	Hyponatremia	Delayed interwave latencies in some patients.
Saito et al. (1997)	1	Spastic tetraplegia	Normal ABR, with marked atrophy of medulla oblongata.
Pal et al. (1999)	26	Olivopontocerebellar atrophy	No ABR abnormalities.
Pal, Taly, Nagaraja, & Jayakumar (1995)	14	Cerebellar ataxia (early onset)	50% of patients with ABR abnormalities.
Benitez et al. (1990)	1	Cogan's syndrome (atypical)	Severe ABR abnormalities; interwave latency delays.

Other authors have also described abnormally increased interwave latencies in children with brainstem gliomas (Davis et al., 1985; Goldie, van Eyes & Baram, 1987; Hecox et al., 1981). Evidence of ABR abnormalities in this population, in combination with unremarkable CT scans, indicates the need for MRI (magnetic resonance imaging) assessment.

Among varied posterior fossa tumors in a pediatric population, Goldie, Van Eyes, and Baram (1987) noted the most severe ABR abnormalities in children with brainstem gliomas, including absence of wave V. They reported that all four patients with brainstem ependymomas also showed ABR abnormalities, whereas over two-thirds of the patients with medulloblastomas (nine out of twelve) had normal ABRs. The other three showed latency delays. The authors conclude that since ependymomas and medulloblastomas present with similar clinical and neuroradiologic findings, ABR findings may be useful in differentiating among them. Normal ABR findings with neurologic and CT evidence of brainstem tumor are most consistent with medulloblastoma versus ependymoma.

TABLE 10.7. Summary of Techniques and Strategies for the Assessment of Brainstem Auditory Function with a Neurodiagnostic ABR

- Obtain an audiogram and analyze. Rule out conductive hearing loss for either ear. Consider diagnostic audiologic assessment for auditory processing disorder. Record uncrossed (ipsilateral) and crossed (contralateral) acoustic reflexes for at least one frequency (e.g., 1000 Hz). Measure acoustic reflex decay.
- Ready equipment, instruct and prepare patient.
- Apply electrodes, verify impedance (reapply electrodes as indicated). Determine the appropriate inverting electrode design for detection of the ABR wave I component (e.g., TIPtrode with mild hearing loss or tympanic electrode with a moderate hearing loss).
- Consider ABR recording with multiple channels (e.g., noncephalic and/or horizontal electrode arrays to better define each ABR component (e.g., wave IV versus V).
- Place insert earphones (transducers), verifying that electrodes and earphones are on the correct side of the head.
- Record an ABR with high-intensity (70 to 90 dB HL) click stimuli presented at conventional rate (e.g., 21.1/sec). Identify waves I, II, III, and V. Calculate absolute and interwave latency values, assess symmetry, and compare to normative data. Use techniques described in Chapter 7 for waveform enhancement.
- Record a replicated ABR as described above, but using a rapid stimulus rate (91.1/sec). Identify and calculate latency for wave V. Compare absolute and interaural wave V latency values to normative data.
- Before the ABR assessment is completed and the patient is disconnected, verify that the ABR is replicable and major components can be confidently identified.
- Plot out replicated waveforms with appropriate labels for ear, stimulus level, and location of peaks. Prepare chart note and/or report.

Benna, Gilli, Ferrero, and Bergamasco (1982) reported delayed wave III–V and wave I–V latencies in patients with supratentorial tumors and clinical signs of increased ICP. Waves VI and VII were not observed. Musiek and Geurkink (1982) presented data obtained with a battery of audiometric procedures, including ABR, from a series of ten patients with brainstem lesions (including three with extra-axial tumors). Each of these three patients showed abnormalities in either latency, morphology, amplitude ratio, and/or latency shift at high stimulus rate. Although latency measures were most sensitive to brainstem tumors, the other response parameters enhanced ABR sensitivity.

Comprehensive studies of ABR in mentally retarded children and adults have been conducted by Nancy Squires and colleagues (Squires, Aine, Buchwald, Norman, & Gal-

braith, 1980; Squires, Buchwald, Liley, & Strecker, 1982; Squires, Ollo, & Jordan, 1986). In the 1986 study (Squires et al., 1986), subjects were thirty-four adults with Down syndrome (eighteen male and sixteen female) and fifty-four adults with non–Down syndrome retardation (twenty-five male and twenty-nine female). Importantly, if patients showed impedance audiometry evidence of middle ear dysfunction, ABR assessment was postponed until the problem cleared, except for chronic pathology. ABR data for the retarded groups were compared to a nonretarded group of adults. The major finding was a reduction (shortening) of ABR interwave intervals in Down syndrome subjects versus non–Down syndrome or normal subjects, confirming previously reported observations by these investigators and others (Folsom, Widen, & Wilson, 1983; Galbraith et al., 1983; Squires et al., 1980, 1982). Specifically, there was a reduction in the wave I–III and wave III–V latency intervals. ABR interwave intervals, although often referred to as a measure of "central or brainstem conduction time," can be also be reduced as a function of peripheral hearing impairment, especially for high-frequency loss. However, Squires et al. (1986) found shortened interwave latency values even in Down syndrome subjects with normal peripheral auditory status. No clear physiologic basis for this paradoxical decrease in ABR interwave intervals has been identified. The authors recommend a test battery approach for hearing assessment in mental retardation.

Demyelinating Diseases

This is a group of diseases that affect the myelin sheath of neurons, sparing the axons of CNS and peripheral nervous system neurons. Two categories are demyelinating diseases (disease process affects normal myelin sheath) and dysmyelinating diseases (defective myelin metabolism). The following diseases fall into the CNS demyelinating category: acute disseminated encephalomyelitis (ADEM), acute hemorrhagic leukoencephalitis, multiple sclerosis, and Schilder's disease. Guillian-Barre syndrome demyelination affects the peripheral nervous system. Dysmelinating diseases encompass leukodystrophies, such as metachromatic leukodystrophy, globoid cell leukodystrophy, sudanophilic (orthochromatic) leukodystrophy, adrenoleukodystrophy, Pelizaeus-Merzbacher disease, and Alexander's disease.

MULTIPLE SCLEROSIS (MS). | MS is the most common type of demyelinating disease and a major cause of neurologic impairment in adults except the elderly. Young adults are usually affected (about 50 to 70 percent of patients have onset between age 20 and 40 years). MS in children is extremely rare. The male: female ratio is about 1:1.7. For reasons not completely understood, it is most prevalent in colder climates. Estimates on prevalence vary from approximately 10 per 100,000 in the southern regions of the United States and from 50 to 70 per 100,000 in the northern regions of the United States. The disease has a slow and progressive course that characteristically is irregular with fluctuating periods of exacerbation and remission of specific symptoms. Plaques, which are large, irregular, discontinuous lesions, may be found anywhere in the CNS on myelin sheaths, but rarely destructing axons. They are especially common in the optic nerves, spinal cord, periventricular brainstem regions, and periventricular cerebral white matter. Symptoms include sensory and motor deficits in the head, limbs, and trunk, sphincter disturbances; visual (quite frequent), tactile, and, less commonly, hearing deficits.

Hearing impairment is typically not an initial symptom or a prominent complaint in MS. Reported incidence of peripheral hearing loss varies markedly, ranging from as low as 1 percent to as high as 86 percent (Djupesland et al., 1981; Fischer et al., 1985; Musiek, Gollegly, Kibbe, & Reeves, 1989; Mustillo, 1984; Noffsinger et al., 1972; Schweitzer & Shepard, 1989). Since the deficit is most often unilateral, it is often not detected during routine physical examination. If present, hearing impairment is high frequency, sensorineural, and bilateral in 85 percent of patients. Sudden onset of hearing loss in MS, although rare, is reported (Schweitzer & Shepard, 1989). Accurate large-scale statistics on the incidence of hearing loss due specifically to MS are not available. Importantly, up to 40 percent of MS patients with normal audiograms may report hearing difficulties in everyday listening conditions (Musiek et al., 1989). Performance for simple speech audiometry procedures is usually good, but deficits are evident for complex speech intelligibility tasks (e.g., dichotic digits and staggered spondaic word test) for up to one-third of patients. Abnormalities are also reported for masking level difference, acoustic reflexes, frequency pattern recognition test, and low-pass filtered speech test (see Musiek et al., 1989; Jerger, Oliver, Chmiel, & Rivera, 1986; Hannley, Jerger, & Rivera, 1983, for reviews). Diplopia (double vision) often results from medial longitudinal fasciculus lesions in the brainstem.

Diagnosis of MS is based on the multifocal involvement of the nervous system, usually in combination with a course that is erratic and periods of intense symptoms (exacerbation) and lessening of symptoms (remission). Whether MS occurs in children is controversial. Although the average age of onset is 30 years, there are reports of patients as young as 2 years meeting the diagnostic criteria (Hausler, Bresman, Reiherz, & Weiner, 1982, in Duquette, 1987). Duquette et al. (1987) conducted a survey in Canada that showed that 125 of 4,632 patients with MS (2.7 percent) were under age 16 at onset. The average age was 13 years, and the youngest child was 5 years. The female to male ratio in children was 3:1. With onset in youth, MS may be more severe than onset in middle age. The etiology of MS is not known. Genetic, infectious, immunologic theories, and a combination of these, have been proposed. Symptoms typically become more apparent with elevation of body temperature. CT, MRI, and sensory evoked responses (auditory, somatosensory, and visual) are useful in making the diagnosis. Among the standard medical therapies for MS is intravenous adrenocorticotropic hormone (ACTH) for ten days followed by oral steroids for three weeks to a month. No therapy is effective as a cure, and none are equally successful for all patients.

Published and widely applied systems for classifying the clinical severity of MS according to information from history and physical examination were introduced by Allison and Millar (1954), McAlpine, Lumsden, and Acheson (1972), McDonald and Halliday (1977), and Rose, Ellison, Myers, and Tourtelotte (1976). Most categorize MS as "definite," "probable," and "possible," but McDonald and Halliday (1977) add "progressive possible" and "progressive probable" categories. Additional clinical data include analysis of cerebrospinal fluid (CSF) for presence of abnormal (elevated) gammaglobulins or an abnormal IgG index and functional disability, according to the Kurtzke (1970) scale. There are numerous texts and reference sources on multiple sclerosis.

Application of sensory evoked responses, including the ABR, in diagnosis of MS has been extensively investigated for many years. As suggested by data in the Table 10.8, ABR results among studies vary widely, even for patients with clinically "definite" MS. Reasons for the variations in the percentage of abnormal ABRs include differences in (1) recording techniques (ipsilateral versus contralateral electrode arrays), (2) stimulus parameters (rate, intensity, monoaural versus binaural), (3) definition of an abnormal response, (4) physiologic characteristics (body temperature), (5) the diagnostic categories and criteria for classification of MS, and (6) the extent of patient disability.

Response abnormalities in MS include prolonged interwave (I–III, III–V, I–V) latencies, decreased amplitude especially of wave V, poor morphology (desynchronization) for later wave components, poor test repeatability, total absence of one or more recognizable wave components after wave I or II (most often wave V), and occasional absence or prolongation of wave I. Although abnormally increased ABR latency, especially for wave V, is the most characteristic finding in MS, this clinical interpretation is compromised in some cases by difficulty in accurately identifying specific wave components, as noted by Parving, Elberling, and Smith (1981). A frequently noted ABR phenomenon in MS is the bimodal distribution for latency values. In some MS patients, ABR latencies are indistinguishable statistically from those of normal subjects. When MS affects the ABR, however, latency values are markedly abnormal (usually 4 or more standard deviations above the mean normal value). The pathophysiologic implication is that the ABR will be normal if MS for a given patient does not involve auditory brainstem pathways, but even a small plaque in the

TABLE 10.8. Summary of Selected Studies of the Auditory Brainstem Response (ABR) in Multiple Sclerosis (MS)

STUDY (YEAR)	N	MS CRIT	ABN CRIT*	ABR CRIT
Robinson & Rudge (1977)	88	McAlpine	1,2	95%ile
Mogensen & Kristensen (1979)	29	McAlpine	1–4	+ 2 sd
Chiappa (1980)	81	McAlpine	1–5	+ 3 sd
Khoshbin & Hallett (1981)	30	McAlpine	1,2	+ 2.5 sd
Parving et al. (1981)	13	McAlpine	1,2	+ 2.5 sd
Matthews et al. (1982)	06	McAlpine	1,2	+ 3 sd
Kjaer (1983)	80	McAlpine	1–4	+ 2 sd
Phillips et al. (1983)	20	Rose	1,4	+ 3 sd
Bartel et al. (1983)	36	McAlpine	1–4	?
Hannley et al. (1983)	20	McAlpine	1–4	+ 2 sd
Tackmann et al. (1984)	49	Schumacher	?	?
Deltenre et al. (1984)	56	McDonald	1,3	+ 3 sd
Cutler et al. (1986)	19	?	?	?
Antonelli et al. (1986)	16	Rose	1–5	+ 2 sd
Jerger et al. (1986)	62	Waksman	1–4	95%ile
Jacobson et al. (1987)	10	Schumacher	1–5	99%ile
Hammond & Yiannikas (1987)	64	Rose	1–5	+ 3 sd
Antonelli et al. (1988)	32	Posner	1–5	+ 2 sd
Musiek et al. (1989)	33	McAlpine	1–5	defined

* Crit = ABR waves analyzed; I, II, III, VI, V = absolute latency for these ABR waves; 1–5 = absolute and interwave latencies; Abn Crit = criteria for upper normal limit of latency

auditory brainstem is enough to radically alter neural conduction along the pathways.

It is important, of course, to document stimulus parameters in study of MS. Monaural, as opposed to binaural, stimulation is recommended because ABR findings may be unilateral in approximately 45 percent of patients. These lateralized lesions would go undetected with stimulation of both ears simultaneously, since a normal response would be recorded from stimulus to the unaffected ear. Comparison of ABR amplitude recorded with binaural versus monaural stimulation may have diagnostic value in MS. In normal subjects, binaural stimulation produces an augmentation of wave V, whereas Prasher, Sainz, and Gibson (1982) found no wave V amplitude increase in the majority of their 18 MS patients. Some investigators suggest that sensitivity of the ABR to MS is enhanced by increased stimulus rates (Elidan, Sohmer, Gafni, & Kahana, 1982; Jacobson, Murray, & Deppe, 1987; Musiek et al., 1989; Robinson & Rudge, 1977; Shanon, Gold, & Himmelfarb, 1981; Stockard, Stockard, & Sharbrough, 1977), although there is also evidence to the contrary (Chiappa, Harrison,

Brooks, & Young, 1980; Chiappa & Norwood, 1977; Jacobson & Newman, 1989). As Jacobson and Newman (1989) point out, ABR outcome may be influenced by interactions between stimulus rate and polarity (see Chapter 6). With rarefaction polarity click stimuli, these authors failed to show further ABR wave I–V latency abnormality for rapid versus slow rates. The authors speculate that the absence of a rate effect on ABR abnormality in MS may reflect "a less severe form of axonal demyelination." Using pairs of clicks as stimuli, Mogensen and Kristensen (1979) recorded ABR abnormalities in 83 percent of their MS group. They noted that abnormality of the negative voltage peak after wave V (referred to by them as the far-field potential 7 or FFP 7, and probably comparable to the SN10) was a common finding in MS.

The literature permits several generalizations about the role of ABR in MS. It appears that among sensory evoked response modalities, the visual evoked responses (VERs) usually have the highest overall sensitivity and specificity, followed by either somatosensory evoked responses (SSERs), stimulated at the median nerve in the arm (upper extremity) and the posterior tibial nerve in the leg (lower extremity) or, in fewer studies, ABR. The electrophysiologically recorded blink reflex appears least sensitive. For example, Deltenre, Van Nechel, Strul, and Ketelaer (1984) reported abnormalities in patients with definite MS of 66 percent for VERs, 23.2 percent for SSERs, 17.8 percent for ABRs, and 12.5 percent for the blink reflex. Also, Giesser et al. (1987) found abnormality rates in patients with possible MS of 63 percent for VERs, 53 percent for ABRs, and 49 percent for SSERs. Tackmann, Ettlin, Wuthrich, and Strenge (1984) and Matthews, Wattam-Bell, and Pountney (1982), among others, ranked VERs and SSERs well above ABRs in sensitivity to MS, especially detecting clinically silent lesions. As an example of the variation in hit rates among modalities from study to study, however, Chiappa (1980) reported abnormality rates in possible MS that were relatively low (37 percent) for VERs, and 49 percent for SSERs and 30 percent for ABRs.

There is agreement that application of a multimodal evoked response battery yields the higher sensitivity (over 85 percent) than any single modality in isolation. Distribution of multimodal sensory evoked response abnormality for different categories of MS as compiled from varied studies by Hart and Sherman (1982) was 97 percent for definite, 86 percent for probable, and 63 percent for possible MS. Also, sensory evoked responses abnormalities can be used to reclassify MS patients—that is, moving a patient from one category (based on history and clinical data interpreted with one of the classification systems noted above) to another category with greater diagnostic probability. For a specific study, however, the percentage of sensory evoked response abnormalities does not necessarily vary systematically among classification categories. It is not always highest for patients with "definite," progressively lower for "probable," and then "possible" MS. Within a category, the extent of patient disability may be an important factor. In patients with definite MS, an increase in ABR abnormality rate may be found among those patients with greater disability (Hammond & Yiannikas, 1987; Hutchinson, Blandford, & Glynn, 1984; Kjaer, 1980). The proportion and degree of evoked response abnormalities increased as body temperature increased (Geraud et al., 1982; Matthews, Read, and Pountney, 1979; Phillips et al., 1983). Monitoring MS clinical status with sensory evoked responses is clinically appealing, but its efficacy is not clearly established. VERs are variable from test to test, even with stable clinical condition and, correspondingly, SSER and ABR findings may vary from assessment to assessment without corresponding worsening or remission in clinical status (Likosky & Elmore, 1982; Matthews & Small, 1979). On the other hand, improvement of symptoms has been related to reversal of sensory evoked response abnormalities by some investigators (Stockard & Rossiter, 1977). This latter relationship suggests that evoked responses could be used to evaluate the effectiveness of medical therapy in MS, perhaps with more sensitivity and objectivity than the neurological examination.

Finally, evoked responses are perhaps most powerful clinically when incorporated into a neurodiagnostic test battery. Jerger, Chmiel, Frost, & Coker (1986) found that a combination of audiometric procedures (ABR, acoustic reflexes, and masking level difference) yielded a higher rate of identification (87 percent) than ABR alone (52 percent). Others have also emphasized the value of interpreting ABR results in MS within the context of an audiometric test battery approach and included such procedures as dichotic digits, staggered spondaic word test, low-pass filtered speech, pitch pattern recognition, and acoustic reflex amplitude measures (Musiek et al., 1989). Reliance on an audiometric test battery that includes assessment of auditory sensitivity is particularly important in view of the possibility that peripheral (eighth cranial nerve) hearing impairment may be a component of MS. As noted above, hearing impairment is traditionally not one of the clinical symptoms associated with MS. However, case reports of MS-related hearing loss have infrequently appeared in the literature for 100 years. The site of lesion is presumed to be the eighth nerve, and perhaps the ipsilateral cochlear nucleus. Parving, Elberling, and Smith (1981) observed intensity-dependent prolongations in the latency for the ECochG AP component and decreases in AP amplitude in nine patients with MS. The authors present this as evidence of a cochlear and eighth nerve site of lesion. Suggested mechanisms for the dysfunction are abnormalities in synaptic transmission in the cochlea/eighth nerve region, plaques on the eighth nerve, and aberrant efferent innervation of the cochlea.

Evoked responses may offer a more sensitive index of MS than CT or more recent neuroradiologic techniques, such as MRI (Giesser et al., 1987; Tramo, Schneck, & Lee, 1985). Evoked response abnormalities may be found in patients with normal MRI. Giesser et al. (1987) reported overall sensitivity rates of 90.5 percent for multimodal evoked responses, as opposed to 71.4 percent for MRI in possible MS patients. In contrast, Cutler, Aminoff, and Brant-Zawadzki (1986) and Bartel, Markand, and Kolar (183) provided evidence that MRI is, in general, more sensitive than evoked responses in detecting MS. ABR did have greater value than MRI in identifying lesions in the brainstem. ABR abnormalities are usually, but not invariably, correlated with more severe plaque lesions as detected by MRI (Pkalnis, Drake, Dadmehr, & Weiss, 1987). Since these two general neurodiagnostic methods evaluate different characteristics of the CNS (functional versus structural and sensory pathways versus entire CNS), they are, in fact, complementary. The relative high cost of MRI, in comparison to evoked responses, is an additional issue to consider in routine clinical use of these two neurodiagnostic approaches in MS (Cutler et al., 1986).

LEUKODYSTROPHIES. | These are rare familial abnormalities of myelination formation that are found in infants and children and affect white matter (gray matter is spared). There is widespread and often symmetrically bilateral failure or degeneration in the formation of myelination in the CNS with some degree of axonal degeneration. Diagnosis is suggested by CT scanning, which shows extensive white matter hypodensity. Metachromatic leukodystrophy is inherited as an autosomal recessive trait and has its onset around 12 to 18 months of age with progressive leg weakness and ataxia and then upper limb involvement, progressive dementia, and speech/language deficits. There are six different types of metachromatic leukodystrophy. Death occurs by age 7 in most cases. Adrenoleukodystrophy is a childhood disease affecting boys only with an onset at approximately 7 years. Long-chain fatty acids are elevated in the CNS. Neurologic and mental deterioration progressively develop secondary to diffuse cerebral sclerosis. There may also be spinal cord or peripheral nerve demyelination. Death occurs within one to four years. Krabbe's leukodystrophy (globoid cell leukodystrophy) has three forms: infantile, juvenile, and adult. Infantile is most common and recognized by failure to thrive, myoclonic seizures, spasticity, macrocrania, loss of acquired skills and early death. Pathology includes multinucleated giant cells in the white matter. There are three leukodystrophies with no known biochemical markers. Pelizaeus-Merzbacher disease is inherited and usually sex linked, affects only males, and has an onset as early as the first months of life. Symptoms include head trembling, roving eye movements, ataxia, and slow motor and mental development that worsen during adolescence. The disease has an extended course, with death occurring in early adulthood. Alexander's leukodystrophy begins in infancy. Symptoms are deterioration of psychomotor functioning, seizures, and spasticity. During the second year, macrocephaly becomes apparent with death by age 6 years. Canavan's sclerosis begins also in infancy. Symptoms are hypotonia, optic atrophy, seizures, spasticity, megalencephaly, and failure to thrive. Another form of this disease begins at age 5 and develops at a slower rate. Along with a variety of diseases, leukodystrophies produce neurological degeneration.

ABR abnormalities are typically found in this white matter disease and are useful in distinguishing white versus gray matter involvement. Prolonged ABR interwave (I–V) latencies characterize adrenoleukodystrophy and a related disease, adrenomyeloneuropathy (Garg et al., 1982; Grimes et al., 1983; Markand et al., 1982; Tobimatsu et al., 1985; Vercruyssen, Martin, & Mercelis, 1982). These ABR findings are associated with increased central conduction times for SSERs and VERs. Absence of ABR waves III or V, or all components after wave I and wave II, are not uncommon (Markand et al., 1982; Yagi, Kaga, & Baba, 1980). Wave I is usually present, but the ABR is rarely normal, and then only in patients with a mild form of the disease. Eighth-nerve pathology has been reported (Igarashi, Neely, & Anthony, 1976). Isolated unilateral absence of wave VI has also been given diagnostic significance in adrenoleukodystrophy (Black, Fariello, & Chun, 1979).

Similarly markedly abnormal ABRs are recorded in most patients with Pelizaeus-Merzbacher disease and both infantile and juvenile onset metachromatic leukodystrophy (Brown et al., 1981; Carlin et al., 1983; Davis, Aminoff, & Berg, 1985; Hecox, Cone, & Blaw, 1981; Markand et al., 1982; Nuwer et al., 1982). Pelizaeus-Merzbacher disease is an X-linked central nervous system dysmyelinating disorder caused by a submicroscopic duplication containing the proteolipid gene (Inoue et al., 2001). Inoue et al. (2001) reported two case reports of patients with Pelizaeus-Merzbacher disease who showed improvement (a decrease) in abnormal ABR interwave latencies over a ten-year period. The authors speculate "that the remarkable clinical improvement is a result of myelin compensation by oligodentrocytes in the formation of central nervous system myelin" (p. 747). In patients with metachromatic leukodystrophy, there may be, in addition, a delayed latency wave I (Carlin et al., 1983; Hecox, Cone, & Blaw, 1981; Markand et al., 1982; Ochs, Markand, & DeMyer, 1979). These types of ABR were normal in carriers of Pelizaeus-Merzbacher disease who were unaffected. ABR aberrations in leukodystrophies are correlated with demyelination and are again useful clinically in differentiating white matter versus gray matter disease.

OTHER DEMYELINATING DISEASES. | Varied ABR findings were reported in other demyelinating diseases. Jacobson, Means, and Dhib-Jalbut (1986) described eighth-nerve involvement evidenced by increased wave I latency and slight high-frequency pure-tone hearing threshold deficit for a 30-year-old male patient with acute inflammatory demyelinating disease. Twelve patients with inflammatory acute transverse myelopathy had normal ABRs. This disease involves neural tracts on both sides of the spinal cord. Yagi, Kaga, and Baba (1980) reported the absence of waves after I in West syndrome.

In an interesting twist on the usual format for a clinical study, Sawaishi, Tomita, and Mito (1990) investigated possible pathologies for seventeen patients with various nonspecific neurological disorders who had no detectable ABR. Neuroradiology confirmed brainstem atrophy for one patient, and five had abnormal laboratory findings and delayed motor development. However, the ABR findings for another five patients with otherwise normal audiologic test results were attributed to "desynchronization" within the auditory pathways.

OPTIC NEURITIS. | There is a considerable likelihood that patients with optic neuritis will subsequently develop multiple sclerosis. Tackmann, Ettlin, and Strenge (1982) measured multimodal sensory evoked responses and electrically stimulated blink reflex in thirty-two patients with isolated optic neuritis. Six patients showed ABR abnormalities. These consisted of a unilateral delay in wave V latency in five patients and unilateral absence of waves II through V in the remaining patient. VER findings were abnormal for thirty-one patients, while SSERs were abnormal for six and the blink reflex for two. Likewise, Robinson and Rudge (1980) and Stockard, Stockard, and Sharbrough (1980) described ABR latency delays in optic neuritis. However, the collective findings of these investigations are not in agreement with data reported by Chiappa, Harrison, Brooks, and Young (1980) indicating normal ABRS (and SSERs) in eighteen patients with optic neuritis.

Cerebrovascular Diseases

Approximately one-half million persons suffer a cerebrovascular accident (CVA), or "stroke," each year, and 200,000 die. Stroke is actually a simple layman's term for a wide range of vascular diseases. Because stroke occurs more often in the elderly and is frequently caused by atherosclerotic vascular disease, it is commonly associated exclusively with this disease. Cerebrovascular disease is the third leading cause of death in the United States. Risk factors for CVA include primarily hypertension, but also include aging (especially after 65 years), heart disease, diabetes, and birth control pills. Cerebrovascular disease is actually damage to brain tissue (parenchyma) due to pathologic changes in blood vessels that serve the brain, among them the internal carotid system (internal carotid artery, middle cerebral artery, anterior choroidal artery, anterior cerebral artery) and the vertebrobasilar system (vertebral artery, basilar artery, posterior cerebral artery). These two systems (carotid and vertebrobasilar) are joined to varying degrees at the base of the brain by the circle of Willis (see discussion of vascular anatomy in Chapter 2). The term "stroke" can, therefore, be used to describe vascular accidents affecting the cerebrum or the brainstem. There are three general mechanisms of strokes: (1) occlusion, resulting in infarction; (2) a subarachnoid artery rupture producing a subarachnoid hemorrhage or an intraparenchymal artery rupture producing an intraparenchymal (within brain tissue) hemorrhage; and (3) hypotension, which leads to various hypoxic or ischemic events. AER findings in neuropathy of vascular basis in each of the general anatomic regions are reviewed below.

In young, normal adults, total cerebral blood flow (CBF) is in the range of 700 to 900 ml/min with two-thirds of the blood reaching the brain via the carotid system and one-third via the vertebrobasilar system. With inadequate CBF, and consequently inadequate oxygen and glucose, there is rapid development of brain ischemia (described further in the discussion of neurointensive unit monitoring with ABR later in this chapter). In addition to clinical signs, the EEG and evoked responses show abnormalities with CBF decreases of

25 to 30 percent below normal levels. These changes reflect progressive deterioration in neuronal metabolism. Irreversible brain ischemia (irreparable neuronal damage) will occur within minutes of complete reduction of CBF. Again, as described previously in Chapter 2, the middle cerebral artery distribution includes portions of the auditory cerebrum cortex contributing to AMLR, ALR, and the P300 response. Within the internal carotid system, middle cerebral artery distribution circulation is impaired (by stenosis or occlusion) more often than any other artery of the brain.

The vertebrobasilar system supplies anatomic structures giving rise to ECochG and ABR. From one person to another, the vertebral arteries may not be of equal size. Branching of both vertebral and basilar arteries, and their distribution, are also variable among normal persons. Consequently, the same site for obstruction of a vessel may produce different signs and symptoms clinically. The effect of impaired posterior cerebral artery blood circulation depends on the status of the circle of Willis. Brainstem, cerebellum, and thalamus infarction and dysfunction may result from stenosis or occlusion of the basilar artery or both vertebral arteries. There is often occlusion of the penetrating branches of the basilar artery, causing brainstem infarction. Impairment of vertebrobasilar circulation results in characteristic clinical signs and symptoms, including cranial nerve palsies, ataxia, vertigo, visual deficits, swallowing dysfunction, Horner's syndrome, gaze deficits, and transient global amnesia (a hippocampal deficit).

TYPES OF VASCULAR NEUROPATHY. | A minor cerebrovascular accident without any residual neurologic deficit is called a transient ischemic attack (TIA) or reversible ischemic neurologic deficit (RIND). The former by definition is a temporary but often repetitive focal CNS dysfunction of limited duration (usually less than 30 minutes) secondary to decreased blood supply. TIAs are more common in males than females. The latter (RIND) develops slower and symptoms may persist for over 24 hours (as long as several months). Other major types of cerebrovascular disease include vascular malformations. Saccular aneurysms are a dilatation of the lumen of the blood vessel caused by weakness and outward deformation of the layers of the wall. The basis in most cases is probably a congenital defect in the blood vessel wall structure. Aneurysms are detected first around puberty. Size may range from small (1 mm) to 3 or 4 cm (average is about 9 mm). Aneurysms are found in major arteries in the base of the brain, usually in the subarachnoid space. Among these aneurysms, 10 percent are in the vertebrobasilar system and 90 percent are in the internal carotid system. There is more than one aneurysm in from 10 to 20 percent of cases. Far more often than not, aneurysms are without symptoms throughout an affected person's lifetime.

Rupture of an aneurysm under the age of 15 years is unusual, while 90 percent rupture between ages 30 and 70 years. Depending on its location, a ruptured aneurysm produces intracranial hemorrhage, such as subarachnoid or intracerebral hemorrhage. This initial hemorrhage is fatal for 30 percent and an equal number of those who survive the first hemorrhage will die from a recurrence within a month to six weeks. When the hemorrhage extends into the brainstem via the cerebral peduncles, clinical signs may include coma, decerebration, abnormalities in pupillary responses, and loss of other brainstem reflexes. A large intracerebral hemorrhage can lead to transtentorial herniation (of the medial temporal lobe or uncus), resulting in brainstem compression with the signs noted above. Pontine hemorrhage is usually a fatal injury. Ocular bobbing is a classic sign. Primary subarachnoid hemorrhage (SAH) most often results from ruptured aneurysm. Typically, at the onset the patient reports a severe headache and a stiff neck, then irritability and sleepiness. Acute management decisions are based on the extent of neurological dysfunction and CT findings. Secondary complications of SAH are cerebral arterial spasm (in approximately 35 percent of cases) and hydrocephalus (either obstructive within two or three weeks of the initial bleed or communicating type at two or three months). Aneurysms are also associated with cerebral infarction due to arterial spasm, embolus, or compression of other blood vessels. Intracerebral hemorrhage is often directly related to hypertension. One theory is that with long-standing hypertension there is the development of microscopic aneurysms of distal cerebral arterioles that then rupture. Hypertensive intracerebral hemorrhage is often limited to the basal ganglia or thalamus. Intracranial (e.g., subarachnoid) hemorrhage may infrequently be due to brain tumor, as well as AVMs, aneurysms, and encephalitis.

Arteriovenous malformations (AVMs) include a wide variety of abnormalities in arteries, capillaries, and/or veins. Most commonly, the malformation is a tangle of blood vessels that consists of both arteries and veins. AVMs are usually found in cerebral hemispheres. Only 7 to 15 percent occur in the posterior fossa (involving brainstem or cerebellum). In contrast to aneurysms, almost 40 percent of AVMs are found in persons under the age of 40 years. The AVM leaves nearby vasculature undisturbed, but leads to CNS dysfunction by hemorrhage (often fatal) or compression and ischemia of surrounding brain tissue. Bleeding from AVMs is usually less severe than from aneurysms and, consequently, prognosis is better. Although uncommon, posterior fossa AVMs are quite relevant to ABR clinical application. Brainstem AVMs tend to be intra-axial (intrinsic) more often than extra-axial (outside confines of CNS). There may be extension to other areas. Acute hemorrhage (subarachnoid, fourth ventricle, or parenchymal) usually leads to clinical signs. Signs and symptoms include chronic and/or progressively severe headache, ataxia, cranial nerve dysfunction, eye movement abnormalities, ocular bobbing, conjugate gaze, and limb weakness. Many of these general symptoms, of course, are associated

with other brainstem pathology, such as neoplasms or multiple sclerosis. In addition, AVMs in the posterior fossa are asymptomatic in from 48 to 77 percent of patients.

Acute infarction of the brainstem may produce a clinical condition referred to as "locked-in syndrome," a term coined by Plum and Posner (1980). The typical etiology is basilar artery occlusion at the caudal pontine region, but locked-in syndrome may also result from traumatic brainstem damage. Reticular activating system in the tegmentum of pons is not involved, and the tegmental corticobulbar tracts that innervate the nuclei of the third (oculomotor) cranial nerve are also not involved, preserving vertical eye movements and blinking. Therefore, the patient is alert but quadriplegic and only able to blink and to move the eyes vertically. There is loss of voluntary movement from destruction of corticospinal pathways in the pontine brainstem. Varied ABR findings have been reported in locked-in syndrome, as described below.

In the following discussion on evoked responses in CNS vascular lesions, it is important to keep in mind that transient ABR abnormalities can be recorded from brainstem structures that are essentially intact and not permanently damaged (e.g., the tegmentum), as reported by various investigators (Seales et al., 1981; Selters & Brackmann, 1977; Starr & Achor, 1975; Stockard & Rossiter, 1977; Stockard, Sharbrough, & Stockard, 1977). The likely pathophysiologic explanation is the effect of reversible local edema, ischemia, or pressure from other brainstem structures on ABR anatomy. And, with the exception of acute CVAs that are accompanied by brain swelling and secondary compressive brainstem effects, AER findings in cerebral vascular disease are reported mostly for AMR, ALR, or P300 components.

BRAINSTEM PATHOLOGY. | Next to brainstem neoplasms, literature on pathologic correlations of ABR in brainstem pathology is probably most extensive for vascular diseases (Fischer et al., 1982; Hashimoto, Ishiyama, & Tozuka, 1979; Møller & Møller, 1985; Musiek & Geurkink, 1982; Stockard & Rossiter, 1977; Stockard, Stockard, & Sharbrough, 1986). Actually, many of the papers just cited report data also for patients with brainstem neoplasms. The discrepancies among studies attempting to relate site and side of lesions to ABR abnormalities, noted earlier in the discussion of brainstem tumors, are at least as commonplace in the literature on vascular disease. In fact, the picture is probably less clear because of the complex blood supply to the brainstem and the often-diffuse nature of vertebrobasilar and brainstem diseases, such as infarctions, hemorrhages, and TIAs. The overall generalization drawn from studies of ABR and brainstem tumors applies as well for vascular pathology. ABR is a highly sensitive measure of brainstem pathology affecting the auditory pathways, and it can sometimes differentiate caudal (pons/medulla region) versus more rostral (mid to upper pons and midbrain) lesions, but is otherwise not particularly site specific. Selected articles on this topic are discussed briefly in this section.

Stockard, Rossiter, et al. (1976) presented a case report of a patient with central pontine myelinolysis showing demyelination of neural fibers in ascending auditory pathways in pons. Seales et al. (1981) described ABR findings for a 76-year-old female with a 48-hour history of episodic dizziness who collapsed and was admitted to the hospital. Right hemiparesis evolved quickly to quadriplegia. Only vertical eye movements and a blink remained. Serial ABRs were recorded on hospital days 10, 14, and 16. Initially, there was prolongation of the wave III–V latency interval bilaterally. Both wave I–III and wave III–V latency intervals on the right ear were abnormal by day 14, but this abnormality entirely reversed and the previously normal wave I–III latencies actually were improved by the 16th day, although the wave III–V latency remained delayed. Wave V amplitude, initially reduced, returned to a value within the normal range. ABR morphology on the 21st hospital day was extremely poor, and it was difficult to identify major wave components. ABR continued to deteriorate through day 45 when even a wave I was not recorded. Autopsy revealed evidence of multiple lesions in the pons and pons/medulla region (infarct, cystic changes, necrosis), including trapezoid body and lateral lemniscus. Eighth nerves, cochlear nuclei, and superior olivary complexes appeared to be normal.

Chang and Morariu (1979) described a case report of a 25-year-old male with transient locked-in syndrome of traumatic etiology. He was found with multiple injuries and loss of consciousness at scene of an automobile accident. Initially, the patient was comatose and then only minimally responsive to sensory stimulation. Complications during this period included temporary respiratory failure, sepsis, and massive urinary bleeding. By post-injury day 10, he showed clinical signs consistent with locked-in syndrome. Status improved thereafter, with return of motor function and speech. CT scans were always normal. During this period, unilateral ABR abnormalities were noted. Amplitude was decreased and the wave III–V latency interval was increased on the left. The patient survived.

Gilroy, Lynn, and Pellerin (1977) presented ABR findings for a 34-year-old male patient with an occlusion of the basilar artery about 7 mm above its origin that resulted in infarction at the junction of the lower one-third and upper two-thirds of pons. Initial symptoms were bifrontal headaches, left-sided weakness, and lethargy. Then, the patient developed bilateral horizontal nystagmus, mild left-sided facial weakness, ataxia of left upper limb, generalized hyperreflexia, and bilateral extensor plantar responses. His clinical status deteriorated to quadriplegia and coma. CT scan was normal, but arteriograms confirmed basilar artery obstruction. ABR wave I, wave II, and wave III were normal in latency, amplitude, and morphology.

Waves IV and V were prolonged in latency and reduced in amplitude.

Varied ABR findings have been reported in locked-in syndrome. Stockard, Stockard, and Sharbrough (1978) found a normal ABR in a patient with massive pontine infarct, but Gilroy, Lynn, Ristow, and Pellerin (1977) and Stockard, Rossiter, Weiderholt, and Koboyashi (1976) described abnormalities in two other patients. The etiology for one of their case reports was a central pontine myelinolysis in which there was demyelination of neural fibers in ascending auditory pathways in the pons. The tegmental location of ABR pathways in the brainstem may be one reason for the normal findings in some cases.

Portnoy et al. (1985) reported ABR data for a 65-year-old male receiving anticoagulation medical therapy for brainstem ischemia. Initially, there was improvement of neurologic status. After ten days, therapy was discontinued with subsequent deterioration of status and ultimately coma. CT initially showed a large pontomesencephalic hemorrhage and later residual hematoma in left pons tegmentum and right midbrain. For a period of time, the patient was alert but locked-in. Initially, ABR waves I through III were normal with right ear stimulus, but later all waves were not replicable. There were never reliable waves on left. Serial ABRs showed some improvement on right, but not on the left.

Buettner, Stohr, and Koletzki (1983) reported abnormal ABR findings for five patients with AVMs in the posterior fossa (involving the verterbrobasilar artery system) and signs and symptoms of trigeminal neuralgia, facial spasm, and facial paresis. The authors do note experience with other patients having this pathology who did not show ABR abnormalities, and are therefore not reported. The characteristic finding was a prolonged wave I–III latency on the side of the AVM.

ABR can be useful in the early localization of a focal brainstem lesion, but not in prognosis. In the above case, neurological condition improved in spite of very abnormal ABR and SSER findings. SERs have especial value in the evaluation of structures in the lower brainstem where CT is less effective and also on occasions when the neurological exam is of limited value. SERs are unlikely to change with lesions that affect the level of consciousness. Survival of brainstem hemorrhage is very rare, with approximately three-fourths of patients reported in the literature dying within 48 hours. This case reported by Portenoy et al. (1985) also demonstrates that the ascending reticular activating system can escape damage in brainstem hemorrhage.

Factor and Dentinger (1987) carried out ABR assessments from eight patients after vertebrobasilar TIAs. Initially (within one to sixteen days after the TIA), all ABR recordings were abnormal. Among the clinical symptoms at the time of TIA or signs observed by a neurologist related to the attack were vertigo, hemiparesis, diplopia, ataxia, dysarthria, blurred vision, and headache. Abnormalities included increased wave I–V latency intervals, decreased wave V/I amplitude ratio, or no response. Importantly, five of these patients showed complete return of the ABR to within normal expectations, and another patient showed significant improvement.

Fischer et al. (1982) and Chiappa and Ropper (1982) reported normal ABRs after vertebrobasilar TIAs. Of the nine patients with vertebrobasilar TIAs presented by Kjaer (1980), only one showed an abnormal ABR (by increased interwave latency criteria). Rizzo et al. (1983) noted in a preliminary report that initial ABRs were abnormal in 36.8 percent of sixteen patients with vertebrobasilar TIAs. Baldy-Moulinier et al. (1984) described ABR abnormalities, particularly the wave III–V latency interval, but also wave I–III and wave I–V latencies and the amplitudes of waves, in ischemic patients. ABR findings recorded from fifty patients within a seven- to twenty-day period after vertebrobasilar TIAs by Rizzo et al. (1983) were abnormal in sixteen (32%). ABR interwave (I–V) latency delays and decreased V/I amplitude ratio were the characteristic abnormalities. Criteria of TIA was sudden onset of at least one symptom, as opposed to the two or more signs or symptoms of Factor and Dentinger (1987). By twelve months, follow-up ABRs showed reversal of abnormalities for five of ten patients. Ragazzoni, Amantini, Rossi, and Bindi (1982) found abnormal ABRs in eight of fifteen patients (53 percent) with vertebrobasilar TIAs during the same post-onset time period. The most common ABR abnormality was increased wave I–V latency, followed by delay of the III–V latency. Repeat ABRs at three months failed to show improvement. According to Baldy-Moulinier et al. (1983), ABR interwave latencies are characteristically delayed in patients with vertebrobasilar TIAs and a high "vascular index" versus those also with TIAs yet a normal "vascular index."

According to the experience of Lynn and Gilroy (1984), patients with vertebrobasilar TIAs assessed between episodes do not typically yield abnormal ABRs unless there is accompanying brainstem infarction in auditory regions. No ABR abnormalities were associated with lesions involving the internal carotid artery distribution either. Discrepancies among studies of evoked responses and vertebrobasilar TIAs, according to Factor and Dentinger (1987), result from differences in the time of ABR recording after the TIA (abnormalities are more likely soon after onset) and minimal symptomology criteria for TIA (more required symptoms and therefore more definite TIAs are presumably related to a higher proportion of ABR abnormalities).

Musiek and Lee (1995) recorded the ABR in a series of thirty-two patients with brainstem lesions, including fifteen with vascular disorders (e.g., cerebrovascular accidents, aneurysms, and "structural abnormalities"). ABR findings were not specified for each type of pathology, but based on an analysis of ROC curves for the ABR, the authors conclude "the ABR may not be as powerful a clinical tool for detecting brainstem disorders as some early reports suggest" (p. 635).

Faught and Oh (1984) described ABRs for forty patients with clinical diagnoses of severe brainstem infarction. Death occurred in twenty percent of the patients. The group was subdivided by physical findings into those with medullary, pontine, or midbrain syndromes that were medial or lateral and unilateral or bilateral. ABRs were abnormal (delayed interwave latencies) for 70 percent of the entire group (abnormalities in twenty of twenty-three with pontine lesions), 73 percent (of eleven) with mesencephalic lesions, and none of the six with lesions at the medullary level of the CNS. As expected, a high proportion of patients with lateral brainstem lesions (twenty-eight of thirty-one) had abnormal ABRs. Ipsilateral ABR abnormalities (for stimulus ear ipsilateral to lesion) predominated (78 percent of eighteen patients with unilateral clinical signs). Importantly, only 27 percent of the patients showed CT evidence of infarction and, conversely, 47 percent of patients with normal CT had an abnormal ABR.

Kjaer (1980) observed ABR latency delay in thirteen of fifteen patients with clinical evidence of brainstem infarction. There was a poor correlation between the level of lesion, as determined by the pattern of clinical signs, versus ABR. Likewise, Robier, Saudeau, Autret, and Reynaud (1981) found that ABRs were sensitive to subclinical dysfunction in brainstem infarcts and were consistently recorded for the stimulus ear ipsilateral to the side of the lesion, but did not adequately indicate the level of lesion. Other European investigators also reported studies of ABR in brainstem stroke (Charachon & Dumas, 1980; Palenga, Valigi, & Bicciolo, 1985).

CNS lesions such as pontomesencephalic brainstem pathology or post-anoxic neuropathy or drug intoxication (benzodiazepines and chlormethiazole) resulting in coma may show evidence of rhythmic, nonreactive EEG activity in the alpha (8 to 12.5 Hz) region. Hari, Sulkava, and Haltia (1982) presented a case report of a 32-year-old male in alpha pattern coma with suspected brainstem infarction. This was confirmed by autopsy that revealed total occlusion of the basilar artery and infarct in the rostral half of the pons, midbrain, and thalamus, but no damage to the caudal pons region. He showed clinical signs of brainstem involvement. CT scan was normal. ABR assessment yielded only a wave I component.

Minami et al. (1984) described a correlation between ABR findings and clinical status in a 13-year-old child with primary brainstem hemorrhage. Often related to systemic hypertension (high blood pressure), primary brainstem hemorrhage usually features abrupt onset of coma and severe neurological damage. Peak incidence is in the 40- to 50-year age region. Death often occurs due to respiratory arrest. These investigators found that the ABR interwave latencies were initially prolonged, but the ABR abnormalities reversed as CT scanning showed resolution of the lesion and as the patient's clinical status improved.

Hashimoto, Ishiyama, and Tozuka (1979) presented ABR findings for patients with varied brainstem pathologies. Although they did not specify ABR patterns for each etiology, these patients were categorized in groups with intrinsic brainstem lesions and midbrain lesions. Group data were presented. Intrinsic brainstem lesions (including fifteen vascular lesions of pons) were associated with abnormally increased latency for waves III, IV, and V, whereas midbrain lesions (among them one patient with a ruptured AVM and another with an undescribed vascular lesion) produced statistically significant delay of wave V only.

Lynn and Gilroy (1984) also reported ABR findings for a series of thirty-three patients with varied vascular CNS disease. Two groups of patients were formed on the basis of site of lesion. There were fourteen with cerebral infarction secondary to occlusion of vessels in the internal carotid artery distribution and nineteen with vertebrobasilar artery occlusive disease (five with significant stenosis but no clinical or radiologic evidence of infarction and fourteen with definite evidence of infarction). All patients in the first group had normal ABRs. Within the second group, the five patients with no clinical signs of infarction each also showed normal ABRs bilaterally. In distinct contrast, thirteen of the fourteen patients with clinical signs of infarction (93 percent) showed ABR abnormalities, including increased wave I–III latency in five, increased wave III–V latency in three, an increase in both of these latency intervals in three, and no identifiable waves III, IV, and V in two patients. Importantly, and somewhat uniquely among published studies in the neurological literature, peripheral hearing function was assessed for all patients whose neurological state permitted valid behavioral audiometry. Finally, Musiek et al. (1988), in summarizing their data and data reported in selected papers (Chiappa, 1983; Rosenhall et al., 1981) on brainstem infarcts, concluded that from approximately 75 to 80 percent of patients have abnormal ABR findings.

Pregnancy toxemia may be a factor in vertebrobasilar system disorder. Nighoghossian et al. (1991) described a case report of a female subject with apparent vasospasm secondary to administration of beta-sympathomimetic agents given two weeks before the onset of toxemia for preterm labor. The ABR wave III and wave V disappeared initially. A CT scan showed substantial hypodensity in the midbrain. Within two days, the ABR returned to normal.

Liu, Lin, and Chang (2001) report a case study of a patient with isolated compression of the vestibulocochlear nerve by a large, dolichoectatic, horizontally oriented vascular loop of the left vertebral artery. Aside from a unilateral (left-side) hearing loss, the patient should no neurological deficits. CT and MRI confirmed a vascular abnormality protruding into the left porus acousticus and displacing the brainstem to the right. ABR findings were consistent with retrocochlear auditory dysfunction (delayed wave I–III and wave I–V latency on the left side). The authors describe the pathological condition as "cochlear vertebral entrapment syndrome."

Ayerbe et al. (1991) also presented a case of a cochleovestibular syndrome with neuroradiological evidence of a calcified dolichoectasis of the basilar trunk and the left vertebral artery. Symptoms resembled those of Ménière's disease. Patterns for an audiologic test battery were consistent with endolymphatic hydrops, including electrophysiological findings.

Schwaber and Hall (1992) report findings for an audiologic test battery, including ABR, for a series of sixty-three patients with symptoms consistent with cochleovestibular nerve compression syndrome (CNCS), also referred to as "vascular loop syndrome." Abnormal ABRs consistent with retrocochlear pathology (e.g., prolongations of the wave I to III latency interval) were found in 75 percent of the patients.

Perez et al. (1997) present a case report of a 40-year-old woman with cochleovestibular nerve compression syndrome. She had a hearing loss on the right side, vertigo, tinnitus, and motion intolerance. MRI confirmed a vascular loop near the right cochleovestibular nerve. ABR measurement showed asymmetrical (right-side) latencies for the wave I to III and wave III to V intervals.

CHRONIC CEREBRAL VASCULAR PATHOLOGY. | Lumenta (1984) recorded ABRs from nineteen patients with spontaneous intracerebral hemorrhage. Determinable etiologies included ruptures of aneurysms (e.g., of anterior communicating artery or posterior communicating artery), hypertension, and AVMs. Thirteen were deeply comatose (Glasgow Coma Score of less than 7) at the time of assessment (Glasgow Coma Score is defined later in this chapter). Before summarizing ABR findings, it is important to point out that Lumenta's (1984) criteria for abnormal latency was atypically lax (only a difference of more than 1 standard deviation from data for forty-three normal subjects). By these criteria, 10.5 percent of the group showed normal ABRs, 31.6 percent showed unilateral abnormalities, and 57.9 percent had bilateral abnormalities.

Ho, Kileny, Paccioretti, and McLean (1987) reported ABR and AMLR findings for a 67-year-old female with sudden deafness following sequential temporal lobe infarcts. Pure-tone and speech audiometry initially showed no behavioral response to sounds, even though acoustic reflexes and ABR were consistent with normal peripheral hearing sensitivity. Over a seven-month period, hearing sensitivity returned to within normal limits. The AMLR during this time evolved from no response to a slightly delayed but reliable Pa component from each hemisphere. AMLR appearance was correlated with improvement of temporal lobe structural status as confirmed by CT scan. Kileny and colleagues (Kileny, Paccioretti, & Wilson, 1987) also reported another comprehensive study of ABR and AMLR in various cortical lesions. All but one of eleven patients had damage involving the temporal lobe related to a cerebrovascular infarct. Normal ABRs were recorded for all patients. Wave Pa amplitudes were significantly reduced when recorded with electrodes over the involved hemisphere versus uninvolved hemisphere. AMLR findings were not related to the stimulus ear (ipsilateral or contralateral to lesion) or the inverting electrode site (ear ipsilateral versus contralateral to lesion). Furthermore, AMLRs were intact in patients with cerebral lesions that did not involve the cortex of the temporal lobe.

Kalayam et al. (1997) describe ABR findings for a series of fifty-three elderly patients (mean age of 74 years) with the diagnosis of "late-life depression with vascular disease" as defined by depressive symptoms, performance on cognitive measures, physical examination findings, formal assessment of disability, and vascular disease (e.g., hypertension, stigmata of arteriosclerosis, history of CVA, and/or previous surgery for vascular disease). In the authors' words "The interaction between depression and vascular disease had a significant effect on change in wave V latency" (p. 970). The effect of the two diagnoses on the ABR was synergistic. Depressed patients with vascular disease showed more ABR abnormalities than depressed patients without vascular disease. The authors' consider the ABR abnormalities as evidence of "demyelination afflicting the pons and mesencephalon."

ACUTE CVA. | An often-fatal consequence of acute CVA (e.g., secondary to subarachnoid hemorrhage, intracerebral hemorrhage, cerebral-embolic infarction) is brain edema (swelling), particularly if it leads to cerebral transtentorial herniation (the related concepts of intracranial pressure, transtentorial herniation, and brainstem compression are described in detail in later in this chapter). Nagata, Tazawa, Mizukami, and Araki (1984) reported ABR findings for forty-one patients with acute stroke and clinical signs of impending transtentorial herniation. Ten of these patients survived, and thirty-one died even with aggressive medical and surgical therapy. On the average, ABR interwave latency values at three days post-onset were prolonged for those patients who eventually died in contrast to survivors (within normal limits). Amplitude was not analyzed. In addition, examples of initial ABR abnormalities that reversed were presented for selected survivors. ABR outcome was related to the stage of transtentorial herniation (Plum & Posner, 1980). All patients with only an ABR wave I (and no brainstem components) were in the medullary stage of transtentorial herniation and died. Evolution of ABR abnormalities corresponded to rostral-to-caudal development of brainstem dysfunction and progressively increased intracranial pressure.

Degenerative Diseases

The term *degenerative disease* is descriptive but does not specify any homogeneous collection of etiologies. A degenerative disease is often hereditary, has an insidious onset and then progresses. Some diseases that lead to CNS degeneration, but have distinct toxic or metabolic causes, are described in a following section. Classification of degenerative diseases is based on the anatomic regions or systems involved. However, a wide range of signs and symptoms are encompassed, including disorders of movement, tone, and coordination and also higher level functions. Diseases other than those cited below may also be associated with degeneration of CNS function and are described elsewhere in this chapter (e.g., demyelinating diseases and miscellaneous neuropathies), whereas papers reporting ABR findings in pediatric neuropathies are reviewed in Chapter 9.

Included within the broad definition of degenerative diseases is dementia. Patients with dementia by definition show memory disturbances and deficits in one or more higher level cortical functions, such as language, mathematical calculations, affect, reasoning, and orientation. Thus, degenerative diseases and dementia can be described anatomically by the locus of the lesion or on the basis of a complex of symptoms. Dementias can have varied etiologies, among them metabolic (e.g., vitamin B-12 deficiency, Addison's disease), toxic (e.g., lead encephalopathy), and vascular (e.g., Binswanger's encephalopathy). These etiologies are reviewed, therefore, under the heading of "Poisons and Toxins" in this chapter.

Dementia is a major health problem. An estimated 15 percent of persons over age 65 need assistance with activities of daily living due to dementia. Life expectancy is abbreviated in different forms of dementia.

ALZHEIMER'S DISEASE AND SIMPLE DEMENTIA. | Alzheimer's disease may be found in persons of any age, but generally in the elderly population. Features of Alzheimer's disease include senile plaques (amorphous material that contains amyloid protein), nonspecific neuronal loss, granulovacuolar degeneration, atrophic CNS changes, and Alzheimer's neurofibrillary degeneration, that is, tangles of neural tissue. The senile plaques are found almost exclusively in the cortex, especially frontal and temporal lobe gray matter, and also the hippocampus. The brainstem is not involved typically, although brainstem or midbrain nuclei can be abnormal. There are also reports of pathologic involvement of the inferior colliculus, medial geniculate body of the thalamus, and both primary and secondary auditory cortex (e.g., O'Mahoney et al., 1994). These changes are not simply a extension of normal physiologic aging, which may be characterized by relatively few plaques and neural tangles but in different anatomic sites. The precise cause for Alzheimer's disease is not known, although it appears to be related to a disorder of metabolism or a slow viral infection. Alzheimer's disease and Down syndrome (trisomy 21) have in common many neuropathologic features.

Simple (senile) cerebral atrophy or dementia is characterized by neuronal loss, nonspecific changes in residual neurons and astrocytosis in the cerebral cortex (frontal and temporal lobes). By definition, the brain is reduced in size. With a loss of brain tissue, ventricles become dilated. The extent of CNS changes varies from patient to patient. The disorder usually occurs after the age of 65 years and may be a variant of normal CNS physiologic aging.

Late response (ALR and P300) abnormalities have been reported most often in Alzheimer's disease (see Chapters 12 and 13). An analysis of ABR data for six demented patients by Harkins (1981b) showed increased wave I–V latency values, in comparison with data for age-matched control subjects. However, there were gender discrepancies between the two groups. Grimes, Grady, and Pikus (1987) performed a comprehensive battery of audiologic procedures with 69 patients with the diagnosis of dementia of the Alzheimer's type. Severity ranged from mild to severe. High-frequency sensorineural hearing loss, greater than expected for patients' age, was not uncommon. Only three patients had ABR wave I–V latency values that were greater than 2.5 standard deviations above the mean value for normal control subjects. The abnormalities were unilateral for two patients and bilateral for one. In this study by Grimes et al. (1987) the AMLR Pa component was of normal latency and amplitude for all subjects with Alzheimer's disease. A possible explanation for these generally normal AER findings in Alzheimer's type dementia is that the responses reflect mostly white matter integrity whereas the disease involves mostly cortical gray matter.

O'Mahoney et al. (1994) recorded the ABR and AMLR in 35 patients with mild-moderate Alzheimer's disease and an age-matched group of health elder control subjects (N = 34). There were significant prolongations in the ABR wave I to V latency interval, as well as for latency of the Pa component of the AMLR.

AMYOTROPHIC LATERAL SCLEROSIS (ALS, CHARCOT'S DISEASE). | ALS is often referred to as "Lou Gehrig's disease" for a great baseball star who is particularly remembered for playing 2,130 consecutive games in fourteen seasons with the New York Yankees. ALS forced Gehrig to retire from baseball in 1939 and was the cause of his death at age 39 in 1941. With ALS, there is degeneration and loss of large motor neurons, which is most apparent in the anterior horns of the cervical and lumbar regions and motor nuclei in the brainstem (with corresponding upper and lower motor neuron dysfunction). Of relevance to AERs, neuronal degeneration in midbrain structures and the pontine tegmentum has been reported. This primary motor neuron disease (sensory deficits are occasionally reported and debated) has no known etiology. Approximately 95 percent of the cases in

the United States are sporadic, and 5 percent are related to family history. It occurs in midlife (mean age for diagnosis of 56 years). The frequency of new cases of ALS rivals that of MS. In infancy, the disease process is termed Werdnig-Hoffmann disease, and in adolescence or young adulthood Kugelberg-Welander syndrome. The usual symptoms are progressive muscular weakness, wasting of the extremities, and widespread muscle fasciculations.

In a series of seventeen patients with ALS studied by Ratke, Erwin, and Erwin (1986), two showed ABR abnormalities on repeated measurements. One had bilateral wave I–V delay (5.0 ms), and in the other there was a unilateral I–V interwave latency of 4.72 ms. CT scans were normal for each of these two patients, but the authors note that each had prominent symptoms of bulbar pathology. In addition, SSERs were abnormally delayed for upper extremity stimulation (two of sixteen patients) and lower extremity stimulation (seven of sixteen patients). VER findings were consistently normal.

Matheson, Harrington, and Hallet (1983) found ABR abnormalities for four of thirty-two patients with ALS. One had prolonged wave I–III latency interval unilaterally, one had a slight overall I–V latency delay unilaterally, one had no wave III on the right side and a delayed I–III latency interval on the other, and the final patient had no ABR bilaterally. In contrast to this report, Chiappa et al. (1980) reported normal ABR findings for nine patients and Tsuji et al. (1981) reported normal ABR findings for twenty patients.

FAMILIAL (HEREDITARY) SPASTIC PARAPLEGIA. | This is one of the hereditary spinocerebellar degenerative diseases affecting corticospinal tracts and posterior columns.

In two patients with familial spastic paraplegia (one 11-year-old and one 22-year-old) reported by Campanella et al. (1984) and Cassandro et al. (1986), the ABR was normal. Pedersen and Trojaborg (1981) described normal ABRs for twelve of thirteen patients with hereditary spastic paraplegia. The remaining patient, however, yielded no detectable response. Most patients also showed normal SSERs and VERs, although these responses were abnormal for the patient with no ABR.

HUNTINGTON'S DISEASE (CHOREA). | Huntington's disease is hereditary (autosomal dominant), with each child of an affected parent having a 50 percent chance of having the disease. Evidence of the disease may not appear until middle life. Huntington's chorea is characterized by diffuse loss of cells in the caudate nucleus and putamen and atrophy of remaining cells. Frontal horns of the lateral ventricles are dilated. These neuronal changes may also be found elsewhere in the brain, especially the substantia nigra and thalamus. Signs and symptoms are abnormal movements (chorea) and progressive loss of intellectual function (dementia).

There are half dozen papers describing SSER or VER findings in Huntington's disease, but few reports that include AERs. Ehle, Stewart, Lellelid, and Leventhal (1984) obtained evoked response data for auditory, somatosensory, and visual modalities from twelve adult patients with the classic clinical signs and symptoms of Huntington's disease. ABR wave I–V latency interval was equivalent to normative data for all subjects. VERs and SSER latency was also normal. The only remarkable evoked response finding was reduced amplitude for the SSER N20-P25 cortical component.

PARKINSON'S DISEASE. | Parkinsonism typically begins in the mid to late fifties. Parkinsonism affects over 200,000 persons in the United States. In the past, the main site of lesion was thought to be the basal ganglia, but the neuronal changes are now localized primarily to the substantia nigra and, on occasion, other nuclei. The etiology, however, is unknown. There is a complex of signs and symptoms including reduction of spontaneous movements, rigidity, tremor, hypokinesia, and gait disturbance. The goal of treatment is to reduce the symptoms and signs, not to effect a cure. L-DOPA is administered as therapy in an attempt to replace dopamine in the brain, which is reduced in the disease. The pathophysiology of Parkinsonism is complex, and a review of general research findings is beyond the scope of this discussion.

Most studies of auditory electrophysiology in Parkinson's disease involved cortical auditory evoked responses (see Chapters 11 through 14). ABR in Parkinson's disease may have increased latency and poor morphology, with normal amplitude (Gawel, Das, Vincent, & Rose, 1981). Muthane, Satishchandra, and Subhash (1993) collected ABR data from twenty-three patients with Parkinson's disease, relating findings to dopaminergic (DA) and serotonergic (5 HT) disturbances, as documented by measurement of homovanillic acid (HVA) and 5-hydroxyindoleactic acid (5-HAA) in cerebrospinal fluid. Six of the subjects (26%) yielded abnormal ABR findings, but no correlation was established between ABR interwave latencies and either HVA or 5-HIAA levels in the CSF.

PICK'S DISEASE. | This is a rare disease consisting of severe but localized atrophy, usually in frontal and temporal lobes of the cerebral cortex and less often other CNS structures such as the caudate, putamen, globus pallidus, and substantia nigra. It is often clinically very similar to Alzheimer's disease. Two histological findings are a combination of neurofilaments/microtubules and Pick cells (called "ballooned cells").

FRIEDREICH'S ATAXIA. | Friedreich's ataxia is classified as one of the spinocerebellar degenerative diseases. It has many clinical variants. Degeneration is found in dorsal root ganglia, dorsal roots, dorsal columns, spinocerebellar tracts, pyramidal tracts, and brainstem nuclei and tracts. Degenera-

tion in the spiral ganglion (in the cochlea) causes auditory impairment. Signs and symptoms include gait disturbances, dysarthria, reflex abnormalities (areflexia), and sensation deficits.

Among the spinocerebellar degenerative diseases, AERs and auditory function in general have been studied most extensively for Friedreich's ataxia. Satya-Murti, Cacace, and Hanson (1980) administered a comprehensive audiometric test battery (pure-tone audiometry, aural immittance measurements, simple and complex [synthetic sentence identification] speech audiometry) and ABR measurements to four patients with early onset progressive ataxia and two patients with late onset ataxia. Auditory deficits included bilateral sensorineural pure-tone hearing deficits, pronounced rollover on performance intensity functions for single-syllable words, bilaterally depressed scores for synthetic sentence identification with an ipsilateral competing message (SSI–ICM), and markedly abnormal ABRs. There was no recognizable ABR in the four patients with early onset of disease, whereas the two patients with late onset ataxia both had unequivocally normal ABRs. The pattern of findings strongly suggested peripheral (eighth-nerve) auditory dysfunction, presumably at the level of the spiral ganglion.

Rossi et al. (1984) also applied an audiometric test battery approach in a study of eight patients with Friedreich's ataxia. The tests included pure-tone thresholds, an adaptation test (Supra-Threshold Adaptation Test), ipsi- and contralateral acoustic reflex measurement, complex speech audiometry, and electronystagmography (ENG), along with ABR. Abnormalities were observed for all measures on some patients, with complex speech audiometry showing the most pronounced deficits and on all patients. Pure-tone thresholds were outside of the normal range for three patients. Seven of the eight patients had ABR abnormalities. Two of these patients had no detectable response, and in two others there was a wave I only.

Cassandro, Campanella, and Italian colleagues (Campanella et al., 1984; Cassandro et al., 1986) presented ABR data for sixteen patients with Friedreich's ataxia. No ABR could be observed for eleven patients. The ABR for the other five patients, however, was normal. ABR abnormality was correlated with score on the Inherited Ataxias Clinical Rating Scale, and consequently severity of the illness. Two of five patients studied by Hecox, Cone, and Blaw (1981) also showed ABR interwave latency prolongation. In contrast, Rossini and Cracco (1987) reported that only one of nine patients with Friedreich's ataxia showed an ABR abnormality (an interaural wave I–V latency difference). SSERs were more likely to show abnormalities than the ABR. Nuwer et al. (1982) also consistently found normal ABR latency, amplitude, and morphology in a series of twenty patients. They conclude that the ABR may characteristically be normal in this disease and when abnormal may reflect peripheral versus central auditory dysfunction. Jabbari et al. (1982) found only a questionably increased wave

I–V latency for a child with Friedreich's ataxia. Peripheral hearing was within normal limits. Among six patients with Friedreich's ataxia, Pedersen and Trojaborg (1981) recorded a normal ABR in two, a unilateral abnormality in one, and a bilateral increase in wave V latency for three. All patients had reliably recorded wave I, wave III, and wave V. Central conduction time delays were found for SSERs and VERs.

The Italian group noted above (Amantini, Rossi, de Scisciolo, Bindi, Pagnini, & Zappoli, 1984) carried out ABR, AMLR, and ALR assessments in nine patients with Friedreich's ataxia. Only one patient showed an AMLR change (delay of Pa component). The ALR N1 component was delayed in four of nine patients, and the P2 component in two of nine. ABR findings were normal. ALR abnormalities in Friedreich's ataxia were also noted by Taylor, McMenamin, Andermann, and Watters (1982). However, despite marked ABR abnormalities, generally unremarkable ALR findings were described by Satya-Murti, Wolpaw, Cacace, & Schaffer (1983). Amantini et al. (1984) had also pointed out the tendency for only mild ALR changes in patients with even undetectable ABRs. These authors suggest that the reduced demand for neural synchrony at the cortical AER level versus different sites of lesion may explain the ABR versus ALR differences.

OLIVOPONTOCEREBELLAR ATROPHY. | Degeneration is located in pontine nuclei, olivary nucleus, pyramidal tract, spinocerebellar tracts, dorsal columns, lower motor neurons, and other CNS structures. The term olivopontine cerebellar degeneration (OPCD) is sometimes used in referring to this disease. The brainstem and cerebellum may show evidence of atrophy, and the prepontine cistern and fourth ventricle are enlarged. Patients present a history of progressive ataxia and dysarthria with onset usually in late childhood or adolescence. There is a hereditary component to the disease.

Gilroy and Lynn (1978) recorded generally well-formed ABRs with subtle increases in interwave latency values from three patients with olivopontocerebellar atropy (degeneration). An interesting finding was prolongation mainly in the most caudal (wave I–II and wave I–III) portion of the ABR. Hammond and Wilder (1983) carried out a three-modality evoked response evaluation on two adults with olivopontocerebellar atrophy. The ABR was normal in one patient. For the other patient, wave III amplitude was unusually small, and waves IV and V were abnormally delayed in latency. SSERs and VERs were more consistently and noticeably abnormal. Pedersen and Trojaborg (1981) reported abnormal ABRs and also VERs in three patients. In the largest series of patients (N = 6) with olivopontocerebellar degeneration reported to date, Chokroverty, Duvoisin, Lepore, and Nicklas (1984) describe no statistically significant increase in ABR interwave latencies. Two patients had an abnormally prolonged wave I component, suggesting a peripheral auditory deficit. Pure-tone audiometry was not done. In contrast,

VERs were clearly abnormal. All five patients with olivopontocerebellar atrophy reported by Nuwer et al. (1982) showed ABR abnormalities, most often decreased amplitude (wave V/I ratio) and/or delayed interwave latencies. In two of three patients with olivopontocerebellar atrophy reported by Rossini and Cracco (1987), there were ABR abnormalities. For one patient no wave components were observed, waves I and V were of small amplitude, and the wave I–V interval was prolonged. In a series of twenty patients with the diagnosis of spinocerebellar degeneration, Fujita, Hosoki, and Miyazaki (1981) recorded consistently normal ABRs. According to data for thirty-seven patients with olivopontocerebellar degeneration compiled by Musiek et al. (1988), and based on studies of Lynn, Cullis, and Gilroy (1983), Satya-Murti, and Cacace (1982), Pedersen and Trojaborg, 1981; Nuwer, Perlman, Packwood, and Kark (1983), just under 50 percent showed abnormal ABRs.

CEREBELLAR ATAXIA. | Cerebellar ataxia usually is due to disease involving the cerebellum. Less often degeneration of spinocerebellar tracts also leads to gait disturbances (ataxia), dysarthria, hyperreflexia, and sometimes impaired sensation. This latter disease is hereditary.

Pedersen and Trojaborg (1981) carried out multimodal sensory evoked response assessments with eleven adult cerebellar ataxia patients. In three patients, wave V latency was prolonged. ABR was normal in the other patients. In combination, however, the multimodal evoked response battery showed evidence of CNS dysfunction in eight of the eleven patients. Musiek, Gollegly, Kibbe, and Verkest (1988) compiled their data for patients with cerebellar tumors, along with data reported by Chiappa (1983) and Rosenhall, Hadner, and Bjorkman (1981). Among a total of eighteen patients, 72 percent (thirteen) showed abnormal ABRs.

HEREDITARY MOTOR SENSORY NEUROPATHY (DEJERINE-SOTTAS DISEASE). | This disease, identified by French physicians in 1893, is classified as a hereditary motor sensory neuropathy HMSN type III. Cranial nerves are involved. It is related pathophysiologically to olivopontocerebellar degeneration (described earlier). Involvement of subcortical auditory pathways would not be predicted in this neuropathology.

Italian neurologists Baiocco, Testa, d'Angelo, and Cocchini (1984) presented ABR, pure-tone and speech audiometry for two patients with Dejerine-Sottas disease. The diagnosis was confirmed with nerve biopsies. Pure-tone and complex speech auditory measures were consistent with retrocochlear dysfunction. The ABR was markedly abnormal with wave I–V latency values of greater than 5.5 ms and the absence of wave III. Rossini and Cracco (1987) studied the ABR in three patients with HMSN Type I, in three patients with HMSN Type II, and in one patient with HSMN Type III. Only one of the patients with HMSN Type III had abnormal ABR findings (markedly increased wave I–V latencies). Likewise, Satya-Murti et al. (1979) found ABR abnormalities, including prolongation of the wave I–III latency interval and poor morphology or absence of wave V in two patients with hereditary motor sensory neuropathy Type II. Behavioral audiometry confirmed normal peripheral auditory status; however, for meaningful clinical interpretation of ABR, it is important to keep in mind that eighth-nerve involvement and related serious hearing deficit may be a feature of this disease. Stockard, Stockard, and Sharbrough (1986) provide further evidence of ABR wave I–V latency prolongations in HMSN. In some cases, the delay was between wave I and wave II, indicating eighth-nerve dysfunction and consistent with polyneuropathy (multiple peripheral nerve lesions) while intrinsic brainstem dysfunction evidenced by wave III to V latency increases were recorded in other cases.

Also, Garg, Markand, and Bustion (1982) found prolongation of the ABR wave I–III latency interval (greater than 3 standard deviations above normal mean value) in three patients with hereditary motor sensory neuropathy Type I. This latency prolongation was, largely, secondary to an increase in the interval between wave I and II. Later latency intervals were normal. These findings imply eighth-nerve dysfunction, perhaps related to deficient Schwann cell myelin.

MYOCLONUS EPILEPSY. | Myoclonus is a movement disorder, an abrupt involuntary contraction of muscles, that is a feature of numerous and varied diseases. The movement may be caused by sensory stimulation, such as a flash of light or a loud sound. Clinical classes of this disorder are myoclonus of idiopathic epilepsy, infantile myoclonic epilepsy, progressive myoclonic epilepsy, viral myoclonus, myoclonus of metabolic encephalopathy, and palatal myoclonus. This final type of myoclonus is somewhat different than the others. It may result from lesions in the brainstem, spinal cord, or cerebral hemispheres that are secondary to neoplasms, vascular accidents, or encephalitis.

CHRONIC ALCOHOLISM AND VITAMIN-DEFICIENCY STATES. | Among these disorders are Wernicke's encephalopathy, Korsakoff's disease, alcoholic cerebral atrophy, Marchiafava-Bignami disease, central pontine myelinolysis, pellagra, and fetal alcohol syndrome. Wernicke-Korsakoff syndrome is a thiamine deficiency state usually related to chronic alcoholism. Patients have severe memory disturbances, but may be alert and communicative. Additional clinical signs are peripheral neuropathy, nystagmus, ataxia, and ophthalmoplegias. Brainstem nuclei are often involved. Leigh disease (subacute necrotizing encephalomyelopathy) is histologically similar to Wernicke's disease. The brainstem is severely involved. Pellegra is a rare disease (in the United States) in which dementia is found along with diarrhea and dermatitis. It may be a component of widespread carcinoma, unsupervised diets, or certain gastrointestinal disorders. In summary, chronic alcoholism produces distinct CNS damage and a variety of neurological deficits. Patients also have

generalized disturbances of brain function, including poor judgment and personality changes.

Central pontine myelinolysis may appear in chronic alcoholics and is characterized by signs of slowly progressive motor suprasegmental system disease. There is paresis of muscles innervated by CNS regions below the level of the pons with intact higher cerebral functions and consciousness (the "locked-in" pattern described earlier). Neurologic status tends to deteriorate even when overall medical condition improves. The neuropathy is localized to the pons, often a demyelination that extends dorsally into the tegmentum of the pons. The auditory pathway in this region may be affected by the demyelination or by secondary effects of edema that can reverse. Vitamin B-12 deficiency is associated with myelopathy in approximately two-thirds of these patients. Neurologic findings central pontine myelinolysis due to posterior and lateral column spinal cord degeneration include spasticity and diminished sensation.

Stockard, Rossiter, Wiederholt, and Kobayashi (1976) recorded serial ABRs from two chronic alcoholics during development and then resolution of central pontine myelinolysis. For one patient, ABR findings were initially normal (wave I–V interval of 4.3 ms), but with progression of the disease the wave I–V interval increased to 7.0 ms while the patient was locked-in. Following resolution of severe neurological deficits, the wave I–V latency interval was again 4.3 ms. Another patient initially had a prolonged ABR wave I–V latency interval (8.4 ms), which returned to within normal limits with improvement of neurological status.

Prolongation of ABR latencies was found in chronic alcoholics without severe neurological deficits (Begleiter, Porjesz, & Chou, 1981; Mabin, LeGuyader, & LeMevel, 1985) and also in alcoholic patients with related but distinct disease processes, including central pontine myelinosis (Stockard et al., 1979; Wiederholt, Kobayashi, Stockard, & Rossiter, 1977), cerebellar ataxia (Rosenhamer & Silverskiold, 1980), and Wernicke-Korsakoff syndrome, dementia, and cerebral degeneration (Chu & Squires, 1980). Some of these latter diseases (Wernicke-Korsakoff syndrome, Marchiafava-Bignami disease) are associated with ABR abnormalities without alcoholism (Komsuoglu, Jones, & Harding, 1981). In a study of fourteen patients undergoing withdrawal from chronic alcohol use, Reilly et al. (1983) found no latency abnormalities when data were compared to a control group. ABR morphology and repeatability, however, was poor in the patient group. SSER latencies, in contrast, progressively shortened during withdrawal, consistent with the notion of CNS hyperexcitability in withdrawal.

Studies of ABRs in patients with vitamin B-12 deficiency have yielded conflicting results. Fine and Hallett (1980) recorded normal ABRs from three patients with subacute combined degeneration of the spinal cord to due vitamin B-12 deficiency. VERs were reported as mildly abnormal and SSERs as moderately abnormal. Although these authors state that the neuropathologic and neurophysiologic pattern in subacute combined degeneration of the spinal cord is similar to that in Friedrich's ataxia and adrenoleukodystrophy, the ABR patterns among these diseases apparently differ. In contrast to the Fine and Hallett (1980) findings, Krumholz, Weiss, Goldstein, and Harris (1981) reported distinct ABR (plus VER and SSER) abnormalities in two of seven patients with definite evidence of vitamin B-12 deficiency (including neurological deficits such as sensory loss and motor loss). The two patients with the ABR interwave latency (I–V) prolongation also had the most pronounced neurological deficits. A follow-up ABR assessment for these patients after one year of parenteral vitamin B-12 therapy revealed reversal of the previously recorded abnormalities.

POISONS AND TOXINS. | Toxins and poisons include anesthetics and hypnotics, carbon monoxide, common household substances (e.g., glue, lacquer), heavy metals (inorganic and organic lead and mercury), and industrial agents (e.g., solvents) and by-products. An example of the latter is hydrogen sulfide, a highly dangerous gas that occurs naturally and is a by-product of many industrial processes. Industrial byproducts are not uncommon. For example, occupations at risk for hydrogen sulfide exposure include:

> asphalt roofing, barium carbonate production, brewery work, caisson work, carbon disulfide production, chemical laboratory work, felt making, glue making, hydrogen sulfide production, industrial waste disposal, industrial fishing, liquid manure storage and production, mining, natural gas production, petroleum refining, phosphorus sesqui-sulfide production, rubber vulcanizing, septic tank cleaning, sewer work, sugar beet processing, sulfur dye production, sulfur monochloride production, sulfuric monochloride production, sulfuric acid purification, tannery work, vicose rayon production, and well digging. (Wasch, Estrin, Yip, Bowler, & Cone, 1989, p. 902)

Clinical symptoms of exposure include nervousness, extremity muscle weakness, light-headedness, problems sleeping, convulsions, agitation, and delirium (Wasch et al., 1989). Before dementia is apparent, toxins typically produce other more clinically notable signs and symptoms. In adults, chronic lead poisoning is very rare. Lead poisoning in children, described in Chapter 9, results in convulsions, lethargy, irritability, papilledema, and projectile vomiting. Chronic paint or toluene sniffing causes toxic neuropathology, including optic nerve lesions, acute muscle weakness, dementia, cerebellar dysfunction, and varied peripheral neuropathies. Some of the many papers describing ABR findings in toxins and poisons are summarized in Table 10.9. A small sample of other publications is now described briefly.

In an interesting clinical paper, Matsuzawa et al. (1997) reported the results of a survey of over 1,000 publications on which tests of function were used in toxicity studies appearing in seven Japanese toxicology journals over a ten-year period. The ABR was among the function tests administered most often, along with visual evoked responses, electroreti-

nography, some general clinical measures (e.g., respiration, heart rate, body temperature) and laboratory studies.

Metrick and Brenner (1982) report markedly abnormal ABRs for two young adult males with neurological deficits caused by inhalation of spray paint (toluene). Only wave components I and II were consistently recorded for each patient. One patient also showed a wave III component unilaterally. Other waves were not recorded. CT scans demonstrated brainstem atrophy. Importantly, despite these ABR and CT findings, the authors reported that behavioral audiometry (pure-tone and speech audiometry) and acoustic reflex measures were normal. In a case report of a 24-year-old male with a five-year history of toluene (lacquer) sniffing, Poungvarin (1991) described abnormal delays in ABR interwave latencies bilaterally. MRI documented diffuse toxic demyelination of white matter and abnormal iron deposits with multiple areas of the brain (e.g., thalamus, basal ganglia, cortex).

Sjogren et al. (1996) investigated the ABR and other electrophysiologic measures (P300 and EEG) in a series of thirty-eight welders exposed for to aluminum and manganese (median time was 7,065 hours). Documentation of blood and urine concentrations of the two substances showed levels seven times higher than concentrations in a control group. ABR latencies were increased in the welders.

Kumar and Tandon (1997) confirmed abnormal ABR absolute and interwave latency values in 47 percent of workers, in comparison to data for control subjects, presumably following exposure to neurotoxic solvents while working in a rubber factory.

Controlled-release carbamazepine (CBZ-CR) is used in the treatment of epilepsy. The effect of CBZ therapy on the ABR in children was noted in Chapter 9. In a double-blind, randomized, placebo-controlled study, van der Meyden et al. (1992) described increased ABR interwave latency values for ten healthy volunteers following administration of three doses of CBZ (800, 1200, and 1600 mg). Changes were also found for other clinical, psychomotor, electrophysiological, and cognitive measures.

Sator et al. (1999) investigated for twelve weeks the effect of tibolone (a synthetic steroid) on the ABR in twenty-four healthy postmenopausal women. Women receiving the tibolone showed a decrease in latencies for ABR wave II, III, and V in comparison to pretreatment values, and to subjects who were given a placebo. Concentrations of hormones were unchanged before and after treatment for the two groups.

Matsuyama, Katayama, and Nakamura (1993) report a case study of a 34-year-old patient who ingested a large amount of sodium bromate (14 grams) in an attempt to commit suicide. MRI and SPECT studies confirmed brain pathology. The patient developed common symptoms within minutes after ingestion of the drug (e.g., vomiting, diarrhea), and a severe-to-profound hearing impairment within twelve hours. ABR interwave latencies were abnormally prolonged before the onset of deafness.

TABLE 10.9.   Summary of Selected Studies of the Effect of Toxins and Poisons on the Auditory Brainstem Response (ABR) in Adults

STUDY (YEAR)	N	TOXIN/POISON	MODE OF EXPOSURE	COMMENTS
Hirata et al. (1992)	75	Carbon disulfide	Work	Rayon factory; latency delays with long-term exposure.
Hirata & Kosaka (1993)	41	Lead	Work	Abnormally prolonged interwave latencies.
Murata et al. (1993)	22	Lead	Work	Gun metal foundry; latency correlated to lead absorption.
Otto & Fox (1993)	NA	Lead	Variable	Review article including ABR findings.
Murata et al. (1995)	36	Lead	Work	Glass workers; no ABR abnormalities.
Counter & Buchanan (2002)	30	Lead	Work	Ceramic glazing; delayed absolute latencies; hearing loss.
Chang, Yeh, & Wang (1995)	26	Mercury vapor	Work	Chlorakali workers; increased interwave latencies.
Musiek & Hanlon (1999)	1	Mercury	Work	Chemistry professor; dimethylmercury; interwave delays.
Anyanwu, Campbell, & High (2002)	5	Molds (toxic)	Home	Abnormal wave I–III latency in all subjects.
Kumar & Tandon (1997)	40	Rubber solvent	Work	47% of subjects showed ABR latency prolongations.
Murata et al. (1997)	18	Sarin	Attack	No ABR abnormalities; prolonged P300 latencies.
Matsuyama et al. (1993)	1	Sodium bromate	Ingestion	Suicide attempt; interwave latency delays; deafness.
Poungvarin (1991)	1	Toluene	Sniffed	Lacquer produced abnormal ABR interwave latencies.
Abbate, Giorgianni, Munao, & Brecciaroli (1993)	300	Toluene	Work	Rotogravure workers; latency delay at 11 & 90 stimuli/sec.

WILSON'S DISEASE. | This is a genetic disorder of copper metabolism. It is inherited (autosomal recessive) and can first appear at any time in life. Liver and CNS pathology cause the clinical manifestations. The regions of the CNS involvement include basal ganglia, caudate, putamen, thalamus, globus pallidus, and substantia nigra. Neurologic signs and symptoms may include tremor, rigidity, cerebellar signs, and abnormal deep tendon reflexes. Excessive copper deposition and demyelination is suggested as a mechanism.

Fujita, Hosoki, and Miyazai (1981) in apparently the first report of ABR in Wilson's disease described increased interwave (III–V and I–V) latencies in three patients with neurologic symptoms and normal ABR latencies in three with no neurological abnormalities. Chu, Yang, and Cheng (1985) presented a case report of an 18-year-old female with hepatic encephalopathy and Wilson's disease who underwent a liver transplantation. ABRs were described as normal on multiple assessments. In contrast, central conduction times for SSERs were initially prolonged and then decreased to within the normal range as the patient's status improved. Chu and Yang (1987) presented more comprehensive data for twenty patients with Wilson's disease. Analysis of group findings revealed a statistically significant increase in the I–V latency interval versus control subject data.

DIABETES MELLITIS. | There are various forms of diabetes, including mellitus, insipidus, pancreatic, renal and others. This discussion will be limited to diabetes mellitus (d. mellitus), a chronic, incurable carbohydrate metabolism disorder. Blood hyperglycemia and glycosuria develops because of inadequate production or utilization of insulin. Prevalence of diabetes mellitus is highest in older adults. Approximately one-half of patients with d. mellitus have peripheral neuropathy. In addition, pathologic studies have shown evidence of diffuse degeneration of ganglion cells and nerve fibers in the cerebellum, brainstem, and cerebrum and severe vascular pathology with consequences for neural structure and function. Major symptoms are elevated blood sugar (hyperglycemia), sugar in urine (glycosuria), excessive urine production (polyuria), excessive thirst, and increased food intake. Complications include eye, kidney, peripheral nerve, and otologic (ear) disorders. The literature on diabetes mellitus and hearing impairment is inconsistent. An incidence of hearing impairment as high as 55 percent, particularly high-frequency progressive sensorineural hearing loss is reported by some investigators (Dejong, 1982; Makashima & Tanaka, 1971; Taylor & Irwin, 1978; Triana et al., 1991). Other authors, however, have found no significant abnormalities among insulin-dependent patients with diagnosed diabetes mellitus (Sieger, White, Skinner & Spector, 1983). Treatment of this disease consists of dietary regulation, exercise, and regular administration of insulin in many cases.

Peripheral, spinal cord, and even other CNS neuropathy is a well-appreciated component of d. mellitus. Sensory nerve conduction and, later, the SSER findings have been studied for over twenty-five years. Diabetic patients showed longer SSER latencies for arm and leg stimulation than normal control subjects. Donald et al. (1981) described audiometric and ABR findings for a group of twenty insulin-treated adult patients with d. mellitus. Patients with other diseases associated with neuropathy, such as uremia, were excluded. There was no serious pure-tone hearing deficit for any of the twenty patients in this study. ABR wave I and wave II latency and amplitude values were equivalent for the two groups, but interwave latencies (I–V) were significantly greater for diabetic group. It is important to observe, however, that ABR morphology was consistently good in diabetics and that the mean wave I–V latency value for the diabetic group (4.21 for the right ear stimulus and 4.26 ms for the left ear) was still well within the accepted clinical normal range.

In contrast, Fedele et al. (1984) studied ABR in thirty normal-hearing insulin dependent patients with d. mellitus and found significant delays in both absolute latency for wave I and interwave (I–V) latency values compared to data for a normal control group. At a click rate of 11/sec, 30 percent of the diabetic subjects showed ABR wave I latency outside of the normal range, and 20 percent showed abnormal wave I–V delays. Amplitude was not significantly reduced. ABR abnormalities were not related to duration of diabetes affliction. Martini, Comacchio, Fedele, Crepaldi, and Sala (1987), in a follow-up study of sixty insulin-dependent diabetic patients, recorded ABR abnormalities (wave I–V latency delays) in 28.2 percent. For thirteen cases, the delay was in the I–III latency interval, for one subject the III–V latency interval, and for five subjects only the overall I–V latency interval was prolonged. Test-retest data available for twenty of the patients showed no significant variation. These findings were both refuted and confirmed by Khardori et al. (1986). That is, this group described in thirty-four subjects with insulin-dependent diabetes normal wave I latency values, but a significant abnormal increase in wave I–V latency in comparison to normal data. Eleven of the thirty-four subjects (32 percent) had ABR wave V and wave I–V latency

values exceeding 2 standard deviations above normal data. The diabetes group average ABR I–V latency value was 4.40 ms for males and 4.15 ms for females.

Harkins, Gardner, and Anderson (1985) provided further evidence of ABR latency delays in d. mellitus. There were ten subjects with insulin-dependent diabetes and ten control subjects. Mean ABR wave I–V latency values were 4.0 ms in the control group and 4.2 ms in the diabetes group. Statistically, the wave I–V latency was longer in the diabetic subjects (p <0.05). Virtaniemi et al. (1993) studied ABR in a series of fifty-three adult patients with type I diabetes and 42 randomly selected nondiabetic control subjects. As a group, the diabetic patients had an abnormally prolonged wave I–V latency interval. ABR abnormalities were correlated with duration of the disease, and microvascular complications (e.g., retinopathy, nephropathy). Furthermore, medical management (intensified insulin therapy with GhbA$_{1c}$) to maintain metabolic control did not alter the ABR abnormalities in diabetic patients (Virtaniemi et al., 1995). Durmus, Yetiser, and Durmus (2004) conducted a prospective investigation of ABR in 17 adult patients with type I DM, twenty-six patients with type II DM, and also an age- and gender-matched control group for each experimental group. Absolute latencies for waves I, III, and V, as well as interwave latency values (wave I–III, wave III–V, and wave I–V) were significantly delayed for the two diabetes groups in comparison to control subjects. Multiple additional reports confirm ABR abnormalities, particularly interwave prolongations, in diabetes mellitus (e.g., Buller et al., 1988; Goldsher et al., 1986; Khardori et al., 1986; Lisowska, Namylowski, Morawshi, & Strojek, 2001; Parving, 1990) and also provide evidence of abnormal brainstem function by ABR in adult diabetics. In a study of twenty patients with another form of diabetes— tropical pancreatic diabetes, Alexander, Thomas, Mohan, and Narendranathan (1995) confirmed abnormal ABR latencies and found a correlation between the ABR findings and duration of the disease. In contrast, Verma, Bisht, and Ahuja (1984) failed to document any differences in ABR latency values between diabetic and normal adult subjects. Comi (1997) presents a concise review of the literature on sensory evoked response (ABR, SSER, VER, and pattern electroretinography, or PERG) and motor evoked potential findings in diabetes mellitus, concluding, "subtle abnormalities of central afferent and efferent pathways are revealed by evoked potential tests in about a quarter of diabetic patients. Interestingly, these abnormalities do not reflect homogeneously the different nervous pathways in the same patient, suggesting a multifocal rather than a diffuse process" (p. 378). Comi (1997) supplemented the review with original data for thirty adult insulin-dependent diabetic mellitus (IDDM) patients. In comparison to a control group of thirty normal subjects, the IDDM patients yielded significantly longer latencies for wave V and the wave I–V interval. Other ABR parameters were not abnormal. Diabetic children may also show ABR abnormalities, as noted in Chapter 9, although findings are inconsistent, as they are in studies of adults with diabetes.

RENAL DISEASE AND UREMIA. | Uremia is a toxic condition occurring secondary to renal insufficiency and retention of nitrogenous substances in the blood that are normally secreted by the kidney. Symptoms include anemia, hypertension, bone abnormalities, and gastroenteritis. Uremic symptoms may be reversed with regular dialysis treatment. Peripheral and central nervous system dysfunction can be associated with severe uremia. Neurological complications lead to nausea, vomiting, headache, drowsiness, convulsions, and coma.

Walser et al. (1984) carried out ABR studies in three groups of patients with a history of primary renal failure. Thirteen patients with severe chronic renal impairment were assessed prior to an initial dialysis treatment. A hemodialysis group consisted of eleven patients on long-term dialysis. Ten patients had undergone successful renal transplant procedures. The main finding was significantly increased wave I–V latency in the pre-dialysis group versus transplant or control groups. Wave I amplitude was reduced for each of the patient groups, consistent with the expectation of some sensorineural deficit in uremic patients. Abnormal findings were also reported for SSERs and VERs in the pre-dialysis group.

Rizzo et al. (1982) recorded ABRs and VERs from twelve adult patients with chronic renal failure who were managed with dialysis. Three patients showed evidence of ABR abnormalities, two patients with wave I–III or III–V latency delays (but no I–V abnormality) and one patient with a significant prolongation of only the wave III–V latency on the right ear and all interwave latencies on the left (wave I–V of 4.67 ms). This latter finding alone exceeded normal clinical expectations for ABR latency. Six of the patients had abnormal latencies for VERs.

Knoll, Harbort, Schulte, and Zimpel (1982) recorded ABRs and AMLRs from forty-three uremic patients on regular dialysis treatment. Although exact numbers of patients showing abnormalities were not stated, approximately one-half of the uremic patients without neurological symptoms noted above had AMLR latencies (for an N30 component) beyond the range for a control group. All patients with these symptoms yielded latency values for this component that fell above the normal region.

Rossini et al. (1984) evaluated with ABRs twenty-eight adult patients with chronic renal failure. ABRs for fifteen of fifty-six ears were abnormal. For two patients, no peaks were observed after wave I. The other thirteen ears yielded ABRs of good morphology but abnormally delayed wave III and/or V latency values (greater than 3 standard deviations above normative data). The latency for ABR wave I, and the wave I–II latency interval, was altered more often in patients with clinical evidence of peripheral neuropathy. Also, abnormal ABRs were more characteristic of patients treated with diet than dialysis.

Hypothyroidism

The CNS features hypothyroidism include mental retardation, memory deficits, depression and, rarely, convulsions and coma. ABR findings reported for hypothyroidism are mixed. Vanasse et al. (1989) described normal ABRs in adult patients. Lai, Tai, Liu, and Howng (1997), however, recorded normal ABRs in an animal (rat) model for hypothyroidism. Khedr, El Toony, and Tarkhan (2000) studied with multiple electrophysiological measures (ABR, P300, VERs, EEG, EMG) twenty-three patients (age range of 17 to 64 years) with the new diagnosis of hypothyroidism, as defined by total thyroxine level below normal limits. Absolute latencies (I, III, and V) and interwave latencies (I–III, III–V, I–V) were prolonged for the group of patients with hypothyroidism in comparison to the control group. Other investigators confirm the presence of ABR abnormalities in patients with hypothyroidism (Di Lorenzo et al., 1995; Hohmann, Kahaly, & Warzelhan, 1990; Huang et al., 1989).

Hypogonadotropic Hypogonadism

Hypogonadotropic hypogonadism is a rare form of hypogonadism (defective internal secretion of the gonads) related to insufficient gonadotropin-releasing hormone from the hypothalamus that can be associated with sensorineural hearing loss and other neurosensory deficits.

Ozata et al. (1996) studied the ABR in a series of fifty-six untreated male patients with idiopathic hypogonadotropic hypogonadism in comparison to an age-matched group of male control subjects. ABR findings (absolute and interwave latencies) were equivalent for the two groups, although the authors did find a delay in SSER latencies for selected patients.

Infections and Inflammatory Diseases

BRAIN ABSCESS. | Approximately 60 percent of brain abscesses result from spread of infections from the middle ear and mastoid or from the paranasal cavities or nasal cavity. In these cases the abscess is located in the adjacent inferior temporal lobe or cerebellar hemisphere, or frontal or anterior temporal lobes. Other sources are metastatic infection, congenital anomalies, trauma, and postsurgical development. Abscesses begin with an infection and inflammation (*Staphalococcus aureus*, *streptococci*, gram-negative bacilli, anaerobes in 80 percent of cases) that destroys brain tissue, forming a cystic mass. A thin layer of compressed brain tissue surrounds the mass. Abscesses are found most often in deep cerebral white matter (versus cortical gray matter) and are distributed in certain sites with the brain. Neurological symptoms and signs are headache, fever, systemic illness, nausea, reduced alertness, and seizures. Diagnosis is based on these clinical findings and CT scanning. In contrast to meningitis, lumbar puncture (LP) in suspected abscess is contraindicated because of the possibility of herniation of brain tissue from the supratentorial compartment due to mass effect and increased intracranial pressure (ICP). The overall mortality for brain abscess is approximately 45 percent. Without surgical intervention, virtually all patients die. With early diagnosis (e.g., by CT scanning), antibiotic therapy is often successful in effecting a cure. There is a male-to-female ratio of occurrence of 3:1.

Goitein, Fainmesser, and Sohmer (1983) describe the relation among ABR findings, clinical findings (neurologic status), physiologic parameters (e.g., mean arterial blood pressure, intracranial pressure, cerebral perfusion pressure), and outcome for a group of children with varied brain pathologies. Within this group are eleven children with meningitis, five with encephalitis, and one with a brain abscess. A potential pathophysiologic process in each of these pathologies, including brain abscess, is increased intracranial pressure that can lead to brain ischemia. Absence of waves IV and V were noted in the child with a brain abscess, presumably because of the effect of supratentorial pressure (due to the mass of the abscess) on upper brainstem functioning.

VIRAL INFECTIONS. | Viral diseases involving the nervous system are varied and include herpes zoster (Ramsay Hunt syndrome), herpes simplex encephalitis, congenital cytomegalovirus (CMV), meningoencephalitis, meningitis, poliomyelitis, rabies, and slow virus infections (Jakob-Creutzfeldt disease), progressive multifocal leukoencephalopathy, subacute sclerosing panencephalitis, progressive rubella panencephalitis, and human immune virus (HIV) or acquired immune deficiency syndrome (AIDS). Congenital and perinatal viruses may affect the nervous system in many ways, producing chromosomal damage, encephalitis, congenital defects, mental retardation, and fetal death. To a large extent, the amount of damage caused by the virus is related to the embryonic time of exposure. In childhood, encephalitis may result from different viral diseases, among them measles, rubella, varicella, and mumps. Herpes zoster infections have been appreciated since 1831. They are now known to result from a virus infection that affects peripheral or cranial nerves, although which anatomic structures are necessarily involved is still debated. The disease more commonly affects persons over age 45 years and males versus females. Patients with the Ramsay Hunt syndrome from herpes zoster can present with skin eruptions on areas of the head and neurotologic pathology including external ear lesions, facial nerve paralysis, eighth-nerve lesions, and inner ear (cochlea) abnormalities, along with related sensorineural hearing impairment. Neurotological findings are usually unilateral.

Abramovich and Prasher (1986) carried out audiometric, ECochG, and ABR assessments with thirteen patients with Ramsay Hunt syndrome. Pure-tone hearing threshold deficits were found in eleven and abnormal tone decay in four patients. Transtympanic ECochG recordings (AP amplitude and the SP/AP ratio) were interpreted as normal for all patients. Seven of the thirteen patients showed evidence of

ABR abnormalities. In six patients, there were prolongations of the wave I–V interval (a value of greater than 2 standard deviations above the normal mean). Another patient yielded an ABR of extremely poor morphology with no identifiable wave components. In one other patient (a 73-year-old), absence of an ABR was attributed to severe sensorineural hearing loss. The authors speculate that the retrocochlear dysfunction by ABR is related to lesions, perhaps inflammation, at the level of the spiral ganglion or eighth nerve and possibly brainstem.

Van Nechel, Deltenre, Strul, and Capon (1982) summarize ABR findings for a group of patients with miscellaneous lesions, including central pontine myelinosis and Jakob-Creutzfeldt's disease, but do not specify outcome for each disease.

Rosenblatt and Majnemer (1984) illustrated the effect of *brainstem encephalitis* on ABR with two case reports (a 10-month-old boy and an 11.5-month-old girl). Typical clinical symptoms in the disease include reduced level of consciousness (lethargy), dysarthria, dysphagia (swallowing problems), cranial nerve deficits, and ataxia. Among proposed etiologies for selected cases are herpes simplex infection, and influenza inoculation. Serial ABRs for each patient initially showed an abnormal delay for interwave latencies. Over time (eight months for case 1 and three months for case 2), the ABR improved substantially. Other abnormalities reported were poor morphology, decreased wave V/I amplitude ratio, and absence of wave components. There was evidence of peripheral auditory deficit for each patient. The authors point out that initial ABR findings in these two patients with brainstem encephalitis were indistinguishable from those of children with brainstem glioma (also discussed in the paper), but that over time the ABRs for brainstem encephalitis improved, whereas those for the neoplasm did not or even worsened.

Watanabe et al. (1999) present a case report of a 36-year-old woman with brainstem encephalitis. Symptoms included facial palsy, ophthalmoplegia, cerebellar ataxia, and rhythmic myoclonus of the neck, following symptoms of a common cold and general fatigue. Findings for the ABR, and also for SSERs, were entirely normal.

Jain and Maheshwari (1984) recorded ABRs from fifteen patients (aged 13 to 51 years), comatose (mean Glasgow Coma Scale score of 8.2) secondary to meningoencephalitis. Etiology was unknown for four patients and included pyogenic meningitis, tubercular meningitis, enteric encephalopathy, and fungal meningoencephalitis for the remainder. Five patients in the group had normal ABRs bilaterally, in comparison to control group data. The other ten patients showed abnormalities (reported only for the most involved ear) that consisted of either delayed interwave latencies (eight patients) or missing wave components (two patients). This proportion of comatose patients with abnormal ABRs is far greater than would be expected for coma due to head injury.

Funakawa et al. (1999) reported a case study of a 23-year-old pregnant woman with Bickerstaff's brainstem encephalitis. Initial symptoms were consistent with an upper respiratory infection, but then the patient became somnolent and had multiple neurological symptoms, including cerebellar ataxia, hyperreflexia, extraocular movements, and spasticity of the lower limbs. The ABR wave III to wave V latency interval was abnormally prolonged. Treatment with plasma exchanges resulted in improved neurological status, including ABR findings.

In another report of a patient with Bickerstaff's brainstem encephalitis, Koyama et al. (1998) described abnormal ABR findings (prolonged interwave latencies), although the CT and MRI results were normal. The 50-year-old woman had a high titer of anti-GQ1b IgG antibody, a finding that the authors related to the pathogenesis of the lesion.

Kalita and Misra (1999) report ABR findings for a series of twelve adult patients (average age 28 years) with Japanese encephalitis, described by the authors as "the commonest human endemic encephalitis in the world and . . . especially prevalent in south east Asia" (p. 24). The average Glasgow Coma Score for the patients was 7. Note: The Glasgow Coma Score is described in a later section of this chapter ("ABR in Neurointensive Care Unit Monitoring"). CT and MRI confirmed lesions among the patients in various regions of the brain, including the thalamus, white matter pathways, putamin, basal ganglia, pons, and cerebellum. All ABR latency measures were reported as normal, including absolute and interwave latencies. However, the wave V/I amplitude ratio was abnormally reduced in five patients. For the group of patients with Japanese encephalitis, the average ABR wave V/I ratio was 1.64, whereas the ratio was 2.96 in a control group. It's relevant to note that the inverting electrode during ABR recordings was located on the earlobe. The authors attribute the reduced wave V/I amplitude ratio to either increased intracranial pressure or brainstem involvement in Japanese encephalitis.

Kalita and Misra (2001) report ABR findings in twenty-four patients diagnosed with tubercular meningitis ranging in age from 10 to 62 years. CT confirmed related neuropathology in some patients, including hydrocephalus, exudates, infarction, and tuberculoma. The ABR was described as abnormal in fifteen patients and not detected in another patient. The ABR abnormalities were not correlated with level of consciousness or the stage of meningitis.

SYSTEMIC LUPUS ERYTHEMATOSIS (SLE). | SLE is an inflammatory disease of connective tissue (membranes around kidneys, joints, lungs, and other structures), but CNS involvement may be a feature. Criteria for the disease were developed by the American Rheumatism Association. Depending on the focus of inflammation and damage, symptoms may include skin rash, bald patches, kidney dysfunction, stiff joints and pain, and shortness of breath. Neuropsychiatric symptoms occur in up to 70 percent of patients. Neurological deficits common in systemic lupus erythematosus (SLE) include cognitive decline, convulsions, peripheral neuropathies, paralysis, and movement disorders. SLE is most likely to affect women aged 30 to 50 years. Diagnosis is made on the basis of blood tests. Medical treatments include steroids, immunosuppressives, and antirheumatics.

In a study of twenty-two patients with SLE, Mongey, Glynn, Hutchinson, and Bresnihan (1987) found ABR interwave latency abnormalities in six patients. Hall (1992) also reported a case study of ABR findings in SLE. Fradis et al. (1989) and Borton et al. (1992) investigated the ABR in patients with SLE. In each study, rate of stimulation was manipulated in an attempt to increase the sensitivity of the ABR to subclinical central nervous system dysfunction. In general, there was no ABR abnormality at low or high rates of stimulation. Borton et al. (1992) conclude, "the usefulness of routine ABR-stimulus-rate tests as a predictor of neuropsychiatric disorder in SLE patients was not demonstrated" (p. 338).

LUES (SYPHILIS). | This is a chronic infection caused by the microorganism *Treponema palidum* (a spirochete). It may be congenital or acquired. Congenital syphilis is due to infection of the fetus during pregnancy. The traditional clinical findings of neurosyphilis (paresis or tabes dorsalis, with delusions, poor judgment, motor and language dysfunction, pains in trunk region, primary optic atrophy, Argyll Robertson pupils) are now very uncommon. Congenital syphilis with onset of symptoms in infancy is more severe and may result in death. Diagnosis is more secure when based on fluorescent treponema antibody (FTA) test than on VDRL (Venereal Disease Research Laboratory) test. Treatment of choice is benzathine penicillin. Auditory deficits in patients with congenital syphilis are usually progressive and occur in from 20 to 40 percent of patients, more often males than females. Hearing impairment may begin in childhood or be delayed until some point in adulthood. Hearing loss associated with acquired syphilis is a less serious clinical problem because of antibiotic medical therapy. Vascular syphilis of the brain is less common today than in the past. Neurological symptoms are also less apparent.

Rosenhall and Roupe (1981) studied ABR in seven men with secondary syphilis and four with latent syphilis and two women (one with congenital syphilis and one with general paresis). Only the patient with general paresis had markedly abnormal ABR findings, specifically prolonged wave I–V interval on one side and no apparent wave V on the other side. A patient with congenital syphilis showed subtle interwave latency delays.

MARCUS GUNN PTOSIS. | Ptosis is a droopy eyelid. Marcus Gunn ptosis is a congenital disorder in which eyelid elevation accompanies speaking, swallowing, jaw movement, or smiling. Although the anatomic origin is not known, an incorrect cranial nerve connection (among oculomotor, trigeminal, and other cranial nerves) is theorized.

Creel, Kivlin, and Wolfley (1984) described ABR abnormalities (delayed or absent wave III component) in three of seven patients with Marcus Gunn ptosis.

ACQUIRED PALATAL MYOCLONUS. | Kurauchi, Kaga, and Shindo (1996) reported ABR abnormalities for three patients with palatal myoclonus that were "correlated with the location of the brainstem lesion."

ACQUIRED IMMUNE DEFICIENCY SYNDROME (HUMAN IMMU-NODEFICIENCY VIRUS). | The acquired immune deficiency syndrome (AIDS) retrovirus, human immunodeficiency virus (HIV), involves T-lymphocytes (HTLV-III) as well as other cell types, such as monocytes. Viral infection results in an alteration of the ratio of T4 to T8 lymphocytes and too many suppressor lymphocytes. HIV-infected patients have reduced host defenses to other infections and to the development of neoplasms (tumors). Those at risk for HIV are homosexuals, bisexuals, hemophiliacs, intravenous drug users, and children born of infected mothers.

HIV (AIDS) is among the major health problems in the United States. Central nervous system infection is often a component of AIDS (in over three-fourths of patients as determined by autopsy), and neurotologic complications may also be a feature (Koenig et al., 1986). Subacute encephalitis is common, with cortical atrophy, abnormal histopathologic findings, myelination degeneration, and both white and gray matter involvement. There are cases of central auditory nervous system lesions by autopsy (Hart, Cokely, Schupbach, Dal Canto, & Coppleston, 1989). CNS-related disorders include dementia and depression. AIDS is a terminal disease. Death is often due to unrelated infection, such as pneumonia.

Markedly abnormal ABR findings are reported in a thorough case report of an adult male with AIDS contracted as a result of a blood transfusion during heart surgery. Inter-wave latency values (I–III, III–V, and I–V) were abnormally prolonged. With this patient, there were also abnormal findings for another central auditory procedure (synthetic sentence identification) and evidence of high-frequency sensorineural hearing impairment by pure-tone audiometry.

Miscellaneous Neuropathy

EPILEPSY. | Seizures can accompany or follow varied types of acute brain injury, such as head trauma, metabolic encephalopathies (e.g., hypoxia), cerebral ischemia, and drug intoxication. They may be focal or generalized cerebral seizures, but they do not usually recur after recovery from the brain injury. Epilepsy is a complex neurological disorder. The term usually refers to convulsive seizures that occur repetitively and chronically, with or without loss of consciousness. The general pathophysiologic basis of epilepsy is abnormal and recurrent discharge of large groups of cerebral neurons. The actual etiology may be metabolic, structural, or genetic and,

within these categories there may be subtypes (e.g., structural causes include tumors, cerebral infarcts, arteriovenous malformations, and cysts). It is important to realize that many classifications for epilepsy have evolved. Among the types of seizures that characterize epilepsy are partial seizures, generalized tonic-clonic (grand mal) seizures or absence (petit mal) seizures, myoclonic seizures, infantile spasms, and status epilepticus. A thorough review of epilepsy is beyond the scope of this book.

Weiner, Erwin, and Weber (1981) found no ABR abnormalities during or after electroconvulsive therapy producing epilepsy for six patients with psychiatric disorders (four with depression and two with schizophrenia). Since epilepsy is a cerebral disorder, ABR abnormalities are not be expected. Cortical auditory evoked response findings in epilepsy are reviewed in Chapters 11 through 14.

PROGRESSIVE SUPRANUCLEAR PALSY. | In this disease, there can be widespread damage of brainstem (pons and midbrain) nuclei, but white matter is not involved.

Since white matter is not damaged, normal ABR findings would be expected in progressive supranuclear palsy. Tolosa and Zeese (1979) studied seven female adults with progressive supranuclear palsy and consistently recorded normal ABRs. They found no correlation between interwave latency values and severity of disease. Stockard, Stockard, and Sharbrough (1980) confirmed these findings.

MYOTONIC DYSTROPHY. | Myotonic dystrophy is a hereditary (autosomal dominant) disease affecting multiple bodily systems. Neurological deficits are myotonia and muscle weakness, personality changes, and impaired cognitive abilities. Other clinical abnormalities include pulmonary and gastrointestinal problems, cataracts, and disturbances in endocrine function.

Seven of fifteen patients with myotonic dystrophy reported by Thompson, Woodward, Ringel, and Nelson (1983) had ABRs equivalent to normal control subjects. Delayed interwave (I–III and/or I–V) latencies were recorded for the remaining eight patients. Pure-tone thresholds were outside the normal region for five of the patients, and each showed an abnormally prolonged ABR wave I component. Most patients (thirteen of fifteen) had normal SSERs as well. There was no correlation between evoked response abnormalities and patient age, but a gender effect was noted. The group consisted of nine males and six females. Evoked response abnormalities were found only for males.

SCHIZOPHRENIA AND DEPRESSION. | The term *schizophrenia* essentially is "split mind." The main symptoms of schizophrenia, disorganization in thinking and emotion, appear first in late adolescence or early adulthood, almost always following a period of extreme stress. Characteristics of the disorder are withdrawal from daily activities, vague speech and poor comprehension of language, inappropriate emotion (e.g., exaggerated happiness or sadness, laughing in time of sadness or crying for no apparent reason, a persistent bland and apathetic affect, and hearing voices, which are often hostile). Schizophrenia is usually differentiated as either paranoid or nonparanoid. Approximately 1 in 1,000 persons has, at some time, been treated for schizophrenia, with men and women equally affected. Schizophrenia is due to a disorder in brain chemistry. Mild cases are treated with psychotherapy. Medical treatment with tranquilizers and antidepressant drugs, which may influence AERs, is not uncommon.

Occasional depression is a common feeling among otherwise healthy persons, but severe depression that persists is an illness. Severely depressed people lose concern for the outside world, even eating and sleeping. They may have hallucinations, acute anxiety, and ultimately be totally withdrawn. Manic depression is characterized by extreme mood changes, ranging from elation to deep depression. Stress may trigger these emotional changes. Depression is often treated with medication or psychotherapy.

There are numerous papers describing abnormalities for cortical evoked responses in schizophrenia, as summarized in Chapters 12 and 13. Among twelve patients with primary depressive disorder and fifteen patients with diagnosed schizophrenia, Bolz and Giedke (1982) found no evidence of ABR abnormality. Likewise, Pfefferbaum, Ford, Roth, and Kopell (1980) and Small, Milstein, Kellams, and Small (1981) reported normal ABRs in patients with schizophrenia. However, components of longer latency auditory evoked responses, particularly the ALR N1 and P2 waves and the P300, are usually reduced in amplitude, as compared with normal control subjects. Abnormal latency delays are observed somewhat less often. These ABR patterns for groups of patients with schizophrenia are not invariably observed in individual patients. For example, St. Clair, Blackwood, and Muir (1989) reported that 46 percent of their schizophrenic group (N=65) had significant latency delays, 35 percent had significant amplitude reductions, and 24 percent were abnormal on both measures, in comparison to data for 119 healthy subjects. P300 differences were unrelated to length of disease, clinical subtype, or effects of medication.

RENAL FAILURE. | Fan, Jiang, and Quian (1994) reported ABR findings for twenty patients with chronic renal failure. Absolute and interwave latencies were markedly increased. Latency values improved with dialysis, although they did not return to normal.

SLEEP APNEA. | Muchnik, Rubel, Zohar, and Hildesheimer (1995) recorded the ABR from seventy-nine patients with obstructive sleep apnea categorized as mild, moderate, and severe. ABR interwave latencies were abnormal in all three groups of subjects in comparison to a control group. Analyzed with respect to clinical normative data, however, only 10 percent of the patients (eight) yielded abnormal ABR latencies. Also, ABR abnormalities remained unchanged

following surgical management of sleep apnea (uvulopalato-pharyngoplasty).

HEPATIC ENCEPHALOPATHY. | This is brain abnormality associated with liver infection.

ABR findings vary among different types of hepatic diseases, according to Chu and Yang (1987). Severity of ABR abnormalities increases from liver cirrhosis, to alcoholic liver disease, to Wilson's disease (see earlier discussion of degenerative neuropathologies). The primary abnormality is excessive interwave latency interval. The pathophysiologic process is unclear, but may involve aberrations in energy metabolism and, in chronic alcoholics, demyelination.

PURE TRIGEMINAL MOTOR NEUROPATHY. | Chiba et al. (1990) present a case of a 57-year-old male with pure trigeminal cranial nerve motor neuropathy. The ABR was entirely normal.

WAARDENBURG SYNDROME. | Waardenburg syndrome is an inherited autosomal dominant mutation, first reported in Dutch populations, characterized by stigmata related to neural crest defects. Major anomalies in Waardenburg syndrome include pigmentation features (hair, eyes, skin) and hearing impairment. There are four types of Waardenburg syndrome categorized according to clinical features. Hearing impairment is most common among type II patients.

Black, Pesznecker, Allen, and Gianna (2001) investigated ECochG and the ABR in twenty-two adult white patients with the diagnosis of Waardenburg syndrome. ABR findings were generally consistent with the degree of sensory hearing loss, with normal interwave latencies. For 77 percent of the patients, there was an enhanced SP/AP ratio (> 40 percent).

BELL'S PALSY. | The etiology of Bell's palsy, a peripheral and often transient facial palsy, is unknown and the site of lesion is disputed.

ABR findings in Bell's palsy are inconsistent (Hanner et al., 1985; Maurizi et al., 1987; Rosenhall et al., 1983; Shanon, Himelfarb, & Zikk, 1985; Uri et al., 1984). ABR findings are mixed. Uri, Schuchman, and Pratt (1984) carried out ABR and audiometric assessment of twenty-four patients within one week of onset of facial weakness. Audiometry was normal, but 25 percent of the patients yielded ABR interwave latencies greater than 2.5 standard deviations above normal mean values. The authors admit that if a normal cutoff of 3 standard deviations had been used, only three (versus six) of the patient ABRs would have been classified as abnormal. Two findings of this study were somewhat unexpected. First, ABR abnormalities were not necessarily on the involved side. Also, for some patients an abnormality was only observed for high stimulus rate (55/sec). Investigators report only infrequent abnormalities (less than 10 percent), although some (Rosenhall et al., 1983; Shanon et al., 1985) describe an abnormality rate as high as 25 percent. Variations in criteria for a normal response and differences among actually etiology for Bell's palsy among reported studies may account for the discrepancies. Maurizi et al. (1987) found normal appearing AMLR Pa components in their thirty patients with Bell's palsy.

Assessment of facial nerve function in Bell's palsy with facial nerve EMG or electroneuronography (ENOG) is discussed in Chapter 15.

VITILIGO. | Vitiligo is a systemic disease of the pigmentary system that may involve cellular components in the nervous system containing melanin. Experimental investigations of animals with pigment abnormalities (e.g., albino cats) show brainstem atrophy in auditory structures. Nikiforidis et al. (1993) recorded the ABR from thirty patients with active vitiligo and a control group of fifty healthy subjects. Interestingly, the authors reported a decrease in latency for ABR wave I, yet an increase in the wave I to III latency interval. Possible explanations offered for these divergent findings include an abnormal decrease in melanocytes within the inner ear (wave I latency decrease) and abnormal synaptic efficiency between the auditory nerve and the superior olivary complex (for the interwave latency delay).

SPASMODIC (SPASTIC) DYSPHONIA. | Spasmodic (spastic) dysphonia is a voice disorder of unknown etiology characterized by vocal spasms that may be either a stoppage of phonation (adductor) or aspirate (abductor). Patients often have other voice abnormalities, among them hoarseness, breathiness, glottal fry, and irregular vibrations.

Abnormal ABRs are reported in patients with spasmodic dysphonia (Finitzo & Freeman, 1989; Finitzo-Hieber, Simhadri, & Hieber, 1981; Hall, 1981; Schaefer, Gerling, Finitzo-Hieber, & Freeman, 1983; Sharbrough, Stockard, & Aronson, 1978). The abnormalities include increase wave I–V latency intervals, especially at high stimulus rates, for some patients, although group patient data is typically not significantly abnormal in comparison to control data. Sharbrough, Stockard, and Aronson (1978) found delays in wave I–V latencies in 39 percent of a series of eighteen spasmodic dysphonia patients. Hall (1981) included ABR with in a central auditory test battery along with acoustic reflex measures and diagnostic speech audiometry. ABR abnormalities included interwave latency delays and an apparent reduction in binaural wave III and V enhancement, in comparison to an age- and gender-matched control group. Schaeffer et al. (1983) reported for nine of twelve patients with spasmodic dysphonia some evidence of ABR abnormality. There was a prolonged wave I–V interval at a standard click rate (20/sec) for three patients. For seven patients, an abnormally large latency shift was noted at a high click rate (90/sec). Amplitude was consistently normal. These findings confirmed the results of an earlier study of six patients by these same authors (Finitzo-Hieber et al., 1981). Then, in a later study

these investigators and additional authors (Schaeffer et al., 1985) expanded the assessment of nineteen spasmodic dysphonia patients to include, in addition to ABR, speech audiometry and magnetic resonance imaging. Ten of the nineteen had abnormal ABRs as previously defined. Also, six patients showed abnormal spin echo MRI findings (each was one of the ten with abnormal ABRs). There was no strong anatomic correlation, however, between ABR and MRI outcome. Among forty-three spasmodic dysphonia patients, Finitzo and Freeman (1989) found an abnormal ABR on the basis of either rate study or interwave latencies for 35 percent (fifteen patients). Middleton, Wilson, and Keith (1997) described entirely normal ABR findings in fourteen patients with the diagnosis of spasmodic dysphonia.

MIGRAINE. | Patients with migraine may have auditory complaints, particularly intolerance to loud sounds and "phonophobia" (e.g., Vanagaite et al., 1998). Sand and Vingen (2000) recorded the ABR, and also longer latency AERs and VERs, in a series of twenty-one migraine patients (sixteen female and five male) with a mean age of 39.3 years. Patients met the International Headache Society criteria for migraine. Consistent with previous reports (Bank, 1991; Podoshin et al., 1987), Sand and Vingen (2000) found no difference in ABR latencies between "migraineurs" and an age- and gender-matched control group. In addition, the patient's sound discomfort level was not related to ABR amplitude. The same findings were reported also for the auditory late response. No clear or consistent relation was found for habituation of ABR or ALR amplitudes in the migraine patients.

CENTRAL TINNITUS. | Tinnitus, perception of sounds in the absence of an acoustic stimulus, is a symptom of numerous otologic diseases. Cochlear (hair cell) dysfunction is a common finding and considered the peripheral source of tinnitus, but the central auditory nervous system and related regions of the brain (e.g., limbic system and autonomic nervous system) clearly play a role in the perception of and physiologic response to tinnitus.

Several investigators report evidence of ABR abnormalities in patients with a central form of tinnitus, including interwave latency delays (Ikner & Hassen, 1990; Maurizi et al., 1985). Rosenhall and Axelsson (1995) recorded ABR from two groups of patients with tinnitus (fifty-six patients with normal or near-normal hearing loss and fifty-seven patients with moderate or more severe sensorineural hearing loss) and a large (N = 220) control group with no complaint of tinnitus matched for age, gender, and hearing loss. ABR latencies for wave I, wave V, and the wave III to V interval, were significantly prolonged for the normal-hearing tinnitus group compared to the control group. Prevalence of ABR abnormalities in the normal-hearing group was 31 to 40 percent. Among the tinnitus subjects with hearing loss, absolute latencies for ABR waves I and V, and the wave III to V latency interval, were prolonged for males, but not for females.

HYPERACUSIS. | In a case study of a patient with hyperacusis (intolerance to everyday sound levels), Gopal, Daly, Daniloff, & Pennartz, (2000) found increased amplitude for ABR wave I, wave III, and wave V in an unmedicated state, and then a decrease in ABR amplitudes associated with treatment consisting of selective serotonin reuptake inhibitors (fluvoxamine and fluoxetine). It is relevant to note that the patient also had withdrawn depression, hypersensitivity to touch, pressure, and photic (light) stimuli, and difficulty understanding speech.

VERTIGO. | Vertigo is a symptom of different neurotologic pathologies. A patient with true vertigo, as opposed to dizziness or light-headedness, senses that either that he or she is spinning or the environment is spinning around. Vertigo may be produced by putting the head in a certain position or may occur spontaneously. As a symptom of Ménière's disease, vertigo is described in the review of clinical applications of ECochG in Chapter 5.

Rosenhall, Pedersen, Johansson, and Kall (1984) analyzed ABR findings for thirty patients with vestibular neuronitis, sixteen patients with epidemic vertigo and sixteen patients with benign positional vertigo. Eight patients with vestibular neuronitis (27 percent) had an abnormal ABR, including two with no wave IV–V complex, six with delayed wave I–V latency intervals, and two with an asymmetry in the wave I–V interval (greater than 0.4 ms). Rosenhall, Pedersen, Johansson, and Kall (1984) reported that only one patient with epidemic vertigo showed an abnormal ABR (I–V latency delay), and only on one ear. Each of the sixteen patients with benign positional vertigo showed normal findings.

VIBRATION-RELATED CNS DISORDER. | Murata, Araki, and Aono (1990) studied the ABR in twelve male forest chain saw operators (mean age of fifty-six years) and eight brush saw workers (mean age forty-three) exposed to excessive hand-arm vibration, and a control group of normal subjects matched by age and gender. The average number of years of exposure was sixteen for the chain saw operators and twelve for the brush saw operators. ABR wave V absolute latency and interwave latency values (wave I–V) were significantly prolonged in chain saw operator group, whereas only the wave I–V latency interval was prolonged for the brush saw operator group. Hearing loss was poorer for the chain saw operators. The findings were in agreement with a previous report of ABR in chain saw operators with "white finger attacks" (Sasaki et al., 1987).

SLEEP APNEA (ADULT). | This is a breathing disorder occurring during sleep and resulting in reduced oxygen content in the blood and hypoxemia (lowered oxygen reaching the brain tissue). With obstructive sleep apnea extra tissue in the nasopharynx (back of the throat) partially or completely blocks the passage of air when the patient is sleeping. Breathing is disrupted and less oxygen gets into the blood. During sleep,

the patient usually snores and breathes irregularly. Surgery to remove the extra tissue in the throat may correct the problem. Central apnea is disruption of breathing during sleep that is not directly related to an obstruction in the throat. The end result is also reduced oxygen in the blood.

Peled, Pratt, Scharf, and Lavie (1983) recorded normal ABRs by latency and amplitude analysis from seven patients with predominantly central sleep apnea, and Mosko, Pierce, Holowach, and Sassin (1981) reported normal ABRs in a series of patients with obstructive sleep apnea by Karnaze, Gott, Mitchell, and Lofton (1984) found normal ABRs (I–V intervals no greater than 4.16 ms even for a subgroup of subjects over age 50) for seventeen of eighteen sleep apneic patients (seven central, six obstructive, and five mixed). In the one patient with an abnormality (prolonged wave I–III and wave I–V latency), central sleep apnea resulted from meningeal leukemic infiltration. This latter study, and data reported by Stockard, Sharbrough, Staats, and Westbrook (1980), suggest that ABR abnormalities found in apparently idiopathic sleep apnea may actually be due to more widespread brainstem dysfunction of which the sleep apnea is a clinical component.

HEMIFACIAL SPASM. | The likely etiology of a subset of cases of hemifacial spasm is compression of the facial nerve at the root entry zone by vascular structures. This produces hyperactive facial nerve dysfunction and involuntary contractions of facial muscles, which is usually unilateral. Hemifacial spasm is found more often in women than men, and more often with increasing age (Jannetta, 1981).

Møller, Møller, and Jannetta (1982) recorded ABRs from each side of thirty-seven patients with hemifacial spasm before surgery to relieve the spasm. Latencies for ABR waves III and V were significantly delayed on the spasm side versus the unaffected side. In a follow-up study of 143 patients with hemifacial spasm, Møller and Møller (1985) confirmed these earlier findings, and also presented evidence of an unusual audiogram configuration (decreased thresholds in the low- and mid-frequency region) presumably secondary to eighth nerve compression by a blood vessel.

PALATAL MYOCLONUS. | This disease is a syndrome that includes twitching movements (rhythmic and voluntary) of the soft palate, often accompanied by movements of other structures in the head and neck (larynx, pharynx, and facial, extraocular, and neck muscles). The exact anatomic locus of the syndrome has not been documented, but a brainstem abnormality is confirmed. Pathologic findings reported in patients with palatal myoclonus are varied, among them diverse brainstem lesions (infarcts, tumor, multiple sclerosis, posterior circulation aneurysm, miscellaneous degenerative processes, syphilis, and trauma), and hypertrophic degeneration of pontine structures.

Westmoreland, Sharbrough, Stockard, and Dale (1983) conducted a study of ABRs in a group of twenty patients with palatal myoclonus with a diverse distribution of etiologies (seven with head injury, five with infarctions, three with tumor, two with degenerative disease, and one each with demyelinating disease, inflammatory disease, and developmental disease). Patients with all but two of these etiologies (a total of six patients, or 30 percent of the group) showed ABR abnormalities. The two exceptions were degenerative and developmental disease. The ABR abnormalities were decreased wave V/I amplitude ratios and increased wave I–V latency intervals (unilateral in five patients and bilateral in one). In a case report of a 30-year-old male with palatal myoclonus (secondary to right-sided infarct in the brainstem), Epstein, Stappenbeck, and Karp (1980) also found prolonged ABR wave V latency and reduced amplitude. On the other hand, two patients with palatal myoclonus reported by Gothgen, Jacobs, and Newman had normal ABRs. Westmoreland et al. (1983) conclude that on occasion the lateral portions of the brainstem may be involved with widespread pathology in palatal myoclonus and then ABR abnormalities are not unexpected, but more discrete lesions in the dentarubro-olivary region or diseases involving brainstem gray matter are associated with normal ABR findings.

GUILLAIN-BARRE SYNDROME. | This is an acute, but uncommon, type of peripheral neuropathy that often follows a viral infection. The exact cause is not known. Symptoms include first a sensation of tingling and then numbness, proceeding to weakness and sometimes paralysis spreading from hands and feet to other regions of the body. Breathing may be affected in severe degrees of paralysis. These symptoms, and the disease, may be only temporary.

Five of six patients with Guillain-Barre syndrome (without Miller-Fisher variant) reported by Schiff et al. (1985) showed ABR abnormalities, mainly in the I–III latency interval. ABR findings for both Guillain-Barre syndrome and the Miller-Fisher variant in children are reviewed in Chapter 9.

ACUTE NUCLEORETICULAR VESTIBULAR SYNDROME. | The chief complaint is vertigo. Patients have spontaneous nystagmus and hyporeflexia. The etiology may be toxic or vascular.

Among twenty-five adult patients with acute nucleoreticular vestibular syndrome reported by Russolo and Poli (1983), 28 percent had unilateral ABR abnormalities and another 28 percent had bilateral abnormalities. The percentage of patients with various types of abnormalities were distributed as follows: unreliable, 22 percent; undetectable wave I, 12 percent; undetectable wave III, 12 percent; undetectable wave V, 10 percent; delayed latency for wave V, 4 percent; delayed wave I–V interwave latency, 22 percent; and decreased wave V/I amplitude ratio, 8 percent. Criterion for abnormal I–V interwave latency (greater than 4.2 ms) and V/I amplitude ratio (less than 1.0) was relatively lax. These patients had normal hearing sensitivity and normal middle ear function. A battery of audiometric procedures, including diagnostic speech audiometry, tests of sound lateralization,

and acoustic reflex measurement, also showed hearing deficits in this subgroup, but correlation among procedures was not high.

SICKLE CELL DISEASE (ANEMIA). | Sickle cell anemia is an inherited disease that is relatively common in the black population, affecting 1 out of every 1,000 black persons in the United States. In sickle cell anemia, red blood cells have abnormal hemoglobin. Blood cells do not flow properly through smaller blood vessels and may clog the vessels. This prevents the blood from reaching bodily tissue and can lead to anoxia. When anoxia occurs, a sickle cell patient is in "crisis." Duration of the crisis may be less than a day or last for three or four days.

Elwany and Kamel (1988) carried out audiologic evaluation, including ABR, in ten sickle cell anemia patients during crisis episodes and then one month after resolution of the crisis. Four of the ten patients showed abnormal ABRs during severe crisis, usually with other neurological signs. The most common abnormality was delayed wave III–V latency. In two of the four patients, the abnormality reversed after resolution of the crisis. ABR wave I latency value was only prolonged in patients with sensorineural hearing loss.

TRAUMATIC HEAD INJURY. | The demographic and pathophysiologic features of traumatic head injury are summarized in the final section of this chapter in a discussion of neuromonitoring with ABR. Since the early work of Greenberg and colleagues in the mid-1970s (Greenberg, Becker, Miller, & Mayer, 1977), many papers have described applications of AERs, and other sensory evoked responses, in traumatic head injury (Hall, 1988; Hall, Hargadine, & Allen, 1985; Hall, Mackey-Hargadine, & Kim, 1985; Hall, Huangfu, & Gennarelli, 1982; Hall et al., 1984; Hall & Tucker, 1985, 1986; Karnaze, Marshall, McCarthy, Klauber, & Bickford, 1982; Linsay, Carlin, Kennedy, et al., 1981; Lutschg, Pfenninger, Ludin, & Fassela, 1983; Narayan, Greenberg, Miller, & Miller, 1981; Seales, Rossiter, & Weinstein, 1979; Tsubokawa, Nichimoto, Yamamoto, et al., 1980; Yagi & Baba, 1983). The initial objective this clinical research effort was estimation of long-term neurological outcome with evoked response measurements made within days after severe injury, while the patient remained comatose. Then, the emphasis of evoked response research shifted to neuromonitoring of patients with severe injury in the intensive care unit (ICU) during the acute period following the injury and also to documentation of peripheral auditory dysfunction requiring medical and/or audiologic management (e.g., Hall et al., 1982; Hall, Hargadine, & Allen, 1985; Lew et al., 2004). The literature on ABR, AMLR, and ALR findings in acute head injury is far too extensive to review in detail here.

ABR findings are normal in over 70 percent of comatose patients with severe traumatic head injury. Patients sustaining severe head injuries with primary (due to the accident) brainstem damage are not likely to survive the initial insult and reach a hospital ICU. Abnormalities of cortical AERs and other sensory evoked responses, however, are not uncommon in the severely head-injured population. Progressive deterioration of the ABR may occur in head injured patients with secondary CNS pathophysiology, such as brainstem ischemia due to increased intracranial pressure (ICP) and transtentorial herniation and brainstem compression or hypotension (low blood pressure), or due to hypoxemia (low blood oxygen). Again, the use of ABR for neuromonitoring of acute CNS status in the neuro-ICU is reviewed toward the end of this chapter. There are reports suggesting that ABR latency increases in patients recovering from moderate or even minor head injury and suffering from suspected "postconcussion syndrome" provide evidence of organic brain dysfunction (Noseworthy, Miller, Murray, & Regan, 1981; Rizzo, Pierelli, Pozzessere, Floris, & Morocutti, 1983; Rowe & Carlson, 1980).

INTRAOPERATIVE NEUROPHYSIOLOGIC MONITORING WITH ABR

Criteria for Intraoperative ABR Alterations

Guidelines used for interpreting the significance of changes in response are lacking most in reports of AER findings obtained intraoperatively. Reported criteria for interpretation of ABR alterations intraoperatively are various, as displayed in Table 10.10. For ABR neuromonitoring, most authors base their criteria on the absolute latency value of wave V. However, the amount of wave V latency change that is considered clinically significant ranges from as little as 0.5 ms to complete disappearance of the response. In ABR interpretation with such criteria, it is assumed that the nonsurgical causes of the ABR changes are ruled out. Examples of these nonsurgical causes would include physiologic fluctuations (e.g., body temperature or blood pressure), equipment problems (e.g., electrode or transducer slippage), modifications in measurement parameters, and effects of anesthesia.

In addition to absolute latency of ABR wave V, criteria for latency and amplitude of ABR wave I (i.e., the ECochG AP), and also the ABR wave I–V latency interval, are recommended for interpretation of intraoperative ABR (Levine, Ojemann, Montgomery, & McGaffigan, 1984; Møller & Jannetta, 1983a, 1984; Ruth, Mills, & Jane, 1986; Silverstein, Wazen, Norrell, & Hyman, 1984). The arguments against reliance on only wave V absolute latency or amplitude in intraoperative ABR monitoring are equivalent to those cited earlier in this chapter in the discussion of ABR in the diagnosis of retrocochlear auditory pathology. That is, absolute wave V latency or amplitude reflects both central *and* peripheral (including middle ear and cochlear) auditory functioning, whereas the wave I–V latency interval measure is predominantly a measure of eighth nerve through auditory brainstem integrity. A reduction in stimulus intensity level, for example, due to slippage of an insert earphone during surgery, would be more likely to affect amplitude and latency of wave V than the wave I–V latency interval, assuming a clear wave I remained present.

The ABR wave I–V latency interval, however, is also not the ideal neurophysiologic index for two reasons: First of

TABLE 10.10. Summary of Reported Criteria for Intraoperative Changes in Auditory Brainstem Response (ABR)

Changes in morphology, including the broadening of wave V, are not uncommon during surgery and are not included among criteria.

STUDY	YEAR	WAVE	CRITERIA*
Little, Lesser, Leuders, & Furlan	1983	V	>0.5 ms latency increase
Raudzens & Shetter	1982	V	>1.0 ms latency increase
Manninen, Lam, & Nicholas	1985	V	>1.0 ms latency increase
Grundy, Jannetta, Procopio, et al.	1982	V	>1.5 ms latency increase
Schwartz, Bloom, & Dennis	1985	?	>2.0 ms latency increase or >50% amplitude decrease
Friedman, Kaplan, Gravenstein, & Rhoton	1985	V	Total disappearance of ABR
Hall**	1992	I–V	>0.5 ms latency increase = alert >1.0 ms latency increase = warning
		I–III	>0.5 ms latency increase = warning

* Change is in comparison to baseline values, unless otherwise indicated

** Analysis made after correction for change in body temperature

all, the wave I–V latency interval does not necessarily limit intraoperative information on auditory system integrity to the specific anatomic region of interest. Second, a clear wave I may not be observed from patients with hearing sensitivity deficits. Optimally, interwave latency for a component immediately distal (peripheral) to and a component immediately proximal (central) to the anatomic region of surgery is analyzed intraoperatively (Levine et al., 1984; Ojemann et al., 1984). If the eighth nerve is at risk, then ABR wave I, wave II, and wave III, and the wave I–II and wave I–III intervals are the most appropriate AER components to monitor. Perhaps the best approach for obtaining this information is a two-channel measurement of ECochG with electrodes located on the promontory and directly on the eighth nerve as it enters the brainstem during eighth-nerve surgery (Møller & Jannetta, 1981, 1983a, 1984; Silverstein et al., 1984).

Friedman et al. (1985) specifically address the issue of criteria for intraoperative interpretation of ABR changes. These authors observe that a simple prolongation in wave V or in the wave I–V latency interval does not appear to be closely related to postoperative hearing status. Using a latency prolongation criterion, then, produces excessive false alarms. Friedman et al. (1985) cite as evidence of this problem the relatively small number of warnings to the surgeon (19%) with their criteria (loss of the response) versus the higher number that would have been reported in their series of twenty-one patients if the criteria of Grundy et al. (1982) and of Raudzens and Shetter (1982) were used (52% and 100%, respectively). There are several relatively new and potentially effective and efficient approaches for intraoperative AER interpretation. Two examples are cross-correlation of response phase and an optimal digital filtering technique, which permits a compressed EP (evoked potential) array, that is, a sequence of waveforms occurring approximately every 10 seconds (Hammerschlag et al., 1986). More clinical documentation of the intraoperative value of such analysis techniques is needed.

Sensitivity and Specificity of Neuromonitoring Information

An important question related to criteria for ABR alterations and often raised in discussions of intraoperative monitoring with sensory evoked responses concerns both the sensitivity and the specificity of the technique. That is, what is the likelihood that surgery-induced auditory dysfunction will be detected by the ABR? And, conversely, what is the chance that patients with normal responses intraoperatively will have postoperative deficits? There is no consensus on this issue and, in fact, there will probably never be a totally satisfactory answer to the question. However, since the early studies of Betty Grundy and colleagues, evidence has accumulated in support of the sensitivity of ABRs (Grundy et al., 1982; Jacobson, 1990). The issue of specificity in intra-operative monitoring is, for the most part, based on our knowledge

of response component generators. Sensitivity to auditory dysfunction is greatest for the later components of the ABR, particularly wave V, because disruption of function at any point distal (peripheral) to the pons-midbrain region of the brainstem will presumably be detected. That is, ABR wave V reflects brainstem, eighth-nerve root entry zone (i.e., the CPA), eighth-nerve, and cochlear dysfunction. Although ABR wave V alterations intraoperatively by definition are evidence of auditory dysfunction, they do not necessarily predict loss of hearing. The ABR wave V change may be a product of desynchronization or (less likely) dysfunction of a specific subpopulation of neurons. Other auditory measures, such as pure-tone or speech audiometry, may show less decrement in performance.

Another confounding variable in the sensitivity of auditory evoked responses in monitoring auditory function intraoperatively is the temporal relationship between a surgical insult to the auditory system and the subsequent detection of ABR changes. Naturally, auditory evoked response changes will not precede a surgical insult, but they may occur at variable time intervals after an insult. That is, a response may appear stable within moments after manipulation of an anatomical structure, yet undergo progressive deterioration minutes or perhaps even hours later (Levine at al., 1984). Also, other intervening events may obscure the precise cause of the change in ABR. Along the same line, in order to facilitate reversal of ABR abnormalities following an insult, a period of surgical inactivity of minutes or more may be necessary (Levine et al., 1984; Ruth, Mills, & Jane, 1986). Morphology and reproducibility of ABRs is also suggested as a sensitive analysis measure intraoperatively (Mokrusch, Schramm, & Fahlbusch, 1985), and it is presumed to reflect synchronization of neural activity.

In contrast, latency and amplitude of ABR wave I (the ECochG AP component) is not sensitive to proximal eighth-nerve or auditory brainstem dysfunction. There are repeated accounts of brainstem dysfunction or inactivity and marked eighth-nerve dysfunction, including complete transection of the nerve, in the presence of a consistently recorded and normal-appearing wave I (ECochG AP) component (Hall, 1992; Hall, Mackey-Hargadine, & Kim, 1985; Levine et al., 1984; Ohashi et al., 1996; Ohashi et al., 2001; Ruben, Hudson, & Chiong, 1963). Cacace and colleagues (1994) refer to this pattern as the "disconnected ear." For preservation of ABR wave I (ECochG AP), blood supply via the internal auditory artery must remain intact. Hearing in these cases of retrocochlear damage is completely lost. Eventually, there is apparently retrograde degeneration of cochlear functioning, or delayed vascular disturbance, and the ABR wave I (ECochG AP) also disappears. Nonetheless, the reliance intraoperatively on cochlear nerve action potentials (ECochG AP or ABR wave I) for preservation of hearing is reported in the literature (Stanton, Cashman, Harrison, Nedzelski, & Rowed, 1989) and is discussed next. Clearly, serious pathophysiology involving major portions of the nervous system (cranial nerves, brainstem, cerebellum, or cerebrum) can develop intraoperatively and yet go undetected by auditory evoked responses, if auditory pathways are not compromised (Piatt, Radtke, & Erwin, 1985). As noted earlier, a combined modality approach (AER and SSER) for monitoring more widespread neuroanatomy may be useful to reduce the likelihood of this outcome.

Preservation of Hearing during Tumor Removal

BACKGROUND. | An attempt to preserve hearing during eighth-nerve tumor removal was reported as early as 1954 (Elliott & McKissock, 1954). The majority of published papers on the topic of hearing preservation by means of intraoperative monitoring with ABR, however, have appeared since 1980. Table 10.11 summarizes published studies of the application of intraoperative monitoring with ABR during surgical removal of retrocochlear tumors. Meaningful comparison of findings among studies is difficult because of differences in the size of tumors (including widely varying techniques for estimating size), the type of tumor (usually a vestibular schwannoma, meningioma, or neurofibroma), criterion for evaluating pre- and postoperative hearing, the surgical approach, and the surgeon's skill. The issue is further confused by the natural tendency to highlight successful hearing preservation in isolated patients (or case reports), especially those with large tumors, or to emphasize occasional patients who actually show postoperative hearing improvement, rather than to base conclusions about hearing preservation on systematic analysis of results for a consecutive series of patients.

In 1984, Levine, Ojemann, Montgomery, and McGaffigan noted that for the majority of patients with tumors on or near the auditory (eighth cranial) nerve, and with preoperative hearing integrity, postoperative hearing is worse or entirely lost, even though surgery spares the structural integrity of the nerve. The exact reason for this discrepancy between apparent structural and functional integrity was not clear. Auditory evoked responses, particularly the ABR, however, have gained a well-deserved reputation for being sensitive to auditory dysfunction in retrocochlear pathology. In a sense, intraoperative monitoring with auditory evoked responses is further exploitation of this sensitivity to eighth-nerve and brainstem function. The objective with neurodiagnosis is early identification of retrocochlear dysfunction, whereas with neuromonitoring, the goal is early detection and avoidance of pathophysiologic processes that might lead to postoperative hearing deficits. Mechanisms underlying surgery-related damage to auditory structures are reviewed in the section of Chapter 5 on the application of ECochG in intraoperative monitoring. The application of intraoperative monitoring for tumors on or near the eighth nerve is now widespread, particular for the middle cranial fossa and retrosigmoid surgical approaches (e.g., Brackmann et al., 2000; Stidham & Roberson, 2001). An international collection of

clinical investigators have reported rates of success in hearing preservation with intraoperative monitoring with auditory evoked responses ranging from 20 percent to as high as 71 percent (e.g., Arriaga, Chen, & Fukushima, 1997; Brackmann et al., 2000; Cohen, Lewis, & Ransohoff, 1993; Dornhoffer, Helms, & Hoehmann, 1995; Fischer, Fischer, & Remond, 1992; Gantz et al., 1986; Hecht et al., 1997; Irving, Jackler, & Pitts, 1998; Josey et al., 1988; Kemink et al., 1990; Nadol et al., 1992; Sanna et al., 1987; Sterkers et al., 1994; Stidham & Roberson, 2001; Tonn et al., 2000).

Some lingering controversy surrounds the benefits of preservation of hearing during surgical treatment of lesions involving the auditory nerve and brainstem. The main concern is whether the benefit of preserving auditory function, especially the practical amount of function preserved, outweighs the potential surgical-medical disadvantage, namely, incomplete tumor removal and possible regrowth of the residual tumor. Thus, there are really five distinct questions to be answered:

- Is there a consistent relation between the size of a tumor and the likelihood of hearing preservation?
- What pre- and postoperative criteria should be used to describe hearing function? Simply put, how good should *pre*operative hearing be in order to warrant attempts to preserve hearing, and how bad should hearing be *post*operatively before it can be concluded that the attempt at hearing preservation was unsuccessful?
- If every attempt is made to preserve hearing surgically by avoiding as much as possible trauma to auditory structures and blood vessels serving auditory structures, what is the likelihood that tumor removal will be incomplete, and how much residual tumor, for a given pathology, justifies concern?
- How can auditory evoked responses recorded intraoperatively provide early warning of impending or reversible surgery-related damage and dysfunction of auditory structures?
- What is the relation between intraoperative AER findings and hearing status after surgery? That is, can auditory evoked responses accurately predict hearing outcome?

The American Academy of Otolaryngology-Head and Neck Surgery (AAOHNS) Committee on Hearing and Equilibrium has offered guidelines for categorizing hearing preservation in surgery for removal of vestibular schwannomas (Committee on Hearing and Equilibrium, 1995). Briefly, the categories in descending order of hearing integrity are labeled alphabetically, as follows: Class A = PTA ≤ 30 dB HL and WR = ≥ 70 percent; Class B = PTA > 30 and ≤ 50 dB HL and WR = ≥ 50 percent; Class C = PTA > 50 dB HL and WR = ≥ 50 percent; Class D = PTA at any level and WR = < 50 percent. PTA refers to pure-tone average (average of the hearing thresholds for test frequencies of 500, 1000, and 2000 Hz) and WR refers to word recognition (percent

TABLE 10.11.   Selected Studies (published since 1990) of the ABR as a Tool for Monitoring Neurophysiologic Status Intraoperatively during Surgical Removal of Retrocochlear Tumors

SURGICAL PROCEDURE STUDY (YEAR)	N	APPROACH*	PATHOLOGY(IES)	COMMENTS
Tumor Removal				
Kemink et al. (1990)	93	??	Vestibular schwannoma	No serviceable hearing for tumors >1.5 cm
Harper et al. (1992)	90	??	Vestibular schwannoma	ABR contributed to hearing preservation
Hsu et al. (1992)	6	??	Vestibular schwannoma	ECochG quicker for detecting wave I
Cohen et al. (1993)	141	RS	Vestibular schwannoma	ABR monitoring not a factor in outcome
	7	RS	Meningiomas	
	6	RS	Neurofibromas	
Aoyagi et al. (1994)	9	MF	Vestibular schwannoma**	Size of tumor not predictive of outcome
Dornhoffer et al. (1995)	93	MF	Vestibular schwannoma	Wave V latency <6.8 ms in good outcome
Harner et al. (1996)	144	RS	Vestibular schwannoma	
Roberson et al. (1999)	22	??	Vestibular schwannoma	Hearing preservation with no ABR pre-op
Jackson & Roberson (2000)	23	??	Vestibular schwannoma	ABR monitoring not related to outcome
Battista et al. (2000)	66	??	Vestibular schwannoma	Direct eighth nerve monitoring valuable
Brackmann et al. (2000)	333	MF	Vestibular schwannoma	Tumor location predictive of outcome
Tonn et al. (2000)	508	RS	Vestibular schwannoma	Improved outcome with ABR monitoring
Tokimura et al. (1990)	3	MF	Vestibular schwannoma	Wave V latency change of <1.5 ms good
	2		Epidermoid	
	1		Meningioma	
Stidham & Roberson, (2001)	30	MF	Vestibular schwannoma	Hearing improvement in 23% of patients
Browning et al. (2001)	36	RS	Vestibular schwannoma	Abnormal ABR predicts poor outcome Supports use of transtympanic ECochG
Microvascular Decompression				
Sindou, Fobe, Ciriano, & Fischer (1990)	17	??	Hemifacial spasm	ABR useful in avoiding traction and vascular injuries to cranial nerves
	17		Trigeminal neuralgia	
Tokimura et al. (1990)	12		Hemifacial spasm	
	10		Trigeminal neuralgia	
Acevedo, Sindou, Fischer, & Vial (1997)	75	RM	Hemifacial spasm	Only 1.6% of patients had hearing change
Van et al. (1999)	13		Hemifacial spasm	ABR was an important surgical guide

* MF = middle fossa approach; RS = retrosigmoid (suboccipital) approach; RM = retromastoid

** Vestibular schwannoma = acoustic tumor

correct score for a list of 25 or 50 single-syllable and typically phonetically balanced words presented most often at a comfortable listening level). Of course, valid comparison of findings among studies of hearing preservation with ABR is confounded because not all investigators follow the AAOHNS guidelines.

FACTORS AFFECTING PRESERVATION OF HEARING. | The success of hearing preservation among the many studies reporting intraoperative AER recording during surgery for tumor removal is dependent on diverse variables. Dozens of investigators have attempted to relate the audiologic outcome of surgery—hearing preservation—to specific factors. The most common three factors reported are the patient's preoperative hearing levels, tumor size, and both preoperative ABR findings and intraoperative ABR changes. However, published papers have collectively attempted to determine whether postoperative hearing status is affected by seven factors: (1) tumor size, (2) postoperative timing of hearing evaluation, (3) tumor type, (4) location of blood vessels, (5) surgical approach, (6) preoperative ABR findings, and (7) exposure of manipulation of the eighth nerve. Unfortunately, meaningful interpretation of the accumulated data from published studies of hearing preservation is constrained by a variety of methodological weaknesses. Most studies report data for a limited number of patients. Not all of the investigators consistently used ABR in monitoring, and there are substantial differences among studies in the criteria used to describe hearing status pre- and postoperatively. For these reasons, an exhaustive listing of the "success rates" for hearing preservation among published studies would have limited value.

Collective experience with surgical management of acoustic tumors at the House Ear Clinic and Institute in Los Angeles is extensive. In a paper entitled "Prognostic Factors for Hearing Preservation in Vestibular Schwannoma Surgery," Brackmann and colleagues from the House Ear Clinic (Brackmann et al., 2000) report results for a series of 333 patients with some hearing and vestibular function who underwent resection of acoustic tumors with the middle fossa craniotomy surgical approach. According to the authors, the middle fossa approach is appropriate for tumors that are ≤ 2 cm in diameter at the largest portion. In the authors' practice, the approach is used for about 45 percent of the patients with vestibular schwannomas. Brackmann et al. (2000) apply conventional audiologic criteria for selection of patients for attempted hearing preservation, that is, a preoperative pure-tone average of ≤ 50 dB HL and word recognition scores of ≥ 50 percent. Based on analysis of data for their large series of patients, Brackmann et al. (2000) reported a "small but significant difference" in preoperative hearing levels and the likelihood of hearing preservation. That is, patients with better hearing before surgery (e.g., a PTA of < 25 dB HL and WR > 85 percent) were less likely to lose their hearing during surgery than patients with somewhat poorer hearing preoperatively. For clinical purposes, however, there was considerable overlap among patients meeting the audiologic criteria for candidacy for hearing preservation surgery. Similarly, preoperative ABR findings, such as the size of the difference in wave V latency between the side of the tumor and wave V latency of the ABR elicited with stimulation of the ear on the opposite (uninvolved) side did not seem to correlate with hearing preservation. In fact, whether the preoperative ABR was normal or abnormal (based on ILD for wave V) was not related to postoperative hearing status. Some patients with normal ABRs before surgery lost hearing, and hearing was preserved for some patients with abnormal ABR findings before surgery. The apparent independence of preoperative ABR findings and postoperative hearing outcome was highlighted a report by Roberson, Jackson, and McAuley (1999) of four patients who had no ABR before surgery and the return of an ABR in the months following surgery. Brackmann et al. (2000) also reported that tumor size, at least among patients with tumors < 2 cm, did not accurately predict the outcome of hearing preservation surgery—that is, "On the basis of our experience, small tumor size does not necessarily predict successful hearing preservation, and large tumor size does not necessarily impact hearing loss" (p. 423). One factor was related to hearing preservation. Patients with tumors that originated from the superior vestibular nerve (see Figure 10.1) were more likely to retain their preoperative hearing levels and word recognition scores than patients with tumors arising from the inferior vestibular nerve. This latter finding confirms the results of earlier comprehensive reports of hearing preservation in surgery for removal of CPA tumors (e.g., Cohen, Lewis, & Ransohoff, 1993).

Tumor Size. First, ABR waveforms are more likely to disappear permanently and postoperative hearing is more likely to worsen in patients with large tumors. Large tumors, with size determined by preoperative CT scanning, are usually defined as 2.0 to 2.5 to 3 cm in diameter, or greater. The relationship between tumor size and the likelihood of hearing preservation has long been considered (House, 1979), but inconsistently confirmed (Glasscock, Dickins, & Wiet, 1979; Jannetta, Møller, & Møller, 1984; Kanzaki, Ogawa, Shiobara, & Toya, 1989; Lenarz, & Sachsenheimer, 1985) although exceptions are noted (Fischer, Constantini, & Mercier, 1980). Hearing preservation is reported in 15 to 60 percent of patients with small- to moderate-sized acoustic neuromas, for both the suboccipital and middle cranial fossa surgical approaches, but rarely for tumors exceeding 2.5 cm (e.g., Harner et al., 1996). Silverstein, McDaniel, Wazen, and Norrell (1985) reported findings for thirteen patients undergoing surgery for tumor removal with an attempt to preserve hearing. Hearing was preserved in three or four patients with tumors of 1.0 cm or less, in two of five patients with 1.5 cm tumors, and in only one out of four with relatively large (>2.0 cm) tumors. These authors further provide a concise summary of the success rates in hearing preservation in relation to tumor size, as reported among other studies.

In a 1989 paper, Kanzaki and colleagues reported that hearing was preserved with a middle fossa surgical approach in 40 percent of patients with tumors of 2 cm or less in diameter, whereas hearing could not be preserved for any patient with tumors greater than 2 cm in diameter. These authors used a 50/50 criterion for hearing integrity. That is, hearing thresholds are better than 50 dB HL and speech-recognition scores are higher than 50 percent. This is another variation on a theme repeated often—the smaller the tumor (and the earlier its identification), the better. A problem in interpreting such statistics, however, is the inconsistency among investigators in definition of postoperative hearing status. Among the most commonly reported indexes of hearing are pure-tone HTLs (hearing threshold levels) for audiometric frequencies, speech-reception (spondee) threshold, and word-recognition scores at a comfortable intensity level. Some investigators employed a comprehensive audiometric test battery, but others reported only a single measure, such as pure-tone audiometry. Vague definitions of hearing, such as "serviceable" or "usable" also complicate matters. Systems proposed for categorizing hearing before and after neurotologic surgery (e.g., Silverstein, McDaniel, Norrell, & Haberkamp, 1986), are at this point not widely used.

Postoperative Timing of Hearing Evaluation. The time of the postoperative and audiometric assessment is also an important variable. Although postoperative improvement in hearing is unusual, occurring in less than 10 percent of patients, there are rather dramatic reports of clearly improved hearing for patients over the course of months after surgery (e.g., Stidham & Roberson, 2001; Tucci et al., 1994). In other cases, hearing may be reasonably intact immediately after surgery, but then deteriorate dramatically, in some cases to total deafness within days, weeks, months, or even years (Kanzaki, Ogawa, Shiobara, & Toya, 1989; Levine et al., 1984; McDonnell, Jabbari, Spinella, Mueller, & Klara, 1990; Palva, Troupp, & Jauhianen, 1985; Shelton, Hitselberger, House, & Brackmann, 1990; Shelton & House, 1990). The reason for delayed postoperative hearing deficits is not clear, although a vascular mechanism must be suspected. Important clinical implications of possible delayed hearing impairment are appropriate during patient counseling and regular otologic/audiologic follow-up in the postoperative period.

Tumor Type. Type of tumor is a very important factor in the preservation of hearing. The vast majority of experience is reported for "acoustic neuromas." Among vestibular schwannomas, hearing outcome is best for patients with tumors arising from the superior vestibular nerve, rather than the inferior vestibular nerve (Brackmann et al., 2000). However, approximately 10 percent of tumors reported in a large series of CPA tumors were not acoustic neuromas (Brackmann & Bartels, 1980). According to these authors, tumor types were distributed as follows: acoustic neuromas (neurinomas), 91.3 percent; meningiomas, 3.1 percent; primary cholesteatomas, 2.4 percent; facial nerve neurinomas, 1.2 percent; neurinomas of other cranial nerves within the posterior fossa, 0.2 percent. Hearing preservation is far less likely with neurofibromas, regardless of the size of the tumor, because of the intimate relationship of the tumor to the nerve and blood vessels (Miyamoto, Campbell, Fritsch, & Lochmueller, 1990). On the other hand, preservation of hearing and sometimes hearing improvement is more likely

in patients with meningiomas and cholesteatomas (Tator & Nedzelski, 1985). Tumors totally within the internal auditory canal (IAC), described also as intrameatal or intracanalicular, may be classified as small yet may produce distinct preoperative hearing deficits.

Location of Blood Vessels. The location of blood vessels, such as the labyrinthine artery, relative to the eighth nerve also may influence hearing outcome. Palva, Troupp, and Jauhianen (1985), for example, note that hearing preservation is more likely if this artery is located anterior to the nerve and, therefore, not in the direct line of tumor dissection when the posterior suboccipital approach is taken. Just touching a blood vessel surgically can produce both vasospasm and serious sensorineural dysfunction secondary to ischemic pathology (Eichlin, 1965). Probably some of the cases of delayed hearing impairment during the postoperative period are due to this vascular mechanism.

Surgical Approach. A translabyrinthine surgical approach, which essentially obliterates the cochlea and is incompatible with hearing preservation, may be taken in patients with no usable preoperative hearing. Some surgeons have routinely taken the translabyrinthine approach when tumor size exceeds 1.5 cm (Glasscock, Hays, Miller, Drake, & Kanok, 1978). Before evidence from AER monitoring experience had accumulated, others argued that the translabyrinthine approach is almost always in the best interest of both the patient and surgeon because it poses less surgical risk of mortality (Maddox, 1982; Tos & Thomsen, 1982). In addition, there is concern that microscopic portions of tumor remain attached to the nerve and/or within the lateral end of the IAC. The concern is that residual tumor may lead to recurrence, although the clinical significance of tiny tumor remnants may be minimal. However, as noted above, Brackmann et al. (2000) regularly use the middle fossa surgical approach in an attempt to preserve hearing of patients with tumors that are ≤ 2 cm, assuming the patient has salvageable hearing.

Some authors maintain that the translabyrinthine approach is routinely indicated because the likelihood for hearing preservation using other approaches is small, and in patients with unilateral tumors, the opposite normal-hearing ear is adequate for communication purposes (Clemis, 1984; Maddox, 1982; Tos & Thomsen, 1982). There is some evidence, however, that if preoperative hearing sensitivity is relatively intact, even though speech discrimination (word recognition) is very poor, hearing preservation may still be a reasonable surgical objective (Abramson, Stein, Pedley, Emerson, & Wazen, 1985). That is, speech audiometry performance may be somewhat improved postoperatively. Nonetheless, substantially improved hearing postoperatively in acoustic tumors is actually very unusual (Anderson, Barr, & Wedenberg, 1970; Shelton & House, 1990; Wade & House, 1984). As a rule, audiologic evidence of retrocochlear dysfunction is greater after surgery than before it.

Preoperative ABR. Preoperative ABR pattern is useful in predicting hearing outcome. Poor preoperative ABR morphology or absence of ABR wave components is associated with postoperative loss of hearing (Kanzaki et al., 1989; Lenarz & Sachsenheimer, 1985; Silverstein et al., 1986). The extent of preoperative ABR abnormalities is also directly, but not invariably, related to tumor size. Reversal of contralateral ABR abnormalities may occur with brainstem decompression following removal of large tumors (Deans, Birchall, & Mendelow, 1990). It is also possible for the ABR to temporarily return during surgery, but this may not be an indicator of permanently improved postoperative hearing status.

These relationships among preoperative ABR alternations and preoperative hearing thresholds, size of tumor, and postsurgical hearing changes were summarized by findings for eighteen patients with eighth-nerve tumors reported by Lenarz and Sachsenheimer (1985). Patients with preoperative hearing impairment of 40 dB or greater tended to also have moderate or severe ABR abnormalities before surgery. These patients were likely to show a postoperative deterioration in hearing. Those with no detectable preoperative ABR, regardless of hearing sensitivity levels, remain severely hearing impaired after surgery.

Exposure or Manipulation of the Eighth Nerve. The eighth nerve is at greatest risk intraoperatively when the IAC is drilled away (in order to expose the eighth nerve and adjacent tumor) and the nerve is manipulated before tumor removal is complete. Intraoperative experience repeatedly shows that auditory evoked responses are typically altered with tumor dissection from the nerve. Probably the second most cited surgical manipulation associated with ABR change is retraction of the cerebellum (Friedman, Kaplan, Gravenstein, & Rhoton, 1985; Grundy et al., 1982; Raudzens & Shetter, 1982; Ruth, Mills, & Jane, 1986). Mechanisms for surgery-related damage to auditory structures were reviewed in Chapter 5 (application of ECochG in intraoperative monitoring).

Laser-induced ABR changes were reported as well (Hammerschlag et al., 1986). Modification of surgery at this precise intraoperative moment, including halting surgery until a waveform returns, is probably the single most important factor contributing to improved outcome. Clearly, total and irreversible loss of the ABR and ECochG during surgery is an ominous sign, consistently associated with poor hearing outcome, whereas unchanged auditory evoked responses imply favorable hearing outcome.

The relationship between intraoperative AER changes and postoperative hearing still requires further description. There are, for example, reports of serious postoperative hearing deficits in patients without AER changes intraoperatively and, conversely, intact postoperative hearing despite distinct alterations of AERs during surgery (Friedman et al., 1985; Grundy et al., 1981; Ojemann et al., 1984; Ruth, Mills, & Jane, 1986; Silverstein et al., 1986). The resolution of these inconsistencies may lie in more sophisticated analysis of latency, amplitude, and (perhaps) other response parameters for all wave components of ECochG and ABR. Stanton et al. (1989), for example, recommend evaluation of ECochG AP threshold, and then monitoring AP status as close to threshold as possible, as opposed to monitoring AP latency or amplitude at a high stimulus-intensity level. Manipulation of stimulus parameters, such as rate or frequency (clicks versus tones), may also be productive.

Conclusions. Aside from the trend of AER findings monitored intraoperatively, then, the postoperative status of hearing is, according to some investigators, related to two preoperative indexes—tumor location and hearing integrity. Hearing outcome is better for patients with tumors arising from the superior vestibular nerve and reasonably intact hearing as defined by pure-tone thresholds and word recognition scores. Tumor size alone does not consistently correlate with the success of efforts intraoperatively to preserve hearing. There is also the suggestion that hearing outcome is more favorable for patients with meningiomas, in comparison to acoustic neuromas or neurofibromas. Reported criteria for the degree of preoperative hearing integrity that is necessary in order to attempt hearing preservation vary considerably among studies. There is consensus, however, that hearing preservation attempts are indicated when the PTA for 500, 1000, and 2000 Hz is 30 dB or less (better) and the word recognition score is better than 70 percent. Still, hearing preservation is sometimes both attempted and successful for patients with poorer hearing sensitivity and discrimination scores (Brackmann et al., 2000; Kanzaki et al., 1989; Ojemann et al., 1984; Silverstein, McDaniel, Wazen, & Norrell, 1985).

The presence of normal ECochG and ABR amplitude and latency at the conclusion of surgery is typically a strong sign of immediate postoperative hearing integrity. For most patients (up to 90 percent or even more), auditory evoked response findings at the close of surgery are related to postoperative hearing status. That is, presence of an ECochG AP component and an ABR is associated with hearing preservation, whereas absence of a detectable response is associated with loss of hearing (Harner et al., 1996; Ojemann et al., 1984; Silverstein et al., 1985; Stanton et al., 1989; Tucker et al., 2001). Specifically, in analysis of data for 312 patients who were monitored with both ABR and cochlear nerve action potentials (direct eighth-nerve recordings), Tucker et al. (2001) found that patients with no ABR invariably had a poor hearing outcome, i.e., usually Class D or, less often, Class C according to AAOHNS system (described above). However, these authors also reported that "patients with positive ABR or CNAP results [i.e.,. no intraoperative change in either response] were just as likely to have a Class C or D results as a Class A or B result (p. 471)." Clearly, an abnormality or a disappearance of ABR wave V is an ominous sign, and the additional disappearance of ABR I (ECochG AP) as well is an almost certain indicator of serious hearing deficit postoperatively, but the reverse is not necessary true. As Tucker et al. (2001) demonstrated, the presence of an ABR or direct eighth-nerve response throughout surgery is only associated with an approximately 50 percent likelihood of hearing preservation.

Preservation of Hearing during Other Surgical Procedures

Intraoperative monitoring with ABR is most often applied during surgical removal of tumors when the auditory system is at risk. The ABR, however, is also contributes to the early detection and prevention of auditory deficits during surgical management of other disorders (see Table 10.12). The principles of neuromonitoring reviewed at the outset of this section are relevant for most examples of neuromonitoring with the ABR when a major objective is preservation of auditory function.

MICROVASCULAR DEPRESSION OF THE COCHLEOVESTIBULAR NERVE. | Efforts to eliminate or reduce with surgical management symptoms associated with compression of cranial nerves date back to the early 1980s—the beginning of the era of intraoperative monitoring. A disorder referred to as the "cochleovestibular compression syndrome" was discussed

earlier in this chapter. In a small proportion of persons, blood vessels within the skull and the cerebellopontine region and appearing as "vascular loops" rest on and sometimes compress cranial nerves, including the cochleovestibular nerve (eighth cranial nerve) and the facial nerve (seventh cranial nerve). Vascular structures most often involved are the posterior inferior cerebellar artery, the anterior inferior cerebellar artery, and the vertebrovascular complex. The symptoms associated with the compression, such as hemifacial spasm, hearing loss, tinnitus, and vertigo, can be pronounced and sometimes debilitating. The presence of a vascular loop can be inferred from the pattern of audiologic findings (e.g., Schwaber & Hall, 1990), including retrocochlear findings for the ABR, and confirmed with neuroradiologic studies (e.g., MRI).

Microvascular surgical procedures are a useful therapy for decompressing cranial nerves affected by vascular loops. One typical approach involves the insertion, after a craniotomy is performed to expose the involved portion of the nerve, of a small pad (e.g., Teflon) between the vascular loop and the nerve (or nerves) to minimize the effects of the compression. Clearly, this is a critical phase during the operation when the cranial nerve is manipulated surgically and is at risk for damage. Continuous monitoring of the ABR during this delicate procedure offers a valuable guide to the surgeon

TABLE 10.12.   Summary of Intraoperative Monitoring with Auditory Evoked Responses

PATHOLOGY	RATIONALE	
	Surgical procedure	AER monitoring
Aortic aneurysm	Clip and/or excise aneurysm; prevent CVA (cerebrovascular accident)	Prevent brain ischemia
Vertebrobasilar artery aneurysm	Clip aneurysm; prevent CVA; artery bypass	Prevent brainstem ischemia
Brainstem tumor	Remove tumor; eliminate mass effect on CNS	Prevent brainstem ischemia and trauma
Brainstem AVM	Excise malformation; prevent CVA; eliminate mass effect on CNS	Prevent brainstem ischemia and trauma
CPA (cerebellopontine angle) tumor[a]	Remove tumor; decompress eighth nerve and brainstem; maintain auditory integrity	Preserve hearing; prevent brainstem ischemia and trauma
Trigeminal nerve neuralgia	Vascular decompression or section for relief of pain	Preserve hearing, prevent eighth-nerve trauma
Vestibular nerve disease[a]	Section off vestibular portion of eighth nerve for relief of vertigo	Preserve hearing
Facial nerve exploration[a]	Middle fossa approach for decompression of facial nerve	Preserve cochlear integrity
Endolymphatic sac decompression/shunt	Decrease excessive cochlear fluid pressure, relief of vertigo	Document cochlear integrity and function during and after decompression

[a] Facial-nerve electrophysiologic monitoring may also be indicated.

This summarizes the rationale for selected neurologic or neurotologic surgical procedures.

for early detection of adverse neurophysiologic changes secondary to the surgical procedure. Possible surgery-induced insults to the cranial nerve(s) include compression, stretching, and disruption of blood flow in nearby vascular structures. Over the years, a number of clinical investigations provided evidence of the benefits for hearing of intraoperative monitoring with ABR during microvascular decompression surgical procedures (e.g., Van et al., 1999).

Combined ECochG and ABR Recording

The conventional ABR recording technique is still important for intraoperative monitoring during neuro-otologic surgery. The main disadvantages of the technique have already been noted. Because amplitude of wave V is relatively small, as recorded with the far-field electrode array, the response must be averaged from as many as 1,000 or more stimuli in order to obtain an adequate SNR (signal-to-noise ratio). A clear response with stable latency throughout surgery is generally considered evidence of auditory integrity. Interpretation of an alteration or loss of the response, however, is less straightforward. Even if an effective stimulus is confirmed and surgery-related pathophysiology is suspected, the precise focus of the abnormality may be anywhere from the cochlea to the brainstem. A two-channel measurement technique, combining promontory ECochG and conventional ABR recordings, is recommended. Steps in simultaneously recording ECochG and ABR intraoperatively during surgical procedures are summarized in Table 10.13. With this technique, the inverting electrode for the ECochG is a short (subdermal) needle placed on the promontory, and the ABR inverting electrode is a TIPtrode®. These two electrode designs were described in Chapter 3, and their application during intraoperative monitoring was discussed in Chapter 5. Schwaber and Hall (1990) provide a detailed discussion of both electrode designs and their applications in recording ECochG and ABR. Waveforms

---

TABLE 10.13. Basic Steps in Intraoperative Monitoring with ECochG and/or ABR

- Place auditory evoked response (AER) equipment in a predesignated location in the OR.
- Plug in AER equipment power cord, or connect it to an approved OR extension power cord, taking care to keep power cords away from OR traffic lanes.
- Boot up AER system, enter date and correct (OR) time, patient demographics, and so forth, and select appropriate test setup. Never turn ER system power on or off with patient connected via electrodes.
- After induction of anesthesia, and after checking with the anesthesiologist and/or surgeon, insert subdermal needle electrodes or apply disk electrodes. Secure all primary and spare electrode wires with adhesive tape or skin staples and lead away from the head. Keep wires and tape a safe distance away from surgical field.
- Surgeon places transtympanic (TT) needle electrode by looking through a microscope and using bayonet forceps (see Chapter 4 for details).
- Place insert transducer cushion or TIPtrode® into ear canal(s) and secure it with tape.
- After the patient is turned and in surgical position, but before the surgical field is prepared, run the electrode box and cable away from the head, secure on the patient or table, and carefully plug in all electrodes, including any spare electrodes.
- Immediately check the impedance of all possible electrode combinations (each channel). Replace faulty electrodes immediately. Attach stimulus tube(s) to insert transducer cushion(s) and secure with tape.
- Immediately record an AER to ensure an adequate stimulus and response. Notify the surgeon if there is no response, and troubleshoot any stimulus, response, or equipment problem at once.

- Obtain replicated baseline AER data, complete the data sheet information, document anesthetic agents and pertinent physiologic parameters (e.g., body temperature, MAP [mean arterial pressure]), and calculate and record baseline latency and amplitude values. Conduct AER threshold search.
- Beginning at opening and ending at closing, continuously record, analyze, and compare to baseline the ongoing AER data. Minimally, keep baseline and most recently averaged waveforms on the oscilloscope at all times for ready comparison. Maintain ongoing calculations of latency and amplitude data for waveforms being averaged. Verify physiologic parameters and anesthesia conditions both periodically and at any time that there is a change in AERs.
- Periodically report AER findings, and immediately report changes in AER findings to surgeon, according to previously decided criteria and protocol.
- Record replicated waveforms prior to closing. Conduct final threshold search. Note the time that data collection ends. Inform surgeon that monitoring is concluded.
- Wait for access to electrode box and transducer, or make arrangements for OR personnel to retrieve them when drapes come off the patient.
- Print selected waveforms, and complete the report if feasible and time permits.
- Turn off equipment power after the patient is disconnected. Prepare equipment for removal (protect disks, secure loose items). Verify that supplies are retrieved.
- Arrange for sterilization of subdermal needle electrodes.

Two-Channel Technique for Simultaneous Intraoperative Recording of ECochG and ABR in Retrocochlear Auditory Dysfunction

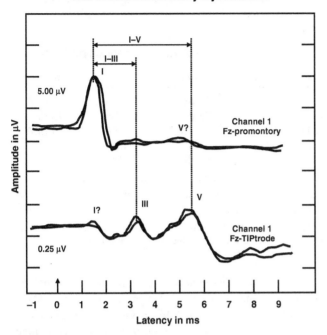

FIGURE 10.4. Waveforms recorded with a combination ECochG and ABR technique.

Waveforms recorded with the two-channel technique were shown also in Figure 4.5.

recorded with such a two-channel technique are illustrated in Figure 10.4. Near-field auditory evoked response recordings, by definition, produce relatively large amplitude responses. The near-field ECochG detected with a promontory electrode, therefore, provides the major clinical advantage of a large response—namely, a very favorable SNR. The operating room environment contains numerous sources of electrical and acoustic noise that can compromise the quality of AER recordings. Strategies for minimizing sources of measurement artifact within the OR setting are summarized in Table 10.14. A clear ECochG AP component (the ABR wave I) is observed with minimal signal averaging with as few as 20 to 25 sweeps. A secondary and related advantage is that a wave I/AP component may be recorded with the near-field TT technique when no response can be detected with surface electrodes, including ear-canal types. As noted earlier, documentation of the ECochG AP component alone appears to be an insufficient intraoperative measure of auditory function. Disappearance of the component must be considered strong evidence of cochlear deficit. However, preservation of the AP component intraoperatively only confirms cochlear function. It does not necessarily imply auditory integrity (Ojemann et al., 1984). Even complete sectioning of the eighth nerve, resulting in profound hearing impairment, does not invariably

TABLE 10.14. Strategies for Decreasing Artifacts in Auditory Evoked Responses Recorded Intraoperatively

- Remove debris and film from skin; abrade skin before applying scalp electrodes.
- Keep electrode impedances at or below approximately 2000 ohms.
- Use short electrode wires.
- Limit interelectrode distances between pairs of recording electrodes.
- Braid the recording electrode wires.
- Insert backup recording electrodes on the patient preoperatively.
- Keep recording versus stimulating wires and cords separated.
- Separate transducer(s) from recording electrodes as much as possible.
- Don't cross cables or wires over other cables, especially power cables.
- Don't touch the wires; separate them from ventilation tubes and anesthesia lines.
- Unplug unused equipment.
- Never use two-pronged power plugs (ungrounded).
- Pause signal averaging whenever amplifiers are blocking (e.g., electrocautery).
- Adjust amplifier sensitivity to produce some artifact rejection.
- Advise anesthesiologist to use neuromuscular junction blocking agents (unless facial nerve is monitored).

Adapted from Kartush J, Bouchard K. *Neuromonitoring in otology and head and neck surgery.* New York: Raven, 1992.

eliminate the ECochG AP component, provided cochlear blood supply remains intact (Ruben, Hudson, & Chiong, 1963; Silverstein et al., 1984).

Recording a response directly from the eighth nerve as it exits the IAC or enters the brainstem offers similar advantages (Battista, Wiet, & Paauwe, 2000; Cueva, Morris, & Prioleau, 1998; Møller & Jannetta, 1983a,b; Møller & Jho, 1989; Ruckenstein, Cueva, & Prioleau, 1997; Silverstein, McDaniel, Norrell, & Haberkamp, 1986; Yamakami et al., 2002). The technique is often referred to as "direct eighth nerve monitoring," or DENM. The near-field response recorded from the surface of the acoustic nerve may be larger by up to four or five times than the promontory ECochG AP and, therefore, also requires little or no signal averaging. Electrophysiological data are collected almost instantaneously, permitting continuously prompt information for the surgeon. With conventional ABR measurement in the OR, signal averaging over 1,000 to 2,000 stimulus repetitions may be required with a data collection time of 1 to 2 minutes. During this period, the AER may be dynamic, not stable. Consequently, the averaged response does not reflect the status of the auditory system at any one time, whereas the response that is recorded directly, with several seconds of averaging at most is essentially time specific. Not surprisingly, therefore, some clinical investigations report higher rates of hearing preservation when patients are monitored with recordings directly from the eighth nerve or other CPA anatomic structures (e.g., Battista, Wiet, & Paauwe, 2000; Cueva, Morris, & Prioleau, 1998; Matthies & Samii, 1997; Roberson et al., 1996). The direct eighth-nerve monitoring technique is reviewed further in the discussion of intraoperative monitoring with ECochG in Chapter 5.

A second and very important advantage of the direct eighth-nerve recording is site specificity. Presumably, the technique provides information on the status of the proximal portion of the nerve, between the porus (opening at the medial end of the IAC) and the root entry zone (REZ) near the brainstem. A major disadvantage of the technique is that an electrode cannot be placed directly on the nerve until the nerve is exposed, and then it often must be removed for periods of time during surgery to prevent its interference with dissection of tumor, transection of the vestibular portion of the nerve, or other manipulations. A fine silver wire with a cotton wick at the end is less obtrusive.

The primary objective of intraoperative monitoring with ABR is the early detection of surgery-related pathophysiologic changes produced by multiple mechanisms, such as direct mechanical and thermal trauma, compression, ischemia, or infarction. However, subject and other nonpathologic factors influencing ABR measurement in general, as reviewed in Chapter 7, must always be taken into account in the analysis of ABR findings in the operating room. A handful of factors are likely to influence the ABR recorded from a patient undergoing surgery, notably, body temperature and focal temperature at the surgical site, anesthetic agents, noise produced by surgical instruments (e.g., drills), electrical artifact, and perhaps transient conductive hearing loss secondary to the collection of fluid in the middle ear space (e.g., Hall, 1992; Hsu et al., 1992; Legatt, 2002).

For the sake of completeness, another technique—otoacoustic emissions—warrants mention in this review of intraoperative monitoring of the auditory system. The presence of OAEs preoperatively in patients with retrocochlear tumors is viewed as a sign of pure neural pathology, thus increasing the likelihood of hearing preservation following surgical removal of the tumor (e.g., Ferber-Viart et al., 1998; Hall, 2000; Kileny, Edwards, Disher, & Telian, 1998). In an investigation of DPOAEs in twenty-four patients with confirmed acoustic tumors, Oeken (1996) found that the typical sensorineural hearing loss was in fact related to a combination of cochlear and retrocochlear auditory dysfunction, i.e., a sensory and a neural hearing loss. There are several reported attempts to record transient and distortion product

TABLE 10.15. Sound Levels in the Operating Room

Sound levels (specified in dBA) generated by several surgical tools as measured at the level of the surgical tools, at the ear of the surgeon, and at the ear of the monitoring personnel during surgery.

	LOCATION OF SOUND LEVEL METER		
SURGICAL TOOL	**Surgeon**	**Tool**	**Monitor**
Pneumatic drill	83 dBA	85 dBA	78 dBA
CUSA	73 dBA	78 dBA	73 dBA
CO2 Laser	71 dBA	79 dBA	74 dBA
PD and CUSA	85 dBA	79 dBA	
CUSA and Laser	86 dBA	80 dBA	

CUSA = Cavitron Ultrasonic Surgical Aspirator
PD = Pneumatic drill
Adapted from Kartush, J., Bouchard, K. *Neuromonitoring in otology and head and neck surgery.* New York: Raven, 1992.

otoacoustic emissions continuously during to detect cochlear changes secondary to surgical manipulations (e.g., Cane, O'Donoghue, & Lutman, 1992). Otoacoustic emissions have appeal as a monitoring tool, or at least as an adjunct approach with ECochG and ABR, because they are very sensitive to cochlear dysfunction. Two practical problems encountered during otologic surgery, however, complicate ongoing intraoperative measurement of OAEs. The level of noise in the operating room in general, and the high levels of noise often generated during surgery by drills and other surgical devices, may compromise the confident detection of OAEs. As displayed in Table 10.15, substantial acoustic noise levels are produced by surgical instruments. In addition, the middle ear is exposed with some otologic surgical procedures and, in time, bodily fluids (e.g., blood or CSF) or saline solution used for irrigation may collect in the middle ear space and obliterate measurement of OAEs. Finally, OAEs have an anatomic limitation shared by ECochG, i.e., they are a strictly a measure of cochlear function. Even serious surgery-induced damage to retrocochlear auditory structures, such as the eighth nerve or auditory brainstem, may go undetected with reliance only on OAEs as a monitoring technique.

NEUROINTENSIVE CARE UNIT MONITORING

The first report describing the use of sensory evoked responses in monitoring neurologic status of acute brain-injured patients appeared in 1976. Since the early 1980s, application of evoked responses in the intensive care unit (ICU) had been regularly reported. The rationale for neuromonitoring with evoked responses in the ICU setting is in some respects similar to that for OR monitoring. In the OR, patients are anesthetized and cannot be assessed by neurological examination. A major objective of evoked response monitoring is early detection of pathophysiologic processes in the peripheral or central nervous system, usually secondary to surgical manipulations. Then, based on this information, surgery is in some way altered so as to preserve nervous system integrity.

The acute, severely brain-injured patient in the neurointensive care unit is typically comatose, with limited physical responsiveness. Medical therapies, such as sedatives and neuromuscular blocking agents, further limit or even invalidate the neurological examination. Sensory evoked response monitoring in the neurointensive care unit, therefore, is useful in early detection of pathophysiologic processes, such as ischemia or hypoxia, in the peripheral or, more often, central nervous system due to primary injury or developing within the days and weeks after severe injury. This information may contribute to decisions on medical and/or surgical management of the patient and ultimately improve neurological outcome. Although there are similarities between OR and neurointensive care unit neuromonitoring, the latter involves unique measurement principles and clinical challenges, as outlined in this chapter.

General Rationale

Rational management of the acute, brain-injured patient requires systematic monitoring of neurological status. Structural central nervous system (CNS) damage can be documented with computerized tomography (CT) or magnetic resonance imaging (MRI). These neuroradiologic studies, however, cannot be done at bedside and are, therefore, not feasible techniques for CNS monitoring. In addition, CT and MRI imaging does not provide information on the functional status of neurons. Continuous measurement of systemic physiologic parameters and CNS physiologic parameters, such as mean arterial pressure (MAP), intracranial pressure (ICP), and blood gases (PaO_2, $PaCO_2$), by means of monitoring devices provides valuable data for determining the status of the neuronal environment and for preventing CNS ischemia and hypoxia (Messick, Newberg, Nugent, & Fanst, 1985). Still, although clinically indispensable, these parameters do not reflect integrity of neurons in specific regions of the CNS but, rather, overall status. Finally, the clinical neurological examination is the mainstay of CNS monitoring in this patient population. Unfortunately, the neurological examination has several crucial limitations. Neurological signs may be invalidated by therapy modalities commonly employed with acute brain-injured patients, such as chemical paralyzing agents (neuromuscular blocking agents) and high dose barbiturates (Marshall, Smith, & Shapiro, 1979; Messick et al., 1985; Nordby & Nesbakken, 1984; Piatt & Schiff, 1984). Furthermore, localization of lesions in the comatose patient is

often not possible solely on the basis of the neurological examination.

There is, therefore, the need for a method of objectively and regularly assessing CNS functional status, a method that meets at least ten clinically important criteria:

1. *Mobility.* Assessment can be carried out at bedside in a neurointensive care unit environment. Transportation of acute brain-injured patients increases the risk of CNS damage and is a clear contraindication for a monitoring technique.
2. *Noninvasiveness.* Serial measurements do not require repeated insertion of needles or catheters.
3. *Safety.* The technique does not pose substantial risk or harm to the patient and does not involve radioactive substances.
4. *Limited time.* Assessment can be completed in a reasonable period of time so as not to interfere with ongoing intensive care of the patient.
5. *Objectivity.* The test data can be stored for later analyses, and be subjected to mathematical and/or statistical, and interclinician, examination.
6. *Sensitivity.* The technique is sensitive to subtle changes in neuronal functional status.
7. *Specificity.* The information obtained may not be limited to a specific anatomical region, yet does provide information on specific regions of the CNS.
8. *Coma/therapy independence.* The test results are not seriously influenced by the level of coma, nor commonly used medical therapy modalities, such as sedatives, chemical paralyzing agents, hyperosmolar drugs, and barbiturates.
9. *Cost.* Monitoring fees must be reasonable.
10. *Automation.* Some degree of automated data collection and preliminary analyses is essential for evoked responses to be clinically and economically feasible as a constant monitoring technique in the neurointensive care unit. (e.g., Hilz et al., 1991)

In the neurointensive care unit, the time frame for monitoring patients is usually days or even weeks, rather than hours as in the OR. It is not cost effective, or even possible, to conduct neuromonitoring in the neurointensive care unit with a dedicated sensory evoked response system operated around the clock by a clinician.

Historical Overview

Auditory evoked responses, in particular the ABR, and sensory evoked responses (SERs) in general, meet the first nine of these clinically important criteria and have multiple applications in acute brain-injured patients. Perhaps the first clinical reports of the application of multimodality sensory evoked responses in acute brain-injured patients were the papers published by Greenberg and his colleagues in the 1970s

(Greenberg & Becker, 1976; Greenberg et al., 1977). These important clinical studies generated considerable interest in the potential value of sensory evoked responses in this population and provided the impetus for the author's initial attempts to measure evoked responses in the neurointensive care unit. In the early studies reported by Greenberg and colleagues, auditory evoked responses were included within a multimodality sensory evoked response test battery (along with visual and somatosensory evoked responses) and the emphasis was on predicting long-term neurological outcome, largely in adults, from the pattern of evoked response findings recorded during the acute period after the injury. Since then, the role of auditory evoked responses in the ICU setting has expanded dramatically. Auditory evoked responses have unique value in early identification and evaluation of peripheral auditory dysfunction, a finding not uncommon in patients with both traumatic and nontraumatic acute brain injury. Auditory evoked responses can be applied in evaluating and monitoring neurological status during the acute period following a severe brain injury, much as they are used as a neurophysiologic monitor intraoperatively. The use of auditory evoked responses in monitoring CNS status in the ICU, and the factors that must be considered for meaningful interpretation of AER findings, are now reviewed. The clinical experiences presented herein for acutely injured adult patients with a variety of brain pathologies were derived from data collected at bedside in a neurointensive care unit environment with commercially available evoked response equipment. The following principles apply as well to neuromonitoring of brain-injured children. Clinical entities found in the pediatric ICU include hypoxic-ischemic encephalopathy, hydrocephalus, meningitis, brain tumors, seizure disorders, and head injury. The exact etiologies of these entities may differ considerably. For example, hypoxic-ischemic insults may result from pulmonary infection, near drowning, smoke inhalation, foreign body aspiration, anesthetic accidents, strangulation, cardiac arrest, or shock. Pediatric application of neuromonitoring is reviewed briefly in Chapter 9.

Rationale for Specific Applications

Patients with acute CNS pathologies usually require intensive medical therapy and close monitoring of vital systemic and neurological parameters. The majority of patients evaluated in the adult neurointensive care unit setting have traumatic head injury from motor vehicle accidents or gunshot wounds. Regardless of the type of CNS pathology, however, a major objective of intensive care is to preserve or improve the physiologic environment for brain function. An adequate and continuous supply of oxygen and nutrients (e.g., glucose) to the brain are essential. Therefore, ongoing physiologic monitoring, medical therapy, and, occasionally, surgical intervention is employed to maintain two major physiologic conditions. First, there must be sufficient oxygen saturation in the blood. Patients are mechanically ventilated and blood gases are determined periodically. Second, adequate blood flow and cerebral perfusion are essential. Either hypotension (reduced mean arterial pressure, MAP) or increased intracranial pressure (ICP) results in decreased cerebral perfusion pressure (CPP), that is:

$$CPP = MAP - ICP$$

Insufficient blood supply to the brain resulting in neuronal dysfunction and subsequently damage is ischemia. Ischemia is usually the common denominator in the neurological deterioration of acutely brain-injured patients. MAP is routinely monitored in a neurointensive care unit setting. ICP is typically monitored in patients with cerebral edema or pathophysiologic processes leading to an increase in ICP, such as hydrocephalus. The goal is to maintain CPP of at least 50 to 60 mmHg (Torr) that is necessary to maintain brain integrity. In either the pediatric or adult ICU, the primary reason for sensory evoked response, including ABR, measurement is to provide information on neuronal integrity. Neuroradiologic studies (CT, MRI, and ultrasonography) describe structural, not functional, status. Standard techniques for evaluating physiologic status of the patient, such as MAP and ICP monitors, are extremely valuable but do not meet this vital clinical need. They do not describe the status of specific regions in the CNS—for example, the brainstem versus cortex. Furthermore, actual neuronal status can only be inferred from MAP and ICP relationships.

The neurological examination is the traditional means of regularly evaluating CNS status in brain-injured patients. While invaluable in many patients, validity of the neurological examination is compromised by some of the common medical therapies used in the ICU, including sedatives and muscular paralyzing agents. The neurological examination is of no value in patients in therapeutic barbiturate coma for management of increased ICP. None of these drugs exert a serious influence on the ABR (Hall, 1985), which is a distinct clinical advantage in this patient population.

Factors Influencing Auditory Evoked Responses in the Neurointensive Care Unit

ARTIFACT IN ABR MEASUREMENT. | Environmental electrical artifact is probably the most troublesome, and commonly encountered, obstacle to obtaining reliable and meaningful and reliable evoked response data in a neurointensive care unit environment. There are many sources of electrical artifact, including 60 Hz line noise and a spectrum of airborne electromagnetic energy. Even though an ICU is a potentially a hostile environment for evoked response recording, it is possible to routinely measure evoked responses for auditory, somatosensory, and visual stimulus modalities from acute, severely brain-injured children and adults with commercially available equipment. Precautions for minimizing the deleterious effects of electrical artifact include reliance on well-grounded evoked response measurement instrumentation, quality electrodes, low interelectrode resistance (less than 5000 ohms), and especially a very good electrical contact for the ground electrode. Guidelines for optimizing auditory evoked response recording in general, as described in Chapters 4 and 9, and troubleshooting techniques outlined for OR recordings summarized elsewhere in this chapter apply also to the ICU. As a last resort, attempt to reduce artifact contamination by restricting filter settings, e.g., from 30 to 3000 Hz to 150 to 1500 Hz for the ABR and, if that technique fails, return to the patient's bedside at another time, perhaps in the evening.

Neuromuscular artifact is a less serious problem in the acute period following brain injury. As noted later in the chapter, the patient is typically sedated, often paralyzed chemically, and sometimes is in deep barbiturate induced coma. During recovery from brain injury, however, increasing movement can contribute to muscular artifact that contaminates or even precludes evoked response recording. Muscle artifact is a more significant factor for the AMLR and SSERs than for the ABR. Sometimes it is necessary to request mild sedation in patients recovering from brain injury in order to successfully carry out testing.

OTOLOGIC PATHOLOGY. | Peripheral auditory abnormalities associated with otologic pathology must be regularly considered in the interpretation of auditory evoked responses recorded from traumatically head-injured patients, and also from brain-injured patients with other etiologies, such as meningitis. The frequent occurrence of auditory dysfunction following head trauma is well recognized (Aguilar, Hall, & Mackey-Hargadine, 1986; Hall et al., 1982). Two-thirds of the patients in an ICU studied by the author and colleagues were found to have otologic pathology by physical examination (Aguilar et al., 1986; Hall, 1988). Hemotympanum (blood within the middle ear space) was most common (33%). Prolonged coma and mechanical ventilation may contribute to the development of middle ear pathology associated with Eustachian tube dysfunction and middle ear pressure abnormalities (Hall et al., 1982) and lead to conductive hearing loss, usually transient. Documentation of middle ear status must be done on an ongoing basis whenever AER changes suggest peripheral otologic pathology during the acute period in the neurointensive care unit. Failure to take peripheral auditory deficits into account in the interpretation of the ABR may confound interpretation of serial findings and result in incorrect inferences about CNS status. Of course, evaluation of peripheral auditory status after head injury and suspected temporal bone fracture may be the primary reason for AER assessment in the neurointensive care unit.

As an example of the importance of peripheral auditory dysfunction in neuromonitoring, Taylor, Houston, and Lowry (1983) presented a case report of a brain-injured child monitored with the ABR. The ABR at one point disappeared and then reappeared. The child survived. The authors offered the case as evidence that the ABR is not a reliable measure of CNS status in this population, and interpretation of the loss of an ABR as a sign of severe neurological dysfunction is not advisable clinically. With close scrutiny of their findings, however, we would conclude that the disappearance of the ABR was not due to dynamic brainstem pathology but, rather, to transient peripheral otologic pathology. Even the wave I was not observed at one point, and this finding occurred after increased wave I latencies were noted. The importance of documenting middle ear function with otologic examination, immittance audiometry, and bone-conduction ABR stimulation as a routine practice in acute brain injury is stressed in the literature (Aguilar et al., 1986; Hall et al., 1982; Hall et al., 1984).

As a rule, AER assessment in the neurointensive care unit is done for evaluation of CNS status. Evaluation of peripheral auditory function can be carried out more effectively in the audiology clinic as the patient's status improves. Therefore, in the neurointensive care unit, auditory stimulation is typically presented first at high intensity levels (75 to 95 dB HL Re: click threshold). Techniques for enhancing AER waveforms in patients with apparent otologic pathology include the use of insert acoustic transducers when bandages cover the ears, bone conduction stimulation when severe middle ear dysfunction is suspected, and multichannel recordings (Aguilar et al., 1986; Hall, Hargadine, & Allen, 1985; Hall, Morgan, et al., 1984; Hall & Tucker, 1985). Among these modifications of standard measurement techniques, multichannel recordings are especially useful.

BODY TEMPERATURE. | The importance of body temperature in ABR measurement was described in Chapter 9. Evaluating a patient with a low body temperature is a condition frequently encountered in the operating room OR and neurointensive care unit. Hypothermia may occur in patients who have suffered a cardiac arrest. Additionally, patients with brainstem pathology often demonstrate an inability to regulate their body temperature. Acute-care therapies, such as barbiturate-induced coma, may also lower temperature. Hypothermia has a profound effect on evoked response testing. Body temperature must always be documented in neurointensive care unit monitoring.

THERAPY MODALITIES. | Therapy modalities commonly used in the management of acute brain injury, as noted above, may compromise the validity of the clinical neurological examination. For the most part, these same drugs do not serious affect the ABR. Among the therapy modalities that do not appear to influence the ABR are chemical paralyzing agents (e.g., Pavulon, Metocurine), sedatives (e.g., Haldol, morphine), and therapeutic doses of anti-convulsants (e.g., Dilantin) and barbiturates, such as high-dose pentobarbital (Hall, 1985; Hall, Hargadine, & Allen, 1985; Newlon et al., 1983; Samra et al., 1985; Sutton et al., 1982). The effects of drugs on the ABR were reviewed in Chapter 7.

Relations among ABR and Other Neurodiagnostic Findings

CLINICAL NEUROLOGIC FINDINGS. | Reports of the ABR and neurologic findings describe good clinical correlations. Uziel and Benezech (1979) found clear-cut relationships among ABR abnormalities and brainstem signs. Patients with di-lated and unreactive pupils, for example, were considered to have pontine or lower CNS lesions and typically showed marked ABR alterations, including wave V and III abnor-malities; Tsubokawa and colleagues (1980) reported similar correlations. That is, although ABR abnormalities were oc-casionally noted in patients without brainstem neurological dysfunction by examination, and therefore in these cases might predict impending progressive brainstem dysfunction, gross ABR abnormalities, such as disappearance of waves III and/or V, were usually found in patients with mesencephalic/pontine or lower CNS clinical signs. The author's experience does not entirely support these relations among the ABR and neurological signs.

The GCS is a widely accepted method for grading depth of coma and severity of brain injury (Jennett & Teas-dale, 1981). The GCS consists of three measures of patient response: an eye opening, a motor, and a verbal response. The scale ranges from a low score of 3 to a high score of 15. Severe brain injury, and coma, is defined as a score of 8 or less. For the purpose of assessing its relationship with other neurodiagnostic findings, the author has categorized the ABR as either normal, abnormal (wave I–V delay or absent wave V), or no response (wave I component only or no observable components). The ABR versus GCS re-lationship was assessed for 133 brain-injured patients (see Table 10.16). Although the greatest proportion of pa-tients with an abnormal or no ABR had GSCs of 3 or 4, there were more patients with a normal ABR at this GCS level. Statistically, there is no correlation between ABR and GCS. A well-formed ABR with brainstem transmis-sion times within normal limits can be repeatedly recorded from patients with no response to deep painful stimuli. This is a common finding in the severely brain-injured population.

For many brain-injured patients in the ICU, particu-larly those managed with sedatives, chemical paralyzing agents, or even low doses of therapeutic barbiturates, the neurological examination is limited to evaluation of the

TABLE 10.16. Relation between Initial Auditory Brainstem Response (ABR) Patterns as Recorded at Bedside in the Neurointensive Care Unit and the Initial Glasgow Coma Score (GCS) Following Head Injury

The GCS is described in the text.

GCS (NUMBER OF PATIENTS)	ABR CATEGORY*		
	Normal	**Abnormal**	**No Response**
3 to 4	26	13	10
5 to 7	36	7	6
8 to 15	13	2	1

Severe head injury is defined by a GCS less than 8.

* ABR grading is as follows: Normal = wave I, wave III, and wave V are reliably recorded with normal absolute and interwave latency values; Abnormal = an abnormal delay in the wave I–V interval or absence of wave V; No response = a wave I component only or no observable ABR components.

pupil response to light stimuli. This neurological param-eter is among the most commonly reported signs reported in patient medical records. In Figure 10.5, the proportion of normal versus abnormal (and no response) ABR find-ings are compared for patients with pupils that are reac-tive versus those with unreactive pupils (total N = 111).

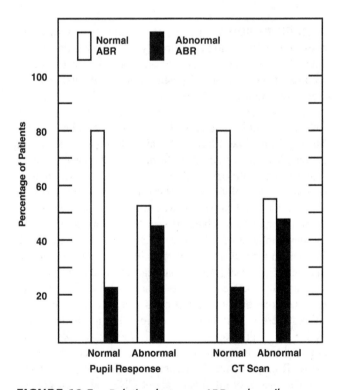

FIGURE 10.5. Relation between ABR and pupil response in a series of adult patients with acute, severe head injury.

Pupil-response findings were noted at the time of ABR testing. Not unexpectedly, a high proportion of patients with normal pupil findings also had a normal ABR (79 percent). But among the patients with abnormal pupils, a majority yielded normal ABRs. There was no statistically significant relation between these two neurodiagnostic parameters. Abnormal pupil responses are not invariably associated with impending neurological decompensation. The ABR may offer evidence of brainstem integrity, a neurophysiologic tool for monitoring during acute brain injury, and may support the rationale for aggressive intensive management.

NEURORADIOLOGY. | Current management of acute, severe brain injury depends strongly on neuroradiological evidence of CNS structural status. The CT or MRI scan is especially crucial in clinical decision making (for reviews, see Toyama et al., 2005; Lee & Newberg, 2005; Kobylarz & Schiff, 2004). Other neuroradiologic techniques employed in brain injury include ultrasonography and nuclear cerebral blood flow, or CBF (e.g., Goodman & Heck, 1977; Goodman, Heck, & Moore, 1985), and functional neuroimaging (e.g., Kobylarz & Schiff, 2004). The author studied the association of ABR outcome (normal versus abnormal) and CT findings (neuroradiologist interpretation of transtentorial herniation or no evidence of herniation). The results of this analysis were similar to the comparison of ABR and pupillary responses just described. Both relationships are illustrated in Figure 10.5. Although one might expect that a normal ABR would be found in patients with no evidence of transtentorial herniation, and vice versa, there were many exceptions to this pattern of findings. For example, over one-fifth of the patients with a "normal" CT scan, as defined by these criteria, had definite ABR abnormalities (usually abnormal delays in the wave I–V latency interval). And, perhaps more surprising, a majority of the patients with evidence of brainstem compression by CT yielded a normal ABR. Among this latter group were patients who survived the injury.

Applications of Auditory Evoked Responses in Acute Brain Injury

MONITORING NEUROLOGIC STATUS WITH SERIAL RECORDINGS. | As noted above, therapy modalities employed in the management of acute brain injury may invalidate the clinical neurological examination. Sensory evoked responses provide a noninvasive means of objectively evaluating CNS functional status over time without contamination by necessary treatment regimens. Early reports of sensory evoked responses in acute brain injury emphasized their possible value in predicting neurological outcome (Greenberg & Becker, 1976; Greenberg et al., 1977). These pioneering studies generated the initial interest and excitement in the potential role

of sensory evoked responses in this challenging population. And prediction of both neurological and cognitive/communicative outcome was introduced as a topic for clinical investigation. Most investigators serially evaluated CNS function over time with sensory evoked responses, rather than attempting to rely on data collected from a single test session three or four days after the injury (e.g., Anderson, Bundlie, & Rockswold, 1984; Hall, 1992; Hall & Mackey-Hargadine, 1985; Hilz et al., 1991; Jordan, 1993; Karnaze et al., 1982; Lindsay et al., 1981; Narayan et al., 1981; Rappaport et al., 1977; Rosenberg, Wogensen, & Starr, 1984; Seales, Rossiter, & Weinstein, 1979). As discussed next, serial evoked response data have varied applications in the acute period following severe brain injury. Maximum exploitation of evoked responses is achieved when recordings are initially made within 24 hours of the injury and then repeated during the period of neurological instability. There is evidence that the auditory middle latency response may be more useful in estimating the quality of outcome than the ABR. In previous reports (Hall, Mackey-Hargadine, & Allen, 1984; Hall, Mackey-Hargadine, & Kim, 1985; Hall & Tucker, 1985), the author has stressed the point that an abnormal ABR almost always implies poor outcome, or death, whereas a normal acute ABR (within 24 to 76 hours post-injury) has little predictive value and may be followed by patient death within the acute stage. Multimodality evoked responses often augment the clinical value of these serial measures.

DIAGNOSIS OF BRAIN DEATH. | Diagnosis of brain death is based on evidence of cerebral and brainstem neuronal inactivity (Korein, 1980). There are numerous criteria for definition of brain death, and there has been considerable medical, legal, and ethical discussion of the topic (Beresford, 1984; Guidelines, 1981). The primary mode of assessment in the determination of brain death has been, and will be, the physical examination. Current therapy modalities in acute severe brain injury, as pointed out already, may compromise the validity of the neurological examination. Also, in the era of organ transplantation, some of the criteria requiring an established time period of physiologic inactivity before brain death can be declared are simply not feasible, since they preclude obtaining viable organs. Sensory evoked responses have, for these reasons, been applied as ancillary procedures in the diagnosis of brain death.

The author and colleagues have reported group data and case reports in support of this application of SERs, mostly in adult populations with traumatic head injury (Hall, Hargadine, & Allen, 1985; Hall, Mackey-Hargadine, & Kim, 1985; Hall & Tucker, 1985). A strong correlation between the ABR and nuclear cerebral blood flow (CBF) measures (Goodman & Heck, 1977; Goodman, Heck, & Moore, 1985) was found for over eighty adults with acute severe brain injury. The majority of these patients were chemically paralyzed or in barbiturate coma at the time of assessment, and some were assessed with the first six hours after injury, with recreational drugs in the blood. The relationship between ABR and nuclear CBF for over 100 patients with traumatic head injury is depicted in Figure 10.6. Not included in this analysis are patients with acute cerebral vascular accidents (CVAs). All of the patients with normal CBF had either a normal ABR, or at least wave I and wave III. None of the patients without CBF had an ABR. In this group, most patients had no response, while one-third had a wave I and no other components. Thus, in traumatic head injury, the relationship between ABR and CBF is very strong and statistically significant (at 0.000001 level of confidence). Other authors have also described the application of ABR in defining brain death (e.g., Goldie, Chiappa, & Young, 1981; Guerit, 1992; Machado et al., 1991; Starr & Achor, 1975; Waters, French, & Burt, 2004). Sensory evoked responses are recognized as confirmatory procedures for the diagnosis of brain death in some European countries (Guerit, 1992).

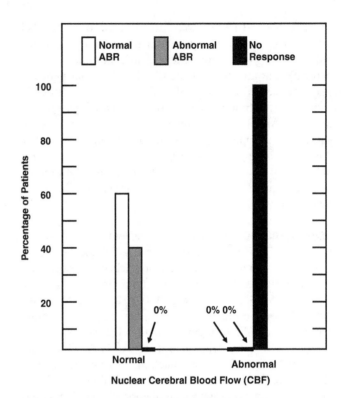

FIGURE 10.6. Relation between ABR and cerebral blood flow (CBF) in a series of adult severely head-injured patients undergoing clinical assessment for brain death.

11

CHAPTER

Auditory Middle-Latency Response (AMLR)

BACKGROUND

In the late 1960s and throughout the 1970s, the AMLR was repeatedly offered as a potential technique for clinically estimating the auditory sensitivity for discrete frequency regions (e.g., Beiter & Hogan, 1973; Goldstein & Rodman, 1967; Lane, Kupperman, & Goldstein, 1971; McCandless & Best, 1966; McFarland, Vivion, Wolf, & Goldstein, 1975; Skinner & Antinoro, 1971; Skinner & Jones, 1968; Thornton, Mendel, & Anderson, 1977; Vivion, Wolf, Goldstein, Hirsch, & MacFarland, 1979). Unfortunately, most of this research was conducted with cooperative, normal-hearing young adults. Subsequent clinical experience with audiogram estimation by AMLR tempered the early enthusiasm. AMLRs can be recorded from young children, but a variety of factors must be considered in measurement, analysis, and interpretation. In young children, the AMLR is less reliable than the ABR, especially when the ABR is recorded with a sedated child. Sedation is not a viable option in AMLR measurement as CNS-suppressant drugs influence the response. For these reasons, the AMLR gave way to the ABR for estimation of auditory thresholds.

During the 1980s, ABR became the preferred technique for electrophysiologic audiologic assessment of infants and young children. A major disadvantage of the ABR soon became apparent—that is, information on auditory function was limited to subcortical pathways and structures. Most clinicians were well aware that the ABR was not a test of hearing. We hear with our brains, not our ears. There was clinical interest in an electrophysiologic measure of auditory function at the thalamic and cortical level, rostral to the brainstem. Within this time frame, as summarized below, several research groups independently demonstrated with human investigations that the AMLR was generated in these suprabrainstem regions.

Typical AMLR waveforms, recorded with a rather conventional three-channel electrode array, are shown in Figure 11.1. The anatomic and physiologic bases of auditory evoked responses, including the AMLR, were reviewed in Chapter 2.

What follows here is a brief overview. Generators of the AMLR are in the thalamocortical auditory pathways. The Na component receives contributions from subcortical regions

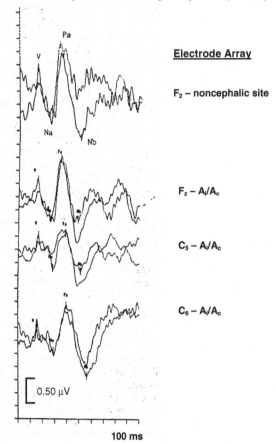

FIGURE 11.1. Auditory middle-latency response (AMLR) waveforms as evoked with 1000 Hz tone-burst stimuli and recorded with a three-channel electrode array (noninverting electrodes at the C3, C4, and Fz locations and linked earlobe inverting electrodes).

of the auditory system, specifically the medial geniculate body of the thalamus (Fischer, Bognar, Turjman, & Lapras, 1995; Kaseda, Tobimatsu, Morioko, & Kato, 1991; Mäkelä, Hämäläinen, Hari, & McEvoy, 1994), and perhaps portions of the inferior colliculus (Hashimoto, 1982). However, evidence from intracranial electrophysiologic recordings and magnetic responses in humans suggests that generation of the Na component also involves the primary auditory cortex within the temporal lobe—Heschl's gyrus (Liegeois-Chauvel, Musolino, Badier, Marquis, & Chauvel, 1994).

In the 1980s, studies of AMLR utilizing scalp electrodes in patients with cortical lesions confirmed the major role of primary auditory cortex in generation of the Pa component (Kraus, Özdamar, Hier, & Stein, 1982; Scherg & von Cramon, 1986). These findings have subsequently been confirmed with intracranial recordings, scalp topography measurements, and magnetic response techniques (Liegeois-Chauvel, Musolino, Badier, Marquis, & Chauvel, 1994; McGee & Kraus, 1996). Based on investigations in patients with temporal lesions, however, subcortical (e.g., thalamic) structures also appear to contribute to the Pa component (Graham, Greenwood, & Lecky, 1980; McGee & Kraus, 1996; Özdamar, Kraus, & Curry, 1982; Parving, Salomon, Elberling, Larsen, & Lassen, 1980; Peronnet & Michel, 1977; Woods, Clayworth, Knight, Simpson, & Naeser, 1987). It is likely, therefore, that the Pa component, as recorded from the scalp, actually is the product of activity within both subcortical and cortical regions of the auditory system (Jacobson, Newman, Privitera, & Grayson, 1991; Polyakov & Pratt, 1994). There is general agreement that the Pb component of the AMLR arises from auditory cortex, perhaps the posterior region of the planum temporale. Finally, the pronounced effects of state of arousal, sedatives, and, especially, anesthetic agents on the Pa and Pb components provide evidence that the reticular activating formation is involved in generation of the AMLR. The relation between the AMLR, consciousness, and CNS suppressants is reviewed below in reference to clinical application of the AMLR in monitoring depth of anesthesia.

What role does, and can, the AMLR play in the electrophysiologic assessment of auditory function today? Given the vital function of the thalamus and primary auditory cortex in hearing and auditory processing, it seems reasonable to expect the AMLR to provide valuable information in the clinical assessment of children and adults at risk for auditory processing disorders (APD). With typical auditory evoked response instrumentation, perhaps purchased for the purpose of recording ABRs, protocols can be developed for measurement of the AMLR. Clinically proven AMLR protocols are described in the next section of this chapter. The audiologist can easily adapt skills learned in ABR applications to measurement of the AMLR, including the analysis of the latency and amplitude values of the major wave components, Na and Pa. With modest changes in the conventional AMLR protocol, as detailed below, it's possible to consistently record clinically both a Pa and a Pb component.

The Pb component of the AMLR is presumably equivalent to the P1 component of the auditory late response (ALR). With the detection of a reliable Pb component, the clinician can extend the anatomic reach of the AMLR beyond the primary auditory cortex to secondary auditory regions within the temporal lobe, regions of the brain that also are important in language functioning. In addition, there is a substantial and rapidly growing literature on a novel approach for recording the Pb component. Since the Pb component is usually detected with a latency of about 50 ms, it is often referred in as a P50 component. When evoked with a pair of identical stimuli, the Pb (P50) component is reduced in amplitude for the second stimulus (S2) versus the first stimulus (S1), a finding that is interpreted as evidence of "sensory gating" within the nervous system. The P50 component represents "preattentive" activity of the brain. The brain recognizes that the second stimulus is the same as the first and, therefore, does not indicate a relevant or meaningful stimulus. Preattentive brain activity is presumably diverted or reserved for the possible appearance of a relevant stimulus. Meanwhile, the brain's response to the second stimulus (S2) is inhibited, and amplitude of the P50 response is reduced. Just the opposite response pattern occurs when the second stimulus is different from the first stimulus, or novel. The P50 component for S2 is enhanced, or larger in amplitude. The AMLR P50 response has in recent years been applied in a variety of patient populations, especially schizophrenia. The fascinating literature on the P50 component as an index of sensory gating is reviewed briefly in this chapter.

The final section of this chapter is devoted to a review of current and potential clinical applications of the AMLR, with one exception. Electrically elicited AMLRs are included within Chapter 15, which is devoted to other AERs evoked by electrical (versus acoustic) signals. For audiologists, the two obvious clinical applications are the electrophysiologic estimation of auditory thresholds of patients who, for various reasons, do not yield valid behavioral audiometric results and the neurodiagnostic use of AMLR as an electrophysiologic index of cortical auditory function in selected patient populations at risk for CNS abnormalities. More than forty-five years after the discovery of the AMLR, innovative clinical applications and research trends continue to be reported. Two will be highlighted here. As noted above, there is evidence that the AMLR is dependent, in part, on the status of the reticular activating system. Within recent years, interest has grown in the AMLR as a method for quantifying the depth of anesthesia. Also, there is increasing investigation of "sensory gating" with the Pb component of the AMLR. In these papers, the Pb component is referred to as the P50, or the P50 EP (Buchsbaum, 1977), and it is viewed as a "preattentive" component. Sensory gating is defined generally as "the ability of the brain to modulate its sensitivity to incoming sensory stimuli . . . including the capacities to minimize or stop responding to incoming irrelevant stimuli (gating out) and to respond when a novel stimulus is presented or a change occurs in ongoing stimuli (gating in)" (Boutros & Belger, 1999, p. 917; Braff & Geyer, 1990; Freedman, Waldo, Bickford-Winner, & Nagamoto, 1991). Initially, research on sensory gating with the Pb (P50) component of the AMLR was conducted with schizophrenia. The growing literature on each of these AMLR applications is reviewed below. It is important to realize that, in the non-audiology literature (e.g., in psychiatry journals), the term "mid-latency evoked potentials" may refer to responses in the latency range of 10 to over 200 ms.

TEST PARAMETERS AND PROTOCOLS

A protocol for clinical measurement of the AMLR is summarized in Table 11.1. Note in this table the distinction among certain parameters for values or settings that are appropriate for recording a conventional AMLR waveform with reliable Na and Pa components versus an AMLR protocol that will result in the consistent detection of the Pb component, in addition to other AMLR waves. AMLR measurement conditions that are important for reliably recording the Pa component are reviewed in more detail at the end of the section on test parameters and protocols. For some of the measurement parameters in Table 11.1, a specific value or selection is not critical for consistent detection of the AMLR, and considerable latitude is acceptable. Examples of these parameters include stimulus transducer (e.g., supra-aural or insert earphone) and stimulus polarity (e.g., rarefaction, condensation, or alternating). Other measurement parameters, however, must be carefully selected to assure that an AMLR will be recorded and/or to minimize the likelihood of contamination of the waveform with artifact or, in some cases, the creation of an artifact that will be inadvertently chosen as an AMLR component. In addition, there are clear interactions among some of the measurement parameters and among measurement parameters and nonpathologic subject factors, such as age, and auditory dysfunction.

A few examples will clarify these clinically important points. When the AMLR is recorded with overrestricted filter settings (e.g., 30 to 100 Hz), a filter-related artifact is sometimes be detected in the same latency region as the Pa component. The artifact can lead to false negative neurodiagnostic AMLR findings. That is, AMLR findings for patients who lack a Pa component due to auditory system dysfunction may be mistakenly interpreted as normal—the artifact is analyzed as a Pa component. Also, for the AMLR there is an interaction between subject age and the rate of stimulus presentation. With adults and older children, a clear AMLR can be recorded for stimulus rates of 7/second and even faster signal presentation rates. As subject age decreases below 10 years, progressively slower stimulus rates must be employed

to record a clear and reliable AMLR Pa component. Even slower rates (e.g., 1 stimuli/second or slower) are required for consistent generation of the AMLR Pb component in children and adults. Another example of the importance of careful selection of measurement parameters, and the interaction among the parameters and subject factors, involves the postauricular muscle (PAM) artifact. The PAM artifact is most likely to be detected under certain measurement conditions, including high stimulus intensity levels (> 70 dB nHL), inverting electrodes on either the mastoid or earlobes near the location of the PAM (behind the ear), and a tense patient whose neck is extended. Naturally, appreciation of the conditions leads to strategies for eliminating the problems with PAM in the clinical measurement of the AMLR, that is, evoking the response from relaxed patients with moderate intensity levels and detecting the response with inverting electrodes at a noncephalic site (e.g., the nape of the neck).

Stimulus Parameters

TRANSDUCER. | The AMLR can be elicited with stimuli presented with either supra aural or insert earphones. Multiple clinical advantages for insert earphones in ABR measurement were cited in Chapter 3, and were listed in Table 3.3. Most of these advantages are not as important in AMLR measurement or, put another way, some disadvantages to the clinical use of supra-aural earphones in recording shorter latency AERs are not relevant for the AMLR. For example, the problems with stimulus artifact interference in the analysis of early latency waves for the ECochG or ABR, associated with the use of supra-aural earphones, are not encountered in AMLR measurement. Even the Na component, the shortest latency wave within the AMLR, occurs 10 to 15 milliseconds beyond the time frame of the most serious stimulus artifact. However, selected advantages of insert earphones versus supra-aural earphones in auditory electrophysiologic measurements remain very important for AMLR recording, among them increased interaural attenuation, heightened attenuation of ambient sounds, aural hygiene permitted by disposable insert cushions, and greater comfort. This last advantage is particularly meaningful for research applications of the AMLR, when recording sessions are lengthy and a relaxed and comfortable subject is essential. Therefore, insert earphones are recommended for AMLR measurement with pediatric and adult patient populations. AMLR can also be validly recorded with bone-conduction stimulation.

STIMULUS TYPE. | Literature shows that the two most common types of stimuli employed in AMLR measurement are clicks and tone bursts. A general definition of each of these terms—click and tone burst—was offered in Chapter 3. Close inspection of the descriptions of signals found in articles published in journals representing different disciplines and scientific or clinical specialties, however, reveals inconsistency in the meanings of the terms. For example, in an

TABLE 11.1. Guidelines for Auditory Middle-Latency Response (AMLR) Test Protocol

Note the modifications in the test protocol required for consistent detection of the Pb component. The rationale for specific measurement parameters is reviewed in the text.

PARAMETER	SUGGESTION	RATIONALE/COMMENT
Stimulus Parameters		
Transducer	ER-3A	Supra-aural earphones are acceptable for AMLR, but insert earphones are more comfortable and, because the insert cushions are disposable, contribute to infection control.
Type	click	For neurodiagnosis only. However, a more robust AMLR is usually recorded with longer duration tone-burst signals.
	tone burst	For neurodiagnosis or frequency-specific estimation of auditory sensitivity.
		Detection of the Pb component of the AMLR is enhanced for lower frequency tone-burst signals.
Duration		
click signal	0.1 ms	Click signals are less effective than tone bursts in evoking the AMLR.
tone-burst signal		
rise/fall	2 cycles	Rather abrupt tone-burst onset is important for AMLR as it is for the ABR.
plateau	multiple cycles	Plateau durations of 10 ms or longer are appropriate for evoking the AMLR, especially the Pb component.
Rate	≤7.1/second	A slower rate of signal presentation is indicated for younger children, or for patients with cortical pathology. Signal presentation rates as low as 1 per second, or 0.5/second (one signal every two seconds) are required to consistently record the Pb component.
Polarity	rarefaction	An AMLR can also be recorded for condensation or alternating polarity signals.
Intensity	≤70 dB nHL	For neurodiagnosis, a moderate signal intensity level is appropriate. Signal intensity is decreased, of course, for estimation of thresholds. High signal intensity levels should be avoided. Tone-burst signals should be biologically calibrated to dB nHL in the space where clinical AMLRs are recorded.
Number	≤1000	Signal repetitions vary depending on size of response and background noise. Remember the signal-to-noise ratio is the key. Averaging may require as few as 50 to 100 signals at high intensity levels for a very quiet and normal hearing patient.
Presentation ear	monaural	For estimation of auditory sensitivity and neurodiagnosis. There is no apparent clinical indication for binaural AMLR measurement.
Masking	50 dB	Rarely required with insert earphones and not needed for stimulus intensity levels of ≤70 dB HL.
Acquisition Parameters		
Amplification	75,000	Less amplification is required for larger responses.
Sensitivity	50 μvolts	Smaller sensitivity values are equivalent to higher amplification.
Analysis time	100 ms	Long enough to encompass the Pa and Pb components.
Prestimulus time	10 ms	Provides a convenient estimate of background noise and a baseline for calculation of the amplitudes for waveform components (Na, Pa, Nb, and Pb).
Data points	512	
Sweeps	1000	See comments above for signal number.

TABLE 11.1. (continued)

PARAMETER	SUGGESTION	RATIONALE/COMMENT
Filters		
band-pass	10 to 1500 Hz	For recording an ABR, and AMLR with an Na and Pa component.
	10 to 200 Hz	For recording an AMLR with an Na and Pa component. Do not overfilter (e.g., high-pass setting of 30 Hz and low-pass setting of 100 Hz) as it may remove important spectral energy from the response, and it may produce a misleading filter artifact.
	0.1 to about 200 Hz	Decrease high-pass filter to 1 Hz or less to detect the Pb (P50) component.
notch	none	A notch filter (removing spectral energy in the region of 60 Hz) is never indicated with AMLR measurement because important frequencies in the response (around 40 Hz or below for young children) may also be removed.
Electrodes		
Type	disc	Disc electrodes applied with paste (versus gel) to secure the noninverting electrodes on the scalp. It is helpful to use red- and blue-colored electrode leads for the right and left hemisphere locations, respectively. Ear-clip electrodes are recommended when an earlobe inverting electrode site is used.
Sites		
Channel 1	C3 to Ai/Ac or C3 to NC	Hemisphere electrode locations are required for neurodiagnosis. A linked earlobe inverting electrode arrangement (Ai = ipsilateral ear; Ac = contralateral ear) or a noncephalic (NC) inverting electrode (on the nape of the neck) is appropriate and reduces likelihood of PAM artifact.
Channel 2	C4 to Ai/Ac or Nc	C3 = right hemisphere site; C4 = left hemisphere site. See comments above.
Channel 3	Fz to Ai/Ac or NC	A third channel (3) is optional for neurodiagnosis. Only the midline noninverting electrode channel is needed for the estimation of hearing sensitivity.
Channel 4	outer canthi of eye	Optional; for detection of eye blinks, and rejection of averages contaminated by eye blinks.
Ground	Fpz	

article entitled "Midlatency Evoked Potentials Attenuation and Augmentation Reflect Different Aspects of Sensory Gating," published in the journal *Biological Psychiatry*, Boutros and Belger (1999) describe three stimulus conditions. All three stimuli are clicks, but the authors claim that one "click" was at a frequency of 1000 Hz, another at a frequency of 1500 Hz, and the third at a frequency of 500 Hz. This explanation is rather puzzling, as transient clicks produce acoustic energy across a broad spectrum of frequencies. Also, in the methodology section of the paper, details of the duration of the click stimuli include reference to a plateau of 4 ms with rise/fall times of 1 ms. Conventional duration for click

stimuli in the auditory research is 0.1 ms. It would appear from these discrepancies in terminology, and the definitions used to explain the terms, that relatively short-duration toneburst stimuli are referred to by some research disciplines as "clicks." It is also interesting to note methodological differences for auditory versus non-auditory researchers with regard to criteria for subject selection. In auditory research, hearing status of subjects is typically assessed rigorously with multiple audiologic procedures, and then described in detail in the published article. In journals representing other disciplines, e.g., neurology and psychiatry, the emphasis in subject selection is, naturally, on neurological status. Again, as an example, the paper authored by Boutros and Belger (1999), subjects were carefully interviewed and examined to rule out neurological and psychiatric problems, head injury, loss of consciousness, and the use of any medications. In contrast, there was no mention in the paper of the hearing of subjects ("healthy adults . . . ranging in age from 19 to 45 years old").

The auditory versus neurological and psychiatric literature is also distinguished by procedures for presenting and calibrating the signals. Invariably, signal calibration is precisely defined in the auditory literature, and signals are delivered to subjects with a type of transducer (earphones) that is widely used in auditory research, e.g., TDH supra-aural or ER-A insert earphones. Referring once more to the above-noted article published in a psychiatry journal as an example, the "click" stimuli were presented through speakers (no further description) placed 1 meter in front of the subject, and "clicks were 90 dB SPL as measured at the ear using a measure and hold digital sound meter (Tandy Corp.)." The foregoing discussion clearly highlights some important distinctions among different disciplines in terminology in journal articles and also, perhaps more significantly, in subject selection and research methodology. In interpreting findings and conclusions from articles published in diverse scientific journals, the reader would be well advised to be aware of, and to take into account, these methodological distinctions.

Until relatively recently, click signals were by far the most popular type of signal in AMLR. Now, however, there is growing appreciation of the value of longer duration tone-burst signals for both clinical applications of AMLR—estimation of auditory thresholds and neurodiagnosis. Distinct differences in AMLR waveforms evoked by click versus tone-burst stimuli are evident in Figure 11.2. Because duration is an important characteristic of the tonal stimuli used in AMLR measurement, the topic will be reviewed in the next section of this chapter. In a study with normal-hearing adult subjects, Woods et al. (1995) reported larger amplitude for the Na-Pa wave complex with click versus tone-burst stimuli (of 250 and 4000 Hz). Also, amplitude was larger for the 4000 Hz versus 250 Hz tone bursts. Previous investigators describe larger AMLR amplitudes for lower versus higher frequency stimuli (e.g., Kraus & McGee, 1988; Picton et al., 1974). Woods et al. (1995) ascribed the difference to their use of ipsilateral masking to minimize the likelihood of evoking an AMLR from frequency regions beyond the stimulus frequency, i.e., from high-frequency regions for high-intensity low-frequency signals.

In a study utilizing tone-burst stimuli and ipsilateral tonal masking, Mackersie, Down, and Stapells (1993) reported that frequency selectivity was similar for the ABR and AMLR. Their findings indicate that equivalent tonotopic tuning within the auditory system extends from the brainstem through the cortex and that either the ABR or the AMLR can play a role in the frequency-specific estimation of auditory thresholds. Nelson, Hall, and Jacobson (1997) reported

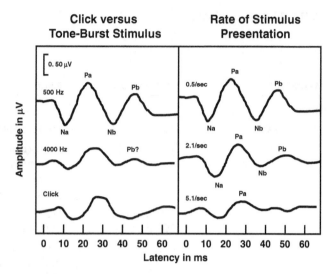

FIGURE 11.2. An example of the effect of the rate of stimulus presentation from 5.1/sec to 0.5/sec (right panel) and stimulus frequency, i.e., click, 4000 Hz, 500 Hz (left panel) on the AMLR. Recordings were made with a young adult, normal-hearing, female subject. Note the enhancement of a consistently recorded Pb component for slower signal rates and lower signal frequencies.

that the Pb component of the AMLR was more consistently detected, and the amplitude larger, for tone-burst than click signals, and also for lower frequency (500 Hz) versus higher frequency (4000 Hz) tone-burst stimuli.

DURATION. | In contrast to relatively limited study of stimulus duration and ABR, there are numerous investigations of stimulus rise/fall and plateau times and AMLR. Beginning in the late 1960s and throughout the 1970s, AMLR was repeatedly offered as a potential technique for estimating auditory sensitivity for discrete frequency regions in some patient populations (e.g., Beiter & Hogan, 1973; Goldstein & Rodman, 1967; McFarland, Vivion, & Goldstein, 1977; McFarland, Vivion, Wolf, & Goldstein, 1975; Skinner & Antinoro, 1971; Skinner & Jones, 1968; Thornton, Mendel, & Anderson, 1977; Vivion, Wolf, Goldstein, Hirsch, & MacFarland, 1979). An important part of this research effort was definition of the effects of stimulus duration on the response.

Constraints in the methodology of earlier studies of stimulus duration and AMLR led to somewhat limited conclusions. Indeed, it is curious, in retrospect, that various investigators repeatedly assessed the effect of rise/fall and plateau times only for tonal stimuli of 1000 Hz and usually only at a single intensity level (40 to 50 dB SL), and they did not attempt to evaluate stimuli of lower or higher frequencies at different intensities (Beiter & Hogan, 1973; Lane et al., 1971; Skinner & Antinoro, 1971; Skinner & Jones, 1968). Stimuli with shorter rise times, over a range from 50 ms down to a click, consistently produce AMLRs of larger amplitude. The rise/fall time effects were greater for later component amplitudes (e.g., Pa-to-Nb, Nb-to-Pb) than for earlier components (e.g., Po-to-Na, Na-to-Pa). No consistent change in AMLR amplitude, in contrast, was observed as stimulus plateau time was varied except for the Nb-Pb component, which was larger for a plateau of 40 ms than a 20 ms plateau.

All of the studies just cited used very restricted filter settings, probably about 30 to 100 Hz, based on the appearance of waveforms displayed in figures published. The importance of electrophysiologic filter settings as a factor in AMLR measurement was apparently not well appreciated by these early investigators. In some published reports, filter settings were not even mentioned in the description of the test protocol (Lane, Kupperman, & Goldstein, 1971; Skinner & Antinoro, 1971).

Vivion, Hirsch, Frye-Osier, and Goldstein (1980) reported perhaps the most comprehensive investigation of the effect of rise/fall times on the AMLR. AMLRs were elicited by tone bursts of 500, 1000, or 3000 Hz with linear-ramp rise/fall times of 3, 5, and 10 ms in combination with "equivalent plateau durations" (Dallos & Olsen, 1964) of 0, 10, or 30 ms. Equivalent plateau was defined as two-thirds of the rise time plus the plateau duration. Filtering was quite restricted (25 to 175 Hz). Previously reported findings for 1000 Hz stimuli were essentially confirmed for 5000 and 3000 Hz. In summary, Vivion et al. (1980) showed a distinct increase in amplitude and a small increase in latency (1 to 3 ms) as rise/fall time was lengthened from 3 to 5 to 10 ms. The authors speculate that because the bandwidth of the stimulus spectrum was greater for the briefer stimuli, differences in the energy content of the different stimuli might have contributed substantially to the apparent rise/fall time effects. Latency and amplitude, as expected, decreased with stimulus intensity. AMLRs were regularly observed for intensities of 10 dB SL. Latency was also decreased, as expected (see preceding discussion of stimulus frequency), for higher frequency stimuli. Peak latencies became longer as equivalent stimulus duration was increased. Vivion et al. (1980) conclude that a short (less than 10 ms) rise/fall time is optimal for clinical recording of AMLR with tonal stimuli. The AMLR is primarily an onset response, as is the ABR, but plateau duration does exert an effect on AMLR. A separate AMLR can be elicited for stimulus offset as well.

Signal duration has also been manipulated in the electrophysiologic investigation of the critical band phenomenon in humans. Fletcher (1940) first proposed the existence of critical frequency bands in the processing of acoustic signals at the level of the cochlea. Since then, numerous psychoacoustic and electrophysiologic studies in animal models and human subjects has confirmed that the concept of critical bands forms a basic principle in understanding frequency resolution within the auditory system. Along with the ABR (Sammeth, Burkard, & Hecox, 1986; Zerlin, 1986) and later cortical auditory evoked responses (Keidel & Spreng, 1965; Skinner & Antinoro, 1971), the AMLR has been applied in

the investigation of the critical band phenomenon (Burrows & Barry, 1990). Consistent with the results reported by Sammeth et al. (1986), Burrows and Barry (1990) failed to show a clear change in ABR wave V as stimulus bandwidth was changed, but they did describe an abrupt increase in the amplitude of the AMLR Na component as the bandwidth of a two-tone complex was altered from 268 to 330 Hz. Nelson, Hall, and Jacobson (1997) reported significantly larger amplitudes for the Pb component of the AMLR as signal duration was increased from 5 ms (rise/fall time of 2 ms and plateau of 1 ms) to 60 ms (rise/fall time of 5 ms and plateau of 50 ms).

INTENSITY. | As click-stimulus intensity level increases from behavioral threshold (for the click) up to about 40 to 50 dB SL, Pa latency systematically decreases. Then, for higher intensity levels, latency remains relatively constant (Goldstein & Rodman, 1967; Madell & Goldstein, 1972; Mendel & Goldstein, 1969; Thornton, Mendel, & Anderson, 1977). Amplitude, in contrast, increases steadily from over the intensity range of 0 to 70 dB SL, but the amplitude–intensity function is not linear. Tucker and Ruth (1996) found consistently higher Pa amplitude and shorter Pa latency for 70 dB nHL versus 40 dB nHL click stimuli recorded in various conditions, including ipsilateral and contralateral electrode arrays, slower and faster stimulus rates (3.3/second and 11.3/second), and for different age groups (newborn infants, children aged 5 to 7 years, children aged 9 to 12 years, teens 13 to 16 years, and adults aged 18 to 35 years). Madell and Goldstein (1972) found a high linear correlation between AMLR amplitude, especially of the Po-Na components, and loudness.

STIMULUS RATE AND INTERSTIMULUS INTERVAL: ADULTS. | Age, body temperature, drugs, and CNS dysfunction interact with stimulus rate in influencing AMLR outcome. The majority of investigators of the AMLR, and clinicians applying AMLR, have used a stimulus rate in the region of 8 to 11 stimuli/second. With normal adult subjects, a well-formed, robust AMLR can be consistently recorded at these rates. Amplitude of the Pa component recorded from normal adult subjects remains stable for rates of 1 stimuli/second to 15 signals/second, but latency is significantly shorter for very slow rates (0.5 and 1 stimuli/second) than for faster rates (Erwin & Buchwald, 1986; Goldstein, Rodman, & Karlovich, 1972; McFarland, Vivion, Wolf, & Goldstein, 1975; Tucker & Ruth, 1996). For rates higher than about 15 Hz in adults, response latency increases and amplitude decreases until the stimulus rate approaches 40 stimuli/sec. The characteristic response at a rate of about 40 stimuli/second, the 40 Hz ERP, is described later in this chapter.

Maximum length sequence (MLS) is a specific electrophysiologic measurement approach that involves the presentation of stimuli at very high rates. The MLS technique has been investigated with ABR (e.g., Thornton & Slaven,

1993) and also otoacoustic emissions (e.g., Thornton, Shin, Gottesman, & Hine, 2001). The goal of MLS clinically is to achieve an adequate signal-to-noise ratio (SNR) with minimal recording time. Bell, Allen, and Lutman (2001) recorded the AMLR with relatively slow click presentation rates often used clinically and also faster rates of 42, 89, and 185 clicks/second over an intensity range of 30 to 70 dB nHL. The authors report enhanced response detection, and a four-fold reduction in test time with a stimulus presentation rate of 89/second, in comparison to the conventional rate.

Stimulus rate is inversely related to interstimulus interval (ISI). By definition, as stimulus rate increases, the time period between stimuli per unit of time (e.g., each second) must decrease. A common explanation for the reduction in AMLR amplitude as signal rate increases involves the refractory period for neurons. That is, with multiple stimulus presentations, a stimulus is presented before the neuron activated by the previous stimulus (stimuli) has totally returned to its depolarized state or, put simply, neuron hasn't recovered fully from responding to an earlier signal. In general, longer latency auditory evoked responses have longer refractory times. As summarized in Chapter 2, there are differences in the neural generators, in the number of neural synapses (the length of the "neural chain"), and in neurotransmitters that are involved in the generation of components appearing within the latency region for the AMLR—15 to more than 50 ms. In addition, there may be differences in the refractory period for neurons that give rise to these components (e.g., Na versus Pb). Clinical studies clearly document a differential effect of stimulus rate and ISI on the early versus later latency components within the AMLR waveform (Cardenas, McCallin, Hopkins, & Fein, 1997; Erwin & Buchwald, 1986; Kodera, Yamada, Yamane, & Suzuki, 1978; McFarland et al., 1975; Onitsuka et al., 2003). Clinical studies in adult populations demonstrate consistency in the latency and amplitude for the Pa (or P30) component with stimulus rates up to at least 10/second and ISIs as short as 100 ms. In contrast, when stimulus rate increases above 1 stimulus every second or even slower rates, i.e., ISIs of ≤ 1.0 seconds, latency of the Pb (or P50) component is prolonged and amplitude reduced. The Pb (P50) component may be markedly reduced in amplitude, or not present, at stimulus rates faster than about 5/second. Remarkably, the maximum amplitude for the Pb (P50) component may be reached until the IDI is as long as 8/second, i.e., a rate of 0.125 stimuli/second (Zouridakis & Boutros, 1992).

The effect of stimulus rate on the AMLR, especially the Pb component, was illustrated in Figure 11.2. Also shown in this figure are effects of stimulus duration (described above). Nelson, Hall, and Jacobson (1997) reported consistent detection of the Pb component of the AMLR in twenty-four adult subjects for click and tone-burst stimuli (500 and 4000 Hz) with a rate of 0.5/second (one stimulus every other second). As stimulus rate was increased modestly to 1.1/second, the Pb component was consistently recorded only for the 500

Hz tone-burst stimulus condition. At faster stimulus presentation rates (2.1 and 5.1/second), the Pb was not consistently recorded and amplitude was reduced. In contrast, the Pa component of the AMLR was detected under all of these stimulus conditions.

STIMULUS RATE AND INTERSTIMULUS INTERVAL: INFANTS AND CHILDREN. | Early investigators applying the AMLR in the assessment of infants and children, even those ages 8 years and older, regularly used rates of stimulus presentation in the 8/second to 11/second range. This practice led to conflicting results and, indeed, prompted a debate about whether the AMLR could even be recorded from children. The effect of age on AMLR in general is reviewed later in this chapter. For AMLR measurement in children, most investigators report a distinct interaction between age and stimulus rate. To record an optimal AMLR, slower stimulus rates should be utilized for younger children, with rates as low as one stimulus every two seconds for newborn infants (Fifer, 1985; Jerger, Chmiel, Glaze, & Frost, 1987; Mora, Exposito, Solis, & Barajas, 1990). In contrast to this previously reported evidence of a clear effect of stimulus presentation rate on Pa latency and amplitude, Tucker and Ruth (1996) did not find statistically significant age versus rate interactions in subjects ranging in age from newborn infants through adults. Several factors may have contributed to this discrepancy in findings. Two rates of stimulus presentation were studied, and the difference was modest (3.3 versus 11.1/second). Also, the lack of statistical significance may have been in part related to the substantial variability in latency and amplitude, a finding that was, in turn, perhaps due to the relatively small number of subjects in each age group (N = 10). As an example, the average amplitude for the Pa component was only 0.77 μV for the newborn infants and almost twice that value for the preteen, teen, and adult groups (1.36, 1.33, and 1.22 μV respectively), yet these differences failed to reach statistical significance.

Among infants, a component that resembles Pa, with a latency of about 50 ms, can be recorded if stimulus rate is as slow as 1 or 2 stimulus/second. With faster rates (of 4 to 10 stimulus/second), the response is usually not observed. The importance of stimulus rate on elicitation of the AMLR in infants is illustrated in Figure 11.3. Jerger et al. (1987) found a pronounced rate effect in their study of eight babies (age range of 2 to 6 months). AMLRs were recorded with filter settings of 3 to 1000 Hz (6 dB/octave) and a midline electrode array set to 500 Hz tone bursts (4 ms linear rise/fall times and 2 ms plateau). For rates of 20 to 50/sec, the AMLR waveform was essentially a series of ABR components, with no apparent middle latency contribution, in agreement with previous reports (Kileny, 1983). From the foregoing discussion, it is clear that stimulus rate is an important factor in AMLR recording from infants and young children, although the topic requires further investigation.

Even though the interactions of stimulus rate and other clinically important factors on AMLR have yet to be systemat-

Influence of Stimulus Rate on AMLR in Newborn Infants

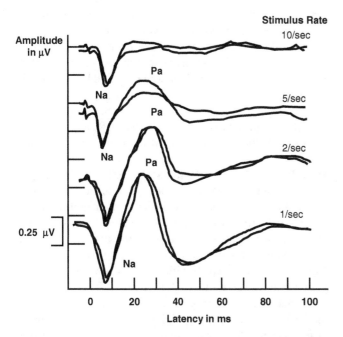

FIGURE 11.3. The importance of the rate of stimulation in evoking an AMLR from infants. As age decreases, slower rates are required for detection of the AMLR Pa component.

ically investigated, there are ample suggestions that they exist. For example, the author has monitored auditory CNS status during *hyper*thermia treatment for advanced cancer while patients undergo whole-body heating up to 42°C (107.6°F) in operating room conditions (anesthesia, mechanical ventilation, physiologic monitoring). Under these measurement conditions, ABR showed expected rate-dependent changes. Wave V latency increased about 0.4 ms from 20 stimuli/second to 80/second. In contrast, AMLR appeared to be profoundly affected by rate. With normal body temperatures, there was an AMLR at conventional rates (11.1 stimuli/second). At high temperatures, no AMLR was observed for stimuli at this rate. A small amplitude response was recorded for a rate of 5.1 stimuli/second, and there was a robust response for a very slow rate (1.1 stimuli/second). Notably, this temperature-versus-rate interaction was comparable for AMLR waveforms recorded from three different electrode sites. It is unlikely that anesthesia or nontemperature factors underlie this rate-versus-AMLR relation because these conditions were constant throughout the treatment session. The variable that changed was body temperature. Whether a slower stimulus rate may be required to record an AMLR in CNS pathology is unclear. Further study is needed regarding AMLR rate effects in normal adult subjects, in contrast with infants, patients under the influence of drugs, or patients with various pathologies.

The effect of stimulus rate on the AMLR Pb component with adult subjects reported by Nelson, Hall, and Jacobson

(1997), and summarized above in the discussion of rate in adults, was also observed for children (all females, aged 10 to 14 years).

40 HZ RESPONSE. | A discussion of the effect of stimulus rate on the AMLR would not be complete without reference to the 40 Hz response. An overview of the 40 Hz-response was provided in Chapter 1. The 40 Hz response is recorded with a conventional AMLR protocol. The rate of signal presentation, however, is approximately 40 per second, or 40 Hz. For adults, the major AMLR components are recorded at latency intervals of about 25 ms (e.g., Pa at 25 ms and Pb at 50 ms), or 40 times per second. Therefore, at 40/sec the rate of stimulation is in synchrony with the response, and the response components are superimposed or overlapping. The 40 Hz response is typically explained as the augmentation of overlapping AMLR components at the signal rate of 40/second (Azzena et al., 1995; Galambos et al., 1981; Santarelli et al., 1995). Since the precise generation of the 40 Hz response is dependent on the latency interval between major AMLR components, the response in adults is optimally recorded for slightly slower or faster rates of stimulus presentation when the latencies are, respectively, longer or shorter than 25 ms. As described later in this chapter, AMLR Pa and Pb components are recorded at progressively longer latencies as age decreases under about 10 years. Therefore, the "40 Hz" response in children actually occurs for variably slower stimulus rates (e.g., 30 or even 20 Hz) depending on the latencies of these components.

NUMBER AND SEQUENCE OF STIMULUS PRESENTATIONS. | With conventional test protocols, an AMLR is evoked with a series of single click or tone-burst stimuli, and the resulting electrophysiological activity is averaged periodically during the process. The discussion of stimulus characteristics reviewed in this section is, for the most part, limited to this mode of stimulus presentation. As noted in the introduction to the chapter, however, innovative applications of the AMLR have been reported in recent years. Investigations of some fundamental auditory system, and central nervous system, processes via the AMLR have utilized atypical stimulus paradigms, such as pairs of clicks, combinations of tone-bursts, trains of clicks, and even the oddball paradigm that is commonly associated with the P300 response (e.g., Ambrosini et al., 2001; Boutros & Belger, 1999; Boutros et al., 1995; Kisley, Olincy, et al., 2003; Kisley, Polk, et al., 2003; Rosburg et al., 2004).

One stimulus paradigm commonly employed in studies of schizophrenia, for example, involves the elicitation of the AMLR Pb (P50) component with a pair of stimuli. The concept, sometimes referred to as the "double-click paradigm" (e.g., Rosburg et al., 2004), is illustrated in Figure 11.4. The waveforms in the top portion of the figure depict an AMLR recorded with a conventional stimulus paradigm in which the response is averaged for a series of identical stimuli presented at a consistent rate (e.g., 1/second) and the patient is not attending to the stimuli. Each stimulus evokes a similar response during the period of signal averaging, and similar responses are recorded for repeated averaging periods or runs. In the simplest version of the sensory gating stimulus paradigm (middle waveform in Figure 11.4), the two identical stimuli, e.g., both of the clicks or both of the tone bursts at the same frequency, are presented as a pair. The first stimulus (S1) is followed relatively soon after (e.g., < 500 ms) by the second stimulus (S2), and then a longer interval (e.g., 8 to 10 seconds) separates the stimulus pair from the subsequent signal pair. Some authors refer to the first and second stimulus as the "conditioning" and "test" stimuli (e.g., Adler et al., 1982; Ambrosini et al., 2001; Kisley, Polk, et al., 2003; Smith, Boutros, & Schwarzkopf, 1994). A fundamental function of the brain is to filter or "tune" out irrelevant, unimportant, or redundant information (e.g., Rosburg et al., 2004). According to investigators utilizing this stimulus paradigm, the ability of the brain to inhibit, or habituate to, irrelevant (repetitive) stimulation is reflected by the reduction in amplitude for the second stimulus in the pair. The amplitude change from the first to the second stimulus is calculated as a ratio (S2/S1) or simple mathematical difference (S1 − S2), with lower ratios and larger differences

consistent with more inhibition or "gating out" of irrelevant sensory input. If the second stimulus is different than the first, or "novel," then larger ratios and smaller differences (or no difference) is consistent with "gating in," or a preattentive response of the brain indicating the ability to identify novel or potentially significant stimuli (Adler et al., 2004; Boutros & Belger, 1999; Rosburg et al., 2004; Smith et al., 1994).

POLARITY. | In contrast to ECochG and ABR, stimulus polarity is not a critical measurement parameter for the AMLR.

MONAURAL VERSUS BINAURAL STIMULATION. | In general, amplitude for the AMLR Pa component is smaller for true binaural recordings than for the sum of monaural responses (Dobie & Norton, 1980; Kelly-Ballweber & Dobie, 1984; Özdamar, Kraus, & Grossmann, 1986; Peters & Mendel, 1974; Woods & Clayworth, 1985). Kelly-Ballweber and Dobie (1984) assessed BI with ABR and AMLR for twelve younger and twelve older adult subjects. The two groups were matched for hearing impairment, and each showed a moderate to severe sloping, high frequency loss. No latency differences in AMLR were found for the summed monaural versus true binaural stimulus conditions, but Na-Pa and Pa-Nb amplitude values in the younger group were significantly reduced for the binaural condition in comparison to the summed-monaural condition. This expected binaural AMLR amplitude reduction was, on the average, not observed for the older subjects.

Woods and Clayworth (1985) found evidence of a binaural difference waveform in AMLR recordings from twelve normal subjects. Wave Pa amplitude values were about 20 percent larger and latencies about 1.5 ms longer for binaural versus monaural stimulation. Na amplitude was larger and latency shorter when recorded with an inverting electrode on the stimulus-contralateral mastoid versus an ipsilateral location. There was little inverting electrode effect on the Pa component amplitude or latency. The actual binaurally stimulated AMLR Pa amplitude was smaller than the amplitude for the summed-monaural condition. A BD waveform was derived (with the same paradigm described for the ABR), and it consisted of a triphasic trace, first observed in the 25 to 30 ms range. There was a positive voltage component with a latency value just earlier than the Pa component in the typical AMLR waveform and a negative voltage component just before the expected latency for Nb.

Debruyne (1984) studied binaural interaction in ABR, AMLR, and ALR for nine normal subjects. BI was defined, as usual, by smaller amplitude for the waveform generated with actual binaural stimulation than for the summation of monaurally stimulated (derived binaural) waveforms. BD waveforms were not generated by digital subtraction of these data because of concerns that AERs in the different time periods (ABR versus AMLR versus ALR) would interact and affect BI magnitude. BI was observed for all wave compo-

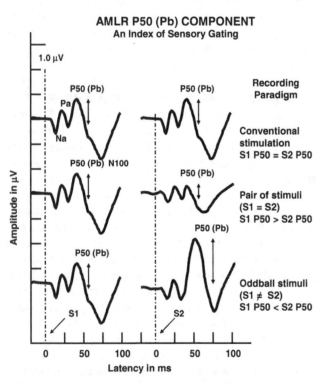

FIGURE 11.4. The "double-click" stimulus paradigm used to elicit a P50 (Pb) component in the AMLR for documentation of "sensory gating", i.e., the capacity of the brain to detect and inhibit or tune out repetitive and irrelevant stimuli. S1 = stimulus 1; S2 = stimulus 2. A pair of stimuli is presented in relatively quick succession, with a longer interval between the stimulus pair.

nents, beginning with ABR wave V, but it was most evident for the ALR N1-P2-N2 complex.

In the measurement of binaural interaction in AMLR recordings, it's important to eliminate the possible influences of PAM artifacts. These artifacts are more likely to be present in the binaural condition, due to greater stimulus intensity, and if present, they will preclude valid monaural versus binaural data analysis. Stimulus intensity does not appear to influence the likelihood or magnitude of AMLR binaural interaction. This is taken as evidence that stimulus crossover effects are not a concern in BI studies of AMLR (Dobie & Norton, 1980). However, masking noise presented to the contralateral ear during monaural stimulation does significantly increase amplitude of major AMLR components, based on experimental findings in guinea pigs (Özdamar, Kraus, & Grossman, 1986). Generalization of animal findings to humans is, of course, not necessarily possible.

Zhou and Durrant (2003) investigated a variation of the binaural interaction or fusion phenomenon with dichotically presented tonal stimulus, i.e., a different tone presented simultaneously to each ear. The interaural frequency difference (IFD) for the tones was manipulated in an attempt to determine the correspondence between electrophysiologic and psychoacoustic measures of binaural fusion. Stimuli were tone bursts near 500 Hz, with a 20 ms duration. As the IFD increased to 57 Hz, subjects first reported that the perception of the sound source moved from the center of the head and then, with further increase in the IFD to 209 Hz, two different frequencies were perceived. These psychoacoustic findings were not confirmed with the electrophysiologic measurements, as the BI component in the AMLR remained constant for IFDs up to 400 Hz (the maximum tested).

RIGHT VERSUS LEFT EAR STIMULATION. | The Na and Pa components of the AMLR are evoked similarly by right and left ear (monaural) stimulation, when recorded with either linked-ear inverting electrodes or a noncephalic electrode. That is, when the AMLR is recorded with noninverting electrodes at various scalp locations, the likelihood of detecting the components, and their latency and amplitude values, are equivalent regardless of which ear is stimulated. In contrast to this relationship between AMLR components and ear of stimulation, the Pb is consistently recorded only for right ear and binaural stimulus conditions, and only inconsistently observed with left ear stimulation (Cacace et al., 1990).

ACQUISITION PARAMETERS

Analysis Time

The term "middle-latency" indicates that the AMLR is described on the basis of analysis time. As noted in the historical review in Chapter 1, this response was referred to as the early response before the discovery of ABR, when the

auditory late response (ALR) was the focus of most research and clinical application. With the emergence of ABR as a clinical procedure, components in the 15 to 60 ms region became known as middle-latency responses. It is important to use the adjective "auditory" because responses within a comparable latency region are also generated by somatosensory stimulation. The term "middle latency response," abbreviated "MLR" is rather imprecise, as it does not specify a sensory modality (visual, somatosensory, or auditory). Although the AMLR now typically refers to a well-defined sequence of four waves including Na, Pa, Nb, and Pb located in time between ABR and ALR, the analysis time in recording AMLR begins with the stimulus, not after the ABR time period. Therefore, with an appropriately wide filter setting, ABR components appear at the earliest portion of the AMLR analysis time and are followed by the negative (N) and positive (P) waves just noted. Some evoked response manufacturers recommend, and investigators report, using an AMLR analysis time of 50 or 60 ms since the major component (Pa) is invariably located within this latency region. However, the second major positive voltage component (Pb) occurs at about 50 to 60 ms. With an inappropriately brief analysis time, portions of the AMLR may, therefore, be truncated or not detected. An analysis time of 100 ms is suggested. All AMLR components are included within this time frame, yet even with a minimal number of data points (256 per channel) latency resolution is adequate for the response. The maximum latency resolution associated with a 100 ms analysis time is approximately 0.4 ms (1000 ms divided by 256 data points for a transient stimulus). Temporal resolution of less than 0.5 ms (the minimum difference in time between data points) is sufficient for accurate latency analysis. The ABR is usually clearly recorded at the initial period of this analysis time period (with filter settings on the order of 10 to 1500 Hz). However, temporal resolution of 0.4 ms is inadequate for ABR recording, as it would not permit the degree of accuracy needed for ABR latency calculations. Doubling the number of data points to 512 cuts in half the time interval between each point (down to 0.2 ms), whereas 1024 data points for the 100 ms analysis time would provide adequate ABR latency resolution and would certainly exceed the requirements for calculation of AMLR latency and amplitude values.

Electrodes

Until the early 1980s, AMLR was invariably recorded with a single channel using the conventional ABR electrode array, with a noninverting electrode located in midline on either the vertex (Cz) or the forehead (in the region of the Fz electrode site). The inverting electrode was located on the mastoid or earlobe on the side ipsilateral to the stimulus presentation. Virtually all AMLR investigations conducted in the late 1960s and throughout the 1970s employed this simple electrode arrangement. There are several likely reasons for this practice. Measurement is easier with a single scalp electrode site, and usually AMLR amplitude is robust for a recording site on the midline of the head. For many investigations just cited, the emphasis was on defining the effects of stimulus parameters (intensity, duration, rate, frequency) or evaluating the usefulness of AMLR in estimating auditory threshold level, rather than neurodiagnosis of cortical auditory dysfunction. That is, the anatomic area of interest was the ear, rather than the brain. For that clinical application of the AMLR, the simple electrode array was adequate. However, there is now convincing evidence that the mastoid electrode is active and contributes substantially to the response and, in fact, a well-formed AMLR can even be recorded with a mastoid to noncephalic electrode array (Kadobayashi, Kira, Toyoshima, & Nishijima, 1984). In this study, a balanced noncephalic electrode arrangement was used (Stephenson & Gibbs, 1951), with linked electrodes located on the seventh cervical vertebra and the right sternoclavicular junction. Technically, this second electrode should be repositioned until both electrodes, when connected to a potentiometer, show minimal detection of the electrocardiogram (EKG).

As detailed in Chapter 2, and summarized above, the AMLR can provide useful information in auditory neurodiagnosis. Landmark human depth electrode investigations and clinical topographic data, mostly from clinical investigations conducted in the 1980s, confirmed that the primary auditory cortex in the temporal lobe contributes to generation of AMLR (Celesia et al., 1968; Kileny et al., 1988; Kraus et al., 1982; Lee et al., 1984; Scherg & von Cramon, 1986). A simple midline electrode arrangement is inadequate for neurodiagnosis with AMLR. The response must be measured with electrodes located over temporal-parietal cortical regions for identification and localization of cortical auditory dysfunction (Kileny, Paccioretti, & Wilson, 1987; Kraus, Özdamar, Hier, & Stein, 1982; Woods et al., 1987). Other researchers have repeatedly observed normal appearing midline-recorded AMLRs in patients with unilateral (right or left) temporal lobe pathology. A protocol with hemisphere specific electrodes yields a different pattern of findings. Characteristically, there is an abnormal AMLR or no response for the recording made with an electrode over the involved hemisphere.

The three noninverting electrode sites best suited for AMLR recording are designated by an 10–20 International Electrode System illustration in Figure 11.5. Although a vertex (Cz) midline site is not inappropriate, a response with comparable latency and amplitude characteristics is recorded from a forehead (Fz) electrode. The other two non-inverting electrode sites are located over the left and right temporal-parietal regions (C3 and C4). AMLR waveforms recorded simultaneously with three non-inverting electrodes were shown in Figure 11.1. Amplitude for the Pa component is largest, usually in the range of 1.0 to 1.20 μV, at the vertex (Cz) or forehead (Fz) and progressively diminishes symmetrically for more lateral (right and left) sites (e.g., Amenedo

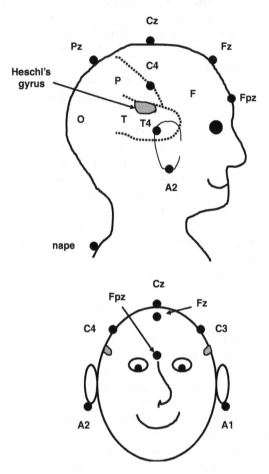

Auditory Middle-Latency Response Electrode Sites

FIGURE 11.5. Electrode sites (noninverting and inverting) used for measurement of the AMLR for neurodiagnostic applications. The inverting electrodes can be located on the ears (e.g., ear lobes) and linked, or on a noncephalic site (e.g., the nape of the neck). Electrode sites are labeled according to the 10–20 International system.

& Diaz, 1998; Kileny, Paccioretti, & Wilson, 1987; Kraus et al., 1982; Özdamar & Kraus, 1983). A Pz noninverting electrode site is not advisable for AMLR recording, and amplitude of all AMLR components is markedly lower that for the Cz or Fz sites. There are slight but clinically unimportant advancing age-related differences for AMLR components recorded at various midline electrode sites, and also differences in the amplitude of specific components for some midline sites, with slightly larger amplitude for Pa at the Fz site and Pb at the Cz site. For a parietal location just above the temporal lobe (C5 and C6), the average amplitude is slightly less than 1.0 μV (0.90 to 1.0 μV). Also, average amplitude among these sites is smallest (0.60 to 0.80 μV) for the electrodes (T3 and T4) in the temporal region corresponding to a location below the Sylvian fissure (not shown). The amplitude difference for responses that are recorded from vertex versus temporal lobe electrode sites is statistically significant. Latency of the Pa component, however, does not vary significantly as a function of electrode site.

Using a coronal electrode array in a study of AMLR in seven normal adult subjects, Cohen (1982) confirmed that maximum amplitude for the Pa component was recorded from just anterior to the vertex. With an inverting ("reference") electrode on the nose, the Pa component polarity underwent a reversal with five of the seven subjects at approximately the same level as the Sylvian fissure, and voltage gradients were steepest over this area. These findings resemble the polarity reversal of the ALR recorded with a similar electrode array by Vaughan and Ritter (1970). Jerger, Chmiel, Glaze, and Frost (1987) provided evidence of a rate versus electrode site interaction in a study of AMLR in infants. At a very slow rate of 1/sec, the Cz-Ai and Cz-Ac electrode arrays yielded equivalent AMLR patterns (a Pa-like response at a latency of about 50 ms). The contralateral (Cz-Ac) array showed a smaller amplitude response for slightly faster stimulus rates (2 to 4/second). These observations confirmed findings noted previously by Wolf and Goldstein (1980).

There is no convention for inverting electrode sites with the multichannel (hemisphere and midline) recording arrangement. Some earlier investigators used a stimulus ipsilateral mastoid or earlobe location (Özdamar & Kraus, 1983), assuming that the mastoid was essentially neutral as evidenced by the absence of AMLR activity with a horizontal (mastoid-to-mastoid) electrode array. With adult subjects, it appears that the AMLR detected with midline noninverting electrodes is similar when recorded with inverting electrodes located on the ear ipsilateral or contralateral to the side of stimulus presentation (Peters & Mendel, 1974). On the other hand, Wolf and Goldstein (1980) found that AMLRs recorded from infants with a midline noninverting electrode array were present only with an inverting electrode on the side of stimulation, and not with a contralateral inverting electrode array. As noted previously, noncephalic electrode recording techniques show that the ipsilateral mastoid is active with respect to AMLR activity. AMLRs are also recorded with a linked-earlobe (or mastoid) inverting electrode arrangement, in order to counterbalance any possible mastoid contribution to the response (e.g., Kileny, Paccioretti, & Wilson, 1987). For clinical AMLR measurements, this is now a commonly employed inverting electrode arrangement. The waveforms shown earlier in Figure 11.1, for example, were recorded with linked earlobe inverting electrodes. Linked earlobe inverting electrodes have also been reported in ABR measurement (Rossini et al., 1980; Terkildsen & Osterhammel, 1981). Given the importance in analysis of the ABR in neurodiagnosis of recording a wave I from the stimulus ear, the linked earlobe technique would seem to have little value clinically. The technique for linking earlobe electrodes in clinical AER measurement is rather straightforward. The inverting electrodes from both ears are connected or linked

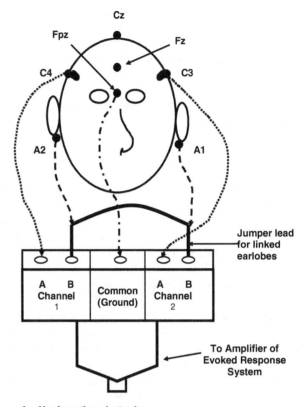

AMLR:
Electrode Sites and Preamplifier Inputs

A = Noninverting electrodes
B = Inverting electrodes

FIGURE 11.6. The arrangement of electrode wires or leads plugged into the preamplifier or electrode box for measurement of the AMLR using two channels. Note that an electrode wire for the left and right hemisphere (see Figure 11.5) is plugged into the first (noninverting) input for each channel (one and two, respectively), and the ear lobe electrode wires are linked together via a small connecting "jumper" cable.

with a "jumper" cable, as illustrated in Figure 11.6. Electrode options were shown in Figure 3.9 (in Chapter 3). A serious potential problem in AMLR recording is interference by postauricular muscle (PAM) artifact (described below). The earlobe and mastoid inverting electrode site is particularly susceptible to PAM artifact contamination. A most effective solution to the PAM artifact problem is reliance on a noncephalic reference electrode.

The arguments presented above for the use of a noncephalic reference electrode in ABR recordings apply as well to the AMLR. One of these arguments, compatibility between clinical recording protocol and the technique employed in studies of the neural generators of the response, is particularly applicable. Lee et al. (1984), in a germinal investigation on neural generators of the AMLR in man, relied on a noncephalic (fifth cervical spinous process) electrode.

Nelson, Hall, and Jacobson (1997) reported that the detection of the Pb component was most often observed for the Fz noninverting electrode site, although the Cz site also yielded a Pb component in most subjects. A Pb was rarely detected for hemisphere electrodes (C3 and C4) and, when present, amplitude was substantially lower. These investigators demonstrated that linked earlobe electrodes do not detect AMLR activity, and that equivalent Pa and Pb components were recorded with noncephalic and with linked earlobe inverting electrode configurations.

Filtering

Filtering in AMLR recordings is employed mostly to reduce the unwanted influence of low-frequency EEG activity as a source of noise in the response. Filter settings, especially the high-pass filter cutoff frequency, are an extremely important variable in AMLR measurement (Izuma, 1980; Jerger, Chmiel, Glaze, & Frost, 1987; Kileny, 1983; Kraus et al., 1987; Scherg, 1982b; Suzuki, Hirabayashi, & Kobayashi, 1984). The majority of early studies of AMLR, as noted in Chapter 1, employed restricted analog filter settings, typically about 30 to 100 Hz. Unfortunately, the sometimes marked distortion of AMLR by restriction of, primarily, the analog high-pass filter cutoff was not appreciated clinically until the early 1980s (Hall, 1992; Hall, Hargadine, & Allen, 1985; Kileny, 1984; Kileny, 1984; Musiek, Geurkink, Weider, & Donnelly, 1984; Scherg, 1982b; Suzuki, Hirabayashi, & Kobayashi, 1983). Filter effects can be pronounced in AMLR measurement, producing phase distortion (latency shifts) and reduced power (diminished amplitude) for certain components (e.g., Pa) and leading to artifactual components in the waveform (Lane et al., 1974; Scherg, 1982b). Scherg (1982b) simulated analog filtering (with the commonly used Butterworth type of filter) digitally using a 24 dB/octave slope and assessed filter effects on AMLR waveform morphology. Low-pass analog filtering, as expected, tended to produce a very smooth waveform and increased latency for components Na, Pa, and Nb. High-pass analog filtering, however, resulted in the most marked distortion of the waveform. Increasing the high-pass filter setting from 1 Hz actually was associated with greater amplitude of some components due to filter oscillations generated by earlier components. Latency of Pa shortened as the high-pass cutoff was reduced from the wide setting (1 Hz), and by 40 Hz there was a polarity reversal of the Pa component. Greater waveform distortion is observed with steeper filter slopes.

At the extreme, with an overly restricted analog filter setting, as used in most of the early investigations of AMLR (band-pass filter setting such as 30 to 100 Hz), it is possible to observe a Pa component at about 30 ms or even an Na-Pa-Nb sequence of components when, in fact, there is no AMLR (Jerger, Chmiel, Glaze, & Frost, 1987; Kileny, 1983; Scherg, 1982b). This spurious "response" represents filter distorted ABR activity ringing into the middle-latency region

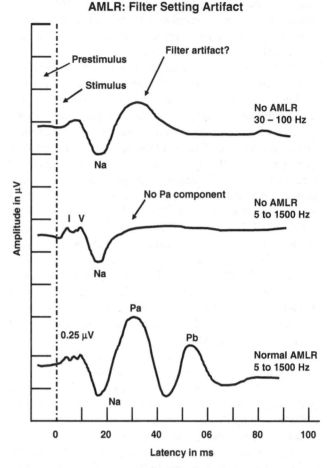

FIGURE 11.7. Illustration of auditory middle latency response (AMLR) measurement from a 2-year-old patient with severe temporal lobe dysfunction bilaterally secondary to a cerebral vascular accident with restricted band-pass filter settings (30 to 100 Hz) and wider band-pass filter settings (10 to 1500 Hz). Note the presence of a spurious Pa component with the restricted filter settings with no apparent response when the AMLR was recorded with wider filter settings.

(Kileny, 1983). The artifact, as illustrated in Figure 11.7, is most often observed when an ABR is recorded, or there is in the waveform at least a large wave I component (Hall, 1988, 1992; Hall, Brown, & Mackey-Hargadine, 1985). The patient in this figure was a 2-year-old child with bilateral temporal lobe infarcts. There is an apparent AMLR Pa component with an analog filter setting of 30 to 100 Hz, but not 5 to 1500 Hz. In this case, when the waveform recorded with filter settings of 5 to 1500 Hz recording was digitally filtered at 30 to 100 Hz, no artifactual component was observed. In the absence of an ABR, the filter-produced AMLR is generally not recorded.

Further extending the cutoff frequency of the high-pass filter downward below 15 Hz may, however, not always be desirable in clinical AMLR measurements. For example,

Kraus, Reed, Smith, Stein, and Cartee (1987) found in a study of AMLR recordings in 217 patients ranging in age from 6 days to 20 years that the likelihood of observing the Na and Pa components was greater for a high-pass filter setting of 15 Hz (12 dB/octave slope) than 3 Hz (6 dB/octave slope). These authors attributed the more favorable findings with the 15 Hz cutoff to effective reduction of unwanted low EEG activity (20 Hz and below), which, in children at least, can obscure the AMLR (Suzuki, Hirabayashi, & Kobayashi, 1983, 1984). Mora et al. (1990) also reported that the likelihood that a Na and Pa component would be detected during AMLR measurement in newborn infants was greater for a high-pass filter setting of 10 Hz than a setting of 5 Hz.

Spectral analysis of the AMLR shows that the major power or energy region, for normal hearing adults, is between 30 to 50 Hz (Kavanagh & Domico, 1986; Kavanagh, Harker, & Tyler, 1984; Suzuki, Kobayashi, & Hirabayashi, 1983). Alterations in high-pass filter settings exert the greatest effects. With digital filtering techniques, all AMLR components are observed with a high-pass cutoff frequency of 30 Hz. As the cutoff frequency is increased from 30 to 50 Hz, amplitude of the Na and Pa components decreases and, at about 40 Hz, the Pb component disappears. As an aside, an AMLR protocol for consistent detection of the Pb component is summarized below. This suggests that latter components of the AMLR are composed of somewhat lower frequency energy. With a high-pass cutoff frequency above 60 Hz, the AMLR entirely disappears. Furthermore, the characteristic intersubject variability in AMLR morphology is considerably reduced with elimination of frequency content below 30 Hz. Energy at about 10 Hz in the AMLR may represent an important contribution from general neurobiologic activity that is not response related. Certainly, based on these studies, there is important AMLR energy in the frequency region below 30 Hz.

One additional noteworthy feature of AMLR spectrum is its apparent variability among normal adult subjects, with peaks for different subjects occurring at different frequencies within the response spectrum. It is quite possible, as demonstrated by Kavanagh and Domico (1986), for two subjects to each have a distinct AMLR with an unfiltered AMLR and yet, with a 30 Hz analog or digital high-pass filter cutoff, for one subject to show no AMLR while the other does. The influence of subject characteristics, such as young or old age or gender, on AMLR spectrum and susceptibility to filter effects is not known.

Detailed discussions of filtering, particularly in AER recording, can be found in several articles (Doyle & Hyde, 1981a; Scherg, 1982b). Practical suggestions for filtering in clinical AMLR measurement would, ideally, include the use of little filtering during online recordings (e.g., 1 to 2000 Hz) and then zero phase shift filtering offline after data collection. Since this is not possible with most commercially available evoked response systems and requires additional time, an alternative is to use an analog filter with a relatively gradual slope (e.g., 6 dB/octave) and a high-pass filter cutoff frequency of no higher than 10 to 15 Hz. Clinical interpretation of AMLR waveforms with higher filter settings, or among studies with differences in filter settings, must be done with extreme caution. The Pb component of the AMLR is best recorded when the high pass filter setting is 5 Hz or less (e.g., Nelson, Hall, & Jacobson, 1997).

ANALYSIS AND INTERPRETATION

Nomenclature

Goldstein and Rodman in 1967 first introduced the labels that are used to describe the AMLR components. The measurement parameters employed by these investigators were quite different than those currently recommended for AMLR measurement. Filters were set at 1 to 50 Hz. The noninverting electrode was located on the vertex, and the inverting electrode was always placed on the ear contralateral to the stimulus. An ear mold was fitted in the nontest ear to reduce ambient noise stimulation. Robert Goldstein chose the labels Na, Pa, and Nb to designate polarity (N for negative and P for positive) of the presumably vertex-recorded response, thus avoiding confusion with ALR peaks, which were already labeled P1, N1, P2, and N2. He further defined the expected normal latency range for each of the AMLR peaks, taking into account increases in latency at lower intensity levels: Na = 16.25 to 30.00 ms; Pa = 30.00 to 45.00 ms; Nb = 46.25 to 56.25 ms. These latencies, recorded with the restricted filter settings used in this study were, of course, longer than those recorded with wider filter settings. Of the three components, Nb was least consistently recorded. The latency regions for each component were referred to as "latency criteria." Another criterion, the interval between Na and Pa (ranging from 7.50 to 18.75 ms) was added in an attempt to further distinguish a response from a control run (no stimulus) waveform. The third criterion did appear to reduce the likelihood of a false positive interpretation (failing to identify a response).

Normal Waveform Variations

A historical perspective on AMLR, including a review of various terms used in referring to the response and nomenclature for labeling wave components, was presented in Chapter 1. At the outset of this discussion, it is important to restate that subject characteristics and stimulus/acquisition parameters exert a marked effect on AMLR. These factors are summarized later in this chapter. The following description of the AMLR is, initially, limited to waveforms recorded with currently accepted measurement parameters from normal adult subjects. Typical adult AMLR waveforms were shown in Figure 11.1. With a filter setting of 10 to 1500 Hz, the ABR is apparent within the initial portion of the waveform, followed by a relatively slow, negative-going component in the 12 to 15 ms region. This is labeled Na (N for negative voltage, and "a" to denote the first component within the middle-latency region). Other components are similarly named. The major AMLR component is wave Pa. As noted below, normal morphology of the Pa component varies. With the recommended analysis time of 100 ms (a prestimulus period is included in the illustrated waveforms), two additional AMLR waves (Nb and Pb) are sometimes seen following the Pa component.

In contrast to ABR and for a combination of reasons, analysis of AMLR waveforms is more concerned with amplitude than latency. Even casual inspection of the AMLR waveforms shown in Figure 11.1 reveals that the response is characterized by relatively gradual, rounded waves rather than the sharp peaks in an typical ABR waveform. Spectral analysis of AMLR confirms that it is composed mostly of energy in the region of 10 to 50 Hz. Because there is no high-frequency energy in the waveform, extremely precise latency resolution is less important than with ABR. Clinically, a latency difference between waveforms for wave Pa of 1 or 2 ms is negligible, whereas an ABR wave V difference of this magnitude between waveforms would be highly significant. Normal latency variability, likewise, is far greater for AMLR components.

There is also a clinically important reason for greater reliance on analysis of amplitude versus latency. Limited clinical experience with AMLR suggests that CNS auditory neuropathology exerts a more pronounced effect on amplitude than latency. That is, amplitude appears to be a more sensitive indicator of auditory dysfunction than is latency. Again, this is in direct contrast to the relative importance of latency versus amplitude in the analysis of the ABR. Presumably, these differences between ABR and AMLR are a reflection of distinct neurophysiologic bases. Since amplitude is important in clinical analysis of AMLR waveforms, the clinician must appreciate methods for amplitude calculation. Two main techniques for amplitude measurement of the prominent Pa component are illustrated in Figure 11.8. Traditionally, in AMLR analysis amplitude was calculated for the Na-to-Pa wave complex. This technique, which is still widely applied, is relatively straightforward because each component tends to be distinct, at least in the normal waveform. In fact, wave Na is usually quite robust even in persons with neuropathology. This is, in turn, also a limitation of the Na-Pa amplitude calculation. In patients showing a Na but no apparent Pa component, apparent amplitude for the Na-Pa complex may be calculated due solely to presence of the Na component. An alternate approach is to calculate the amplitude of the Pa-to-Nb components (Figure 11.8). It is possible, however, that this approach may produce just the opposite problem. Auditory dysfunction at higher levels in the central nervous system may eliminate the Nb component and spare the Pa component, yet Pa amplitude calculated as Pa-Nb is typically reduced. A third possible AMLR amplitude analysis approach, the difference between the Pa peak

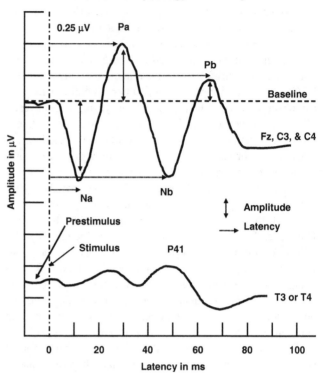

FIGURE 11.8. Techniques for calculation of the latency and amplitude of AMLR waves Na, Pa, Nb, and Pb as recorded conventionally with midline inverting electrodes (top portion) and electrodes over the temporal lobe (lower portion).

and a measure of baseline activity, has rarely been reported, probably because of the difficulty in defining a valid index of baseline.

DETERMINING RESPONSE PRESENCE VERSUS ABSENCE. | Since AMLR amplitude and morphology are more important clinically than latency, it is not surprising that morphology of the AMLR waveform has been systematically described (Fifer & Sierra-Irizarry, 1988; Kraus, Smith, Reed, Stein, & Cartee, 1985; McGee, Kraus, & Manfredi, 1988; Özdamar & Kraus, 1983). The first objective in waveform analysis is, of course, confirmation that a response is present. While on the surface this would seen to be a simple task, it can be rather difficult and time consuming for AMLRs recorded clinically. Response reliability is as important in AMLR analysis as it is for ECochG and ABR. However, the AMLR is more likely to be altered or simply not detected due to methodologic factors than these shorter latency responses. Selected nonpathologic factors influencing the interpretation of AMLR clinically are summarized in Table 11.2. Essentially, one must rule out each of these factors before concluding that there is no response for a given patient. Kraus et al. (1985) presented two sets of criteria for judging response presence or absence.

TABLE 11.2. Nonpathologic Factors Influencing AMLR Measurement

FACTOR	COMMENT
Test Parameters	
Filtering	Restricted high-pass filter setting (e.g., 30 Hz versus 5 or 10 Hz) can produce artifact components in the AMLR waveform; lowering the high-pass filter setting to 1 or even 0.1 Hz is required to consistently record the AMLR Pb component.
Stimulus intensity level	High intensity levels, e.g., > 70 dB nHL can produce postauricular muscle (PAM) artifact in the latency region of 12 to 20 ms.
Stimulus duration	Longer stimulus durations (e.g., > 10 ms) are preferred to highly transient signals, e.g., clicks, especially in recording the AMLR Pb component.
Stimulus rate	Slower rates (< 5 signals/second) are advised for children under the age of 10 years; in pathology, rates as slow as 1 signal/sec are required to consistently record the AMLR Pb component.
Subject Factors	
Age	
children	The AMLR can be recorded in newborn infants (see notation above regarding slower signal rate) with the Na component initially most prominent. Reflecting CNS maturation, the likelihood of recording an AMLR consistently increases with age up to 10 years, with a progressive decrease in latency and increase in amplitude for the Pa component.
adults	AMLR Pa and Pb latency and amplitude values increase with advancing age in elderly adults.
Gender	To date, studies have provided no consistent evidence of are statistically significant differences between males and females for AMLR components. The latency values of AMLR waves appear to be longer for males in comparison to females, consistent with the general influence of gender on the ABR.
Sleep	Sleep is an important factor in the analysis of AMLR recordings for children and, to some degree, for adults. The AMLR is most consistently recorded in REM sleep, generally not detected in sleep stage 3, and not recorded in sleep stage 4.
Myogenic	Postauricular muscle (PAM) activity can seriously interfere with the recording of the AMLR under certain measurement conditions, e.g., high signal intensity, tense subject, and inverting electrode on the mastoid or earlobe (near the PAM). Other muscle activity associated with body movement or tension in the jaw and neck muscles can also confound AMLR recordings, with unwanted muscle artifact affecting mostly activity recorded under 500 Hz.
Hypobaric oxygen	No apparent effect on AMLR Na and Pa components recorded from normal adult male subjects with ambient oxygen partial pressure of 84.5 mm Hg compared with typical atmospheric pressure (159.2 mm Hg) (Lucertini, Ciniglio-Appiani, Antonini, & Urbani, 1993).
Sedation	The AMLR is highly affected by conscious sedation, with a reduction in amplitude and variability in waveform morphology.
Anesthesia	Anesthetic agents typically suppress AMLR activity, although the effects of anesthesia on the AMLR varies considerably for different drugs.

With criteria in set I, an AMLR was present if electrical activity corresponding to the Na and Pa components (but not necessarily limited to any region in the analysis time) was observed below (Na) or above (Pa) relative to a baseline defined by ABR. Criteria set II criterion was a characteristic AMLR waveform appearance, that is, a broad negative trough (Na) followed by a vertex-positive Pa component.

One rather unique problem in AMLR analysis is assuring that apparent components are neurogenic (true responses from the auditory nervous system) and not artifacts that are unrelated to brain activity within the auditory system. Generally, artifacts are not time locked to the stimulus or reliably recorded. These artifacts can be detected by comparing several successive averaged waveforms. With adequate averaging or other manipulations of measurement parameters, they can be minimized or eliminated. Ruling out the presence of two types of artifact in AMLR waveforms, however, can be especially troublesome as they tend to be highly reliable. Perhaps the most serious measurement problem encountered clinically is a *myo*genic response—postauricular muscle

(PAM) activity. PAM artifact appears as a sharply peaked component in the 13 to 15 ms region. Amplitude of the PAM activity is much greater than for the Pa component. PAM activity is more likely to be recorded with a high-intensity stimulus, with an electrode on the ipsilateral ear, and from a tense patient.

Another type of "reliable" artifact is caused by overly restricted filter settings and steep filter slopes. With a filter bandwidth of 30 to 100 Hz and/or slopes of 24 to 48 dB/octave, for example, a filter distortion component that resembles the Pa component may be observed in the same general latency region as the Pa component (Osterhammel, 1981; Scherg, 1982b). This nonphysiologic component can be eliminated by using appropriately wide filter settings and, particularly, by extending the high-pass filter setting downward, e.g., a high pass filter setting of 10 Hz rather than 30 Hz. Filter settings for AMLR measurement were reviewed earlier in this chapter and summarized with other stimulus parameters in Table 11.1.

MORPHOLOGY VARIATIONS. | The first peak traditionally described in the AMLR waveform is often referred to as P_0. In early studies of AMLR, P_0 was thought to be a reflection of the ABR wave V component, on the basis of analysis of AMLR waveforms recorded with restricted filter settings. With less restricted filtering, however, there is a clear distinction between ABR wave V and P_0, and the P_0 peak is not consistently observed. When present, it consists at least in part of postauricular muscle (PAM) artifact (Kileny, 1983). Waves Na and Pa are identified most consistently in normal subjects, whereas waves P_0 and Pb are observed far less than 50 percent of the time (Özdamar & Kraus, 1983). Although Pa is the dominant peak for AMLR analysis, its normal morphology may vary considerably among subjects under identical measurement conditions, and even between ears and electrode locations in a single subject. Some general morphologic variations for AMLR waveforms with a normal Pa component are illustrated in Figure 11.9, and include:

- A sharp single peak for wave Pa and Pb, separated by a distinct trough
- A broad Pa component with two rounded peaks with a minimal trough between the two, and with the second peak well before the expected latency for wave Pb, and
- A clear wave Pa which may be sharply peaked or rounded with a broad base, and may be followed with either a deep Nb trough or no apparent negative voltage trough. It is not followed by a Pb component (McGee, Kraus, & Manfredi, 1988; Özdamar & Kraus, 1983).

Clinical experience suggests that there are additional normal variations for AMLR waveform morphology.

McGee, Kraus, and Manfredi (1988) systematically applied a set of analysis parameters in a study of AMLR waveforms in eleven normal subjects. One objective was

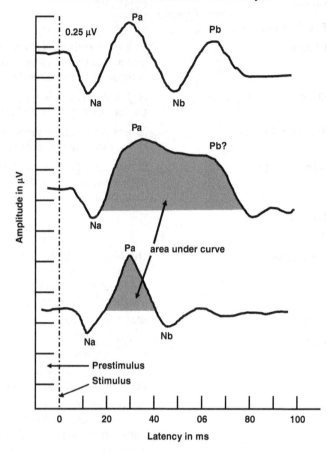

**AMLR
Normal Waveform Variations with Analysis**

FIGURE 11.9. Variations in AMLR waveform morphology, especially the Pa wave, with the "area under the curve" technique for calculation of amplitude of the Pa wave. Integrating the area under the Pa wave takes into account the width of the component, in addition to the amplitude.

to develop an analysis technique that encompassed all the normally diverse waveforms. In part, this was an attempt to quantify what the clinician interprets as "good or poor morphology". More importantly, it extended with two additional parameters—width of Pa and area under Pa—the conventional strategy for analysis of AMLR latency and amplitude. This analysis approach was illustrated in Figure 11.9. The rationale for this analysis approach was stated succinctly by the authors:

> It is our reasoning that these are meaningful parameters under the hypothesis that Pa latency assesses time of peak neural activity, while Pa amplitude indicates the amount of activity at that time and Pa width describes the length of time that the neural activity is sustained. Under this reasoning, Pa area is an indication of the total neural activity involved in Pa. (McGee, Kraus, & Manfredi, 1988, p. 121)

This explanation, however, assumes that all dipoles underlying the AMLR are stationary throughout the time course of the response. As noted in the following discussion on dipole localization techniques, this is unlikely.

Musiek et al. (1999) published a detailed account of a technique for analysis of the AMLR, and validated the analysis approach with a series of patients with confirmed and anatomically defined brain lesions. Waveform analysis began with identification of peaks within acceptable time frames, i.e., an expected latency region following the stimulus. AMLR analysis included calculation of latency for the Na component (within the region of 12 to 21 ms) and the Pa component (within the latency region of 21 and 38 ms), and amplitude from the trough of the Na component to the peak of the Pa component or wave complex.

Analysis Techniques for the Pb (P50) Component: Sensory Gating

As noted above in the discussions of the effect of stimulus repetition on the AMLR, and also in the sections below reviewing the effects of attention and the effects of drugs (cocaine) on the AMLR, the Pb (P50) component is used by some investigators as a measure of preattentive sensory gating within the central nervous system. For example, Boutros and colleagues (Boutros & Belger, 1999; Boutros, Campbell, et al., 2000; Boutros, Torello, et al., 1995) first calculate the amplitude of the Pb (P50) component for individual stimuli presented in a series or "train," for a pair of identical stimulus (S1 and S2) presented as a pair (e.g., two tone bursts of 1000 Hz) and separated by an interval of 500 ms (the "paired signal paradigm") or for an oddball stimulus paradigm in which two different signals (S1 and S2) are presented, e.g., a 500 Hz and a 1000 Hz tone burst. These authors determine the presence of the Pb (P50) component with two criteria: (1) The wave is the second positive component within the latency region of 30 and 80 ms after a stimulus, following the Pa component (the first positive component) that appears in the region of 15 to 40 ms, and (2) the Pb (P50) is consistently recorded from one noninverting electrode array in addition to the Cz noninverting electrode array.

In applying the AMLR P50 (Pb) component as an index of sensory gating, the authors then calculate either a ratio for the amplitude of S1 versus S2 (S2/S1) or a simple mathematical difference in the amplitudes for S2 – S1. This process was illustrated above in Figure 11.4. With two identical signals (i.e., S1 = S2), with preattentive processing, the brain "gates out" the second identical signal (S2) because it is irrelevant and contains the same information as the first signal. Thus, S2 produces a smaller Pb (P50), with attenuated amplitude, and the S2/S1 amplitude ratio and the S2 – S1 difference is smaller. With a pair of different stimuli (the oddball paradigm), the second novel or "deviant" stimulus produces a Pb (P50) component with higher amplitude. The

brain, with preattentive processing, "gates in" the S2 because it represents new or significant information. Relative amplitude calculation for the stimuli will show an increase in the S2/S1 ratio and in the S2 – S1 difference.

ABNORMAL PATTERNS. | For the most part, analysis of AMLR waveforms has been limited to latency and amplitude parameters, especially amplitude. However, abnormal patterns for AMLR are, for several reasons, not as clear-cut as for the ECochG or ABR. First, as noted above, there is considerable normal variability in waveform morphology. The P_0, Nb, and Pb components are present only inconsistently in normal subjects and are, therefore, not useful clinically. Second, in contrast to the numerous published and unpublished databases for ABR, normative data for AMLR analysis are scarce. Finally, patterns of AMLR abnormalities for a patient are based on relative differences in waveforms recorded from multiple electrode arrays versus in a single waveform.

Imaging AMLR findings with computer evoked potential topography (brain mapping) techniques also may prove clinically valuable (Kraus & McGee, 1988). Meanwhile, analysis of AMLR latency and amplitude as a function of multiple electrode arrays, or for a single midline electrode array, dominates clinical applications of the response and will be emphasized in the following discussion.

NONPATHOLOGIC FACTORS IN AMLR ANALYSIS

Age

INFANCY AND CHILDHOOD. | The literature on AMLR in infancy and childhood dates back at least thirty years (e.g., McRandle, Smith, & Goldstein, 1974; Mendel, Adkinson, & Harker, 1977). The influences of age (in children and adults) and other nonpathologic factors in AMLR analysis and interpretation are summarized in Table 11.2. Unfortunately, conclusions drawn from some of the earlier studies are open to question when considered in the light of current knowledge of the effect of certain measurement conditions on AMLR. Developmental AMLR findings reported over the years are conflicting. Some investigators did not consistently observe the Pa component in normal neonates and young children who were apparently normal (Davis, 1976). Others, however, appeared to demonstrate that AMLRs could be reliably recorded from newborn infants and young children (McRandle et al., 1974; Mendel, Adkinson, & Harker, 1977; Mendelson & Salamy, 1981; Wolf & Goldstein, 1980). Curiously, latency of the major component (wave Pa) either did not change as a function of age or was even shorter in infants than in adults.

In retrospect, what the authors' interpreted as a highly reliable AMLR in infants was in many cases probably an artifact and the product of extremely restrictive filtering. As the high-pass filter setting (the low-frequency cutoff) is shifted upwards from 5 Hz to, for example, 30 Hz, and when the low pass (the high-frequency cutoff) is reduced from, for example, 1500 Hz to 100 Hz, a wave component that resembles Pa may be recorded even when a true response is not present (Hall, Brown, & Mackey-Hargadine, 1985; Kileny, 1983; Kraus, Reed, Smith, Stein, & Cartee, 1987; Scherg, 1982b; Suzuki, Hirabayashi, & Kobayashi, 1984). An example of the AMLR artifact produced by overly restrictive filter settings was depicted in Figure 11.7.

Stimulus rate was another confounding variable in the early studies of AMLR in children. Then, a rate of 10 stimuli/sec or a slightly faster rate was typically used, in part because it facilitated speedy data collection. It is now known, however, that this rate is excessively rapid for recording AMLRs from children (Fifer, 1985; Hall, 1992; Kraus et al., 1987). Indeed, this is simply another example of the general relationship of signal rate to latency of any auditory evoked response—slower stimulus rates are required for longer latency of responses. The same point will be raised again in the review in the next chapter of stimulus rate for the auditory late responses. As illustrated above by waveforms in Figure 11.3, a stimulus rate as slow as 1/second may be necessary before the AMLR becomes apparent in infants and young children. When stimulus rate is relatively high (11/second) and held constant, the proportion of children, and even adolescents through age 15 to 20 years, yielding a detectable AMLR declines directly as age decreases.

Finally, noninverting electrode location appears to be an important factor in recording AMLR activity. Until approximately 1982, virtually all studies of AMLR in children, or adults for that matter, used a midline (vertex or high forehead) electrode site to record the response when either ear was stimulated. Evidence from animal and clinical research, however, indicates that a response may be detected from a midline electrode when there no response is recorded from a electrode located over the temporal-parietal region of the brain (Kileny et al., 1988; Kraus, Ozdamar, Hier, & Stein, 1982; Kraus et al., 1988). Recall from an earlier discussion that the Na wave of the AMLR originates mostly from subcortical anatomic auditory pathways, whereas the Pa component arises at least in part from the primary auditory cortex (Heschl's gyrus). Presumably, then, electrodes located over each hemisphere detect activity in the auditory temporal lobe, while the midline electrode detects activity in subcortical structures (e.g., thalamus).

Under appropriate measurement conditions, namely a slow stimulation rate (1 to 2/second) and appropriate filter settings (e.g., 10 to 300 Hz), a true AMLR can usually be recorded in neonates and young children. In term and also preterm infants, the Pa component in the AMLR is not reliably recorded for stimulus rates exceeding 5/second (Fifer & Sierra-Irizarry, 1988; Jerger, Chmiel, Glaze, & Frost, 1987; Kraus et al., 1989; Pasman et al., 1991). At the slower stimu-

lation rate, latency of the Pa component is usually in the 50 ms range, or twice the expected adult latency value. It may be even further delayed in very young normal infants (Fifer & Sierra-Irizarry, 1988). In addition, the morphology of Pa recorded from infants tends to be broader, rather than the sharply peaked wave often observed in adults. Wave Na of the AMLR tends to be the most consistently recorded AMLR component and may be present even if waveforms lack the Pa component (Kraus, Reed, Smith, Stein, & Cartee, 1987). Amplitude of Pa increases steadily from infancy through late childhood, and then decreases with advancing age, following the pattern observed for ABR amplitude. AMLR findings in children under the age of 8 to 10 years must analyzed and interpreted with extreme caution. In addition to this potential age effect on AMLR, it is important to take into account other nonpathologic subject characteristics that might affect the response, including state of arousal, sedatives, and other drugs. These factors are discussed below.

As reviewed in Chapters 12, 13, and 14, there is tremendous research interest in application event-related potentials as a tool for the study of postnatal brain development and an early indicator of disruption in the brain development of children at risk for various central nervous system disorders, such as schizophrenia, alcoholism, and dyslexia. It is theorized that a disruption in sensory gating function is a characteristic of selected disorders (e.g., schizophrenia). The Pb component of the AMLR, also referred to as the P1 or P50 component, has attracted attention as a possible neurophysiologic marker for preattentive auditory functioning and sensory gating. The literature on the AMLR Pb component in clinical populations, including the above-noted disorders, is reviewed later in this chapter.

Kisley et al. (2003a,b) reported an investigation of the Pb (P1 or P50) component in eleven healthy infants, aged 1 to 5 months. The evoked responses were recorded while the infants were in REM sleep during a daytime nap. An additional nine subjects were enrolled in the study, but data were not included in the analysis because the infants did not remain within REM sleep during the AMLR recording. Sleep as a factor in AMLR recording and analysis is discussed in the next section of this chapter. In the study, responses were evoked with paired click signals presented at an intensity level of 85 dB peSPL, with a gap of 500 ms between the two clicks in a pair, and an interval of 10 seconds between the click pairs. The Pb component (called P1 by the authors) was recorded with a noninverting electrode at the Cz site using a band-pass filter setting of 0.5 to 100 Hz. The authors defined as evidence of sensory gating the difference in amplitude of the Pb component between the first and second click of the pair, described as a ratio. The first click was referred to as a conditioning (C) signal and the second click as the test (T) signal. The Pb component for the conditioning signal was identified within the latency region of 50 to 100 ms, and the response for the second (test) click was the peak occurring within 10 ms of the initial Pb component. Amplitude was measured from the trough preceding the Pb to the peak of the Pb component. An amplitude ratio, i.e., a T/C ratio, was calculated for the two stimuli. Sensory gating was considered robust if the response to the second "test" click was entirely suppressed by the first "conditioning" click, and the T/C ratio was 0. Citing work reported by Siegel, Waldo, Mizner, et al. (1984), the authors state that T/C ratios of < 0.4 in adult subjects imply intact sensory gating, whereas ratios > 0.5 suggest an impairment in sensory gating. The average latency for Pb (P1) evoked by the conditioning stimulus was 86.6 ms (standard deviation of 5.5 ms), and the average amplitude was 2.22 μV (s.d. of 1.73 μV), whereas the latency and amplitude values for the test stimulus were 87.6 μV (s.d. of 8.5 ms) and 0.90 μV (s.d. of 0.85 μV), respectively. In the study, the infants showed statistically significant suppression and the amount of suppression increased with subject age. This finding was interpreted as evidence that "the neural circuits underlying sensory gating are functional very early in postnatal development" (Kisley et al., 2003a,b, p. 693). The authors do acknowledge the possibility that changes in sleep status during the AMLR data collection could be a variable in the interpretation of the findings. This interesting study illustrates the influence of neural maturation (age) on the AMLR and also highlights a creative approach for applying the AMLR in the description of higher level auditory functions.

Curtis Ponton and colleagues (Ponton, Don, Eggermont, Waring, & Masuda, 1996) reported maturational changes in the latency of the P1 (Pb) component. The rate of maturation was different for normal subjects versus those with auditory deprivation prior to cochlear implantation. For normal-hearing subjects, latency of the P1 (Pb) component reached adult values by age 15 years, whereas maturation was not complete for subjects with a long period of auditory deprivation (over 8 years) until they were over 30 years old. Subjects with shorter periods of auditory deprivation, e.g., 1 or 5 years, showed intermediate delays in maturation of P1 (Pb) component latency. The authors conclude from these findings that the anatomic generators of the P1 (Pb) component require the effects of auditory stimulation for maturation. With the introduction of even intermittent auditory stimulation, even after years of deprivation, the auditory cortex is capable of maturation, an observation consistent with maintenance of neural plasticity in the auditory system despite childhood deafness.

ADVANCING AGE. | There is less attention in the literature of AMLR to the effects of advancing age. Woods and Clayworth (1986) compared AMLR data for a group of twelve young (20 to 40 years) versus twelve old (60 to 80 years) subjects. Stimuli were rarefaction clicks presented at a rate of 13/second at intensity levels of 50 and 60 dB sensation level (SL) above hearing threshold in monaural and binaural conditions. Both subject groups consisted of equal numbers of males and females. Latency of the Pa component was longer (by 2.3 ms on the average) in older versus younger

subjects. More striking, however, was the amplitude difference between groups. For each of three electrodes arrays, the Pa component was significantly larger in amplitude for the older subjects than the younger subjects. For example, with right ear stimulation at 60 dB SL, average Pa amplitude recorded at the vertex (Cz) electrode was 0.82 μvolts for the young group and 1.76 μvolts for the older group. The stimulus sound pressure level (at the 60 dB sensation level) was presumably higher for at least some of the older subjects than younger subjects because the average of 1000, 2000, and 4000 Hz pure-tone thresholds was 45 dB for the older group and only 6 dB for the younger subject group. However, ABR wave V and the AMLR Na component, in comparison, were equivalent between the two groups. Although AMLR components tended to be shorter in latency and larger in amplitude in female versus male subjects (Hall, 1992; Palaskas, Wilson, & Dobie, 1989), the differences do not always reach statistical significance (Özdamar & Kraus, 1983).

Other investigators (e.g., Amenedo & Diaz, 1998; Azumi, Nakashima, & Takahashi, 1995; Chambers, 1992; Lenzi, Chiarelli, & Sambataro, 1989; Pekkonen, Rinne, & Näätänen, 1995; Woods & Clayworth, 1986) have confirmed age-related changes in the AMLR, including poorer waveform morphology, as well as increased latency and amplitude. The effects of aging on latency and amplitude of the Na and Pa components of the AMLR are displayed in Figure 11.10. Yamada et al. (2003) recorded magnetic AMLRs from eleven younger (21 to 38 years, mean 30.5 years) and fifteen older (56 to 84 years, mean 70 years) subjects. Subject hearing status was not precisely defined. Rather, the authors' note "all subjects showed unimpaired hearing sensitivity within the frequency range 1000 to 2000 Hz." One would expect poor hearing sensitivity in an unselected group of healthy older subjects, in comparison to younger subjects, a suspicion supported by other publications on the AMLR in aging (e.g., Amenedo & Diaz, 1998). However, it would appear that poorer hearing sensitivity in the elderly group is not compatible with the overall findings of the study by Yamada et al. (2003), i.e., larger Pa amplitudes under certain measurement conditions yet no age-related difference in latency. The AMLR was evoked with 1000 Hz toneburst signals of 100 ms duration and at an intensity level of 95 dB SPL. All signals were presented only to the right ear. Recording were made with a 74-channel system, using an analysis time of 600 ms (prestimulus time of 100 ms) and band-pass filter settings of 1 to 100 Hz. Interstimulus intervals were randomly "jittered" between 610 and 1010 ms, corresponding roughly to signal rates of 1 to 2/second. The authors analyzed latency, amplitude, and neural source of the AMLR components using a single equivalent current dipole (ECD) model. Neurophysiologic and neuroanatomic factors possibly contributing to changes in the AMLR with age are listed in Table 11.3. Consistent with a previous report of a MEG study (Pekkonen et al., 1995), Yamada et al. (2003) recorded larger Pb (P50) components from the older

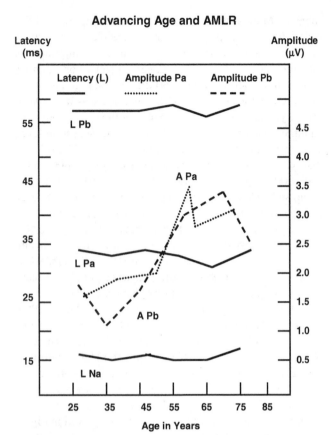

FIGURE 11.10. Effect of advancing age on latency and amplitude of the Na, Pa, and Pb components of the AMLR.

subject group and, among the older group, responses were larger as recorded over the left versus right hemisphere with contralateral (right ear) stimulation. No age differences or inter-hemispheric asymmetries were found for latency of the

TABLE 11.3. Summary of Neuroanatomic and Neurophysiologic Changes That Are Thought to Play a Role in the Changes in the AMLR with Advancing Age

- Alterations in cortical "folds" (and possibly the orientation of the scalp distribution of cortical AERs
- Cortical atrophy, including loss of functioning neurons in the auditory cortex (e.g., superior temporal gyrus)
- Reduced communication and feedback between the auditory cortex and subcortical structures (e.g., inferior colliculus in brainstem and medical geniculate body in the thalamus; decrease in the number of neurons projecting caudally from the temporal lobe)
- Decrease in gamma-aminobutyric acid (GABA) levels within thalamic auditory centers (i.e., decreased capacity for inhibition of cortical activity)
- Reduction in white matter in prefrontal cortex

From Amenedo & Diaz, 1998; Creasey & Rapoport, 1985.

P50 component. The N100m component findings, in distinct contrast, showed increased latency for the contralateral (left hemisphere), but no intergroup or interhemisphere difference in the amplitude of the N100m component.

Amenedo and Diaz (1998) also conducted an investigation of aging effects on AMLR. Subjects were seventy-three persons aged 20 to 86 years who "had subjective auditory thresholds that were normal for their age." The authors, however, documented behavioral thresholds for the click stimulus among age groups and took hearing status into account in the statistical analysis of their findings. The AMLR was evoked with rarefaction polarity clicks (0.1 ms duration) and at an intensity level of 60 dB SL (above behavioral threshold for the click). All signals were presented binaurally. Recordings were made simultaneously with twenty scalp electrodes, using an analysis time of 110 ms (prestimulus time of 10 ms) and band-pass filter settings of 1 to 300 Hz. The click presentation rate was 1.1/second. Among the age groups, there were no differences in the latency of AMLR components Na, Pa, Nb, and Pb. Gender differences for this study are described below. Taking into account subject hearing levels, age had a significant effect on the amplitude of all major AMLR components (Na, the Na-Pa complex, and Pb but not Pa amplitude), with enhanced amplitude for subjects over the age of 50 years. Again, trends in Pa and Pb latency and amplitude as a function of advancing age were illustrated in Figure 11.10 (adapted from Amenedo & Diaz, 1998).

Rasco, Skinner, and Garcia-Rill (2000) describe effects of aging on sensory gating, as measured with the conditioning/test stimulus paradigm of the AMLR P50 response. Subjects were in age groups from 12 to 78 years. Absolute amplitude of the P50 (Pb) component was equivalent across the age range (and for males versus females). Sensory gating, however, was reduced for only the adolescent age group (12 to 19 years) and for only an ISI of 250 ms (not for ISIs of 500 and 1000 ms). There was no change in sensory gating (the S2/S1 ratio for P50 amplitude) for younger versus older subjects.

Amenedo and Diaz (1998) and Yamada et al. (2003) make reference to previously suggested neurophysiologic explanations (e.g., Creasey & Rapoport, 1985; Woods & Clayworth, 1986) for the increased P50 amplitude in advance aging. One possible mechanism for the increased amplitude from cortically generated AMLR components is the reduction in the inhibition of auditory cortex function by subcortical regions (inferior colliculus in the brainstem and especially medial geniculate body in the thalamus) due to diminished gama-aminobutyric acid (GAMA) in aging. Conversely, there may be in advancing age diminished downward inhibition from layer VI of the auditory cortex to the inferior colliculus or from layer V to the medial geniculate body within the thalamus. A third potential neurophysiologic mechanism is the well-documented age-related reduction in white matter within the prefrontal regions of the cortex that plays a role in modulating or inhibiting activation of sensory cortical regions.

AUDITORY 40 HZ RESPONSE IN INFANCY AND CHILDHOOD. | For a period time in the 1980s, the auditory 40 Hz response (Galambos, Makeig, & Talmachoff, 1981) showed promise as a procedure for estimation of auditory thresholds in infants and young children. Experience with the auditory 40 Hz response confirmed, however, a strong relationship between age and signal rate. There is little question that for young children a slower stimulus rate than 40 per second is optimal for eliciting the so-called 40 Hz ERP. Perhaps the easiest way to view the effect of age on the auditory 40 Hz ERP is to consider the AMLR waveform and spectral composition for infants versus adults. In adults, AMLR peaks (i.e., Pa, Pb) appear at 25 ms intervals, or the occurrence of a positive peak 40 times per second (a rate of occurrence of 40 Hz). In addition, the most pronounced frequency component in the spectrum of the AMLR is around 40 Hz. In infants, AMLR peaks, especially Pa, occur about 50 ms after the stimulus, or at a rate of 20/second (40 Hz) and the greatest spectral energy in the infant AMLR is close to 20 Hz (Suzuki, Hirabayashi, & Kobayashi, 1983; Suzuki, Kobayashi, & Hirabayashi, 1983). For the superimposition of AMLR peaks to take place, they must be "driven" by the appropriate stimulus rate. The effectiveness of stimulation at 20 versus 40 stimuli/sec in evoking an auditory 40 Hz ERP in children versus adults was demonstrated by Suzuki, Hirabayashi, and Kobayashi (1983), Suzuki and Kobayashi (1984), and Stach (1986). The 40 Hz ERP is less likely to be recorded in newborn infants than in older children and adults, perhaps due to inconsistencies of EEG patterns in newborns (Fifer & Sierra-Irizarry, 1988). The clinical implication of the foregoing discussion is that the 40 Hz ERP may not be detectable in newborn infants, and even when present may not provide an accurate measure of auditory threshold (Kileny, 1984; Shallop & Osterhammel, 1983).

AUDITORY 40 HZ RESPONSE AND ADVANCING AGE IN ADULTS. | In a study of the topographic distribution of the 40 Hz auditory response, Johnson et al. (1988) found no significant differences in either amplitude or phase of the response for a group of elderly subjects (mean age of 70 years) versus younger subjects (mean age of 38 years). These authors did note reversal of the potential in the region of temporal auditory cortex, suggesting that this region contributes bilaterally in the generation of the response and confirming previous magneto-encephalographic investigations (Johnson et al., 1988; Mäkelä & Hari, 1987).

Gender

Given the pervasive influence of gender on the central nervous system in general, and specifically on in the region of the temporal lobe (e.g., Kulynych, Vladar, Jones, Weinberger, 1993; Witelson, 1991) and in auditory function (e.g., McFadden, 2002), a difference in AMLR findings for males versus females would not be surprising. It should be noted that gender differences in auditory anatomy and function are interactive with aging effects (e.g., Cowell et al., 1994). Researchers conducting investigations involving the AMLR often include both males and females among their subjects, and in most cases, examine statistically possible gender effects. Careful experimental design and subsequent analysis of data to rule out the influence of gender, and age, is advisable with an AER investigation, even if these two subject factors are irrelevant to the objective of the study. Clinical investigations to date have, in general, failed to demonstrate a clear and statistically significant gender affect in AMLR recordings (e.g., Özdamar & Kraus, 1983; Palaskas, Wilson, & Dobie, 1989; Phillips, Connolly, Mate-Kole, & Gray, 1997; Rodriguez-Holguin, Corral, & Cadaviera, 2001; Stewart, Jerger, & Lew, 1993). Some investigators, however, describe an apparent trend toward longer latencies and smaller amplitudes for selected components for males in comparison to females. This tendency is in agreement with the well-appreciated gender effect for ABR, i.e., shorter latencies and larger amplitudes for females versus males. According to findings reported by Amenedo and Diaz (1998), gender was a factor for the latency of the Na component, with average latency values that were longer for male versus female subjects, whereas latencies for other components and amplitude values for all AMLR components were equivalent for adult male and female subjects across the age span of 20 to 86 years. Phillips et al. (1997), in a study of elderly patients with Alzheimer's disease and a matched control group, found that the area under the Pb component was twice as large for females as for males.

Two features of the study might be factors in the apparent effect of gender on the AMLR Pb component. The authors reported that males in the control group were less likely than females to show a repeatable Pb component. Also, hearing status was not specified for any of the subjects in the study. In an elderly population (average age of 70 years), it's reasonable to expect a greater degree of hearing loss for male versus female subjects, especially in the higher frequency region that is important in generating AERs for click stimulation. Arguing against hearing status as a factor in the study, however, was the absence of a gender factor in the analysis of the Pa component. In a figure in the Phillips et al. (1997) paper, grand average AMLR waveforms were compared for the male and female subjects in the control group. Visual inspection showed reduced Pa amplitude for the male versus female subjects. Also, the Pa component was quite robust, whereas the Pb component was markedly smaller for both males and females. This observation is confirmed by the gender distribution for average amplitude values in the control group for the Pa and Pb components summarized in a table, i.e., average Pa amplitude was 0.83 μV for males and 1.35 μV females. Average amplitude for the Pb component, on the other hand, was − 0.21 μV for the males and + 0.21 μV for the females. The modest Pb amplitude data for the control group reported by Phillips et al. (1997) are curious, given the trend toward larger Pb amplitude values in normal aging. Phillips et al. (1997) acknowledged "difficulty in observing readily identifiable Pb responses in elderly control subjects . . ." (p. 131). Selected parameters of the AMLR protocol may help to explain the authors' findings and concerns. Nelson, Hall, and Jacobson (1997) found that tone-burst signals with relatively long durations were considerably more effective in evoking the Pb component than transient (0.1 ms) click signals. Also, the likelihood of consistently observing a Pb component is enhanced by extending the high-pass filter setting downward to 5 Hz, or even a setting used typically for recording the ALR, e.g., 1 Hz or 0.1 Hz. In the protocol described by Phillips et al. (1997), the AMLR was evoked with click signals, and the high-pass filter setting was 10 Hz. Phillips et al. (1997) displayed in figures in their paper replicated AMLR waveforms for all control and Alzheimer's disease subjects. Criteria for definition of the Pb component included the requirement that latency fall within the region of 50 to 68 ms. Close inspection of the waveforms in the figure showed control subjects with clear waves of positive voltage with peaks at the upper end of this range, or beyond the 68 ms limit. It's possible that data for some subjects with delayed Pb components, perhaps secondary to the effect of unknown hearing loss, were not included in the calculation of Pb amplitude.

In a study of aging (noted above), Rasco, Skinner, and Garcia-Rill (2000) also assessed possible gender effects on sensory gating using the conditioning/test stimulus paradigm of the AMLR P50 response. Absolute amplitude of the P50 (Pb) response was equivalent for males and females across the age span of 19 to 78 years. In addition, there was no significant difference in sensory gating, as indexed by the S2/S1 amplitude ratio for the P50 component.

STIMULUS EAR (RIGHT VERSUS LEFT). | The Pb component is more reliably recorded with right ear or binaural stimulation than signals presented to the left ear (e.g., Cacace et al., 1990). In an elderly population, Phillips et al. (1997) found no difference in AMLR Pa components evoked by right- versus left-ear stimulation, but the Pb component was observed with greater consistency and at higher amplitude for left- versus right-ear stimulation.

Handedness

With any electrophysiological response arising from cortical regions, it's reasonable to question whether handedness might affect latency or amplitude. There is, indeed, evidence of differences increased latency values for the AMLR Pa and, particularly, the Pb component for left- versus right-handed normal-hearing persons (Hood, Martin, & Berlin, 1990; Stewart, Jerger, & Lew, 1993). Stewart, Jerger, and Lew (1993) conducted an investigation of possible handedness effects on the AMLR with thirty-two normal-hearing (hearing thresholds of 15 dB HL or less) young adult (20 to 29 years)

subjects equally divided into those who were right handed and left handed. A preferred hand response on seven of the twelve items of the Annett Hand Preference Questionnaire (Annett, 1970) was used to define handedness. The AMLR was evoked with 1000 Hz tone bursts (2 ms rise/fall and 1 ms plateau) presented at a rate of 2.4 signals/second and an intensity level of 80 dB SPL. AMLR activity was recorded with a collection of 20 scalp electrodes, plus electrodes to detect eye-blink artifacts, and then band-pass filtered from 5 to 120 Hz. Approximately 2.5 hours were required for AMLR data collection for each subject. Analysis time was 100 ms, with a 14 ms prestimulus baseline. The global field power (GFP) technique was used for waveform analysis (Skrandies, 1990). For waveforms recorded at the Fz electrode site, there was no difference in Pa latency as a function of handedness. Confirming the findings published previously by Hood, Martin, and Berlin (1990), latency for the Pb component, however, was significantly longer in left-handed versus right-handed subjects. The average latency difference for the groups (left- minus right-handed subjects) was 2.4 ms for right-ear stimulation, 4.6 ms for left-ear stimulation, and 3.9 ms for binaural stimulation. Stewart, Jerger, and Lew (1993) did not comment on amplitude findings in their report. There was no statistically significant group interaction for gender and handedness effects and AMLR latency. When the gender effect was assessed with no regard to handedness (right- and left-handed subjects collapsed into one group), females showed longer Pb latencies values than males. There was no gender effect on the Pa component.

Muscle Interference (Artifact)

High-frequency muscle, and electrical, artifact is usually not a serious problem in AMLR recordings because the low pass (high-frequency limit of the recommended filter setting—200 to 1500 Hz) is effective in minimizing these types of measurement contamination. Low-frequency muscle artifact is, on the other hand, very troublesome since it often occurs within the same frequency region as the response. Elimination of this low frequency artifact by filtering is, therefore, not an alternative. The most effective clinical strategy for minimizing muscle artifact in the measurement of the AMLR is to verify that the patient is motionless and resting comfortably, with the head supported and the neck neither flexed nor extended. Best results are obtained when the patient is resting in a recliner or lying supine on a bed or gurney. For measurement of the AMLR, it is not advisable for the patient to be sitting upright in a straight-back chair with no head support.

Postauricular Muscle (PAM) Activity

As noted earlier in this chapter, PAM activity is elicited with a sound and recorded with an electrode near the ear (e.g., earlobe) and, especially, behind the ear (e.g., mastoid). The PAM response is one of numerous "sonomotor" or myogenic responses (Davis, 1965) that are described by the final efferent component, i.e., the muscle involved. The acoustic stapedial reflex is another sonomotor response well known to clinical audiologists. Since the PAM muscle activity is comparatively diminished in humans, averaging is usually required to observe the PAM response, but it is clearly visible in certain animals (such as dog) following an intense sound. An example of PAM activity in a normal young adult is shown in Figure 11.11. Postauricular muscle (PAM) artifact is sometimes apparent toward the end of an ABR waveform if an analysis time of 15 ms or longer is used, and it is not uncommon in AMLR measurement. PAM artifact is more likely to occur in patients who are tense and is usually observed when the inverting electrode is located on the earlobe or mastoid that is ipsilateral to the stimulus and at high (70 dB nHL or greater) intensity levels. However, PAM can also be recorded under other measurement conditions. Interestingly, PAM activity may be recorded from electrodes located on the side that is ipsilateral to the stimulus, contralateral to the stimulus, or even bilaterally with a monaural stimulus. The most effective electrode array for minimizing PAM activity includes a noncephalic reference electrode (Figure 11.11).

The clinician recording AMLR in the assessment of peripheral or central auditory nervous system function naturally views PAM as an annoyance, at the least, to be circumvented if at all possible. Indeed, initially there was a debate as to whether the AMLR was really a neurogenic response (arising from the nervous system) or, instead, a myogenic (arising from muscle) response from the postauricular muscles (Bickford, Galbraith, & Jacobson, 1963; Geisler, Frishkopf, & Rosenblith, 1958). Only after an AMLR was reliably recorded from persons during chemical paralysis (under the influence of neuromuscular blockade agents) was it considered a true neurogenic response (see Kileny, 1984). Interestingly, not long ago PAM activity was a desired response (versus an artifact) recorded intentionally as a measure of auditory function, much as the acoustic reflex is today. Ironically, the PAM response was proposed for essentially the same clinical purpose as the AMLR, namely as "objective" technique for auditory assessment in patient populations that were difficult to test by behavioral audiometry. The PAM response was also referred to as the crossed acoustic response (with its own acronym, CAR). This is a distinctly different response than the crossed (contralateral) acoustic reflex. The PAM response has been studied rather extensively (Cody & Bickford, 1969; Douek, Gibson, & Humphries, 1973; Humphries, Gibson, & Douek, 1976; Kiang, Crist, French, & Edwards, 1963; Thornton, 1975; Yoshie & Okidura, 1969). Clinical applications of the PAM response ranged from estimation of auditory threshold in children to evaluation of brainstem integrity in patients with neurological disorders (e.g., multiple sclerosis).

Knowledge about PAM is useful for the clinician who is intent on eliminating it as a factor in measurement of the

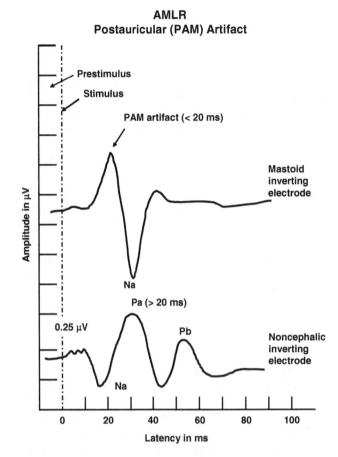

AMLR
Postauricular (PAM) Artifact

FIGURE 11.11. Effect of filter artifact on an AMLR recording (bottom portion). Filter artifact (artifactual Pa component) is eliminated with less restrictive filter settings. Waveforms in the upper portion of the figure show postauricular muscle (PAM) artifact. PAM is eliminated by the use of a noncephalic (nape of neck) inverting electrode, rather than an electrode near the ear (earlobe or mastoid).

AMLR. Anatomically, the PAM response is a brainstem reflex that is somewhat similar to the acoustic stapedial reflex. The optimal stimulus has an abrupt onset (e.g., a click) and is presented at a suprathreshold (usually high) intensity level. Stimuli with slow rise times may be ineffectual. The exact pathways are not known in man. The PAM response is equivalent, however, to the Preyer reflex in some animals (e.g., cat and guinea pig). On this basis, anatomic structures underlying the PAM response are thought to include the cochlear nuclei, superior olivary complex, nucleus of the lateral lemniscus, and possibly inferior colliculus (Gibson, 1975). The reticular formation, however, is an unlikely component (Galambos, 1956).

The triphasic response occurs in the 13 to 20 ms range and is optimally detected with an electrode on or in (via a needle electrode) the PAM lying over the mastoid region of the temporal bone, behind the ear. Amplitude ranges from 2 to 4 μvolts at low intensity levels to 20 μvolts or greater for high intensity levels (90 dB and above). As a rule, a larger response is detected with the inverting electrode located nearby (e.g., mastoid or earlobe). Under the appropriate recording conditions, a sound-elicited muscular response can also be detected from the posterior cervical muscles, frontalis muscles and temporalis muscles (Cody & Bickford, 1969), and from an electrode on the inion. The afferent portion of the PAM pathway is, of course, the eighth cranial nerve. A monaural stimulus produces bilateral contraction of the post-auricular muscles (Gibson, 1975; Kiang et al., 1963) with innervation of the muscles via the seventh (facial) cranial nerve. The researchers noted above who were engaged in purposeful measurement of the PAM response used a filter setting of approximately 1 to 200 Hz. Unfortunately, this is a common setting for AMLR recordings as well. Power spectral analysis of PAM response shows an energy peak mainly at 600 Hz, but the spectrum ranges from 100 through 1600 Hz (Thornton, 1975).

The likelihood of observing a PAM artifact is increased if the patient is anxious, tense, smiling or in a head-down position (flexion of the neck). With these maneuvers, Dus and Wilson (1975) recorded PAM activity to clicks from 89 percent of a group of thirty-seven adults. PAM artifact is diminished or eliminated by neck extension (Bickford et al., 1963; Kiang et al., 1963), anesthesia, muscle relaxants, alcohol and tranquilizers, and facial nerve paralysis (Cody, Jacobson, Walker, & Bickford, 1964; Gibson, 1975). There are reports of reduced or absent PAM activity during natural sleep (Erwin & Buchwald, 1986; Kileny, 1983; Yokoyama, Ryu, Uemura, Miyamaoto, & Imamura, 1987), but it is possible to record from comatose patients a distinct PAM from electrodes in the region near the ear that is on the same side or the opposite side from the signal, or bilaterally (Hall, Hargadine, & Allen, 1985; Hall & Tucker, 1986). Yokoyama et al. (1987) suggest that the No and Po components variably seem in AMLR recordings during light sleep are remnants of PAM activity.

Robinson and Rudge (1977) found that the PAM response was absent when recorded from an electrode ipsilateral to the stimulus in 15 percent of normal subjects and absent bilaterally in 40 percent of normal subjects (all of whom showed clear AMLRs). Inconsistency in recording the PAM response is not unexpected, since the rapid stimulation could lead to muscle fatigue, a common component of muscle physiology. However, little recovery time is apparently needed since the response can be observed for stimulus rates as high as 200/sec (Kiang et al., 1963). The effect of repetitive stimulation on the PAM is unclear (e.g., Davis, 1964). Kiang et al. (1963) found that an electrical shock to the foot was useful in resuscitating a flagging PAM response. Amplitude of the PAM response is somewhat variable (usually in the range of 5 to 15 μvolts), but latency is remarkably constant (estimated at approximately 8 ms by Gibson, 1975) and bilaterally symmetrical, with an interside difference of less than 0.6 ms (Clifford-Jones, Clarke, & Mayles, 1979).

The neuromuscular junction transmission accounts for 0.7 ms of this latency for a high (80 dB SPL) intensity level (Totsuka, Nakamura, & Kirikae, 1954). In contrast to the experiences reported by Robinson and Rudge (1977), these investigators described PAM response evaluation as quick and easy and were able to obtain a clear response in fifty-two of fifty-three normal subjects, although with some they found it necessary to resort to special techniques, such as neck flexion against resistance. As with other AERs, differences in stimulus parameters (e.g., rise time, intensity) and subject characteristics probably contributed to discrepancies among studies. In their study of sensory evoked responses in MS, Clifford-Jones et al. (1979) found that 73 percent of their patients yielded abnormal PAM response findings, a higher proportion than for other tests of brainstem function and for somatosensory evoked responses (SERs) or visual evoked responses (VERs). Douek et al. (1973) also noted the diagnostic value of PAM response in MS, and also in patients with brainstem lesions. Remarkably, abnormal findings for the PAM response were present for thirty-four out of forty-nine MS patients who had no clinical signs. Gibson (1975) presented preliminary data for three patients with acoustic tumors (vestibular schwannomas) indicating abnormally small PAM responses.

Artifact related to movement in general can interfere with AMLR recording, and postauricular muscle (PAM) activity can obscure or distort components in the 12 to 25 ms latency region (e.g., Na, Pa), or actually be mistaken for an AMLR (Kileny, 1983). There was, as noted above, a debate among early investigators of AMLR (Bickford, 1964) about whether the response was actually neurogenic (arising from the auditory nervous system), partly neurogenic and partly myogenic (a muscle potential), or entirely myogenic, prompted by reports offered in support of the latter theory (Bickford, Jacobson, & Cody, 1964) and the second theory (Mast, 1965).

Patuzzi and O'Beirne (1999) systematically investigated in four adults and two infants the interrelationships between signal intensity level and the enhancement of PAM response amplitude with variables such as voluntary contraction of the muscle, electrode location, eye rotation, and electromyographic (EMG) noise in an attempt to define optimal recording conditions. These authors also discussed techniques for averaging the response and performing various statistical analysis strategies, e.g., a correlation measure. A detailed review of the paper is beyond the scope of this chapter. Readers who are interested in the PAM response as a potential measure of auditory sensitivity or a neurodiagnostic tool are encouraged to review this paper.

Attention

Repetitive acoustic stimulation has no apparent effect on the ECochG and ABR. That is, the response does not diminish with ongoing presentation of a repetitive signal, e.g., clicks or tone bursts. In addition, neither of these short-latency responses is affected by subject attention. In contrast, components of the AMLR show habituation with ongoing repetition of the signal. Specifically, the amplitude of the AMLR Pb (or P50) component decreases with repetitive auditory stimulation. This is not an adaptation of the response due to neural fatigue or the inability of the neurons to continue firing at a constant rate. The effects of repetition are considered evidence of an automatic inhibition of irrelevant sensory input, also referred to as "sensory gating." On the other hand, when the AMLR is recorded with an oddball paradigm, i.e., the occasional and random presentation of a different signal, there is an increase in Pb (P50) amplitude as the brain detects a novel and potentially meaningful signal. These contrasting responses to either repetitive or changing signals can also be viewed as, respectively, inhibitory and excitatory.

Habituation

As reviewed earlier in this chapter (in the section on "stimulus number and repetition"), there is a growing literature on the application of the AMLR P1 (Pb) component in clinical investigations of short-term habituation (e.g., Rosburg et al., 2004). With the "double-click paradigm," two transient signals are presented with a relatively brief interval of about 500 ms, and then the pair of signals is separated by a longer interstimulus interval (e.g., 8 to 12 seconds). Normally, amplitude of the P1 (Pb) component is reduced for the second signal in the pair, a finding interpreted as "sensory gating" within the brain. Sensory gating is taken as evidence of inattention to irrelevant and repetitive (redundant) stimulation, permitting the brain to focus on important and meaningful external stimulation. According to Rosburg et al. (2004), there are several methodologic differences between studies of sensory gating and habituation. For example, sensory gating experiments employ shorter and more consistent intervals between the pairs of signals (in the click train) than habituation studies. Also, transient signal durations (e.g., 0.1 ms clicks) are used with sensory gating measurements, whereas in habituation studies the signals are typically longer duration tones (> 30 ms). Finally, studies of sensory gating involve analysis of amplitude for the P1 (Pb) component of the AMLR, while the N100 wave of the ALR is often employed in studies of short-term habituation.

State of Arousal and Sleep

In adult subjects, the AMLR can be reliably recorded in light sleep and after mild sedation and in different states of subject attention (Kupperman & Mendel, 1974; Mendel & Goldstein, 1969; Mendel & Hosick, 1975; Mendel, Hosick, Windman, Davis, Hirsh, & Dinges, 1975; Okitsu, 1984; Osterhammel, Shallop, & Terkildsen, 1985; Özdamar & Kraus, 1983; Picton & Hillyard, 1974; Skinner & Shimota, 1975; Suzuki, Hirabayashi, & Kobayashi, 1983). However, sleep, sedation and attention exert clinically important influences on the AMLR, especially in infants and children, and must be

considered in interpretation of the response (Jerger, Chmiel, Frost, & Coker, 1986; Jerger & Jerger, 1985; Okitsu, 1984).

Stages of sleep are summarized in Table 11.4. Sleep is not a major factor the interpretation of findings in adults

TABLE 11.4. Key Features of the Five Stages of Sleep
Additional information on sleep is reviewed in the text.

STAGE	FEATURES
1	Best described as falling asleep (or dozing during a class), sleep stage 1 is the 1- to 5-minute transition between wakefulness and true sleep. The relative proportion of alpha waves in the EEG (8 to 12 Hz) decreases. Theta EEG waves (4 to 7 Hz) become apparent. During a normal night of sleep, approximately 2 to 5 percent of time is spent in sleep stage 1.
2	During the night, a person repeatedly completes cycles of sleep lasting about 1.5 hours (90 minutes). Sleep stage 2 is the beginning of the true sleep cycle, with no awareness of external events. During a normal night of sleep, up to one-half of the time or a little more (45 to 60%) is spent in sleep stage 2. The EEG is characterized by the theta rhythm or frequency, along with K-complexes and spindles.
3	Sleep stage 3 takes about 10 to 20 minutes and leads to the deepest type of sleep (stage 4). During sleep stage 3, the EEG rhythm or frequencies begin to slow down to only 1 or 2 Hz, and EEG amplitude increases markedly (> 75 μV). Hence, sleep stage 3 (and stage 4) are often referred to as "slow wave sleep (SWS)."
4	Sleep stage 4 is commonly known as "Delta sleep" because it is characterized by a slow and large wave EEG rhythm. Stage 4 is the most restful and restorative phase of the sleep cycle (not REM sleep). Arousal is most difficult for persons in sleep stage 4—deep sleep. Children are in this deep sleep stage for up to 40 percent of total sleep time.
5	The fifth stage is REM (rapid eye movement) sleep. Sleep stages 1 through 4 are, therefore, described as "non-REM sleep." It's characterized by increased physical activity, including more rapid breathing, heart rate, brain (EEG) activity, and also vivid dreams. An adult is in the REM stage up to about 25 percent of a normal night, or about every 90 minutes during the night and for progressively longer durations. A person generally returns to stage 2 after REM sleep. Auditory evoked responses recorded during REM sleep are most similar to those recorded during wakefulness. Paradoxically, large muscles in the body are most relaxed (muscle atonia) during REM sleep, even though the small ocular muscles and the brain are very active. For this reason, sleep stage 5 is sometimes described as "paradoxical sleep."

(Okitzu, 1984; Osterhammel et al., 1985). Amplitude of the Pa component may be modestly reduced, particularly in sleep stages 3 and 4, but stability of the AMLR Pa component is expected in sleep states 1 and 2 and in rapid eye movement (REM) sleep. Age interacts with sleep in the detection of the AMLR. Age as a factor in AMLR analysis and interpretation was reviewed earlier in this chapter. As a general rule, for all stages of sleep, the detection of the AMLR is more likely as the rate of signal presentation is reduced. With relatively slow rates of 1 signal per second, the AMLR is typically detected even in sleep, but the amplitude of the Pa component decreases substantially for faster signal rates up to 20/second and higher (Erwin & Buchwald, 1986; Jerger, Chmeil, Frost, & Coker, 1986; McGee & Kraus, 1996).

Given this discussion of the effects of state of arousal on the AMLR, one might anticipate considerable problems in AMLR measurement with children and, in particular, newborn infants. Indeed, with pediatric applications of AMLR, sleep is a critical factor to consider in the analysis and interpretation of findings. And, the effects of sleep interact with the influence of another factor, chronological age or, more precisely, maturation of the primary sensory (thalamocortical) pathways underlying the response. Within the first two to three weeks after birth, newborn babies are in a REM sleep state much of the time (Thomas, Davis, & Denenberg, 1987). Thus, for newborn infants it's not as critical to document sleep stage as for older children and, fortunately, the AMLR is usually recorded without a decrement in Pa amplitude. Beyond the newborn period, and through the first few years after birth, the proportion of time each day that a child is in REM sleep continues to decrease to less than 20 percent and the likelihood of recording an AMLR in sleep also decreases (McGee et al., 1993). Specifically, the presence of a detectable AMLR Pa component is inversely related to presence of delta EEG activity in sleep.

For infants and young children, the effects of sleep state on AMLR are now well recognized and must be taken account to accurately analyze and interpret the response (e.g., Hall, 1992; Kraus, Kileny, & McGee, 1994; Kraus, McGee, & Comperatore, 1989; Okitzu, 1984; Stapells et al., 1988). The AMLR can be clearly recorded in REM sleep and also sleep stage 1, but the AMLR is more variable and inconsistent in sleep stage 2. The AMLR is rarely detected in sleep stage 3, and it's altogether absent in sleep stage 4. The effect of selected sleep stages on the AMLR is illustrated in Figure 11.12. These rather dramatic effects of sleep on the AMLR are a good example of the dependence of the response for activation on the reticular formation, as reviewed in Chapter 2. Clearly, ongoing documentation of sleep stage during AMLR measurement provides information that is useful for the analysis and interpretation of AMLR findings in pediatric populations. There is an interaction in the effects on the AMLR between age and state of arousal. The likelihood that an AMLR will be consistently recorded increases both as a function of chronological age, from infancy through adolescence, and also with heightened state of arousal (e.g., from sleep to the awake state).

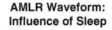

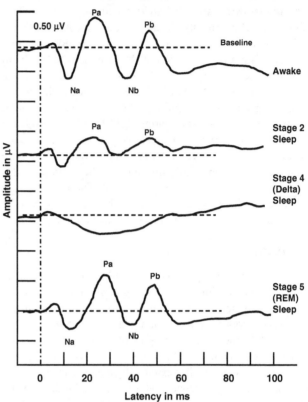

FIGURE 11.12. An example of the effect of sleep on the AMLR. AMLR amplitude is markedly reduced when a person is falling asleep and during sleep stages 2 through 4. However, a normal-appearing AMLR waveform can be recorded during rapid eye movement (REM) sleep (stage 5).

Kadobayashi and Toyoshima (1984) found decreased amplitude for the Pa component of the AMLR when subjects paid no attention to click stimuli. On the other hand, the Pa component in adults was stable across sleep conditions (wakefulness, slow wave sleep and rapid eye movement sleep), according to Erwin and Buchwald (1986). In general, wave Pa amplitude tends to be reduced during sleep in comparison to the awakened state, by up to 40 percent of maximum in stage IV sleep. Latency, on the other hand, remains stable in sleep (Mendel & Goldstein, 1971; Osterhammel, Shallop, & Terkildsen, 1985).

Before the full clinical potential of the response is exploited clinically, additional information on the interactions among drugs, age, and the AMLR is needed. The investigations must be carried out with humans, since it appears the AMLR in some animal models (e.g., cat) is resistant to the effect of sleep and drugs, such as anesthesia, probably because there are different anatomic generators for the AMLR components in man versus animal (Kaga, Hink, Shinoda, & Suzuki, 1980).

Auditory 40 Hz ERP

State of arousal can definitely influence the auditory 40 Hz response (Dauman, Szyfter, Charlet de Sauvage, & Cazals, 1984; Jerger, Chmiel, Frost, & Coker, 1986; Kankkunen & Rosenhall, 1985; Linden, Campbell, Hamel, & Picton, 1985; Palaskas, Wilson, & Dobie, 1989; Sammeth & Barry, 1985; Shallop & Osterhammel, 1983; Szyfter et al., 1984). The exact effect of sleep on estimations of thresholds with the auditory 40 Hz response, however, is not clear. Although Linden et al. (1985) noted reduced amplitude (but not phase) during sleep they found no difference in auditory SSEP threshold values in awake vs. sleeping subjects. Likewise, Jerger, Chmiel, Frost, and Coker (1986), in a study of auditory 40 Hz ERP elicited by a 500 Hz tone pip during natural and sedated sleep in nine normal-hearing subjects, showed a sleep-related decrease in amplitude, little change in phase variability (phase coherence) and no difference in auditory threshold estimates as a function of sleep. Decreased amplitude and increased threshold levels are reported for subjects who are asleep versus awake (Dauman et al., 1984; Kankkunen & Rosenhall, 1985; Szyfter et al., 1984). The overall effects of sleep tend to be similar for the 40 Hz response and the conventional AMLR. That is, amplitude is reduced by 50 percent or more during sleep (Davis, Hirsh, & Turpin, 1983; Jerger, Chmiel, et al., 1986). The attention to acoustic signals does not appear to play a role in measurement of the auditory 40 Hz response (Linden, Picton, Hamel, & Campbell, 1987; Spydell et al., 1985).

Body Temperature

In contrast to the substantial literature on effects of temperature, especially hypothermia, on ECochG and ABR, there are few studies of AMLR and temperature. Kileny et al. (1983) monitored hypothermic patients undergoing open-heart surgery with AMLR. (Hall, 1992; Hall, Ball, & Cronau, 1988) applied AMLR in monitoring patients undergoing hyperthermia (increased body temperature) treatment for advanced cancer. There is evidence of decreased latency yet reduced amplitude of the Pa component in some patients as body temperature is elevated from normal levels (about 37 degrees Centigrade) to 42.2 degrees C. This is not, however, a consistently observed finding.

Drugs

An overview of the terminology and mechanisms of sedatives and anesthetic agents is provided toward the end of Chapter 8. The following discussion is limited, for the most part, to the effect of drugs on the AMLR.

SEDATIVES. | Although accumulated clinical experience and published reports confirm that chloral hydrate does not affect ABR (Mokotoff, Schulman-Galambos, & Galambos, 1977;

Palaskas, Wilson, & Dobie, 1989; Sohmer & Student, 1978), amplitude of the Pa component of the AMLR is decreased and latency may be increased (Okitsu, 1984; Osterhammel, Shallop, & Terkildsen, 1985; Palaskas et al., 1989). Changes in the AMLR with chloral hydrate sedation are more pronounced when the stimulation rate is increased (from 4 stimuli/second to 10 stimuli/second). This experimental finding has obvious clinical implications for AMLR evaluation of children. Chlorate hydrate sedation (2 grams) also reduces the amplitude, and increases the latency, of the auditory 40 Hz response (Palaskas et al., 1989). In addition, threshold level of response detection is increased by 9 to 12 dB HL in the sedated state.

Meperidine is an IV opioid analgesic, like morphine, that has no apparent effect on early or late latency AERs. Droperidol (dehydrobenzperidol) produces a latency prolongation of about 10 m for AMLR Pb component (and the ALR N1 component) and amplitude reduction (Pfefferbaum, Roth, Tinklenberg, Rosenbloom, & Kopell, 1979).

Anesthetic Agents

During the past twenty-five years, an increasing number of papers have described the application of AMLRs during surgical procedure as an index of the depth of anesthesia. The characteristic effect of anesthetic agents on the amplitude and latency of AMLR components is shown in Figure 11.13. The

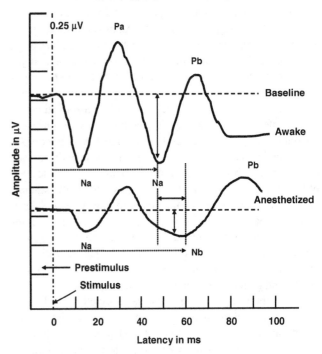

FIGURE 11.13. Illustration of the effect of anesthesia on latency and amplitude of the AMLR. The AMLR can be used as a neurophysiologic index in monitoring depth of anesthesia during surgery.

literature on this relatively new application of the AMLR is discussed below (under Clinical Applications). An appreciation of the effects of anesthetic agents on AERs is essential for any clinician involved in neurophysiologic intraoperative monitoring during surgery. Anesthesia is defined as loss of sensation (partial or complete), with or without loss of consciousness, that may be drug-induced or due to disease or injury. The following discussion will be limited to general anesthesia that affects the brain and produces loss of sensation and consciousness. Local anesthesia of nerves serving a specific anatomic region may be used in AER measurement. An example would be Phenol (89 percent) that effectively numbs the tympanic membrane for transtympanic needle ECochG recordings. The ECochG response is, of course, not affected.

Depth or stage of general anesthesia may be described according to different schema. According to one description, there are three stages. In stage one, the patient is first excited until voluntary control is lost (hearing is the last of the senses to become nonfunctional). The corneal reflex is still present in the second stage of anesthesia, although loss of voluntary control persists. The third stage of anesthesia is defined as complete relaxation, deep regular breathing, and a sluggish corneal reflex. There are four stages of anesthesia according to another schema, including: (1) analgesia (no feeling), (2) delirium, (3) surgical anesthesia, and (4) medullary depression. From these terms, it is clear that the patient should be maintained in stage 3 during surgery. Stages 1 and 2 represent inadequate anesthesia, while anesthesia is excessive in stage 4.

Before anesthesia, drugs are administered to decrease anxiety, relieve pre- and postoperative pain and provide amnesia for the perioperative period. Examples of these drugs are benzodiazepines (e.g., Valium), conscious sedatives (e.g., Versed), barbiturates, and neuroleptics. There are three major components to anesthesia. The purpose of the first component, induction, is to produce a rapid loss of consciousness. Drugs used to induce anesthesia include benzodiazepines, barbiturates, narcotic analgesics, etomidate, ketamine, and inhalation agents. The second, and longest lasting, component is maintenance of anesthesia. The purpose of this phase, which persists throughout surgery, is to produce a stable state of loss of consciousness and loss of reflexes to painful stimuli. Among the drugs often administered to during maintenance of anesthesia are inhalational agents (gases), narcotic analgesics, ketamine, muscle relaxants, and anti-arrhythmic agents. Finally, anesthesia must be reversed so the patient will wake up and return to the preanesthetic state. This is achieved with opioid antagonists and anticholinesterase agents.

Anesthetic agents are often categorized according to their mode of administration. Some are intravenous (IV) agents, infused directly into the bloodstream via a line inserted into a vein (at the wrist or ankle). Examples of IV agents are barbiturates (thiopental/Sodium Pentothal, methohexital/Brevital, thiamylal), benzodiazepines (diazepam/Valium, midazolam), etomidates (amidate), opioid analgesics (morphine, fentanyl, meperidine), neuroleptics (droperidol + fentanyl), and dissociative anesthetic agents (ketamine). With IV anesthetics, there is fast action and fast recovery. The brain receives one-tenth of the dose within 40 seconds following IV administration. Other anesthetic agents are administered as a gas by inhalation. Inhalational agents, in contrast to those administered IV, are slower acting and are measured by partial pressure (tension) in the blood (brain). One commonly used inhalational agent is nitrous oxide, a gaseous anesthetic that is a good analgesic and induction agent, but has low anesthetic potency. Others are called volatile anesthetics (e.g., halothane, isoflurane), which are potent even at low concentrations.

As noted in Chapter 8, anesthetic agents produce differential effects on AERs. ECochG components, which are dependent on the end organ (cochlea) and eighth nerve, are not seriously influenced by anesthesia. The ABR is generated by the eighth cranial nerve and by primary (lemniscal) sensory pathways within the brainstem. The ABR is, however, influenced by selected drugs, e.g., enflurane and halothane. In contrast, so-called "extralemniscal" responses (e.g., AMLR, ALR), which involve multisynaptic nonlemniscal pathways, are highly sensitive to the effects of anesthetic agents on the central nervous system (refer to Figure 11.13. These responses are also affected to a greater degree by sedatives, such as chloral hydrate. Unfortunately, much of the information on the relationship between the anesthesia and these latter AERs was obtained from animal experiments versus clinical experience (e.g., Pradhan & Galambos, 1963; Smith & Kraus, 1987).

HALOGENATED INHALATIONAL AGENTS. | The halogenated inhalational drugs, such as desflurane, enflurane, halothane, isoflurane, and sevoflurane, are commonly used clinical in various types of surgery. In general, the halogenated inhalational agents depress the EEG and produce increases in AER latency and decreases in amplitude (Sloan, 1998, 2002), including AMLR parameters.

FENTANYL. | Fentanyl is a popular narcotic analgesic. In adults anesthetized with fentanyl, Kileny et al. (1983) observed only slight alterations in AMLR latency and, as with chemical paralysis, noted improved waveform quality as muscle activity subsided. In general, however, even high doses of fentanyl do not appreciably affect the AMLR and, in fact, fentanyl is recommended as an anesthetic when the AMLR is applied intraoperatively (e.g., Sasaki, 1991). There are a growing number of reports of monitoring depth of anesthesia that is induced or maintained with fentanyl (e.g., Nishiyama, Matsukawa, & Hanaoka, 2004; White et al., 2004).

SUFENTANIL. | Sufentanil is a narcotic anesthetic that is ten times more potent than fentanyl, but provides a greater margin of safety because is produces less hemodynamic stress than fentanyl.

ENFLURANE. | With therapeutic doses of enflurane, significantly increased latency and reduced amplitude of AMLR and ALR are expected. Enflurane produces marked dose-dependent reduction in the amplitude of the AMLR Pa and Nb components and increased latency (Thornton et al., 1981, 1984). The response is observed, however, with end-tidal concentrations of over 2.5 percent.

SEVOFLURANE. | Weber, Hahne, Friedrich, and Friederici, (2004) reported in a study of twenty children undergoing eye surgery that the AMLR showed predictable effects by the inhalational agent sevoflurane.

DESFLURANE. | Christine Thornton and colleagues from the United Kingdom have conducted many of the germinal studies on monitoring depth of anesthesia with the AMLR. Recently, these authors and others (e.g., Dutton et al., 1999) have confirmed that the effects of the volatile inhalational anesthetic agent desflurane are similar to those for other anesthetic agents (Thornton, Heyderman, Thorniley, et al., 2002; White et al., 2004).

FLUOROTHANE. | AMLR recorded from nine children ages 1 to 4 years under general anesthesia with fluorothane was characterized by abnormally increased latency, reduced amplitude, and instability (greater variability in peak latency and lack of replicability) according to Prosser and Arslan (1985).

PROPOFOL. | Propofol is a commonly used anesthetic agent that is administered intravenously. Studies in neurologically normal adults (Cagy & Infantosi, 2002; Struys et al., 2002; Tooley, Stapleton, Greenslade, & Prys-Roberts, 2004) confirm that anesthesia with propofol is associated with a dose-dependent delay in latency and reduction in amplitude for the AMLR Nb component. Tooley et al. (2004) reported that the addition of alfentanil lowers the propofol infusion rate needed to produce an unconscious state without affecting the relation between propofol and the AMLR. Other investigators (e.g., White et al., 2004) have also reported the use of AMLR as an index of depth of anesthesia induced or maintained during surgery with propofol.

REMIFENTANIL. | Wright et al. (2004) conducted a placebo-controlled study of the effect of remifentanil on the AMLR. There was an intubated and nonintubated group of subjects. A control group received a bolus of saline. All subjects were anesthetized with isoflurane and nitrous oxide and then randomized into different groups (based on intubation and the placebo). The authors conclude that remifentanil affects the AMLR by reducing the arousal generated by tracheal intubation. Weber et al. (2004) confirmed that remifentanil has no direct effect on the AMLR.

ETOMIDATE. | Etomidate is an IV anesthetic agent that has no effect on ABR but, for AMLR, produces significant increases in component Pa and Nb latency and reductions in amplitude. These changes are dependent on serum concentration. The effects on AMLR were comparable to those of halothane and enflurane on ALR peaks (Navaratnarajah, Thornton, Heneghan, Bateman, & Jones, 1983).

THIOPENTAL. | Sodium pentothal is an IV barbiturate. Effects of thiopental on late AERs were demonstrated by Abrahamian, Allison, Goff, and Rosner (1963).

PENTOBARBITAL. | Pentobarbital, a fast-acting barbiturate, severely or totally suppresses AMLR and ALR (Hall, 1985).

KETAMINE. | Ketamine (hydrochloride) is a dissociative IV anesthetic that works by altering limbic system activity, but not medullary structures. In the guinea pig, AMLR latency is increased with ketamine, while the amplitude of early components is made larger, and later components are made smaller or are not observed (Smith & Kraus, 1987). Importantly, AMLR changes were more pronounced as stimulus rate was increased. In the cat, ketamine likewise produced mixed effects on AERs recorded directly from electrodes placed in inferior colliculus and mesencephalic reticular formation (Dafny & Rigor, 1978). Lower doses reduced amplitude while higher doses increased amplitude and also latency. Activity in the inferior colliculus showed the greatest sensitivity to ketamine effects. However, ketamine appears to have no significant effect on the AMLR (Sasaki, 1991; Weber et al., 2004).

NITROUS OXIDE. | This drug is a gaseous, inhalation agent that is a good analgesic. It is used to induce anesthesia, but has low potency (strength) for maintaining anesthesia. ABR is resistant to the effects of nitrous oxide. AER components with latency values beyond 50 ms show dose dependent reduction in amplitude, yet latency is not affected (Lader, 1977).

Neuromuscular Blockers (Chemical Paralyzing Agents)

These drugs produce paralysis by interrupting transmission of neural impulses at the skeletal neuromuscular junction. Examples of neuromuscular blockers used in the operating room and intensive care unit are pancuronium (Pavulon), Metocurine, succinylcholine, and curare. All AERs can be reliably recorded during chemically induced muscle paralysis with such agents as Pavulon, Metocurine, and succinylcholine (Hall, 1988; Hall, Hargadine, & Allen, 1985; Hall, Mackey-Hargadine, & Kim, 1985; Harker, Hosick, Voots, & Mendel, 1977; Kileny, 1983; Kileny, Dobson, & Gelfand, 1983; Smith & Kraus, 1987). Waveforms are, in fact, often enhanced in patients under the influence of chemical paralysis due to the lack of muscle-related noise or artifact.

Tranquilizers and Psychotherapeutic Agents

Tranquilizers are referred to as neuroleptic drugs that are thought to block postsynaptic dopaminergic receptors in the mesolimbic region of the brain. Minor tranquilizers are anti-anxiety and sleeping drugs, such as diazepam and Librium.

Major tranquilizers are used as antipsychotic agents. Other psychotherapeutic agents are lithium-based drugs, used to treat manic disorders. The mechanism is unknown, but alteration of neuronal and neurotransmitter function is suspected. There is a long list of antipsychotic drugs. All are, by definition, psychotropic and may affect longer latency AERs, including possibly the AMLR Pb component.

Other Drugs Influencing AERs

ALCOHOL. | Although alcohol-related brain damage and dysfunction is well appreciated and documented, there are few studies of chronic alcohol abuse on the AMLR (Ahveninen et al, 1999a; Diaz, Cadaveira, & Grau, 1990; Katbamma, Metz, Adelman, & Thodi, 1993). This is in contrast to the hundreds of publications on the effect of chronic alcohol use on the P300 and MMN responses (reviewed in Chapters 13 and 14). The AMLR studies in withdrawal or detoxification from alcoholism have produced conflicting results, including decreased latencies (Diaz, Cadaveira, & Grau, 1990) and prolonged latencies (Katbamma, Metz, Adelman, & Thodi, 1993). Confounding factors in the subject groups, e.g., other drug use, may have contributed to the discrepancies.

Ahveninen et al. (1999a) studied the influence of chronic alcoholism on the AMLR Pa component in a group of fourteen male alcoholics who were within one to six weeks of a period of abstinence, and a control group of thirteen age-matched male social drinkers. The AMLR was evoked with click signals presented binaurally at an intensity of 60 dB SL (above hearing threshold). The authors did not specify either the signal rate or signal duration. The response was detected with noninverting scalp electrodes located at Cz, C5, and C6, and band-pass filtered with settings of 10 to 250 Hz. Amplitude of the Pa component was significantly larger in the alcohol subject group. Average latency values for the Pa components were about 3 ms shorter for the alcohol group, but the difference was not statistically significant. The results are interpreted as evidence of brain hyperexcitability that characterizes withdrawal from chronic alcohol abuse.

Rodriguez-Holguin, Corral, and Cadaveira (2001) applied the AMLR in an investigation of children at risk for alcoholism. Subjects were fifteen children in a high-risk group (seven males and eight females with an average age of 12 years) with an alcoholic father and strong family history of alcoholism (two or three close alcoholic relatives) and a control group consisting of seventeen children (seven male and ten female with an average age of 12 years) matched in terms of socioeconomic status and education who had no family history of alcoholism, including their fathers and close relatives according to findings for the Semi-Structured Assessment for the Genetics of Alcoholism (SSAGA). All subjects were also carefully screened for factors such as psychological disorders, prenatal exposure to alcohol, developmental or academic disorders, any medications, sensory deficits, and a family history of mental disease. Subjects sat in a comfortable chair in a electrically isolated and sound-treated room during AMLR measurements. As is typical for AMLR investigations, subjects were instructed to focus their gaze to a point 1 meter in front of their eyes (to minimize the potential contamination of eye movements). AMLRs were evoked with rarefaction polarity clicks (0.1 ms duration) presented binaurally at a rate of 1.1/second at an intensity of 60 dB SL (above behavioral threshold for the click signal). The responses were recorded with noninverting electrodes located at Cz and Fz and linked earlobe inverting electrodes, with band-pass filter settings of 1 to 300 Hz and an analysis time of 100 ms and a prestimulus time of 10 ms. The authors reported significantly smaller amplitude for the Pa component and shorter latency for the Pb component in the group at high risk for alcoholism versus the control group. In addition, there was an interaction between age and alcohol risk for the AMLR. Latency of the Pa component decreased with age in this pediatric population, and the effect was relatively greater for the alcohol risk group than the control group. Rodriguez-Holguin et al. (2001) are apparently the first investigators to report an effect of alcohol risk in children on the AMLR Pb component. The finding of relationship between age and decreased Pa latency in alcohol risk is consistent with previous reports (e.g., Diaz, Cadaveira, & Grau, 1990). On the other hand, the authors did not expect to find decreased Pa amplitude in children at risk for alcohol abuse since abstinent adult alcoholics show increased Pa amplitude (e.g., Diaz, Cadaveira, & Grau, 1990). It may be relevant to note that larger Pa amplitudes also have been reported in the elderly, as noted above, and with selected patient populations, such as Alzheimer's disease and prefrontal lobe cortical pathology (Phillips, Connolly, Mate-Kole, & Gray, 1997).

NICOTINE. | Harkrider and Champlin (2001a) investigated the possible effect of nicotine on the AMLR. Previous basic research has shown that regions of the CNS that contribute to the generation of the AMLR are affected by the cholinergic mechanisms that are associated with nicotine. Subjects were twenty nonsmoking young adults (ten male and ten female). The AMLR and the 40 Hz response was evoked with click signals with negative polarity presented at two rates (8.1/second and 39.9/second) and at an intensity level of 70 dB nHL (104 peSPL). A double-blind, controlled experimental design was used for counterbalanced four-hour administration of the placebo or the nicotine with a patch on the arm. Nicotine levels were documented by blood plasma analysis. Harkrider and Champlin (2001a) reported an increase in the Na-Pa amplitude with nicotine administration. This finding is consistent with the neural stimulation effect (excitability), via release of Ach secondary to cholinergic agonists, on projection pathways from subcortical structures to the cortex.

Nicotine also works within the reticular activating system in releasing Ach and, therefore, increasing arousal and physiological activity. Thus, both primary (cortical) and secondary (subcortical reticular formation) regions were stimulated by nicotine. Gender was a factor in the effect of nicotine, as the Na-Pa amplitude was augmented more in male than female subjects. This finding was also consistent with the basic research literature on gender differences in the density of nicotine acetylcholine receptors in the brain. There was also an apparent ear effect, with a greater nicotine effect on AMLRs evoked by left versus right ear stimulation.

MARIHUANA. | Patrick and colleagues (Patrick, Straumanis, Struve, Fitz-Gerald, & Manno, 1997) described increased amplitude for the AMLR P50 component in thirty-six chronic marihuana users versus a group of forty-five control subjects. There was no significant difference between groups for other AERs (ABR, P300), nor visual or somatosensory evoked responses. Marihuana in this paper, and others, is also referred to as TCH. This group of investigators had previously presented preliminary data for chronic marihuana users suggesting increased latency for ABR wave I, increased amplitude for the AMLR P50 component, and decreased amplitude with increased latency for the auditory P300 response, as well as increased P50 amplitude (Patrick, Straumanis, Struve, Nixon, Fitz-Gerald, Manno, & Soucair, 1995). The authors cite more rigorous medical and psychiatric screening of normal subjects, more stringent subject exclusion criteria, careful control for subject age, and the inclusion of blind data collection and analysis methods in their explanation of the clear discrepancy in the findings for the preliminary versus later investigations. This rather distinct difference in AER findings for normal subjects versus marihuana users and specifically, the failure to replicate positive (abnormal) findings in the experiment group, is a valuable reminder of the importance of sound experimental design in clinical investigations.

COCAINE. | Boutros et al. (2000) studied the AMLR P50 (Pb) and N100 components in a group of fifteen cocaine-dependent subjects (twelve men and three women) aged 23 to 45 years (mean of 38) and a control group (thirteen subjects). The authors evoked the AMLR with two stimulus conditions or paradigms, described above in the sections on stimulus repetitions and Pb (P50) analysis. One paradigm consisted of different series (or trains) of click signals presented with varying ISIs (500 ms, and 2, 5, and 8 seconds). The other condition was a paired-click stimulus paradigm with the first signal (S1) of the pair followed after a 500 ms interval by a second signal (S2). In other publications, Boutros and colleagues have described two versions of the pair signal paradigm. With one paradigm, the two signals in the pair are identical (each signal is a click), whereas with the other paradigm the pair consists of two different signals (e.g., 1000 Hz and 500 Hz tone bursts). There was no difference between the cocaine versus control groups in the ampli-

tude of the AMLR Pb (P50) component evoked by repeated click presentations with short ISIs. With longer ISIs, however, P50 amplitudes were larger for control subjects than for the cocaine-dependent subjects. The authors interpreted these findings as evidence of intact inhibition in preattentive sensory processing for both subject groups. With the paired-click paradigm, the N100 component (but not the P50 component) was significantly decreased for the S2 signal among the cocaine-dependent subjects. The authors interpret this finding as consistent with an inhibitory deficit in preattentive information processing for the cocaine subject group. Thus, according to Boutros et al. (2000), chronic cocaine use appears to have an adverse effect on information processing.

Miscellaneous Factors Influencing the AMLR

ALTERNATIVE MEDICINE. | Acupuncture is among the more unusual medical management techniques. Actually, acupuncture is an alternative medical treatment option that has been applied, or at least evaluated, for relief of many and diverse diseases and disorders from rheumatoid arthritis to tinnitus. Liao, Nakanishi, and Nishikawa (1993) formally evaluated the effect of acupuncture stimulation on the AMLR as recorded from nineteen normal male subjects with an array of 21 electrodes. With acupuncture stimulation, the polarity of several AMLR components (the Po and the Na) reversed to what the authors described as N12 and P17. The amplitude of major AMLR wave complexes (Na-Pa and Nb-Pb) increased significantly with acupuncture stimulation of the ipsilateral site, whereas there was no change in latencies. Changes in the AMLR with acupuncture stimulation occurred for postauricular muscle (PAM) activity and also for components (Pa and Pb) arising from the auditory cortex within the temporal lobe.

CLINICAL APPLICATIONS AND POPULATIONS

Assessment of Auditory Sensitivity

The AMLR offers at least three advantages for electrophysiologic estimation of auditory thresholds. First, amplitude of the major component (Pa) is relatively large—about twice as big as the ABR wave V. The larger amplitude enhances the signal-to-noise ratio and, in comparison to the ABR, contributes to response detection at lower signal intensity levels with less signal averaging. Second, the AMLR is easily evoked by frequency-specific tone-burst signals with relatively long durations (e.g., 10 ms or more). Low-frequency signals are quite effective in evoking the AMLR, in contrast to the difficulty of generating a frequency-specific ABR with low-frequency tone bursts. Third, the type of instrumentation and the simple electrode array used for recording the ABR is appropriate also for AMLR measurement. However, the application of the AMLR in auditory assessment is not without constraints. Muscle and movement interference is a practical problem for infants and young children who are either awake or sleeping naturally. The use of conscious sedation, a logical and effective solution to this problem for ABR measurement, is not really an option for the AMLR. As reviewed in more detail above, both sleep and sedation can have marked effects on AMLR analysis, and even the consistent detection of AMLR components. The clinical dilemma is apparent. With young and restless children, it's impossible to record the AMLR without sedation or an extended period of natural sleep, and yet it's also difficult or impossible to detect a reliable AMLR with sedation or in most sleep states.

The AMLR can be elicited with electrical signals, as well as sounds. Because the main components within the AMLR waveform appear at least 15 to 20 ms after the signal, electrical stimulus artifact is not a concern for the AMLR, as it is with electrical ABR measurements. Applications of electrical AERs—including the EAMLR—are reviewed in Chapter 15.

CLINICAL FINDINGS. | Historically, the application of the AMLR in estimation of hearing sensitivity in pediatric populations was inversely related to the same application for ABR. That is, there was considerable interest in the clinical application of the AMLR as an electrophysiologic index of auditory sensitivity in infants and difficult-to-test children until the emergence of ABR in the early 1970s. As clinical ABR instrumentation was introduced toward the end of the 1970s and early 1980s, most audiologists began to rely exclusively on the ABR for electrophysiologic estimation, or confirmation, of auditory status in children (e.g., Hall, 1992; Jerger & Hayes, 1976). The major reason for this rapid replacement of the AMLR by the ABR as the technique of choice for pediatric electrophysiologic auditory assessment was the independence of the ABR from the effects of sedation. The use of the AMLR for electrophysiologic auditory assessment of infants and behaviorally difficult-to-test children was seriously compromised by problems with movement interference and the effect of sleep. And, unfortunately, sedation was not an option as the AMLR was highly susceptible to the effects of sedation and anesthesia. Thus, the ABR offered the audiologist a clinically feasible and attractive—actually irresistible—alternative to the AMLR for electrophysiologic assessment of auditory sensitivity in infants and young children. This clinical application of the AMLR was confined, then, to adult populations and, often, mostly for the estimation of low-frequency hearing sensitivity. The advent of the auditory steady-state response (ASSR) further minimizes the relevance of the AMLR as a technique for frequency-specific estimation of auditory sensitivity in young children, particularly for signals at frequencies of 1000 Hz and below. The ASSR is reviewed in Chapter 8.

With most adult patients, auditory thresholds can be determined accurately with conventional behavioral techniques for hearing assessment, e.g., pure-tone and speech audiometry. The purposes for applying the AMLR in the estimation of auditory threshold in adult patients are limited, typically, to cases for which the findings for behavioral audiometry are incomplete or considered inconclusive or unreliable due to malingering, i.e., nonorganic hearing loss (Musiek et al., 1984), low cognitive status (e.g., mentally handicapped), or inadequate state of arousal (e.g., lethargic, comatose). The Pa component of the AMLR is most often used as the index of a response to auditory stimulation. Tone-burst signals with relatively long duration are employed, and signal intensity is progressively decreased until there is no detectable response. A logical question at this juncture is, How closely is detection of the AMLR Pa related to behavioral threshold? That is, at what signal level (in dB) above behavioral pure-tone hearing threshold is the AMLR Pa component first observed? With adults, the performance of the AMLR in threshold estimation is, at least, equivalent to the accuracy of frequency-specific ABR measurements (Musiek & Geurkink, 1981; Palaskas et al., 1989). A reliable Pa component is typically detected when the signal intensity level is within 10 dB of the pure-tone threshold for the same frequency region (Musiek & Geurkink, 1981; Scherg & Volk, 1983; Zerlin & Naunton, 1974). In selected patients, with minimal electrophysiologic noise, the AMLR may be more accurate for threshold estimation than the ABR. The AMLR is less dependent on synchronous firing of afferent nerve fibers in the auditory system. Short-duration (transient) signals are required to evoke the ABR, whereas longer duration signals are effective as signals in AMLR measurement. Therefore, patients with compromised neural synchrony due to neurologic disease produce an AMLR even when the ABR is grossly abnormal, or no activity can be detected (Kraus, Özdamar, & Stein, 1982). Whether this clinical advantage for AMLR applies also to patients with auditory neuropathy is not yet clear.

The AMLR can be applied in the assessment of conductive, sensory, and mixed types of peripheral hearing loss (e.g.,Hall, 1992; McFarland, Vivion, & Goldstein, 1977) and, of course, pseudohypacusis (malingering). Of course, as with any auditory electrophysiologic procedure, the accuracy with which the AMLR estimates auditory threshold is increased when recordings are made with the optimal test protocol and, especially, when noise (physiologic and ambient acoustic) levels are low and when a robust and highly reliable response is recorded at suprathreshold intensity levels. It bears repeating that the pronounced effects on the AMLR of age in infants and young children (e.g., CNS immaturity) coupled with the challenges associated with recording an AMLR in either an awake active child (with movement interference) or a child who is asleep or sedated (with response suppression) serve to limit the pediatric application of the AMLR in electrophysiologic estimation of auditory thresholds.

Neurodiagnosis

Since the early 1980s, the AMLR has attracted clinical interest as an electrophysiologic measure of auditory function for regions rostral to the anatomic limits of the ABR, i.e., from the thalamus to the primary auditory cortex. The investigations defining the anatomic generators of the AMLR (e.g., Kileny et al., 1987; Kraus et al., 1982; Lee, Lueders, et al., 1984; Scherg & Von Cramon, 1986) provided clinicians with the minimal information needed to apply the AMLR in the neurodiagnosis of central auditory dysfunction. A fundamental concept in neurodiagnostic AMLR application is the analysis of latency and, particularly, amplitude values for the Pa component as recorded with different scalp electrode locations. Of these two simple response parameters—latency and amplitude—there is general agreement that latency is less useful clinically in detection of auditory system dysfunction (Hall, 1992; Kileny et al., 1987; Shehata-Dieler, Shimizu, Soliman, & Tusa, 1991). Although the AMLR is characterized by considerable intersubject variability, there is reasonable normal intrasubject consistency in the amplitude of the Pa component for recordings of the AMLR from electrodes located over the auditory temporal lobe region (e.g., C3 and C4) and, often, a frontal midline electrode site (e.g., Fz). The goal of AMLR waveform analysis is to ascertain symmetry of Pa amplitude among these two or three electrode arrays. Reduction in amplitude of the Pa component common to a single electrode site over, for example, the right or the left temporal lobe is viewed as consistent with auditory dysfunction in this region. Musiek and colleagues (1999) have referred to the interelectrode differences in Pa amplitude as the "electrode effect." Guidelines for the analysis of the AMLR were described earlier in this chapter. Briefly, amplitude for the AMLR Pa component under one measurement condition, e.g., a recording with the noninverting electrode over hemisphere (C3 or C4), is considered abnormally reduced when it is less than 50 percent of the amplitude for other recording conditions, e.g., the response recorded with a midline (Fz) or opposite hemisphere noninverting electrode. Amplitude of the wave V component can also be used in the analysis of the AMLR. That is, amplitude for an AMLR Pa component can be considered abnormally reduced when, with stimulation of the same ear, it is smaller than the amplitude for the ABR wave V.

AMLR findings reported for various disorders and pathologies are summarized in Table 11.5. In general, the analysis of the AMLR in neurodiagnosis involves the calculation of the latency and, more importantly, amplitude of the Pa component as recorded by a midline electrode site and also electrode sites located over each temporal lobe (C3 and C4). As discussed in more detail earlier in this chapter, abnormally reduced amplitude for a hemispheric electrode array, regardless of which ear is stimulated (right or left ear), is interpreted as consistent with thalamo-cortical auditory dysfunction on that side (left or right side). That is, the basis of AMLR interpretation in neurodiagnosis is the analysis of a possible interhemispheric amplitude difference, usually for the Pa component. Findings for selected studies will now be reviewed briefly.

BRAIN TUMORS. | Some of the early papers on AMLR in cerebral pathology included findings for patients with intracranial tumors lesions, although the specific diagnosis or site of lesion was not always defined. Yokoyama, Ryu, Uemura, Miyamaoto, and Imamura (1987) described AMLR findings in four adult patients with "well localized" cerebral gliomas. The tumors were located in the hypothalamus in one patient, the thalamus in another patient, and within the cerebral hemispheres for the remaining two patients. AMLR Na, Pa, and Nb components were severely attenuated or absent in each of the patients.

CEREBROVASCULAR PATHOLOGY. | Patients with cerebrovascular pathology are the most common clinical population described in the literature on neurodiagnostic application of the AMLR (e.g., Ho et al., 1987; Kileny et al., 1987; Kraus et al., 1982; Musiek & Baran, 2004; Musiek et al., 1999; Musiek, Charette, Morse, & Baran, 2004; Ozdamar et al., 1982). Ho et al. (1987) reported ABR and AMLR findings for a 67-year-old female with sudden deafness following sequential temporal lobe infarcts. Pure-tone and speech audiometry initially showed no behavioral response to sounds, even though acoustic reflexes and ABR were consistent with normal peripheral hearing sensitivity. Over a seven-month period, hearing sensitivity returned to within normal limits. The AMLR during this time evolved from no response to a slightly delayed but reliable Pa component from each hemisphere. The appearance of the AMLR was correlated with an improvement of the structural status of the temporal lobe as documented by CT scan. Kileny and colleagues (Kileny, Paccioretti, & Wilson, 1987) reported another comprehensive study of the AMLR in various cortical lesions. For all but one of eleven patients with damage involving the temporal lobe, the etiology was a cerebrovascular infarct. Normal ABRs were recorded for all patients. Wave Pa amplitudes were reduced significantly when recorded with electrodes over the involved hemisphere versus uninvolved hemisphere. The AMLR findings were not related to the stimulus ear (ipsilateral or contralateral to lesion) or the inverting electrode site (ear ipsilateral versus contralateral to lesion). Furthermore, AMLRs were intact among patients with cerebral lesions that did not involve the cortex of the temporal lobe. AMLR findings in patients with CVAs are typified by the waveforms in Figure 11.14.

In a series of twenty-five patients with CT documented cortical lesions involving temporal lobe (unilateral or bilateral), Özdamar, Kraus, and colleagues (Kraus et al., 1982; Özdamar et al., 1982) found evidence of grossly abnormal AMLRs (reduced amplitude or no detectable wave Pa component bilaterally) when the response was recorded with electrodes located over the damaged hemisphere. Midline recorded AMLRs were characteristically normal. All but three patients had lesions secondary to cerebral infarcts. In contrast, a patient described in a case report by Parving et al. (1980) showed normal AMRs despite bilateral infarcts

TABLE 11.5. Summary of Auditory Middle-Latency Response (AMLR) findings in Selected Clinical Populations, Arranged Alphabetically

CLINICAL ENTITY	STUDY(S)	SUMMARY OF FINDINGS
Alcoholism (chronic)	Ahveninen et al., 1999 Diaz et al., 1990	Larger Pa amplitude in abstinent alcoholics.
Alcoholism (risk)	Rodriguez-Holguin, et al., 2001	Smaller Pa amplitude in children at risk for alcoholism.
Alzheimer's dementia	Buchwald et al., 1989 Jessen et al., 2001 Phillips et al., 1997 Green et al., 1997 Cordone et al., 1999	Abnormality of the AMLR Pb (P50) component. Deficit in Pb (P50) component and "sensory gating." No difference in Pa or Pb latency or amplitude versus control group.
Auditory processing disorder (learning disability)	Purdy et al., 2002	Delayed Na component in LD group versus control group.
Autism	Buchwald et al., 1992	Abnormality of the AMLR Pb component.
Cerebrovascular disease	Kileny et al., 1987 Hall, Brown, & Mackey-Hargadine, 1985	Cerebral pathology can be localized with AMLR. Documentation of temporal lobe dysfunction in children.
Cocaine users	Boutros et al., 2000	Pb (P50) difference in cocaine users versus control subjects for a paired-click stimulus paradigm.
Diabetes mellitus	Martini, Comacchio, & Maguavita, 1991	
Down syndrome	Diaz & Zurron, 1995	Longer latency for the Na component.
Head injury	Hall et al., 1982 Hall & Tucker, 1985 Hall, Hargadine, & Allen, 1985	Abnormal Pa component in temporal lobe injury. AMLR findings in acute head injury useful in predicting long-term cognitive and communicative outcome. AMLR sensitive to sedatives and anesthetic agents, e.g., barbiturates.
Learning disabilities	Jerger & Jerger, 1985 Kraus et al., 1985 Purdy et al., 2002	Smaller Pa amplitude or absent Pa component in LD. AMLR findings showed no significant difference versus control subjects.
Malingering	Musiek et al., 1984	Analysis of the AMLR Pa component at progressively lower intensity levels for tone-burst signals can provide electrophysiologic estimation of auditory thresholds in nonorganic hearing loss.
Mania	Adler et al., 1990	Deficit in the S2/S1 ratio of the P50 response.
Marijuana users	Patrick et al., 1997	Larger Pb amplitude in users than in control subjects.
Multiple sclerosis	Jerger & Jerger, 1985 Celebisoy et al., 1996	Abnormal findings (Na or Pa) for over 70 percent of twenty-two patients.
Parkinson's disease	Mohamed, Iacono, & Yamada, 1996	Abnormally delayed Pb (P50) latency and reduced amplitude and return to normal values with surgical treatment (posterior ansa-pallidotomy).
Post-traumatic stress syndrome	Neylan et al., 1999	Abnormal findings for Pb (P50) in sensory gating paradigm.
Schizophrenia	Erwin, Mawhinney-Hee, Gur, & Gur, 1991 Freedman et al., 1983 Adler et al., 1982 Grillon, Ameli, & Braff, 1991 Bramon et al., 2004	Abnormality of the AMLR Pb (P50) component. Meta-analysis of twenty studies of AMLR Pb (P50) component.
Stuttering	Hood et al., 1990	Abnormality of the AMLR Pb component.
Temporal lobe disorders	Shehata-Dieler et al., 1991 Woods, Clayworth, Knight, Simpson, & Naeser, 1987 Kraus et al., 1982 Ibanez, Deiber, & Fischer, 1989	

AMLR in Patient with Left Temporal Lobe Cortical Disorder

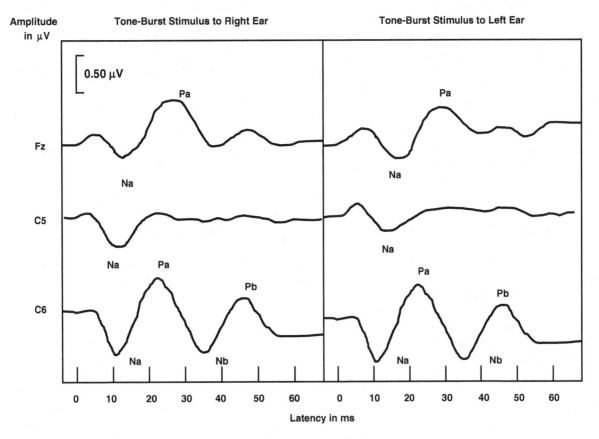

FIGURE 11.14.   AMLR waveforms recorded from a 50-year-old male following cerebrovascular accident (stroke) affecting the left cerebral hemisphere.

of the temporal lobe. Importantly, however, AMLRs were recorded with a midline, rather than hemisphere specific, electrode array. During the 1980s, other investigators also confirmed in various pathologies the neurodiagnostic value of comparing AMLR amplitude values for different electrode arrays (Ibanez, Deiber, & Fischer, 1989; Woods, Clayworth, Knight, Simpson, & Naeser, 1987).

Musiek and colleagues (1999) reported a comprehensive and meticulous investigation of AMLR findings in cerebrovascular pathology. Subjects were twenty-six people (fourteen women and twelve men) ranging in age from 16 to 64 years (average 41.5 years) with confirmed lesions within the central auditory nervous system. For eighteen of the subjects, the lesion was secondary to a cerebrovascular accident within the right or left temporal lobe region of the brain. Sites of lesions for each subject were further defined, e.g., superior posterior temporal gyrus or right basal ganglia hemorrhage involving the internal capsule. The control group consisted of healthy subjects (sixteen women and ten men) ranging in age from 17 to 64 years (average 41.3 years). Hearing status was well defined for each group, with most subjects having normal hearing sensitivity. AMLR was evoked with click signals of 0.1 ms duration, presented monaurally via insert

earphones at a rate of 9.8/second and an intensity level of 60 dB nHL. The response was detected with hemispheric non-inverting electrodes located at C3 (left side of head) and C4 (right side of head), and inverting electrodes located on the ear lobes (A1 for left ear lobe and A2 for right ear lobe), with an analysis time of 72 ms and band-pass filtered from 20 to 3000 Hz. Waveform analysis included calculation of latency for the Na component (within the region of 12 to 21 ms) and the Pa component (within the latency region of 21 and 38 ms), and amplitude from the trough of the Na component to the peak of the Pa component or wave complex.

Utilizing these latency and amplitude data, Musiek et al. (1999) analyzed interhemispheric symmetry for ipsilateral (C3 to A1; C4 to A2) and contralateral (C3 to A2; C4 to A1) electrode arrays. Ipsilateral versus contralateral symmetry was quantified with the following equation:

$$\text{Percent difference} = \frac{\text{larger amplitude} - \text{smaller amplitude}}{\text{smaller amplitude}}$$

Data analysis in the investigation by Musiek et al. (1999) included the creation of receiver operating characteristics (ROC) curves for subjects in the experimental and control groups for each of the AMLR parameters noted above. With the information available from the ROC curves derived from latency and amplitude data, the authors then described AMLR rates for hits (correct identification of the site of lesion) and false-positive errors (suspicion of a lesion in a control subject). In addition, the authors evaluated the diagnostic utility of two other AMLR parameters. Musiek et al. (1999) compared the diagnostic sensitivity of absolute versus relative amplitude measures, i.e., amplitude values for a patient relative to normative data versus amplitude values for a patient in one measurement condition to another (e.g., ipsilateral versus contralateral measurements). They also examined the diagnostic accuracy of several categories of the relative (ipsilateral versus contralateral) differences in AMLR amplitude, e.g., a 20 percent decrease versus a 50 percent decrease in the Na to Pa amplitude among measurement conditions.

Consistent with previous reports of AMLR in neurodiagnosis (e.g., Ho et al., 1987; Kileny et al., 1987; Kraus et al., 1982; Musiek et al., 1994; Shehata-Dieler et al., 1991), latency for the Pa component was a more sensitive measure of brain pathology than latency for the Na component. In addition, analysis of the ROC curves for latency data showed greater sensitivity to pathology for the contralateral versus ipsilateral recordings. Neither latency measure, however, equaled the accuracy of Na to Pa amplitude in determining the presence of central auditory nervous system pathology. Again, the contralateral measurement condition was superior to the ipsilateral condition. It's important to clarify at this juncture that the contralateral condition refers to AMLR recordings with the noninverting electrode over one hemisphere (e.g., C3) and the inverting electrode on the opposite ear lobe (e.g., A2), rather than the location of the inverting (ear lobe) electrode relative to the site of lesion. Consistent with the literature (e.g., Musiek et al., 1999), amplitudes were typically reduced for the AMLR Pa components recorded when the noninverting electrode was on the side of the lesion (e.g., over the involved hemisphere). Bilateral AMLR abnormalities, however, may also occur with apparently unilateral brain lesions (e.g., Baran, Bothfeldt, & Musiek, 2004).

With regard to the diagnostic power of the amount of asymmetry in AMLR amplitude for the Pa component, there was an expected improvement in hit rate when an abnormality was defined by a modest versus marked difference in AMLR amplitude for the ipsilateral versus contralateral conditions. For example, in the analysis of relative AMLR amplitude (Na to Pa) difference with the noninverting electrode over the involved versus uninvolved hemisphere, and with the contralateral measurement condition, a > 20 percent difference in amplitude yielded a hit rate of about 75 percent and a false-positive rate of about 15 percent. By increasing the criterion for a clinically significant asymmetry in amplitude to > 50 percent (involved side amplitude is less than half of the uninvolved side), the hit rate dropped to about 43

percent, but there were no false positives. Applying a similar approach to the examination of test performance for absolute amplitude values, again in the most favorable (contralateral) measurement condition, an asymmetry criterion of 0.2 mV yielded a hit rate of about 65 percent and a false-positive rate of about 12 percent, whereas increasing the criterion for asymmetric amplitude to 0.5 µV produced a false positive rate of 0 percent (no false positives) but decreased the hit rate to only about 30 percent. Citing the high degree of variability in AMLR findings among patients due to differences in the "nature, size, and locus of CNS lesions," and the need for further investigation, the authors refrain from recommending a specific criterion for AMLR amplitude analysis. There are at least two constraints to the generalization of the conclusions of the study by Musiek et al. (1999) to the application of the AMLR in other patient populations, such as children with APD. The subjects were, for the most part adults (not children) and auditory dysfunction was secondary to relatively localized and acquired pathology (e.g., cerebrovascular accidents), rather than developmental disruptions in auditory processing.

ALR abnormalities have long been associated with temporal parietal cerebral damage producing aphasia, although the precise site of lesion was often not documented (Gerull, Giesen, Knupling, & Mrowinski, 1981; Greenberg & Metting, 1974; Jerger et al., 1969; Knight, Hillyard, Woods, & Neville, 1980; Liberson, 1966; Papanicoulaou, Levin, & Eisenberg, 1984; Peronnet et al., 1974; Rapin & Graziani, 1967; Rothenberger, Szirtes, & Jurgens, 1982). Many of these studies employed speech stimuli, as well as meaningless click and tone-burst stimuli. Careful study of the relationship among confirmed and localized vascular lesions and results for the AMLR and ALR revealed complete loss of the AMLR Pa when acoustic radiations are involved and ALR components when cortical auditory regions (e.g., AI and AII) are involved (Scherg & von Cramon, 1986).

ALZHEIMER'S DISEASE. | Abnormal AMLR findings are found in patients with Alzheimer's disease, also referred to as dementia of the Alzheimer's type or DAT (Buchwald et al., 1989; Green, Flagg, Freed, & Schwankhaus, 1992; Grimes, Grady, & Pikus, 1987; O'Mahoney et al., 1994; Phillips et al., 1997). The patterns of findings for different AMLR components reported in Alzheimer's disease, however, vary among the studies. The latency and amplitude for the Pa component are typically within normal limits in patients with Alzheimer's disease. In a study with a modest number of male patients with Alzheimer's disease (N = 6) and an equal number of control group subjects, Buchwald et al. (1989) reported smaller Pb amplitude among the patient group, whereas the latency and amplitude of the Pa component was similar for both groups. Appropriately slow stimulus presentation rates (0.5 and 1.0/second) were used for consistent detection of the Pb component (e.g., Nelson, Hall, & Jacobson, 1997). Two other groups of investigators

(Green et al., 1992; O'Mahoney et al., 1994), in studies of larger subject samples of patients with Alzheimer's disease (approximately thirty subjects for each study) and with binaural signal presentation, also reported reduced amplitude or absence of the AMLR Pb component. Green et al. (1992), found that the Pb component was actually absent (less than 1 μV by their criterion) for a higher proportion of patients with Parkinson's disease (58%) than Alzheimer's patients (39%). This pattern in AMLR findings with Alzheimer's disease was not, however, replicated by Phillips et al. (1997). These researchers studied fourteen patients with Alzheimer's disease and an age (about 70 years) and gender (about 55% male) matched control group. The AMLR was evoked with rarefaction polarity click signals (duration of 0.1 ms) presented to each ear separately at an intensity level of 90 dB SPL and a rate of either 1/second or 0.5/second. According to the authors, "there was no history of hearing impairment in any of the patients except for one 78-year-old male who exhibited a slight hearing impairment in the left ear," but no details were provided on how hearing status was documented, nor on the criteria (if any) for subject exclusion. The AMLR was detected with a noninverting electrode located at the Cz site and linked ear inverting electrodes with band-pass filter settings of 10 to 300 Hz and an analysis time of 150 ms (50 ms prestimulus time).

AUDITORY PROCESSING DISORDERS (APD) AND LEARNING DISABILITIES. | The AMLR has for years been investigated as an electrophysiologic measure of auditory dysfunction in children and adults with APD and in children with learning disabilities (e.g., Arehole, 1995; Chermak & Musiek, 1997; Fifer & Sierra-Irizarry, 1988; Hall, 1992; Jerger & Jerger 1985; Marvel, Jerger, & Lew, 1992; Mason & Mellor, 1984; Musiek et al., 1999; Purdy, Kelly, & Davies, 2002; Squires & Hecox, 1983). Over the years, with accumulated clinical experience and formal investigations, the methodology for AMLR measurement has evolved and improved with regard to the consistent and optimal detection of each component, e.g., Pa and Pb. Unfortunately, based on information produced by reported clinical experience and research findings, it is clear that the protocols followed in many of the earlier investigations included parameters that were not ideal for the neurodiagnostic application of the AMLR, especially in children. Common methodological weaknesses in the earlier studies included reliance on only transient (0.1 ms) click signals versus tone bursts, inappropriately high-signal presentation rates (e.g., > 5/second) and high-pass filter settings (> 5 Hz), and detection of the AMLR with only midline versus hemispheric noninverting electrode sites. Some of these studies (e.g., Grillon et al., 1989; Kraus, Smith, Reed, Stein, & Cartee, 1985; Mason & Mellor, 1984) reported no significant difference in the detection, or the latency and amplitude values, of the Pa component in children with LD or language impairment. One observation noted by a number of these investigators is the failure to consistently record the

AMLR Pb component (e.g., Purdy, Kelly, & Davies, 2002). The most likely explanation for the apparent absence of the Pb component lies in the use of inappropriate settings for one or more of the first three measurement parameters just cited. The results of the above-noted studies of AMLR in children with APD can be generalized as follows. A typical finding is latency prolongation and, particularly, amplitude reduction for the Na and Pa components. Indeed, among auditory evoked responses, the AMLR and the P300 response are abnormal most often, i.e., in approximately 40 percent of patients referred for an APD assessment (Hall & Mueller, 1997). Several of the more recent papers will now be reviewed.

Purdy, Kelly, and Davies (2002) conducted an investigation of multiple AERs (ABR, AMLR, ALR, and P300) in a small sample (N = 10) of children aged 7 to 11 years with the diagnosis of learning disabilities (LD). AMLR was evoked with click signals (0.1 ms duration) presented monaurally and also binaurally with insert earphones at a rate of 8.7/second and an intensity level of 70 dB nHL (99.7 dB peSPL). The AMLR was detected with noninverting electrodes located at midline (Cz), hemisphere (C5 and C6) electrodes, and linked earlobe inverting electrodes with an analysis time of 100 ms (prestimulus time of 2 ms) and band-pass filtered at 3 to 300 Hz. This protocol is an example of the statement in the preceding paragraph about the absence of the Pb component. Given the use of transient click rather than longer duration tone-burst signals presented at the relatively fast rate of 8.7/second rather than 1 per second or even 1 every other second, it is not surprising that the authors failed to record a Pb component. LD "and a possible APD" was defined by performance on psycho-educational procedures (e.g., *Learning Efficiency Test, Detroit Tests of Learning Aptitude-2, Following Oral Directions* test, the *Selective Reminding Test*, and the *Lindamood Auditory Conceptualization (LAC)* test. For all subjects, cognitive function was normal by the *Weschler Intelligence Scale for Children-Revised (WISC-R)*, and attention deficit was ruled out. APD assessment was limited to two procedures: the SCAN screening test battery and the staggered spondaic word (SSW) test. The control group consisted of ten children matched in age and gender with normal educational history. For LD and control subjects, normal hearing sensitivity was confirmed with pure-tone thresholds of < 15 dB HL, normal tympanometry, and normal ipsilateral and contralateral acoustic reflexes. The authors reported AMLR differences for the LD versus control group, including delayed Na latency and smaller amplitude (less negativity) for the Nb component. Trends for other AMLR components, e.g., Pa latency prolongation, were not statistically significant.

AUTISM. | Grillon, Courchesne, and Akshoomoff (1989) reported a study of AMLR (and ABR) in eight subjects with infantile autism with an average age 23 years. Findings were compared to another eight subjects with receptive language impairment (mean age of 16 years) and a normal control group. AMLR findings (Pa latency and amplitude) were comparable among the three groups. Kemner, Oranje, Verbaten, and van Engeland (2002) applied the AMLR P50 in a study of sensory gating in twelve children with autism and a control group. There was no difference between groups in the suppression of the P50 for the second stimulus.

DOWN SYNDROME. | Kavanagh, Gould, McCormick, and Franks (1989) reported ABR and AMLR findings for forty-eight subjects with "mental handicaps," including seven with Down syndrome. Average subject age was 8.5 years (range of 8 months to 32 years). Notably, sedation was required with AER measurement for all of the subjects. In this study, AMLR was studied as a potential measure of auditory sensitivity, rather than in neurodiagnosis. Not unexpectedly, test–retest reliability was higher for the ABR than the AMLR. Diaz and Zurron (1995) applied the ABR, AMLR, and ALR in a study of twelve subjects with Down syndrome and a control group age of matched (11 to 19 years) subjects. The status hearing sensitivity was "estimated" only with the signals used for each of the three types of AERs, with average hearing thresholds of 61 dB SPL for the Down syndrome group versus 47 dB SPL for the control group. The AMLR was evoked with 500 Hz tone bursts presented at an intensity level of 65 dB SL and at a rate of 10/second. The AMLR was detected with a noninverting electrode located at the Cz site, inverting electrodes on the ear lobes, and band-pass filter settings of 5 to 250 Hz. The significant AMLR finding for the study was prolongation of the Na latency for the Down syndrome group versus the control group, whereas Pa latency was equivalent for the two groups. Interestingly, the Na latency was in distinct contrast to the predominant ABR abnormalities in the Down syndrome subjects, i.e., shorter absolute latencies for waves II, II and V, and also shorter interwave latencies (wave I–II, wave I–III, and wave I–V). The authors note as a possible factor in this discrepancy in findings for the ABR versus AMLR the difference in signal characteristics and site of activation along the cochlea (click versus 500 Hz signals).

EPILEPSY. | Rosburg, Trauter, Korzyukov, (2004) investigated intracranially recorded P50 (Pb) components in patients with epilepsy. Since their findings for the P50 are closely linked with those for the ALR N100 wave, the study is reviewed in the section on epilepsy within the next chapter (Chapter 12 on the ALR).

SCHIZOPHRENIA. | There are more studies of AMLR studies of the Pb (P50) component in schizophrenia than any other clinical population (e.g., Adler et al., 2004; Freedman et al., 2003). Selected publications describing the AMLR P50 component in schizophrenia are summarized in Table 11.6. Many of the papers also report findings for the P300 response, as reviewed in Chapter 12. One abnormal finding reported in schizophrenia is the lack of the normal suppression of the P50 wave with the presentation of paired signals (a train of signals). This AMLR has been interpreted as evidence of an abnormally long "recovery cycle" in schizophrenia (Freedman, Adler, Myles-Worsley, et al., 1996; Yee, Nuechterlein, Morris, & White, 1998) that may, for some patients, have a hereditary or genetic basis (Clementz, Geyer, & Braff, 1997; Waldo, Cawthra, Adler, et al., 1995). Bramon et al. (2004), in a literature review in preparation of a meta-analysis of the P50 (Pb) and the P300 response in schizophrenia, found seventy-five articles that included data for the AMLR P50 (Pb). The authors cite as a reason for the considerable ongoing research interest the anticipation that these two auditory evoked response components will be useful as a biological marker in identifying a specific genetically determined type of the disorder. Measurement criteria for inclusion of studies reporting data for the AMLR P50 component included the auditory conditioning paradigm (see discussion under the stimulus presentation section above) for evoking the response and a noninverting electrode at the Cz location for detecting the response. Other experimental design criteria were also used in the decision to include or exclude studies from the meta-analysis. Since antipsychotic drugs are commonly used for medical management of schizophrenia, the authors carefully analyzed data for studies with patients in the unmedicated versus medicated condition. The authors included twenty studies in the meta-analysis of the AMLR P50 wave, reporting data for a total of 421 patients with schizophrenia and 401 control subjects. There was no difference for P50 latency, but the S2/S1 ratio for the P50 was significantly larger (1.56 standard deviations larger) for the schizophrenia patients than the control subjects. This finding was interpreted as evidence of a sensory gating deficit in schizophrenia. To determine whether selected test parameters or subject factors contributed to the variability in the size of the effect of schizophrenia on the P50, the authors performed random effects regression with the following factors: age, gender, task difficulty, duration of the illness, severity of the psychopathology, duration of the signals, and the high-pass and low-pass filter settings. The latter three factors (test parameters) significantly influenced the P50 ratio findings. Antipsychotic medications also did not have a significant influence on the S2/S1 ratios for the P50 response.

More recently, Adler et al. (2004) conducted an investigation of the relation between medication and sensory gating in schizophrenia. Subjects were 132 patients with schizophrenia and a control group of 177 healthy subjects. The authors cited previously reported data showing that genetically determined sensory gating impairments are found in patients with schizophrenia (e.g., Freedman et al., 2003) and also about one-half of their close relatives. The typical AMLR pattern in schizophrenia is an S2/S1 ratio of greater than 50 percent. In the study reported by Adler et al. (2004), groups selected from among eighty subjects were treated with one of several unconventional neuroleptic drugs (e.g., clozapine, olanzapine, risperidone, and quetiapine). Another thirty-four patients received typical neuroleptics, and then ten patients were not medically treated. Only clozapine produced S2/S1 amplitude ratios for the P50 component that were within the normal range. Subjects who were untreated or treated with any of the other drugs showed poorer than normal inhibition (i.e., lower S2/S1 ratios). This study confirms the role of the AMLR P50 component in the verification of neurophysiologic dysfunction in schizophrenia, and illustrates the application of this measure of sensory gating in documenting the therapeutic value of medical management in schizophrenia.

MACHADO-JOSEPH DISEASE. | Ghisolfi and Brazilian colleagues (Ghisolfi et al., 2004b) described abnormalities of the AMLR P50 (Pb) component in twelve patients with Machado-Joseph disease (MJD), twelve patients diagnosed with schizophrenia, and twenty-four normal subjects. MJD is an autosomal dominant degenerative disorder that involves multiple sensory and motor systems and is associated with a variety of neurological findings. Abnormalities were reported for other auditory evoked responses in MJD, including the auditory brainstem response (e.g., Kondo et al., 1990). Ghisolfi et al. (2004b) investigated suppression of the P50 component with a pair (train) of stimuli, as described elsewhere in this chapter (see sections on signal parameters and AMLR application in schizophrenia). Stimuli were two 0.1 ms clicks presented with an interpair interval of 500 ms interval, and an intertrial time difference of 10 seconds (the conditioning paradigm) and an intensity level of 60 dB SL. Responses were recorded with a Cz noninverting electrode and linked ear inverting electrodes, and band-pass filter settings of 10 to 10,000 Hz and an analysis time of 1000 ms. The authors reported a reduction in sensory gating (less suppression of the P50 component indicated by higher S2/S1 P50 amplitude ratios) in the MJD patient group, in comparison to the normal subjects. In addition, latency for the P50 component elicited by the first stimulus (S1) was prolonged for the MJD group.

MULTIPLE SCLEROSIS. | Multiple sclerosis (MS) is the most common type of demyelinating disease and one of the major causes of neurological impairment in adults, except the elderly. Prevalence varies according to climate, with an estimated 10 per 100,000 patients in the southern regions of the United States and 50 to 70 per 100,000 in northern regions. Young adults are usually affected, with 50 to 70 percent of patients reporting onset of symptoms between the ages of 20 and 40 years and only rare cases in children. The female to male ratio is 1.7:1.

In contrast to thee extensive literature on the ABR in MS, there are few papers describing AMLR findings (Celebisoy, Aydogdu, Ekmekci, & Akurekli, 1996; Robinson & Rudge, 1977, 1980; Versino et al., 1992). Latency delay of the AMLR Pa component was the most common abnor-

mality reported in MS, with amplitude values typically not affected. Robinson and Rudge (1977), for example, reported abnormal AMLR Pa component latency for 45 percent of a group of sixty-six patients with MS. Versino et al. (1992) described ABR and AMLR results for thirty-four patients with MS (seven classified as early probable and twenty-seven with definite MS) and a control group of thirty-five patients. Hearing status was not described for group of subjects. Stimuli were clicks (alternate polarity) presented at an intensity level of 65 dB HL and a presentation rate of 8/second. AMLR was recorded with a Cz noninverting electrode, an analysis time of 100 ms, and band-pass filter settings of 5 to 1500 Hz. Abnormal findings were reported for 47 percent of the subjects for the AMLR versus 37 percent of the subjects for ABR. The AMLR abnormality in MS consisted of delayed latency for the Pa component, where as Pa amplitude and Na latency were normal.

Stach and Hudson (1990) described AMLR and ALR findings for a series of 118 patients with the diagnosis of MS (eighty male and thirty-eight female) ranging in age from 17 to 64 years (average of 42 years). Hearing sensitivity, as defined by the pure-tone average for frequencies of 500, 1000, and 2000 Hz, ranged from −12 to 42 dB HL. A normal subject group consisted of twenty patients matched for age and hearing thresholds, ranging in age from 24 to 66 years, with an average of 45 years. The AMLR was evoked with 500 Hz tone-burst signals (duration 10 ms) presented monaurally at a rate of 10/second and an intensity level of 70 dB nHL. The response was detected with a Cz noninverting electrode and an inverting electrode located on the ipsilateral ear lobe, band-pass filtered at 10 to 1000 Hz, using a 100 ms analysis time. Stach and Hudson (1990) described abnormal AMLR findings for 47 percent of the MS subjects. The most common abnormality was absence of a repeatable Pa component (72%), followed by delayed Pa latency (16% of the MS subjects), and then poor morphology or "hemispheric asymmetry." Citing the close correspondence between abnormalities for the ABR and AMLR, these authors noted the possibility that the AMLR abnormalities are secondary to the effects of demyelination on the synchrony required for generation of the ABR rather than pathology specifically within the generator sites of the AMLR. This interpretation of findings is in agreement with a study of AMLR in MS by Celebisoy et al. (1996) that documented predominantly latency delays (for the Na and Pa components). Arguing against this mechanism as the only explanation for the findings of the study, however, was the observation that specific abnormalities of the AMLR were documented for twenty-one patients with normal ABRs.

DEGENERATIVE DISEASES. | Amantini, Rossi, de Scisciolo, Bindi Pagnini, and Zappoli (1984) applied the AMLR in an AER test battery in the assessment of nine patients with the diagnosis of Friedreich ataxia, a spinocerebellar degenerative disease. One of the patients reportedly showed an abnormal delay in Pa latency. Ghisolfi et al. (2004b) applied the AMLR P50 response with the conditioning/test stimulus paradigm in a study of sensory gating in of twelve patients with Machado-Joseph disease (MJD), an autosomal dominant spinocerebellar degenerative neurologic disease. Subjects also included twelve schizophrenic patients and twenty-four normal subjects. Higher S2/S1 amplitude ratios for the P50 component were found for the patients with MJD and schizophrenia than the normal subjects, confirming a sensory gating deficit in these two patient populations. Uc, Skinner, Rodnitzky, and Garcia-Rill (2003) investigated the AMLR P50 (Pb) component l in Huntington's disease (HD), a hereditary (autosomal dominant) disorder often appearing in mid-life and characterized the diffuse loss of cells in the caudate nucleus and putamen, and sometimes in thalamus. The authors cited in their rationale for the study evidence that the AMLR Pb component is, at least partly, generated by the neurons in the cholinergic pedunculopontine nucleus (PPN) than contribute to the reticular activating system. The AMLR was recorded from eleven patients with HD and thirteen control subjects using the paired (conditioning versus test) stimulus paradigm applied in studies of sensory gating. Patients with HD showed two patterns of AMLR abnormalities. In comparison to the control group, the HD group has smaller P50 (Pb) amplitude values for the first (conditioning) stimulus (S1). In addition, the HD group demonstrated a deficit in sensory gating characterized by a reduction in the S2/S1 ratio with ISIs of 250 and 500 ms.

POSTTRAUMATIC STRESS DISORDER (PTSD). | A common feature of PTSD is enhanced responses to cues specific to the person's previous trauma and sometimes other signals, such as the startle response to sounds. Smaller amplitudes for the P300 response were found in patients with PTSD (McFarlane, Weber, & Clark, 1993), reflecting an overall impairment of attention processing and suggesting the possibility of a deficit in the discrimination of relevant versus irrelevant signals. Using the conditioning/test paradigm with pairs of stimuli, Neylan et al. (1999) investigated the P50 response as an index of sensory gating in a group of fifteen male subjects with PTSD secondary to combat (Vietnam veterans) and a control group (twelve subjects). There was no difference between groups in the P50 (Pb) amplitude for the first (conditioning) stimulus (S1). However, the second (test) stimulus (S2) yielded significantly larger amplitude for the P50 component in the PTSD group in comparison to the control group. The increased S2/S1 ratio for the PTSD subjects was evidence of diminished inhibition or impaired sensory gating to auditory stimuli. Findings were consistent with previous reports of the AMLR P50 in PTSD and in schizophrenia (see summary of studies in Table 11.6). However, Neylan et al. (1999) demonstrated that the impairment in sensory gating in combat veterans was for the P50 component evoked with "neutral non-provocative stimuli," that is, "innocuous auditory stimuli" not related to trauma sounds. Ghisolfi et al. (2004a) reported impaired sensory gating also for patients with PTSD who were victims of urban violence.

TABLE 11.6. Selected Studies of the Auditory Middle-Latency Response P50 (Pb) Component with the Conditioning Signal Paradigm as a Measure of Sensory Gating and Habituation, Including Investigations in Different Clinical Populations

STUDY	CLINICAL POPULATION	COMMENT
Freedman et al., 1983	schizophrenia	effect of medication
Reite et al., 1988	normal findings	study of anatomy
Jerger, Biggins, & Fein, 1992	normal findings	not affected by attention
Cardenas, McCallin, Hopkins, & Fein, 1997	normal findings	no effect on state of arousal
Freedman et al., 1996	schizophrenia	impaired habituation
Fein, Biggins & MaKay, 1996	alcoholics	reduced suppression
Erwin et al., 1991	schizophrenia	
Boutros, Overall, & Zouridakis, 1991	schizophrenia	sensory gating deficit
Judd, McAdams, Budnick, & Braff, 1992	schizophrenia	sensory gating deficit
Waldo et al., 1992	normals	noradrenergic effects
Johnson & Adler, 1993	normals	stress and suppression
Ghisolfi et al., 2002	normals	study of neurotransmitters
Adler et al., 1998	schizophrenia	sensory gating deficit study of neurotransmitters
Neylan et al., 1999	PTSD*	deficits in combat veterans
Metzger et al., 2002	PTSD*	Vietnam combat nurses
Ghisolfi et al., 2004a	PTSD*	deficits in victims of violence
Ghisolfi et al., 2004b	Machado-Joseph disease	sensory gating impairment

* PTSD = posttraumatic stress syndrome

TRAUMATIC BRAIN INJURY. | Most studies of AERs in traumatic head (brain) injury are limited to the ABR (e.g., see Hall, 1992, for review), some investigators have applied the AMLR in this clinical population (Hall, 1992; Musiek, Baran, & Shinn, 2004). Auditory dysfunction secondary to diffuse brain pathophysiology in the acute period following severe head injury can be documented with the AMLR (Hall, 1992; Hall & Tucker, 1985). One specific application of the AMLR in this patient population—predicting outcome following head injury—is reviewed in the next section of this chapter.

In a recent study, Musiek et al. (2004) demonstrated the value of AMLR in documenting electrophysiologically the benefit of rehabilitation of central auditory processing in a patient with traumatic brain injury. The patient was a 41-year-old female who suffered brain injury when she was thrown from a horse. The initial comprehensive diagnostic audiologic assessment was completed thirteen months after the injury. The AMLR was recorded, along with a battery of behavioral measures of auditory processing. Before therapy, the AMLR amplitude was abnormally reduced for right-ear stimulation and normal for left-ear stimulation. There were no differences in the AMLR waveforms among electrode arrays (C3, C4, or Fz) for right- or left-ear stimulation. Following an intensive program of auditory training, the AMLR was again recorded. Amplitude was increased and morphology improved post-therapy. This finding was consistent with the patient's subjective impression of an improvement in communication abilities.

Abnormalities in the AMLR are also described for patients with mild traumatic brain injury (MTBI), including prolonged latency and reduced amplitude for the Pa component (Drake, Weate, & Newell, 1996; Soustiel, Hafner, Chistakov, Barzilai, & Feinsod, 1995). On the other hand, Gaetz and Weinberg (2000) reported normal AMLR findings in persistent postconcussion syndrome.

Recognizing that brain injury can be associated with attention and memory impairment, Arciniegas et al. (2000) applied the sensory gating paradigm with the AMLR P50 component in a group of twenty brain-injured patients and a control group (also twenty subjects). The reader is referred to Figure 11.4 for a display of the two-click stimulus paradigm often used to elicit the P50 response in neuropsychiatric disorders. Amplitude for the P50 component was significantly larger for the test stimulus (S2) in the brain injury group than in the control group. Interpreting the increased S2/S1 ratio for the brain-injury subjects as evidence of impaired sensory, the authors discuss the diagnostic and therapeutic implications of the findings.

COMA. | An AMLR with normal latency and amplitude values for the Na and Pa components can be recorded in post-traumatic coma if the auditory cortical regions are intact (e.g., Hall, 1992). There is no relation between the AMLR and depth of coma, as indicated by the Glasgow Coma Scale.

This finding is not necessarily characteristic of other forms of coma. For example, Thornton et al. (2002) reported findings for the ABR, AMLR, and somatosensory evoked responses in six Zimbabwa patients with malarial coma. Malarial coma is associated with diffuse and symmetrical encephalopathy. These authors consistently recorded a normal ABR. AMLR components (Na, Pa, Nb, Pb) were present during malarial coma, but latencies shortened with emergence from coma. The authors noted similarities in the effects of malarial coma on the AMLR and previously collected data on the effect of anesthetic agents on AMLR.

Predicting Cognitive and Communicative Outcome in Head Injury

Greenberg and colleagues at the Medical College of Virginia in Richmond (Greenberg & Becker, 1976; Greenberg et al., 1977) published the first reports of AERs in head injury. The goal of these investigations was the estimation with multimodality sensory evoked responses, evoked by auditory, visual, and somatosensory stimulation, of long-term outcome following severe head injury. The outcome of these germinal studies provided the motivation for further research on the clinical applications of AERs in this challenging population and led to ongoing interest and clinical research by others (Anderson et al., 1984; Karnaze et al., 1982; Narayan et al., 1981; Rappaport et al., 1977; Rosenberg, Wogensen, & Starr, 1984; Seales et al., 1979).

In the 1980s, the author examined the relationship between serial AER data obtained within the first week after injury and cognitive and communicative outcome at six months as described with the Ranchos Los Amigos Hospital Scale (RLAHS) (Hagan et al., 1979) in seventy-four survivors of severe head injury (Hall, 1992). All of these patients had normal ABRs. None were in barbiturate coma at the time of testing. Mean Glasgow Coma Score (GCS) was 5.7. Severe head injury is defined conventionally as a GCS of 8 or less. Data for patients dying within the first post-injury week were not analyzed. ABR was, as expected, not related to long-term outcome. AMLR was, therefore, selected as the AER measure for estimating cognitive/communicative status. One reason for this decision was the possibility that the AMLR receives contributions from regions of the auditory cortex that are closely related to speech recognition and language function. To simplify data analysis and this potential clinical application of AMLR, cognitive/communicative outcome as assessed with the Ranchos Scale was reduced to four categories, as described below. AMLR waveforms were defined as follows:

- *Normal.* A reliable Pa component bilaterally with amplitude (Pa-Nb) equal to or greater than 0.30 µV.
- *Abnormal.* A reliable Pa component unilaterally or bilaterally with an amplitude of less than 0.30 µV, or only a unilateral AMLR Pa component (regardless of amplitude).

• *No response.* No reliable Pa component is recorded from noninverting electrodes over either cerebral hemisphere.

Patients with excellent recovery (RLAHS level VIII) invariably had a consistently normal AMLR during the first week post-injury (see Table 11.7). All but 5 percent of the patients with good recovery (RLAHS level VII) and 19 percent of those with fair recovery (RLAHS levels IV–V) also yielded normal AMLRs in the acute period. Among the patients with poor recovery (RLAHS levels I–IV), a majority produced either an abnormal response (low amplitude) or no AMLR within the first week after injury. While these findings are only preliminary, they do appear to suggest that a complete recovery depends on integrity of the neuroanatomic region generating the AMLR, perhaps in part the primary auditory cortex (Celesia, 1976; Kaga et al., 1980; Lee et al., 1984).

Not unexpectedly, some (32%) of the patients with very unfavorable outcome, at least at three months after the injury, had normal AMLRs bilaterally. Other neuroanatomic regions are, of course, vital for normal speech/language/ cognitive functioning, not just the primary auditory cortex, and these regions may have sustained substantial damage. In addition, it is likely that in many cases significant further cognitive/communicative improvement occurred after the month limit of this study.

Monitoring Depth of Anesthesia

Physicians routinely monitor depth of anesthesia during surgical procedures using clinical signs and general physiologic parameters, such as hemodynamic variables (e.g., arterial blood pressure), the frequencies for heart activity (e.g., pulse) and respiration (e.g., breathing rate), and arterial oxygen saturation (SaO_2). Some anesthetic agents, particularly neuromuscular blockers and "vaso-active" drugs, can influence or even suppress these conventional physiologic parameters, leading to inaccurate description of the depth of anesthesia. Depth of anesthesia was defined in Chapter 8. The consequences of inappropriate or suboptimal depth of anesthesia are not trivial. With inadequate depth of general anesthesia, the patient may remember intraoperative events with, understandably, a negative impact on behavior, quality of life, or postoperative recovery. Awareness during anesthesia is determined by several factors, including the type and dose of anesthetic agents and the surgical procedure. At the other end of the anesthesia spectrum, suppression of important physiologic parameters can be associated with acute (intraoperative) medical crises and poor postoperative neurological outcome, or even death. In addition, with unnecessarily deep anesthesia during surgery, the patient is more likely to demonstrate slower postoperative recovery and to show adverse cognitive outcome. The relation between excessive anesthesia and negative cognitive outcome is strongest in older patients or those with compromised neurological or cognitive status before surgery. And, monitoring depth of anesthesia is particularly challenging for children (Weber et al., 2004).

Neither the earlier latency AERs nor the later latency AERs are suitable, in isolation, as electrophysiologic indices of depth of anesthesia. Both the ECochG and ABR are resistant to the effects of even deep anesthesia, showing

TABLE 11.7. The Relation between Acute Findings for the Auditory Middle-Latency Response (AMLR) and the Rancho Los Amigos Scale (RLAS) of Cognitive/Communicative Function

AMLR categories are defined in the text.

	AMLR CATEGORY					
	Normal		**Abnormal**		**No Response**	
RLAS*	N	%	N	%	N	%
1 Month						
Good	5	13	0	0	0	0
Fair	20	53	0	0	0	0
Poor	13	31	9	100	3	100
3 Months						
Good	13	31	0	0	0	0
Fair	24	63	2	22	0	0
Poor	1	3	7	78	3	100
6 Months						
Good	30	79	0	0	0	0
Fair	7	18	2	22	2	67
Poor	1	3	7	1	1	33

* RLAS categories: Good = Level VIII; Fair = Levels V through VII; Poor = Levels I through IV.

TABLE 11.8. Summary of Studies of the Auditory Middle-Latency Response (AMLR) in Monitoring Depth of Anesthesia (arranged chronologically)

STUDY(S)	RESPONSE(S)	SUMMARY OF FINDINGS
Sasaki, 1991	ABR, AMLR	Neuroleptanesthesia (fentanyl, ketamine, althesis) had least effect on the AMLR.
Cagy & Infantosi, 2002	AMLR	AMLR amplitude reduction is reliable as an index of unconsciousness in propofol anesthesia.
Struys et al., 2002	AMLR	AAI calculated from the AMLR predicted loss of consciousness and depth of anesthesia with propofol but not the arousal response to noxious stimuli.
Tooley et al., 2004	AMLR	Latency of the AMLR Nb component is useful in determining level of unconsciousness in propofol anesthesia. Alfentanil assists in lowering propofol infusion rate without further affecting the AMLR.
Bell et al., 2004	AMLR	A description of techniques for recording the AMLR while monitoring depth of anesthesia.
White et al., 2004	AMLR	AMLR monitoring during anesthesia with desflurane can be used to achieve desired depth of anesthesia and can contribute to improved outcome following ambulatory surgery.
Heinke et al., 2004	AMLR, MMN	The MMN response is more sensitive to the effects of propofol sedation, whereas the AMLR Pb component is a more effective index of anesthesia (unconsciousness).

no change with most anesthetic agents at even high doses. At the other extreme, the later cortical AERs (e.g., the ALR and P300) are affected by conscious sedation (e.g., chloral hydrate) and may be entirely suppressed by even light anesthesia. The AMLR is exquisitely sensitive to the effects of commonly used anesthetic agents. By virtue of its graded sensitivity to the influences of CNS acting drugs and the relatively straightforward recording technique, the AMLR has for about twenty years been the object of intense investigation as a tool for monitoring depth of anesthesia, as summarized earlier in Table 11.8. (Bell, Smith, Allen, & Lutman, 2004; Iselin-Chaves, Moalem, Gan, Ginsberg, & Glass, 2000; Jensen, Lindholm, & Henneberg, 1996; Litvan, Jensen, Revuelta, 2002; Schwender, Kaiser, Klasing, Peter, & Poppel, 1994; Schwender et al., 1995; Thornton et al., 1992; Thornton et al., 1989; Tooley et al., 2004; Trillo-Urrutia, Fernandez-Galinksi, & Castano-Santa, 2003).

What follows here is a brief review of the substantial literature on monitoring the level of unconsciousness and depth of anesthesia with the AMLR.

AMLR Protocol for Monitoring Depth of Anesthesia

Although AMLR measurement parameters are not consistent among studies, the following test protocol is typical. The AMLR is usually evoked with click signals presented binaurally at a moderate intensity level (e.g., 70 to 75 dB

nHL or SL) at a presentation rate somewhere in the range of about 4 to 6/second. As in other clinical applications of AERs, an odd presentation rate, e.g., 5.7 or 6.1/second is advisable to avoid the likelihood of an interaction between the averaging process and electrical power frequency (60 Hz in the United States and some other countries and 50 Hz in England and other countries). It is important to avoid common integer multiples for the stimulus presentation rate and the frequency of electrical interference. Although a seemingly minor component of the AMLR test protocol, it is important to select an odd stimulus presentation rate and to modify the rate if electrical inference is encountered in the operating room. Acquisition parameters include a noninverting electrode at the vertex (Cz) or forehead (Fz) and inverting electrodes at the mastoid, ear lobe, or the inion. Recall that selected electrode sites for the 10–20 International system were shown in Figure 11.5. Predictably, there is less interference with the AMLR by postauricular muscle (PAM) activity with a noninverting electrode located away from the ear, e.g., the inion (Tooley et al., 2004) or a true reference site located at a noncephalic site, such as the nape of the neck (Bell et al., 2004; Hall, 1992). A disadvantage of the nape of neck location is difficulty accessing the site when a patient is lying in the supine position and cannot move voluntarily due to anesthesia. Electrodes serve as antennae for unwanted airborne electrical artifacts. Therefore, electrode leads should be as short as possible in the operating room setting and braided to further reduce electrical interference. The ideal placement for the electrode box (preamplifier) is near the patient's head (e.g., underneath that end of the table). There are multiple and serious sources of electrical artifact in the operating room environment (see discussions of intraoperative monitoring with ECochG and ABR in Chapters 5 and 10, respectively). Typically, muscle artifact and movement interference is minimal or nonexistent in the operating room setting because the patient is anesthetized and, often, chemically paralyzed for surgery. Band-pass filter settings should be selected to minimize possible interference from unwanted external electrical signals, e.g., 10 to 250 or 300 Hz. Enabling the notch filter (60 Hz) option will remove critical energy from the averaged AMLR and may distort latency and/or amplitude, and thus is strongly discouraged.

AMLR Analysis Techniques during Anesthesia

The results of clinical studies show that the AMLR Nb component is most useful in monitoring depth of anesthesia (Thornton et al., 1992). Specifically, progressively deeper anesthesia is reflected by prolongation in Nb latency and reduction in Nb amplitude, as well as Pa latency. Conversely, shortened latencies indicate lighter anesthesia. This general relation between the AMLR and anesthesia is common to most anesthetic agents used during surgery. Mantzaridis and Kenny (1997) introduced simplified analysis of the AMLR during anesthesia with the use of a single numerical variable, referred to as the auditory evoked potential index. The index is calculated by a proprietary algorithm for analysis of the averaged AMLR waveform that involves mathematical analysis and comparison of different segments of the waveform. A practical disadvantage of this technique is the time required (about 40 seconds) for averaging a response to 256 signal presentations (sweeps). Other investigators have developed different techniques for the intraoperative measurement and analysis of AMLR data during anesthesia (e.g., Bartnik, Blinowska & Durka, 1992; Haig, Gordon, Rogers, & Andersen, 1995; Jensen, Nygaard, & Nenneberg, 1998), among them maximum length sequencing or MLS (Eysholdt & Schreiner, 1982). One of the more recent techniques, known as the A-Line ARX Index (AAI), involves an autoregressive statistical approach permitting the identification of the AMLR signal after less than 25 sweeps over an analysis time of 110 ms, or a data collection time of only 6 seconds.

Recently, Heinke et al. (2004) investigated the combined use of an AMLR component (Pb) and the mismatch negativity (MMN) response to monitor the depth of propofol anesthesia. Level of sedation was classified into four categories: awake state, light sedation, deep sedation, and unconsciousness. The authors demonstrated that the MMN was more sensitive to sedation than the AMLR, but disappeared entirely with loss of consciousness, whereas amplitude of the AMLR Pb component was not influenced by sedation (the first three categories), yet progressively decreased in amplitude with loss of consciousness and depth of anesthesia.

Benefits of Monitoring Depth of Anesthesia with AMLR

There is accumulating evidence confirming the value of AMLR monitoring during anesthesia in improving titration of intravenous and inhalational anesthetic agents during general anesthesia, in reducing the likelihood of unexpected awareness during surgery, and in improving quality of recovery after surgery (e.g., Bonhomme et al., 2000; Nishiyama, Matsukawa, & Hanaoka, 2004; White et al., 2004;). Titration of the anesthetic agents refers to the ongoing adjustment of the dose of the drug to maintain a target status for the AMLR. Anesthesiologists with immediate access to information from cerebral monitoring indices (e.g., the AMLR) utilize lower concentrations of volatile anesthetic agents (e.g., Recart et al., 2003; White et al., 2004). In a randomized clinical trial, White et al. (2004) showed, for example, that patients monitored with the AMLR received 28 percent less volatile anesthetic (desflurane) than another subject group that was not monitored. In this study, none of the twenty patients assigned to the group monitored with AMLR recalled intraoperative events. Speed of postoperative recovery and a reduction in side effects can also be applied as parameters in assessing the benefits of monitoring depth of anesthesia with the AMLR. Initial findings (White et al., 2004) appear to confirm fewer side effects (e.g., nausea, vomiting, headache, dizziness) and higher postoperative scores on the Quality of Recovery scale. It is likely that further research on this clinically and, potentially, financially important issue will be published soon. As noted above, monitoring depth of anesthesia is especially challenging in children. There is some evidence (Weber et al., 2004), that the AMLR can be applied for this purpose, as it is in adults, for preschool children older than 2 years.

Changes in the AMLR associated with the depth of anesthesia and depression of the central nervous system are influenced by surgical stimulation, e.g., skin incision. That is, while the anesthetic agents work to suppress arousal, surgical manipulations produce an opposite effect and serve to increase arousal. Consequently, along with the type and dose of anesthetic agent(s) administered in the operating room, the type of surgical procedure and associated amount of physical stimulation is a variable to consider when monitoring depth of anesthesia with the AMLR. Tracheal intubation at the beginning of a surgical case is a good example of the type of physical stimulation that produces an arousal reaction.

CONCLUDING COMMENTS

The AMLR can be recorded with conventional evoked response systems used for ABR measurement. The AMLR is underutilized as a clinical measure. Advantages for clinical application of the AMLR include (1) origin in auditory cortex, (2) value in lateralizing auditory cortical dysfunction, (3) presence in young children, (4) feasibility of evoking the response with tonal and other complex stimuli (e.g., speech), (5) sensitivity to nonlemniscal auditory pathways (e.g., reticular activating system), and (6) suitability for assessing sensory gating mechanisms.

Auditory Late Responses (ALRs)

BACKGROUND

Terminology for the description of auditory evoked responses is rather inconsistent, ambiguous, confusing, arbitrary, and especially troublesome with longer latency responses. At least two general approaches are taken to describe these responses. One approach is based on latency and the temporal sequence of components. With this schema, the traditional ALR components that occur within the 50 to 200 ms latency region are distinguished from the event-related P300 component by shorter latency values and, therefore, a relatively earlier occurrence after an appropriate acoustic stimulus. An immediate problem with the temporal sequence approach is that, under certain stimulus conditions and subject states, there may be additional event-related evoked response components within the traditional ALR region, and these may alter the usual ALR components. Components recorded under event-related response conditions, such as N1 and P165 components, may not follow the ALR but, instead, may appear at an earlier latency.

The other general approach for describing AERs is to categorize them as either exogenous or endogenous (Donchin, Ritter, & McCallum, 1978). Exogenous AERs are a product primarily of stimulus characteristics and, normally, are recorded invariably without regard to the subject's attention to the stimuli (see Chapter 1 for additional features that differentiate endogenous versus exogenous evoked responses). ECochG, ABR, and AMLR are classified as exogenous responses. Longer latency components are, for the most part, generated in higher regions of the auditory CNS. AERs are found within the same latency region and arise presumably from the same general level of the CNS. Endogenous AERs are less dependent on stimulus characteristics, but highly dependent on the stimulus context, a change in the ongoing stimulation, subject state, especially attention to the stimulus and cognition, or a task required of the subject. Relatively small alterations in any of these variables may result in the appearance, or the disappearance, of compo-

nents (positive or negative waves) within a waveform from one test to the next, or even within a single data collection period.

The endogenous AERs also are complex with regard to their anatomic origins. The generation involves dynamic physiologic interactions among structures found in the auditory cortex within the temporal lobe, the frontal lobe, the limbic system, and subcortical regions (e.g., thalamus and reticular formation). The term "event-related response or potential" is sometimes used interchangeably with term "endogenous" in describing this category of auditory evoked response. Thus, exogenous responses are determined mostly by external factors, such as physical stimuli presented to the nervous system, while endogenous responses are determined mostly by internal factors, such as the state of the nervous system when stimuli are presented. The distinction between exogenous and endogenous AERs is, however, not clear and not consistent. One could even argue that the terms exogenous and endogenous are confusing and misleading. That is, the responses defined as *exo*genous do not, as the term would imply, arise from outside of the body of the subject. By this definition, all AERs are endogenous. Similarly, the responses of AERs referred to as *endo*genous are clearly as dependent on an external stimulus for their generation as are the exogenous responses.

The scope of the present chapter encompasses, with three exceptions, the many and diverse auditory evoked responses occurring with latencies greater than 50 ms. One of the exceptions is the auditory P300 response. Since it was discovered forty years ago, the P300 has been the focus of intense clinical research interest and the topic of many hundreds of publications. Therefore, a separate Chapter (13) is devoted to the auditory P300 response. The same general argument can be made for the second exception—the mismatch negativity (MMN) response. Within recent years, there has been an explosion of research internationally on the MMN response. The review in Chapter 14 barely makes a dent in the vast amount of information that has been published about the MMN response since its discovery in 1978. Without doubt, innovative clinical and basic research on the MMN will continue unabated in the years to come, to the benefit of our understanding of normal and disordered auditory perception and auditory processing across the age spectrum. The final exception pertains to the application of AERs in patients before, during, or after cochlear implantation. Chapter 15 includes a discussion of responses electrically evoked from one end of the auditory system to the other—cochlea to cortex. Given the rather unique features of AER measurements in patients with cochlear implants, it seemed logical to also locate within Chapter 15 a review of all AER information regarding this clinical population, including responses evoked with auditory signals that are then processed by the cochlear implant and delivered to the afferent auditory fibers of the eighth cranial nerve as electrical stimulation.

The sequence of topics in the present chapter adheres to the format followed in the previous chapter on the AMLR. That is, a clinical test protocol is first presented, along with the rationale for stimulus and acquisition parameters and a reference to innovative or sophisticated techniques for evoking or recording the ALR that have research merit, even though they all may not at this time be clinically feasible or possible with clinical instrumentation. A historical perspective on the ALR was presented in Chapter 1. Next, factors influencing the analysis and interpretation of the ALRs are delineated. Analysis and interpretation of the ALR is, in many respects, far more complicated than it was for the earlier latency responses. Whereas early AER peaks reflect sensory processing of the stimulus in relatively discrete anatomic regions, the later waves (e.g., N1, P2, P3, N400) and their multiple subcomponents are products of diverse factors ranging from stimulus characteristics to cognitive processing that integrates the acoustic information extracted from stimuli. The relation between the numerous ALR waves and subcomponents of waves and cognitive processing is only now being investigated intensely, and our knowledge of the link between the ALR waves or components and cognition is sketchy at best. The review of ongoing research on the ALR in this chapter, and the similar reviews of the P300 and MMN response in the next two chapters, should be viewed as introductions to the topics. Space constraints for the book do not permit a definitive or detailed synopsis of the literature on these three categories of auditory evoked responses. Given the rapid proliferation of research information on them, a detailed literature review would be outdated even as the book was published.

The final section of the chapter addresses clinical applications of the ALR, or clinical research that is likely to lead to new applications in various patient populations. Now, over sixty-five years after the initial report on the ALR by Davis et al. (1939), there certainly appears to be renewed interest in the clinical value of information extracted from the analysis of components within the auditory late response time domain, e.g., the N1 and P2 waves. ALRs are now the target

of investigation as potential electrophysiological probes of fundamental brain processes (e.g., memory and habituation), and mechanisms underlying the neural representation of speech processing in young children (including infants) and also in advancing age. ALRs are also applied now in the investigation of auditory processing disorders (APD) in diverse patient populations. One particularly exciting potential application of the ALR is the electrophysiological description of brain plasticity and documentation of the clinical value, benefit, or outcome from the intervention for auditory disorders. The growing literature describing changes in ALR components associated with intervention with cochlear implantation is an example of this application. Electrically evoked auditory responses are reviewed in Chapter 15, along with a discussion of the measurement of ALR components with acoustic signals that are processed by a cochlear implant and then evoked by the resulting electrical stimulation of fibers within the auditory nerve.

Nomenclature for the ALRs

Nomenclature for describing ALR waveforms according to vertex positive and negative peaks was proposed by Williams, Tepas, and Morlock in 1962. An ALR waveform as recorded clinically consists usually of gently sloping and broad components, in contrast to the sharp and narrow peaked components characterizing shorter latency responses. The first negative voltage component, N1, occurs in the 90 to 150 ms region (average latency value of about 100 ms). It is followed by a positive component, P2, between 160 and 200 ms (see Figure 12.1). An earlier positive component in the region of 40 to 50 ms (P1) occurs less consistently than N1 and

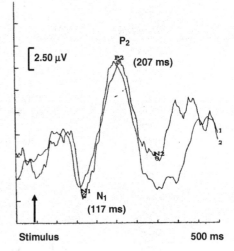

FIGURE 12.1. Auditory latency response (ALR) waveform as evoked with a tone-burst signal and recorded with a single channel electrode array (noninverting electrode at the Fz or Cz location and an inverting electrode on the nape of the neck).

P2. As discussed Chapter 11, the ALR P1 wave appears to be the same electrophysiological component as the AMLR Pb wave. A second negative component, N2, follows the P2 component with a latency value in the region of 275 ms. The N2 wave is not invariable and may or may not be present in normal subjects. Finally, as described further in Chapter 13, the P300 response as conventionally recorded with the oddball stimulus paradigm is a special component within an extended ALR time frame. The simplest measurement condition consists of an infrequent (rare) stimulus presented randomly within a series of frequent and predictable stimuli. The response is sometimes referred to as P300, because it's observed in the 300 ms region, and sometimes the P3 wave, because it forms a third major positive voltage component appearing after ALR waves P1 and P2. In fact, however, the P300 may be recorded in normal subjects as early as 250 ms or as late as 400 ms and may not necessarily be the third major component in the ALR waveform.

TEST PROTOCOLS AND PROCEDURES

Stimulus Parameters

STIMULUS TYPE: TONES. | Since early investigations in the 1960s by Davis and colleagues, tonal stimuli have typically been used to elicit the ALR (Davis, Bowers, & Hirsh, 1968). Whereas shorter latency responses generally are not effectively evoked with stimuli having rise/fall times longer than 5 ms, optimal ALR stimuli have rise/fall times and plateau times of greater than about 10 ms (Onishi & Davis, 1968;

Rothman, 1970; Ruhm & Jansen, 1969; Skinner & Jones, 1968). Rise/fall times of over 20 ms and durations of hundreds of milliseconds are even effective in eliciting the ALR. As a rule, amplitudes for the N1 and P2 components of the ALR are larger, and latencies longer, for low-frequency tonal signals in comparison to higher frequency signals (Alain, Woods, & Covarrubias, 1997; Antinoro, Skinner, & Jones, 1969; Jacobson et al., 1992; Sugg & Polich, 1995). In terms of the acoustic stimulus, therefore, the ALR is the ideal response for frequency-specific electrophysiological auditory assessment. Clinical challenges arise, however, with response reliability and the susceptibility of the ALR to changes in state of arousal of the subject. As discussed below, ALR components are influenced by subject attention. As a rule, amplitude increases directly with attention. Indeed, with manipulation of stimulus and subject-related factors, it is possible to elicit a variety of wave components within the same general latency region. Selected waves or wave complexes are listed in Table 12.1. A number of investigators have examined the negative ALR waves evoked with complex signals consisting of multiple tonal frequencies. With this stimulus paradigm, a stimulus block of two, three, or more different tones of different frequencies is presented at the same intensity level and with the same level of probability. The subject is instructed to attend to one of the frequencies and to ignore the others. This is a form of the "oddball stimulus paradigm" described in more detail in the review of the P300 response in the next chapter. The Nd wave complex is also referred to as the "processing negativity" or PN (Näätänen, Gaillard, & Mantysalo, 1978; Näätänen & Michie, 1979).

TABLE 12.1. Selected Auditory Evoked Responses That Occur within the Latency Region from of 50 to 1000 ms (1 second)

RESPONSE	LATENCY REGION (MS)	COMMENT
P1	50	Also referred to as AMLR Pb wave.
N1 (N100)	100	An obligatory component of the ALR.
N1b	100	Wave detected with a midline electrode.
N1c	150	Detected with temporal lobe electrode.
N1d	100–???	Negative wave that persists beyond the signal.
N150	150	
N250	250	A wave particularly robust in children.
P165	165	
P2	200	
MMN	150–275	Mismatch negativity response
P3a	≤300	Passive oddball paradigm response.
P3	300	Recorded with oddball paradigm.
Nc	400–700	
Nd	60–700	Referred to as processing negativity (PN).
N400	400	Evoked with semantic signals.
Sustained negativity	50 to 1000 ms	Recorded for duration of the stimulus.

N = negative component or wave; P = positive component or wave.

More information on the Nd wave, and other components of the ALR, can be found later in the chapter under the heading "waveform analysis." With the multiple-tone stimulus paradigm, amplitude of the Nd (processing negativity) wave is greatest for the target tone, that is, the tone that the subject is listening for. Attention during ALR measurement is usually verified by asking the subject to count silently the number of target stimuli presented and to keep a mental or written record of the number until the averaging run is complete. The Nd wave (processing negativity) is recorded, however, even for the ignored tones. Amplitude of the negativity to the nontarget tones is greater for those that are closer in pitch to the target tone pitch and less for those nontarget tones with frequencies that are more dissimilar (Alho, Paavilainen, et al., 1986). Näätänen and colleagues submit the proposition that "the processing negativity reflects a matching process between the sensory input and a hypothesized 'attentional trace' characterized as a voluntarily maintained cerebral neuronal representation of the physical features of the stimulus to be attended" (Alho, Sams, Paavilainen, & Näätänen, 1986, p. 190; Näätänen, 1982). Alho, Paavilainen, et al. (1986, 1990) presented evidence in support of this explanation for the generation of the Nd wave complex to attended and ignored tonal stimuli. These authors also demonstrated that the negativity was enhanced (larger in amplitude) as the difference in frequency (pitch) was decreased. Later, Alho, Näätänen, and colleagues further showed that the processing negativity (Nd) wave was smaller as the probability of the irrelevant (nontarget) tonal stimuli decreased. Smaller pitch separation makes for a more difficult discrimination task and, therefore, demands closer attention.

Some components of the ALR (e.g., P100 and N250) show larger amplitude and shorter latency for complex tones than for single-frequency (sinusoidal) tonal stimuli. In addition, the amplitude for these ALR components and other components with the late-latency region (e.g., N1, P2, and N4) vary as a function of the nature of the stimulus, such as complex tonal signals versus acoustically rich speech sounds (Čeponiene et al., 2001; Čeponiene et al., 2005). Two major ALR components—N1 and P2—can also be elicited by the modulation of amplitude or frequency of a tonal signal and by acoustic manipulations of features of speech stimuli (e.g., amplitude, spectrum, formant frequencies), reflecting neural detection of the acoustical changes (Kaukoranta, Hari, & Lounasamaa, 1987; Näätänen & Picton, 1987; Ostroff, Martin, & Boothroyd, 1998).

STIMULUS TYPE: SPEECH. | Unlike earlier latency auditory responses (e.g., ECochG, ABR, and AMLR), speech stimuli are quite effective in eliciting the ALR. ALR findings have been reported for different types of speech signals, including natural and synthetic vowels, syllables, and words (e.g., Čeponiene et al., 2001; Kurtzberg, 1989; Martin & Boothroyd, 1999; Näätänen & Picton, 1987; Ostroff, Martin, & Boothroyd, 1998; Sharma, Marsh, & Dorman, 2000;

Steinschneider et al., 1999; Tiitinen et al., 1999; Tremblay, Friesen, Martin, & Wright, 2003; Whiting, Martin, & Stapells, 1998).

In general, amplitude of the N1 to P2 complex is larger for speech sounds than for single frequency tonal stimuli, but latency values for the N1 and P2 are usually earlier for tonal versus speech stimuli (e.g., Čeponiene et al., 2001; Tiitinen et al., 1999). In these studies, investigators carefully verify equivalency of overall intensity and temporal onset for the two types of stimuli. In contrast, as noted above, complex tonal stimuli generate ALR components P100 and N250 with larger amplitudes than speech (vowel) sounds (Čeponiene et al., 2001). There are other differences in ALRs evoked by simple tonal versus speech signals. Latency of the ALR N1 component, for example, varies with the frequency of tonal signals (e.g., Crottaz-Herbette & Ragot, 2000; Roberts, Ferrari, Stufflebeam, & Poeppel, 2000), whereas for natural speech sounds the N1 latency is consistently about 120 ms (Mäkelä et al., 2001). The ALR can be applied in the electrophysiological assessment of the representation of speech cues in the central auditory nervous system. For example, latency of the ALR N1 wave evoked by speech sounds varies with voice onset time (Kurtzberg, 1989; Sharma et al., 2000; Steinschneider et al., 1999; Tremblay, Piskosz, & Souza, 2003). The effects of other speech cues on the ALR have also been reported for normal subjects (e.g., Kaukoranta et al., 1987; Martin & Boothroyd, 1999; Ostroff et al., 1998), in studies of auditory function in aging (e.g., Tremblay, Piskosz, & Souza, 2003), and in the clinical application of ALR in varied patient populations. Clinical applications of the ALR are summarized in the final segment of this chapter.

Tremblay, Piskosz, and Souza (2003) provide a description of speech sounds that is typical of those used in more recent investigations of the ALR evoked by changes in voice onset time (VOT). Synthetic speech sounds (tokens) were generated with a Klatt digital speech synthesizer. Equivalent intensity level for each stimulus was carefully verified digitally. VOT ranged from 0 to 60 ms in 10 ms increments for a /ba/ to /pa/ continuum. Starting frequencies for five formant-frequency transitions were defined, each with a constant duration of 40 ms for the formant transition. Temporal characteristics for a simulated burst (10 ms duration, 60 dB amplitude, and a spectrum from 2500 to 4000 Hz) and the steady-state (vowel) part of the stimulus, including five formant-frequency bandwidths, were also defined. Other stimulus and acquisition parameters were similar to those described later in this chapter in the section on ALR test protocol. Age effects on the ALR, reported by Tremblay and colleagues (Tremblay, Billings, & Rohila, 2004; Tremblay, Piskosz, & Souza, 2003), are summarized below in the section on subject factors.

Natural vowel sounds generate ALR components (N1 and later waves) that are detected with considerably larger amplitude from the left hemisphere, whereas tonal stimuli produce symmetrical brain activity (Szymanski et al., 1999).

Most investigators of speech-evoked ALRs utilize synthetically created speech sounds (e.g., syllables /ga/, /da/). Tremblay, Friesen, Martin, and Wright (2003), however, describe ALR findings for natural speech. The stimuli were four consonant-vowel syllables (/bi/, /pi/, /si/, and /shi/), each a token from the *Nonsense Syllable Test (NST)*. Taken together, the stimuli include a variety of acoustic features of speech, such as place of articulation, fricative phonemes with high-frequency energy, low-frequency vowel energy, and voice onset time. An external trigger initiated averaging by the evoked system coincided with speech sound presentation. Stimuli were presented in the sound field at an intensity level of 64 dB SPL (at the ear) and with an ISI of almost 2 seconds (1910 ms). The ALR was recorded with a 31-channel electrode array (Neuroscan™ Quik-Cap system) over a 1400 ms analysis time (prestimulus time of 100 ms), and then band-pass filtered from 0.15 to 100 Hz. Averages containing possible eye-blink activity were rejected. Although the ALR was recorded with a multichannel technique, results were described mostly for a mid-line (Fz or Cz) electrode site, as maximum amplitudes were detected at these scalp locations. During ALR measurement, subjects watched a video of their choosing after being instructed to ignore the stimuli. There is long-standing evidence that tonal stimuli and synthetic speech sounds produce repeatable ALRs (Pekkonen, Rinne, & Näätänen, 1995; Tremblay et al., 2001). Tremblay, Friesen, Martin, and Wright (2003) demonstrated that natural speech sounds also elicit reliable ALR components (P1, N1, and P2). Intersubject test–retest reliability was high, and the ALR was stable within subjects from one test session to the next. ALR morphology varied as a function of the speech stimulus. That is, speech sounds with different acoustic features generated differences in ALR waves, including smaller or larger amplitudes for specific negative and positive waves (e.g., N130 or P217) and shorter or longer latencies for waves (e.g., N345 and P413). There were also reliably distinctive ALR findings (e.g., neural patterns) when natural speech sounds differed according to important acoustic dimensions, such as two fricative sounds with different places of articulation or two stop constants that differed in voice onset time. Previous investigators found, for example, that synthetically generated voiced speech sounds evoked ALR waves (N130 and P217) with larger amplitudes than waves evoked by voiceless speech sounds (Steinschneider et al., 1999). Tremblay, Piskosz, and Souza (2003) confirmed this response pattern for natural speech sounds. Given the stability of the ALR to natural speech sounds, and its sensitivity to changes in acoustic properties of speech, we can anticipate investigations of the potential clinical application of the ALR in documenting auditory processing in various patient populations, including children with hearing aids and cochlear implants.

STIMULUS TYPE: OTHER. | Speech stimuli at the word level are effective in eliciting the N400 wave within the ALR.

Words with semantic content (e.g., common names and proper names), specifically those that are semantically anomalous or incongruent, are particularly effective in eliciting the N400 response. Amplitude of the response increases directly with the extent of semantic incongruence (e.g., Kutas & Hillyard, 1980). As summarized in the discussion of sleep factors later in this chapter, the N400 can be recorded in this way during certain sleep stages, as well as during wakefulness (e.g., Bastuji, Perrin, & García-Larrea, 2002; Brualla, Romero, Serrano, & Valdizan, 1998; Perrin, Bastuji, & García-Larrea, 2002; Perrin, Bastuji, Mauguiere, & García-Larrea, 2000; Perrin, García-Larrea, Mauguiere, & Bastuji, 1999).

Jerger and Estes (2002) studied in subjects of different ages auditory late responses evoked by *simulated auditory motion,* that is, the apparent movement of sound along a horizontal plane of space. Previous investigations of dynamic sound movement (e.g., Chandler & Grantham, 1992; Grantham, 1986) employed psychoacoustic (behavioral) methodology, rather than auditory electrophysiology techniques. Detection of sound movement versus stationary sound, or changes in the velocity of sound movement, is influenced by different cues and signal factors, such as signal frequency, intensity, interaural time differences, and subject factors or variability (Grantham, 1986). Experimental investigation in animals, and clinical studies in patients with pathology, confirm that the detection of sound motion involves processing in brainstem and cerebral regions of the central nervous system. Subjects in the Jerger and Estes (2002) study were thirty male, right-handed normal hearers, including eleven children (9 to 12 years), ten young adults (18 to 34 years), and nine older adults (65 to 80 years). The oldest group of subjects had, on the average, mild to moderate sensory hearing loss attributed to presbycusis (hearing loss with aging). Auditory evoked responses were evoked with recorded stimuli presented so as to simulate sound motion, using a technique described by Grantham (1986). Broadband noise stimuli delivered from one speaker placed 1.5 meters from the right ear and another speaker the same distance from the left ear were changed (linear ramping) in intensity over time to simulate the motion of the signal from the midline (toward the right or toward the left side) to a position about 80 degrees to the right or left. Jerger and Estes (2002) produced a velocity of 160 degrees/second for the apparent sound movement. Auditory responses were recorded with 30 scalp electrodes attached within an elastic cap, plus electrodes around the eye, over an analysis time of 1400 ms after the signal presentation, with a 200 ms prestimulus time. The brain activity was band-pass filtered from 0.15 to 70 Hz. The authors confirmed for each subject group a high degree of accuracy for behavioral responses to the apparent sound movement. Auditory late response components (waves in the latency regions for N1, P2, and N2) were recorded for a stationary stimulus and, with larger amplitudes, for sound movement to the right and to the left. Composite (global field power) waveforms displayed for each of the three subject groups consistently showed greater amplitude in the movement conditions in the latency region of 500 to 600 ms, but no difference in amplitude for sound movement to the right versus left side. The amplitude of auditory evoked responses evoked by sound movement was greatest in the children and decreased as a function of age for the young and older adult subject groups. Jerger and Estes (2002) acknowledged the possible effect on the findings of peripheral hearing loss in the older subjects. Consistent with previous reports and hemispheric specialization for spatial processing, topographic mapping of the auditory evoked response data showed an asymmetric pattern, with more activation over the right versus the left hemisphere.

DURATION. | As early as the 1960s, Davis and colleagues conducted extensive studies of the effects of duration (rise/fall and plateau times) on the ALR in normal-hearing subjects (Davis & Zerlin, 1966; Onishi & Davis, 1968). In the second study, the stimuli were 1000 Hz tone bursts with linear onset-offset ramps. Varying rise/fall and plateau times produced somewhat complex effects on ALR latency and amplitude. For example, at a fixed rise/fall time (30 ms), there was no change in latency (of N1 or P1 components) or of amplitude (N1 to P1) as duration was varied from 0 through 300 ms. However, with a relatively brief rise/fall time of 3 ms, a progressive reduction of the plateau time from 30 ms down to 0 ms produced a corresponding reduction in ALR amplitude. Also, with a relatively long fixed-plateau time, ALR amplitude remained constant as rise/fall time was decreased from 50 to 300 ms. Steeper slopes for the rise/fall time resulted in shorter ALR latencies.

Temporal integration time, as assessed with auditory evoked responses, corresponds to the minimum duration of a signal that produces maximum AER amplitude. Among AERs, temporal integration times are directly related to latency of the response. For example, temporal integration times are short (less than 2 ms) for the short latency ABR (e.g., Hecox et al., 1976), longer (about 5 ms) for the AMLR (Lane et al., 1971; Skinner & Antinoro, 1971), and longer yet ($\geq$30 ms) for the ALR (Forss, Mäkelä, McEvoy, & Hari, 1993; Onishi & Davis, 1968). More recently, investigators of the ALR have extended these findings to include more detailed analysis changes in ALR waves' subcomponents associated with changes in duration for pure-tone and noise signals and trains of click signals (Alain, Woods, & Covarrubias, 1997; Forss et al., 1993; Ostroff, McDonald, Schneider, & Alain, 2003). As an example, Alain et al. (1997) examined with the ALR the effects on temporal integration of stimulus duration features (e.g., rise time) and frequency (low versus high). Notably, the authors also evaluated temporal integration times for different waves and subcomponents of the ALR, such as N1a, N1b, and N1c. Alain et al. (1997) presumed that the subcomponents reflect functionally different neural populations (e.g., onset neurons, neu-

rons specialized for complex signals) that, in turn, are likely to have different temporal integration times. To test this assumption, the authors subtracted ALR waveforms elicited by 24 ms tones from those elicited with 72 ms tones. The remaining N1 wave (a duration difference wave) presumably was not a product of the onset response common to each of the signals but, rather, a reflection of the neural process associated with the duration difference between the two signals. The authors interpreted this finding as evidence that neurons other than simply onset detectors are involved in the generation of the ALR N1 wave, perhaps primary, pauser, or off response neurons. In addition to confirming the general temporal integration time findings reported by previous investigators, Alain et al. (1997) discovered that changes in signal duration produced different scalp distributions for the ALR N1 wave (fronto-central region) and the P 2 wave (posterior electrode sites). Changes in stimulus duration also differentially influenced subcomponents of the N1 wave (N1a, N1b, N1c).

Alain et al. (1997) provided some evidence, consistent with well-recognized patterns for psychophysical data, of longer temporal integration times for lower stimulus frequencies and vice versa. Eddins and Peterson (1999) investigated temporal integration with the ALR N1 and P2 components. Subjects were five audiometrically normal (thresholds of 15 dB HL or better) hearing adults (four female and one male) aged 21 to 34 years. The ALR was elicited with tonal stimuli of 1000 and 4000 Hz presented via insert earphones at a rate of 1.1/second with rise and fall times of 4 ms, and with total durations of 8, 16, 32, 64, and 128 ms. Stimulus intensity was varied in 2 dB increments from 20 dB above behavioral threshold, for the same stimulus, to –4 dB sensation level (relative to behavioral threshold). Recordings were made with an Fz noninverting electrode site and a right mastoid inverting electrode site, an analysis time of 500 ms, and band-pass filter settings of 1 to 30 Hz. Eddins and Peterson (1999) found a significant reduction in ALR threshold as a function of signal duration, a pattern consistent with the conclusions of numerous psychophysical studies of temporal integration. In addition, the slope of the threshold improvement with duration was higher for the 1000 Hz versus 4000 Hz signal. Also, consistent with long-standing findings for the ALR (e.g., Onishi & Davis, 1968; Skinner & Jones, 1968), latencies for N1 and P2 waves decreased with increasing duration, although the latency changes were mostly for the change in signal duration from 8 to 32 ms. Amplitude of the ALR waves did not change notably with signal duration. Durations of less than 8 ms were not employed in the study. These two studies demonstrate the potential value of the ALR in exploring with humans neurophysiologic mechanisms underlying basic auditory processes, such as temporal processing.

Rosburg, Haueisen, and Sauer (2002) investigated the effect of signal duration on habituation with the auditory evoked neuromagnetic field (AEF) N100m component.

The N100m component is the neuromagnetic counterpart to the ALR N1 (N100) component that is typically recorded with electrophysiological measures. Signals were 1000 Hz tones with durations of 50, 100, or 200 ms, presented monaurally in three blocks of 210 trials/block. Duration of the tonal stimuli employed in the study had no effect on habituation. However, in another paper published in the same year, Rosburg, Haueisen, and Sauer (2002) found within the time course of the N100m component a shift in the dipole equivalent source. The shift in detection of the response from superior to inferior electrode sites, and from posterior to anterior electrode sites, was affected by stimulus duration.

Ostroff, McDonald, Schneider, and Alain (2003) applied the ALR in a study of the effect of advancing age on sound duration processing. Subjects consisted of three groups: young (average age of 27 years), middle aged (average age of 47 years), and older (average age of 69 years). Stimuli of different durations (8 to 18 ms) were created from 2000 Hz pure tones. Amplitude for the N1 wave increased linearly as a function of stimulus duration, and the change was the same for in all subject age groups. Amplitude changes were noted with stimulus duration differences of 2 to 4 ms. An age-related effect, however, was observed for the P2 component. Young and middle-aged subjects showed an increase in amplitude with longer durations, whereas duration changes did not produce a significant amplitude change for the older adults. The authors interpreted this finding as evidence of impairment in the encoding of signal duration with advanced age.

Numerous investigators have for many years analyzed in detail the ALR and P300 elicited by the end of a stimulus, that is, the "off response" (Davis, Davis, Loomis, Harvey, & Hobart, 1939; Davis & Zerlin, 1966; Hillyard & Picton, 1978; Papanicolaou, Lorring, & Eisenberg, 1985; Pfefferbaum, Buchsbaum, & Gips, 1971; Rose & Malone, 1965). Both off response morphology and latency tend to be comparable to that elicited by stimulus onset, but amplitude is generally smaller.

INTENSITY. | As with other AERs, one of the first observations made about the ALR was that amplitude increased in an essentially linear fashion as stimulus intensity increased, whereas latency decreased over the same intensity range (Antinoro, Skinner, & Jones, 1969; Beagley & Knight, 1967; Davis, Mast, Yoshie, & Zerlin, 1966; Davis & Zerlin, 1966; Onishi & Davis, 1968; Picton et al., 1977; Rapin, Schimmel, Tourk, Krasnegor, & Pollak, 1966; Rothman, 1970). Changes in amplitude as a function of stimulus intensity function tended to level off, or saturate, for moderate to high intensities (above approximately 70 dB). This basic relation between ALR amplitude and stimulus intensity is illustrated in Figure 12.2. Amplitude in these earlier studies was typically calculated from the trough of N1 to the peak of P2 (for vertex-positive voltage recordings) because that was the most stable ALR measure. In retrospect, information from the lit-

erature on stimulus intensity and the ALR is constrained by the analysis convention at the time of viewing the N1 and P2 waves as an N1-P2 wave complex. It is now recognized that the N1 and P2 waves have different anatomic generators. Furthermore, the two waves do not always co-vary with changes in stimulus characteristics, such as intensity, frequency, duration, or more subtle acoustic properties (e.g., Adler & Adler, 1989; Crowley & Colrain, 2004; Hari et al., 1987). With regard to signal intensity alone, amplitude for the N1 and P2 waves does increase in parallel for low and moderate levels. For higher signal intensity levels (70 to 90 dB), however, P2 amplitude continues to increase while, curiously, latency and amplitude for the N1 wave actually decrease (Adler & Adler, 1989; Picton, Woods, Baribeau-Braun, & Healey, 1977). The differential effects of low- to moderate- versus high-stimulus intensity levels on ALR waves, and amplitude versus latency measures, can be clearly defined with clinical measurement protocols, such as tone-burst stimuli and simple electrode configurations (e.g., noninverting electrode at Cz and linked ear inverting electrodes).

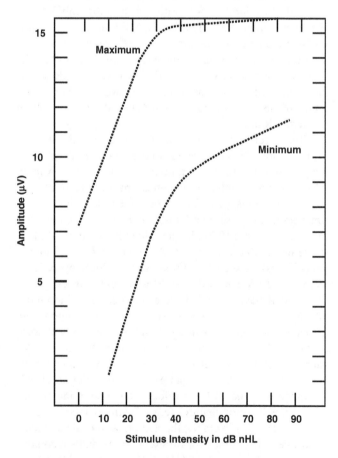

Effect of Stimulus Intensity on Amplitude of the N1-P2 Wave Complex of the ALR

FIGURE 12.2. Effect of signal intensity on the P2 component of the ALR compiled from multiple published studies (see text for references).

The general conclusion that latency of the ALR N1 and P2 components decreases systematically and in parallel as a function of stimulus intensity, reported in early studies cited above, has also undergone revision. Adler and Adler (1989) described a nonlinear change in latency with stimulus intensity, with a more pronounced decrease in latency for lower intensity levels (< 45 to 50 dB) than higher signal intensity levels and relatively greater effect of intensity on latency for the P2 wave than for the N1 wave at low intensity levels. As intensity approximates behavioral threshold for the same stimulus (e.g., 1000 Hz), the P2 wave disappears first, and then the N1 wave. ALR latency changes with intensity vary for clicks versus tonal stimuli (Rapin et al., 1966). For an ALR evoked by a click stimulus, latency for the N1 or P2 components changes relatively little as stimulus intensity increases, except at intensity levels very close to auditory threshold. As Rapin et al. (1966) point out, ALR latency has limited potential for estimation of audiometric threshold. In contrast, latency for N1 and P2 systematically decreases as tone stimulus intensity increases (Adler & Adler, 1989). Variability in response latency occurs with intensity levels near threshold, but it decreases as stimulus intensity level is increased to about 40 dB or higher levels. ALR can be elicited by intensity (amplitude) modulation of an ongoing (carrier) tone, as well as by presentation of a transient stimulus (Butler, 1968; McCandless & Rose, 1970; Picton, Hillyard, & Galambos, 1976). Eddins and Peterson (1999), in the study of the time-intensity relationship for the ALR with five normal-hearing young adults (cited above in the review of duration effects), noted that the N1 wave was detected for signal intensity levels that were an average of 8 dB higher than behavioral thresholds for 1000 Hz (standard deviation of 3.7 dB) and 7 dB higher for 4000 Hz (standard deviation of 3.2 dB). ALR threshold is clearly influenced by signal duration, reflecting an electrophysiological version of the psychophysical process of temporal integration or "time-intensity trading." The relation between signal duration and intensity was discussed also in the previous section on signal duration.

There was, early on, debate as to whether the amplitude–intensity relationship was better described by a power law (i.e., a straight line plotted on double-logarithmic coordinates) or a linear function of absolute amplitude in microvolts and intensity in dB (Antinoro, Skinner, & Jones, 1969). The decibel is, by definition, a logarithmic unit, so this method of plotting results is actually done by converting amplitude to a logarithmic unit. Keidel and Spreng (1965) found that the slope of the log-log intensity-amplitude plot agrees with a power-law (Stevens, 1961) relationship. With different experimental designs, research has failed to support such a strong association (Davis, Bowers, & Hirsh, 1968; Davis & Zerlin, 1966; Tempest & Bryan, 1966). Also, the effects of signal intensity on the ALR interact with non-inverting electrode site. ALRs recorded from midline site (e.g., Fz and Cz) are more dependent on signal intensity and the order of signal presentation (of different intensities) than those for lateral scalp electrode sites over the temporal lobe regions (Carrillo-de-la-Pena & Garcia-Larrea, 1999).

As noted above, early studies confirmed that the largest amplitude increase occurs within the first 20 to 30 dB above auditory threshold, and then amplitude increases more gradually with increasing intensity levels, in some persons actually reaching a plateau or "saturation" above approximately 75 dB (Beagley & Knight, 1967; Davis & Zerlin, 1966; Onishi & Davis, 1968; Picton et al., 1977; Rapin et al., 1966; Spink, Johannsen, & Pirsig, 1979; Spoor, Timmer, & Odenthal, 1969). Although considerable intra- and interindividual variability characterizes the amplitude–intensity relationship, the changes in amplitude are more regular for tonal versus click stimuli. There is an interaction among stimulus frequency, intensity, and ALR amplitude. As intensity level is increased, females show greater overall amplitude and a steeper slope in the intensity-amplitude function. Amplitude increases as a function of intensity are steeper for lower frequency stimuli (e.g., 500 Hz) than for higher frequencies (e.g., 8000 Hz), according to Antinoro, Skinner, and Jones (1969). However, Rapin et al. (1966) found the largest amplitude changes with intensity for 1000 Hz, less for 250 Hz, and least for 6000 Hz. In related studies, Shimizu (1968) reported larger ALR amplitude in patients with clinical evidence of loudness recruitment, as well as smaller responses in those with tone decay. Clayton and Rose (1970), however, did not confirm the connection between the ALRs and loudness recruitment.

RATE AND INTERSTIMULUS INTERVAL (ISI). | The ALRs are highly dependent on ISI (Budd et al., 1998; Davis et al., 1966; Fruhstorfer, Soveri, & Jarvilehto, 1970; Hari, Kaila, Katila, Tuomisto, & Varpula, 1982). The duration of monaural signals used in eliciting the ALR is often about 50 or 60 ms (e.g., 20 ms rise and fall times, plus a 20 ms duration), or even longer. Consequently, the total accumulated duration constitutes a considerable portion of the analysis time. This is in distinct contrast to the relation between stimulus duration and ISI for transient (e.g., 0.1 ms) click signals. Even when the total time occupied by multiple click signals is accumulated, it occupies a negligible portion of the analysis time and has a minimal impact on ISI. Importantly for the ALR, recovery times (e.g., neural refractory periods) are also longer. For this reason, ISI is a more accurate and straightforward way of describing the rate factor in ALR measurement than simply noting the number of stimuli presented per second. Another related term encountered in the literature on the late auditory responses is "stimulus onset asynchrony," abbreviated SOA. A short SOA condition implies smaller ISIs (e.g., a time interval of 700 ms from the onset of one stimulus to the onset of the next stimulus), whereas with a long SOA the time between onsets for successive stimuli is on the order of seconds, not milliseconds (e.g., 8 seconds). Often, the term SOA is used with rather complex stimulus conditions involving the presentation of a series of signals that vary along one or more dimensions, such as frequency and/or duration, hence the reference to "asynchrony."

Some of the early ALR studies confirmed that longer ISIs and, concomitantly, slower stimulus rates produced substantially larger amplitudes for N1 and P2 components, but had little effect on the latency of these ALR components (Davis et al., 1966; Fruhstorfer, Soveri, & Jarvilehto, 1970; Hari et al., 1982; Keidel & Spreng, 1965; Nelson & Lassman, 1968; Picton, Woods, Barbeau-Braun, & Healy, 1977; Rothman, Davis, & Hay, 1970). The effect of ISI on the ALR amplitude was interpreted as linear relation with the refractory period of neurons in the auditory cortex. That is, after being activated by a stimulus, the neurons require time to return to their normal resting state before they are capable of responding maximally to the next signal. The refractory time is directly related to the latency of the evoked response, but also to response amplitude. Presentation of a signal during the neuronal recovery process (i.e., when the ISI is shorter than the refractory time) results in smaller than optimal amplitude. Conversely, with increases in the ISI there are predictable increases also in ALR amplitude (e.g., Davis et al., 1966; Davis & Zerlin, 1966). The increased ISI required for production of maximum amplitude ALR waves is not necessarily related temporally, or neurophysiologically, to the refractory period for individual neurons (Umbricht et al., 2004). Refractory times for neurons are considerably shorter than the "refractory" period for the N1 and P2 waves of the ALR. Other nonstimulus factors, such as memory, also affect the generation of ALRs (e.g., Näätänen & Winkler, 1999), perhaps exclusively the ALR and not other responses.

Longer latency AERs are dependent on longer refractory times and vice versa. The general relationship between the ISI and the combined amplitude of the N1 ad P2 components of the ALR is illustrated in Figure 12.3. At a moderate intensity level (60 to 70 dB peSPL), ALR amplitudes are very modest (e.g., less than 2 μVolts) for stimulus presentation rates of greater than 1/sec, i.e., ISI times of less than 1 second. Amplitudes of the N1 and the P2 components increase markedly as the signal rate is slowed, and ISI time is increased. The most pronounced effect of longer ISI times is within the range of 1 to 6 seconds. However, further increases in amplitude may be observed by lengthening ISI times to 10 seconds or even longer. At these slower stimulus presentation rates (longer ISI times), the amplitude of the N1 or the P2 components of the ALR are, on the average, 6 to 8 μVolts when evoked with a similarly moderate stimulus intensity level. Again, later investigation prompted a revision of some of the conclusions from the initial ALR studies from the 1960s. For example, Roth, Ford, Lewis, and Kopell (1976) reported differential effects of ISI for the amplitude of N1 versus P2. The amplitude for P2 did increase rather systematically with stimulus rate, whereas N1 ampli-

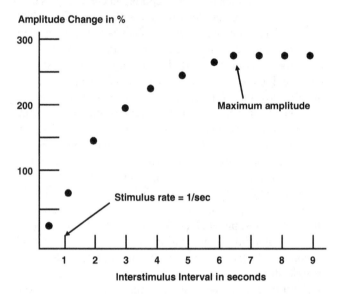

Effect of Interstimulus Interval on the Combined Amplitude for ALR N1-P2 Waves

FIGURE 12.3. An illustration of the effect of interstimulus interval (ISI) on the auditory latency response (ALR) N1 and P2 component.

tude remained relatively stable for ISIs within the range of 0.75 to 1.5 seconds. Latency of the Nd wave ("processing negativity") is highly dependent on signal presentation rate. With slow stimulus presentation rates, and ISIs of 1250 ms and longer, the Nd wave is first detected at a latency beyond the N1 wave. At faster signal presentation rates and shorter ISIs, the Nd wave latency decreases until it overlaps with N1 wave. With a decrease in ISIs down to 800 ms, the processing negativity (Nd) begins during the initial negative slope of the N1 wave (Hansen & Hillyard, 1984; Hillyard, Hink, Schwent, & Picton, 1973; Näätänen et al., 1978).

The clinical implication of the well-appreciated relationship between stimulus presentation rate and ALR amplitude is to employ slow stimulus rates (longer ISIs) in recording the ALR in patient populations. Of course, in the clinical application of longer latency AERs, other factors (e.g., test time, patient compliance and age, habituation) must also be taken into account in determining the optimal and most clinically feasible rate of stimulation.

Stimulus intensity also interacts with rate. The amount of amplitude increase associated with lengthened ISIs—that is, the amplitude-versus-ISI slope—is steeper for higher intensity levels. Davis et al. (1966), for example, found a slope of 19.1 μV amplitude/log 10 ISI in seconds at 85 dB HL. At 60 dB SL, Nelson and Lassman (1968) reported a slope of 5.6 μV amplitude/log 10 ISI in seconds. Examining the relationship from another perspective, there is also evidence that the amplitude-versus-intensity slope is steeper for longer ISIs (Keidel & Spreng, 1965).

Stimulus rate and ISI are also interactive with multiple additional variables, including stimulus, acquisition, and subject factors (nonpathologic and pathologies). For example, there is an interaction among ALR amplitude, stimulus rate, stimulus laterality (monaural versus binaural), ALR electrode site, age and, perhaps, pathology. For ISI values of less than 4 seconds, ALR wave N100 amplitude is comparable for frontal versus central electrode recordings. With longer ISIs (greater than 4 seconds), vertex electrode recordings yield larger amplitudes. Hari et al. (1982) speculated that frequent-versus-infrequent stimuli activate different anatomic generators for the ALR. Although a prominent N1 component is detected from fronto-central electrode sites (e.g., Fz), with increased ISIs (slower signal rates) larger amplitudes for the N1 wave are recorded at more posterior electrode sites, with maximum amplitude at the vertex (Cz) location (e.g., Hari et al., 1980; McCallum & Curry, 1981; Näätänen & Picton, 1987). Longer ISIs (e.g., > 1 second) are required to consistently record an N1 component from children (Bruneau et al., 1997). For children, stimulus rate in general is an important factor in the amplitude of the N1 component, with decreases in amplitude on the order of 50 percent or more when the ISI is reduced from 4 seconds to 1 second (Picton et al., 1974). In children, the refractory period for the N1 component (and perhaps its generators) decreases as a function of age. The ALR N2 wave, other hand, appears to be relatively unaffected by comparable increases in signal rate (decreases in ISI).

Recent investigations have focused on the interaction of ISI and mode of stimulation—monaural versus binaural. The discussion herein is limited to those studies that utilized binaural presentation of stimuli, tones for example, to each ear in the measurement of ALRs with one stimulus serving as the target stimulus evoking the ALR and the other signal as competition. Clinical studies in patient populations are reviewed later in the chapter. One paper is noted here to illustrate the potential value of manipulating stimulus parameters in the clinical investigation of ALR in brain pathology. Knight, Hillyard, Woods, and Neville (1980) recorded ALRs from patients with confirmed cerebral lesions. Frontal lesions did not produce ALR (N1 and P2) abnormalities, regardless of stimulus rate (ISIs of 0.5 to 3 seconds). The N1 component had poor morphology, however, among patients with temporoparietal lobe lesions. Furthermore, increasing the ISI over this range did not produce the amplitude increase expected for normal subjects. This study also supports the concept that N1 and P2 receive contributions, in part at least, from different neuroanatomic sources. Clinical applications of ALR are discussed in greater detail in the final section of this chapter.

STIMULUS REPETITION. | Late AERs have been elicited with various patterns of stimulus repetition, including presentation of single stimuli at regular intervals, single stimuli at irregular intervals, and trains of stimuli (a cluster of one or more signals separated by relatively short intervals) followed by longer (intertrain) intervals. There are also studies of the ALR elicited with frequent and predictable stimuli presented in combination with infrequent (e.g., improbable, rare, or deviant) stimuli—the oddball stimulus paradigm commonly associated with the P300 response. As noted in a discussion of stimulus repetition patterns for the AMLR (Chapter 11), analysis of the differences in the amplitude of auditory evoked responses for the first stimulus (S1) versus a second stimulus (S2) in a train has been applied in the investigation of higher level brain processes, such as "sensory gating." For the AMLR, an amplitude change for the P50 (Pb) component from the first to the second stimulus is calculated as a ratio (S2/S1) or simple mathematical difference (S1 − S2), with lower ratios and larger differences consistent with more inhibition or "gating out" of irrelevant sensory input. If the second stimulus is different than the first, or novel, then larger ratios and smaller differences (or no difference) are consistent with "gating in," or a preattentive response of the brain indicating the ability to identify novel or potentially significant stimuli (e.g., Boutros & Belger, 1999; Rosburg, Trautner, Korzyukov, et al., 2004). Recall that the Pb (P50) component of the AMLR is most likely the P1 wave of the ALR.

The phenomenon of short- and long-term habituation to acoustic signals has been investigated with the ALR. Crowley and Colrain (2004) reported decreased N1 amplitude for signals within a train, indicating short-term habituation, and decreased N1 amplitude from train to train as an indication of long-term habituation. In a study of neuromagnetic auditory evoked fields (AEF), Rosburg, Marinou, et al. (2004) applied the ALR N1 (N100m) wave and the MMNm as an index of habituation. Results of previous studies of habituation with the auditory evoked neuromagnetic response N100m component were inconsistent (e.g., Budd et al., 1998; Fruhstorfer, Soveri, & Jarvilehto, 1970; Ritter, Vaughn, & Costa, 1968; Soininen et al., 1995). The "m" descriptor for the waves specifies an auditory evoked neuromagnetic response, rather than a conventional electrophysiologic response. Subjects in the Rosburg, Trautner, Korzyukov, et al. (2004) study were sixteen young healthy males (N = 6) and females (N = 10) ranging in age from 21 to 28 years. The AEF was elicited under two different stimulus conditions. In the "habituation" condition, Stimuli were five identical 1000 Hz tones with rise/fall times of 5 ms and a total duration of 50 ms, presented at an intensity level of 85 dB SPL. The stimulus onset asynchrony (SOA) within the train of tones was 1000 ms (1 second), whereas the interval between the sequences (trains) of tones was 7000 ms (7 seconds). In the other "mix" condition, there were ten different tones that varied in frequency from 800 to 1250 Hz in 50 Hz increments. Duration was the same (50 ms with 5 ms rise/fall times) for each of the stimuli. The stimuli were delivered with an SOA of 1000 ms in a pseudorandomized sequence, although every tenth stimulus was repeated and each of the stimulus patterns was repeated with the same probability. A complete description of the AEF recording technique is beyond the scope of this discussion. For technical details, the reader is referred to the reviews of methodology in the many published papers on neuromagnetic auditory evoked responses. Neither amplitude nor latency of the AEF N100m component was affected by permanently varying signal (tone) repetition. Interestingly, the dipole location for the N100m component varied during the first four stimulus repetitions. It's unclear whether this pattern for habituation to repeated stimulus presentations occurs also with the P2 wave of the ALR (Fruhstorfer, 1971; Kenemans, Verbaten, Roelofs, & Slangen, 1989; Lutzenberger, Elbert, Rockstroh, & Birbaumer, 1979; Megala & Teyler, 1979; Rust, 1977).

There are rather complex interactions among stimulus rate (ISIs), stimulus repetition, age, ALR waveform morphology, and topographic distribution of the ALR waves. The interactive influences of multiple measurement and subject factors on the ALR contribute to difficulty in comparing results among published investigations. Karhu et al. (1997) conducted an ALR study with 9-year-old children and with adult subjects. The ALR N1 component was evoked with repeated trains (sequences) of four tones presented with ISIs of 1 second and separated by an interval of 12 seconds. In children, amplitude of the N1 wave decreased by about 50 percent from the first to the fourth successive tones within the sequence, and N1 latency increased. During the stimulus repetition, the N2 wave in children increased in amplitude. With continued recording of the ALR from children, there was a gradual dominance of the N2 wave and loss of the N1 wave. Although signal repetition with the four tone sequences also produced smaller N1 amplitude in adults, the decrease was less than in the children, and the N1 wave clearly remained.

Tremblay, Billings, and Rohila (2004) reported findings highlighting the effects of stimulus complexity and stimulus presentation rate, and the role played by age, in the N1 -P2 complex of the ALR. Subjects were adults grouped according to age as younger (21 to 33 years) and older (63 to 79 years). Although all subjects were described as "normal hearing" based on pure-tone hearing thresholds of 25 dB HL or better, hearing for audiometric frequencies above 500 Hz was better for the younger subjects. For example, average hearing thresholds for the younger subject group were about 5 dB better at 1000 Hz and about 15 dB better at 8000 Hz. Stimulus intensity was 74 dB SPL for both groups. At an ISI of 910 ms (for tonal and for speech stimuli), latencies for the N1 and the P2 components of the ALR were significantly delayed for older subjects, but there was no age effect when the ISI was increased to 1510 ms (i.e., stimulus presentation rate was slowed down). Tremblay, Billings, and Rohila (2004) offer as a possible explanation for the findings "age-related refractory differences in younger and older auditory systems. Specifically older auditory systems might require a longer period of time than younger systems to recover from the initial excitation before neurons are able to fire again" (p. 235).

CONTRALATERAL SIGNALS. | The ALR may be altered by sounds presented to nonstimulus ear. The contralateral sounds may be tones, some type of noise (e.g., white noise), or speech (e.g., multitalker babble, meaningful discourse). Competing sounds presented to one ear appear to interfere with subject attention to signals presented to the other ear. Cranford and colleagues (Krumm & Cranford, 1994; Martin & Cranford, 1991) reported amplitude reduction for the N1 to P2 wave complex with the presentation of a speech signal (babble) to the nonstimulus ear. Follow-up topographic AER studies showed that the effect of the contralateral sound was different for the N1 versus P2 waves. In addition, the effect of the competing speech signal varied as a function of the interaction of various factors, including the characteristics of the target stimulus (e.g., tones versus speech), difficulty of the listening task (i.e., discrimination of the target signal), and subject factors, such as age (Fisher et al., 2000; Hymel, Cranford, & Stuart, 1998).

Cranford, Rothermel, Walker, Stuart, and Elangovan (2004) further investigated the effects of the difficulty of a listening task and a competing signal on the N1 and P2 components of the ALR. In this study, subjects were ten young normal-hearing female adults (age 20 to 35 years). The tasks involved discrimination of two frequencies that were separated by either an octave (1000 versus 2000 Hz) or only 100 Hz (1000 versus 1100 Hz), and these tasks were performed in quiet (with no competing signal) and then with speech competition presented to the nontarget ear. Amplitude for the N1 wave was the same for each discrimination task (easy versus difficult) and in the quiet versus competition signal conditions. In contrast, there was a reduction in amplitude for the P2 component for the difficult versus easy task and with the competing signal in comparison to the quiet condition. These findings are another example of the independence of the N1 and P2 waves and argue against simple analysis of the N1 -P2 complex within the ALR waveform. The work of Dr. Cranford and colleagues also points to some potential clinical applications, such as measurement of the ALR with competing sounds in children with auditory processing disorder (APD).

Acquisition Parameters

ANALYSIS TIME. | The ALRs are long latency responses with major components (P1, N1, P2, N2) and other waves (e.g., N400) beginning or persisting long after the "middle-latency" region. The ALR analysis time should extend for at least for 500 ms after the stimulus. Poststimulus analysis times of 1000 to 1500 ms (1 to 1.5 second) in ALR measurement are often reported in literature, almost always with a prestimulus analysis period (e.g., 100 ms). In the interest of consistency among protocols, and for simultaneous measurement of more than one AER within the same time frame, equivalent analysis periods can be used for measurement of both the ALR and P300 response.

ELECTRODES. | Much of the current information on the different effects of electrode location on the ALR was generated by investigators attempting to determine the neural sources of the response (Goff, Allison, & Vaughan, 1978; Kooi, Tipton, & Marshall, 1971; Picton, Hillyard, Krausz, & Galambos, 1974; Simson, Vaughan, & Ritter, 1976; Vaughan, 1982; Vaughan & Ritter, 1970; Wood & Wolpaw, 1982). Pauline Davis (1939), in the first description of ALR, noted that the response was largest when recorded at the vertex. Many other investigators have subsequently presented evidence confirming that the vertex, or a location within two or three centimeters lateral or anterior, is an optimal electrode site (Abe, 1954; Cody & Bickford, 1965; Cody, Jacobson, Walker, & Bickford, 1964; Davis & Zerlin, 1966; Picton, Hillyard, Krausz, & Galambos, 1974; Ruhm, 1971; Teas, 1965; Vaughan & Ritter, 1970; Walker, Jacobson, & Cody, 1964). The figure adapted from the classic Vaughan and Ritter (1970) study showing ALR waveforms recorded from different coronal electrode arrays offers a concise illustration of the influence of recording site on the response (see Figure 1.12 in Chapter 1). There is diminishing response amplitude at greater distances from midline and then clear reversal of the waveform polarity in the region or plane of the temporal lobe (the Sylvian fissure).

The ALR can, therefore, be reliably recorded with a noninverting electrode located anywhere over the frontal portion of the scalp of the head, especially along the midline (see Figure 12.4). The ALR components usually have maximum amplitude with a vertex site. Major ALR components (e.g., N1 and P2) have smaller amplitudes when recorded with hemispheric electrodes over coronal (e.g., C3 and C4) and temporal regions (T3 and T4). However, some ALR components, such as the Nc wave with a latency of about 150 ms, are recorded with noninverting electrodes over the temporal lobes. Wolpaw and Penry (1975, 1978), for example, provided evidence of a difference in waveform morphology in the 80 to 200 ms region for Cz versus T3/T4 electrode sites that they referred as the "T complex." The T complex was composed of a positive voltage peak at about 105 to 110 ms and then a negative peak at about 150 to 160 ms. These investigators further showed that the conventional N1-P2 complex and new T complexes were greater in amplitude when recorded from electrodes located on the scalp contralateral to the stimulus, and greater for T4 (the right side) than T3 (the left side). A right hemisphere dominance in brain activity (and sometimes a left ear effect) is often observed for nonverbal stimulation. Components in the early portion (0 to 80 ms) and late portion (200 to 250 ms) of the analysis period are generally comparable as recorded with vertex versus temporal electrodes. ALR generation, at least for the N1 component, involves in part the posterior superior temporal plane and nearby parietal lobe regions. Amplitude of the N1-P2 complex is influenced by an interaction of signal intensity, the order of signal presentation, and the noninverting electrode site (Carrillo-de-la-Pena & Garcia-Larrea, 1999).

Auditory Late Response Electrode Sites

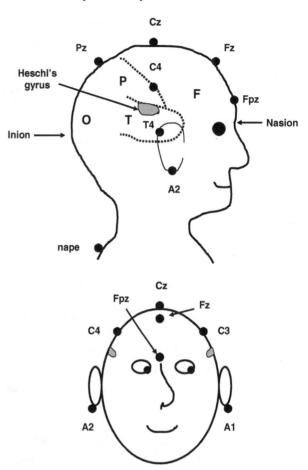

FIGURE 12.4. Minimal electrode sites (noninverting and inverting) used for clinical measurement of the ALR. The inverting electrodes can be located on the ears (e.g., earlobes) and linked or on a noncephalic site (e.g., the nape of the neck). Electrode sites are labeled according to the 10–20 International system.

ALRs recorded from frontal-central electrode sites (e.g., Fz and Cz) are more dependent on signal intensity and the order of signal presentation (of different intensities) than ALRs detected with lateral scalp electrode sites over the temporal lobe regions. In addition, amplitude of the N1 component is larger when it is recorded from an electrode over the frontal or temporal lobe contralateral to the side of stimulation, whereas amplitude of the P1 and P2 components is diminished for a contralateral (versus ipsilateral) noninverting electrode array (Näätänen & Picton, 1987). Hemispheric differences in amplitude for the N1 versus P1 and P2 components have also been reported in the effects of auditory training on the ALR (Tremblay & Kraus, 2002). The general topic of auditory training and the ALR is reviewed later is this chapter.

The inverting electrode for ALR measurements, as reported in the literature, is usually located either on the

TABLE 12.2. Guidelines for an Auditory Late Response (ALR) Test Protocol

PARAMETER	SUGGESTION	RATIONALE/COMMENT
Stimulus Parameters		
Transducer	ER-3A	Supra-aural earphones are acceptable for ALR, but insert earphones are more comfortable for longer AER recording sessions. Insert earphones also serve to attenuate background sound in the test setting. In addition, since the insert cushions are disposable, their use contributes to infection control.
Type	Tone burst	Highly transient click signals are inappropriate for the ALR. Longer duration tonal signals are preferred.
	Speech	The ALR can be effectively elicited with speech signals (natural or synthetic), such as /da/ and /pa/. Various characteristics of speech signals, e.g., voice onset time, can be used in ALR stimulation.
Duration		
Rise/fall	~10 ms	Longer onset times are feasible for signals used to elicit the ALR.
Plateau	~50 ms	Extended plateau durations are effective in eliciting the ALR.
Rate	≤ 1.1/second	A slow rate of signal presentation is essential for the ALR, due to the long refractory time of cortical neurons. ALR amplitude may increase with progressively slower signal presentation rates to 0.125/sec and longer interstimulus intervals, or ISIs, up to 8 seconds.
Polarity	Rarefaction	Signal polarity is not an important parameter for ALR measurement.
Intensity	≤ 70 dB HL	Modest signal intensity levels are typical for ALR measurement.
Number	≤ 200	Signal repetitions vary depending on size of response and background noise. Remember the signal-to-noise ratio is the key. Averaging may require as few as 20 to 50 signals at high intensity levels for a very quiet and normal-hearing patient.
Presentation ear	Monaural	Binaural signals are often used.
Masking	50 dB	Rarely required with insert earphones and not needed for stimulus intensity levels of ≤ 70 dB HL.
Acquisition Parameters		
Amplification	50,000	Less amplification is required for larger responses.
Sensitivity	25 or 50 μvolts	Smaller sensitivity values are equivalent to higher amplification.
Analysis time	600 ms	An analysis epoch long enough to encompass the later (e.g., N400) components.
Prestimulus time	100 ms	The extended prestimulus time provides a stable estimate of background noise and a baseline for calculation of the amplitudes for negative and positive waveform components (N1, P2, P3).
Data points	≤ 512	
Sweeps	1000	See comments above for signal number.
Filters		
Band-pass	0.1 to 100 Hz	The ALR consists of low-frequency energy within the spectrum of the EEG.
Notch	none	A notch filter (removing spectral energy in the region of 60 Hz) should always be avoided with ALR measurement because important frequencies in the response will be removed.
Electrodes		
Type	Disc or disposable	Disc electrodes applied with paste (versus gel) are useful to secure the noninverting electrodes on the scalp. Red- and blue-colored electrode leads for the right and left hemisphere locations, respectively, are suggested. Disposable electrodes or a multiple-electrode cap are also appropriate with ALR measurement.

TABLE 12.2.   (continued)

PARAMETER	SUGGESTION	RATIONALE/COMMENT
Electrode sites		
	Noninverting	The Fz or Cz sites are appropriate for recording the ALR clinically, although many published studies include twenty or more electrode sites.
	Inverting	Linked earlobes are commonly used for inverting electrodes. A noncephalic electrode site (e.g., nape of the neck) is also appropriate.
	Other	Ocular electrodes (located above and below or to the side of an eye) are required for the detection of eye blinks and rejection of averages contaminated by eye blinks.
Ground	Fpz	The common (ground) electrode can be located anywhere on the body, but a low forehead or nasion (between the eyes) location is convenient and effective.

mastoid or on the earlobe ipsilateral to the stimulus ear, or electrodes linked between both ears. Wood and Wolpaw (1982) studied relative activity of cephalic versus noncephalic reference sites with human ALRs. They did not detect voltage gradients at the neck or below, whereas there were large voltage gradients for varied electrode locations on the head. These studies confirmed that the commonly used reference sites (e.g., mastoid, nose, ear) in ALR measurement are highly active. The authors recommended a noncephalic reference site, such as the balanced sterno-vertebral (SV) reference because it is both inactive and is minimally affected by EKG (heart activity) artifact. Giard et al. (1988) also presented data suggesting that a nasal inverting electrode site was active with regard to the detection of brain activity underlying the ALR N1 and Nd waves. With differential amplification, amplitude of any AER wave will be attenuated by the use of an electrode array that includes two active electrodes. The role of differential amplification AER measurement is reviewed in Chapter 3. As indicated in the test parameters summarized in Table 12.2, the nape of the neck is a practical and effective option for a noncephalic inverting, and true reference, electrode site. When the noninverting electrode serves as a true reference (i.e., inactive with regard to the AER activity being recorded), all of the brain activity contributing to the response is detected with the noninverting electrode and amplitude is maximal.

FILTER SETTINGS. | Frequency composition or spectrum for the ALR response and the P300 response are mainly in the frequency region under 30 Hz (Sayers, Beagley, & Henshall, 1974; Yamamoto, Sakabe, & Kaiho, 1979). Band-pass filter settings of less than 1 Hz (e.g., 0.1 Hz) to 30 or 100 Hz are typically employed in ALR and P300 measurement, with commonly reported values for the roll-off of 24 dB/octave for the high-pass filter (e.g., the 0.1 Hz setting) and 12 dB/octave for the low-pass filter (e.g., the 100 Hz setting).

Clinical Protocol for ALR Measurement

Stimulus and acquisition parameters for clinical measurement of the ALR, and their rationale, are summarized in Table 12.2. Some of these parameters, such as band-pass filter settings and electrode arrays, are appropriate for detection of the many ALR waves, are utilized for virtually all of the clinical applications of the ALR, and are shared with other long-latency cortical responses. Other parameters, such as stimulus type (e.g., one tone or multiple tones, tonal stimuli versus speech sounds), are varied to record or enhance the detection of specific ALR waves, such as subcomponents of the N1 wave complex. One of the most important variables in ALR measurement—subject state—is neither a stimulus nor acquisition parameter. Yet, manipulation of the listening task required of the subject, and inherent subject factors such as attention and memory, can have a profound impact on ALR measurement.

Analysis and Interpretation

NORMAL VARIATIONS. | As Donchin and Heffley (1978) noted, ALR components are not necessarily the same as ALR peaks. Although this issue of terminology may appear to be simply a matter of semantics, the point is rather fundamental and related to the anatomic source of the ALR. That is, a wave may in fact include more than one individual component, perhaps multiple components arising from different neural sources and affected differentially by manipulation of stimulus parameters (Hari, Sams, & Jarvilehto, 1979; Lehtonen, 1973), or even neuropathology. This basic concept in ALR measurement was emphasized in the discussion of ALR anatomy and physiology in Chapter 2. Indeed, the distinction between waves and components is only one of the clear conceptual differences between the early AERs and the late responses. Another distinction is related to the nature of the waveform. Waveform morphology for earlier latency AERs, such as ECochG, ABR, and even the AMLR, is remarkably consistent from one subject to the next and within subjects, for most variations of stimulus characteristics. Subject factors, such as state of arousal or attention to the signals, are negligible for the early latency responses. When subject factors do exert an influence on the earlier responses, each of the waves tends to be involved. Just the opposite is true for measurement of the late responses, including wave complexes within the ALR time frame. Relatively minor alterations in the acoustical properties of the signal(s) and subtle variations in subject behavior markedly influence morphology of the late responses and even the presence or absence of specific ALR waves or components with a single wave. The diverse wave components recorded within the late latency period were summarized in Table 12.1. Put another way, individual waves in the ALR do not always covary with changes in the stimulus or with subject factors. To some degree, each wave within the ALR time frame can be viewed as a "mini-response" that differs from its neighbors in terms of development, topographic distribution, and often other dimensions. In general, the morphology of auditory late response waveforms is complex and highly variable, especially for certain types of signals (e.g., speech sounds) and for demanding listening tasks. The complex interactions among multiple stimulus and acquisition parameters and subject characteristics were noted earlier in the present chapter.

The ALR N1 (N100) wave, really a wave complex, is usually a well-defined and sharp wave occurring within the latency region of 75 to 150 ms (Figure 12.5). Parameters of the N1 component (including its presence, latency, and amplitude) and the presence of subcomponents or other negative waves within the same time frame, are determined by the physical properties of the stimulus, such as the type (e.g., tone-burst or speech stimulus), the frequency for tonal stimuli, the intensity, the duration, and the rate of presentation), and also subject factors, such as state of arousal and sleep, attention, and memory (Alain, Woods, & Covarrubias, 1997; Picton, Woods, Baribeau-Braun, & Healy, 1977). Indeed, the N1 wave is enhanced (made more negative) when a subject selectively attends or listens to a specific stimulus. Researchers have debated whether the N1 is actually increased in amplitude during selective attention or whether the negativity in the region of N1 is really made greater by an overlapping processing negativity (the Nd component). Variations or components of the N1 wave complex include the N1b and N1c components, although it is not always easy with modification of measurement parameters to clearly differentiate the two waves (Perrault & Picton, 1984). The Nb component is recorded with a latency of about 100 ms with a noninverting electrode at a midline (e.g. Cz or Fz) site, whereas Nc is recorded with electrodes sites over the temporal lobe (e.g., C3 and C4). The N110 response, another variant or component of the N1 wave complex, can be evoked with speech stimuli or by specific acoustic properties or features of speech stimuli.

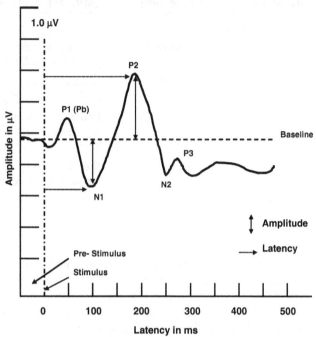

FIGURE 12.5. Analysis of latency and amplitude for the N1 and P2 components of the ALR.

The Nd wave, referred to as the "processing negativity" or PN (Näätänen & Michie, 1979), is a broad wave that follows and persists after presentation of a stimulus (Hillyard & Kutas, 1983; Näätänen, 1982). The Nd wave usually begins at a latency of about 150 ms, although with alterations in stimulus parameters (e.g., the ISI) or specific characteristics of subject attention to the stimuli, processing negativity may coincide with the earliest portion of the N1 wave. Attention to, and recognition and memory of, the stimulus is required for generation of the Nd wave (Hillyard, Hink, Schwent, & Picton, 1973). The processing negativity is considered an "attentional trace" that is influenced not only by selective attention or listening, but also such stimulus variables as "sensory reinforcement" (Alho et al., 1990) by a variety of stimulus-related factors, such as stimulus relevance, the probability of stimulus presentation, and the magnitude of the difference between stimuli (e.g., frequency separation for tones). In general, greater negativity (larger amplitude) of the Nd wave complex is associated with less probable stimuli and by smaller differences among stimuli that impose more challenging discrimination tasks.

The Nd component is not the same as the N1 component but, rather, contributes to the recording of negative voltage amplitude of the N1 component within the same latency region. The Nd wave or processing negativity really consists of early and late components with different scalp distributions (e.g., Hansen & Hillyard, 1980; Näätänen, 1982). By varying the specific requirements or stimulus features in a complex attention task that are required of a subject during ALR measurement, earlier and later latency subcomponents of the Nd wave (e.g., Nd_1, Nd_2, Nd_3) can be detected (see Giard et al., 1988, for review). These subcomponents of the Nd wave vary in latency, amplitude, and stability (reliability). The Nd can be differentiated from the conventional N1 component in three ways. First, the N1 component is essentially an onset response, whereas the Nd persists considerably beyond the latency of the N1 component. Second, when the N1 component for an attended signal is subtracted from the Nd elicited by an unattended signal, a negative wave remains, i.e., the Nd component. And, finally, topographic mapping of the evoked responses over the time domain shows that the persistent Nd component is generated in the region of the frontal lobe, whereas the initial negativity (N1 component) arises from the superior temporal gyrus region of the auditory cortex in the temporal lobe (Hansen & Hillyard, 1980; Hillyard & Picton, 1978; Näätänen, 1975; Näätänen & Michie, 1979; Okita, 1979).

The N400 response, as the label implies, is a negative wave in the region of 400 ms. The auditory N400 response is evoked with speech stimuli, but a comparable component can also be generated with visual linguistic stimuli, including sign language signals (Kutas, Neville, & Holcomb, 1987; McCallum, Farmer, & Pocock, 1984). The typical stimulus paradigm for the auditory N400 response involves semantic properties of language for single words, e.g., related versus nonrelated or for words within sentences. For example, the subject listens to sentences that are either semantically congruous or incongruous. A sentence that is semantically appropriate and expected—that makes sense (e.g., "I like my beer in a glass")—does not elicit an N400 response, whereas a sentence that is, unexpectedly, not semantically appropriate (e.g., "I like my beer in a shoe") produces an N400 response.

The P2 component is a robust, positive wave in the latency region of 180 to 250 ms. In normal persons, P2 may appear as a rather sharply peaked wave, as a broad wave with no distinct peak, or as a wave complex with multiple peaks. As noted in the preceding discussion about the N1 component, it's likely that major waves of the ALR as recorded from the scalp, are really wave complexes. Much of our information about the ALR dates back to investigations conducted in the 1960s and 1970s, cited throughout this chapter. As noted by Crowley and Colrain (2004), there was a tendency in the early studies to view the N1 and P2 waves not as independent components but, rather, as an N1-P2 wave complex. Amplitude, for example, was usually calculated from the trough of the N1 to the peak of P2, and not from the extreme amplitude of each wave to a prestimulus baseline. The effects of changes in stimulus characteristics, subject state (awake versus asleep, attending versus ignoring) and other manipulations of measurement conditions were assessed for the N1-P2 complex, and not for the individual waves or their subcomponents.

The N2 wave, the negative wave following P2, is substantially influenced by stimulus intensity, stimulus probability, the difficulty in determining a difference between two stimuli, and subject attention. Related to these variables affecting the N2 component is observation that the N2 component of the ALR is recorded within the same latency region as the MMN response.

Finally, underlying components of the ALR N1 wave (e.g., N1, Nb, Nc, and Nd) is a general negative voltage shift in brain electrical activity referred to as the "sustained negativity potential." The sustained negativity potential has negative voltage relative to the prestimulus baseline and is maintained throughout the duration of a stimulus.

Even in subjects that are normal audiologically and neurologically, ALR morphology, latency, and amplitude may vary substantially. The normal variations between subjects and within subjects from one averaged waveform to the next in a single test session are, to some extent, due to the susceptibility of the response to fluctuations in subject state. Waveform morphology, for example, may be very different if a subject is awake and alert versus awake and drowsy. Clinically, as noted below, it is important to take into account the effects of young age and sleep, including sleep stage, in interpreting ALR waveforms. Indeed, normal intersubject variations are a characteristic feature of the late (i.e., endogenous or event-related) responses. Often, late response waveforms are dependent on details of the test paradigm and subtle variations in subject attention to stimuli. Response parameters are closely related to subject state and only rarely are the relationships between subject state and response morphology all or none. For example, amplitude of the later latency components (e.g., N2 and P300) can be closely related to the degree to which a subject expects the stimulus to occur (Duncan-Johnson & Donchin, 1977; Roth, Ford, Lewis, & Kopell, 1976; Squires, Donchin, Herning, & McCarthy, 1977). That is, amplitude will be larger if the subject is not expecting to hear the stimulus and smaller if the stimulus is expected. Also, there is a direct relationship between processing time and the latency of some late response components. Latency of the response increases as the time taken by a subject to perceive a stimulus and determine certain characteristics increases (Ritter, Simson, & Vaughan, 1982; Roth, Ford, & Kopell, 1978).

Finally, in children up to at least adolescence (about 16 years) ALR waveform morphology varies remarkably as a function of age (development or maturation), a variety of stimulus parameters, such as the type (e.g., tone versus speech), number of repetitions, especially rate and ISI, and also acquisition parameters, e.g., recording electrode site (scalp distribution). The prominence, amplitude, latency, and even the detection of individual ALR waves and subcomponents of waves in children are influenced by very complex and dynamic interactions among these factors. A complete discussion of the myriad permutations in waveform morphology across childhood is far beyond the scope of this review.

Indeed, the findings of developmental investigations of the ALR that examine the multiple interactions among measurement factors are regularly reported in the literature (e.g., Čeponiene, Rinne, & Näätänen, 2002).

ABNORMAL PATTERNS. | Abnormal ALR findings include reductions in amplitude and prolongations in latency, polarity reversal for selected components, and total absence of one or more components (e.g., Kileny, 1985; Kileny & Berry, 1983; Knight, Hillyard, Woods, & Neville, 1980). Because of the inherent normal response variability, the rather strict type of criteria used in analysis of shorter latency responses, such as ABR, are not appropriate for ALR. Even interaural (between ear) differences in response parameters are not applicable in most cases because binaural stimulation is often employed.

NONPATHOLOGIC SUBJECT FACTORS

Age

INFANCY AND EARLY CHILDHOOD. | Throughout the 1960s and into the 1970s, numerous researchers demonstrated that ALR could be recorded from premature and full-term newborn infants and older children. In the pre-ABR era, clinical interest in an "objective" measure of auditory sensitivity in children was the primary motivation for the investigations (Barnet & Lodge, 1966; Rapin, Ruben, & Lyttle, 1970; Taguchi, Picton, Orpin, & Goodman, 1969), although later papers focused more on monitoring CNS maturation (e.g., Barnet, Ohlrich, Weiss, & Shanks, 1975). Individual ALR waves mature at distinctly different rates (e.g., Čeponiene, Rinne, & Näätänen, 2002). In general, the ALR in children is characterized by prominent P1 and N2 waves, in contrast to the sequence of P1, N1, and P2 waves typically recorded from adults. Developmentally, the P1 wave appears first, followed in the age period of 3 to 6 years by emergence of an almost adult-like P2 wave and a clear and often robust N2 wave. The N1 wave isn't observed until after 3 years, and then only with long ISIs (slow signal rates).

For all ALR waves, latency decreases and amplitude increases as a function of age during childhood. However, the age-related changes are distinctly different for major ALR waves, with the P2 wave leading the N1 wave in maturation. Prominent changes in ALR waves occur within the first year of life, and to a lesser extent within the 2 to 5 year age range as documented initially by many early investigators (Akiyama, Schutze, Schulte, & Parmalee, 1969; Barnet & Goodwin, 1965; Cody & Bickford, 1965; Davis, 1965; Davis, Mast, Yoshie, & Zerlin, 1966; Davis & Onishi, 1969; Ohlrich & Barnet, 1972; Rapin & Graziani, 1967; Suzuki & Taguchi, 1968; Taguchi, Picton, Orpin, & Goodman, 1969; Weitzman, Fishbein, & Graziani, 1965) and since confirmed by more sophisticated ALR measurements (e.g., Kushnerenko et al., 2002; Paetau, Ahonen, Salonen, & Sams, 1995; Pang & Taylor, 2000; Ponton et al., 2000; Sharma, Kraus,

McGee, & Nicol, 1997). The N1 is not present in infants and young children, and for children age 3 to 10 years it is recorded only with extended ISIs of 1 second or longer (Paetau, Ahonen, Salonen, & Sams, 1995; Ponton et al., 2000; Sharma et al., 1997). For example, Barnet, Ohlrich, and colleagues (Barnet et al., 1975; Ohlrich et al., 1978) reported the following latency changes during the age range of 15 days to 3 years: The latency of P2 shortens from 230 to 150 ms; N2 from 535 to 320 ms; and P3 from 785 to 635 ms.

The rate of maturation varies among the different ALR components and for selected measurement conditions (e.g., ipsilateral versus contralateral electrode array), with developmental changes for selected components (e.g., N1) under some conditions (e.g., ipsilateral electrode array) continuing into adolescence. Latency and amplitude values for all of the ALR components do not reach adult values until 16 to 18 years (e.g., Courchesne, 1978b; Ponton, Eggermont, et al., 2000; Ptok, Blachnik, & Schonweiler, 2004; Sharma, Kraus, McGee, & Nicol, 1997). The reliability with which these auditory late response components are recorded also increases throughout childhood up to adolescence and the onset of puberty. There are also differences between children and adults in the composition of major ALR wave complexes (e.g., N1) and the effects that alterations of signal characteristics (e.g., intensity and rate) have on subcomponents of ALR waves (e.g., N1b, N1c), the scalp distributions, and probably anatomical generators of these subcomponents (Bruneau, Roux, Guerin, Barthelemy, & Lelord, 1997; Čeponiene, Rinne, & Näätänen, 2002). In contrast, other waves within the same general latency region (e.g., the P3a response and the MMN response), can be recorded consistently in infants (Kraus, McGee, Littman, & Nicol, 1992; Kurtzberg et al., 1986). Auditory late responses recorded from the midline (e.g., Fz) mature at a more rapid rate than those recorded from temporal (lateral) sites (Kurtzberg, Vaughn, Courchesne, Friedman, Harter, & Putnam, 1984). It is noteworthy that some of the reports just cited were based on well-designed, yet uncommon, longitudinal studies of normal-hearing infants. ALR measurement in young children is often conducted during sleep. The differential effects of sleep and sleep stage on late auditory response components, discussed in a subsequent section of this chapter, must be taken into account in the evaluation of the literature on maturation of the auditory late responses. Developmental trends for selected ALR components are shown in Figure 12.6. The latencies in children are in contrast to expected ALR latency values for normal adult subjects of just under 100 ms for N1, about 200 ms for P2 and 300 ms for the P300 component. The P3 described in the study by Barnet and colleagues (1975), however, was defined differently than the traditional P3 measured in adult subjects. Age differentially affected various components of the ALR in children. Generally, ALR amplitude increases as a function of age, but decreases are reported for the N1 to P2 amplitude measure. Again, for comparison purposes,

Effect of Maturation on Latency and Amplitude of the Auditory Late Response

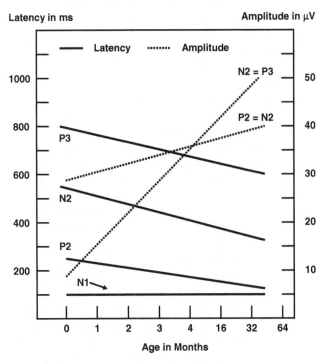

FIGURE 12.6. Developmental trends for the ALR in children.

ALR amplitude (N1 to P2) in adults is in the range of 5 to 20 μV.

McIsaac and Polich (1992) recorded auditory late responses in an investigation of the passive P300 response with ten normal infants (five male and five female) ranging in age from 6 to 10 months. ALR data were compared with findings for a control group of ten young normal adults (18 to 22 years). The test protocol included standard (frequent) tones of 1000 Hz and target (rare) tones of 2000 Hz with 9.9 ms rise/fall times and a plateau of 50 ms presented via a speaker located 1.5 m in from the subject. A block of 10 of these stimuli was presented, with the target tone occurring randomly at one of the positions between the seventh and the tenth tone. There was then a 4 to 6 second silent interval before the next block of tones was represented, with the target tone occurring in a different position. The authors did not specify stimulus intensity. Infants sat in their parents' laps and remained awake during the auditory evoked response recording. Data collection was performed only when the infant was still. Auditory evoked responses were recorded with midline noninverting electrodes (Fz, Cz, and Pz) and linked-earlobe inverting electrodes using band-pass filter settings of 0.01 to 30 Hz over an analysis time of 1100 ms with a 110 ms prestimulus time. Electro-ocular activity was monitored with electrodes as per conventional protocol, and trials with eye blink activity were rejected before signal averaging.

Normative ALR data reported by McIsaac and Polich (1992) are summarized in the appendix. Latency and amplitude values for ALR components N1, P2, and N2 were generally longer and smaller for infants than for adults.

In keeping with the principle that shorter latency responses mature or become adult-like at earlier chronological ages that longer latency responses, ALR is not fully developed until at least school age, in contrast to 18 months for ABR as an example. Published estimates on when ALR becomes adult-like range from about 6 years up to adolescence, or about 15 years (Goodin, Squires, Henderson, & Starr, 1978; Polich, Howard, & Starr, 1985), in part because individual ALR components mature along different age gradients. As with other AERs, interaction of stimulus parameters and maturation must be considered for ALR. As reviewed in an earlier section of the chapter, types of stimuli effective in eliciting ALR include speech sounds (Kurtzberg, Stone, & Vaughan, 1986), in addition to clicks and tones. This approach for neurophysiologic evaluation of cortical processing of speech sounds has obvious clinical possibilities, particularly in newborn infants at risk for communicative disorders, as reviewed in the final section of the chapter.

In addition to published descriptions of maturational changes in the auditory late responses, the literature contains a sizable number of papers describing the application of these responses, along with the P300 and MMN responses, in the evaluation of cognitive processes, such as the development of memory. For example, the ability of an infant to recognize the maternal voice is uniformly appreciated, and well documented with formal behavioral studies and also with electrophysiologic investigation (e.g., DeCasper & Fifer, 1980). The P2 wave of the ALR is greater in amplitude and longer in latency when elicited by a word (e.g., baby) recorded from the mother's voice than with someone else's voice (deRegnier et al., 2000). The findings of these investigations confirm that recognition memory can be evaluated with the ALR. Interestingly, recognition memory in newborn infants as documented by the P2 wave of the ALR is correlated with cognitive (mental) development at one year (deRegnier et al., 2000). Normal infants also produce during the presentation of a stranger's voice (not the mother) a prolonged negative wave throughout ALR recording time frame, indicating the recognition of a novel acoustic signal after the ongoing processing of a familiar signal. The literature on ALR in infants at risk for central nervous system dysfunction is reviewed in the final section of this chapter.

ADVANCING AGE IN ADULTS. | There are inconsistencies in published descriptions of ALR changes in aging. Some investigators have described for ALR waves a general increase in latency and decrease in amplitude advancing age (Callaway, 1975; Callaway & Halliday, 1973; Goodin, Squires, Henderson, & Starr, 1978a), However, there are reports (e.g., Spink, Johannsen, & Pirsig, 1979) of shorter P2 latencies for older subjects (average age of 63 years) versus younger subjects (average age of 22 years), and other investigators maintain that P2 wave latency doesn't change with aging (e.g., Amenedo & Diaz, 1998; Brown, Marsh, & LaRue, 1983; Pfefferbaum, Ford, Roth, & Kopell, 1980). Similarly, confusion surrounds the possible effect of aging on P2 amplitude. There are published studies in support of age-related amplitude decrease (e.g., Czigler, Csibra, & Csontos, 1992) and of amplitude increase (e.g., Amenedo & Diaz, 1998; Pfefferbaum et al., 1980). And, consistent with the preceding discussion about P2 latency, others studies failed to demonstrate a change in amplitude with aging (e.g., Barrett, Nehshige, & Shibasaki, 1987; Picton et al., 1987). In a study of three cortical AER waves (N200, P300, N3) in a population of 224 elderly subjects (ranging in age from 60 to over 90 years), Stenklev and Laukli (2004) found an age-related decrease (60.5% to 38.9%) in the prevalence of the N200 wave, with an overall prevalence of 46.9 percent for the group. The responses were evoked with an oddball paradigm. The frequent stimulus was a 1000 Hz tone with rise/fall times of 10 ms and a plateau of 40 ms presented at a rate of 0.7/second and an intensity level of 70 to 110 dB HL ("adjusted according to the subjects' best pure-tone hearing threshold at 2K Hz"). Among 105 subjects with an N200 wave, latency increased significantly over the age range but, curiously, there was no difference in the average N400 latency for the elderly group in comparison to data for a young (19 to 26 years) control group (N = 22). Also, N200 latency was not significantly related to hearing threshold at 2000 Hz. N400 amplitude showed no change with age within the elderly group, and no difference between the elderly and young (control) groups.

Some of the discrepancies in studies on aging and the ALR may be related to the state of arousal of the subjects. Sleep is a factor in the interpretation of ALR findings in aging. Crowley, Trinder, and Colrain (2002) reported differential effects of sleep on the P2 wave for older (65 to 80 years) versus younger (18 to 31 years) subjects. During sleep, P2 wave amplitude was larger and latency was prolonged for the older subjects. In addition, these authors observed a "long-lasting late positive waveform (LLP) in the older group that was not apparent in younger subjects" (Crowley et al., 2002; Crowley & Colrain, 2004).

Tremblay, Piskosz, and Souza (2003) studied the effect of age on the P1, N1, and P2 components of the ALR evoked with synthetic speech sounds and compared the electrophysiologic findings to those obtained with behavioral measures. Characteristics of the speech sounds used in this study were summarized above in the section on ALR signals. Subjects consisted of a group of ten young normal hearers (average age of 26 years), ten older normal hearers (average age of 68 years), and ten older subjects with a high frequency sensory hearing loss due to presbycusis (average age of 71 years). Older subjects were intact cognitively. Age-related perceptual problems with VOT discrimination were demonstrated with the behavioral measures and confirmed electrophysi-

ologically with the ALR. Specifically, latency for the N1 wave (an onset response) was longer for the two older subject groups as VOT duration increased. The authors raise the possibility that the initial burst in the speech signal affects the subsequent response to the onset of voicing in the older subjects because of an age-related increase in neural recovery time (a forward masking effect). Tremblay et al. (2003) also offer other possible explanations for the N1 latency delay in older subjects, and for the confounding effect of hearing loss on speech processing. In any event, the study confirms previously reported behavioral evidence of difficulty in the perception of temporal acoustic cues in aging adults.

Fisher, Hymel, Cranford, and DeChicchis (2000) and, a few years later, De Chicchis, Carpenter, Cranford, and Hymel (2002) studied possible age effects on the ALR N1 and P2 waves under different conditions for attention, task difficulty, and contralateral competing signals. With the study reported by Fisher et al. (2000), subjects were young (age 20 to 27 years) and elderly (age 60 to 79 years) normal-hearing adults. The ALR was evoked while subjects attempted to discriminate between two signals in a oddball stimulus paradigm. The signal condition was either two tones (an easy task) or two natural speech signals (/da/ and /ga/), a more difficult task. The ALR was recorded topographically with nineteen scalp noninverting electrodes using band-pass filter settings of 1 to 70 Hz, and an analysis time of 1000 ms plus a –100 ms prestimulus baseline. As with other studies reported by these investigators, maximum ALR amplitude for the N1 and P2 components was distributed around the midline region represented by the Cz electrode site. For the easy listening task, subjects in each group showed a reduction in amplitude for the ALR N1 and P2 components with a competing (contralateral) speech signal. The amplitude reduction for the N1 wave, however, was greater for the elderly subjects. For the more difficult listening task (with speech signals), neither group showed a change in amplitude of the N1 wave with the competing speech signal, but amplitude for the P2 wave was significantly reduced for the elderly subjects versus the young subject group. The effects of age on the ALR with contralateral competing signals, therefore, were different for the N1 versus P2 waves, and varied with the level of difficulty for the listening task. For elderly subjects, more difficult tasks seem to affect the later latency P2 component more than the N1 component. Comparing their findings to the extensive literature on attention and the ALR N1 component, Fisher et al. (2000) speculate that the competition produces an inverse effect on neural activity. That is, the effects of attention versus competition may reflect two different brain mechanisms, with selective attention to signals enhancing amplitude of the N1 wave and competition or a distracting signals diminishing N1 wave amplitude.

De Chicchis, Carpenter, Cranford, and Hymel (2002) extended this line of research on aging effects with a study of the influence of selective attention versus contralateral competition on the ALR N1, P2, and N2 waves of in young versus elderly subjects. Waveform analysis included differentiation of the N2e and N2i components of the N2 wave complex. Confirming the findings of the earlier study (Fisher et al., 2000), N1 amplitude in both age groups was enhanced by attention to signals, whereas amplitude for the P2 wave was reduced in the attend (versus ignore) condition. The authors acknowledge the possibility that P2 amplitude was diminished by the ongoing attention-related processing negativity component within the same latency period. Competition exerted a more pronounced effect on the ALR.

GENDER. | A gender effect has long been suspected, but rarely investigated, in ALR measurements. Gender differences in brain structure and function, especially in the temporal-parietal regions and corpus callosum, are well documented (e.g., Cowell, Turetsky, Gur, Grossman, Shasel, & Gur, 1994; Witelson, 1991). Onishi and Davis (1968) noted that ALR amplitude in general tended to be larger and the amplitude versus intensity function steeper for females than males. In a series of studies of the ALR recorded within a background of complex verbal or nonverbal auditory stimulation in infants, children and adults, Shucard and colleagues (Shucard, Shucard, & Cummins, 1981) found in both verbal and nonverbal conditions that females produced higher amplitude responses from the left hemisphere than male subjects, whereas males showed higher amplitude responses than females from the right hemisphere. These data were interpreted as consistent with expected lateralization of language and spatial functions for males versus females, in children and adults. The results of these studies also serve to emphasize the complexity of interactions among ALR, stimulus conditions, age and gender.

McIsaac and Polich (1992) recorded auditory late responses in an investigation of the passive P300 response with ten normal infants (five male and five female) ranging in age from 6 to 10 months. Details of the test protocol are noted above in a review of the auditory late response in infants and, for the P300 response, in Chapter 13. There was no consistent gender effect for the ALR N1, P2, and N2 components.

Handedness

Alexander and Polich (1997) investigated the possible influence of handedness on the P300 response (reviewed in Chapter 13) and the N1, P2, and N2 components of the auditory late response. Subjects were twenty left-handed males and twenty right-handed males. Although there was no handedness effect for N1 amplitude, latency of the N1 component was shorter for left-handed versus right-handed subjects, particularly for lateral scalp electrode sites. P2 amplitude values were smaller for the left-handed subjects, whereas latency was not related to handedness. Handedness was not a factor in N2 amplitude, but for anterior electrode locations N2 latency was shorter for left- versus right-handed

subjects. Similar handedness findings were reported for the P300 response.

State of Arousal and Sleep

In contrast to shorter latency AERs, sleep has a pronounced effect on the responses in the late latency range. The influence of sleep was recognized by some of the earliest investigators of ALR (Cody, Klass, & Bickford, 1967; Williams, Tepas, & Morlock, 1962), but the complexities of the sleep effects became appreciated only later. The reader will recall that stages of sleep were summarized in Table 11.4 (in Chapter 11). In sleep, the intensity at which the ALR is first observed in normal hearers is elevated by approximately 20 to 30 dB, and ALR latency is increased (Cody, Klass, & Bickford, 1967; Mendel, Hosick, Windman, et al., 1975; Osterhammel, Davis, Wier, & Hirsh, 1973). Amplitude generally becomes more variable in sleep (Rapin, Schimmel, & Cohen, 1972; Weitzman & Kremen, 1965; Williams, Tepas, & Morlock, 1962). Early investigators of the ALR recognized that individual waves are differentially affected by sleep. For example, amplitude of the N2 component is markedly increased during sleep (Ornitz, Ritvo, Carr, et al., 1967; Picton et al., 1974; Williams, Tepas, & Morlock, 1962). There are clear changes in patterns of EEG activity during various sleep stages, e.g., alpha, theta, and delta frequencies, sleep spindles, K-complexes. Probably, some of the sleep-related changes in the ALR waveform are related to the underlying fluctuations in EEG activity (Colrain, Di Parsia, & Gora, 2000). In any event, the importance of the influence of sleep stage on later latency auditory evoked responses is now well appreciated. Variability in findings of early studies on ALR and sleep is probably due, in part, to the failure to carefully document the stage(s) of sleep during the ALR measurement session.

There are significant but differential changes in the major ALR waves as a person becomes drowsy and falls asleep (see Figure 12.7) and two conflicting explanations for them. One explanation of the changes in the N1 versus P2 components invokes sleep-related decreases in negative activity, whereas the other explanation suggests that positive voltage activity is enhanced. According to the first line of thinking, a gradual reduction in a subject's ongoing attention to the signals, and the related disappearance of slow negative wave activity, i.e., a general processing negativity found in the awake state (Campbell & Colrain, 2002; Campbell, Bell, & Bastien, 1992), results in progressively diminished amplitude of the N1 wave from the wake state to sleep stage 4 (delta or deep sleep). During this transition to deep sleep, P2 amplitude may actually increase, although agreement on this trend is lacking (e.g., Campbell et al., 1992; Nielsen-Bohlman, Knight, Woods, & Woodward, 1991; Ogilvie et al., 1991; Salisbury & Squires, 1993; Winter, Kok, Kenemans, & Elton, 1995). Because the changes in the amplitude for the N1 and P2 components are inversely related (just

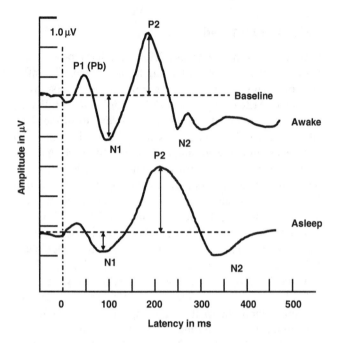

ALR Waveform:
Awake versus Asleep

FIGURE 12.7. Illustration of the effect of sleep on the ALR waveform. Note the apparent smaller amplitude for the N1 and the larger amplitude for P2 during sleep, relative to the prestimulus baseline (adapted from Crowley & Colrain, 2004).

the opposite), the overall amplitude of the N1-P2 complex (trough of N1 to peak of P2) may remain reasonable stable across sleep stages (de Lugt, Loewy, & Campbell, 1996). According to the alternative interpretation for changes in ALR amplitudes with sleep, decreased amplitude for the N1 wave and increased amplitude for the P2 wave are due to a general increase in positive voltage activity throughout the waveform (e.g., Näätänen & Picton, 1987).

There is auditory electrophysiologic evidence (mostly P300 response) of brain processing and reactivity to external acoustic signals during sleep (e.g., see Bastuji & García-Larrea, 1999). Brualla et al. (1998) and later Perrin and colleagues (Bastuji, Perrin, & García-Larrea, 2002; Perrin, Bastuji, & García-Larrea, 2002; Perrin et al., 1999; Perrin et al., 2000) have shown that semantic discrimination, as documented by the ALR N400 response to incongruous words, persists during sleep stage 2 and stage 5 (REM sleep). Auditory evoked responses can be recorded during sleep especially well when the signal is the subject's own name (e.g., Perrin et al., 1999; Pratt, Berlad, & Lavie, 1999). Although sleep stage is an important factor in the response, the effect of specific type and level of the discrimination (e.g., phonologic versus semantic) is not clear (Bastuji et al., 2002). With more complex variations of speech signals, e.g., pseudowords versus incongruous words, there are differences in

processing during sleep stage 2 versus REM sleep (Bastuji, Perrin, & García-Larrea, 2002). The P300 response has been extensively investigated in sleep, as summarized in the next chapter.

Attention

Consistent with the effects of sleep, amplitude of the N1 and P2 waves of the ALR are altered differentially when the subject is paying close attention to the stimulus or listening for a change in some aspect of the stimulus. That is, for the N1 wave an increase in attention to the eliciting signals is associated with a prominent increase in amplitude (particularly for the N2 or processing negativity component), i.e., on the order of up to 50 percent (Davis, 1964; Hillyard, Hink, Schwent, & Picton, 1973; Keating & Ruhm, 1971; Näätänen, Gaillard, & Mantysalo, 1978; Okita, 1979; Okita & Ohtani, 1977; Parasuraman, 1978; Picton & Hillyard, 1974; Picton, Hillyard, & Galambos, 1971; Roth, Krainz, & Ford, 1976; Schwent & Hillyard, 1975; Schwent, Snyder, & Hillyard, 1976; Wilkinson & Morlock, 1967). The P2 wave, however, appears to diminish with increased attention by the subject on the signals (Michie, Solowij, Crawford, & Glue, 1993; Näätänen & Picton, 1987). The Nd wave complex (the "processing negativity" or PN wave) overlaps to some extent with the P2 wave, as well as the N1 component. Characteristically, the Nd wave is enhanced (greater negativity) when the subject's level of attention to a signal, or even some aspect of the signal, increases (Alho, Sams, Paavilainen, & Näätänen, 1986), whereas the superimposition of this negativity in the latency region of 175 to 250 ms has just the opposite effect on the positive voltage P2 component, i.e., smaller amplitude.

Auditory Training

Kelly Tremblay, Nina Kraus, and colleagues (Tremblay & Kraus, 2002; Tremblay, Kraus, McGee, Ponton, & Otis, 2001) demonstrated changes in the P1 (AMLR Pb), N1, and P2 components of the ALR with auditory training. In these studies, responses were evoked by synthesized speech signals ("tokens") with different voice onset times (VOTs) of 10 ms, over the range of –50 ms (pre-voicing) to +50 ms (voicing after release of closure). Before auditory training, the subjects (normal-hearing, adult native English speakers) perceived the signals simply as /ba/. That is, subjects did not distinguish differences in VOT on the order of 10 ms and, instead, perceived the two acoustic signals as within the same phonemic category. The ALR was recorded with electrodes at midline (Fz, Cz, Pz) and electrodes over the right and left frontal and temporal lobe regions. Filter settings were 0.1 to 100 Hz and the analysis time was 500 ms plus a 100 ms prestimulus time. Perceptual identification of the VOT differences improved with training, as assessed behaviorally. Training was associated with a decrease in amplitude for the ALR P1 (AMLR Pb) component as recorded for midline noninverting electrodes. The training-related amplitude decreased progressively and markedly from anterior (Fz) to posterior (Pz) electrode sites. In contrast, the authors described increases in amplitude for the N1 and, especially, P2 components of the ALR with training. The marked increases in P2 amplitude with midline electrodes (Fz and Cz) are promising for clinical application of the ALR in documenting the benefits of auditory training for patients with auditory processing disorders. Tremblay, Kraus, Carrell, and McGee (1997) have also documented the effect of auditory training on neural activity with the MMN response, as reviewed in Chapter 14.

Drugs

Background information on drugs commonly administered during sedation or anesthesia was reviewed in Chapters 5 (ECochG), 8 (ABR and ASSR), and especially 11 (AMLR). The following discussion is limited to the influence that the drugs have on the ALR, based on published evidence.

SEDATIVES. | During sedation with chloral hydrate, as with natural sleep, ALR variability is increased (Hosick & Mendel, 1975; Skinner & Antinoro, 1969; Skinner & Shimota, 1975). Measurement of the ALR and P300 response under sedation is ill advised, as validity of findings may be compromised. Mendel, Hosick, Windman, Davis, Hirsh, and Dinges (1975) reported that secobarbital-induced sleep was associated with increased variability in ALRs and, in turn, less accurate auditory threshold estimations. ALR N1, P2 and N2 component amplitude is reduced by benzodiazepines, but latency is not affected (Lader, 1977). Meperidine, an opioid analgesic like morphine, has no apparent effect on early or late latency AERs (Pfefferbaum, Roth, Tinklenberg, Rosenbloom, & Kopell, 1979). Droperidol (dehydrobenzperidol) produces a latency prolongation of about 10 ms for the P1 and N1 components of the ALR and amplitude reduction.

ANESTHETIC AGENTS. | Anesthetic agents produce very diverse effects on different types of AERs (e.g., short versus late latency) and even between components of a group of AERs, such as the auditory late responses. Halliday and Mason (1964) found no significant decrease in ALR amplitude during hypnotic anesthesia. The effects of etomidate on AMLR were comparable to those of halothane and enflurane on ALR peaks (Navaratnarajah, Thornton, Heneghan, Bateman, & Jones, 1983). Effects of Thiopental on late AERs were demonstrated by Abrahamian, Allison, Goff, and Rosner (1963). With nitrous oxide anesthesia, AER components with latency values beyond 50 ms show dose dependent reduction in amplitude, yet latency is not affected (Lader, 1977).

Tranquilizers and Psychotherapeutic Agents

Tranquilizers are referred to as neuroleptic drugs that are thought to block postsynaptic dopaminergic receptors in the mesolimbic region of the brain. All are, by definition, psychotropic and may affect longer latency AERs. Because of this relationship, and the fact that patients for whom late latency AER testing may be indicated (e.g., schizophrenics) are often treated with psychotherapeutic medications, there are literally hundreds of published papers describing changes in ALR, the P300 response, and the contingent negative variation (CNV) response following administration of this category of drugs.

Different tranquilizers produce mixed effects on ALR components. For example, chlorpromazine increases latency of waves P2 and N2 without affecting the latency of the N1 component, nor the amplitude of any components (Lader, 1977). In contrast, phenothiazine in schizophrenics produced a dose-dependent decrease in ALR amplitude (Roth & Cannon, 1972). Lithium increases ALR latency without affecting amplitude.

Haloperidol is an antipsychotic drug commonly used in the medical management psychiatric disorders. Quetiapine is an atypical antipsychotic drug. Graham et al. (2004) reported in a study of twenty healthy adult (19 to 38 years) males that neither drug affected amplitude of the ALR N1-P2 wave complex. Rosburg, Marinou, et al. (2004) reported on the effects of lorazepam (benzodiazepine lorazepam), a GABA agonist, on the auditory evoked magnetic field N100m component. Subjects were twelve healthy adults who, in a single blind trial research design, were given the lorazepam, caffeine, or a placebo. The AEF measurement technique used by the authors is described in detail in this and other recent publications (e.g., Rosburg, 2004; Rosburg, Haueisen, & Sauer, 2002), and summarized in the review of other papers by the authors in this chapter. One of the main findings of the Rosburg, Marinou, et al. (2004) study was a decrease in the source of the N100m component associated with the administration of lorazepam.

Other Drugs Influencing ALRs

ALCOHOL. | Amplitude ALR is decreased by acute alcohol intoxication (Gross, Begleiter, Tobin, & Kissin, 1966; Kopell, Roth, Tinklenberg, 1978; McRandle & Goldstein, 1973; Pfefferbaum et al., 1979, 1980; Porjesz & Begleiter, 1981; Wolpaw & Penry, 1978). In general, primary sensory regions are more resistant to the effects of alcohol and association areas are quite susceptible, based on visual and somatosensory evoked response data. The relationship between blood alcohol level (BAL) and AER alteration is not well defined. Amplitude of the N1-P2 complex of the ALR is decreased by acute alcohol consumption (Krough, Khan, & Fosuig, 1977). The medications may therefore also influence AERs. Studies of the N1 component of the ALR (and the P300) in abstinent and medication-free chronic alcoholics suggests that patterns of abnormalities are similar to those found during acute alcohol ingestion (Porjesz & Begleiter, 1981). This is taken as evidence that subcortical (hippocampus) deficits are also a feature of chronic alcoholism. In a study that also included the P300 response, Murata, Araki, Tanigawa, and Uchida (1992) investigated the effect of acute alcohol (200 ml of Japanese spirits) ingestion on the ALR N1 and P2 waves. Subjects were thirteen healthy male medical students who reportedly "consented readily to become volunteers for this study" (Murata et al., 1992, p. 958). ALR measurement was also made at the same time in the late afternoon or evening for subjects. Body temperature was not noted in the description of the study. ALR components were recorded also in a control condition (water ingestion). Latency of the N1 (N100) component was significantly prolonged when recorded two hours after alcohol ingestion, whereas P2 latency was unchanged. Findings are consistent with previous reports on the effects of alcohol on the ALR (e.g., Teo & Ferguson, 1986).

Brain Mapping

In the late 1970s computer-processed analysis of evoked response (and EEG) activity was introduced in clinical neurophysiology. A word about terminology is in order at this juncture. Frank H. Duffy of Boston reported some of the earliest work in the area, including clinical application (e.g., Duffy, 1982; Duffy, Burchfield, & Lombrosco, 1979). Duffy's technique for computerized topographic evoked response analysis became known as "brain electrical activity mapping, or BEAM." This term is now a trademark of a manufacturer of evoked response instrumentation. Simply "brain mapping" or "topographic (T) mapping" are terms often used to describe computerized evoked response topography. The descriptive and rather generic computed evoked response (or evoked potential, EP) topography is the term that will be used in the following discussion. It might be easier to understand the concepts underlying this analysis technique if the term is first explained. The word "computed" is very important because the display of large amounts of EP data over space and time is dependent on computer power. The technique requires an adequately powerful and fast computer, along with sophisticated software programs. Traditional EP topography, in contrast, can be carried out with most evoked response systems that have capacity for multichannel recording. The term "evoked response" hopefully does not require further definition for the reader. Topography is a term borrowed from geography that, literally, means to graph or map the physical features of a place or region. In the case of computed EP topography, the features are amplitudes of evoked response peaks and troughs, rather than the amplitudes of hills and valleys. These three topographic displays, which are usually shown in color, may also be illustrated by shading. In color displays, different colors along the spectrum indicate different amplitudes. For example, red may represent higher amplitude than blue. EP topography can also be displayed numerically, or with figures depicting dipole sources of evoked responses (Scherg & von Cramon,

1984). This latter display essentially focuses on the areas of greatest AER amplitude on the scalp. While peak to trough amplitude calculations are typical in conventional AER measurement, peak to baseline values are incorporated into computed EP topographic data analysis. It is likely that computerized EP topography technology will have a profound impact on clinical application of AERs.

Computed EP topography is distinguished from the traditional AER topographic measurement approach not so much by differences in stimulation or recording techniques, but by a fundamentally different means of processing and displaying AER information, and in the case of some techniques, unique approaches for distinguishing patient data vs. normative data. A direct and appropriate analogy can be made with traditional EEG vs. EEG mapping. Virtually any AER can be displayed topographically and computer analyzed. Most early investigations were based on the ALR, but subsequent research utilized topography of the ABR (Grandori, 1986), AMLR (Kraus & McGee, 1988), and P300 (Baran, Musiek, Long, & Ommaya, 1988).

Several recording features are common to all techniques for computed EP topography. The principles of AER stimulation and acquisition reviewed in earlier chapters generally apply in computed EP topography, with a few exceptions. A slower stimulus rate than even the 1 or 0.5/second used for ALR measurement may be necessary for the computer to perform analog-to-digital conversion and averaging for the numerous channels used in computed EP topography. Computed EP topographic recording is done with many electrodes (from 16 to over 90) located at well-defined (10-20 system) sites on the scalp. Since a thousand or more data points are required for construction of topographic maps, voltages between the limited number of electrodes on the scalp must be interpolated. That is, voltages between electrode sites are estimated according to known information on brain electrical fields. A noncephalic inverting ("reference") electrode site is recommended in computed EP topographic recording. Subject characteristics and other factors in conventional AER measurement must also be taken into account for meaningful interpretation of computed EP topography.

There are at least six major advantages of computed EP topography versus traditional AER topographic recordings. First, even though AER data are really detected at discrete electrode locations, the electrical activity between electrode sites is estimated (interpolated) so that there is a more continuous response pattern over the scalp. Second, the degree of activity at any location in a computed EP topographic display is usually depicted in color, or by shades on a black-to-gray-to-white spectrum. Even the novice viewer, without experience in analyzing AER waveforms, can thus immediately note differences in activity across the scalp. Third, this image of scalp-detected AER activity is ongoing and dynamic. That is, it develops as the AER is recorded, not just after the averaging process is completed. This facilitates detection of changes in activity over time and space, adding a new (spatial) dimension to traditional multichannel AER measurement. Finally, these visual images (analog data) of AER activity are, in fact, a reflection of actual AER voltages (digital data) stored in computer memory over time and at the different electrode sites. The computer can then be used to further analyze these raw data in many ways. For example, patient data can be statistically compared to normative data that is also stored in the computer. Or, patient data can be subjected to spectral analysis (discussed above) and other forms of offline (after data collection) analysis.

Routine clinical application of computed EP topography is by no means straightforward. At the very least, another four factors can seriously affect clinical feasibility, reliability, and validity of computer EP topography. First of all, the technique is more time consuming. For example, it requires more time to place as many as ten to thirty electrodes than the three electrodes used, for example, in routine ALR recording. Second, computed EP topography is considerably more sophisticated than traditional ALR measurement, both in terms of instrumentation design and cost and in technical demands on the tester. Even though waveform interpretation is not necessary, the tester certainly needs a firm grounding in EEG electrode placement techniques and a broad knowledge of the underlying response. For computed ALR topography, this would include an appreciation of subject and measurement factors influencing the response. Some authors (Finitzo & Poole, 1987) have expressed serious concerns about the appropriateness of brain mapping by persons without extensive preliminary education and training clinical neurosciences. According to these authors, for example, eighteen months is necessary to acquire adequate background in EEG measurement and analysis, plus special computed EP topography instruction.

Third, the relation between computed EP topographic findings at the scalp to underlying AER neurophysiology in the brain is extremely complex and dependent on numerous theoretical concerns and assumptions. Some understanding of these technical and anatomic concepts, such as dipole generator models and the influence of scalp, skull, and nonbrain intracranial contents on surface recordings, is a prerequisite. Fourth, problems associated with adequate normative data for conventional AER interpretation are compounded for computed EP topography. Fifth, although data are displayed over the collection time, the component within an AER waveform for which amplitude information will be analyzed and the method of analysis must be determined beforehand. In computed topography of the ALR, for instance, voltages for the P2 component would be a logical selection. The P2 latency region must be defined so that a map can be generated in this region. A problem arises because latency for a certain component (e.g., P2 of ALR or Pa of AMLR) will vary from subject to subject. Therefore, the map of this component may be blurred by analysis of offpeak data. Computed EP topography analysis techniques may include many of the sophisticated approaches noted above for conventional AERs, including principal component analysis, spectral analysis, discriminant analysis, and others.

Last, definition of logical clinical applications and additional documentation of the diagnostic value of brain mapping is needed before the technique becomes fully accepted and widely applied clinically. A wide range of potential clinical applications have been suggested or actually attempted. Among the clinical entities studied with computed EP topography are Alzheimer's disease, dyslexia, spasmodic dysphonia, stuttering, traumatic brain injury, cerebrovascular accidents, and various neuropsychiatric disorders. Clearly, application of computed EP topography will always be limited by certain clinical constraints. It is, for example, inappropriate as an approach for auditory screening in newborn infants. There is excitement, yet also considerable skepticism, regarding the unique benefits of the computed topographic approach versus traditional AER measurement in neurodiagnosis of higher level CNS dysfunction with ALR offering a highly sophisticated and quantifiable mode of analysis.

CLINICAL APPLICATIONS

As noted in the overview of AERs in Chapter 1, and in the introduction to the present chapter, the early audiologic application of the ALR in the 1960s, before the discovery of the ABR, was electrophysiological estimation of hearing sensitivity in infants and young children. Then, for about forty years, publications describing clinical applications of the ALR were few and far between. Occasionally, papers highlighting the application of the ABR in clinical populations also noted ALR findings. Often, the emphasis in these publications was the divergence of results for the ABR versus the ALR. For example, Starr et al. (1977) in one of the initial studies of the ABR in neurologic pathology showed that ALR components could be recorded in patients with no detectable ABR. Other authors made just the opposite point, that is, the ALR could be used to document high level central auditory dysfunction in patients with normal ABR findings (e.g., Kileny & Berry, 1983). Clinical investigations of the ALR were also occasionally reported for diverse clinical populations, such as children with autism (Ciesielski, Courchesne, & Elmasian, 1990; Loiselle, Stamm, Matininsky, & Whipple, 1980; Novick, Vaughan, Kurtzberg, & Simpson, 1980; Satterfield, Schell, & Backs, 1987), Down syndrome (Dustman & Callner, 1979), reading disorders (Kutas, Van Petten, & Besson, 1988), cochlear implants (Oviatt & Kileny, 1991), and auditory processing disorders (Jirsa & Clontz, 1990) and adults with schizophrenia (Hink & Hillyard, 1978). There appears to be a resurgence of basic research and clinical studies of the ALR in audiology. The growing number of publications on the ALR has paralleled the markedly increased clinical investigation of the P300 and, especially, MMN response (reviewed in Chapters 13 and 14). With the new information produced by this research effort, coupled with advances in clinical instrumentation, it is likely that clinical interest in the ALR as an electrophysiological audiologic measure of auditory processing will continue to grow.

Sensorineural Hearing Loss

Tremblay, Piskosz, and Souza (2003) investigated with speech signals the effects of hearing loss in advancing age on the P1 component (AMLR Pb), the N1, and the P2 waves. Hearing loss was sensorineural and characterized by a sloping configuration with average hearing thresholds of about 15 dB HL at 250 and 500 Hz and then decreasing rather systematically to 60 dB HL at 8000 Hz. For all subject groups, speech signals were presented via insert earphones to the right ear at an intensity of 74 dB peSPL with an interstimulus interval of 910 ms. Responses were detected with a noninverting electrode at the Cz location and band-pass filter settings of 0.1 to 100 Hz (filtered offline again from 1 to 40 Hz), using an analysis time of 500 ms poststimulus and 100 ms prestimulus. Changes in latencies for these ALR components produced by different voice onset time durations occurred as a function of aging, i.e., for young (average 26 years) versus old (average 68 years) subject groups, rather than hearing loss. In general, ALR findings were similar for the normal-hearing and hearing-impaired older subjects, even though the signal intensity level was only 74 dB peSPL. Tremblay, Piskosz, and Souza (2003) offer as an explanation previously reported larger amplitudes for ALR waves, e.g., the N1 wave, in response to lower versus higher frequency signals (Picton, Woods, & Proulx, 1978). There are, however, inconsistencies among studies of the ALR in hearing loss in young and elderly subjects (e.g., Martin, Kurtzberg, & Stapells, 1999; Oates, Kurtzberg, & Stapells, 2002). More research is needed to clarify the effects of hearing loss and related variables, e.g., age, on different ALR waves.

Auditory Processing Disorders (APD) and Learning Disabilities (LD)

The focus of most studies of cortical evoked responses in children with APD is the P300 response or the MMN response. There are, however, a handful of papers on the ALR in APD (e.g., Arehole, 1995; Tonnquist-Uhlen, 1996) and other pediatric populations with APD as a possible co-existing disorder (Bernal, Harmony, Rodriguez, et al., 2000; Bruneau, Roux, Adrien, & Barthelemy, 1999; Seri, Cerquiglini, Pisani, & Curatolo, 1999). Purdy, Kelly, and Davies (2002) included ALR components in an investigation of cortical auditory evoked responses in ten children diagnosed by a psychologist "with learning disability and a possible APD" (p. 370) and a control group of children with no history of learning or auditory problems. Hearing sensitivity was within normal limits (< 15 dB HL), normal tympanometry, and normal acoustic reflexes. All of the children had normal cognitive function, and none had attention deficit disorder. The suspicion of APD

was raised by poor performance on auditory processing and phonemic awareness components of psychoeducational tests of the *WISC-R* (*Weschler Intelligence Scale for Children-Revised*), the *Detroit Tests of Learning Aptitude–2,* and the *Lindamood Auditory Conceptualization (LAC)* test. Children were also evaluated with measures of word recognition, the SCAN subtests, and the staggered spondaic word (SSW) test. There were significant differences between the two groups for the SSW test and the competing words subtest of the SCAN. Auditory evoked responses were elicited with 300 1000 Hz tone-burst signals with rise/fall times of 5 ms and a plateau of 20 ms, presented at a rate of 1.1/sec and an intensity level of 70 dB HL (70 dB SPL). The responses were recorded with noninverting electrodes located on the vertex (Cz), left and right temporal lobes (C5 and C6), with inverting electrodes on the earlobes (A1 linked to A2), and with band-pass filter settings of 1 to 30 Hz over an analysis time of 750 ms (–100 ms prestimulus time). The following ALR components were analyzed: P1, N1, and P2. Purdy et al. (2002) also reported findings for the ALR and P300 response, as reviewed in the next chapter. The P2 component of the ALR was not consistently recorded and typically small in amplitude. There were significant group differences for the ALR P1 (shorter latency in the APD group) and the N1 component (smaller amplitude in the APD group).

Nina Kraus and colleagues have conducted a series of investigations of late auditory evoked responses (i.e., P1, N1, P2, and N2 waves of the ALR, and the MMN response) in children with "auditory learning problems" (Cunningham, Nicol, Zecker, & Kraus, 2001; King, Nicol, McGee, & Kraus, 1999; Kraus, McGee, Carrell, & Sharma, 1995; Kraus, McGee, Carrell, Zecker, Nicol, & Koch, 1996; Kraus & Nicol, 2003; Tremblay, Kraus, McGee, Ponton, & Otis, 2001; Wible, Nicol, & Kraus, 2002). Most of the studies employed speech signals to elicit the auditory responses. As stated by Kraus and Nicol (2003), "we take a behavioral-neurophysiological, acoustic-phonetic approach to the investigation of biological processes involved in speech-sound perception" (p. 36). Research questions guiding the line of research were also clearly articulated by the authors, among them "how speech sounds are represented in the brains, how that representation is related to perception in a normal system and in clinical populations, and . . . how experience and speech-sound training alters the biology of sound perception" (Kraus & Nicol, 2003, p. 37). The reader is referred to the original publications for details on measurement parameters and outcomes of the studies, and for articles describing experimental studies in animals. Literature on the P300 and MMN response is reviewed in the next two chapters. What follows here is a brief summary of selected clinical findings in normal subjects and children with deficits in auditory processing (learning problems). Auditory electrophysiological investigations show left versus right asymmetries in the auditory responses evoked by speech sounds at subcortical and cortical regions within the brain. The lateralization of activity is observed for auditory responses elicited by speech sounds, but not for pure-tone signals, and appears to be independent of conscious attention to the signals.

One of the well-recognized challenges encountered by children with auditory processing disorders (APD) is difficulty with speech perception in the presence of background noise and competing speech signals (Jerger & Musiek, 2000, 2002). Kraus and colleagues (Cunningham et al., 2001; Hayes et al., 2003; Warrier, Johnson, Hayes, Nicol, & Kraus, 2004; Wible et al., 2002) found smaller amplitude for the P2 and N2 wave complex recorded from children with auditory learning problems when the speech signal /ga/ was presented in the presence of background noise (0 dB SNR) in comparison to ALR amplitude for a control group under the same conditions. The P1 and N1 waves were not analyzed because they were consistently recorded in fewer than one-half of the subjects in the study. This is in contrast to the findings for the quiet test condition with the /ga/ speech signal (see summary in the next paragraph). Of relevance to the management of APD, auditory late responses for the group of children with auditory learning problems were improved (more normal) when a "cue enhancement strategy" was used to facilitate speech perception.

Warrier et al. (2004) reported a larger follow-up study of the ALR in noise. Subjects were eighty children with learning problems and thirty-two normal children. All subjects passed a hearing screening at 20 dB HL for octave frequencies from 500 through 4000 Hz. Learning problems were defined by performance below one standard deviation on a psychoeducational test battery that consisted of the reading and spelling components of the *Wide Range Achievement Test–3 (WRAT)* and portions (incomplete words and sound blending) of the *Woodcock-Johnson-Revised*. The ALR was averaged for 1,000 presentations of the synthetic speech sound /da/ presented to the right ear with insert earphones with ISIs of 590 ms and at a intensity level of 80 dB SPL. Broadband noise was used in the noise condition to create a SNR of 0 dB. The ALR was recorded with a noninverting electrode located at Cz, with an inverting electrode on the nose and a ground electrode on the forehead. A bipolar electrode array (supra-orbital to lateral canthus) was used to monitor eye blinks. Three approaches were taken for analysis of the ALR: conventional measurement of amplitudes and latencies of peaks, a cross-correlation technique, and the calculation of root-mean-square (RMS) amplitude.

A strong theme in the work reported by Kraus and colleagues is the documentation with auditory evoked responses of perceptual learning, including the effect of intensive auditory training. Auditory cortical responses evoked by speech signals are less mature, i.e., smaller amplitudes, earlier latencies, and poorer morphology, for children with learning disabilities characterized by auditory processing weakness in comparison to normal children (Cunningham, Nicol, Zecker, & Kraus, 2000). Again, of particular interest to those professionals involved in the assessment and management of

children with APD, some of the studies examined the auditory late response parameters before and after completion of a commercially available computer-based auditory training program (Earobics).

Hayes et al. (2003) conducted an investigation of children with normal hearing sensitivity aged 8 to 12 years, including twenty-seven with learning problems who underwent a training program, fifteen children with learning problems who received no training (learning problem control subjects), and a control group (N = 7). The training consisted of an eight-week enrollment period in the Earobics computer-based program for development of auditory, phonologic awareness, language, and other prereading skills. The auditory late response was evoked with synthesized speech signals /da/ and /ga/, selected for the study because they are distinguished by differences within the initial (onset) portion in brief transitions of spectral and temporal information. The authors had previously demonstrated that children with auditory learning problems experience difficulty in discriminating these differences as well as normal children (Kraus, McGee, Carrell, et al., 1996). Details on the synthesized speech signals are provided in several publications (e.g., Cunningham, Nicol, Zecker, & Kraus, 2001; King et al., 2002). The /ga/ signal was utilized for the measurement of the ALR in quiet, whereas the /da/ signal was used in the noise condition (see summary above). The signals were delivered with an ISI of 490 ms at an intensity level of 75 dB SPL. The ALR was recorded from midline noninverting electrodes (Fz and Cz) with an analysis time of 500 ms, plus a 90 ms prestimulus period, with band-pass filter settings of 0.1 to 100 Hz. Notably, waveforms were averaged for a total of 2,000 to 2,500 sweeps. With the stimulus parameters, i.e., /ga/, used in the quiet condition, the P1 and N1 peaks were most prominent. Comparison of the pre- versus posttraining ALR data showed a decrease in the P1 to N2 amplitude, and shorter N2 latency values, consistent with maturational changes (Cunningham et al., 2000; Sharma et al., 1997).

Visual inspection of the composite grand averaged waveforms for all subjects in each group displayed in the article published by Hayes et al. (2003) revealed modest differences in the pre- versus posttraining measurements and apparently well-formed composite waveforms for all groups. It is reasonable to question, therefore, whether the ALR findings for an single patient with auditory learning problems would be clearly outside of a normal region and whether ALR findings before training, again for a single patient, would be significantly different than pretraining findings for the same patient. This challenge will be regularly encountered in the analysis and clinical interpretation of ALR findings in children with auditory learning problems. Another practical question for audiologists is whether the children in these studies who are categorized with learning problems are equivalent to those with evidence of auditory processing disorders in conventional diagnostic assessments (Jerger & Musiek, 2000, 2002) with procedures such as dichotic tests (staggered spondaic word test, dichotic digits), auditory figure-ground tests, measures of temporal sequencing, etc. In the articles by Kraus and colleagues, the experimental groups were children with "attention deficit disorder and/or learning disability," and the learning problems are defined by performance below at least one standard deviation on "measures of mental ability and reading, spelling, phonologic awareness or auditory processing on the psycho-educational test battery" (Hayes et al., 2003, p. 674). The test battery consisted of the reading and spelling components of the *Wide Range Achievement Test–3 (WRAT)* and portions (incomplete words and sound blending) of the *Woodcock-Johnson-Revised.* Subject enrollment criteria also included an IQ score of ≥85. The subjects in the studies, therefore, appear to be somewhat heterogeneous and not consistently children with auditory specific processing deficits. Nonetheless, the findings of the series of papers by Kraus and colleagues certainly suggest the potential of the auditory late response as an electrophysiologic index of auditory processing and a tool for documenting objectively the outcome of treatment for APD.

In a retrospective study of children 142 children with auditory processing disorders, Ptok, Blachnik, and Schonweiler (2004) were unable to differentiate with the N1 and P2 waves ninety-nine children with the diagnosis of ADHD and forty-three children without ADHD. Also, APD could not be distinguished from ADHD based on ALR findings.

Down Syndrome

Reports of larger amplitudes for ALR waves in Down syndrome date back to the 1960s (e.g., Barnet & Lodge, 1967; Dustman & Callner, 1979; Yellin, Lodwig, & Jerison, 1980). A common explanation for the larger amplitude was a reduction in the normal habituation of cortical function with repeated stimulation. Diaz and Zurron (1995) reported a study of twelve subjects with Down syndrome and twelve normal subjects (average age of 14 years for both groups). The ALR was elicited with a passive oddball signal paradigm. Frequent stimuli were 500 Hz tone bursts (80% probability) and infrequent stimuli were 2000 Hz tone bursts (20% probability) with a duration of 10 ms presented in four blocks with an ISI of 1.25/second and 5 seconds between blocks and at an intensity level of 100 dB SPL. The ALR was recorded with a noninverting electrode at Cz, band-pass filter settings of 1 to 30 Hz, and an analysis time of 750 ms. Among the Down syndrome subjects, latency was significantly delayed for the ALR N1, P2, and N2 components elicited by infrequent signals. In contrast to previously studies, Diaz and Zurron (1995) found no difference in the N1 to P2 amplitudes between the two groups. The authors did report increased amplitude for the N2 -P3 measure, consistent findings for earlier studies, and the explanation that persons with Down syndrome fail to habituate to repetitive auditory stimulation.

Epilepsy

Along with the P300 and MMN responses, the ALR has been investigated in epilepsy. In contrast to findings in schizophrenia (summarized below), there is no decrease in the amplitude for the N100 wave in epilepsy (Ford, Mathalon, Kalba, Marsh, & Pfefferbaum, 2001; Verleger, Lefebre, Wieschemeyer, & Kompt, 1997). Halford (2003) published a concise review of the literature on AERs and epilepsy. The review also includes a readable general introduction to traditional electroencephalography (EEG) techniques, and the more recently developed quantitative EEG (QEEG) methods for estimating the power spectral density in different EEG frequency regions and for quantifying other EEG parameters, e.g., absolute and relative power, coherence of activity among different channels (electrode locations), and interhemispheric symmetry of power for as detected with corresponding electrodes located over each hemisphere.

Rosburg, Marinou, and colleagues (2004) investigated the AMLR Pb (ALR P1) component and the N100 wave in twenty-nine adult (ages 16 to 57 years) patients with epilepsy and "no evidence of a hearing deficit." Notably, the auditory responses were recorded intracranially, with subdural and depth electrodes, rather than conventional scalp electrodes. Signals were tone bursts of 1500 Hz with a duration of 6.6 ms (1.5 ms rise/fall and 3.6 ms plateau), presented in a train of five repetitions with an intersignal duration of 500 ms, and then another tone burst at a different frequency (2000 Hz) and with a different duration (12.8 ms), separated from the preceding train by 8000 ms (8 seconds). It's of interest to note that the authors, who are affiliated with academic departments of "epileptology," psychiatry, and neurosurgery, refer to these tonal stimuli as "clicks." Confusion in terminology among disciplines involved in studies and clinical application of auditory evoked responses was first discussed in this book in the section on AMLR signals (Chapter 11). ALR data were described for an electrode location, "over or close to the auditory cortex, as verified from axial and coronal, magnetic resonance images routinely acquired after electrode implantation" (Rosburg, Marinou, et al., 2004, p. 246) associated with the most prominent P50 (P1 or Pb) component and N100 wave. Measurement parameters included post-averaging band-pass filter settings of 10 to 50 Hz (slope of 12 dB/octave) and an analysis time of 4000 ms poststimulus and 500 ms prestimulus. ALR wave amplitude was calculated from the prestimulus baseline, and amplitudes and latencies of the P50 and N100 waves elicited by different signal locations (e.g., first, second, deviant, etc.) were compared statistically. The P50 component and the N100 wave were reliably recorded for only twelve of the twenty-nine subjects. Amplitude for the P50 (AMLR Pb) and the N100 components were substantially larger for the initial signal within the train versus subsequent signals in the train—that is, the responses for signals 2 through 5 were suppressed. The authors interpret this finding as consistent with the effects of neuronal refractory period, rather than habituation. With habituation, one would expect a continued decrease in amplitude for signals 2 through 5. Amplitudes for the 6th (isolated and different frequency) signal recovered—i.e., they were larger than the preceding signals (2 through 5) in the train. In contrast to these amplitude differences associated with signal position, latencies were unchanged for P50 and N1 (N100) components.

Depression

One mechanism offered for clinical depression is abnormally low levels of serotonin (5-hydroxytryptamine or 5-HT), a neurotransmitter. Clinically, selective serotonin reuptake inhibitors (SSRIs) are used for medical manipulation of serotonin in the treatment of depression. As noted also in the discussion below of hyperacusis, the primary auditory cortex is a major brain site for serotonin synthesis, high levels of serotonin, and for serotonergic activity (Gallinat et al., 2000; Hegerl & Juckel, 1994). Increased intensity dependency (steeper amplitude–intensity functions) is considered by some investigators (e.g., Hegerl, Wulff, & Muller-Oerlinghausen, 1992) to be a feature of depression and other serotonin-related disorders, e.g., abnormally diminished serotonin activity. However, Dierks et al. (1999) failed to confirm this ALR amplitude–intensity pattern. Conflicting findings were also reported for the experimental manipulation of serotonin on ALR latency in animal models (e.g., Concu et al., 1978). Gopal, Bishop, and Carney (2004) conducted a study of loudness dependency with thirty-six subjects with the diagnosis of clinical depression and a control group consisting of twelve subjects. The ALR was evoked with binaural 1000 Hz tone-burst stimulation at a rate of 1.1/second over an intensity range of 15 to 55 dB SL (sensation level). Responses were recorded with a noninverting electrode at the Fz location and an inverting (reference) electrode on the nape of the neck, using an analysis time of 300 ms and band-pass filter settings of 1 to 100 Hz. ALR amplitude growth, as defined by the increase in absolute amplitude for the N1 to P2 peak from 15 to 55 dB nSL, was comparable for control subjects (2.0 μV) and medicated patients with depression (2.07 μV), whereas the unmedicated patients with depression showed significantly higher intensity dependency (growth of 3.4 μV).

Head Injury

There are varied clinical applications for AERs in acute and severe head injury, as reviewed for the ABR (Chapter 10), the AMLR (Chapter 11), the P300 response (Chapter 13), and the MMN response (Chapter 14). AER investigations are reported also for patients with mild traumatic brain injury (MTBI). MTBI will, for this discussion, be defined according to current criteria as "very mild injuries, resulting in any alteration in mental state, to more severe injuries associated with loss of consciousness of less than 30 minutes and post-traumatic amnesia of less than 24 hours" (Gaetz & Bernstein, 2001, p. 388). Although MTBI is not associated with death nor accompanied by severe acute neurophysiologic dysfunction, it can have clear and significant long-term physical, emotional, and cognitive consequences. The latter include deficits in memory, attention, judgment, and the speed for processing sensory and other information.

Mazzini and Italian colleagues (Mazzini et al., 2001) recorded the ALR N1 and P2 waves from twenty-one young (average age of 27 years) patients (nineteen male and two female) with severe TBI, and a control group eleven healthy normal subjects (average age of 32 years). Severity of injury was defined by a Glascow Coma Score of 6 to 10 (average of 8.2). Importantly, none of the patients were treated with sedatives during ALR measurement. The ALR was elicited with three different oddball signal paradigms in which the frequent signal was always a 1000 Hz tone and the rare (deviant) signal was a 2000 Hz tone, a word of an object that was not relevant to the subject, and the subject's first name. For control subjects and those patients who had recovered sufficiently to participate, Mazzini et al. (2001) required in a fourth condition active attention to the rare (deviant) targets. Recordings were made from three midline noninverting electrode locations (Fz, Cz, Pz) with a 1000 ms analysis time (300 ms prestimulus time), using band-pass filter settings of 0.2 to 30 Hz. In the active listening paradigm, all control subjects consistently produced an N1 wave (average latency of 99 ms) and a P2 wave (average latency of 174 ms) with no change in latency or amplitude as a function of the signal condition or age and gender of the subjects. For control subjects in the passive paradigm (not actively attentive), the N1 was always observed and the P2 was detected 82 percent of the time. In comparison to the control subjects, the latency for the ALR N1 and P2 waves was delayed for the brain injury patients only in the passive listening paradigm and amplitudes for the N1 and P2 components were smaller. In commenting on the significance of the findings, the authors note that an ALR can be recorded from patients unconscious following severe traumatic brain injury in a passive measurement paradigm and that the use of a relevant rare (deviant) signal, e.g., a person's name, produces an enhanced the N1 and P2 waves. ALR findings were not correlated with depths of coma, as defined by the Glasgow Coma Score.

Infant Patient Populations

As noted in Chapter 1, auditory late responses have for over forty years been recorded from infants in an attempt to describe auditory or cognitive function. There is now unparalleled interest in the exploration of infant auditory and cognitive processes with cortical auditory evoked responses and in the application of auditory late responses clinically in infants and young children at risk for central nervous system dysfunction. Selected literature on the topic is reviewed here.

Similar investigations with the auditory P300 and MMN responses are discussed in the next two chapters.

PREMATURE INFANTS. | Infants born prematurely with very low birth weight are at increased risk for neurodevelopmental delay and abnormalities and a variety of disorders, among them auditory dysfunction, blindness, language impairment, lower cognitive status, learning disabilities, cerebral palsy, and developmental delay (e.g., Saigal, Hoult, Streiner, Stoskopf, & Rosenbaum, 2000). It is not surprising, therefore, that a number of investigators have applied cortical auditory evoked responses in the at-risk infant population. The literature on the P300 and MMN response findings in infants is reviewed in the next two chapters. Fellman et al. (2004) recorded late auditory evoked responses from three groups of infants, including fifteen described as small for gestational age (SGA), twenty whose weight was appropriate for their gestational age (AGA), and twenty-two control subjects (full-term infants). The authors provided details on clinical characteristics for each group, such as APGAR scores, gestational age, and arterial pH, and also the proportion of children with various perinatal complications (e.g., need for medications, respiratory distress, mechanical ventilation). Auditory evoked responses were recorded in multiple sessions from birth to 12 months corrected age after birth for the premature infants and to 15 months for the control subjects. Signals were presented in a "frequency oddball paradigm" at an intensity level of 70 dB SPL. The frequent or standard signal was a tone at 500 Hz of 100 ms duration (with harmonics at 1000 and 2000 Hz), while the rare or deviant signal was a 750 Hz tone presented with a probability of 15 percent. The ISI (from onset of one signal to onset of the next signal) was 800 ms. A main focus of the study was the P300 and MMN response, as summarized in Chapters 13 and 14. However, the authors recorded components for the standard signal, including the P2 component and a P350 component and also two negative components within the ALR time frame (the N250 wave and the Nc (650 ms) wave). There was no difference in the amplitude of the P2 and P350 peak for preterm infants at the age of 40 gestational weeks versus term infants (at two to four days after birth, although morphology was generally poorly defined for the preterm group. When data were compared, however, for the premature infants and the control infants at the same postnatal age (3 months), amplitudes for the P2 and P350 waves were significantly smaller for both of the preterm infant groups. Also, amplitude for the P2 component was largest at the age of 3 months. For the control group, the N250 component consistently appeared in the waveform between six and nine months after birth. There were differences in the appearance of the N250 wave for the SGA versus AGA premature infant groups. Changes in ALR latency and amplitude during infancy are, presumably, associated with nervous system maturation, including the number of synapses, synchrony of synaptic activity, and the efficiency of synaptic transmission (Fellman et al., 2004).

INFANTS OF DIABETIC MOTHERS. | DeRegnier et al. (2001) extended early investigations of the normal development of cognitive function with auditory late response to infants born of diabetic mothers. The rationale for study of this population, as stated by the authors, was the documented relation between diabetes in mothers and infant cognitive impairments and, specifically, dysfunction within brain regions that are important for recognition memory, e.g., the hippocampus. The auditory late response was recorded at 38 to 42 weeks postmenstrual from carefully selected infants of diabetic mothers (N = 25) and a control group (N = 32). Infants were in "active sleep" during the recordings. Importantly, in the selection of subjects the authors relied on an experienced audiologist to verify integrity of the cochlea (outer hair cells) with otoacoustic emissions. One of the signals was the speech sound /ba/ spoken by a woman's voice. There were two versions of the speech signal, one with the mother's voice and the other with a stranger's voice. Another signal used to elicit the ALR was a nonspeech sound ("computer chime"). Signals were digitized and presented at an intensity level of 80 dB SPL and with an ISI of approximately 4000 ms. The ALR was recorded with midline electrode sites (Fz, Cz, and Pz) and two lateral sites over the temporal lobe (T3 and T4) over an analysis time of 2000 ms (plus a 100 ms prestimulus time). ALR analysis included calculation of P2 amplitude and latency values and an "area under the curve" measure. As an aside, for both subject groups the ALR P2 amplitudes were greater for recordings made with the Cz versus the Fz noninverting electrode. There was a comparable increase in amplitude and latency, and area under the curve, for the P2 wave for the ALR elicited with the maternal versus stranger's voice. ALR findings in neonates (both groups) were correlated with cognitive development at 1 year of age, when none of the subjects showed evidence of abnormal or delayed cognitive development.

Schizophrenia

ALR abnormalities are reported for patients diagnosed with schizophrenia (Adler, Pachtman, Franks, Pecevich, Waldo, & Freedman, 1982; Shelley, Silipo, & Javitt, 1999). Amplitude of the N100 wave evoked by external signals is reduced in schizophrenia (Ford, Mathalon, Marsh, et al., 1999; Frodl, Meisenzahl, Gallinat, Hegerl, & Møller, 1998; Shelley, Silipo, & Javitt, 1999). Normally, the N100 wave is decreased in amplitude during speaking in comparison to amplitude values elicited by an external signal, even if it's a tape recording of the subject's voice. Patients with epilepsy, however, show no decrease in amplitude of the N100 wave that is elicited by self-produced sounds (Ford, Mathalon, Kalba, Whitfield, Faustman, & Roth, 2001). The N100m is the most stable and detectable component among the auditory evoked magnetic field (AEF) responses. Rosburg et al. (2004) investigated the N100m component of the AEF in twenty male patients (average age of 35 years) with the diagnosis of schizophrenia. General features of the methodology for the study were reported in other publications (e.g., Rosburg, 2004) reviewed in this chapter. The mean global field power (MGFP) of the N100m component decreased with repeated presentations of blocks of 1000 Hz tonal signals, while there was a modest increase in latency. In addition, the authors noted a habituation-related change in dipole location. These findings were observed in the control group as well as the patients with schizophrenia.

Tinnitus and Hyperacusis

TINNITUS. | Kadner et al. (2002) investigated intensity dependence of the ALR N1 (N100) wave in eight patients with tinnitus and twelve control subjects. The authors' rationale for application of the midline recorded N100 wave was based on the assumption that it is generated in the primary auditory cortex and, citing the neurophysiologic model of tinnitus of Pawel Jastreboff (Jastreboff, Gray, & Gold, 1996), "it reflects stimulus properties as well as attention and the psychological state of the subjects, both of which are presumed to contribute to tinnitus" (p. 453). Tinnitus subjects showed modestly steeper intensity/amplitude functions at the frequency (4000 Hz) that was matched to the tinnitus pitch, whereas at a stimulus frequency of 2000 Hz, the tinnitus subjects demonstrated less intensity dependence than the control group, and at 1000 Hz the intensity/amplitude functions were equivalent between the two groups. Kadner et al. (2002) speculate that the findings were consistent with lateral inhibition within the auditory cortex.

HYPERACUSIS. | Hyperacusis is an abnormal intolerance to loud sounds. Alterations in serotonin (5-hydroxyindoleacetic acid, or 5-H) levels and neurotransmission are included in suspected mechanisms for hyperacusis. Consistent with findings for all AERs, amplitude of the N1 and P2 components of the ALR grows with increased stimulus intensity. For the ALR, the intensity–amplitude relationship, referred to as "loudness dependency," has been investigated as an index of serotonin-based neurotransmission within the nervous system and a reflection of the responsiveness of serotonin neuropharmacologic influences to antidepressant medication (Hegerl & Juckel, 1993). High concentrations of serotonin and of serotonin synthesis are normally found in primary auditory cortex (Brown, Crane, & Goldman, 1979; Campbell, Lewis, Foote, & Morrison, 1987). There may be an indirect relation between ALR amplitude growth with increased acoustic stimulus intensity level and the level of serotonin (5 -H) in cerebral spinal fluid. Loudness dependency of the ALR components is increased in patients with low serotonin levels and, conversely, decreased with high serotonin activity (Hegerl, Bottlender, Gallinat, Kuss, Ackenhein, & Møller, 1998). Examples of patients with disruption in serotonin

levels include those with migraine headaches and depression (Gallinat et al., 2000; Wang et al., 1999). In animal studies, the loudness dependency of ALR components recorded directly from the primary and secondary auditory cortex is increased by serotonin antagonists and decreased by serotonin agonists (Juckel, Molnar, Hegerl, Csépe, & Karmos, 1997). It is important to note at this juncture that the site of effect for serotonin neurotransmission is within primary auditory cortex, rather than secondary auditory cortex (Juckel et al., 1997). Some authors suggest that a high degree of loudness dependency of the ALR components may, in selected patient populations, be indicative of their responsiveness to medical treatment with selective serotonin re-uptake inhibitors, or SSRIs (Gallinat et al., 2000; Mulert, Juckel, Augustin, & Hegerl, 2002). This finding is supported indirectly by evidence that lower concentrations of serotonin are associated with greater stimulus intensity dependence of visual evoked response amplitudes (von Knorring & Perris, 1981). There apparently are no published studies of the ALR specifically in patients with hyperacusis, although this line of research certainly seems promising.

CONCLUDING COMMENTS

The promise of the ALR as a clinical electrophysiological measure of cortical auditory processing is evidenced by findings of recent studies in children and adults. Unlike the P300 and MMN auditory responses, the ALR can be recorded with clinical evoked response systems currently available and employed in performing ECochG and ABR assessments. Despite the relative simplicity of ALR instrumentation, test protocol, and analysis strategies, the response can be elicited with complex stimuli (e.g., speech sounds) and applied in the electrophysiological documentation of complex auditory processes. Recognizing the clinical potential of the ALR, manufacturers of evoked response equipment are beginning to offer software options permitting ALR measurement with more diverse stimuli. The ALR appears to be sensitive to normal developmental plasticity of the central auditory nervous system in young children, and age-related deterioration of cortical function in older adults. Also, as revealed by the literature review in this chapter, there are investigations of the ALR as an electrophysiological probe in a diverse selection of patient populations, including auditory processing disorders. The ALR, in addition, can serve as an objective index of changes in auditory processing associated with training and other forms of intervention. Although the ALR was first described more than sixty-five years ago (Davis, 1939), and intensive investigations of the ALR as a potential clinical tool date back to the early 1960s, there is reason to suspect that we are on the threshold of the most exciting and productive period of ALR research.

13 CHAPTER

P300 Response

BACKGROUND

Since the P300 response was first identified in the mid-1960s (Davis, 1965; Sutton et al., 1965), well over a thousand published papers have described measurement techniques, especially the effects of alterations in stimulus characteristics in normal subjects and clinical applications in pediatric and adult populations. Space does not permit a thorough review of the voluminous literature on the P300 response. What follows is a discussion of techniques for measurement of the P300 response in a clinical setting with clinical instrumentation. Rationale for the use of specific stimulus and acquisition parameters, and the effect of selected changes in these parameters on the P300 response, are supported by selected published research findings. However, findings for many other investigations would be cited in an exhaustive review. Trends in the clinical application of the P300 response are discussed, with some published studies summarized in tables within the chapter. The reader must realize, however, that many hundreds of publications on the P300 were not referenced in this chapter.

Actually, the term "P300 response" is not entirely accurate. Within the 300 ms latency region are a variety of different components or peaks that may reflect different neurophysiologic or cognitive processes. Also, a P3 component—the third positive peak in an event-related waveform—may be recorded as late as 600 ms with certain speech signals (e.g., those distinguished by semantic properties). Donchin and Coles (1988) outline some prerequisites for classification of the auditory P300 response, including the general latency expectation (about 300 ms), the optimal electrode array for recording the response (maximum amplitude when recorded over the midline), and greater amplitude with lower probability of the rare signal (Picton et al., 2000). The P300 is conventionally recorded with the oddball measurement paradigm that typically involves two different acoustic signals. Terminology used in describing the P300 response is summarized in Table 13.1.

The P300 response is essentially a component within an extended ALR time frame that is recorded under special stimulus conditions. The simplest of these conditions is the oddball paradigm. One stimulus, a frequent and predictable stimulus (the *standard* signal), generates an auditory late response. The other stimulus, which is infrequent (rare), unpredictable (presented randomly), and different (deviant) in some way from the first signal—the oddball or *target* signal—produces a positive wave in the latency region of 300 ms. The response is sometimes referred to as P300, because it is observed in the 300 ms region, and sometimes as the P3 wave, because it forms a third major positive voltage component after ALR waves P1 and P2. In fact, however, the P300 may be recorded in normal subjects as early as 250 ms or as late as 400 ms, and may not necessarily be the third major component in the waveform.

A typical P300 response is shown in Figure 13.1. The rare and random signal can be distinguished from the frequent signal along various parameters of sound, such as intensity, frequency, duration, and, for speech signals, different phonemes or acoustic characteristics of phonemes (e.g., voice onset time). The P300 response can even be elicited by a missing rare or deviant signal (i.e., silence at the time the rare signal would be randomly presented). As concisely explained by Goldstein, Spencer, and Donchin (2002), "the detection, and processing, of deviance is almost by definition among the roles of an executive control system that is mobilized into action when a change in the environment is detected" (p. 781). Since the presence of the P300 response depends on the detection of a difference between frequent versus rare signals, i.e., a cognitive process, it is often described as a "cognitive evoked response." A host of cognitive processes may be involved in generation of the P300 response, among them discrimination of the characteristics of sound, temporal auditory processing, attention, and memory. As reviewed in Chapter 2, diverse regions of the brain contribute to the generation of the P300 response, including subcortical structures (e.g., the hippocampus and

TABLE 13.1. P300 Response Terminology

See the text for details.

TERMINOLOGY	DESCRIPTION
Stimulus	
Oddball paradigm	In the oddball paradigm, there are at least two stimuli. One stimulus is presented frequently, whereas the other is presented infrequently (the "rare" or oddball stimulus).
Standard	The frequent signal in the oddball stimulus paradigm. Standard stimuli are predictable, accounting for about 80 percent of the stimuli presented in the oddball paradigm.
Target	The infrequent, unpredictable, and rare stimulus. Sometimes referred to as "deviant" stimuli (especially in reference to the MMN response), target stimuli are presented in a pseudo-random fashion, accounting for about 20 percent of the stimuli presented in the oddball paradigm.
Novel	Novel stimuli are highly deviant and usually presented along with standard and target stimuli in a three-stimulus paradigm. Even without subject attention to the novel stimuli, they generate a P300 response (the novelty P3).
Response	
Novelty P3 (P300)	The P300 response elicited by highly deviant (very unusual) stimuli (see novel signal above).
P3a (passive)	A shorter latency P3 wave that is evoked independent of attention to the rare (deviant) stimuli.
P3b	The conventional wave in the P300 response that appears about 300 ms after the presentation of a rare stimulus in the traditional oddball paradigm (with attention to the rare stimulus).

Auditory P300 Response

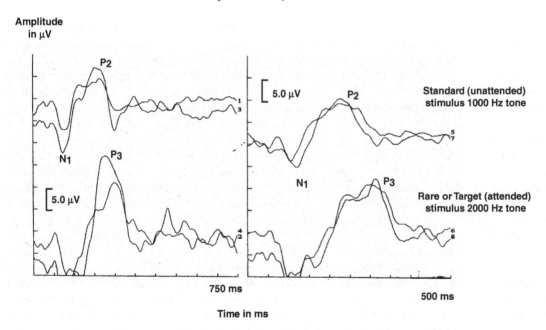

FIGURE 13.1. Auditory P300 response waveform as evoked with a tone-burst signal and recorded with a single-channel electrode array (noninverting electrode at the Fz or Cz location and an inverting electrode on the nape of the neck). The standard signal is a 1000 Hz tone burst (producing the auditory late response in the top portion of the figure) and the target (rare) signal is a 2000 Hz tone burst producing the large amplitude P3 component (lower portion of the figure). The P3 (P3b) response is recorded with subject attending to the target stimulus, whereas the P3a (passive P3) is recorded with the subject's attention diverted from the stimuli (e.g., watching a video or reading).

other centers within the limbic system and the thalamus), auditory regions in the cortex, and the frontal lobe. The relation between signal characteristics and the P300 response is discussed in considerable detail later in the present chapter. Although only the auditory P300 response is reviewed in this chapter, a P3 component can also be elicited with visual and somatosensory stimulation.

With the conventional oddball measurement paradigm, the subject is required to attend to the rare stimulus and to ignore the frequent stimulus. Close vigilance or ongoing attention to the possibility of a rare stimulus enhances the size of the P300 response. A robust P300 response can be recorded with relatively few stimulus presentations (e.g., less than 25). Subject attention to the rare stimulus is sometimes verified by asking the subject to respond actively (e.g., raising a finger, pressing a button) when the stimulus is heard. A P300 response, usually referred to as the P3a component, can also be recorded with a *passive* measurement paradigm (see Figure 13.2). That is, the subject does not attend to the rare stimulus but, rather, ignores both frequent and rare stimuli. In this respect, the *passive P3a* component is an "automatic" response. As a rule, the P3a component is shorter in latency (about 250 ms), smaller in amplitude, and habituates more rapidly than the traditional P3 (P300) wave (Courchesne, Hillyard, & Galambos, 1975; Katayama & Polich, 1998; Polich, 1986; Rugg et al., 1993; Squires et al., 1975). The passive P3a response is prominent when recorded with fronto-central (Fz or Cz) electrode versus more posterior central-parietal (e.g., Pz) scalp locations and with very novel ("colorful") and unexpected stimuli. The P3a component appears to be related to an early component of the P300 response, an "alerting response that most likely originates from neural sources related to initial attention allocation" (Katayama & Polich, 1998, p. 24). With the engagement of memory and more attention processing and resources, the later latency and conventional P300 (P3b) is generated with maximum amplitude in the parietal region (Katayama & Polich, 1998). McIsaac and Polich (1992) showed that the passive P300 response is reliably recorded from normal infants and adults. Details of the test protocol for the McIsaac and Polich (1992) study are noted in discussions of the response in infants in this chapter, and normative data are summarized in the appendix.

The *novelty P300* is yet another response within the same time frame (Figure 13.2). Variations of the P300 response with different deviant or rare stimulus conditions and recorded in different "experimental contexts" (Goldstein, Spencer, & Donchin, 2002) are often referred to as belonging to a "P300 family." Goldstein, Spencer, and Donchin (2002), however, argue that the term family is not appropriate because it implies that the members of the family are variations of the same wave (component), yet waves in the "family" are elicited by different experimental conditions and are recorded with different scalp distributions. Furthermore, Goldstein, Spencer, and Donchin (2002) applied "spatial and temporal event-related potential decomposition techniques" to "disentangle" components that occurred within a common

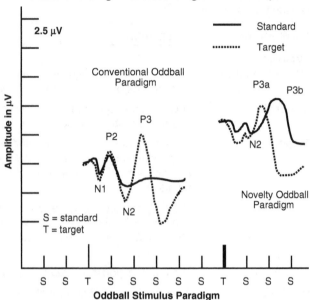

FIGURE 13.2. Conventional oddball stimulus paradigm with standard (S) and target (T) stimuli used in evoking the P300 response (waveforms in left portion of the figure). A variation of the oddball stimulus paradigm (the novelty stimulus paradigm) is depicted in the right portion of the figure.

time frame (p. 786). Initially described by Courchesne, Hillyard, and Galambos (1975), the novelty P300 response is a robust wave elicited by highly unusual (deviant) stimuli, e.g., complex environmental sounds or the subject's name. Presented within a three-stimulus oddball paradigm, the novel stimuli are considered nontarget stimuli. That is, the subject is attending to a target stimulus, not the standard stimulus or the novel stimulus. The novel stimuli produce a P300 response similar to other rare but nontarget stimuli, i.e., stimuli that are not novel (Goldstein, Spencer, & Donchin, 2002; Katayama & Polich, 1998). The novelty P300 can be elicited with any deviant stimulus. According to Goldstein, Spencer, and Donchin (2002), "for an event to elicit the Novelty P3 it has to: (a) be salient relative to the stimuli (or stimulus qualities) that are relevant to the task at hand; (b) not require an overt or covert response, or be irrelevant to the current task (Courchesne et al., 1975); and (c) have low probability of occurrence. Furthermore, the Novelty P3 habituates over time . . . is diminished in patients with various types of brain lesions, including dorsolateral prefrontal cortex (Knight, 1984), posterior hippocampus (Knight, 1996), and the temporal-parietal junction (Knight, Scabini, Woods, & Clayworth, 1989), and is enhanced in other patient populations with attentional deficits . . ." (Goldstein, Spencer, & Donchin, 2002, p. 789). In short, these authors conclude that the Novelty P3 response is not the same as the conventional P300 response, that is, they are "independent and dissociable components." Continuing the family analogy, Goldstein,

Spencer, and Donchin (2002) further clarify the relationship of the Novelty P3 response to the P300 response by stating that they are "certainly not twins . . . they should be considered just acquaintances or neighbors in the same temporal vicinity" (Goldstein, Spencer, & Donchin, 2002, p. 789). In this chapter, therefore, various waves in the general latency region of 300 ms will be considered individuals with unique characteristics each recorded under specific measurement conditions residing in the same temporal neighborhood.

Selected subject and measurement factors are equally important for multiple "event-related potentials (responses)," including the P300 response. To avoid redundant reviews of these factors for the P300 response, the MMN response, and other so-called event related responses in the late latency region, e.g., N400), principles that apply in general to the measurement of event-related potentials are summarized in Chapter 3.

Nomenclature

Normal variations are a characteristic feature of endogenous evoked responses. Morphology of and specific components within endogenous response waveforms are dependent on details of the test paradigm and subtle variations in subject attention to stimuli. Response parameters are closely related to subject state, and rarely are the relationships all or none. For example, P300 amplitude is closely related to how much a subject expects the stimulus to occur (Duncan-Johnson & Donchin, 1977; Roth, Ford, Lewis, & Kopell, 1976; Squires, Donchin, Herning, & McCarthy, 1977). That is, amplitude will be larger if the subject is not expecting to hear the stimulus and smaller if the stimulus is expected. Also, there is a direct relationship between P300 latency and processing time. Latency of the response increases as the time required by a subject to perceive a stimulus and determine certain characteristics increases (Ritter, Simson, & Vaughan, & Friedman, 1979; Roth, Ford, & Kopell, 1978).

ABNORMAL PATTERNS. | As with the conventional ALR, P300 abnormalities are typically described in terms of delayed latency and/or reduced amplitude (e.g., Hillyard, Picton, & Regan, 1978; Papanicolaou et al., 1984; Roth et al., 1981; Squires & Hecox, 1983). Also, in P300 measurement, the above noted defects of normal subject state must be taken into account for meaningful interpretation of such changes. Absence of a P300 component, for example, may be directly related to transient subject inattention to the rare stimulus, rather than to the subject's inability to selectively attend to auditory stimuli presented in the presence of competing background information. The latter finding would be evidence of higher level auditory CNS dysfunction, whereas the former would be simply an example of poor measurement conditions. With the application of P300 in describing higher level CNS functioning, it is also important to take into account the effects of aging and perhaps unrelated medical conditions, such as dementia.

TEST PROTOCOLS AND PROCEDURES

Stimulus Parameters

A word about terminology for P300 stimuli is in order at the outset of this discussion. The oddball stimulus paradigm is typically used to evoke or elicit the P300 response, with two different stimuli presented randomly and one stimulus presented much less frequently than the other. Among guidelines offered by Picton et al. (2000) for research involving event-related responses (see Table 13.2) are stimulus and subject factors. The frequent, predictable, and nontarget signal is often referred to as the *standard* stimulus. The infrequent (relatively rare) and unpredictable (random) stimulus is referred to as the *target* stimulus or, usually in the measurement of the MMN response, the *deviant* stimulus. In the common oddball paradigm for eliciting the auditory P300, one frequent (standard) and one rare (target) signal are distinguished by a difference in frequency (e.g., Alho, Sainio, Sajaniemi, Reinikainen, & Näätänen, 1990; Fein & Turetsky, 1989; Goodin, Squires, Henderson, & Starr, 1978a; Goodin, Squires, & Starr, 1983; Hillyard, Hink, Schwent, & Picton, 1973; Picton, Stapells, Perrault, Baribeau-Braun, & Struss, 1984; Polich et al., 1985; Squires & Hecox, 1983; Syndulko et al., 1982; Winkler, Paavilainen, Alho, Reinikainen, Sams, & Näätänen, 1990). For example, the standard signal may be a 1000 Hz tone burst and the target signal a 2000 Hz tone burst. The subject (or patient) is typically required to attend carefully for the target stimulus and to respond to it by pressing a button or counting silently the number of target stimulus presentations. This paradigm characteristically elicits a positive peak in the latency region of 300 ms—the P300 response—and also increased negativity of the N2 component and a slow wave component. In general, as the difficulty of detecting the rare stimulus is increased, for example by decreasing the frequency difference between the frequent versus the rare stimuli, N2 and P3 latencies increase and amplitudes decrease (Ford, Roth, & Kopell, 1976; Polich, Howard, & Starr, 1985). Differences in hearing threshold levels at the two frequencies, as in some elderly subjects, must be accounted for in P300 interpretation (Pollock & Schneider, 1989). No auditory ERP is elicited if the frequency difference for target versus standard stimuli is smaller than the threshold for discrimination. There are simpler and more complex variations of the two-stimulus oddball paradigm for measurement of the P300 that involve presentation of a single stimulus or, conversely, three different stimuli.

Selected generalizations from the above investigations of one-, two-, and/or three-tone oddball paradigm are as follows:

- P300 latency is shortest for a one-stimulus oddball paradigm in comparison to the two- and three-stimulus paradigm, perhaps an easier task and more processing of less information.
- Changes in probability and interstimulus interval (ISI) for the standard versus target stimuli yield similar

TABLE 13.2. Guidelines for Clinical Investigation with the Auditory P300 Response and Other Event-Related Responses*

GUIDELINE	COMMENT
Planning the study	
Clear rationale	The specific gaps or clarification in knowledge to be addressed by the study must be specified.
Clear hypothesis	The hypothesis must be well defined, in positive terms, with details about the link between event-related response measurements and experimental manipulations.
Task elicits a specific cognitive process	A clear link exists between the subject task and the cognitive process being studied. Established experimental paradigms are most likely to meet this goal.
Monitor subject behavior	When possible, the subject's behavioral responses should be monitored, assessed, and described during the measurement of physiologic responses. When the subject is not required to attend to the stimulus, his or her activity during the measurement should be described, e.g., subject was reading a book. Event-related responses of language processing are an exception to this guideline, as concomitant monitoring of behavioral responses is likely to have a negative impact on physiologic responses.
Subject strategy is controlled	A research publication should include a detailed description of the instructions to the subject, the activity required of the subject during evoked response recording, and the method used to assure subject compliance with the instructions.
Order of experimental conditions	The sequence of experimental conditions (blocks of trials for different conditions) must be described, including the time allotted for each block of trials.
Subjects	
Informed consent	Human subjects enrolled in clinical studies must provided informed consent in compliance with Institutional Review Board (IRB) policies and procedures.
Number	The number of subjects should be described; this number should be adequate to demonstrate a statistically significant effect for the evoked response measurement studied. Homogeneous subject samples are recommended. Reasons for exclusion of subjects should be noted.
Sensory status	Measurement of auditory evoked responses by definition involves the auditory sensory modality. The author's review of the literature (mostly publications in nonaudiology journals) shows multiple examples of vague or inadequate definition of subject hearing status, even in studies of aging in which hearing deficits are likely. Subject self-report of "normal hearing" is inadequate for documenting auditory status. Given the critical importance of sensory detection, and often perception, of the acoustic signal in auditory evoked response measurement, formal audiologic assessment or (minimally) screening of subjects at 15 or 20 dB HL is essential prior to subject enrollment in the study and evoked response data collection. Subject motor status and handedness should also be assessed and defined as indicated for selected auditory evoked response tasks.
Age	The average age and range of ages for subjects should be noted. An acceptable definition for "adult" is age ranging from 18 to 40 years. Age effects are possible for younger or older subjects. Smaller increments for age categories are necessary with children (<18 years) as evoked responses change considerably with maturation. For example, ranges as limited as one month are advised for subjects <24 months, whereas one-year ranges are appropriate between 2 and 8 years, and two-year age groups for subjects >8 years.
Gender	Given the potential influence of gender on auditory evoked responses, the number of males and females must be specified and, preferably, matched. The effect of gender on auditory evoked responses can be assessed as an experimental variable.
Cognitive status	Subject cognitive abilities and ability to perform the task should be described. Documentation of educational level (e.g., subjects are undergraduate or graduate students) is adequate for normal subjects, but formal assessment of mental status is necessary for many clinical subject populations, e.g., children or elderly.
Subject selection criteria	For clinical studies involving patient populations, diagnostic criteria for subject selection must be defined and carefully applied. That is, the investigator must specify how the subjects were categorized into a specific diagnostic group, e.g., schizophrenia, language

TABLE 13.2.   (continued)

GUIDELINE	COMMENT
Subject selection criteria (continued)	impaired, auditory processing disorder. In clinical (not normative) studies, the control subjects should be distinguished from the experimental subjects on by the parameter under investigation. For example, the control and experimental subject groups should be equivalent for age, gender, hearing, intelligence, and socioeconomic status.
Medications	Unless the effect of a drug on evoked response is the focus of the investigation, subjects who are taking drugs that might influence mental status or cognitive processing should be excluded from participation in the study.

Stimulus Factors

Properties of stimuli	The three basic properties of sounds—frequency, intensity, and duration—must be defined for stimuli used to elicit the P300 response. Stimulus calibration techniques and procedures and intensity definitions (e.g., dB SPL, dB nHL) must be described.
Stimulus timing factors	The rate of stimulus presentation and the duration of intervals between stimuli (interstimulus interval, or ISI) must be defined. For ISI, the description must include details on how the interval is defined, e.g., from the beginning (onset) of one stimulus to the onset of the next stimulus. Also, for the oddball P300 stimulus paradigm, the probability and other rules governing presentation of the standard and target stimuli (e.g., random, pseudorandom with details) should be noted.
Speech stimuli	Characteristics of speech stimuli should be delineated, including all important features to permit replication of the stimuli by other investigators, e.g., duration of speech units (phonemes, formants), semantic relatedness among words, familiarity with words.

Acquisition Factors

Subject response	Details of an overt (voluntary) subject response during auditory evoked response measurement should be described, e.g., for pressing a button, which finger was used on which hand. When subject attention was not required during auditory evoked response recording, strategies for assuring inattention to stimuli should be described.
Electrodes	Description of the methodology for auditory evoked response measurement should include details on the type of electrode, e.g., "nonpolarizable Ag/AgCl electrodes," and the technique used for attachment, e.g., adhesive conductive paste, collodion, or an electrode cap. Interelectrode impedance values and maximum limits must be reported. Interelectrode impedance should be <10 K ohms and, preferably, <5 K ohms, and balance among electrodes (<2 K ohm difference).
	The location of the electrodes should be described according to the well-accepted 10–20 system, with locations defined relative to several clear reference points, e.g, nasion, inion, and external ear canals. Multiple noninverting electrode scalp locations are generally preferred for P300 measurement, ranging in number from two or three mid-line electrode sites (e.g., Fz, Cz, and/or Pz) to as many as 75, 128, or even 256 electrode sites. At least one electrode pair should be dedicated to detection of eye blinks that are then rejected from signal averaging. The reference(s) and common (ground) electrode sites should be defined for differential auditory evoked response recordings.
Filter settings	High- and low-pass filter cutoffs (–3 dB points) should be specified, as well as the slope per octave for the analog filters. As stated by Picton et al. (2000) "aliasing occurs when signals at frequencies greater than twice the A/D [analog to digital] conversion rate are reflected back into the sampled data at frequencies equal to sub-harmonics of the original frequencies . . . Rough rules of thumb are to set the high cut-off frequency to approximately one quarter of the A/D rate and the low cut-off to approximately the reciprocal of four times the sweep duration" (p. 135). Any digital filtering after data collection should be noted. Notch filters may distort or diminish recordings of cortical brain activity should not be enabled during measurement of the P300 or, for that matter, any auditory evoked responses.
Amplification	The amplification gain should be described (e.g., ×25,000). Common mode rejection with amplification should be >100 dB, essentially eliminating from averaging electrical noise that is detected equally at each of the electrodes in a pair (noninverting and inverting). The rate of A/D conversion should be adequate for detection of frequencies contributing to the auditory evoked response that is measured.

(continued)

TABLE 13.2. (continued)

GUIDELINE	COMMENT
Signal averaging	The number of stimulus presentations (repetitions or sweeps) must be adequate to produce a signal-to-noise ratio that permits confident detection of the auditory evoked response. The amount of signal averaging needed for response detection depends on the size of the signal (the evoked response) and the level of background noise (nonresponse electrical signals). When measurement artifacts can be traced to the subject, e.g., eye blink, muscle tension, jaw movements, then the subject should be instructed to minimize the source of the artifacts. According the recommendations of Picton et al. (2000), "any trials showing electrical activity greater than a criterion level (e.g., +/− 200 µV) in any recording channel should be rejected from averaging" (p. 138). The number of trials rejected because of excessive artifact should be specified. As a rule, recordings from adult subjects are difficult to interpret when the number of averages rejected due to excessive noise is more than one-third of the total number of averages (Picton et al., 2000). Information should be provided on the temporal ("time-locked") relation of the stimulus to the response.

Data Analysis

Latency and amplitude calculations	A consistent approach should be followed in identifying and labeling the peaks and troughs within a waveform and in calculating latency and amplitude values for each component (wave or part of a wave). Authors (and clinicians) should describe the system followed for labeling waveforms and for calculating latency and amplitudes for each component. Latency calculations can be made from the stimulus onset to the peak amplitude value (the typical approach), to a midpoint in the wave (if the wave consists of multiple smaller peaks), or to the onset or offset of the wave. For amplitude calculations, Picton et al. (2000) recommend measurements from baseline-to-peak, rather than peak-to-adjacent-peak, and a prestimulus baseline period of ≥100 ms to minimize the influence of background noise in amplitude calculations. Peak-to-peak or trough amplitude calculations are suitable when baseline drift or a slow wave shift in the baseline confound its use and when the peak-to-trough value reflects the neurophysiologic process of interest. Amplitudes for auditory evoked response components can be determined at the maximum (for peaks) or minimum (for troughs) voltage if appropriate, or by using a mid-point (intersect) approach. Again, consistency in data analysis within an investigation is essential, with clear description of the analysis method that was followed. When waveforms for a single subject are available for different electrode arrays or different experimental conditions, comparable peaks within each waveform should be measured at the same latency. Composite (summed) grand-mean waveforms should be generated only from individual waveforms with consistent peak latencies and among waveforms combination of different auditory evoked components within a summed wave complex. It is also important to compare amplitude values from one waveform to another only when the waveforms were recorded with similar numbers of stimulus presentations (sweeps or averages). Waveforms recorded with fewer trials will be more greatly affected by background (residual) noise and, usually, will have greater amplitudes. Picton et al. (2000) also recommend caution in calculating area amplitude measurements ("area under the curve") because they are very dependent on accurate definition of the onset and offset of waveform components.

Data Reporting

Waveform display	Guidelines reported by Picton et al. (2000) mandate that authors of research papers display in figures representative actual averaged auditory evoked response waveforms for individuals and/or grand-mean (composite) waveforms, not schematic versions of the waveforms. The waveform display should include the electrode array used in the recording, and information (calibration lines) for temporal (latency) and voltage dimensions, and a clear indication of response polarity, i.e., whether positive voltage is upward or downward. Including the "+" and "−" symbols at appropriate ends of the calibration lines is preferred for defining the voltage direction for evoked response waveforms. Also, original waveforms should be displayed whenever analysis has included the addition or subtraction of data, e.g., summed or difference waveforms.
Scalp distribution of data	In addition to reporting auditory evoked response data in the temporal domain (a waveform is a display of voltage over a period of time), auditory evoked response data should be displayed spatially (scalp topography) in either a figure or a table.

---

* Picton et al. (2000) devote considerable space to the review of guidelines for sophistical event-related response analysis strategies not summarized in this table, among them principal component analysis (PCA), source analysis, statistical analysis of auditory evoked response data, and the discussion of the results of an investigation with respect to previously published findings.

Adapted and abridged from Picton et al., 2000.*

effects on the P300 response elicited by the three different stimulus paradigms.

With adequately long ISI, amplitude of the P300 response is comparable among the three stimulus paradigms.

SINGLE STIMULUS PARADIGM. | The P300 response can be evoked with a *single auditory stimulus,* that is, the measurement paradigm includes a target stimulus but no standard stimulus (McCarthy, 1992; Polich, Eischen, & Collins, 1994). Put another way, the place within the sequence of stimuli typically occupied by the standard stimulus is, instead, "replaced by silence" (Polich, Eischen, & Collins, 1994). A potential clinical advantage of the single stimulus P300 paradigm is simplicity, in terms of both instrumentation and subject task. In combination, these features may permit expansion of single stimulus P300 measurement into new clinical settings and populations, such as young children and persons with serious cognitive deficits (e.g., intellectual disabilities and dementia). The passive P300 paradigm, described below in the subject factors section on "attention," also offers the advantage of simplicity in subject task. However, the single stimulus approach is attractive for another reason. As noted by Polich et al. (1994) "by requiring a response to a stimulus versus a passive presentation, the subject is coerced to allocate attentional resources to the stimulus so that a robust P3 is produced consistently in a fashion similar to the oddball paradigm" (p. 254). P300 amplitude for the single stimulus paradigm was slightly less for the conventional two-stimulus paradigm, whereas peak latencies were equivalent and amplitudes for the single versus oddball paradigm were similar for target probabilities from 0.20 to 0.80 and for different interstimulus intervals, e.g., 2 sec and 6 sec (Polich et al., 1994). Based on their research, Polich and colleagues (Polich et al., 1994; Katayama & Polich, 1996) argue that the same mechanisms play a role in generation of both of the single stimulus and conventional oddball P300 response. In addition, they conclude that the "1-stimulus task can provide the same information as the typical 2-stimulus or oddball paradigm" (p. 38) and, because the task is less demanding, "the 1-stimulus paradigm can be easily performed by young children, demented, or retarded subjects" (Katayama & Polich, 1996, p. 38).

MULTIPLE STIMULUS PARADIGM. | In contrast to the single stimulus paradigm, and at the other end of the stimulus complexity spectrum, the three-stimulus paradigm may yield information on "automatic" cognitive processing not available from the one- or two-stimulus paradigm. With the 3-stimulus paradigm, there are two standard or "nontarget" stimuli and one target stimulus, rather than one standard and one target (Courchesne, Hillyard, & Galambos, 1975; Fein & Turetsky, 1989; Katayama & Polich, 1996, 1998; Polich, Eischen, & Collins, 1994). The subject is still required to attend to, and attempts to identify, the target stimulus. A decrease in the frequency of presentation and predictability of occur-

rence for one of the standard stimuli elicits a P300 response, even though the changes in frequency or occurrence are not the stated target stimulus in the oddball paradigm. Similar P300 responses may be evoked by the "official" target (rare) stimulus and the infrequent standard stimulus. Therefore, the response elicited by the infrequent standard stimulus is thought to reflect "automatic cognitive processes" (Katayama & Polich, 1996).

A variation of the three-stimulus paradigm includes a novel or "alerting" stimulus (e.g., a noise or dog bark) as a "distractor" within the sequence of standard and target stimuli (e.g., tones of different frequencies). The resulting P300 waveform contains a P3a component, elicited by the novel distractor stimulus, and the conventional P300 (also referred to as the P3b component), elicited by the target stimulus. The P3a component is distinguished from the P3b component by shorter latency (see Figure 13.2), largest amplitude for frontal (anterior) and central electrode sites (versus more parietal sites for Pb), and rapid habituation. As noted in the neuroanatomical review in Chapter 2, lesions within the frontal lobe and/or hippocampus are associated with abnormalities of the P3a component (Knight, 1984), as confirmed also by neuroradiologic (functional MRI) findings (McCarthy, Luby, Gore, & Goldman-Rakic, 1997). In contrast, intact temporal-parietal cortical function is important for generation of the P3b (conventional P300) component (Knight, Scabini, Woods, & Clayworth, 1989). As noted by Polich (2004), event-related response "measurement of neurologic and psychiatric disorders suggests that a clinically applicable P3a task could be of considerable benefit because P3a measures may be more sensitive than P3b to clinical status" (p. 139).

STIMULUS PROBABILITY. | Probability of occurrence for the standard and target stimuli affects P300 response characteristics. Within certain limits, amplitude of the P300 response decreases as the probability of the target stimulus increases (e.g., Duncan-Johnson & Donchin, 1977), whereas the effect of target stimulus probability on P300 latency is minimal (e.g., Polich & Bondurant, 1997). However, there is little change in the P300 response when probability of the target stimulus is decreased below 20 percent (0.20). Given this limitation in the effect of decreased probability, and the increase in test time associated with signal averaging of a response for very infrequent target stimuli, the probability in P300 measurement is usually 80 percent for standard and 20 percent for target stimuli.

STIMULUS REPETITION. | There is ample documentation in the literature that P300 amplitude decreases with ongoing stimulus repetition, a finding attributed to habituation (e.g., Lammers & Badia, 1989; Polich & McIsaac, 1994; Romero & Polich, 1986). Decreased P300 amplitude with repeated signal presentation is attributed to habituation and related to the response task, e.g., counting the rare stimuli versus pressing a button upon perceiving a rare stimulus (Ivey & Schmidt, 1993; Lew & Polich, 1993). Generally, habituation or fatigue in the oddball paradigm P300 response is apparent when the number of signal repetitions exceeds 80 to 100 (Polich, 1989). Temporal measurement factors influencing P300 habituation include the interstimulus interval (ISI), the intertarget interval (ITI), and the interval between blocks of stimulus trains (IBI). Larger P300 amplitudes, i.e., less habituation, are associated with longer values for these temporal parameters including ISI, ITI (>13 seconds), and IBIs (>2 minutes). Carrillo-de-la-Peña & García-Larrea (1999) reported that latency of the P300 response and N1, P2, and N2 components were not affected by stimulus repetition. With an oddball counting task, P300 amplitude was generally not influenced by stimulus repetition except for a difficult task that required the subject to perform mental exercises such as counting backwards in threes when upon hearing the target stimulus or "update the week and the month" after each stimulus was presented.

STIMULUS TYPES: TONES. | The most common distinction between frequent (standard) versus rare (target) stimuli employed in the oddball paradigm is a difference in frequency. For example, the standard stimulus might be a 1000 Hz tone and the target stimulus is a 2000 Hz tone. In applying stimulus-frequency-based oddball paradigms clinically, one must first ensure that the patient's hearing sensitivity is comparable for each of the two frequencies. Unfortunately, review of the literature suggests that hearing status for subjects enrolled in P300 investigations is not invariably, or even regularly, evaluated using accepted audiologic techniques. If hearing sensitivity is depressed in the higher frequency region and the rare stimulus in P300 measurement is a tone within this region, then hearing-related P300 response latency or amplitude changes might be expected. Indeed, Pollock and Schneider (1989) showed prolonged P300 latency for a 2000 Hz rare stimulus frequency in older subjects with age-related hearing deficits. The P300 response for young versus old subjects was comparable when the rare (target) stimulus frequency was 500 Hz. Negative and positive auditory ERP components, including the P300, can also be recorded when the target stimulus is omitted or missing (Perrault & Picton, 1984; Picton & Hillyard, 1974; Ruchkin & Sutton, 1978a; Simson, Vaughan, & Ritter, 1976; Sutton et al., 1967).

Amplitude for the P300 response increases directly with the frequency difference between the standard and target stimulus. For example, larger P300 amplitudes would be expected with a standard stimulus frequency of 500 Hz and a target stimulus frequency of 2000 Hz than if the standard and target stimulus frequencies were 1000 Hz and 1100 Hz. The task of detecting the target stimulus is easier for large frequency differences between the standard and target tones and, therefore, the subject will identify the target tone more readily, and with more confidence. The predictable result of these factors is larger P300 amplitude (e.g., Polich & Hoffman, 1998).

STIMULUS TYPES: SPEECH SOUNDS. | There are hundreds of papers describing the use of speech stimuli for evoking the auditory P300 response, even in infants and young children. For example, Kurtzberg and colleagues (Kurtzberg, 1989; Kurtzberg, Hilpert, Kreuzer, Stone, & Vaughan, 1986), in a series of studies during the 1980s, topographically recorded auditory evoked responses in the 200 to 750 ms latency region with speech sounds that differed on the basis of voice onset time (/da/ versus /ba/). Response components included negative and positive peaks, including the P3 wave, detected from electrodes over the frontal and temporal lobes. These authors describe age-related changes in the responses to speech features and in the topographic distribution of the response. Literature on the application of speech stimuli in evoking auditory late response components other than the P300 and the mismatch negativity (MMN) response was reviewed in Chapter 12.

The P300 response can be recorded during REM sleep with frequent versus rare speech stimuli differing in acoustic characteristics and, using the oddball paradigm, probability of occurrence (Bastuji, Perrin, & García-Larrea, 2002). Relevance of speech stimuli influences the P300 response. There is some question as to whether the presence of a P300 response to speech stimuli during sleep is evidence of actual discrimination of the different meaning of the two stimuli (frequency versus rare) or detection of the basic difference in the acoustic characteristics and probability of presentation alone (e.g., Bastuji, Perrin, & García-Larrea, 2002). With speech stimuli in a passive, e.g., sleeping, recording condition, P300 amplitudes are larger when elicited with a personally significant word—the subject's name—than with other ("irrelevant") words (Berlad & Pratt, 1995; Perrin et al., 2000; Pratt, Berlad, & Lavie, 1999). Also, measurement of the P300 response is enhanced, or facilitated, by first familiarizing the subject to the rare speech stimuli (Bastuji et al., 1995). As noted by Bastuji, Perrin, and García-Larrea (2002) in a comprehensive review of speech-evoked "event-related" responses during sleep, "the reasons to choose this type of stimulus were, firstly, that a person's own name, because of its emotional content and repetition along life, appears as one of the most relevant stimulus for any human subject. Secondly, there is evidence that hearing one's name during wakefulness produces cognitive brain responses, including a P300, even in the absence of explicit instructions, thus suggesting that a subject's name is automatically and implicitly processed as a target stimulus" (pp. 244–245).

Syntactically anomalous words presented in the oddball stimulus paradigm generate a positive wave in the 600 ms region (e.g., Osterhoot, Allen, McLaughlin, & Inoue, 2002). Kotchoubey and Lang (2001) investigated the P3 response elicited by words selected from among two of five different word classes, e.g., tools, animals, jobs, body parts, and household objects. There were fifteen German language words in each class, and the eighty normal and healthy subjects were native German speakers. The authors attempted to isolate semantic differences as the factor in P3 response measurement, rather than the high probability of detecting a frequent standard stimulus versus the low probability of the rare target stimulus, as in the typical oddball stimulus paradigm. As stated by the authors, "the words [fifteen nouns in the five classes] were presented in a pseudorandom order, so that each word was repeated four times during the experiment but one and the same word was never presented twice in a row. Thus, the frequency of occurrence was equal for all words (1.33% each) and all classes (20% each)." The semantic difference between the standard and target stimuli evoked a large positive peak in the 500 to 800 ms region, but not for earlier latencies. The response was recorded at parietal and central scalp electrode sites, but not over frontal areas.

Another approach in investigations of specific semantic features in auditory cortical response measurement involves "contextual and priming effects" (Brown, Marsh, & Smith, 1973, 1976; Kutas & Hillyard, 1980, 1982, 1983, 1984; McCallum, Farmer, & Pocock, 1984; Squires, Squires, & Hillyard, 1975). One semantic feature examined extensively is *incongruity,* based on the observation that a linguistic expectancy develops while hearing or reading a sentence. When the last word in a sentence is highly likely (expected), the speed with which it is recognized is facilitated. Contextual cues in the sentence act to prime the processing of the final word. There is no facilitation, however, if the final word forms an acceptable, but unlikely, completion of the sentence, and, in fact, an inhibitory effect occurs if the word is *incongruent*— that is, it makes no sense in the context of the sentence. An incongruous or unpredictable final word may generate a late negative ERP component, referred to as "N400." McCallum, Farmer, and Pocock (1984) found that an N456 component was observed in averaged auditory ERPs when stimuli were semantically incongruous final words in sentences. This response showed an inhibitory effect. In contrast, when stimuli were final words unexpectedly spoken by a female versus a male voice (physical incongruity), a late positive component (P416) was observed in the auditory ERP waveform. There are also reports of ERP patterns recorded while the subject engages in a reading or a listening task (Hink & Hillyard, 1976; Neville, Kutas, & Schmidt, 1982).

The P300 response elicited by speech signals can be recorded in parallel with behavioral neuropsychological assessment instruments. D'Arcy and Connolly (1999) reported measurement of the P300 response evoked with items from the *Token Test,* an established tool for assessing speech comprehension. The overall goal of this research group is to create electrophysiological versions of such standardized neuropsychological tests of language and cognitive function and "to analyze neural responses within the context of existing standardized measures of language" (D'Arcy & Connolly, 1999, p. 1487).

SIGNAL TYPES: SOUND ENVIRONMENT. | Distinct differences in the P300 response are found when recordings are made with stimuli presented in a silent environment (quiet) versus in background sound. Furthermore, the nature of the background sound, e.g., white noise versus culturally significant music, can also exert an important influence on the P300 response (e.g., Arikan et al., 1999). As noted in the section below on clinical applications, the P300 response can be used to electrophysiologically assess auditory processing in the presence of background noise, i.e., auditory figure-ground performance. When the P300 is recorded with frequent versus rare stimuli presented in competing noise, amplitude is usually reduced directly as a function of the signal to noise ratio. That is, the smaller the signal-to-noise ratio (the signal is the rare sound and the noise is background sound), the smaller the P300 amplitude. With a sufficiently adverse signal-to-noise ratio, no P300 can be evoked by the rare stimulus.

Background sound doesn't invariably reduce P300 amplitude. Arikan et al. (1999) recorded the P300 response evoked with the oddball paradigm by two tones (frequent stimulus of 1000 Hz and rare stimulus of 2000 Hz) presented in four different background conditions. As the authors stated, "the stimuli were presented either in a silent environment, or superimposed on white noise, on violoncello improvisations of David Darling or on ney improvisations of Sadreddin Ozcimi. The ney is a reed flute. Ney (Mevlevei) music is popular in the Turkish culture. Subjects were ten young Turkish adults who were "musically naïve." The intensity of the stimuli was 80 dB (an intensity dimension was not noted), whereas background sounds were 60 dB. The P300 response was recorded from multiple electrode sites representing frontal, coronal, temporal, parietal, and occipital scalp locations. No differences in P300 latency were found among the four background conditions. Amplitude for the P300 response, however, varied depending on the background sound condition. In comparison to the quiet condition, amplitude was reduced with white noise and violoncello music. Amplitude for the P300 response recorded from frontal electrode locations with ney music in the background was equivalent to amplitude in the quiet condition, and significantly larger than P300 amplitude was recorded in the other two background sound conditions. The authors interpreted these findings as evidence that the ney music enhanced information processing (selective attention and memory updating) within frontal regions of the brain and, further, demonstrated the influence of cultural factors on cognitive processes.

FREQUENCY. | For the P300 response, stimulus frequency can be considered in absolute and relative terms. The same concept holds for signal intensity. Absolute stimulus frequency applies to both the frequent and rare signals. For example, the P300 can be recorded by two 500 Hz tone bursts that differ in their duration or intensity, or by two 2000 Hz tone bursts that differ along the same dimensions. The absolute frequency is considerably different for the two stimuli. Relative frequency is not a factor with this example. Or, the P300 response may be elicited by a relative difference in stimulus frequency of the stimuli. Actually, in clinical measurement of the P300 response, a frequency difference between the frequent and rare stimuli, e.g., a frequent stimulus of 500 Hz and a rare signal of 2000 Hz, is common employed to elicit the P300. There is some evidence that P300 amplitude is smaller and latency longer for low versus high stimulus frequencies (Sugg & Polich, 1995).

INTENSITY. | The effect of stimulus intensity on the P300 response can be considered in two ways. Absolute stimulus intensity has an influence on the P300 response that is characteristic of all auditory evoked responses. That is, P300 wave amplitude increases and latency decreases as stimulus intensity increases for both the frequent and rare stimuli (e.g., Papanicolaou et al., 1985; Polich, Howard, & Starr, 1985; Sugg & Polich, 1995; Vesco, Bone, Ryan, & Polich, 1993). Relative intensity levels for the frequent versus rare stimuli are also a potential factor in P300 measurement. Although not applied as often as the frequency dimension, intensity differences between rare versus frequent stimuli can form the basis of the oddball paradigm in eliciting auditory ERPs. A paper describing the intensity-difference oddball paradigm in P300 assessment of recovering brain-injured patients (Harris & Hall, 1990) is discussed later in this chapter.

RATE AND INTERSTIMULUS INTERVAL (ISI). | Similar to the ALR, the P300 response is optimally recorded with slow stimulus rates and, therefore, relatively long ISIs. Rates of 1 or 0.5 stimulus/second are commonly employed, but even slower stimulus rates produce larger P300 amplitudes. Amplitudes of P300 components decrease as stimulus rate is increased above these values. Put another way, latency of the P300 response increases and amplitude decreases as the ISI increases (Johnson, 1988; Polich, 1986).

Acquisition Parameters

ANALYSIS TIME. | The P300 response is a long latency response. Therefore, to include the rather broad P300 wave, an analysis time of about 450 to 500 ms is required. The response consists entirely of low-frequency (less than 30 to 40 Hz) energy, and a minimum time period between data points of 1 ms or even more provides adequate temporal resolution and accuracy for amplitude calculations. In the interest of consistency, an equivalent analysis period can be used for measurement of both ALR and P300.

Electrode Location

The P300 response can be reliably recorded clinically with a noninverting electrode located anywhere over the frontal portion of the scalp of the head, especially in the midline. The P300 response has maximum amplitude with a frontal/central (e.g., Fz or Cz) or frontal/parietal (Pz) sites (Cody & Bickford, 1965; Cody & Klass, 1968; Cody, Klass, & Bickford, 1967; Davis & Zerlin, 1966; Goff, Allison, & Vaughan, 1978; Horovitz et al., 2002; Kooi, Tipton, & Marshall, 1971; Picton, Hillyard, Krausz, & Galambos, 1974; Polich et al.,

1997; Vaughan & Ritter, 1970). The P300 evoked by conventional tonal signals (one, two, or three signals in the oddball paradigm) is largest for the midline parietal (Pz) electrode site and decreases as the noninverting electrode is placed at more anterior sites (Cz or Fz), whereas the P3a response is maximal with electrodes at frontal-central (e.g., Fz) sites. Whenever possible (e.g., available instrumentation includes enough channels), the P300 response should be recorded with noninverting electrodes at three midline sites (Fz, Cz, and Pz). Comparison of responses for each of the three electrode arrays, especially in patient populations, helps with proper identification of the P300 component and contributes to measurement of maximum amplitude values. With right-handed normal subjects, larger amplitudes for the P3 wave are recorded with noninverting electrodes over the right versus left hemisphere, especially for anterior-medial locations, such as the frontal sites F3/4 and the central sites C3/4 (e.g., Alexander, Bauer, Kuperman, Morzorati, O'Connor, Rohrbaugh, Porjesz, Begleiter, & Polich, 1996; Polich et al., 1997). P300 latency values are symmetric for scalp electrodes located laterally on the right and left hemispheres.

The inverting electrode for P300 measurement, as reported in the literature, is usually located either on the mastoid or earlobe ipsilateral to the stimulus, or electrodes linked between both ears (A1/A2). The common (ground) electrode is generally located on the forehead with P300 recordings. In addition to the above-noted electrode arrays for detection of auditory evoked brain activity, one or two pairs of electrodes should be located around the eyes. Eye blink artifact must be excluded from P300 recordings. Optimally, vertical ocular activity is detected with a pair of electrodes above and below an eye (sub- and supra-orbital) and horizontal ocular activity is detected with electrodes located on each side (outer canthus) of the eye. Trials with electrical activity that exceed a value of 100 or 200 μV are excluded (rejected) from averaging, thus eliminating the likelihood of response contamination with eye blink artifact.

FILTER SETTINGS. | Band-pass filter setting for measurement of the P300 response are, of course, the same as those used for ALR recordings. Spectral power of normal auditory late responses is within the region of 1 to 15 Hz, most evident below 8 Hz, and typically maximum at approximately 5 Hz (Davis, 1973; Nishida, Tanaka, Okada, & Inoue, 1995; Sayers, Beagley, & Henshall, 1974; Yamamoto, Sakabe, & Kaiho, 1979). This is well within the traditional EEG spectrum. The frequency composition of the P300, including the region of maximum energy, may vary somewhat as a function of scalp distribution. Therefore, filter settings of 1 to 30 Hz were typically employed in early studies of the P300 response. A review of hundreds of more recent P300 response studies reveals typical high-pass filter settings in the region of 0.01 to 0.25 Hz and low-pass filter settings on the order of 30 to 50 Hz (e.g., Polich, 2004). The slope of analog filters used for measurement of the P300 response is typically about 3 dB down at the cutoff (–3 dB), and then a slope of 12 dB/octave.

AVERAGING. | One of the principles of event-related response measurement, specifically "signal analysis," stated in the guidelines of a Committee of the Society for Psychophysiological Research and reported by Picton et al. (2000), was that "averaging must be sufficient to make the measurements distinguishable from noise" (p. 136). There are, however, papers describing the detection of the P300 response from a single trial, that is, following the presentation of one stimulus (Demiralp, Ademoglu, Schürmann, Başar-Eroglu, & Başar, 1999; Nishida, Nakamura, Suwazono, Honda, Nagamine, & Shibasaki, 1994; Nishida, Nakamura, Suwazono, Honda, & Shibasaki, 1997). The rationale for utilizing a single stimulus versus the conventional signal averaging of many stimuli has to do with the well-appreciated variations during measurement of event-related response characteristics (latency and especially amplitude) that are associated with ongoing changes in a subject's cognitive or attention state. Several different analysis techniques have been applied for detecting the P300 response elicited by a single stimulus, including adaptive filtering (Woody, 1967), correlation techniques (Suwazono, Shibasaki, Nishida, Nakamura, Honda, Nagamine, Ikeda, Ito, & Kimura, 1994), the "discriminant function approach" (Squires & Donchin, 1976), and with an artificial neural network (Nishida, Nakamura, Suwazono, Honda, Nagamine, & Shibasaki, 1994). According to Nishida and colleagues (1994), the neural network technique permits detection of the P300 response elicited by a single stimulus with accuracy equivalent to visual inspection of the averaged P300 waveform by experienced persons. An adequate signal-to-noise ratio, larger than about 0.8 according to Nishida et al. (1997), may be required for application of some single stimulus mathematical analysis techniques. Confident identification of the P300 response with statistical verification is achieved with sophisticated waveform analysis strategies, such as the wavelet composition or wavelet transform (WT) approach that represents the response in time and frequency domains. Evoked response waveforms can be decomposed into individual components or stimuli varying in time and frequency characteristics, often arising from different neural structures. Specifically, as described by Demiralp et al. (1999) "the application of a 5 octave quadratic B-spline-WT on single sweeps yielded discrete coefficients in each octave with an appropriate time resolution for each frequency range. The main feature indicating a P300 response was the positivity of the 4th delta (0.5–4K Hz) coefficient (310–430 ms) after the stimulus onset" (p. 108).

CLINICAL TEST PROTOCOL

A test protocol for clinical measurement of the P300 response is summarized in Table 13.3. Rationale for inclusion

of each parameter is also stated. Recommendations for the parameters in Table 13.3 are based on research evidence cited in the preceding section and on P300 methodology as reported in the literature.

ANALYSIS AND INTERPRETATION
Normal Waveform Variations

As a supplement to the brief review that follows here, the reader is referred to guidelines for calculation of P300 latency and amplitude and analysis in general, such as Pfefferbaum, Ford, and Kraemer (1990) and Picton et al. (2000). In contrast to earlier "exogenous" evoked responses, P300 latency and amplitude vary considerably as a function of various signal factors, such as complexity, and subject factors, such as memory and speed of information processing.

LATENCY. | The initial step in the calculation of P300 latency, or timing, is to identify a peak within the appropriate latency region. A generally accepted criterion for the definition of the P300 response (e.g., Verleger, 1998) is a positive deflection in the waveform within a latency region of 250 to 400 ms, and up to 800 ms for selected subject populations (e.g., infants). As reviewed elsewhere in this chapter, actual latency values for individual subjects differ due to intersubject variability and a host of measurement parameters, such as the test paradigm (e.g., passive or attending, task difficulty, stimulus intensity, similarity or difference between the standard and target stimuli, relevance or novelty of stimuli, and recording electrode site) and subject-related factors (e.g., age, cognitive status). Calculation of P300 latency is invariably made, in ms, from the stimulus onset to the peak (point of largest amplitude) of the P300 wave. Given the longer durations for stimuli used to evoke the auditory late responses and the P300 response, it's important for accuracy to calculate latency from the onset of the stimulus, rather some other stimulus-related time. P300 latency estimation is illustrated in Figure 13.3. General techniques for enhancing the accuracy of latency calculations for auditory evoked responses, e.g., adding replicated waveforms and smoothing waveforms, can be used also for the P300 response.

Unlike the waveforms for earlier latency responses, e.g., the ABR, the P300 wave is often broad (see Figure 13.1) and characterized by multiple positive peaks (Dalebout & Robey, 1997; Kileny & Kripel, 1987; Sklare & Lynn, 1984; Wall, Davidson, & Dalebout, 1991). Different strategies have evolved for the calculation of amplitude and latency measures when this occurs. Dalebout and Robey (1997) describe the "intersect method" used by the above authors for P300 analysis. Essentially, latency is determined for the midpoint of the wave, as calculated from the latency point where the initial (leading) portion of the peak crosses the baseline to the corresponding latency point at the final (trailing) portion of the peak.

TABLE 13.3. Parameters for an Auditory P300 Response Clinical Test Protocol

PARAMETER	SUGGESTION	RATIONALE/COMMENT
Stimulus Parameters		
Transducer	ER-3A	Supra-aural earphones are acceptable for P300 measurement, but insert earphones are more comfortable for longer AER recording sessions. Insert earphones also serve to attenuate background sound in the test setting. In addition, since the insert cushions are disposable, their use contributes to infection control.
Type	Tone burst	Highly transient click signals are inappropriate for P300 measurement. Longer duration tonal signals are preferred.
	Speech	The P300 response can be effectively elicited with speech signals (natural or synthetic), such as /da/ and /pa/. Various characteristics of speech signals, e.g., voice onset time, can be used in P300 stimulation.
Duration		
Rise/fall	~10 ms	Longer onset times are feasible for signals used to elicit the P300 response. As noted below, the distinction between frequent and rare signals may be a duration difference.
Plateau	~50 ms	Extended plateau durations are effective in eliciting the P300 response. See comment above about duration as a distinction between the frequent versus rare signals.
Rate	≤1.1/sec	A slow rate of signal presentation is essential for the P300 response, due to the longer refractory time of cortical neurons. P300 response amplitude may increase with progressively slower signal presentation rates to 0.125/sec and longer interstimulus intervals, or ISIs, up to 8 seconds.
Oddball signal paradigm		With P300 measurement, there are two different signals, each generating a response. The *frequent* (aka *standard*) signal, presented at regular and predictable intervals, evokes a conventional late response waveform. The *infrequent* (aka *target* or *deviant*) signal is presented unpredictably (in a pseudorandom manner) usually with a probability of occurrence of about 0.15 to 0.2 (15 to 20% probability).
Signal difference		The distinction between frequent and rare signals may involve various features of sound, including frequency (e.g., 1000 Hz versus 2000 Hz), intensity, or duration. Features of the sound other than this distinction are usually the same for the sound. That is, if the frequent versus rare distinction is a frequency difference, the intensity and duration of the two types of signals are the same.
Probability		The probability of signal presentation is, typically, 100 percent for the frequent signal and 20 percent for the rare signal. The presentation of the rare signal is actually pseudorandom, rather than truly random. There are two constraints for signal presentation. The rare signal cannot be presented as the first signal as averaging of a P300 begins. Also, two rare signals can occur in succession, i.e., there must always be one or more frequent signals presented between any two rare signals.
Number		Since the probability of the rare signal presentation is typically 20 percent (only one in five signals is rare), the P300 response is recorded with relatively few rare signal presentations (as few as 20 or less). The appropriate number of signals depends largely on the amount of averaging necessary to achieve an adequate signal to noise ratio.
Polarity	Rarefaction	Signal polarity is not an important parameter for ALR measurement.
Intensity	≤70 dB HL	Modest signal intensity levels are typical for ALR measurement. As noted above, the distinction between frequent and rare signals may be an intensity difference. Remember the signal-to-noise ratio is the key. Averaging may require as few as 20 to 50 signals at high intensity levels for a very quiet and normal-hearing patient.
Presentation ear	Monaural	Binaural signals are often used for measurement of the P300 response.
Masking	50 dB	Rarely required with insert earphones and not needed for a stimulus intensity level of ≤70 dB HL.

TABLE 13.3.   (continued)

PARAMETER	SUGGESTION	RATIONALE/COMMENT
Acquisition Parameters		
Amplification	50,000	Less amplification is required for larger responses.
Sensitivity	25 or 50 μvolts	Smaller sensitivity values are equivalent to higher amplification.
Analysis time	600 ms	An analysis epoch (time) must be long enough to encompass the P300 wave and the following trough.
Prestimulus time	100 ms	An extended prestimulus time provides a stable estimate of background noise and a baseline for calculation of the amplitudes for negative and positive waveform components.
Data points	≤512	
Sweeps	<500	See comments above for signal number.
Filters		
Band pass	0.1 to 100 Hz	The P300 response consists of low-frequency energy within the spectrum of the EEG.
Notch	none	A notch filter (removing spectral energy in the region of 60 Hz) should always be avoided with P300 response measurement because important frequencies in the response will be removed.
Electrodes		
Type	Disc or disposable	Disc electrodes applied with paste (versus gel) are useful to secure the noninverting electrodes on the scalp. Disposable electrodes or a multiple-electrode cap are also appropriate with P300 response measurement.
Electrode sites		
	Noninverting	The Fz, Cz, and/or Pz sites are appropriate for recording the P300 response clinically, although many published studies include 20 or more electrode sites (as many as 128). With some measurements conditions and subject tasks, P300 amplitude may be maximum at the Pz site.
	Inverting	Linked earlobes are commonly used for inverting electrodes. A noncephalic electrode site (e.g., nape of the neck) is also appropriate.
	Other	Ocular electrodes (located above and below or to the side of an eye) are required for detection of eye blinks and rejection of averages contaminated by eye blinking.
Ground	Fpz	A common (ground) electrode can be located anywhere on the body, but a low forehead or nasion (between the eyes) location is convenient and effective.

There is a direct relation between latency of the P300 response and the speed of information processing (Courchesne, 1978a). With faster information processing, including quicker recognition and categorization of the stimulus, P300 latency is shorter. Conversely, P300 latency increases directly with complexity of the processing task and with short-term memory demands (e.g., Polich, Howard, & Starr, 1983). The more confidence a subject has that the rare stimulus is different from the frequent stimulus, the shorter the P300 latency. As noted below, confidence in the perception of stimuli also directly influences P300 amplitude.

AMPLITUDE. | Amplitude of the P300 response varies as a function of many different measurement and subject variables. However, response amplitude is generally within the range of 10 to 20 μV. There are two common approaches for determining P300 amplitude or size, as illustrated in Figure 13.3. One is calculation of the amplitude in μV from the P300 peak to the trough (negative wave) that immediately precedes or follows the peak. Although apparently straightforward, this technique yields a relative value that is really combination of amplitudes for two peaks (the P300 wave and the other negative wave). The problems associated with this "peak-to-peak" amplitude calculation approach, reviewed in some detail with reference to the AMLR and AMR, apply also to the discussion of P300 analysis. The other preferred amplitude estimation approach involves calculation of the difference (in μV) from a prestimulus baseline period to

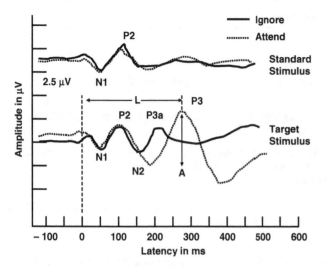

Analysis of P300 Recorded with Oddball Paradigm

FIGURE 13.3. Analysis of P300 response latency and amplitude measures.

the maximum positive voltage point, or peak, of the P300 wave. The result is an absolute value that reflects the amplitude of a single peak. Of course, this approach presumes that the prestimulus baseline activity is a stable reference point.

The intersect method (e.g., Dalebout & Robey, 1997) described for latency calculation is generally not applied in the analysis of P300 amplitude. Instead, amplitude is calculated for the highest of the smaller peaks superimposed on the broad P300 wave. The question for amplitude analysis has to do with what reference point should be used. Two common reference points are the trough of the preceding negative component (usually wave N2) or the baseline (determined from the prestimulus baseline analysis time). Each amplitude analysis approach is characterized by advantages and disadvantages. Calculations of the N2 to P3 amplitude excursion appear to be more stable (Segalowitz & Barnes, 1993). However, the resulting value is not a pure reflection of P300 response activity but, rather, a hybrid measure of both N2 and P3 amplitude. It is not difficult to imagine a scenario in which the P3 peak is actually absent, yet amplitude for the P3 peak (e.g., N2 to baseline) could still be calculated. A comparable analysis dilemma applies to amplitude for the P2 wave of the auditory late response, as discussed in Chapter 12. Laboratory instrumentation and evoked response systems that are commercially available and designed for measurement of cognitive and event related responses often include software for "computer assisted score" or waveform analysis. Thus, waveform analysis is performed with a combination of visual inspection and "machine scoring."

Amplitude of the P300 response is also influenced by factors noted above for P300 latency. In fact, some of the factors, such as the recording electrode site (i.e., scalp distribu-

tion or topography), have more pronounced effects on P300 amplitude than latency. P300 amplitude is generally largest when recorded with electrodes located in frontal/central sites (e.g., Fz or Cz). For example, P300 amplitude is higher with subject anticipation of an impending or probable rare signal presentation (Johnson, 1986). There is long-standing evidence that P300 amplitude is larger when a subject has correctly detected a rare stimulus, as indicated by an overt response, e.g., pressing a button or raising a finger (Ruchkin, Sutton, Kietzman, & Silver, 1980). Likewise, the subject's degree of confidence in the perception of a difference between the frequent and the rare stimulus is associated with larger P300 amplitude (Pritchard, 1981; Squires, Squires, & Hillyard, 1975).

Reliability

Variability is characteristic of all auditory electrophysiological responses, including the P300 response, and a feature of the P300 response that must be defined and understood to exploit the response clinically. Most variability in the P300 response can be attributed or traced to manipulation of measurement conditions (e.g., stimulus intensity, frequency, salience) and intersubject subject factors or traits, such as age, gender, cognitive capacity, state of arousal, clinical status (e.g., dementia, learning disability, auditory processing disorder). Inconsistency and difficulty in analysis of the P300 response—measurement error—also introduces variance in the calculations of amplitude and latency (Dalebout & Robey, 1997; Segalowitz & Barnes, 1993). In addition to these sources of measurement and analysis variance, the P300 response is characterized by an inherent decrement in reliability (increase in variance) that is not secondary to the factors just listed. This intrasubject consistency can be referred to as "the basic reliability of the response itself" (Segalowitz & Barnes, 1993, p. 451) and is thus a fundamental indicator of the extent to which the P300 response can be considered a valid index of cognitive function, such as memory and information processing. The reader is referred to the review paper authored by Segalowitz and Barnes (1993) for a critical summary of the rather modest literature on P300 reliability. As a rule, the P300 has good test–retest reliability, whether the interval between sessions is a few minutes, months, or even years. Correlation coefficients are on the order of 0.5 to 0.8 for amplitude and 0.4 to 0.7 for latency measures (Polich, 1986a,b, 2004; Segalowitz & Barnes, 1993). Kileny and Kripal (1987) reported a high degree of test-retest reliability for the P300 response elicited with tonal signals from young normal-hearing adults. Other authors (Kinoshita, Maeda, Nakamura, Kodama, & Morita, 1995; Polich, 1986; Segalowitz & Barnes, 1993; Sklare & Lynn, 1984) have confirmed the reliability of the P300 response.

Dalebout and Robey (1997) specifically addressed the topic of inter- and intrasubject variability for the P300 response and compared the findings to those for the auditory middle latency response (Pb or P1) and the auditory late response (P1, N1, and P2). The P300 response was recorded in six separate weekly test sessions from eight healthy, normal-hearing, and neurologically normal female college students (age 21 to 24 years). Notably, data were collected at the same time of day for each subject, and both hearing and middle ear status were reassessed prior to P300 measurement. The P300 was elicited with a 1000 Hz tone as the standard stimulus (85% probability) and a 2000 Hz tone (15% probability). The duration of both stimuli was 90 ms, and stimuli were presented at a rate of 1.1/sec. The P300 response was recorded over an analysis time of –50 to 738 ms with a noninverting electrode at the Cz site and earlobe inverting electrodes. The subject was tasked with pressing a button whenever she heard a target stimulus. Three persons performed P300 analysis independently by visual inspection of the waveform.

Dalebout and Robey (1997) compared standard deviations for P300 amplitude and latency for their study (8.24 µV and 20.6 ms) respectively with those from other studies of young adult subjects, including Kileny and Kripal (1987) (5.67 µV and 35.0 ms), Polich (1986a,b) (4.8 µV and 30.0 ms), and Segalowitz and Barnes (1993) (8.6 µV and 24.0 ms). As expected and consistent with previous reports for the P300 response and auditory measurements in general, intersubject variability exceeded intrasubject variability. Regarding other auditory measures, intrasubject variability for the P300 response was greater for the P300 than the ABR, whereas intersubject variability in peak latency and amplitude was equivalent for the two responses. Curiously, Dalebout and Robey (1997) reported greater P300 latency differences within subjects (intrasubject variability) than from one subject to the next (intersubject). The authors noted that variability from one test session to the next for a single subject is expected to fall within +/– 1 standard deviation. Thus, in studies attempting to document the influence of intervention with the P300 response changes in the latency or amplitude beyond this limit could reflect treatment effects and a beneficial outcome.

Alexander et al. (1994) took analysis of P300 reliability one step further by systematically investigating interlaboratory consistency in response amplitude, latency, and scalp distribution. In a multi-site (laboratory) study, P300 data were reported for ninety normal adult subjects from six different laboratories (N = 15 per laboratory) scattered from Connecticut to California. Identical instrumentation and software were used at each site, and the conditions and parameters for the oddball paradigm P300 measurement protocol were consistent among the laboratories. No significant differences were found for P300 response parameters among the laboratories. However, the authors acknowledge that variation in P300 values and waveform morphology within each sample of fifteen subjects (inter- and intrasubject variability) may have contributed to the inability to demonstrate inter-laboratory differences.

NONPATHOLOGIC SUBJECT FACTORS
Age

INFANCY AND CHILDHOOD. | An understanding of developmental P300 characteristics is essential for application of the response in electrophysiological evaluation of children with higher level auditory dysfunction, such as speech and language impairment. Although this application is suggested for the P300 response (Squires & Hecox, 1983), there is relatively less normative data on the P300 response in children than, for example, the ABR. This paucity of data can readily be appreciated if one considers the difficulty of following the typical P300 test paradigm with infants and young children.

A novel stimulus paradigm—the "passive P300 response"—can be used with infants and young children. McIsaac and Polich (1992) applied the passive P300 response measurement paradigm with ten normal infants (five male and five female) ranging in age from 6 to 10 months. Infant P300 data were compared with findings for a control group of ten young normal adults (18 to 22 years). Interestingly, infants were paid for their participation in the study, whereas the adult subjects (students) received course credit. For the benefit of the reader who is interesting in performing P300 recordings with infants, the measurement protocol followed by McIsaac and Polich (1992) will now be reviewed. The P300 test protocol included standard (frequent) tones of 1000 Hz and target (rare) tones of 2000 Hz with 9.9 ms rise/fall times and a plateau of 50 ms presented via a speaker located 1.5 m in from the subject. A block of 10 of these signals was presented, with the target tone occurring randomly at one of the positions between the seventh and the tenth tones. There was then a 4- to 6-second silent interval before the next block of tones was represented, with the target tone occurring in a different position. The authors did not specify signal intensity. Infants sat in their parents' laps and remained awake during the P300 recording. Data collection was performed only when the infant was still. The P300 response was recorded with midline noninverting electrodes (Fz, Cz, and Pz) and linked-earlobe inverting electrodes using band-pass filter settings of 0.01 to 30 Hz over an analysis time of 1100 ms with a 110 ms prestimulus time. Electro-ocular activity was monitored with electrodes as per conventional protocol, and trials with eye blink activity were rejected before signal averaging.

The age period examined with most developmental studies of the conventional attention-dependent P300 (P3b) is school age (6 years) to late adolescence, as depicted in Table 13.4. During this age range, P300 latency decreases and amplitude increases, and morphology improves (Courchesne, 1978b; Goodin, Squires, Henderson, & Starr, 1978a; Pearce, Crowell, Tokioka, & Pacheco, 1989; Polich, Howard, & Starr, 1985; Squires & Hecox, 1983). Martin, Barajas, and Fernandez (1989) also studied P300 response development, utilizing a tone-burst oddball stimulus paradigm, in sixty-eight normal-hearing subjects ranging in age from 6 through

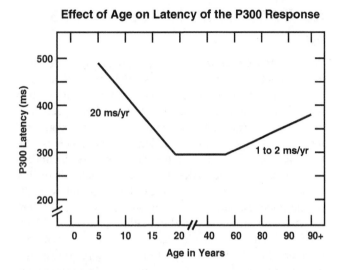

Effect of Age on Latency of the P300 Response

FIGURE 13.4. The effect of development (maturation) and advancing age on latency of the P300 response.

23 years. As illustrated in Figure 13.4, there is a significant negative correlation between development age (up to about 20 years) and P300 latency. The relation between age (up to age 15 years) and latency is defined by an average change in P300 latency as a function of age of approximately –19 ms/year. Pearce et al. (1989) confirmed this age-related trend, reporting P300 latency changes of 20 ms/year over the age range of 5 to 13 years. Maturation of the P300 response, as inferred from latency decreases, is considered electrophysiological evidence of increased efficiency in information processing, that is, the time required to detect or recognize and to categorize the signals (e.g., Pearce et al., 1989).

Kurtzberg and colleagues in a series of publications described the P300 response to speech sounds in awake infants (Kurtzberg, 1989; Kurtzberg, Hilpert, et al., 1986). Stimuli in these studies consisted of stop consonant-vowel (CV) syllables, such as /ta/, /da/, and /ba/, presented in the usual odd-

ball paradigm. A distinct P300 response to speech sounds can be recorded from newborn infants. There are clear changes in response morphology with development. What begins as a negative wave in the preterm infant progressively becomes a positive wave, although morphology may differ as a function of the speech sound stimulus and the developmental course may vary depending on electrode site (midline versus lateral temporal). These P300 data clearly suggest an exciting new avenue for assessing higher level central auditory function in infants and young children. As an example of a practical application of the speech sound P300, Kurtzberg and colleagues have also demonstrated differences in the response with and without amplification (hearing aid use) in hearing-impaired infants.

ADVANCING AGE IN ADULTS. | The effects of aging on the P300 response have been repeatedly reported for over a decade (Ford, Roth, Mohs, Hopkins, & Kopell, 1979; Goodin, Squires, Henderson, & Starr, 1978a,b; Kugler, Taghavy, & Platt, 1993; Pfefferbaum, Ford, Roth, & Kopell, 1980; Pfefferbaum, Ford, Wenegrat, Roth, & Kopell, 1984; Picton, Stapells, Perrault, Baribeau-Braun, & Stuss, 1984; Polich, 1996; Smith, Michalewski, Brent, & Thompson, 1980; Stenklev & Laukli, 2004). The reader is referred a report by Polich (1996) describing a meta-analysis of studies of the effects of aging on the P300 response. Although aging clearly affects P300 latency and amplitude, there is considerable variability among studies in the specific findings for different age groups. Variability in findings among studies result from differences in methodology, including subjects (number, gender, age range, intellectual level, hearing status, general health) and subject tasks (e.g., counting vs. button-pressing response), stimulus parameters, and a host of "moderator variables" (Polich, 2004). Average normal P300 latency over the age range of 10 to 90 years steadily increases from 300 ms to about 450 ms (a change of 1 to 2 ms/year), while amplitude decreases at the average rate of 0.2 μvolt per year (see Figure 13.4). With a narrower subject age range (22 to

TABLE 13.4. Selected Published Findings for the Effect of Age on P300 Latency in Children and Adolescents

Studies are ordered chronologically. Studies with larger changes in latency/year included more subjects under the age of 10 years.

STUDY	NUMBER OF SUBJECTS	AGE RANGE	CHANGE IN LATENCY MS PER YEAR
Finley, Faux, Hutcheson, & Amstutz, 1985	35	5 to 16	3.6
Johnson, 1989	40*	7 to 20	13.8
Enoki, 1990	88	4 to 16	9.4
Polich, Ladish, & Burns, 1990	26	??	7.8
Goodin, Desmedt, Maurer, & Nuwer, 1994	48	??	18.4
Naganuma et al., 1991	53	? to 15	9.8
Zgorzalewicz, Gala-Zgorzalewicz, & Nowak, 2001	80	8 to 18	6.7

* Subjects were all girls.

34 years), Sklare and Lynn (1984) found by linear regression analysis a latency increase of 2.01 ms/year. In addition, there appears to be an interaction between age and scalp topography in P300 measurement.

Polich (1997) investigated the relation between EEG findings and the auditory P300 response in 120 normal adults ranging in age from 20 to over 80 years. In confirming the above-noted expected age-related increase in latency and decreased in amplitude for the P300 response, the author found a positive correlation between spectral power of the delta, theta, alpha, and beta energy bands of the EEG with P300 amplitude. No such correlation was found for EEG spectral power and P300 latency. Polich (1997) comments on the possible connection between the reduction in EEG power and "event-related de-synchronization" (Pfurtscheller, 1992) produced during the cognitive task required for P300 measurement, and the relative independence of P300 latency and EEG frequency.

There is an interaction between aging and scalp topography of the P300 response, with a posterior-to-anterior age-related shift in the region of maximum activation (Anderer, Semlitch & Saletu, 1996; Fjell & Walhovd, 2001; Vesco, Bone, Ryan, & Polich, 1993). However, the neuroanatomic, neurophysiologic, or cognitive explanations for the age-related changes in scalp distribution of the P300 response are unclear. The strongest relationship between age and changes in P300 latency and amplitude values are found for central/parietal electrode sites (Cz and Pz); relationships are relatively weak for the midline Fz site and for lateral electrode locations. That is, less change in latency and amplitude with aging (from 20 to over 90 years) was observed for the Fz site than for the Cz or Pz sites (Fjell & Walhovd, 2001).

The P300 is recorded less reliably with advancing age. Stenklev and Laukli (2004) recorded a reliable P300 response in only 52 percent of 232 subjects age 60 years and older. Notably, prior to P300 measurement the authors documented peripheral auditory status with careful audiologic assessment, including pure-tone and speech audiometry. The P300 was elicited with frequent signals of 1000 Hz and rare signals at 2000 Hz. The authors noted that "stimulus level was adjusted according to the subjects' best pure-tone hearing threshold at 2K Hz," although details were not provided. Subjects were instructed to attend to the rare signals and to press a button when a rare signal was detected. The response components (N2, P300, and N3) were identified with visual inspection of the waveform by an author who did not collect the data. The P300 component was defined as the largest positive peak within the time frame of 250 to 450 ms after the signal presentation. Latency of the P300 response increased from, on the average, 318 ms in the young (control) group to 365 to 366 ms in the 90-year and over 90-year group. In contrast to these age-related changes in P300 latency, the authors found no significant differences in P300 amplitude with age. The likelihood of the presence of a P300 response decreased systematically from the control

group (subjects aged 19 to 26 years) to older subjects aged 60 to over 90 years, a finding predicted statistically by hearing threshold at 2000 Hz and word recognition scores. Stenklev and Laukli (2004) suggest that age-related changes in hearing sensitivity were a factor in the decreased occurrence of the P300 response with age. This point should be emphasized for all investigations of auditory evoked responses that include older subjects. Peripheral auditory status should always be carefully documented with formal assessment techniques, at least pure-tone audiometry, in an appropriate test setting (e.g., sound-treated room).

Young adults have a pronounced parietal distribution, whereas P300 becomes distributed from the parietal region (Pz) to frontal region (Fz) as a function of advancing age (Pfefferbaum et al., 1980, 1984). In a related study, Harbin, Marsh, and Harvey (1984) evaluated the effect of age on a late ERPs elicited by semantic versus nonsemantic tasks. ERPs were generated by the last word in a string of five words that was either in the same semantic category as the other words or a different category. Young subjects showed a larger potential for matched words (versus mismatched), and older subjects showed the opposite pattern.

Gender

In contrast to age, gender does not appear to be an important factor in P300 measurement. In a comprehensive study of normal variation of P300 using a conventional two-tone standard versus target stimulus paradigm, Polich (1986a) found no significant effect between fifty males versus fifty females in latency or amplitude of the P3 wave. There are, however, some reports of greater amplitude of the P3 wave and shorter latency for females than males over the age of 15 years (Deldin, Duncan, & Miller, 1994; Geisler & Polich, 1990; Martin, Barajas, Fernandes, & Torres, 1988; Morita et al., 2001), but other investigators failed to confirm gender differences in P3 wave latency or amplitude values (Polich, 1986a; Sangal & Sangal, 1996; Stenklev & Laukli, 2004). The lack of a clear gender influence on the P300 response is curious given evidence from MRI studies of a gender difference in the area of the corpus callosum. Larger area for the corpus callosum in left versus right-handed subjects has been invoked in the explanations for a handedness effect in P300 amplitude measures (Polich & Hoffman, 1998).

Handedness

Given the contributions of different regions of the cerebral hemispheres to the P300 response, and the sensitivity of the P300 response as a measure of information processing, it is reasonable to question whether the response differs for right-versus left-handed subjects. Alexander and Polich (1997) investigated the influence of handedness in a group of twenty right-handed and twenty left-handed normal young (average age 22.6 years) male subjects. Handedness was verified with a formal questionnaire about hand preference on six different tasks and family history. The protocol used to record the P300 response in this study was similar to the measurement approach reported by Dr. John Polich in dozens of other papers. The P300 was elicited with standard (frequent) signals of 600 Hz and target (rare) signals (probability of 0.125) of 1600 Hz with rise/fall times of 10 ms and plateaus of 60 ms binaurally presented at an intensity level of 60 dB SPL. Recordings were made from multiple scalp electrode locations, with band-pass filters of 0.02 to 50 Hz and an analysis time of 1500 ms (prestimulus time of 187 ms). P300 amplitude was larger for left-handed subjects at anterior electrode sites. (e.g., Fz, F⅞, F¾) and larger for right-handed subjects at posterior electrode sites. P300 latency was shorter for left- versus right-handed subjects. The authors review a variety of possible explanations for the handedness effect, including anatomical differences, such as in brain morphology, size of the corpus callosum, skull thickness, and also cognitive differences (e.g., short-term memory and attention). In a follow-up investigation one year later, Polich and Hoffman (1998) confirmed that the same handedness effects apply to male and female subjects. Also, as noted above, the authors noted a gender difference in the P300 response, i.e., smaller amplitudes for males versus females. Electrode topography also was a factor in the handedness effect. For example, P300 amplitude was larger for left-handed subjects when recorded from central and medial electrodes, while there was no clear difference for left- versus right-handed subjects for the P300 recorded with lateral electrode sites. As Polich and Hoffman (1998) point out, investigations of hemispheric asymmetry in the P300 response should account for other subject variables that may also involve differences between electrophysiological measures from the right and left hemisphere. MRI investigations (e.g., Dennenberg, Kertesz, & Cowell, 1991) confirm that differences between right- and left-handed persons in other neuroanatomic structures, (e.g., the corpus callosum) may also be related to handedness. Corpus callosum areas are larger for left- than right-handed persons (Witelson, 1992).

Attention

With the conventional P300 oddball stimulus paradigm, the subject must listen to the target stimulus and must respond behaviorally to targets either covertly (by silently counting the stimuli) or overtly (by pressing a button or raising a finger). Although normal subjects follow instructions to silently count target stimuli without difficulty, this approach does not assure adequate subject attention in patient populations characterized by cognitive dysfunction. Such patients may be confused by instructions and may require simpler and repeated instructions to maintain an acceptable rate of missed target stimulus presentations (less than 5%). In any event, subject task performance should be monitored closely to verify that the P300 response results from the intended cognitive status. To enhance attention and alertness to target stimuli during P300 measurement, the sub-

ject typically should sit upright or recline in a comfortable chair.

McPherson and Salamat (2004) examined the relation between the auditory P300 response and performance on an auditory continuous performance test, or CPT. An auditory continuous performance test quantifies vigilance or sustained attention during an auditory task. There are analogous versions of the test procedure for visual tasks. In fact, the relation between visual P300 findings and visual CPT performance was the topic of a number of published studies (see McPherson & Salamat, 2003 for review). In the study reported by McPherson and Salamat (2004), subjects were normal-hearing, right-handed, young adults. Subjects with possible attention deficit disorder or other neuropsychiatric disorders were excluded from investigation. The P300 was elicited with binaural tone bursts of 250 Hz (rare) and 1000, 1500, and 2000 Hz (frequent) presented with random interstimulus intervals (ISIs) of 1, 2, or 4 seconds. The authors recorded behavioral (button pushing) reaction times for the presentations of frequent (common) signals. Subjects were instructed to not press the button when they heard the rare (75% probability) signals. McPherson and Salamat (2004) found a direct relation between ISI and both behavioral reaction time and P300 latency. That is, longer ISIs were associated with longer reaction times and P300 latency values. The latter finding is further evidence that P300 latency is a reflection of information processing time. Also, amplitude of the P300 response decreased as ISIs increased.

The P300 response is affected by "dual task" paradigms. Singhal, Doerfling, and Fowler (2002) found that subject performance of a visual task during auditory P300 measurement involving a dichotic listening task was associated with decreased amplitude of the P300 response. In the study reported by Singhal et al. (2002) the auditory P300 response was recorded in combination with a visual task that put a considerable attention workload on the subject, namely, performing a simulated instrument flying task with difficulty manipulated by two levels of turbulence. As difficulty of the visual task increased, and attention allocated more to the visual modality, amplitude of the auditory P300 response decreased.

The nature of the subject's behavioral response during P300 measurement exerts an important effect on the neurophysiologic response. Polich (1987) demonstrated that P300 latency was longer and amplitude larger when the subject silently counted the target signals versus when the subject pressed a button with a thumb or tapped an index finger when detecting a target signal. The author speculated that different methods for subject indication of the occurrence of a target signal might be associated with varying amounts of processing and attention demands.

State of Arousal

A thorough review of the relationship of state of arousal and P300 would in essence be a treatise on the response itself.

Attention to stimulation is the fundamental measurement condition distinguishing P300 from the traditional ALR. In addition to the well-known oddball paradigm, a listening condition that is almost synonymous with the P300 response, P300 findings for both ignore and passive subject conditions and a go/no-go signal paradigm have been described. In general, P300 amplitudes are larger and latencies shorter with conscious and focused attention to the rare (infrequent) signal. The P300 response in the passive condition, actually labeled the P3a wave, typically has smaller amplitudes and even shorter latencies than those for the P300 response in the oddball stimulus paradigm (Pfefferbaum, Ford, Weller, & Kopell, 1985). These P300 trends, however, are not consistently confirmed in published studies (e.g., Iwanami, Kamijima, & Yoshizawa, 1996). Readers are referred to review articles on the general topic of attention, arousal, and the P300 response. The attention factor is, furthermore, virtually inseparable from stimulus factors. Unlike coverage of other AERs, the discussion here will not be limited to effects of sleep and general state of arousal but, rather, will encompass also the influence on the P300 response of selective attention to a certain stimulus. Selective attention "is an important brain function that allows a person to process some types of stimulus events in preference to others" (Hillyard, 1984, p. 52). The multiple stimulus parameters that influence P300, along with other AERs, such as rate, interstimulus interval (and habituation), frequency (in Hz), frequency of occurrence, intensity, task difficulty, are also reviewed in this chapter. A sizable number of well-known neurophysiologists have for over twenty years intensively investigated myriad aspects of endogenous ERPs. Due to space constraints, the vast literature—thousands of articles and several textbooks—cannot be thoroughly reviewed here.

A characteristic feature of the P300, and other "endogenous, cognitive, or event-related" responses, is selective attention to one stimulus versus another. Higher level (CNS) processing implies active participation in the testing, although as illustrated in the beginning of the chapter by P300 waveforms in Figures 13.1 and 13.2, this is not necessarily a requirement for detection of endogenous responses. As the Polich (1989) findings indicate, it is possible to record a reliable P300 from subjects who are not adhering to the conventional "selective attention" test paradigm. And, it's long been recognized that a response can be generated when an expected stimulus is, in fact, absent or a "missing stimulus" (Ruchkin & Sutton, 1978a; Sutton et al., 1967). By far, the most common P300 test strategy includes the presentation of infrequent (rare or deviant) stimuli within a background of predictable and frequent (recurrent) stimuli, the so-called oddball paradigm or procedure. Attention to the rare stimuli may produce a variety of alterations in the evoked response waveform, including both negative and positive voltage components. The P300 was among the first of these evoked responses to be recognized (Sutton et al., 1965), although there are additional attention-related positive voltage peaks

in the waveform in the 165 ms region (e.g., Goodin et al., 1978b). Other endogenous or attention-related responses include a prolonged negativity beginning about 50 ms and lasting beyond 200 ms (Hansen & Hillyard, 1980; Näätänen & Michie, 1979; Okita, 1979), the contingent negative variation (CNV).

Passive P300 Paradigm

Clearly, as reinforced by much of the discussion in this chapter, attention is an important factor influencing the P300 response. Although active attention is not required for generation of the P300 response, conscious detection and discrimination of the target (rare) signal is necessary. As noted earlier in the chapter, there are two general types of P300 response based on the role of attention. The P3a auditory evoked response, recorded with a passive test paradigm and occurring with a latency of about 250 ms, is "automatic" and not dependent on active subject attention (e.g., McIsaac & Polich, 1992; O'Donnell, Friedman, Squires, Maloon, Drachman, & Swearer, 1990; Polich, 1987, 1989; Polich & McIsaac, 1994; Squires et al., 1986). Rather, it appears to be a reflection of automatic detection of a different signal, e.g., signal novelty. Test parameters—stimulus and acquisition—are generally equivalent for measurement of the passive versus active P300 response. The passive P3a response can be recorded with different variations of the oddball paradigm, including the conventional two-stimulus (standard and target) format, a single (novel) stimulus, or a three-stimulus (standard, target, and distractor) paradigm. There is usually one common feature in measurement of the P3a versus P300 (P3b) response. Highly unusual and alerting stimuli, such as dog barks or the subject's name, are employed to elicit the "novelty P3a" response (Courchesne, Kilman, Galambos, & Lincoln, 1984; Knight, 1984; Polich, 2004). Subject instructions and the subject task are, however, different. The attention and response to target stimuli required for the conventional oddball task are lacking for measurement of the passive P300 response. The subject may be instructed to listen to all the sounds without making a voluntary motor (e.g., finger raising or button pressing) response or, especially for young children, simply encouraged to watch a silent video (e.g., cartoon or movie) and to ignore all of the sounds.

There are differences in the P300 recorded with the passive paradigm versus conventional attention paradigm. For example, amplitude for a P300 response recorded with the passive paradigm is distinctly smaller, and latency shorter versus conventional oddball measurement paradigms. Also, the passive paradigm produces a P3 component with a more fronto-central scalp distribution. As with the conventional P300 oddball paradigm, habituation is evident for the passive P300 response, although not initially with stimulation. That is, habituation for the passive P300 response (P3a) is not rapid. Under some electrode conditions (e.g., frontal recording location), the passive response may decrease in amplitude with fewer repetitions than the usual oddball para-digm requiring an attention task (e.g., Polich & McIsaac, 1994). In contrast to the passive P300 response, the tradi-tional P300 response, often referred to as the P3b component, is dependent on relatively slow and conscious information processing, and not immediate and automatic processing. Some authors have also described a component recorded at a latency of about 350 ms, even beyond the P3b latency re-gion, that does not depend on active attention to the signal. Recorded best at more frontal electrode locations, and with highly unexpected signals (e.g., dog barking), it is referred to as the "novel P3" response.

Sleep

It's quite amazing that we know so little about an activity that consumes roughly one-third of our time throughout most of our life. To eliminate any misinterpretation of this statement for readers who might be confused, I'm referring to sleep and not your job. There are really two distinct per-spectives on the topic of sleep and the P300 response. Clini-cians applying the P300 response for electrophysiological assessment of high-level central auditory function in various patient populations must appreciate the influence of sleep on the response. Information on the effects of different stages of sleep on the P300 is essential for meaningful analysis and interpretation of clinical findings. Most of the follow-ing discussion is oriented toward this clinical perspective, with citation of studies designed and conducted by auditory electrophysiologists to define the effect of sleep on the P300 response. Another body of literature, however, is concerned with application of the P300 response as a tool to better un-derstand the basic mechanisms or nature of sleep. For cur-rent and detailed information on the relation between sleep and the P300 response, the reader is referred to review ar-ticles by researchers in several sleep laboratories, including Dr. Helene Bastuji and her colleagues in Lyons France (Bas-tuji, Perrin, & García-Larrea, 2002) and by Kimberly Cote of St. Catharine's Canada (Cote, 2002). That is, sleep scientists "probe awareness during sleep with the auditory odd-ball paradigm" (Cote, 2002, p. 227) to answer questions about such fundamental issues as consciousness, awareness of external events, cognition, and information processing dur-ing sleep. To quote Dr. Cote again, "the P300 is especially critical to defining consciousness within sleep, a period in which behavioral responses are rare" (Cote, 2002, p. 236). Literature on the nature of sleep and, particularly, the status of awareness, consciousness, and memory during sleep, is fascinating. The review articles cited above and, especially, an article entitled "Forensic Sleep Medicine and Nocturnal Wandering," published in the journal *Sleep,* are offered as examples of the interesting research on sleep.

Variable P300 findings characterize different stages of sleep, and some authors have suggested that the P300 cannot be reliably recorded during sleep (e.g., Campbell, Bell, &

Bastien, 1992). The reader may wish to refer back to Table 11.4 in Chapter 11 for a summary of the stages of sleep. There is ample evidence that the P300 response can be re-corded during sleep. The P300 recorded in stage 1 and REM sleep with posterior electrode locations is similar than the response recorded in the awakened state, particularly when evoked by salient signals. Sleep stage is a critical factor in P300 findings. For example, with the oddball paradigm, the P300 response is not apparent during sleep stage 2. Scalp topography in P300 recordings is also an important factor interacting with sleep, as the P300 recorded with frontal electrode sites is absent during these sleep stages. There is also marked variability in the effect of sleep among individu-als (Cote, 2002). Amplitude of the P300 response decreases, and amplitude increases, during the transition from an alert, awake state to drowsiness and then sleep stage 1 (Koshino et al., 1993). A P300 response can be detected in sleep stages 2, 3, and 4, although relative amplitude and latency values for the frequent versus rare signals change in comparison to wakefulness. In REM sleep, the P300 response may be essentially unchanged from the awake state (Bastuji, Gar-cía-Larrea, Franc, & Mauguiere, 1995). The P3a response can consistently be recorded in sleep (Atienza, Cantero, & Escera, 2001).

Sleep deprivation is associated with alteration of the P300 response (Danos et al., 1994), including increases in la-tency and reduced amplitude. However, related factors (e.g., body temperature and fatigue) influence recordings and, in-deed, a variety of subject and everyday factors, such as age, fatigue, time of day, and even food, may interact with sleep in affecting the P300 response (Geisler & Polich, 1992).

Task Difficulty

There is considerable evidence that P300 latency becomes longer and amplitude smaller as the difficulty of the listening task increases (e.g., Ford, Roth, & Kopell, 1976; Katayama & Polich, 1998; Polich, 1986b). That is, when the standard and target signals are similar, reaction time and P300 latency are prolonged and the response is less robust. Conversely, highly novel target (deviant) signals produce large responses with short latency, consistent with shorter evaluation time required to determine that the target signal was different than the standard signal (Hillyard & Kutas, 1983; Ritter, Simp-son, Vaughan, & Macht, 1982).

Other Factors

The effects of other factors on P300 measurement have been investigated, among them memory, circadian rhythms, sea-sonal effects, time within a menstrual cycle, exercise, and fatigue.

MEMORY. | There is a relation between P300 response char-acteristics and the subject's *memory* of the signal (Howard & Polich, 1985). The P300 response appears to reflect the "contextual updating" of working memory (Donchin & Coles, 1988). That is, the frequent signal produces are relatively well formed, but representation in the brain of the infrequent rare signal requires memory updating. Medications that affect memory (e.g., anticholinergics) also have a negative effect on the P300 response (Potter, Pickles, Roberts, & Rugg, 1992). However, memory of the signal is not essential for eliciting a P300 response, as a subject can generate the response during REM sleep and later, when awake, not recollect the signal (Bastuji, Perrin, & García-Larrea, 2002).

MOTIVATION. | Given the dependence of the P300 response on cognitive function and information processing, it's not surprising that a direct relation exists between subject motivation and response amplitude. The positive influence of subject motivation, and feedback to the subject regarding performance, on P300 outcome is occasionally cited in studies involving older persons (Verlegere, Kompf, & Nukater, 1992) and clinical populations, such as patients with depression (e.g., Diner, Holcomb, & Dykman, 1985) and schizophrenia (e.g., Louza, Maurer, & Neuhauser, 1992). In addition, subject incentive clearly influences P300 amplitude, but not latency. There is long-standing appreciation that P300 amplitude increases when the a monetary value is attached to correct identification of the target stimuli, and more reward produces larger amplitudes (Begleiter, Porjesz, Chou, & Aunon, 1983; Hombeg, Grünewald, & Grünewald-Zuberbier, 1981; Johnson, 1986). Carrillo-de-la-Peña and Cadaveira (2000) conducted a formal study of the effect of motivation on the P300 response. The P300 response was elicited from twenty healthy university students eight male and twelve female) with 1000 Hz standard signals and 1100 Hz target signals following either neutral instructions or motivational instructions. The neutral instructions were "Now you will hear two types of tone; some of them are high-pitched ('bip') while the others, which are more frequent, are low-pitched ('bop'). Whenever you hear a 'bip' you must press the button as fast as possible. Please try to avoid unnecessary movements or blinking during the test" (p. 234). The other set of instructions were "Now you have to accomplish the same task as before, but this time it is particularly important that you do well. We are recording your performance on the computer, and your data will be compared with the classroom standards. Remember that it is important to avoid unnecessary movement or blinking during the test" (p. 234). The P300 response was recorded with midline electrodes (Fz, Cz, and Pz). P300 response amplitudes for target signals were larger during run two (motivational instructions), whereas latency was not affected. Interestingly, P2 amplitude for standard signals was also increased as a function of subject instructions. Latency of the N2 component was shorter with the motivational instructions than the neutral instructions. The authors conclude that instructions to motivate the subject to perform the task correctly, and the subject's subsequent increased involvement in the task en-

hanced efficiency of the signal evaluation process and decision making in detecting relevant signals.

EXERCISE. | With the assumption that cognitive function could be enhanced by regular physical exercise (Dustman, Emmerson, & Shearer, 1994; Spirduso, 1980) and previous reports of EEG changes as a function of physically fitness Polich and Lardon (1997) examined the P300 response in two groups of young adults (30 to 40 years) differentiated only by the amount of time they devoted to vigorous aerobic physical exercise. Time spent in exercise was, on the average, 3.1 hours per week for the low-exercise subjects and 18.6 hours per week for the high-exercise group. Although there was considerable intersubject variability, findings confirmed a direct relation between exercise and amplitude of auditory and visual evoked P300 responses, but not for P300 latency. As an aside, exercise did not affect other components (e.g., N1, P2, and N2 waves) in the late latency region.

PREGNANCY. | Tandon, Bhatia, and Goel (1996) reported longer P300 latencies (average of 356 ms) and smaller amplitudes (average of 7.2 μV) for the P300 response in a group of eighteen pregnant women than a control group of twelve nonpregnant women (average latency of 302 ms and amplitude of 14.8 μV). The authors speculate on neuroendocrine explanations for the effect of pregnancy, including the influence of changes in estrogen and progesterone on the generators of the P300 response and an inhibitory effect of pregnancy on cognitive processing.

FACIAL AFFECT RECOGNITION. | In follow-up to other studies of the influence of emotion on the P300 response (e.g., Johnston, Miller, & Burleson, 1986; Lang, Nelson, & Collins, 1990; Yee & Miller, 1987), Morita and colleagues (2001) recorded the response with the conventional oddball paradigm from thirteen men and thirteen women with and without the presentation of faces showing various emotion conditions (sadness, pleasure, anger, and no emotion). Stimuli were 1000 Hz standard tones and 2000 Hz target tones, and the P300 response was detected with electrodes located at midline (Fz, Cz, Pz, Oz) and lateral (C3 and C4) sites. Consistent with previous findings (e.g., Yee & Miller, 1987), peak P300 amplitude was smallest when stimuli were coupled with a facing showing pleasure and then progressively larger with faces showing anger, sadness, and no emotion. Interestingly, Morita et al. (2001) reported that gender was a clear factor affecting the influence of sadness or anger emotions on the P300 response. These authors described a distinct gender difference for the conventional oddball stimulus paradigm (no facial emotion), with larger P300 amplitude and greater area for females versus males.

Central Nervous System Drugs

There are a large number of drugs that affect CNS activity and, therefore, may influence cortical AERs. During sedation with chloral hydrate, as with natural sleep, variability is increased for auditory evoked responses within the latency region of the P300 component (Hosick & Mendel, 1975; Skinner & Shimota, 1975). Measurement of the P300 response under sedation is ill-advised, as validity of findings may be compromised. Phenobarbital and secobarbital are also sometimes used as CNS depressants and, therefore, as sedatives for AER measurement. Phenobarbital is a long-acting barbiturate that depresses the CNS. The typical dose for sedation of children is 2 mg/kg/day (by mouth) in four divided doses. Phenobarbital is also used as an anticonvulsant, that is, in medical management of epilepsy in children. It should not be confused with pentobarbital, a barbiturate agent sometimes applied in management of severely brain-injured patients. Secobarbital is a short-acting barbiturate. Pediatric dosage is the same as for phenobarbital. Mendel, Hosick, Windman, Davis, Hirsh, and Dinges (1975) reported that secobarbital-induced sleep was associated with increased variability in cortical auditory evoked responses and, in turn, less accurate auditory threshold estimations. P300 latencies are increased in children receiving phenobarbital in management of epilepsy (Chen, Chow, & Lee, 2001). Meperidine is an IV opioid analgesic, like morphine, that has no apparent effect on early or late latency AERs (Pfefferbaum, Roth, Tinklenberg, Rosenbloom, & Kopell, 1979).

Other Drugs

ACUTE ALCOHOL INGESTION. | There is an extensive literature on the relationship between alcohol and cortical auditory evoked responses. Studies conducted up through 1980 are thoroughly reviewed in a paper by Porjesz and Begleiter (1981). Three overall alcohol-related issues—acute ingestion, chronic abuse, and withdrawal—have been studied. Acute ingestion of alcohol, without hypothermia, affects the P300 responses. It is important to recall that intoxication with alcohol can be accompanied by lowered body temperature and that a temperature effect must be ruled out in study of alcohol effects on AERs. P300 latency is only slightly increased following alcohol ingestion (Pfefferbaum et al., 1980). In general, primary sensory regions are more resistant to the effects of alcohol and association areas are quite susceptible, based on visual and somatosensory evoked response data. The relationship between blood alcohol level (BAL) and AER alteration is not well defined. Murata and colleagues (1992) investigated the effect of acute alcohol (200 ml of Japanese spirits) ingestion on the ALR N1 and P2 waves and the P300 response. As noted in Chapter 12, subjects were thirteen healthy male medical students who reportedly "consented readily to become volunteers for this study" (Murata et al., 1992, p. 958). P300 measurement was also made at the same time in the late afternoon or evening for subjects. Latency of the P300 component was significantly prolonged when recorded 2 hours after alcohol ingestion.

Miscellaneous Drugs and Substances

In a study of thirty-five healthy subjects (males and females), Dimpfel, Todorova, and Vonderheid-Guth (1999) reported a "tendency toward latency reduction in comparison with placebo values" for the P300 response in single blind clinical trials of repeated administration of commercially available extracts of St. John's wort. The authors interpreted the finding as electrophysiologic evidence of improved (faster) mental performance. However, statistical confirmation of a treatment effect of St. John's wort on P300 latency was not provided, and average latency values on day 1 and day 22 presented in tabular form in the article did not document the trend. For example, with a Cz noninverting electrode recording array, the average P300 latency value for the placebo subject group was 263 ms on day 1 and 256 ms on day 22, whereas the values for one brand of St. John's wort extracts was 281 ms on day 1 and 291 ms on day 22, and the latencies for the other brand of extract on the two days were, respectively, 270 ms and 250 ms.

CLINICAL APPLICATIONS

Some generalizations can be made from literature on clinical applications of the P300 response (summarized in Table 13.5). Investigations in normal subjects show clearly that P300 latency is directly related to the speed with which a subject classifies signals, updates memory, and allocates attention. Patient populations with progressive deficits in cognitive function characteristically show increases in P300 latency (e.g., Goodin et al., 1978b; Hömberg et al., 1986; O'Donnell et al., 1990; Polich et al., 1986; Polich & Herbst, 2000). Not unexpectedly, the sensitivity of the P300 response to cognitive decline and dysfunction (i.e., decrements in information processing, short-term memory, attention allocation) associated with various neurological and psychiatric diseases and disorders is accompanied by a general lack of specificity. That is, similar patterns of P300 abnormalities are found in diverse patient populations. The P300 response is useful in differentiating a group of patients with a common disorder, e.g., schizophrenia, from normal control subjects, but not typically from patients with another disorder, e.g., dementia. Furthermore, even within a relatively well-defined diagnostic entity, such as schizophrenia, there are inconsistencies in P300 findings among studies as a result of differences in, and interactions among, a variety of pathologic and nonpathologic subject factors (e.g., severity of disease, age, gender, intellectual status, and educational level) and test variables (e.g., stimulus parameters, subject task, and instructions). Nonetheless, changes in cognitive status (decline and improvement) for most neurological and psychiatric diseases can be tracked with the P300 response, and the P300 response has value in documenting the therapeutic effectiveness of medical management of selected central nervous system diseases.

TABLE 13.5. Selected Clinical Applications of the Auditory P300 Response
with Representative Published Papers

CLINICAL ENTITY	STUDY(S)	COMMENT
Attention-deficit/ hyperactivity disorder (ADHD)	Lazzaro et al., 1997	No difference in P300 latency or amplitude in 17 unmedicated children with ADHD vs. a control group.
	Rothenberger et al., 2000	P3b amplitude was equivalent for a group of 11 children with ADHD and a control group.
Alcoholism (risk)	Polich, Pollock, & Bloom, 1994	Meta-analysis of P300 response in males at risk for alcoholism. Males with family histories of alcoholism have smaller P3 amplitudes than control subjects.
Alzheimer's disease (AD)	Frodl et al., 2002	Abnormal P300 latency and amplitude values in 30 patients with AD vs. control group.
	Polich et al., 1990	
Amnesia	Polich & Squire, 1993	No P3 differences for 5 amnesic patients vs. control group.
At-risk infants	Fellman et al., 2004	The P300 response (a positive peak in the 350 ms region) was similar in preterm infants and newborn control subjects. The peak was, however, smaller in the preterm infants than infants of a comparable postnatal chronological age (3 months old).
Auditory processing disorder	Jirsa & Clontz, 1990	Delayed latency in APD.
Autism	Bomba & Pang, 2004	Review of the literature on cortical auditory evoked responses in autism (including the P300 response).
Brain injury	Kotchoubey et al., 2001	Abnormalities in the P300 response to speech and tone signals were reported for 33 patients with severe diffuse brain injury (traumatic and nontraumatic), but the authors did not report data for a control group.
Cardiac surgery	Grimm et al., 2001	Prolonged P300 latencies were associated with neurocognitive damage secondary to mechanical replacement of the mitral valve and coronary bypass surgery.
Cerebrovascular disease	Korpelainen et al., 2000	The P300 response was absent at three months following minor ischemic stroke, and present but delayed in latency during post-stroke depression (at twelve months).
Chronic fatigue syndrome (CFS)	Polich, Moore, & Wiederhold, 1995	No differences were found for P300 latency or amplitude for 25 patients with CFS vs. a control group.
Corpus callosum section	Kaga et al., 1990	The P300 response elicited by speech stimuli from an adult patient was affected by section of the posterior half of the truncus of the corpus callosum.
Depression (geriatric)	Kalayam et al., 1998	Longer P300 latencies were reported in 43 elderly patients with unipolar depression vs. a control group.
	Bruder et al., 1995	
Dyslexia	Duncan et al., 1994	
Epilepsy	Verlegere et al., 1997	Increased P300 latencies yet normal amplitudes in patients diagnosed with epilepsy.
Head injury: mild	Potter et al., 2001	No difference in the P3a component for 24 subjects with mild head injury versus a control group.
	Werner & Vanderzandt, 1991	No evidence of P300 abnormalities in mild head injury.
	Haglund & Persson, 1990	P300 latency increased in boxers who were "knocked out," with no change in P300 amplitude.

(continued)

TABLE 13.5. (continued)

CLINICAL ENTITY	STUDY(S)	COMMENT
Head injury: severe	Campbell, Suffield, & Deacon, 1990	Review.
Hypoxia	Fowler & Lindeis, 1992	Hypoxia produces an increase in P300 latency and a decrease in P300 amplitude.
Lead exposure	Solliway et al., 1995	Chronic exposure to lead is associated with increased P300 latency and decreased amplitude.
Marijuana users	Patrick et al., 1995	No difference in P300 latency and amplitude for 32 marihuana users vs. control group.
Migraine headache	Wang & Schoenen, 1998	Habituation of the P300 response is deficient in 24 persons with migraine.
	Ambrosini et al., 2001	Review of electrophysiological studies in migraine, including P300 response confirming reduced habituation.
Narcolepsy	Aguirre & Broughton, 1987	
Parkinson's disease	Iijima et al., 2000	P300 latency was delayed in 30 percent of 20 patients with PD vs. a control group.
	Maeshima et al., 2002	P300 response latency was correlated with *Mini Mental State* findings in predicting daily living problems for 30 patients with Parkinson's disease.
	O'Donnell et al., 1987	
PCBs (poly-chlorinated biphenyls)	Chen & Hsu, 1994	Prolonged P300 latency was found in patients exposed to PCBs.
Premature ejaculation (PE)	Ozcan et al., 2001	Auditory P300 latency was significantly longer in 20 patients with PE vs. control group, whereas there was no difference in amplitude.
Schizophrenia	Ford, 1999	A concise review paper concluding that the "P300 is both a state and trait marker of the disease."
	Jeon & Polich, 2001	Meta-analysis of 50 independent data sets.

Prior to reviewing literature on the clinical application of auditory evoked responses, particularly cortical and event-related evoked responses, the reader is encouraged to consult "Guidelines for Using Human Event-Related Potentials to Study Cognition: Recording Standards and Publication Criteria" (Picton et al., 2000). This paper and/or other publications on appropriate methodology for cortical evoked response measurement, analysis, and interpretation are really essential reading for those planning clinical investigations with the P300, MMN, or other event-related responses. Selected information from the detailed guidelines reported by Picton et al. (2000) was summarized in Table 13.2. The information will assist the reader in critically evaluating the quality and clinical value of published investigations of the P300 response. As noted elsewhere in the book, some of the guidelines offered in this paper are relevant to measurement and analysis of other auditory evoked responses and really of direct value to those professionals—clinical practitioners or clinical scientists—who measure auditory evoked responses with patients or human subjects.

The following discussion of the clinical P300 response investigation is merely an introduction to a voluminous literature on the topic. For more comprehensive information on the topic, the reader is referred to review articles or textbooks, as noted in Table 13.5. A computer-assisted literature search (e.g., PubMed or Medline search via the National Library of Medicine website [www.nlm.nih.gov]) will instantly reveal a plethora of articles describing clinical investigations of the P300 response. Many hundreds of published papers describe P300 response findings in diverse clinical populations, with early reports appearing during the same years as initial clinical investigations of the ABR. Since the late 1970s, the clinical value of P300 has been with a variety of disease entities and patient populations, such as schizophrenia, dementia (including Alzheimer's disease), Huntington's disease, Parkinson's disease, multiple sclerosis, depression, and chronic alcoholism. A thorough review of the literature on the P300 in documenting neurophysiologic and cognitive dysfunction in neurological and psychiatric disorders is far beyond the scope of this book. What follows is a summary of selected psychophysiologic research trends and published clinical findings. The relative brevity of the following discussion is consistent with the theme articulated initially in the Preface to the Book, namely, that the space devoted to information on auditory evoked responses will parallel the extent of their clinical application. Even though there are many articles describing the P300 response in different patient populations, the response is not routinely applied clinically by any discipline of health care provider, e.g., audiologists, psychologists, or medical specialists (neurologists, psychiatrists).

Alcoholism

Genetic factors in the risk for alcoholism are well known, as is the difference in the effects of alcohol ingestion on performance measures, such as motor abilities and the perception of intoxication (e.g., Schuckit, 1980). These observations have led to research on possible "biologic markers" for alcoholism. Investigations of the P300 response amplitude and latency in groups of subjects with a positive family history of alcoholism versus a negative family history have yielded conflicting findings (e.g., Begleiter, Porjesz, Bihari, & Kissin, 1984; Polich & Bloom, 1987). Schuckit, Gold, Croot, Finn, and Polich (1988) reported equivalent P300 latency findings for sons of alcoholic fathers and control subjects (sons) of nonalcoholic fathers before acute alcohol ingestion (baseline measures) and after low dose (0.75 ml/kg) and high dose (1.1 ml/kg) ethanol ingestion (challenge). P300 latency was increased for both groups with the ingestion of alcohol. However, P300 latency returned to baseline values faster for the group with a positive family history of alcoholism than for the control (no family history) group, an outcome consistent with previous reports for behavioral and motor response parameters. In a meta-analysis of data for thirty published studies reporting data on P300 amplitude in males at risk for alcoholism and subjects with no family history of alcoholism, Polich, Pollock, and Bloom (1994) confirmed that "individuals with a positive family history of alcoholism generally demonstrated smaller P3 amplitudes than individuals without a family history of alcoholism" (pp. 64, 65). P300 latency was not evaluated. Factors such as subject age, task difficulty, and stimulus parameters affected findings among studies. The meta-analysis was limited to men because too few P300 data exist for women with a positive family history for alcoholism.

Chronic alcohol abuse, according to animal and clinical research, is associated with significantly prolonged ABR latency values (Begleiter, Porjesz, & Chou, 1981; Chu et al., 1978; Squires et al., 1978). Amplitude of the N1-P2 complex is decreased by acute alcohol consumption (Krough, Khan, & Fosuig, 1977). Investigation of P300 changes with chronic alcohol abuse is difficult because during abstinence

patients may be relying on psychotropic medications. The medications may therefore also influence AERs. Studies of event-related potentials in abstinent and medication-free chronic alcoholics (N1 and P300 ERP) suggests that patterns of abnormalities are similar to those found during acute alcohol ingestion (Porjesz & Begleiter, 1981). This is taken as evidence of subcortical (hippocampus) deficits in chronic alcoholism. During alcohol withdrawal, ABR latency values (for later waves) may be unusually decreased, a possible reflection of CNS hyperexcitability (Chu et al., 1978). Shortened latencies and increased amplitudes for AERs during withdrawal tend to be more pronounced with longer alcohol exposure (Pfefferbaum, Horvath, Roth, & Kopell, 1979).

Alzheimer's Dementia

For over twenty years, evidence has accumulated that the P300 response, with the appropriate measurement approach, can differentiate patients with Alzheimer's disease from age-matched normal control subjects (Brown, Marsh, & Larue, 1982; Holt et al., 1995; Polich & Herbst, 2000). The characteristic pattern of findings is prolonged P300 latency and reduced amplitude (e.g., Goodin, Squires, & Starr, 1978; Pfefferbaum et al., 1990). Although most of the dozens of investigations of the P300 response in Alzheimer's disease report data for modest numbers of subjects (as few as seven subjects and rarely more than thirty subjects), a statistically significant prolongation in P300 latency is a consistent finding. In contrast, less than half of published studies of P300 in Alzheimer's disease report decrements in amplitude. Measurement of the P300 response can contribute to confirmation of earlier diagnosis of Alzheimer's disease and prompt perhaps more effective therapy. Applying a technique for localizing the generator region of P300 components, Brain Electrical Source Analysis (BESA), Frodl et al. (2002) found reduced P300 amplitudes for a temporal-basal (TB) component (generated in the temporal-parietal region) and increased latencies for a temporal-superior (TS) component.

Attention-Deficit/Hyperactivity Disorder (ADHD)

There are some reports of decreased P300 amplitude in persons with attention-deficit/hyperactivity disorder, mostly preadolescent children (Frank, Seiden, & Napolitano, 1994; Holcomb, Ackerman, & Dykman, 1986; Johnstone & Barry, 1996; Loiselle, Stamm, Matinsky, & Whipple, 1980; Oades, Dittman, Schepker, Eggers, & Zerbin, 1996). Other authors, however, found no significant difference between children with ADHD and normal control subjects (Jonkman et al., 1997; Winsberg, Javitt, & Silipo, 1997; Rothenberger et al., 2000). Despite this inconsistency in amplitude findings, a return of P300 amplitude to normal levels has been associated with medical therapy for ADHD (Klorman et al., 1983; Michael, Klorman, Salzman, Borgstedt, & Dainer, 1981; Taylor, Voros, Logan, & Malone, 1993; Verbaten et al., 1994). In contrast to these positive findings, Lazzaro et al. (1997) failed to demonstrate a difference in either P300 amplitude or latency for a group of seventeen unmedicated children versus a control group. Published findings for P300 latency in ADHD are even less consistent. Klorman and colleagues showed no difference in P300 latency for children with ADHD in comparison to control subjects (e.g., Klorman, Brumaghim, Fitzpatrick, & Borgstedt, 1992), yet the same research group reported decreased P300 latency with stimulant medications, in comparison to baseline measures and placement treatment (e.g., Coons, Klorman, & Borgstedt, 1987; Klorman, Brumaghim, Fitzpatrick, & Borgstedt, 1991).

Auditory Processing Disorders (APD)

Given the potential clinical value of the P300 response for assessment of auditory processing and cognitive function, there are surprising few formal published investigations in groups of children with auditory-specific processing disorders (e.g., Hall, 1992; Jirsa & Clontz, 1990). Most papers describe P300 response findings in children with other disorders that sometimes include auditory dysfunction, e.g., autism (Bruneau, Roux, Adrien, & Barthelemy, 1999; Seri, Cerquiglini, Pisani, & Curatolo, 1999), language impairment (Tonnquist-Uhlen, 1996), and learning disabilities (e.g., Arehole, 1995; Purdy, Kelly, & Davies, 2002). Published studies of the P300 response in learning and language disorders are summarized below. Figure 13.5 shows a sampling of abnormal finding in children with APD (data were collected by the author).

Autism

A substantial number of studies have described the P300 response in persons diagnosed with autism, including children as young as 5 years (Oades, Walker, Geffen, & Stern, 1988) and continuing through adulthood (e.g., Ciesielki, Courchesne, & Elmasian, 1990; Courchesne et al., 1984; Dawson et al., 1988; Lincoln, Courchesne, Harms, & Allen, 1993;). The amplitude of the P300 response, as elicited with a variety of sounds (e.g., clicks, tones, novel sounds, and phonemes), is typically reduced in autism (Ciesielki, Courchesne, & Elmasian, 1990; Courchesne et al., 1984; Novick, Vaughan, Kurtzberg, & Simson, 1980), whereas latency is unaffected (Ciesielki, Courchesne, & Elmasian, 1990; Courchesne et al., 1984; Dawson et al., 1988; Lincoln et al., 1993; Oades et al., 1988). Various mechanisms have been offered to explain the reduction of P300 amplitude in autism, but none are uniformly endorsed.

Brain Injury (Head Injury)

Abnormal latency and amplitude for the P300 (Pb) response, as recorded with the oddball paradigm, are a common finding in severe head injury (e.g., Campbell & de Lugt, 1995; Curry, 1980; Duncan, Kosmidis, & Mirsky, 2005; Elting

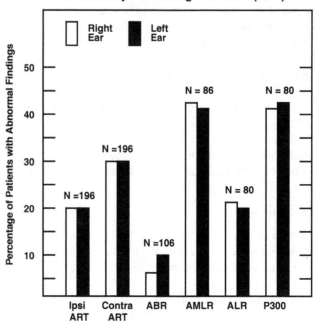

FIGURE 13.5. Proportion of children undergoing assessment for auditory processing disorder (APD) demonstrating an abnormal P300 response, in comparison to acoustic reflex measures and other auditory evoked responses.

et al., 2005; Rugg et al., 1993). The literature is less consistent for the P3a component in severe head injury (Kaipio et al., 2000; Rugg et al., 1993), although Elting et al. (2005) reported that 43 percent of twenty-one patients with mild to moderate head injury had abnormal P3a findings in comparison to a matched control group. Conclusions from studies of the P300 response in mild head injury are mixed, with some authors describing amplitude and/or latency abnormalities (Harris & Hall, 1990; Pratap-Chand, Sinniah, & Salem, 1988; Solbakk, Reinvang, Nielsen, & Sundet, 1999), yet others describing no differences in P300 latency or amplitude with respect to control groups (e.g., Potter & Barrett, 1999; Potter, Bassett, Jory, & Barrett, 2001).

Cerebrovascular Lesions (Stroke)

P300 abnormalities are commonly reported in patients following cerebral ischemic insult, but the nature of the abnormalities (latencies versus amplitudes) is inconsistent (Ebner, Haas, Lucking, Schily, Wallesch, & Zimmerman, 1986; Gummow, Dustman, & Keaney, 1986; Korpelainen et al., 2000; Onofrj et al., 1992; Onofrj, Thomas, Paci, Scesi, & Tombari, 1997; Tachibana, Toda, & Sugita, 1992). Findings range from delayed latencies and/or reduced amplitudes to apparently normal P300 responses. P300 response discrepancies among studies are presumably associated with differences in the severity and type of stroke, e.g., middle cerebral artery, thalamic hemorrhages, lacunar brain infarcts, basilar artery thromboembolism, and internal carotid artery. Korpelainen et al. (2000) showed that minor brain infarction and resulting ischemia, even for patients without hearing loss, psychiatric disorders, prestroke depression, and aphasia affect P300 latency but not amplitude within three months after onset. The authors reported comparable P300 findings for patients with hemispheric and brainstem infarction, and right- versus left-sided lesions. Furthermore, Korpelainen et al. (2000) found a correlation between P300 latency and outcome of a formal depression scale. Alonso-Prieto, Alvarez-Gonzalez, Fernandez-Concepcion, and Jiminez-Conde (2002) found evidence of P300 abnormalities in patients with CVA. In the authors' words, "These results provide new data on the cognitive mechanisms that are affected during a right parietal lesion and demonstrate the sensitivity of P300 in detecting alterations in sustained attention in individuals that differ as regards not only the localization of the lesion but also the type of etiopathogenic mechanism involved" (p. 1105).

Dementia

P300 investigations in dementia date back to the late 1970s (Goodin, Squires, & Starr, 1978) and are ongoing. In comparison to normal effects of aging on the P300 response, P300 latency is prolonged in patients with dementia and the latency delays are progressively greater as cognitive function declines (Polich et al., 1986). As noted in the introduction to this section, the P300 response lacks specificity necessary for differential diagnosis of diseases. There is compelling evidence, however, that the P300 response is a sensitive index of the level of cognitive function in various diseases, including dementia (Polich & Herbst, 2000). In addition, analysis P300 response latency contributes to the diagnostic distinction between patients with dementia versus pseudodementia secondary to depression (Brown, Marsh, & LaRue, 1982; Patterson, Michalewski, & Starr, 1988).

Depression

Varied P300 findings are reported for patients with depression, presumably because the term encompasses a heterogeneous patient population, e.g., geriatric depression, melancholic depression, depression secondary to cerebral infarction, etc. As an example, Roschke et al. (1998) and Karaaslan et al. (2003) reported decreased P300 amplitudes and/or increased latencies in patients with depression disorders, findings that were not confirmed by other investigators (e.g., Bruder et al., 1991; Kaustio et al., 2002). In contrast to previous investigations (Brown, Marsh, & LaRue, 1982; Kraiuhin, Gordon, Coyle, et al., 1990), Kalayam et al. (1998) found longer P300 latencies in a group of forty-three undemented older (> 60 years) patients with a diagnosis of major depression. P300 latency findings were associated with "deficits in initiation and errors in preservation." Although the authors speculated

that the P300 abnormalities were secondary to dysfunction of cortico-striato-pallido-thalamo-cortical pathways, further investigation is warranted.

Epilepsy

Although findings among studies are consistently in agreement, there is some evidence that cognitive processing deficits in adults with epilepsy are reflected by P300 abnormal latencies (Drake et al., 1986; Fukai et al., 1990; Rodin, Khabbazch, Twitty, & Schmaltz, 1989). Also, multiple authors have reported scalp asymmetries in P300 amplitude recorded over the affected versus unaffected medial temporal lobe (e.g., Daruna, Nelson, & Green, 1989; Meador, Loring, King, Gallagher, et al., 1988; Nelson, Collins, & Torres, 1991; Puce, Donnan, & Bladin, 1989). In a study of 108 patients diagnosed with epilepsy, Caravaglios et al. (2001) found a "significant relationship between P300 latency prolongation and epilepsy duration, seizure frequency and polytherapy." Abubakr and Wambacq (2003) conclude from a clinical investigation of P300 in epilepsy, "These findings suggest that postictal ERPs are of localizing value in patients with TLE [temporal lobe epilepsy] while interictal ERPs are not" (p. 692).

Huntington's Disease

An early study of the P300 in Huntington's disease found abnormalities, but "an abnormality of the P3 latency did not correlate with an abnormality in results from computed tomography, electroencephalography, or neuropsychological testing" (Rosenberg, Nudleman, & Starr, 1985, p. 987). The P300 response is useful in differentiating between neurologic diseases with a subcortical substrate, e.g., Huntington's and Parkinson's disease, and cortical pathologies, e.g., Alzheimer's disease (see Polich & Herbst, 2000).

Language Impairment and Learning Disabilities (LD)

Kurtzberg and colleagues (Schafer, Morr, Datta, Kurtzberg, & Schwartz, 2005) have applied tone- and speech-evoked P300 and other responses in the investigation of infants at risk for language impairment. Purdy, Kelly, and Davies (2002) describe findings for a variety of auditory evoked responses (ABR, AMLR, ALR, and P300) recorded from ten children with learning disabilities and "possible APD." The possibility of "APD" was determined by a psychologist based on difficulties experienced by the children on a series of language and cognitive tasks as assessed with psycho-educational test batteries (e.g., *WISC-R, Detroit Tests of Learning Aptitude-2, Lindamood Auditory Conceptualization* test), including measures of phonemic synthesis, speech sound discrimination, auditory "short- and long-term memory" and auditory attention. From the authors' description of psychoeducational test findings for the subjects, it was not possible to verify the presence of auditory specific processing disorders and to rule out common coexisting disorders, i.e., learning and language deficits. The P300 response to standard and to target stimuli was significantly smaller in amplitude and longer in latency for the children with learning disabilities versus the control group.

Magnetic Resonance Imaging (MRI) and the P300 Response

A rapidly growing literature describes the relation between findings for neuroimaging measurements, e.g., functional MRI, and the scalp-recorded P300 response. As noted by Thomas (2003), "when used in combination with structural and functional MRI methods, electrophysiological measures may provide an additional layer of information regarding the temporal dynamics of brain activity" (p. S49).

Multiple Sclerosis

P300 abnormalities are reported for some patients with the diagnosis of multiple sclerosis (e.g., Newton, Barrett, Callanan, & Towell, 1989; Polich, Romine, Sipe, Aung, & Dalessio, 1992).

Parkinson's Disease

Parkinson's disease is characterized by progressive subcortical (substantia nigra) degeneration of no known cause. Deficiency in the neurotransmitter dopamine is a well-known feature of Parkinson's disease. Cognitive decline in Parkinson's disease can be documented by an increase in P300 response latency. P300 latency prolongation is related to duration and severity of the disease and may be documented even for patients with no clinical signs of dementia (Goodin & Aminoff, 1987; Hansch, Syndulko, Cohen, Goldberg, Potvin, & Tourtellotte, 1982; Iijima et al., 2000; Maeshima et al., 2002; O'Donnell, Squires, Martz, Chen, & Phay, 1987; Tachibana, Aragane, Miyata, & Sugita, 1997). Also, there is evidence of a relationship between P300 latency prolongation and performance on activities of daily living, as quantified with the *Mini Mental State* test and cognitive items of the *Functional Independence Measure* (Maeshima et al., 2002).

Schizophrenia

There are perhaps more published papers on the P300 response in schizophrenia than any other single disease, probably because the P300 response is "sensitive to the state, the trait, and the degenerative course of schizophrenia" (Ford, 1999, p. 678). Schizophrenia consists of both positive and negative symptoms. In the words of Ford (1999), "the positive symptoms are the psychological features that *are* present but should not be, such as hallucinations and delusions. The negative symptoms are those that are *not* present, but should be, resulting in blunted affect, emotional withdrawal,

and motor retardation" (p. 674). In the early 1970s, less than a decade after the discovery of the P300 response, the pioneering P300 work of Roth (Roth & Cannon, 1972) and Sutton and colleagues (Levit, Sutton, & Zubin, 1973) provided preliminary evidence in support of the then underappreciated concept that schizophrenia had a biologic basis. These investigations showed lower P300 amplitudes in patients with schizophrenia in comparison to matched control subjects. During the 1960s, prior to these early clinical P300 publications, a major segment of the public viewed schizophrenia as a "psychological disorder," or even a myth (Ford, 1999). Neuroradiologic studies with CT scans and then functional MRI have since unequivocally confirmed brain abnormalities in schizophrenia, specifically diminished gray matter in the frontal and temporal lobes (e.g., McCarley et al., 1999).

P300 findings in schizophrenia are, however, highly dependent on methodology. To be sure, the traditional oddball paradigm utilizing standard stimuli with 80 percent probability and target stimuli with 20 percent probability, in which the oddball stimulus occurs (on the average) after five standard stimuli, typically reveals smaller-than-normal P300 amplitudes in patients with schizophrenia. With other measurement paradigms (e.g., the single stimulus paradigm with long ISIs, the P300 response to an alerting or startle stimulus), or when the target stimulus is presented after a long string of standards, the P300 response from schizophrenic patients may be normal (see Ford, 1999, for review). These findings suggest that the mechanism for abnormal P300 responses in schizophrenia is related to a prolongation in the "cognitive refractory period" (Gonsalvez et al., 1995). Reduced motivation, a characteristic feature of schizophrenia, has also been implicated as a factor contributing to reduced P300 amplitude. However, deficits in the P300 response remain even with clever measurement strategies that minimize the possible effects of motivation, such as automatic elicitation of the P300 or monetary incentives to enhance motivation (e.g., Brecher & Begleiter, 1983; Pfefferbaum, Ford, White, & Roth, 1989). Interestingly, the P300 response amplitude reflects severity of the disease and is sensitive to fluctuations in the clinical presentation or state of schizophrenia, with decreases in amplitude when positive symptoms are more prominent and increased amplitude associated with improvement in symptoms (Ford, 1999; Ford, Mathalon, Marsh, Faustman, Harris, Hoff, Beal, & Pfefferbaum, 1999). Abnormalities in P300 amplitude are also directly related to the duration of the disease and, presumably, progressive neurologic degeneration (Mathalon, Ford, Rosenbloom, & Pfefferbaum, 2000). The complexity of interpreting abnormal P300 responses in schizophrenia is well described by Ford (1999). Following an investigation of possible explanations for reduced P300 amplitude in schizophrenia, she

> concluded that persons with schizophrenia generate fewer P300s than controls, suggesting waxing and waning of attention; that the P300s they do generate are smaller than those of

controls, suggesting reductions in resources allocated, whether due to neuro-anatomical limitations or to enduring attentional limitations; and that the P300s of persons with schizophrenia are more variable in latency, again suggesting fluctuating attention or strategies. (p. 671)

In a meta-analysis of fifty data sets involving investigations of P300 cerebral asymmetry in schizophrenia, Jeon and Polich (2001) confirmed significant differences in P300 amplitude as a function of electrode site along the midline and for lateral (temporal) scalp locations. Topographic analysis of the P300 response in schizophrenia is of interest because some symptoms (e.g., reasoning, executive function deficits, and negative affect) are associated with frontal lobe dysfunction, whereas other symptoms (e.g., hallucinations and delusions) are related to temporal lobe dysfunction. The authors found that P300 amplitude differences between schizophrenic and normal subjects were most pronounced for the Pz midline electrode site and, for lateral electrodes, greatest for left-hemisphere scalp locations. That is, patients with schizophrenia showed P300 amplitudes were more consistently smaller when recorded from these electrode sites. Bramon, Rabe-Hesketh, et al. (2004) also performed a meta-analysis of forty-six papers published in peer-reviewed journals reporting P300 response data for a combined total of 1,443 patients with the diagnosis of schizophrenia and 1,251 control subjects. Only amplitude and/or latency P300 data for the most commonly used electrode sites (Cz and/or Pz) were included in the analysis.

The "pooled effect size (PES)" for P300 amplitude was 0.85 (a reduction), whereas for latency it was –0.57 (a prolongation). In agreement with Jeon and Polich (2001), the authors concluded that unmedicated patients with schizophrenia have marked reductions in P300 amplitude and clear, but less pronounced, delays in latency. The meta-analysis showed no relation between P300 findings and duration of the schizophrenia.

CONCLUDING COMMENTS

The P300 response is an electrophysiological measure of cognitive functioning that can be recorded in most clinics equipped with auditory evoked response instrumentation that includes a common software option. Measurement of the P300 only requires the equipment capacity for presentation of two or more types of stimuli with different probabilities of occurrence. The literature on P300 in various neuropsychiatric disorders is vast. In comparison, there are relatively few formal investigations of the P300 response in children with auditory processing disorders or other types of auditory dysfunction. Two measurement approaches—the passive P300 (P3a) response and the P300 evoked by a single stimulus—are particularly appealing as clinical procedures in children and other challenging patient populations due to their technical simplicity and independence from demands on subject attention.

14

CHAPTER

Mismatch Negativity (MMN) Response

BACKGROUND

The mismatch negativity (MMN) response is a negative wave elicited by a combination of standard and deviant stimuli, and occurring in the latency region of about 100 to 300 ms. A typical MMN response waveform and stimulus paradigm are illustrated in Figure 14.1. The MMN response can be evoked by a vast array of sounds, ranging from simple tones to complex patterns of acoustic features to speech stimuli. Best detected with scalp electrodes over the frontal-central region of the brain, generation of the MMN is a reflection

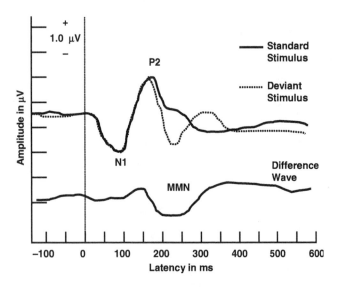

Mismatch Negativity (MMN) Response

FIGURE 14.1. Mismatch negativity (MMN) response waveform as evoked with standard and deviant stimuli. The standard stimulus generates one waveform, and the deviant stimulus generates another waveform. The MMN component is visible within the 100 to 300 ms region in the difference waveform, calculated by subtracting the standard waveform from the deviant waveform.

of several simultaneous or sequential and fundamental brain processes, including preattentive analysis of features of sound (e.g., frequency, intensity, duration, speech cues), extraction or derivation of the invariance within multiple acoustic stimuli, a sensory memory trace in the auditory modality that represents the sound stimulation, and ongoing comparison of the invariant (standard) stimuli versus the different (deviant) stimuli. Serious measurement problems must be solved before the MMN response is regularly applied clinically in the diagnosis of auditory dysfunction and neurological disorders and in the documentation of developmental and intervention-induced changes in neural function. Technical challenges in MMN recording to be addressed include development of a test protocol that is relatively brief and clinically feasible, enhancement of the signal (MMN) to noise (background electrical activity) ratio for confident detection of the MMN wave, proven analysis strategies to assure statistically the presence of a response, and improved reliability of MMN recordings in the clinical setting with various patient populations, including young children.

The relative brevity of the MMN response review in this chapter is commensurate with the uncommon application of the MMN in clinical practice, rather than the extent of literature on the topic. Indeed, the volume of published papers on the MMN warrant an entire book on the topic. Since its discovery by Risto Näätänen and colleagues in 1978 (Näätänen, Gaillard, & Mäntysalo, 1978), many hundreds of articles have described MMN measurement for myriad combinations of experimental (signal and subject) conditions across the age spectrum from infancy to aging adults and in diverse clinical populations. A historical perspective on the MMN response can be found in Chapter 1. The reader is referred for more detailed information to original literature on the MMN response and, in particular, to recent review articles and monographs on the topic (e.g., Näätänen, 1995, 2000; Näätänen & Ahlo, 1997; Näätänen, Pakarinen, Rinne, & Takegata, 2004; Näätänen & Winkler, 1999). A special issue of *Audiology & Neuro-Otology,* guest edited by Dr. Risto Näätänen in 2000, offers a particularly comprehensive review of the MMN response.

MMN Principles and Potential Clinical Practices

The MMN response is often categorized as an event-related response (potential), a cognitive evoked response, or a discriminative cortical evoked response, in contrast to so-called obligatory earlier latency responses (e.g., ECochG, ABR, AMLR). Much of this chapter is devoted to a review of contributions of the MMN response to knowledge of auditory processing, speech sound representation at the cortical level, and other fundamental mechanisms of hearing and cognition. Whether the MMN response is exclusively evoked by auditory stimulation is not clear. There is a substantial literature on visual evoked cortical responses, but the existence of a visual counterpart to the auditory MMN response is open to question (see Pazo-Alvarez, Cadaveira, & Amenedo, 2003, for a review). Selected research strengths and potential clinical advantages of the MMN response are summarized in Table 14.1. The list of MMN response features is impressive and rather unique in that many of the advantages of the MMN response are not shared by other auditory evoked responses. Two characteristics of the MMN response, in combination, are highly attractive from a clinical perspective. One is the independence of the MMN response from conscious attention to acoustic signals, an especially appealing feature for clinical assessment of auditory processing in very young children and other patient populations that are challenging to assess with behavioral audiologic techniques due to deficits in state of arousal, motivation, attention, cognition, and other subject variables. Whether the subject is attending or ignoring a deviant stimulus has little effect on amplitude of the MMN response (e.g., Näätänen, Simpson, & Loveless, 1982), when the possible contribution of the N2 wave is excluded. Indeed, a pure MMN response is best recorded in a passive condition with the patient paying no attention to the stimuli (e.g., reading, watching a video, or even sleeping). Furthermore, a clear MMN can be recorded from infants in deep sleep and from patients in deep coma (Kane, Curry, Rowlands, Manara, Lewis, Moss, Cummins, & Butler, 1996). The other exciting feature of the MMN response is the feasibility of eliciting it with very fine distinctions between the standard and target stimuli, such as acoustic cues within speech signals. Indeed,

TABLE 14.1. Advantages and Strengths of the Mismatch Negativity Response (MMN) as an Electrophysiologic Measure of Auditory Function and, Potentially, a Clinical Procedure

ADVANTAGE	COMMENT
An early cognitive response	The MMN response is present in newborn infants and is, therefore, "ontologically the first cognitive event related potential" (Näätänen & Escera, 2000).
Anatomical substrate	Generators of the MMN response are reasonably well defined anatomically and functionally.
Not dependent on attention	Overt subject task is not required, e.g., paying attention and pressing a button as a response to target stimulus. Attention variables, including deficits, do not contaminate MMN response findings.
Independent of subject state	A MMN response can be recorded during sleep and even in coma. Minimal subject cooperation is required (the subject must remain relatively still).
Approximates behavioral discrimination	The MMN response is generated by a person's discrimination of small differences between repetitive sounds that are on the same order as behavioral discrimination thresholds.
A response to different sound stimuli	The MMN can be elicited by, and is an objective index of a person's perception of, a variety of sound stimuli, ranging from simple tones to complex speech sounds.
An electrophysiologic (objective) measure of normal brain processes	Central auditory processing. Duration of auditory memory. Short-term sensory (auditory) memory. Acoustic, including speech sound, memory. Auditory temporal integration.
An electrophysiologic (objective) measure of abnormal brain processes	Brain and cognitive degeneration. Effect of central nervous system disease on brain function. Acoustic, including speech sound, memory. Auditory temporal integration.

Adapted from Näätänen, 1995; Näätänen & Escera, 2000.

discrimination of sounds as reflected by the MMN response is equivalent to behavioral discrimination of just noticeable differences in the features of sound. There appears to be almost no limit to the sophistication of stimuli used to evoke the MMN response and the ability to evaluate electrophysiologically, and objectively, the brain's processing the sound under varying stimulus conditions. Of particular relevance to potential clinical applications in audiology, the MMN is an objective reflection or index of automatic central auditory processing.

The MMN response is a relatively small amplitude (several μvolts or less) negative wave within the latency region of 100 to 300 ms that is generated passively when some feature of sound is discriminated from the memory of a different sound within the central auditory nervous system (Figure 14.2). Put another way, the MMN reflects a preconscious or preperceptual detection of a change in acoustic stimulation, even a very slight change that is barely greater than the perceptual, and behavioral, discrimination threshold (i.e., the just noticeable difference). The stimulus processing underlying the MMN response is not an esoteric phenomenon but, rather, of critical importance to our life within an acoustic environment. As described vividly by Jääskeläinen and eleven colleagues (2004),

> Life or death in hostile environments depends crucially on one's ability to detect and gate novel sounds to awareness, such as that of a twig crackling under the paw of a stalking predator in a noisy jungle. . . . Survival of higher organisms depends on their ability to automatically distinguish novel ("deviant") sounds amongst background environmental noise. Because conscious attention can dwell on but few events at a time, it is clear that scanning the entire auditory scene bit-by-bit for novelty would be highly inefficient. Instead, novelty needs to be gated to awareness in a fast "bottom-up" manner. (p. 6809)

Evidence supports a link between behavioral ability to discriminate properties of sound (e.g., pitch or speech sound category) and the presence of a MMN (Kraus, McGee, Carrell, & Sharma, 1995; Lang et al., 1995). The MMN also faithfully reflects more psychoacoustic discrimination performance in rather complex tasks involving backward masking (Winkler, Reinikainen, & Näätänen, 1993). The time required between the masking signal and the deviant signal for generation of a MMN response parallels the time needed for recovery of the behavioral discrimination of the deviant (and standard) stimuli. Anatomic origins of the MMN response include the supratemporal plane and posterior regions of the auditory cortex and regions within the frontal cortical lobe. The memory trace underlying the MMN response is not an unchangeable (hard wired) representation of the acoustic stimulation but, rather, a memory trace than can be modified with auditory experience (i.e., exposure to new and perhaps complex information) or during formal training. New memory traces can rapidly form during intense stimulation, as in

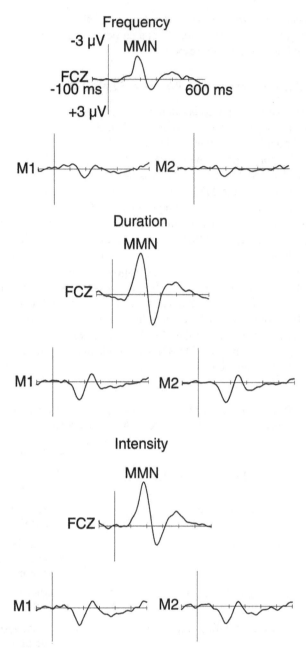

FIGURE 14.2. Group grand average difference waveforms (N = 30) at Fcz for tone stimuli under three deviant conditions (frequency, duration, and intensity). Details on the stimulus characteristics are noted in the text.

Courtesy of Dr. Catharine Pettigrew, with acknowledgment also to colleagues B. M. Murdoch, C. W. Ponton, J. Kei, H. Chenery, R. Sockalingam, and P. Alku. The figure is adapted with permission from Dr. Pettigrew's unpublished doctoral dissertation, University of Queensland, Australia.

a foreign language environment. An initial and essential step in the measurement of the MMN response is the presentation of a sequence of standard—repetitive, unchanging, and "matched"—stimuli. The standard "stimulus stream" produces a sensory (auditory) memory trace, or echoic memory, in neurons within auditory regions of the brain (Näätänen,

1995). Näätänen and colleagues (Näätänen, 1992; Näätänen & Michie, 1979) also proposed, initially, that the MMN response is associated with a brief, involuntary orienting, or attention switching, response. The MMN response is generated by any infrequent change in the stimulus stream—a deviant stimulus—that can be discriminated by the subject, even automatically and before conscious attention or perception of the stimulus. The sensory (auditory) memory trace formation, and the above-noted processing of auditory information, whether it consists of tones, speech, or even music, apparently takes place within a 200 ms "temporal window of integration" (Näätänen, 1990). The MMN response reflects information processing that precedes and may be a prerequisite for behavioral (conscious) attentive processing of auditory changes in the environment.

Differentiation of the MMN versus Other Responses

The MMN response may be influenced by, related to, or even confused with and contaminated by other AERs within the same general latency region, such as the N1, N2, P300, and N400 waves, or components of these waves, e.g., N2b. Any change in an acoustic stimulus, including the onset and offset, may evoke either an N1 or MMN response, or both. Indeed, the N1 wave and the MMN response are closely related both in terms of their elicitation by stimuli and in their latencies. The MMN emerges as a distinct wave when a different stimulus follows a sequence of similar, or identical, stimuli. Picton et al. (2000) identify five findings that differentiate the N1 from the MMN wave, while acknowledging that the literature on the topic is not entirely consistent and "not without some controversy." First, and perhaps most obvious, the MMN will be elicited by any change between the standard and the deviant stimuli, even when the change is a decrease in intensity. The typical effect of decreased stimulus intensity on auditory evoked responses, including the N1 wave, is a reduction in response amplitude. Similarly, the MMN can be elicited by a change in stimulus duration, whereas the N1 is not affected by changes in duration. Second, according to Picton et al. (2000), with the N1 wave, as with other cortical auditory evoked responses, there is an expected decrease in amplitude as the rate of stimulation increases (ISI decreases). The MMN response, on the other hand, is relatively unaffected by ISI and may actually begin to decrease in amplitude or disappear for very long intervals (10 seconds) between deviant stimuli. The maximum interval between successive deviant stimuli that is effective for generation of the MMN is related to the duration of auditory sensory memory (Näätänen, 2003). Third, the MMN is effectively evoked by small (fine) differences between the standard and the deviant stimuli, whereas the N1 is more likely to be generated by large differences. Fourth, there is for the MMN a relationship for differences between the standard and deviant stimuli and response latency, while N1 latency remains essentially unchanged. And, finally, studies using

magnetic and electrical techniques, and clinical investigations in patients with pathology of the central nervous system, reveal differences in the neuroanatomic origins for the N1 wave versus the MMN response. Lesions in the temporal-parietal region affect the N1, whereas MMN abnormalities are expected with pathology of more anterior regions of the temporal lobe and also lesions in the frontal lobe. As Picton and colleagues (2000) go on to note, the MMN can also be distinguished from other waves with similar latencies (e.g., the N2 wave) by the effects of subject attention. With close subject attention to the stimuli, and with highly relevant stimuli, the N2 wave (actually the N2b component) may be superimposed on the MMN response. Assuring that the subject is not attending to stimuli, however, highlights the MMN response and minimizes the likelihood of influence by the N2 wave. The N400 response, as noted in Chapter 12, is evoked by in incongruity in the meaning of words, i.e., by semantically unpredictable words. Thus, both the MMN and N400 are a response to detection of a difference or "mismatch" between what the subject was "primed to process" (Picton et al., 2000) and the stimulus that was actually detected. By definition, the N400 response can be distinguished in part from the MMN by later latency (maximum in the region of 400 ms) and, as expected, the MMN is best elicited in conditions requiring no subject attention to the stimuli.

Consideration of the relation between the N1 and MMN responses involves a fundamental concept regarding the neural mechanisms underlying generation of the MMN response. Review of the literature yields two distinct and alternative neural explanations for the auditory processes contributing to the MMN response. Briefly, one explanation or model is based on an "adaptation hypothesis" (Jääskeläinen et al., 2004). The N1 (N100) response is attenuated in amplitude with repeated stimulation (with standard stimuli) secondary to adaptation of auditory neuronal activity. The MMN response, according to this explanation, appears with transient (short-term) adaptation of the N1 response to repetitive presentation of an acoustic feature and the presentation of stimulus with another acoustic feature. With the other model (the change-specific neural hypothesis), the MMN response to deviant stimuli arises from a separate and independent population of neurons in auditory cortex that respond exclusively to change in acoustic stimulation. Jääskeläinen et al. (2004) present evidence in support of the adaptation theory.

At least four rather simple measurement strategies can be employed to increase the likelihood of recording a "pure MMN" that is not contaminated by other auditory evoked responses superimposed within the same time frame. One typical approach in MMN measurement is calculation of the difference waveform by subtracting the response elicited by standard stimuli from the response elicited by deviant stimuli. Auditory evoked response waves elicited by and common to both sets of stimuli, e.g., N1 and P2, are eliminated or at least minimized by with this process. Unfortunately, deriving the MMN waveform from the difference between two averaged waveforms introduces additional noise into the MMN and may, therefore, decrease the signal-to-noise ratio (SNR). Another effective technique for isolating the MMN response, and minimizing interference by other auditory evoked responses, is to increase the rate of stimulation. With simple stimuli, e.g., standard versus deviant stimuli that differ in frequency or duration, the MMN is enhanced when the standard ISI (the interstimulus interval for standard stimuli) is decreased to, for example, one stimulus per second. This, of course, is the same as increasing the repetition rate of for the standard stimuli. The amplitude of certain auditory evoked response waves, e.g., N1, P2, N2, and even the P300, decreases with shorter ISIs (faster stimulus rate). Fortuitously, increasing the rate of the standard stimuli also strengthens the memory trace that is essential for generation of the MMN response. Increasing the stimulus rate may also shorten the test time. The overall result is simultaneous augmentation of MMN amplitude and diminution of other auditory evoked response components within the same latency region. Subject inattention to stimuli is a third important measurement condition associated with enhancement of the MMN and reduction of other responses, e.g., P300. Subject attention can be directed away from the deviant stimulus during MMN measurement by engaging the subject in an interesting nonauditory task, e.g., watching a video, or with a somewhat demanding auditory task, e.g., directing attention away from the deviant stimuli in one ear and toward stimuli in the other ear with a dichotic listening task. Finally, small differences between the standard and the deviant stimuli will contribute to less interference in the MMN by an N1 wave and a passive P3 (actually P3a) wave.

Among the late event-related responses, similarities are probably greatest with measurement of the MMN response and the P300 response. For example, each response is evoked with a combination of frequent (standard) and unpredictable (rare) signals. One of the main distinctions between the P300 response and the MMN response is the name and the nature of the rare stimulus. The term "target" is appropriate in describing the rare stimulus that elicits the P300 response as, typically, the subject is expected to direct his or her attention to it and to ignore the standard stimulus. In measurement of the MMN response, however, the subject is not actively listening for the rare stimulus. Rather, the MMN response is recorded with the subject in a passive state, i.e., with attention directed away from the stimuli or sleeping. The MMN response is automatically generated by a deviation in a sequence of standard stimuli, hence the term "deviant" for the rare stimulus.

Indeed, one of the potential pitfalls in MMN measurement is the unintended and perhaps inadvertent recording of the P3a component. As a general rule, it is desirable to eliminate the likelihood of P3a contamination in recording the MMN response. One approach for achieving this objective is to rely on fine (small) differences between the standard and the deviant stimuli (e.g., very close in frequency or whatever

acoustic dimension distinguishes the two stimuli). Although MMN responses can be recorded for relatively small differences in speech signals at the phonemic, semantic, and lexical levels, the use of such stimuli to evaluate speech processing introduces a quantum increase overall complexity of MMN measurement and analysis. Extensive study of phonemically elicited MMN responses has prompted the coining of a new term—"phonologic mismatch negativity or PMN." The PMN reflects a prelexical stage of speech analysis that can then be modified by linguistic context and subsequent linguistic experience. In fact, the MMN response can even be elicited by within category acoustic differences in speech sounds, i.e., the acoustic differences are within the acoustic boundaries of a phoneme and the subject does not hear a different phoneme. Also, the "automatic, preconscious auditory analysis" detected by the MMN can be elicited not by physical differences between standard and deviant stimuli but, rather, by abstract deviations in a sequence of acoustic signals. That is, the standard stimuli may not all be the same, but there is a pattern in the frequency direction of the sequence. For example, the standard sequence of stimuli may consist of set of tones with the second tone higher in frequency than the first tone, and the deviant stimulus is actually a descending frequency pair of tones.

What are the differences in test protocols for the P300 response versus the MMN response? And are there also differences in the anatomic generators for each response? There is no simple answer to the first question. However, the dominant differences in test protocols for the two responses center on stimulus features and the task required (or for MMN not required) of the subject. Selected differences in measurement of the P300 and MMN responses are summarized in Table 14.2. The short answer to the second question is yes, with details provided in Chapter 2.

Clinical Application of the MMN Response: Potential and Problems

At the conclusion of the preface to the Special Issue of *Ear and Hearing* devoted to the MMN response published in 1995, Dr. Terry Picton commented "The MMN discovered by Näätänen almost 20 years ago has now become ready for clinical applications. The papers in this issue will provide you with the information necessary to embark upon these clinical applications. More importantly, they suggest the combination of enthusiasm and caution needed for your journey" (Picton, 1995, p. 5). Many of us were ready then to pack the Special Issue into our bags and willing to ride the MMN wave into the clinical arena. The possible clinical and other practical applications of an objective and automated measure of auditory processing and neural plasticity are legion and well appreciated, among them evaluation of speech perception, prelanguage function, or auditory processing disorders in infants; objective documentation of neural plasticity with auditory, phonologic, and language intervention; assessment

TABLE 14.2. Differences in the Measurement and Generation of the P300 versus MMN Response

P300 RESPONSE	MMN RESPONSE
Typically requires conscious attention to the stimulus.	Involves preperceptual detection of a change in the stimulus.
Response amplitude is directly related to subject attention.	Amplitude of the response is independent of subject attention to deviant stimuli.
Response amplitude is directly related to the task and to stimulus relevance.	Amplitude of the response is unaffected by subject task and stimulus relevance.
Response has a latency of about 300 ms.	Latency of the MMN is in the 100 to 300 ms region.
Generators are in limbic system and auditory cortex.	There are frontal lobe contributions to the response.
Larger differences between standard and target produce larger response amplitudes.	Smaller differences between standard and deviant stimuli produce clearest MMN and minimize contamination with other late responses.

of benefit from hearing aids and cochlear implants in children; determination of the capability or talent for music and learning foreign languages; diagnosis of a variety of psychoneurological disorders (e.g., schizophrenia, Alzheimer's disease and other dementias, Parkinson's disease); and prognosis of outcome in comatose patients.

Given the many potential assets of the MMN response and the extensive investigation in normal subjects and patient populations, why almost thirty years after its discovery (Näätänen, Gaillard, & Mäntysalo, 1978) is the MMN response not regularly applied clinically as a technique for the assessment of auditory function in children and adults? There are concerted and international efforts underway to provide answers to this question (e.g., European Union CO-BRAIN project).

Serious measurement and analysis problems must be addressed before the MMN is a feasible clinical procedure, for example:

- The MMN is a small response (no larger than a few microvolts) that must be detected within substantial background noise.
- The MMN is averaged for a limited number (fewer trials) of deviant stimuli, relative to the greater number of standard stimuli.
- The signal (MMN) to noise (background electrical activity) ratio is typically very modest.
- Measurement noise is increased (not reduced) by the process of calculating a difference waveform by subtracting the response to standard stimuli from the response to deviant stimuli.
- With repeated continuous MMN measurement, MMN amplitude may decrease.
- In comparison to calculations for other AER waveforms (e.g., ABR), latency of the MMN is not precise.
- Analysis techniques employed to differentiate the MMN versus background noise are extremely complex and computer intensive.

- There are inconsistent experimental findings on intrasubject reliability of the MMN, with some authors reporting adequate reliability (e.g., Kathman, 1999), yet others questioning MMN reliability (e.g., Dalebout & Fox, 2001).
- Normal MMN amplitude variations reach zero in some subjects. Therefore, as noted by Picton et al. (2000), "it will not be possible to consider any MMN abnormality small or absent" (p. 132).
- Most clinical studies of the MMN are limited to a comparison of a group of patients to a group of normal subjects, whereas in clinical application of the MMN it is necessary to distinguish an abnormal MMN finding for an individual patient from normative data.
- The diagnosis of a specific disorder in a patient presumes that the MMN in a group of patients with that disorder differs from the MMN for patients with another disorder.
- MMN amplitude in patients is typically smaller than for normal subjects, while noise levels are often higher. Consequently, more averaging will be needed to produce an adequate signal-to-noise ratio.
- Intersubject variance, predictably, exceeds intrasubject variance. Differentiation of an individual patient from normal intersubject variance is not straightforward.
- Test performance of the MMN (sensitivity and specificity) has not been described for clinical entities (different patient populations). That is, there are no data on the effectiveness of the MMN in correctly identifying a patient with specific disease or ruling out a specific disease for a patient and no data on false-positives and false-misses for the MMN in different disorders.

Further complicating clinical application of the MMN, a response is not invariably recorded from adult subjects under all stimulus conditions. In fact, for certain contrasts in stimuli the response is detectable in less than 50 percent of normal adult subjects, even when the difference between stimuli can be discriminated behaviorally (e.g., Dalebout & Fox, 2001; Wunderlich & Cone-Wesson, 2001). Reliability of the MMN response within subjects from one test session to the next is also a practical problem.

TEST PROTOCOLS AND PROCEDURES

Most acquisition parameters of the MMN test protocol, such as electrode array and analysis time, are indistinguishable from those for measurement of other late auditory responses. The major and rather unique differences in the measurement of the MMN response have to do with stimulus factors (and complexity) and subject state or attention. Indeed, even the terms used to describe the MMN are not found in descriptions of other auditory evoked responses. A sample of the terms is listed in Table 14.3. A fundamental stimulus condition for elicitation of the MMN is the presentation of a series (or train) of standard (unchanging) stimuli followed by the presentation of a rare (only occasional) different (deviant) stimulus. That is, a "repetitive sound stream" (Sinkkonen & Tervaniemi, 2000) is interrupted by a change or irregularity in some feature(s) of the stimuli. The repetitive standard stimuli create a memory trace for features of the stimulus, and the deviant stimulus activates "an automatic change-detection process" (Näätänen, 2003) that underlies generation of the MMN. The difference between standard and deviant stimuli may be quite simple, such as a small difference in frequency for two pure tones, some acoustic feature of speech, or multiple highly complex and abstract differences. Importantly, the memory trace that is an essential factor in generation of the MMN is highly dependent on the dynamic changing temporal properties of the stimulation, rather than simply features of static stimuli. Examples of these temporal features of stimulation include duration,

the sequence or order of the stimuli, a combination or pattern of spectral and temporal features, the rhythm produced by a pattern of stimuli (e.g., tones), and the direction of frequency change over time for a stimulus. Indeed, no other auditory evoked response has been recorded with as many variations in stimulus features, and with as much stimulus complexity, as the MMN response. Myriad, and often subtle, differences between standard (invariant) and infrequent deviant stimuli in MMN measurement have been reported in hundreds of published papers.

An essential subject condition for MMN measurement is inattention to all stimuli (standard and deviant). In fact, it is desirable in MMN recordings for subject attention to be directed away from the stimuli by requiring nonlistening activities such as reading or watching a video. A wake state is not necessary for measurement of the MMN. The MMN can also be recorded successfully in a deep sleep state, especially in infants, and even in coma.

Stimulus Parameters

Selected variations in stimulus parameters used to elicit the MMN response are summarized in Table 14.4. Stimuli used to elicit the MMN vary from a simple difference between one frequency for the standard stimulus and another frequency for the deviant stimulus to multiple and highly complex sets of standard and deviant stimuli. Selection of the most appropriate stimulus is important for all auditory evoked responses. The options are, however, somewhat limited for the early and so-called "exogenous" responses, such as the ECochG, ABR, and AMLR. The choices are usually either clicks or short tonal signals (e.g., tone bursts), and rarely is more than one type of stimulus presented at the same time. That is, the response is elicited exclusively by one specific stimulus with largely invariant properties, for example, one frequency

TABLE 14.3. Key Terms Used in the Description of the Mismatch Negativity (MMN) Response

- Standard stimulus: Typically, a repetitive invariant sound that forms a sensory memory trace in the brain.
- Deviant stimulus: A sound that differs in some feature (e.g., frequency, intensity, duration, temporal or spectral pattern) from the standard stimulus.
- Stimulus onset asynchrony (SOA): The time or interval between the onset of two adjacent stimuli (inversely related to stimulus rate).
- Temporal window of integration: A time frame of about 200 ms, shifting backward and forward in time, within which auditory information is integrated as a single perceptual event.
- Auditory sensory memory: Immediate auditory memory.
- Memory trace: An immediate sensory memory formed by repeated presentation of the standard stimuli.

TABLE 14.4. Selected Variations or Differences in Stimulus Features (Standard versus Deviant) That Are Used for Generation of the MMN Response

- Frequency difference between two pure tones, e.g., 1000 Hz standard versus 1100 Hz deviant stimuli.
- Intensity difference between two or more stimuli.
- Duration difference between two or more stimuli.
- Gap within a tonal or noise stimulus.
- Sound source difference between two stimuli.
- Missing deviant stimulus.
- Temporal pattern in standard versus deviant stimuli, e.g., pattern of rising or descending tone frequencies.
- Musical chords.
- Rhythm patterns for multiple tones.
- Small acoustic changes in vowel or consonant speech sounds, e.g., voice onset time.
- Syllables and words, including pseudowords and nonwords.

with a fixed duration. In almost all cases, intensity is the only stimulus parameter varied by the tester. The stimulus repertoire for MMN measurement is essentially limitless, with a complete review of all possibilities far beyond the scope of this discussion and perhaps impossible.

The MMN can be elicited by differences between the standard and deviant stimuli that approach the behavioral just noticeable difference (JND) for the sounds. For a simple frequency difference between standard and deviant stimuli in the region of 1000 Hz, the JND is on the order of only 1 or 2 Hz (e.g., Tiitinen, Sinkkonen, May, & Näätänen, 1994), whereas with spectrally complex speech stimuli a JND for, as an example, absolute formant frequency is about 4 to 5 percent (e.g., Aaltonen et al., 1994). The property differentiating standard versus deviant stimulus and the magnitude of the difference in some acoustic property of the standard versus deviant stimulus are important variables for clinical investigation of the MMN response and for differentiation between

normal and patient populations (see Figure 14.3). Baldeweg, Williams, and Gruzelier (1999), for example, reported no difference in the MMN response for normal subjects versus dyslexic patients with relatively large frequency differences (e.g., 90 Hz) between standard and deviant stimuli. However, as the frequency change decreased to 15 Hz, control (normal) subjects continued to show a robust MMN response, whereas the MMN response was significantly smaller in amplitude among dyslexic subjects. In contrast, the authors found equivalent amplitudes in control and dyslexic subjects for the MMN response elicited by a duration difference between standard and deviant stimuli (ranging from a change of 160 ms to a change of 40 ms). The work of Kujala and Näätänen (2001) offers another example of the same phenomenon for tonal standard versus deviant stimuli presented in different patterns. When the standard stimulus was a series of identically spaced tones (same ISI), and the deviant stimulus was a pair of tones (closely spaced), the MMN response was equivalent

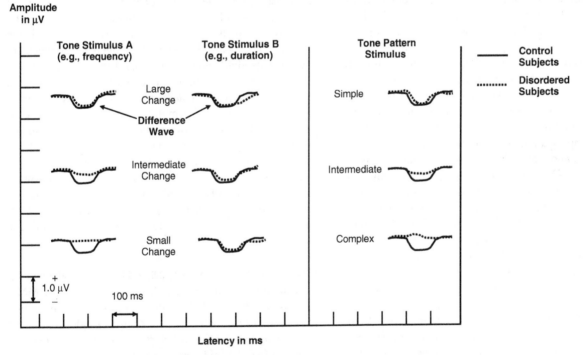

FIGURE 14.3. Interaction among the type of change or difference (e.g., frequency or duration), size of change (e.g., frequency difference of 100 Hz versus 15 Hz), or complexity of difference (e.g., simple tones versus pattern of tones) between standard and deviant stimuli and disorder (e.g., dyslexia). Under some relatively simple stimulus conditions (duration change in this example), the MMN does not differentiate between normal and disordered subjects, whereas another similar change (frequency in this example) produces a clear abnormality in the MMN for disordered subjects for smaller stimulus differences. The complex stimulus (patterns of tones) clearly differentiates between normal and disordered subjects. The diagram does not, of course, reflect adequately the complexity of stimulus variables in MMN measurement in normal subjects and persons with auditory or other disorders.

for the control and dyslexic subjects. For a more complex set of stimuli (a pattern of tones rather than a simple pair), there was a clear MMN response among control subjects and no apparent MMN response for the dyslexic subject group. Similar findings, that is, normal MMN as elicited by simple stimuli yet abnormal MMN responses for complex stimuli (e.g., music) are reported also in other pathologies, such as severe brain injury (Kotchoubey et al., 2003).

These papers highlight at least three pertinent variables in clinical MMN response measurement: (1) the size of the difference or change between standard and deviant stimuli, (2) the nature of the difference (e.g., frequency versus duration, simple versus more complex), and (3) subject factors (e.g., normal versus dyslexic and, presumably, the exact clinical entity represented by the experimental subjects). Figure 14.3 illustrates in a highly schematic fashion the interaction of the three variables in clinical study of the MMN response.

The complexity of the stimuli that can be presented in MMN measurement matches the many variations in perceptual processes evoked by the stimuli. What appear to be slight changes in the acoustic or temporal properties of the standard versus deviant stimuli may produce distinctly different physiologic events at the neuronal level and activity in different anatomical regions. That is, manipulation of the stimulus features, and also the acoustic context (e.g., simple versus complex collection of sounds) within which the stimuli are presented, will affect the anatomic pathways and centers involved in generation of the MMN response and left versus right hemisphere symmetry. Subtle changes in stimuli may also generate highly divergent neuropsychological events, involving complex alterations and interactions in auditory perception, attention, and memory. Much remains unknown about the relation between standard and deviant stimulation and both the resulting brain mechanisms and the subsequent or coincident perceptual and cognitive activity within the brain as reflected by the MMN. The reader is referred to the article entitled "Mismatch Negativity: Different Water in the Same River" by Picton, Benton, Berg, et al. (2000) for a stimulating and thought provoking review of the physiological and psychological underpinnings of the MMN response.

STIMULUS TYPE: TONES. | The MMN is often recorded with a straightforward frequency difference between the standard and deviant stimuli, much as when Näätänen, Gaillard, & Mäntysalo first described the response in 1978. The traditional frequency-difference stimulus paradigm is shown schematically in Figure 14.4. The memory trace is formed by repetitive presentation of a tone at one frequency, e.g., 1000 Hz. This standard stimulus evokes a waveform that consists of a N1 and P2 complex. A second tone at another frequency, e.g., 1100 Hz, generates a negative wave (or wave complex) reflecting the brain's detection of a change in stimulation (neuronal mismatch). The actual MMN response (difference waveform) is usually derived by subtracting

waveform evoked by the standard stimulus from the waveform evoked by the deviant stimulus, as illustrated earlier in Figure 14.1. Any change in the acoustic stimulus will generate the N1 component within the same general latency region. The MMN, however, is specifically associated with the deviation of a stimulus not from silence to sound but, rather, a change in some feature of the previous acoustic stimulation, previous stimulation that has created a sensory memory trace. The repetitive stimulation produces a representation of "invariance," which is in contrast, of course, to the variant (deviant) stimulus. Picton, Benton, Berg, et al. (2000) present a rather detailed review of the categories of stimulus invariance that have been employed in MMN measurement. Some of the characteristics of each category of invariance are summarized in Table 14.5. The invariance may consist of a simple difference in some feature of the stimuli (e.g., frequency or duration) or a rather abstract collection of features ("substandards") that are generalized into a single combined standard stimulus complex. As Picton, Benton, Berg, et al. (2000) point out "the distinction between the different kinds of invariance is important from more than a theoretical point of view. The different kinds of invariance need to be represented in different neuronal circuits" (p. 118). As an example, the MMN response can be effectively elicited by differences in the frequency pattern of series of tones (shown in Figure 14.4), as well as a simple frequency difference between the standard and deviant tones. The standard stimulus in this example is repetition of a sequence of three ascending frequencies, whereas the deviant stimulus is a variation in the pattern. Each set of stimuli (standard and deviant) consists of the same number of absolute frequencies (i.e., lower, middle, and higher). The standard and deviant stimuli, however, differ randomly in the pattern with which these three frequencies are presented. Invariance in standard stimuli is represented in this example by the consistent pattern of change in frequency. There are, as summarized in Table 14.5, multiple types of stimulus variation, ranging from simple to quite abstract.

STIMULUS TYPE: SPEECH SIGNALS. | There is abundant experimental and clinical evidence demonstrating that the MMN response can be evoked by different units of speech, including at one extreme acoustic cues within a single speech, and progressing to phonological units (phonemes), larger speech segments (words), and even prosody and the semantic (grammatical) features of speech and language (e.g., D'Arcy et al., 2004; Newman, Connolly, Service, & Mcivor, 2003; Pulvermüller et al., 2001; Shtyrov, Pulvermüller, Näätänen, & Ilmoniemi, 2003; Weber et al., 2004). The MMN is in a class by itself as an objective "preconscious" measure of speech perception and as a technique for studying in humans the neurobiologic mechanisms and processes that take place during speech perception. Earliest investigation of the MMN response evoked by speech stimuli dates back to the late 1980s (Aaltonen, Niemi, Nyrke, & Tukhanen, 1987). One of the

**Standard versus Deviant Stimuli in Measurement
of the Mismatch Negativity (MMN) Response**

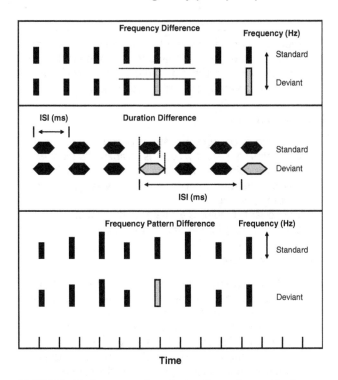

FIGURE 14.4. Examples of stimuli used to evoked the MMN response. The top portion shows a typical frequency stimulus paradigm. The standard stimulus is a repetitive tone of the same frequency (low- or high-frequency difference is represented by the vertical arrow), whereas the deviant stimulus is a randomly presented tone at a higher frequency. The middle portion of the figure depicts the same rather simple type of difference between standard and deviant stimuli for duration, rather than frequency. The deviant stimulus is slightly longer in duration (see vertical dotted lines) than the standard stimulus. Another, perhaps unintended, duration-related difference between the standard and deviant stimuli is the longer interstimulus interval (ISI) for the deviant versus standard stimuli. In the bottom portion of the figure, the pattern of frequency presentation differentiates standard versus deviant stimuli. The subject hears the same frequencies and the same number of each frequency within the train of standard and deviant stimuli, but the temporal pattern for the frequencies is different for the standard versus deviant stimulus.

main findings of the study was the larger MMN amplitude for standard and deviant speech stimuli representing two different phonemes (vowels) in the Finnish language than speech sounds within a single phoneme category. Within a few years, Kraus and colleagues (Kraus et al., 1993a,b) and other researchers (e.g., Csépe, 1995; Maiste et al., 1995; Sams, Aulanko, Aaltonen, & Näätänen, 1990) confirmed and extended these general findings to include MMN recordings

with stimuli that included, in different languages and in children as well as adults, categorical and within-category consonant speech sounds. Differences in the scalp distribution, including hemispheric asymmetries, and stimulus ear differences (e.g., frequency differences elicited larger MMN responses when the stimulus is presented to the left than the right ear) were also demonstrated for speech versus nonspeech stimuli (Csépe, 1995; Jaramillo, Paavilainen, & Näätänen, 2000; Mathiak et al., 2002; Paavilainen et al., 1991). The left hemispheric laterality of the MMN with speech signals appears to be reduced, eliminated, or even reversed (right hemisphere lateralization) when speech stimuli are presented within background noise (Shtyrov et al., 1998)

Kraus and Cheour (2000) cite six advantages of the MMN response as a tool for learning more about neural mechanisms of speech perception. The MMN response is an objective index of memory and the rapidly changing and just noticeable properties of stimuli, and it yields information on corresponding underlying brain function at the neuronal level. The neural activity of the brain generating the MMN response can be modified with experience, learning, and formal training, with corresponding changes in the response.

Differences between categorically distinct speech sounds (e.g., /da/ versus /ga/) are often used in eliciting the MMN response (e.g., Kraus et al., 1992; Kraus et al., 1996; Kraus, McGee, & Koch, 1998; Kraus & Nicol, 2003; Maiste et al., 1995). Persons highly adept at distinguishing behaviorally between /da/ and /ga/ (i.e., "just-perceptibly different variants") yield correspondingly clear MMN responses to the same speech sound differences, whereas no reliable MMN response is detected in "poor /da/-/ga/ perceivers" (Kraus, McGee, & Koch, 1998). Kraus and colleagues have repeatedly demonstrated that children with auditory language learning problems require larger acoustic contrasts between speech sounds for elicitation of the MMN response, a finding of "a biological basis for speech-sound perception deficits" (Kraus, McGee, & Koch, 1998). Clearly, the MMN response in most normal subjects can be evoked by acoustic differences that are close to the psychophysical threshold for detection and can barely be discriminated behaviorally. The MMN response to such stimuli, such as speech sound variations along a continuum from /da/ to /ga/ or /ba/ to /wa/, reflects what is referred to as "fine-grained perceptual discrimination" (Kraus et al., 1999). Interestingly, for a specific change in the stimulus (e.g., a frequency change), the MMN that is generated and its neural generator (Alho et al., 1996) may vary depending on whether the stimulus change is presented in isolation versus within a pattern of sounds, such as a sequence of frequencies or a combination of frequencies (a chord). As noted by Kraus and Cheour (2000), three factors clearly influence the MMN response to speech stimuli: (1) the physical properties, e.g., frequency, duration, intensity and changes in the properties over time; (2) the acoustic context, e.g., the sounds and acoustic conditions surrounding

TABLE 14.5. A Summary of Five Categories of MMN Stimulus Invariance

Invariance is the way that the standard stimuli are similar or grouped together as acoustical information is evaluated and processed by the brain.

Simple Invariance

- The conventional oddball stimulus paradigm.
- All standard stimuli are identical with respect to all acoustic features (e.g., frequency, intensity, same speech sound).
- Deviant stimuli differ from the standard stimuli in one acoustic parameter that can be discriminated behaviorally.
- Example: A simple frequency (pitch) difference between standard (e.g., 1000 Hz) and deviant (1100 Hz) stimuli.

Complex Invariance

- Technically, there are no true "standard" stimuli, as defined above, because the standard stimuli are not identical.
- Some feature is common to all standard stimuli and is identical for each standard stimulus. The deviant stimulus differs from the standard in that one dimension.
- The MMN response reflects a memory trace for the consistent feature within the standard stimuli and is elicited by the deviation from that feature.
- Example: Standard tones consistent of different frequencies and intensities, but only one duration. Deviant stimuli differ from standard stimuli in duration.

Hypercomplex Invariance

- The standard stimuli consist of multiple features and vary in a consistent manner along more than one dimension, perhaps in a pattern or sequence. A particular combination of features (e.g., frequencies, intensities, durations, locations in sound space) is invariant (consistent).
- The deviant stimulus is distinguished from the hypercomplex invariant standard stimuli by differing along

more than one dimension (e.g., the frequency of one of the standards and the duration of another). The pattern of features represented in the deviant stimulus never occurs among the standard stimuli.

Pattern Invariance

- A pattern of changes in features of sounds repeats or alternates consistently, i.e., it is invariant. As many as 8 tones may alternate between two frequencies, intensities, or durations, or even the ISI can vary regularly or in some pattern.
- The deviant stimulus is a change in the pattern of features, or timing, for the standard stimuli.

Abstract Invariance

- Similar to pattern invariance, except that abstract invariance is dependent on relationships among stimulus features rather than on a specific pattern.
- Invariance is not determined by the absolute physical properties or features of the standard stimuli, e.g., a specific frequency or pattern of specific frequencies, but rather some relationship among the standard stimuli.
- An example of abstract invariance used in MMN studies is a decrease in the frequency of tones used as the standard stimulus, where the absolute frequencies are numerous (e.g., up to ten) and are constantly changing. The deviant stimulus might be an increase in the progression of tones or tones that do not change in frequency.
- As noted by Picton et al. (2000) "For abstract invariance, the logic requires the inference of a relationship between stimuli (or between stimulus features) independently of the specific stimuli or features." (p. 118).

Adapted from a description by Picton et al., 2000, pp. 116–118.

---

the speech stimulus; and (3) the perceptual and linguistic experience of the subject.

A speech sound apparently creates a strong memory trace, and clearly generates a larger MMN response when it is from the subject's native language rather than from a foreign language (Näätänen et al., 1997). Differences among languages (native versus foreign) in the MMN response for speech stimuli can be documented within months after birth (Cheour et al., 1998a; Dehaene-Lambertz & Dehaene, 1994).

The MMN response can be elicited with speech stimuli at other points along the complexity and linguistic continuum

in addition to contrasts between speech sounds. For example, there are multiple reports of MMN measurement in children and adults with standard and deviant stimuli consisting of real words and pseudowords in different languages, among them Finnish, English, and French (Korpilahti, Krause, Holopainen, & Lang, 2001; Shtyrov & Pulvermüller, 2002a; Wunderlich & Cone-Wesson, 2001). For example, Pulvermüller et al. (2001) reported that MMN amplitude was larger when evoked by a syllable that completed a real word rather than a pseudoword. Pseudowords are meaningless words that are phonetically equivalent to real words and spoken by the same voice (speaker) as the real words. Typically, one phoneme distinguishes the real versus pseudoword. Words and pseudowords, consisting of equivalent acoustical properties and elements, appear to be equally effective in eliciting the MMN response.

From the foregoing review, it is clear that generation of a MMN response with speech sound stimuli is clinically feasible. However, Dr. Catharine Pettigrew and an international collection of co-authors (Pettigrew et al., 2004a) provide compelling and sobering evidence "that when confounding variables such as acoustic/physical differences between deviant and standard stimuli are appropriately controlled for by the methodology design of the study, MMN responses to fine-grained CV speech stimulus contrasts are not always robust" (p. 63). In this study, simple frequency differences between standard and deviant stimuli elicited an MMN response "significantly different from zero") in from two-thirds to virtually all adult subjects, whereas only 10 percent of the subjects yielded an MMN response for speech stimuli. For example, it was difficult to differentiate with confidence the MMN response evoked by CV syllable contrasts involving voiced plosive sounds (e.g., /d/ versus /g/) from background noise. Other investigators have also described inconsistencies in detecting the MMN response with speech sound contrasts, even though the same speech stimuli were readily identified with accuracy in behavioral tasks (e.g., Dalebout & Stack, 1999; Pettigrew et al., 2004a). The challenges inherent in the careful control of all physical features of speech stimuli in MMN measurement are, of course, greater for naturally spoken versus synthetically or semisynthetically created speech sounds or tokens.

Other measurement variables that must also be taken into account in speech sound MMN investigations include the SOA (stimulus onset asynchrony), i.e., the time interval between consecutive stimuli, MMN measurement with simple versus multiple deviant stimulus paradigms, the possible deleterious influence of backward masking of relatively long duration speech stimuli, and the nature of the distraction task employed during MMN measurement, especially when the task involves possible language processing, such as reading, or a video with subtitles or an audible soundtrack (e.g., Dalebout & Fox, 2000; Pettigrew et al., 2004c; Wunderlich & Cone-Wesson, 2001). The possible influence of subtitles in the silent video used to distract the subject from the acoustic stimuli (i.e., to facilitate the optimal passive listening condition in MMN measurement) is not trivial. As noted earlier in the present chapter, shifting the subject's attention away from the stimuli is important for prevention of unintended and undesirable elicitation of auditory evoked response components (e.g., the N2b or P3a components) that may "contaminate" the MMN and compromise response detection and analysis (e.g., Muller-Gass & Campbell, 2002; Picton et al., 2000). Pettigrew et al. (2004a) found that subtitles on silent videos did not influence the MMN evoked by tonal stimuli, consonant vowel nonwords, and consonant vowel words. Neural mechanisms associated with repetitive

presentation of spectrally complex speech stimuli, including "adaptation and lateral inhibition" (May et al., 1999; Pettigrew et al., 2004b,c) may also play a role in the difficulty of consistently eliciting the MMN response with stimuli consisting of fine grain acoustic differences. The importance in MMN measurement, including the analysis and interpretation of MMN findings and rigorously identifying and controlling with methodological design all acoustic (physical) features for standard and deviant is discussed further in the subsequent section in this chapter on "Analysis and Interpretation."

STIMULUS TYPE: MUSIC. | Uniquely among auditory evoked responses, music is an effective stimulus for eliciting the MMN response. There is almost no limit to the diversity of musical stimuli that can be, and have already been, used in the elicitation of the MMN response including, for example, tones, chords (musical intervals), chord sequences, and even Mozart and Bach melodies (e.g., Lopez et al., 2003). The literature on music and the MMN response is remarkably large and growing rapidly. The application of the MMN response in the study of neuronal mechanisms underlying music perception in musicians and nonmusicians is clearly yielding much basic knowledge about the brain function and, in addition, is of considerable interest to persons on a professional spectrum from the arts to the sciences. Indeed, studies of music, an international language understood and much appreciated by persons around the world, no doubt attract most nonprofessionals as well. The diagnostic value of music-evoked MMN responses in patient populations, however, is not yet documented and may never be. The following review, therefore, will be brief in length and superficial in depth. The reader is referred to original papers cited below and, particularly, to review articles such the one entitled "From Sounds to Music" by Mari Tervaniemi and Elvira Brattico (Tervaniemi & Brattico, 2004), two researchers from among the highly productive group at the Cognitive Brain Research Unit in the Department of Psychology at the University of Helsinki, directed by Dr. Risto Näätänen.

A quote from Tervaniemi and Brattico (2004), in an introduction to the relevance of research on the MMN response (versus other auditory evoked responses) and music puts the importance of and fascination with music into perspective:

> . . . neurophysiological research on late attentive brain responses, though interesting in many aspects, still left it open whether conscious attention towards music is necessary for forming and activating musical neural mechanisms. In other words, it remained unresolved at which neuronal and attentional levels musical percepts and tonal hierarchies are generated. This is a crucial question since the effortless ability to encode and integrate sounds over time, even when we are not focusing our attention and mental resources on them, intuitively enables us to appreciate music. In other words, neural mechanisms underlying preattentive sound processing may trigger the attention switching towards musical events that might be of interest to the listener. (p. 11)

And, commenting on promising research directions for the MMN response and music,

> From a musical perspective it would be of great interest to probe the development of auditory perception by using MMN responses in childhood. For instance, MMN experiments could help disentangling the role of learned knowledge and innate predispositions for our musical preferences. (p. 14)

The relation between behavioral, electrophysiological, and neurometabolic or neuroradiological measures of speech sound and music perception is often described in terms of separate neuronal networks specialized for processing speech versus music (see Tervaniemi & Brattico, 2004; Zatorre & Krumhansl, 2002).

The MMN response is effective not only for evaluating electrophysiologically simple differences in the frequency (pitch) of tones or other basic properties of sounds, but it also reflects preattentive perception of the complex and harmonically rich properties of sound that are inherent in music, e.g., a "multidimensional sound attribute such as timbre" or musical intervals (pitch relations between notes) underlying consonant (tonal) and dissonant (atonal) qualities of music (Brattico et al., 2003; Tervaniemi & Brattico, 2004). As an aside, timbre is defined as the quality of a sound that distinguishes it from another sound, even of the same frequency and intensity. Examples of such features investigated with the MMN response include the direction of pitch change within a sequence of tones and the contour of sound patterns resembling melodies (Saarinen et al., 1992; Tervaniemi et al., 1994b; Tervaniemi, Rytkonen, et al., 2001).

Citing a very limited sample of published findings may whet the readers' interest in the literature on music and the MMN response. A number of studies have confirmed a relationship between MMN response measures of the neural representation of sounds and musical competence and skills of subjects, including professional musicians and nonmusicians and, among musicians, those who play different instruments and even conductors (Munte et al., 2003; Nager et al., 2003a; Tervaniemi & Huotilainen, 2003; van Zuijen et al., 2004). At the extreme, musicians produce a MMN response under certain stimulus conditions (e.g., "good continuation of pitch" or impure chords) when the MMN response for the same musical stimuli is not detected in nonmusicians (Koelsch, Schröger, & Tervaniemi, 1999; van Zuijen et al., 2004). Related to this line of research, plasticity in cortical organization for music is greater in musicians and is related to the length of training and age at which musicians begin to practice (Fujioka et al., 2004; Pantev et al., 2003), but not necessarily by familiarity with the sounds (Neuloh & Curio, 2004). In fact, cortical representations for different notes and timbre as evidenced by the MMN response is even correlated with the instrument played by professional musicians, e.g., violin versus trumpet versus drums (Munte et al., 2003; Pantev et al., 2003). As suggested at the outset of this section, MMN response investigations have been conducted with stimuli representing a variety of musical properties and features, among them timbre, rhythm, and melody (Jongsma, Desain, & Honing, 2004; Lopez et al., 2003; Tervaniemi et al., 2001).

STIMULUS TYPE: OTHER. | The MMN response can be elicited by deviant stimuli that differ from standard stimuli by more than one feature, e.g., duration, frequency, and/or intensity. In general, MMN amplitude is greater for deviant stimuli with multiple differences, in comparison to amplitude for single feature deviants (Kurtzberg, Vaughan, Kruger, & Fliegler, 1995; Levänen, Hari, McEvoy, & Sams, 1993; Schröger, 1994).

DURATION. | As noted elsewhere in the chapter, duration may be the acoustic feature distinguishing standard versus deviant stimuli.

INTENSITY. | MMN responses are typical elicited with stimuli at moderate intensity levels. Intensity may be the acoustic feature distinguishing standard versus deviant stimuli.

STIMULUS REPETITION. | In the conventional MMN measurement paradigm, a series of standard stimuli precede the presentation of a deviant stimulus. Indeed, the sensory memory formed by the standard stimuli is strengthened, and amplitude of the subsequent MMN response to the deviant stimulus enhanced, by increasing the number of standard stimulus repetitions. Jääskeläinen et al. (2004), on the other hand, demonstrate conclusively that the MMN response can (in normal-hearing young adults) be effectively generated during a passive attention state (subjects watched a silent movie) by a deviant stimulus (tones of 1020, 1127, or 1320 Hz) that followed a single standard stimulus (a tone of 1000 Hz). The single standard stimulus condition produced MMN responses that were shorter in latency and smaller in amplitude than those elicited when two to four standard stimuli preceded the deviant stimulus.

It is possible to elicit a MMN response from two deviant stimuli that occur successively. There are, however, conflicting findings on the effect of two successive deviant stimuli on the MMN response. The differences among studies are, at least partly, related to the feature of the deviant stimulus that is manipulated (e.g., frequency, intensity, or duration). Sams, Alho, & Näätänen (1984) reported smaller MMN amplitude for the second of two consecutive and identical deviant stimuli than for the first of the deviant stimuli when frequency was the distinguishing feature. Winkler and Näätänen (1995), however, found no amplitude difference for the second identical deviant stimulus with a duration difference.

In a clever reversal of the typical paradigm for evoking the MMN, some investigators have employed a consistently varying sequence of tones as the standard stimuli and repetition of the tones as the deviant stimuli (e.g., Rosburg, 2004). That is, ironically, a context of permanently varying tones constitutes the invariant (standard) stimulus, and the non-varying repetition of the tone is actually the deviation from the invariance. The generation of a MMN response by a tone repetition, even though it occurs in only about 50 percent of subjects, is a good example of what Näätänen postulated as the "automatic rule extraction" (Näätänen et al., 2001). As described by Rosburg (2004), "These abstract rules govern the relationship between attributes of acoustic events and model not only the immediate auditory past but also extrapolate future events on the basis of extracted rules" (p. 904).

RATE AND INTERSTIMULUS INTERVAL (ISI). | The relation between rate, ISI, and the MMN is more complicated than for other cortical auditory evoked responses. In discussing the effect of rate and ISI on the MMN, one should consider intervals for both the standard and the deviant stimuli. There are really three possible ways of describing the ISI in stimulation of the MMN, i.e., the ISI between standard stimuli, the ISI between deviant stimuli, and the ISI between a standard and a deviant stimulus. Probability of the deviant stimulus is another variable to consider in calculating the effects of rate and ISI on the MMN. The multiple permutations of alterations in ISI in MMN measurement, and the possible effect on the MMN waveform of ISI manipulation, can be readily appreciated. Changing any one of the two stimulus parameters—ISI or probability—for either of the stimuli—standard or deviant—will influence the relationship among them and, in turn, their influence on the MMN. There is another rate and ISI distinction between the MMN and other auditory cortical evoked responses. For other cortical auditory evoked responses, slower stimulus rate and increased ISI enhances amplitude and generally produces desirable changes in the response. For the MMN response, in contrast, increasing stimulus rate and decreasing ISI helps in the identification of the MMN and in differentiating it from other cortical wave components. For example, as ISI is shortened, N1 wave amplitude decreases, while the MMN remains unchanged.

A few generalizations can be made about ISI and the MMN response. MMN amplitude decreases as the interval between the deviant and the preceding standard stimulus increases, at least for simple stimuli (Näätänen, 1992; Näätänen et al., 1987; Ritter et al., 1998). When this interval approaches 10 seconds, there is a possibility that the MMN will not be generated. Presumably, this phenomenon is related to the duration of the sensory memory trace produced by the repetitive standard stimuli. In addition, MMN amplitude increases directly with the ISI. However, an increase in the interval between deviant stimuli introduces probability of the deviant stimulus as a possible factor in the amplitude change.

PROBABILITY. | Among the variables just described—ISI for the standard or deviant stimuli or probability—manipulations of the latter appears to have the most pronounced effect on the MMN response. Amplitude of the MMN is larger

as probability of the deviant stimulus decreases (Javitt, Grochowski, Shelley, & Ritter, 1998) and as the number of standard stimuli preceding the deviant stimulus increases (Sams, Alho, & Näätänen, 1983). More repetitions of the standard stimulus serve to strengthen the memory trace underlying the MMN response.

Acquisition Parameters

ANALYSIS TIME. | A lengthy time window is required for recording the MMN response, just as it is for other cortical event-related responses. MMN latency values for various speech and nonspeech stimuli fall within the region of 100 to 300 ms. To encompass the rather broad wave, analysis times of 500 to 750 ms are commonly used in MMN measurement, with a prestimulus baseline period of 50 to 100 ms. Instrumentation and software currently available for MMN measurement permit adjustment of the poststimulus bioelectrical activity relative to the prestimulus baseline ("baseline adjustment").

ELECTRODES. | Electrode types and location in MMN measurement are similar as those for other cortical evoked responses, e.g., auditory late response (N1 and N2 components) and the P300 response. The electrode composition (metal) should be consistent among all the electrodes, with silver-silver chloride most commonly used in published investigations. Scalp electrode locations in MMN recording are defined in accordance with the 10–20 International system (Jasper, 1958). Studies of the MMN response often employ 21, 30, or even more scalp electrodes, with noninverting and inverting electrodes interconnected on the scalp, or with an inverting electrode(s) on forehead, the earlobes, or each mastoid region. Typical locations for electrodes in MMN measurement with a 32-channel array with an electrode cap (e.g., the Neuroscan Quikcap) according to the 10–20 International Electrode System (Jasper, 1958) include: FP1, FP2; Fpz, Fz, Fcz, F3, F4, F7, F8, FC3, FC4, FT7, FT8, Cz, Cpz, C3, C4, CP3, CP4, TP7, TP8, T5, T6, PZ, P3, P4, and PZ. Earlobe or mastoid electrodes (one on each side) are sometimes linked or "averaged." The MMN response can be recorded, however, with only a few inverting electrodes along the midline (e.g., Fz, Cz, and/or Pz), with inverting electrodes as just noted. To a large extent, MMN has a fronto-central scalp distribution that can be detected adequately with midline electrodes. Some authors (e.g., Lang et al., 1995), however, cite diagnostic value in MMN recordings from lateral electrodes (off the midline), with recommendations for at least seven noninverting electrode sites (e.g., Cz, C3, C4, Fz, F3, F4, and Fpz). Different locations (e.g., Fpz on forehead) are used for the ground (common) electrode. There are also mandatory electrodes located around the eyes (above and below and at each side of one eye) to detect horizontal and vertical eye movement during blinking.

As noted elsewhere in the present chapter, it is often challenging in MMN measurement to obtain a favorable signal-to-noise ratio due to the modest amplitude of the MMN wave and the rather high level of background electrical noise. Careful selection of electrode sites may have a positive influence the SNR in MMN measurement. As noted by Sinkkonen and Tervaniemi (2000), "Traditionally, the electrode locations are chosen on the basis of the signal amplitude rather than the SNR. These two goals are not necessarily equal, for electrodes close to each other share, roughly speaking, a larger amount of common noise than electrodes further apart" (p. 240). "For some non-conventional electrode locations, this reduction in noise may well exceed the reduction in the signal amplitude, thereby leading to improved SNR" (p. 240).

FILTER SETTINGS. | Filtering out unwanted and meaningless electrical activity that has spectral characteristics dissimilar from the response is an immediate and effective step toward enhancing the signal-to-noise ratio in MMN measurement, just as it is with other auditory evoked responses. Filtering optimally eliminates energy at frequencies below and above the spectrum of the MMN response. Methodology described in most published studies of the MMN response over the years includes a reference to band-pass filter settings of 0.1 to 30 Hz. However, the first question to be asked in selecting the *optimal* filter settings for MMN measurement is, of course, where is most of the MMN energy in the frequency domain, i.e., what is the spectrum of the MMN? MMN energy is, as one might intuitively suspect from a cursory inspection of the extended latency slow negative MMN difference wave, limited to very low frequencies—within the 2 to 5 Hz region.

The spectrum of the MMN response, therefore, is dominated by lower frequencies than other cortical auditory evoked responses. It would be reasonable, then, to adapt the filter settings for MMN measurement to these spectral characteristics. Nonetheless, the same band-pass filter settings that are used in recording auditory late responses (e.g., N1 and P2 waves) and the P300 response, namely, about 0.1 to 30 Hz, are typically employed in MMN measurement. There is some evidence that a more restricted band-pass filter region is useful in minimizing unwanted electrical activity and improving the signal-to-noise ratio in MMN measurement (e.g., Tervaniemi et al., 1999). The concomitant distortion of other cortical auditory evoked responses associated with the limited band-pass filtering poses no concern for MMN recording and, in fact, might help with differentiating the MMN from other wave complexes.

AVERAGING. | The concepts of signal averaging reviewed in Chapter 3 and for other auditory evoked responses throughout the book apply as well to measurement of the MMN. In terms of the MMN response, the signal-to-noise ratio is the magnitude of the MMN amplitude divided by the amount of noise during measurement. Remember, the noise level in an evoked response recording is inversely proportional to the square root of the number of samples (stimulus repetitions or sweeps). This statement assumes that the MMN is a constant signal tightly time-locked to the stimulus, and the noise is invariant, stationary, and equivalent (a stochastic process) across sweeps. Another assumption, often not considered, is that an amplifier itself is not the source of some measurement noise. This assumption is, of course, rarely tested and probably rarely valid. A reasonable and common approach for enhancing the signal-to-noise ratio of an evoked response is to increase the number of stimulus repetitions (sweeps). Signal averaging for a sufficient number of standard stimuli does not present a problem, given the relatively short ISI and the essential constant presentation of standard stimuli. The challenge is to perform adequate signal averaging for the waveform evoked by the deviant stimuli without overly prolonging test time. With the MMN response, there is an inevitable trade-off between conducting sufficient signal averaging and a clinically feasible test period. One obvious strategy to achieve this goal would be to reduce the interval between deviant stimuli, permitting presentation of more stimuli (and more signal averaging) within the same time frame. Unfortunately, increasing the rate of deviant stimulus presentation (reducing ISI) has the predictable effect of reducing MMN amplitude. This, of course, results in a smaller signal-to-noise ratio and, counterproductively, the need to continue with more signal averaging with no time savings or even a prolongation in test time. During averaging, the ongoing EEG for the relatively leisurely MMN wave can be sampled at a relatively slow rate (e.g., 40 Hz or 100 Hz), although much faster sampling rates (e.g., 1000 Hz) are often used along with analog-to-digital (A/D) conversion of minimally 10 to 12 bits. Finally, after completion of online real-time MMN response data collection, the waveform for single sweeps may be "baseline corrected" relative to the prestimulus period and then processed with an algorithm for automatically rejecting artifact. Very low-frequency "noise" from the EEG contributes to a shift or drift in the averaged waveform. The noise may be removed by selective high-pass filtering within the frequency region of, for example, 0.01 to 0.2 Hz. Also, before response analysis, the sweeps remaining (after those with artifacts are removed) are further corrected for contamination by eye blink artifact, and then waveforms are averaged separately for the standard and the deviant stimuli. In short, current averaging and signal processing techniques fail to yield the robust SNR for the MMN required for its confident detection and application clinically in the diagnosis of diseases and disorders affecting auditory processing (e.g., Cacace & McFarland, 2003).

Test Protocol for Measurement of the MMN Response

A starting point for a test protocol for MMN measurement is displayed in Table 14.6. Most parameters are selected on

TABLE 14.6.   Guidelines for an Auditory Mismatch Negativity (MMN) Response Test Protocol

PARAMETER	SUGGESTION	RATIONALE/COMMENT
Stimulus Parameters		
Transducer	ER-3A	Supra-aural earphones are acceptable for MMN measurement, but insert earphones are more comfortable for longer AER recording sessions. Insert earphones also serve to attenuate background sound in the test setting. In addition, since the insert cushions are disposable, their use contributes to infection control.
Type	Tone	A variety of differences between standard and deviant tonal stimuli are effective for evoking a MMN response, including frequency, intensity, duration, source in space. Differences in the patterns of some feature of tones, e.g., frequency, also are used in MMN measurement.
	Speech	The MMN response can be effectively elicited with speech signals (natural or synthetic), such as /da/ and /pa/. Various characteristics of speech signals, e.g., voice onset time, can be used in MMN stimulation.
Duration		
Rise/fall	~10 ms	Longer onset times are feasible for signals used to elicit the MMN response. As noted below, the distinction between standard and deviant stimuli may be a duration difference.
Plateau	~50 ms	Extended plateau durations are effective in eliciting the MMN response. See comment above about duration as a distinction between the frequent versus rare signals.
Rate	≤1.1/second	A relatively slow rate of signal presentation is important in measuring the MMN response, but extended intervals between successive deviant stimuli (e.g., 10 seconds or longer) are associated with a reduction in or even absence of MMN activity.
Oddball signal paradigm		With MMN response measurement, there are invariably at least two stimuli, each different and each generating a response. The *standard* stimulus, presented at regular and predictable intervals, evokes a conventional late response waveform. The *deviant* stimulus is presented unpredictably (in a pseudorandom manner) usually with a probability of occurrence of about 0.05 to 0.2 (5 to 20 percent probability).
Signal difference		The distinction between standard and deviant signals may involve various features of sound, including frequency (e.g., 1000 Hz versus 1100 Hz), intensity, or duration. Relatively small (fine grain) differences are optimal for MMN measurement. This is in contrast to guidelines for P300 measurement that call for larger differences between frequent and target stimuli. Features of the sound other than the feature distinction are usually the same for the sound. That is, if the standard versus deviant distinction is a frequency difference, the intensity and duration of the two types of signals are the same.
Probability		The probability of signal presentation is, typically, 100 percent for the standard stimuli and from 5 to 20 percent for the deviant stimuli, but many variations in stimulus probability are possible. A probability of 10 percent for the deviant stimulus is commonly reported. The presentation of the deviant stimuli is actually pseudorandom, rather than truly random. There are at least two constraints for stimuli presentation. The deviant stimuli cannot be presented as the first stimuli as averaging of an MMN response begins. Also, two deviant stimuli cannot occur in succession, i.e., there must always be one or more standard stimuli presented between any two deviant stimuli.
Number		Since the probability of the deviant stimulus presentation is typically 5 to 20 percent (one in five signals is rare), the MMN response is recorded with relatively few deviant stimulus presentations (as few as 20 or less). The appropriate number of stimulus depends largely on the amount of averaging necessary to achieve an adequate signal-to-noise ratio.

(continued)

TABLE 14.6. (continued)

PARAMETER	SUGGESTION	RATIONALE/COMMENT
Polarity	Rarefaction	Stimulus polarity is not an important parameter for MMN measurement.
Intensity	≤70 dB HL	Modest stimulus intensity levels are typical for MMN measurement. As noted above, the distinction between standard and deviant stimuli may be an intensity difference.
		Remember the signal-to-noise ratio is the key. Averaging may require as few as 20 to 50 stimuli at high intensity levels for a very quiet and normal-hearing patient.
Presentation ear	Monaural	Monaural or binaural stimuli can be used for measurement of the MMN response.
Masking	50 dB	Masking is rarely required with insert earphones and not needed for a stimulus intensity level of ≤70 dB HL.
Acquisition Parameters		
Amplification	50,000	Less amplification is required for larger responses.
Sensitivity	25 or 50 μvolts	Smaller sensitivity values are equivalent to higher amplification.
Analysis time	600 ms	Analysis epoch (time) must be long enough to encompass the broad MMN wave (and difference wave) and the auditory late response to the standard stimuli and the MMN response to the standard stimuli.
Prestimulus time	100 ms	Extended prestimulus time provides a stable estimate of background noise and a baseline for calculation of the amplitudes for the negative MMN wave.
Data points	≤512	
Sweeps	<500	See comments above for signal number.
Filters		
Band-pass	0.1 to 30 Hz	The MMN response consists of low-frequency energy (as low as 50 to 10 Hz) within the spectrum of the EEG. Even more restricted band-pass filter settings (0.1 to 20 Hz) might enhance the signal-to-noise ratio (Picton et al., 2000).
Notch	None	A notch filter (removing spectral energy in the region of 60 Hz) should be consistently avoided with MNN response measurement because important frequencies in the response will be removed.
Electrodes		
Type	Disc or disposable	Disc electrodes applied with adhesive paste (versus gel) are useful to secure the noninverting electrodes on the scalp. Disposable electrodes or a multiple-electrode cap are also appropriate with MMN response measurement.
Electrode sites	Noninverting	The Fz, Cz, and/or Pz sites are appropriate for recording clinically the MMN response, because it is prominent for the frontal and central scalp electrode locations. However, many published studies include twenty or more electrode sites (as many as 128). With most measurement conditions and patient populations, MMN response amplitude may be maximum at the fronto-central (Fz) site.
	Inverting	Linked earlobes are commonly used for inverting electrodes. Noncephalic (e.g., nape of the neck) or nose (tip) site inverting electrode sites have also been reported.
	Other	Ocular electrodes (located above and below or to the side of an eye) are required for detection of eye blinks, and rejection of averages contaminated by eye blinking.
Ground	Fpz	A common (ground) electrode can be located anywhere on the body, but a location low on the forehead or at the nasion (between the eyes) location is convenient and effective.

the basis of evidence produced by published laboratory or clinical investigations. Some, like electrodes and filter settings, are quite straightforward and consistent among most investigations. A practical problem with outlining a clinically feasible test protocol for the MMN response is what parameter(s) to list for the stimuli. As emphasized elsewhere in this chapter, there are myriad stimulus options for MMN measurement that include simple and single properties of sound (e.g., frequency, duration, and intensity), missed deviant stimulus elements, combinations of these properties, speech stimuli, music stimuli, temporal and spectral patterns for multiple stimuli, and two or more rather abstract collections of sound that form an overall acoustic impression ("gestalt") that differs in some way from others.

Sinkkonen and Tervaniemi (2000) identified in a critical examination of current MMN methodology important "conceptual and practical issues" that need to be addressed for "optimal recording and analysis of the mismatch negativity" response. Their MMN measurement paradigm is reviewed briefly here and in the following section on MMN analysis. The authors define "optimality" of MMN measurement in terms of the combination of costs (e.g., any discomfort to the patient and the actual cost of the equipment and professional time and effort in performing the procedure) and benefits (what is learned about the patient). MMN variables that must be considered in describing the optimal recording paradigm include, of course, test performance factors (reliability of the response, including inter- and intra-subject variability), the signal-to-noise ratio (SNR), and the ability to discriminate or differentiate between two or more groups (normal versus pathology or pathologies). A parallel set of variables play an important role in optimizing MMN analysis.

Consideration of the complexity and interactive nature of stimulus parameters in the measurement of the MMN response cannot be avoided. However, the MMN response has for many years been successfully recorded with standard and deviant stimuli that differ in a relatively simple feature, such as frequency or duration. For example, a MMN response can be elicited with a standard stimulus of 1000 Hz and deviant stimuli of 1100 Hz, with other measurement parameters as summarized in Table 14.6. Can a clinician with instrumentation for recording the P300 response also perform MMN response measurement? The P300 software permits generation of two separate stimuli, that is, frequent and rare for P300 measurement and standard and deviant for MMN measurement, with different probabilities for presentation of each. Unfortunately, stimulus options are quite limited for the P300 software marketed with most commercially available evoked response systems. For example, tonal stimulus choices are usually limited to octave frequencies with a few interoctave frequencies, precluding selection of standard and deviant stimuli that differ only slightly in frequency. As detailed in the introduction to this chapter, small or fine differences in features between standard and deviant stimuli are important

for minimizing contamination of the MMN response identification with other auditory evoked response components (e.g., the N1 or P300 waves). With P300 software, it's also possible to record two separate waveforms, one evoked by the standard and the other by the deviant stimuli and to then derive a difference wave by digitally subtracting the standard waveform from the deviant waveform.

So, why can't an evoked response system with the P300 option be used as a diagnostic tool in recording and analyzing the MMN response from patients in clinical settings? At least five auditory evoked response design challenges must be addressed before the MMN response can be confidently measured, analyzed, and ultimately applied routinely for neurodiagnostic purposes in a typical clinical setting by nonexperts in the MMN. First, instrumentation must include multiple and sophisticated options for stimuli, including the capacity for, and flexibility in, selecting virtually any tone frequency or tone frequencies for both the standard and deviant stimuli, as well as a wide array of selections for nontonal stimuli, e.g., synthetic speech sounds, combinations and patterns of tones, and other stimuli that are effective for elicitation of the MMN response and have proven diagnostic value. Second, evidence-based guidelines for the clinician are needed for each MMN test parameter, but especially for all aspects of the stimuli used in evoking the MMN response and for the number and location of scalps electrodes used in detecting the MMN response. Third, MMN recording techniques must employed that consistently produce an MMN wave in normal subjects and, particularly, a negative wave that can be reliably distinguished from background electrical noise. That is, MMN recordings in a clinical setting with actual patients must routinely be characterized by an adequate SNR. Fourth, to be clinically feasible, it is essential for MMN test protocols to yield interpretable results within an acceptable time frame. Finally, clinical application of the MMN response requires the availability on commercial evoked response systems of user friendly, yet statistically rigorous, algorithms for MMN analysis, with software developed with evidence on efficacy from laboratory research. For routine clinical use of the MMN response, the clinician must have confidence in the accuracy of MMN detection and the probability that the response for an individual patient is normal or abnormal.

Several recent papers by Näätänen and colleagues (Näätänen, Pakarinen, Rinne, & Takegata, 2004; Takegata, Roggia, & Näätänen, 2003) present guidelines for the development of an efficient, effective, and possibly clinically feasible MMN test protocol. The overall strategy, explored also by other investigators (Deacon et al., 1998; Levänen et al., 1996), is to include more than one type of standard-deviant difference within a sequence of stimuli. Näätänen and colleagues (2004) articulated the rationale for their work relative to research to date as follows: "One practical problem in these MMN studies is, however, their relatively long duration when more than just one type of MMN is to obtained.

Each type of MMN is usually recorded in a separate block in order to rule out any contamination that might occur when several types of deviants are presented in the same stimulus block" (p. 141). In other words, an MMN measurement session totaling an hour or more is required to record responses separately for different variations of differences between the standard and deviant stimuli, e.g., various sizes of frequency difference, plus the same sequence of MMN recordings for other distinctions between standard and deviant stimuli, such as duration, intensity, sound-source location, or temporal manipulations of stimuli. In their study of fourteen normal adult subjects, Näätänen and colleagues (2004) evaluated the test time and quality of MMN findings for three sets of stimulus conditions. One stimulus condition was the conventional oddball condition paradigm in which each standard versus deviant feature was applied in eliciting the MMN response in sequential measurement blocks (three 5-minute sequences for five different stimulus features). Total recording time for the conventional oddball condition was 75 minutes. In one of the other conditions (the most efficient), the five types of deviant stimuli (D1 = frequency, D2 = duration, D3 = intensity, D4 = perceived sound source, and D5 = a gap within a tone) were presented in a single sequence. Uniquely, in each sequence the first fifteen tones were standards, and then every other tone was alternately either a standard stimulus or one of the five types of deviant stimuli. Stimulus onset asynchrony (interval) was 500 ms. Total recording time for this "optimum–1 condition" was only 15 minutes. MMN response latencies and amplitudes were equivalent for "optimum–1" and conventional sequential oddball stimulus conditions. The authors conclude by stating, "we propose a new paradigm (Optimum-1) in which every other tone is a standard and every other a deviant. . . . the proposed paradigm might, for instance, enable one to form multi-attribute 'profiles' of a subject or patient's sound-discrimination abilities and their abnormalities in a time short enough to avoid vigilance, motivational, and other problems associated with too long recording conditions" (p. 143).

In a follow up study, Takegata, Roggia, and Näätänen (2003) reported another approach for minimizing MMN test time without sacrificing quality of the responses. Essentially, the MMN response was measured in a group of ten normal young (Finnish) adults with speech stimuli (phonetic changes reflecting either voicing or place of articulation) presented to the right ear and tone stimuli (standard of 1000 Hz and deviant of 1100 Hz) presented simultaneously to the left ear. The MMN responses for both ears and types of stimuli were recorded in parallel. Although MMN response amplitude was somewhat smaller for the parallel recording approach, the overall outcome was comparable for the conventional separate recording versus the parallel recording and confirmed the feasibility of combined and time-efficient MMN measurement for phonetic and acoustic stimulus changes.

For full exploitation of the MMN response clinically, a simple, single-stimulus paradigm is not desirable, even if it were to yield a robust response and optimum test performance in normal subjects or select patient populations. Indeed, evaluation of different perceptual abilities or cognitive functions or increasing MMN sensitivity to various disorders or pathologies is dependent on varying stimulus conditions. The selection of specific stimulus conditions, e.g., the type of deviant stimulus, and systematic manipulation of critical stimulus parameters, e.g., ISI, is and should be made a priori, that is, before measurement depending on the objectives of the MMN assessment and accumulated clinical experience with the patient disorder of interest. As a rule, stimulus parameters are employed that minimize the likelihood of recording a wave, or waves (e.g., N1, P3, N2) other than the MMN that may contaminate detection or analysis of the MMN. Unfortunately, a tradeoff or a conflict enters into decisions about stimulus parameters, and the tester must settle on a compromise. For example, the same set of stimulus characteristics that produce a robust MMN also increases the chances of recording an overlapping component of another response, with possible contamination of the MMN response. An example of a fundamental, and common, tradeoff in selecting stimulus parameters in MMN measurement involves the relation between stimulus probability and the SNR. Decreasing the probability of the deviant stimulus—making the deviant stimulus more rare—invariably increases the size of the MMN response. Specifically, "the size of the mismatch response is directly proportional to the logarithm of the stimulus probability" (Sinkkonen & Tervaniemi, 2000, p. 239). On the other hand, averaging the response for fewer deviant stimuli (less signal averaging) will almost always increase noise in the recording (smaller SNR). If the probability of the deviant stimuli is decreased (to generate a larger MMN response) and the number of deviant signals presented is increased (for more signal averaging and a more robust SNR), then the inevitable tradeoff is lengthened test time and, perhaps, a methodology that is clinically not feasible in some patient populations or clinical settings. Contributing more complexity to the design or implementation of MMN test protocols, an "MMN additivity phenomenon" may occur when deviant stimuli are different from the standard stimuli along more than one dimension (e.g., frequency, intensity, duration) or, to use a term stated by Sinkkonen and Tervaniemi (2000) there are "simultaneous deviances" or "complex deviance types."

The effect of subject attention on the MMN response is discussed below in the section on nonpathologic factors. A word on the topic, however, is required in the review of an appropriate test protocol for clinical measurement of the MMN response. Defining precisely the subject's task during MMN measurement is an essential part of the test protocol and should be fully described in MMN methodology, along with stimulus and acquisition parameters. Accumulated experience as reported in the literature supports the practice of formal procedures for directing the subject's attention away from the stimuli during MMN measurement to achieve a passive listening condition. Non-MMN auditory evoked responses are minimized when the subject's attention is directed away from the stimuli, thus reducing the possibility of contamination of the MMN and increasing confident identification of the MMN. Pettigrew et al. (2004a) present a brief but comprehensive summary of investigations of various "distractor tasks" and techniques, including videos with and without sound tracks, videos with subtitles, reading books, and playing video games. The goal is to minimize the likelihood of recording an auditory evoked response that is attention-dependent, e.g., N2b or the P3 components. Minimally, the subject should be engaged in an interesting nonauditory activity, such as reading interesting printed material or watching a video. A reading task, while minimizing subject attention to the stimuli, may introduce eye movements that interfere with confident detection and analysis of the MMN wave.

The preferred technique for drawing the subject's attention away from the stimuli is reliance on videos and movies with the sound track either muted or at a low volume level. The mere presence of low-intensity dialog and music from the video will not affect MMN recording when the stimuli are at a moderate intensity level because the background sound is random relative to the standard and the deviant stimuli. According to Lang et al. (1995), requiring the subject to watch a video during MMN measurement has the additional benefit of lowering slow electrical activity, including alpha rhythm, in averaging the waveform. However, more recent investigations provide evidence that audible video and other auditory attention tasks may have a deleterious influence on MMN amplitude and reliability (e.g., Dittman-Balcar, Thienel, & Schall, 1999; McArthur, Bishop, & Proudfoot, 2003; Müller et al., 2002). Of course, effective distractor tasks should not also introduce other variables in MMN measurement, such as the effects of visual processing (e.g., during book reading or with video subtitles), audibility of the sound track for a video distractor, and language-based distractor strategies. Dichotic listening tasks, or tasks involving visual discrimination, offer more rigorous control over attention. The dichotic task was used in the initial paper on the MMN response (Näätänen, Gaillard, & Mäntysalo, 1978). With the dichotic task, different deviant signals are presented to each ear, and the subject attends to the stimuli for one ear. The response evoked by the stimuli presented to the attended ear will typically consist of an N2 wave and a P3 wave, as well as the MMN response, whereas the response evoked by deviant stimuli for the unattended ear will be limited to the MMN response. Implementation of the dichotic stimulus paradigm, however, is more challenging for the tester and not feasible with children or in some adult patient populations.

ANALYSIS AND INTERPRETATION

The MMN response can be detected with visual inspection of the difference waveform, produced by subtracting the waveform elicited by the standard stimulus from the waveform elicited by the deviant stimulus. However, given the relatively small amplitude of the MMN negative wave, more comprehensive, objective, and quantitative analysis approaches are advisable. One rather straightforward and clinically feasible technique is computation of the area of the MMN response (e.g., Dalebout & Fox, 2001; McGee, Kraus, & Nicol, 1997; Sharma et al., 2004). The "area under the curve" of the deviant minus standard difference waveform (actually the area over the curve for the negative wave) is calculated in μV and then analyzed with respect to an established normative criterion (e.g., 100 to 225 μV) for an appropriate measurement protocol, that is, same stimulus contrast. Ponton, Don, Eggermont, and Kwong (1997) suggested another quantitative MMN response analysis strategy, the "integral distribution technique." Many subaverages of the MMN response for an individual subject are collected. The distribution of these responses is defined and then the integrated deviant responses are evaluated in the context of the integrated standard responses.

Derivation of the MMN Waveform

The conventional approach for derivation of the MMN waveform—the difference waveform—is to subtract the response evoked separately by the standard stimuli from the response evoked by the deviant stimuli. The general subtraction of one waveform from another is sometimes subject to certain qualifications or constraints. For example, the composite response for the standard stimuli and the composite response for the deviant stimuli may not be utilized in the derivation process. Rather, the MMN "subtraction curve" may be derived by the subtraction of the response to the standard stimulus that immediately precedes the deviant stimulus from the response evoked by the deviant stimulus. Or the responses to the initial stimuli presented (e.g., the first ten) are not included in the averaged waveform to minimize the effects of the beginning of stimulation on the auditory evoked response components, such as alterations in the amplitude of the N1 component (e.g., Lavikainen, Tiitinen, May, & Näätänen, 1997; Pekkonen et al., 1995). Other routine manipulations of the MMN data before completion of data analysis include exclusion of eye blink artifacts, baseline correction with reference to the prestimulus portion of the waveform, or a secondary referencing process to the inverting electrodes. With the conventional approach for derivation of the MMN response with a subtraction process, portions of the auditory evoked response elicited by both types of stimuli, e.g., the N1 and P2 waves of the ALR, are minimized. Unless care is taken to record responses for a fixed and equal number of standard and deviant stimuli, the response evoked by deviant stimuli will involve considerably fewer sweeps than the response evoked by standard stimuli. Under most measurement conditions, derivation of the MMN waveform from the difference between two averaged waveforms introduces additional noise into the MMN and may decrease the signal-to-noise ratio (SNR).

Another process for derivation of the MMN response—the difference waveform—requires an additional step. Waveforms are averaged separately in the typical oddball paradigm for standard and deviant stimuli. In addition, a response is evoked by a sequence of a specific number of just deviant stimuli—the deviant-alone condition. The waveform averaged in the deviant-alone condition is then subtracted from the response evoked by deviant stimuli in the oddball paradigm, i.e., the conventional difference waveform just described above. Grand average MMN waveforms are then analyzed under the different measurement conditions.

MMN Reliability

The importance of MMN reliability to its value as an electrophysiological measure for the diagnosis of disorders is well appreciated, but clear and consistent information on the reliability of the MMN response in various clinical applications and populations is scarce. Picton et al. (2000) offer a straightforward description of reliability as "the closeness of multiple measurement in a particular subject in a particular state" (p. 132). Test–retest reliability of the MMN response has been modeled mathematically and statistically, with a "semi-experimental heuristic approach, utilizing both small experiments and the available knowledge of the properties of the different paradigms" (Sinkkonen & Tervaniemi, 2000, p. 245). Experimental findings are varied on MMN reliability, with correlation coefficients ranging from below 0.50 to 0.78 (e.g., Frodl-Bauch, Kathmann, Moller, & Hegerl, 1997; Joutsiniemi et al., 1998; Kathmann, Frodl-Bauch, & Hegerl, 1999; Pekkonen et al., 1995; Tervaniemi et al., 1999). In general, published data on reliability of the MMN response as measured in clinical settings are based on small numbers of patients and are rather discouraging. The reliability of the MMN response and its stability over time remain a concern in clinical populations (e.g., Cacace & McFarland, 2003; Pekonnen, Rinne, & Näätänen, 1995). According to some authors (e.g., Dalebout & Fox, 2001; Wunderlich & Cone-Wesson, 2001), the MMN response is, under certain stimulus conditions, not detectable for the majority of normal adult subjects, even when the difference between standard and deviant stimuli can be reliably discriminated behaviorally. Clearly, the signal-to-noise ratio in MMN recordings is a major factor in reliability of the response, with test-retest variability increasing indirectly with the signal-to-noise ratio from one recording run to the next. The SNR, of course, will change with the size of the MMN itself and the amount of background electrical noise (EEG and also various sources of artifact). The detectability and reliability of the MMN response is markedly influenced by fluctuations in the SNR. Serious efforts to develop optimal, or at the least improved, stimulating and recording conditions, test protocols, analysis strategies, and statistic treatment approaches in measurement of the MMN response have been underway for over ten years (e.g., Kurtzberg et al., 1995).

Reasonably high test–retest reliability (intrasubject variance), although essential for clinical application of the MMN response, is not the only aspect of test performance that must be considered in determining the diagnostic value of the response. The ability of the MMN to categorize an individual patient as normal or abnormal, or to differentiate an individual patient with one disorder from patients with other disorders is also critical for confident clinical application of the response. Exact and positive data on the sensitivity and specificity of the MMN in various clinical populations is not plentiful, as suggested below in the review of MMN in different disorders.

Waveform Analysis

For at least six reasons, confident detection of the MMN is considerably more challenging than identification of other cortical auditory evoked responses. First, the response is relatively small in amplitude (only 1 or 2 μvolts), in comparison to other cortical auditory evoked responses (sometimes 10 μvolts or greater), whereas background bioelectric noise is substantial. Second, the process of subtracting the standard waveform from the deviant waveform contributes noise to the MMN difference waveform. Typically, background noise is greater for the deviant waveform than for the standard waveform as the latter is averaged from more stimulus repetitions. Indeed, overall noise in the MMN response can be decreased modestly by increasing the number of standard stimuli, rather than attempting to adjust the number of standard stimuli closer to the number of deviant stimuli. However, as the MMN difference waveform is calculated, noise from the waveform evoked by the standard stimuli is compounded with noise from the deviant waveform. In combination, these two features of the MMN response measurement (smaller amplitude and greater noise) result in an inherently smaller signal-to-noise ratio (SNR). Third, due to the infrequent presentation of deviant stimuli, the MMN is typically averaged for a small number of trials or stimulus repetitions. By virtue of the fundamental MMN paradigm (establishing a memory trace with repetitions of the standard stimulus), the number of standard stimuli always greatly exceeds the number of deviant stimuli. Fourth, the MMN wave is not characterized by a repeatable and distinct peak or trough within a restricted latency region but, rather, a broad slightly negative deflection in the waveform that continues over an extended latency region of 100 ms or more. Other auditory evoked responses, including cortical waves (e.g., N1, P2, N2, P3), can usually be identified by visual inspection because there is a clear, repeatable, and often very pronounced peak or trough, in a specified and predictable latency range and with an absolute voltage value above (positive voltage) or below (negative voltage) a baseline and with a relative voltage that is the opposite of the preceding or following peak or trough. For example, the N1 is a reliable and rather sharp negative deflection from the baseline, whereas the P2 is a positive deflection with the same characteristics. The MMN response, however, is not consistently time locked or stationary relative to the stimulus (Cacace & McFarland, 2003). Fifth, the absolute amplitude of the MMN response is not always constant during a prolonged recording session or from one recording session to the next. Instead, the MMN response may decrease during a lengthy recording period (e.g., Lang et al., 1995) and, on the other hand, increase in amplitude within a recording session with transitions from one block of stimuli to another block of stimuli (Baldeweg et al., 1999). And, finally, response reliability in normal subjects and, particularly, patient populations is generally lower for the MMN in comparison to other cortical auditory evoked responses. The overall objective for MMN analysis is to verify the presence of a neurophysiological response within a background of electrical noise. The first step in achieving the goal is to enhance the SNR by maximizing the signal (the MMN wave) within the constraints of the appropriate stimulus conditions and by minimizing all other electrical activity (noise). Generic strategies for reducing noise in measurement of any auditory evoked response are useful, of course, for MMN measurement. The two most effective approaches—filtering and averaging—were discussed in the preceding section on test protocol (acquisition parameters). The following analysis techniques offer different approaches for meeting with the MMN response this basic objective—enhancing response detection.

VISUAL INSPECTION OF DIFFERENCE WAVEFORM. | Old-fashioned and simplistic visual inspection of replicated averaged waveforms, coupled with manual calculations of latency and/or amplitude of major waves, is a time-tested analysis approach for some auditory evoked responses, among them ECochG, ABR, and the AMLR. Manual calculation of the values for various parameters of the MMN response has been, and can be, performed in the same general fashion. It is important to include more than a single parameter in MMN analysis, since different neural generators appear to be represented by different parameters (e.g., latency, amplitude and duration of the MMN response). As shown in Figure 14.5, MMN latency is defined from the onset of the deviant stimulus to the beginning of the negative trough that constitutes the MMN wave. Amplitude analysis is a little more challenging because during MMN measurement there are often drifts or variations from one sweep or run to the next in the absolute voltages of the waveform. The problem, therefore, is how to define the baseline or reference for calculation of the maximum MMN amplitude. Two other MMN response parameters subject to visual analysis are the rise time of the negative wave (the time from the onset to the peak in ms) and the total duration of the wave (from the onset to the offset). Calculation of each of these response parameters is also

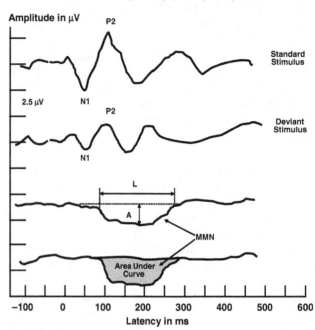

FIGURE 14.5. Schematic summary of some techniques used for analysis of the MMN response following visual inspection.

shown schematically in Figure 14.5. The above-noted MMN response calculations appear to be rather straightforward when reviewed in theory, but confident analysis of the MMN response parameters by visual inspection is not always possible in practice. Unlike other auditory evoked responses, the MMN waveform is characterized not by sharp and highly repeatable peaks and troughs but, rather, a single broad negative wave within the latency region of 100 to 300 ms. Variations in measurement noise can masquerade as negative peaks, and the presence of noise can obscure detection of the real MMN wave. In addition, as noted in a preceding section of this chapter, less than optimum or generally poor intrasubject reliability from one block, run, or session to the next, and considerable intersubject variations in the patterns of MMN waves, particularly amplitude, contribute to the difficulty in analysis by visual inspection. Further complicating analysis of the MMN response performed with visual inspection of the waveform are the somewhat unpredictable effects on the waveform of the subject's state of attention, age, and perhaps even the disorder to be diagnosed.

It is safe, therefore, to conclude that visual inspection is inadequate as the sole technique for analysis of the MMN response. The lack of a distinct and sharp peak or trough certainly limits the usefulness of visual analysis and calculations of peak latency or amplitude. Normal latency values for the MMN response are more variable than for the aforementioned auditory evoked responses, and the duration of the MMN wave is considerably more elongated. There is often no clear and consistent "local minimum or maximum" voltage within the MMN waveform. Measurement parameters, such as signal averaging and filtering (and filtering biases), can exert marked effects on MMN latency, amplitude, and other response characteristics, such as zero (0 voltage) crossings that are incorporated into visual inspection decisions. Several analysis strategies applied with the MMN response are reviewed next. There is, however, no consensus on the best approach for MMN analysis clinically nor much data on the relative accuracy of these techniques.

Beginning with the first report of the MMN response (Näätänen, Gaillard, & Mäntysalo, 1978), calculation of a difference waveform by subtracting the standard waveform from the deviant waveform is a conventional step in MMN measurement and analysis. The rationale for the difference wave is to remove from the MMN waveform those components evoked by both standard and deviant (versus only the deviant) stimuli and common to both waveforms. The subtraction approach is also based on the assumption that non-MMN components, e.g., N1, are not influenced by the acoustic differences between standard and deviant stimuli. That is, all of the acoustic (physical) features differentiated the standard and deviant stimuli are recognized and accounted for in the MMN measurement paradigm, and the deviant stimuli exclusively affect generation of the MMN and not other auditory evoked response components (e.g., N1). For simple stimuli, for example, pure-tone sounds, a small frequency difference between the standard and deviant stimuli, accounting for the acoustic features of the stimuli is straightforward and complete. For complex sound stimuli, however, the assumption is not necessarily valid (e.g., Pettigrew et al., 2004b; Schröger & Wolff, 1998; Shtyrov & Pulvermüller, 2002b; Wunderlich & Cone-Wesson, 2001). As an example, the focus of the investigation might be on differences for standard and deviant stimuli centering on the formant features of speech sounds, yet the standard and deviant stimuli differ also along some other dimension (e.g., fundamental frequency or an unrecognized temporal feature). Some investigators have specifically attempted to control for all differences between standard and deviant stimuli with a "counterbalanced oddball paradigm" in which the role of the standard and deviant stimuli were reversed and mathematically removed from the final derivation of the MMN response (Wunderlich & Cone-Wesson, 2001). In fact, without rigorous control of physical features of the stimuli or differences in the control of the features among studies, there is the likelihood of inconsistent or conflicting MMN findings among studies, misinterpretation of MMN data or even the presence versus absence of an MMN response under apparently similar measurement paradigms (e.g., Pettigrew et al., 2004b; Wunderlich & Cone-Wesson, 2001). Another basic problem with the difference wave strategy in MMN measurement and analysis, noted earlier in this chapter, is the introduction of noise in the final waveform and subsequent undesirable reduction in the SNR and difficulty in identification of the MMN wave.

AREA UNDER (OVER) THE CURVE. | Appreciating the absence of a clear peak or trough in the MMN difference wave, some authors suggest an approach that calculates the "area under the curve" or, since the MMN wave is negative, the area above the curve. With this analysis approach, the amplitude throughout the region defined by the onset and the ending latency of the MMN is estimated and then compared statistically to either data for normal subjects or to values for the waveform before or after the latency region encompassing the "curve" (wave).

INTEGRATED MMN ANALYSIS TECHNIQUE. | Ponton and colleagues (1997) at the House Research Institute developed a formal technique for measuring, quantifying, and verifying statistically the MMN wave. The "integrated MMN technique" differs from other analysis techniques in various ways. Amplitude is not calculated for a specific latency point within the waveform but, instead, is integrated over a time period. The latency region analyzed is determined in advance, based on expectations, rather than after the waveform has been averaged. This "a priori" approach eliminates tester bias in MMN detection with visual inspection. Also, the integration of waveforms is not performed for the MMN difference wave. The amplitude integration technique is applied separately for the waveform for standard stimuli and the waveform for deviant stimuli, and then the integrated amplitudes for these two waveforms are compared statistically using a Monte Carlo method for data sampled from single sweep standard responses. That is, the null hypothesis (there is no MMN) is tested statistically.

PRINCIPAL COMPONENT ANALYSIS. | The principal component analysis technique, long used with replication of other complex waveforms from electrophysiological recordings, can be applied also with replications of the MMN difference wave. The goal is to find the component within the waveform that best identifies the variance (difference) between replicated waveforms, or the most consistent response within the replicated waveforms. A common statistical procedure (the two-tailed t-test) is applied to assess the likelihood that a response is present. Noise (no MMN response) is randomly distributed, whereas the MMN will show a tendency is a single voltage direction (e.g., negative polarity). This analysis process is applied to the entire waveform, and not within a predetermined latency region.

Nonpathologic Subject Factors Influencing MMN Response Recording

MEMORY. | There is an inherent connection between memory and MMN. Put simply, sensory memory of the features of invariant (standard) stimulus is requisite for recording the MMN response. The very presence of an MMN implies that the deviant stimulus generated a neural response due to the detection of a change in incoming information—information that was stored in sensory memory. As noted by Ritter et al. (1995), however, the absence of an MMN response should not be viewed as evidence that memory is lacking. A sizable proportion of the voluminous literature on the MMN response addresses the role of memory in the generation of the MMN response. The invariant (standard) stimuli over a time course of milliseconds to seconds establish a memory trace that, in turn, persists for at least 10 or more seconds (Böttcher-Gandor & Ullsperger, 1992; Cowan, 1984; Sams, Hamalainen, Hari, & McEvoy, 1993). The deviant stimuli elicit a neuronal mismatch in the context of the memory trace. Memory underlying the MMN is apparently not strongly related to attention or to other high-level mental processes. Put another way, the MMN offers an objective and reasonably clear-cut index of memory.

Memory can be probed with the MMN response elicited by deviant stimuli that differ from the standard stimuli along a single dimension (e.g., frequency or duration) or sets of multiple stimuli with subtle variations in multiple dimensions and a more prominent "gestalt" difference (Picton, Alain, Otten, et al., 2000; Ritter et al., 1995). Experimental findings support the notion that information related to the deviant stimuli is stored in memory on the basis of the gestalt representation of the stimulus features, and not simply simple differences for one or more single deviant stimuli (e.g., Ritter et al., 1995; Winkler et al., 1990).

The capacity of the memory as assessed by the MMN response has also generated some research interest. It is clear that more than one stimulus can be held in the short-term sensory memory underlying the MMN response (e.g., Winkler et al., 1990), but the maximum number is not yet known. There is experimental evidence that the capacity of memory with MMN responses evoked by complex deviant stimulus patterns extends to at least seven stimuli (e.g., Ritter et al., 1992; Saarinen et al., 1992; Schröger, 1994; Schröger, Näätänen, & Paavilainen, 1992).

As noted above, amplitude of the MMN response is decreased for the second of two consecutive deviant stimuli when the feature distinguishing the deviant from standard stimulus is frequency, whereas amplitudes are comparable for the MMN response elicited by two successive duration deviants. According to Ritter et al. (1995), these findings imply that memory mechanisms underlying the MMN response vary as a function of the properties of the stimulus.

ATTENTION. | Subject attention to acoustic stimulation is not required in measurement of the MMN response. This rather unique aspect of the MMN response—independence from subject attention—was an immediate attraction for investigators of sensory perception and cognition and also appealing to clinical researchers who were interested in the objective assessment of higher level auditory processing in traditionally difficult to test populations, e.g., infants. Not only is attention not essential for measurement of the MMN, attention to stimulation—both standard and deviant stimuli—actually has undesirable effects on MMN recordings. At first glance, amplitude of the MMN response elicited by simple differences in stimulus properties (e.g., frequency, intensity and duration) appears to decrease without attention to the stimulation (e.g., Alain, Woods, & Ogawa, 1994; Alho, Woods, Algazi, & Näätänen, 1992; Näätänen, Jiang, Lavikainen, et al., 1993). The inclusion of components of the N2 wave in calculation of the MMN difference wave, however, is a likely explanation for this apparent influence of attention on MMN. That is, amplitude of the MMN response is enhanced when the N2 wave to attended stimuli is superimposed (Picton, Alain, Otten, et al., 2000).

Attention to acoustic stimulation during MMN recording, even if it's incidental and inconsistent, may result in contamination of the response by other cortical auditory evoked responses, such as the N1 wave, the P300, and components within the N2 complex. The practical implication of this principle is that a subject, during MMN measurement, should not simply passively listen during stimulus presentation but, rather, purposefully attend to something else.

Findings for studies of the MMN response as a measure of involuntary attention and distractibility (e.g., Escera, Alho, Schröger, & Winkler, 2000) have direct relevance to potential MMN applications in an assortment of pediatric and adult patient populations, such as attention-deficit/hyperactivity disorder (ADHD), autism, dementia, and brain injury. Distraction, as stated by Escera et al. (2000), "denotes the involuntary redirection of one's attention from some goal oriented behavior to other aspects of the environment. Lack of distractibility points to dominance of the top-down control of attention, whereas increased distractibility suggests an abnormally low threshold for breakthrough of the unattended (in most cases irrelevant) information" (p. 152). The article by Escera et al. (2000) is a good review of the literature on the relation among attention, distractibility, and the MMN response. The MMN response is not influenced importantly by top-down processes related to a task that the subject is performing during measurement, as evidenced by the presence of the response at normal amplitudes when subject attention is directed away from the stimuli (Alain & Woods, 1997; Näätänen, Paavilainen, et al., 1993; Ritter et al., 1999) or, in the words of Escera et al. (2000), "the MMN is elicited when the incoming sound does not fit the series of the previous stimuli even when these stimuli fall outside the focus of the subject's attention" (p. 153).

One technique for controlling attention during MMN measurement involves the dichotic listening paradigm in which attention is selectively directed to one ear, and MMN response findings are analyzed for the other (unattended) ear.

STATE OF AROUSAL AND SLEEP. | Coma is at one extreme of state of arousal. There is long-standing evidence that the MMN response can be present in coma and, importantly, that the emergence of a negative wave in the frontal-central region of the brain during serial MMN recordings is an early indicator of recovery of consciousness (Kane, Curry, Butler, & Cummins, 1993; Reuter & Linke, 1989). Later investigations also suggested a relation between appearance of the MMN response and the likelihood of "awakening" (e.g., Kane et al., 1996; Kane, Butler, & Simpson, 2000). In contrast, Fischer and colleagues (Fischer et al., 1999; Fischer, Morlet, & Giard, 2000) in relatively large groups of comatose patients (e.g., N = 128) described poor sensitivity of the MMN response as a predictor of return to consciousness. MMN response was often not detected among patients who later recovered from coma. Accuracy of the MMN in predicting awakening to consciousness improves as the patient nears the time when he or she does regain consciousness. Guerit et al. (1999) questioned whether the negative wave recorded previously in coma was actually an MMN response or, perhaps, another source of negativity, a possibility also suggested by Kane et al. (2000). These different groups of investigators are in agreement that the MMN response is characterized by poor test performance in coma. That is, there is a high false negative rate for the prediction of recovery (patients with no apparent MMN response still go on to recover consciousness) and also false positive outcomes (patients with normal MMN findings may not survive their brain injury). Furthermore, MMN response findings in the acute period after brain injury do not contribute to prognosis of neurological or cognitive outcome following awakening from coma (Kane, Butler, & Simpson, 2000). A variety of other variables, including integrity of other regions of the brain and the status of other systems within the body, also play important roles in ultimate outcome during recovery from brain injury.

As noted by Atienza, Cantero, and Dominguez-Marin (2002) in the introduction of a review article on the MMN and sleep, "automatic detection of an discernable change in the surrounding auditory environment is an adaptive function of the auditory nervous system that persists to some degree under different states of consciousness" (p. 215). Since generation of the MMN response clearly reflects an involuntary attention-switching mechanism with sound stimulation (Näätänen, 1990), it is reasonable to expect the MMN response to be present during sleep. The MMN response is inconsistently recorded or not apparent from subjects in sleep onset and non-REM (rapid eye movement) sleep (e.g., Atienza, & Cantero, 2001; Campbell & Colrain, 2002; Nashida et al., 2000; Nielsen-Bohlman, Knight, Woods, & Woodward, 1991; Sabri, Labelle, Gosselin, & Campbell, 2003; Sallinen & Lyytinen, 1997). The likelihood of detecting the MMN response increases in REM sleep (Atienza & Cantero, 2001; Campbell et al., 1992; Loewy, Campbell, & Bastien, 1996). Factors possibility influencing MMN

findings in sleep include the magnitude of the difference between standard and deviant stimuli and the ISI or SOA (Atienza et al., 2002). Also contributing to inconsistencies among studies of sleep and the MMN are confounding sleep-related effects of other late auditory evoked responses, such as the K-complex, the N350 and the N550 waves. Atienza and colleagues (2002) posit that bottom-up mechanisms (reticular activating system and other subthalamic plus thalamic structures) play a role in the reduced MMN response during sleep, i.e., "inhibition of sensory input prior to entry in the MMN generators located in the temporal lobe" (p. 221), with influence also by top-down mechanisms (e.g., memory of previous experiences).

DEVELOPMENTAL EFFECTS (AGE IN CHILDREN). | Beginning with a pioneering study by Alho and colleagues in 1990, evidence has accumulated that, with appropriate measurement conditions, the MMN response can be consistently recorded from infants, including neonates (Alho et al., 1990; Csépe, 1995; Csépe et al., 1992; Kurtzberg et al., 1995; Pang et al., 1998; Ponton et al., 2000). Indeed, among cognitive evoked responses, the MMN response is the first to be detected in infancy. The earliest studies were conducted with frequency differences between the standard and deviant stimuli, but the presence of the MMN response in infants was soon documented as well for more complex nonspeech sounds and for speech sounds. The finding of a robust and rather well-formed MMN response in newborn infants was not entirely expected, because other cortical auditory evoked responses are either not detectable or, at the least, are very immature in infancy. Also, the MMN has been detected in 50 to 70 percent of infants studied when elicited by frequency changes and speech-sound stimuli, including durational changes within speech sounds (Kushnerenko et al., 2002; Kushnerenko et al., 2001; Tanaka, Okubo, Fuchigama, & Harada, 2001), even in premature neonates at 30 to 34 weeks gestational age (Cheour-Luhtanen et al., 1996; Cheour-Luhtanen et al., 1997). Prematurity and other neonatal risk factors may have long-term consequences for the MMN response. For example, Jansson-Verkasalo et al. (2004) found reduced MMN amplitude for a group of twelve children (average age 5 years 7 months) who were born prematurely and with very low birth weight. The presence of the MMN response essentially at birth raises the possibility of detecting in infancy developmental disruption of higher level cortical functions related to speech perception, speech and language acquisition, and reading. Maturation of the MMN response evoked with speech sound stimuli (e.g., /da/ and /ga/) appears to proceed through the preschool years (e.g., Cheour et al., 1998a; Korpilahti & Lang, 1994; Morr, Shafer, Kreuzer, & Kurtzberg, 2002; Ponton et al., 2000; Shafer, Moor, Kreuzer, & Kurtzberg, 2000). The MMN response elicited with simple stimuli (e.g., frequency differences between standard and deviant stimuli) is remarkably stable in childhood, with only minor maturational changes in response latency from infancy

(241 ms) to school age (207 ms) children (e.g., Kurtzberg et al., 1995).

Although the MMN response elicited by simple stimuli is adult-like by age 6 years with no further changes through age 16 years (Kraus et al., 1999), developmental trends in the MMN for speech sound stimuli occur throughout school-age years (Shafer, Morr, Kreuzer, & Kurtzberg, 2000). In addition, scalp topography (scalp current density) of the MMN response shows maturational changes during the 4-to-11-year age range (Gomot et al., 2000; Martin et al., 2003; Maurer, Bucher, Brem, & Brandeis, 2003b), presumably reflecting developmental shifts in the locus of neural activity evoked by MMN stimulation. The adult MMN response is prominent in midline frontal regions (and smaller laterally), whereas in children lateral (temporal lobe) MMN recordings are larger than those recorded with frontal electrodes. Maturational differences and inconsistencies also are seen in the laterality of activity (left versus right hemisphere) for tonal and speech stimuli, in comparison to expectations for adults. Furthermore, these MMN findings in children imply differential maturational trends for specific mechanisms underlying MMN response generation, e.g., detection of a change in stimulation versus the attention switching process (Martin et al., 2003). Latencies for the MMN responses evoked by speech sounds become shorter by about 11 ms/year between 4 and 11 years, but amplitude remains relatively stable (Shafer et al., 2000). The effects of maturation are different for MMN latency versus amplitude, and even the developmental findings for latency and amplitude are not clear cut, consistent among subjects, or consistent among studies (e.g., Kraus et al., 1993c; Kraus et al., 1992; Kurtzberg et al., 1995).

As reviewed below, evidence is accumulating that the MMN can indeed serve as an early biologic marker or index for developmental disorders, such as auditory processing disorders, language impairment, and dyslexia (Leppänen & Lyytinen, 1997; Schulte-Körne, Deimel, Bartling, & Remschmidt, 1998).

Children with congenital profound hearing impairment present an opportunity to learn more about the impact of auditory deprivation on development of the auditory system. The MMN response, in turn, can in such investigations be employed as a neurophysiologic maturation of the central auditory system and the impact of altered auditory experience on neural function in general and, in particular, such high-level functions as attention and short-term auditory memory.

Advancing Age

Age-related declines for some persons in information processing speed and efficiency, capacity for learning, memory, and cognitive function in general, are well appreciated. It is not surprising, therefore, that clinical investigations have documented changes in the MMN with advancing age (e.g., Czigler, Csibra, & Csontos, 1992; Jääskeläinen, Hautamaki,

Näätänen, & Ilmoniemi, 1999; Karayanidis, Andrews, Ward, & Michie, 1995; Pekkonen, 2000; Pekkonen et al., 1996; Schroeder, Ritter, & Vaughan, 1995). When ISIs are short (e.g., < 1 second), MMN amplitude is reduced with aging for duration differences between standard and deviant stimuli, but not for frequency differences. With long ISIs (e.g., 4 to 5 seconds), on the other hand, there are age-related decrements in MMN amplitude for frequency differences in stimuli, a finding presumably related to a deficit (or decay) in sensory memory (the memory trace) in the elderly. The literature on the MMN response in aging is not entirely consistent, perhaps due to differences in measurement protocols (e.g., stimulus characteristics, subject attention demands, acquisition parameters) and the influence of age-related changes in other auditory evoked responses (e.g., N2 and P3) on analysis of the MMN response findings. The effect of aging on the MMN response, just summarized, is more consistently reported when duration is the difference between standard and deviant stimuli than for frequency differences. Another possible factor in the discrepancies in findings for the MMN response in aging is the relatively small number of older subjects enrolled in the majority of the studies (usually less than twenty subjects). Some of the existing information on the MMN response in normal-aging adults is derived from findings for the control subjects in studies of the MMN in various neuropsychiatric disorders affecting elderly persons, e.g., Parkinson's disease and Alzheimer's disease.

Gender

There are for adult subjects no clear gender differences in latency or amplitude of MMN responses elicited by simple tonal stimuli, when the gender-related changes in other auditory cortical responses (e.g., P2 and N2) are removed (e.g., Nagy, Potts, & Loveland, 2003). Gender differences are also not consistently evident in the scalp distribution and hemispheric symmetry of the MMN response for more complex stimuli, such as speech sounds and music stimuli (e.g., Koelsch, Maess, Grossmann, & Friederici, 2003).

Drugs

Studies describing the effects of psychotropic drugs on the MMN are summarized in Table 14.7. Effect of medications on the MMN response, when present, are mostly characterized by a reduction (attenuation) of amplitude.

CLINICAL APPLICATIONS AND POPULATIONS

Introduction: Pushing Back the AER Frontier with the MMN Response

Although the potential clinical applications of the MMN are plentiful and diverse, and well supported by extensive literature, the challenges to reliable MMN measurement and

TABLE 14.7. Summary of Investigations of the Effect of Selected Drugs on the MMN Response

Many of the papers report studies on the possible effects of antipsychotic medications in studies of schizophrenia.

DRUG	STUDY(IES)	COMMENT
Ketamine	Kreitschmann-Andermahr et al., 2001 Umbricht et al., 2000 Umbricht, Koller, Vollen-weider, & Schmid, 2002	Based on studies of schizophrenia, ketamine reduces MMN response amplitude.
Lorazepam	Rosburg, Marinou, et al., 2004	Benzodiazepines, a GABA agonist, produced a decrease in the moment dipole of the neuromagnetic MMN (MMNm) response. Results were related to reduced signal detection as measured behaviorally.
	Murakami et al., 2002	No effect on the MMN in patients with schizophrenia.
Psilocybin	Umbricht et al., 2003	The 5-HT$_{2A}$ agonist had no effect on the MMN response.
Halperidol	Kähkönen et al., 2001 Kähkönen et al., 2002 Pekkonen et al., 2002	The dopamine D$_2$ receptor antagonist had no influence on MMN response amplitude.
Scopolamine	Pekkonen et al., 2002	A cholinergic antagonist with no clear or direct effect on the MMN response amplitude.
Chlorpheniramine	Serra et al., 1996	Histamine H1-receptor antagonist with no effect on MMN response amplitude.

meaningful analysis in clinical populations are substantial. Picton et al. (2000) succinctly stated this problem: "In order for a physiological measurement to be used clinically, it must reliably and accurately discriminate between patients with a particular disorder and those without" (p. 132). Clinical studies have demonstrated some success in differentiating with the MMN response under laboratory conditions groups of normal subjects from groups of patients with documented diseases and disorders, as reviewed herein. For the MMN to emerge as a true clinical procedure, like ECochG and ABR, fundamental questions about test performance must be answered positively. In addition to reliability, more information is needed on MMN response sensitivity and specificity, cost effectiveness (cost-benefit ratio), and the time required to perform a clinically useful MMN measurement. Even the most enthusiastic proponents and investigators of the MMN response, however, concede (perhaps reluctantly) that the accurate and consistent diagnosis of individual patients with these same diseases and disorders is not yet a reality.

Hundreds of publications describe MMN response findings for a wide range of disorders and diseases. Space permits only a cursory review here. An Internet search will reveal an ever-increasing volume of publications on the clinical investigation of the MMN response. The reader is referred to review articles summarizing clinical research and clinical applications of the MMN (e.g., Näätänen, 2003). One of the most exciting and practical clinical applications of the MMN response is in the objective documentation of the effects of experience, learning, treatment, and training.

New examples of this application of MMN appear regularly in the literature. Published studies on changes in the MMN associated with brain plasticity secondary to intervention, including medical therapy, auditory training, and treatments of any kind, are cited within this chapter in sections pertaining to the general topic of interest, e.g., foreign language or music education or on the disorder of interest, e.g., dyslexia, auditory processing disorders, schizophrenia. A good example of this body of literature on measuring training effects with MMN is the series of studies conducted by Nina Kraus and colleagues clearly demonstrating that parallel changes in the MMN response and behavioral measures among children enrolled in formal programs for developing auditory and speech-sound processing (e.g., Kraus, McGee, Carrell, & Sharma, 1995; Tremblay, Kraus, & McGee, 1998). The MMN response can be applied in confirming improvement in speech perception abilities for persons learning a foreign language.

The following discussion of studies of the MMN response in various patient populations does not include a review of MMN findings for patients with cochlear implants. That topic is covered included within the overview in Chapter 15 of electrical evoked responses and other measures in cochlear implants.

PERIPHERAL AUDITORY DYSFUNCTION (HEARING LOSS). | Along with other cortical evoked responses, the MMN response evoked by speech stimuli has been investigated in patients with sensory hearing loss (Oates, Kurtzberg, &

Stapells, 2002; Tremblay, Piskosz, & Souza, 2003; Wall, Dalebout, Davidson, & Fox, 1991). Other researchers have used ipsilateral masking noise, including broadband noise (BBN), to simulate the effect of sensory hearing loss on the MMN response (Martin & Stapells, 2005; Müller-Gass, Marcoux, Logan, & Campbell, 2001). The results are consistent with expectations for reduced audibility produced by the masking noise, namely, increased latencies and reduced amplitudes for the MMN response. Specifically, the effects of noise on MMN latency and amplitude are progressively greater as the cutoff for low-pass noise is increased, as would be expected for low-frequency sensory hearing loss.

AMPLIFICATION. | The MMN response would have unique clinical value if it could be applied in the objective confirmation of hearing aid benefit for speech perception in infants and young children. Dr. David Stapells and colleagues (Korczak, Kurtzberg, & Stapells, 2005; Oates et al., 2002) demonstrated the benefit of amplification of speech-sound stimuli with the MMN response. Subjects were fourteen young adults with hearing loss ranging in degree from moderate to severe-profound and twenty young normal-hearing adults. MMN responses elicited with /ba/ and /ga/ consonant vowel speech stimuli presented a fixed intensity levels (65 and 80 dB peak-to-peak equivalent SPL) were recorded in the unaided condition and with appropriately fit hearing aids. The MMN response difference wave was analyzed with visual inspection and presence of a response defined by the largest negativity within the 80 to 400 ms latency region. In general, MMN amplitude was increased and latency decreased with amplification, although values did not typically reach the normal range, and there were for individual hearing-impaired subjects exceptions to these trends. In some subjects with severe hearing impairment, no MMN response was detected in the unaided condition yet, with amplification, latency and amplitude of the MMN response was consistent with values for the normal subjects. Korczak, Kurtzberg, and Stapells (2005) speculate that event-related response findings reflect activation of more neurons with amplification and verify neurophysiologic changes associated with speech-sound perception with amplification. However, the paradoxical decrement in event-related response outcome with amplification (i.e., longer latency and smaller amplitude) was observed most often for the MMN versus other responses (e.g., N1, N2b, and P300). It appears from this study that the MMN response, along with other cortical responses (e.g., Kurtzberg, 1989) can be applied in documenting the benefit of hearing aid use for patients with hearing loss in the moderate through severe range. Although amplification may consistently improve audibility to sound, the variability in benefit among individual subject, as documented with the MMN response, suggests that some patients had residual deficits in speech perception and discrimination with hearing aid use.

APHASIA/DYSPHASIA. | Abnormal MMN responses elicited by speech stimuli appear to be a characteristic finding in patients with aphasia, whereas the MMN response is normal for nonspeech stimuli (e.g., Aaltonen, Tuomainen, Laine, & Niemi, 1993; Csépe, Osman-Sagi, Molnar, & Gosy, 2001; Ilvonen et al., 2004). Other authors, however, described abnormal MMN findings for frequency and duration differences between tonal standard and deviant stimuli (Alain et al., 1998).

Jacobs and Schneider (2003) describe MMN findings for a 42-year-old man with pure word deafness and a history of multiple neurosurgical procedures for arteriovenous malformations. The authors define pure word deafness as "a deficit in comprehending and repeating spoken language in the context of relatively intact spontaneous speech production and auditory acuity" (Jacobs & Schneider, 2003, p. 125). The MMN response was abnormal as elicited with speech stimuli (standard /ga/ and deviant /da/ syllables) in comparison to simple pitch differences.

AUDITORY PROCESSING DISORDERS (APDs). | In recent years, a number of investigators have reported abnormalities in auditory cortical evoked responses for children and adults with APDs (e.g., Jerger, Martin, & McColl, 2004; Liasis et al., 2003b). The application of the MMN response in auditory processing disorders (APDs) is a natural outgrowth of the basic investigations of auditory processing mechanisms with the MMN. Case reports and group studies on the clinical use of MMN in the diagnosis of APDs date back to the early 1990s (Kraus et al., 1993). Additional papers on MMN in APDs are cited in the following section on dyslexia.

ATTENTION-DEFICIT/HYPERACTIVITY DISORDER (ADHD). | Barry, Johnstone, and Clarke (2003) published a comprehensive review of event-related responses in ADHD, including the ABR, auditory late response components (N1, P2, and N2), the P300 response, and the MMN response. As noted in the review of these responses in ADHD elsewhere in the book, Johnstone and Barry have published original research findings on auditory evoked responses in ADHD. No clear and consistent MMN response findings are associated with the diagnosis of ADHD. Some investigators describe a trend toward smaller MMN response amplitudes in ADHD (Kemner et al., 1996), whereas others (Oades et al., 1996) reported just the opposite trend (larger amplitudes). In neither of the studies, however, were differences between experimental and control groups statistically significant. A single group of researchers (Winsberg et al., 1993; Winsberg et al., 1997) even reported contradictory MMN findings in ADHD for two separate studies, prompting the overall conclusion that the MMN cannot confidentially differentiate children or adolescents with confirmed ADHD from control subjects (Rothenberger et al., 2000; Winsberg et al., 1997).

AUTISM. | Čeponiene, Lepisto, Shestakova, and colleagues (2003) conducted a study of the MMN response in nine "high functioning" children with autism and ten control subjects using three stimulus conditions: simple tones, complex tones, and vowels. The experimental group showed intact sound processing performance, e.g., processing spectral characteristics of sound, even for complex stimuli. The authors reported an impairment in "attentional orienting to sound changes" for vowel sounds, but not for the other stimuli used to elicit the MMN response. Kemner et al. (1995) found normal MMN response findings (latency and amplitude) in a group of high-functioning autistic children. In contrast, Gomot et al. (2002) and Ferri et al. (2003) reported significantly shorter MMN response latency for children with autism versus a control group. Shorter latency for the MMN recorded was topographically related, i.e., mostly as recorded over the left cerebral hemisphere (Gomot et al., 2002), and Ferri et al. (2003) reported larger MMN amplitude. In contrast, Seri et al. (1999) described longer latency and smaller amplitudes for children with autism, and Jansson-Verkasalo et al. (1993) reported similar findings in children with Asperger's syndrome.

NON-NATIVE LANGUAGE LEARNING. | Shestakova, Huotilainen, Čeponiene, and Cheour (2003) correlated changes in the MMN response to second-language learning in a group of seventeen Finnish children (age 3 to 6 years) who enrolled in a French school and an equal number of age-matched control subjects. The findings confirmed the authors' previous report of progressive decreases in MMN latency and increases in amplitude associated with improvement in the ability to discriminate non-native (also French language among Finnish speakers) speech sounds (e.g., Cheour et al., 2002b).

PREMATURE BIRTH. | Long-term deficits in auditory processing, language, learning, reading and writing among children born preterm and at low birth weight are well appreciated. Follow-up of infants born prematurely and with very low birth weight shows abnormally reduced MMN response amplitude and, curiously, shorter MMN latency, for speech-sound stimulation, in comparison to a control group and to expectations for chronological age (Jansson-Verkasalo et al., 2003a; Jansson-Verkasalo et al., 2004).

DYSLEXIA. | Dyslexia is a reading disorder. Different theories and mechanisms have been offered for dyslexia, with some authors emphasizing visual deficits and involvement of regions of the brain such as the occipital lobe and the magnocellular system (e.g., Habib, 2000) and many others highlighting auditory temporal and/or phonologic processing deficits involving central auditory pathways and the temporal lobe of the cortex (e.g., Habib, 2000). As typically used, the term *dyslexia* implies a reading disorder secondary, or related, to an auditory and/or language deficit. A complete review of the extensive literature on dyslexia, including theories on underlying mechanisms and neurobiologic bases, is far beyond the scope of this discussion. For more information, the reader is referred to a review article by Michel Habib entitled "The Neurological Basis of Developmental Dyslexia: An Overview and Working Hypothesis" (Habib, 2000). It is very important, however, to point out two competing auditory theories on the nature of dyslexia. With one theory, deficits in phonological awareness and linguistic (speech-language) processing are cited in the explanation of dyslexia, whereas the other view hypothesizes a more general deficit in auditory processing of both speech and nonspeech signals. A reconciliation of these two apparently divergent explanations for dyslexia—auditory processing versus phonologic/linguistic processing—is likely to emerge from clinical data reported in the rapidly expanding literature on the MMN response in dyslexia (see Table 14.8). Dyslexia is probably best explained by possible deficits in multiple modalities and conditions, with dyslexia in some persons arising from one modality (auditory or visual), in others primarily the auditory system, and still other persons a phonologic and/or language impairment with or without an auditory processing disorder. In the following discussion, dyslexia will be defined as an auditory-based reading disorder. Difficulty perceiving speech-sound differences (including vowel and consonant sounds requiring precise perception of rapid timing changes) and in phonologic awareness (the ability to detect and manipulate speech sounds in words) is a characteristic feature of dyslexia. The MMN response for speech stimuli can be detected in infants before it's possible to evaluate speech perception behaviorally. The early appearance of the MMN response, and the feasibility of measurement in sleep, has led to fascinating investigations of auditory processing and speech-sound perception in infants at familial risk for auditory-based reading disorders.

Leppänen and Lyytinen (1997) reported differences in the MMN response for infants with a family history of delayed speech acquisition and dyslexia versus a control group. Using nonspeech (pure tones) and speech stimuli, Schulte-Körne et al. (1998) continued this line of investigation with children in adolescence. Speech stimuli were /da/ for the standard stimulus and /ba/ for the deviant stimulus. The authors reported a difference between the dyslexic and control groups in the MMN (smaller amplitude) evoked by speech stimuli, but not for tonal stimuli. However, Baldeweg et al. (1999) described abnormal MMN response findings in persons with dyslexia, with pure-tone standard stimuli (1000 Hz) and deviant stimuli (different frequencies from 1015 to 1090 Hz or frequency differences from 15 to 90 Hz). Smaller differences between the standard and deviant stimuli were more effective in differentiating the dyslexic subjects from the control group (refer to Figure 14.3). In addition, the authors reported a correlation between the MMN findings and behavioral performance in processing the stimuli. Kujala et al. (2000) also reported abnormal MMN results in dyslexia, with stimuli consisting of different rhythmic patterns

TABLE 14.8. A Chronological Summary of Investigations and Publications on the Topic of Dyslexia Involving the Mismatch Negativity (MMN) Response

STUDIES	COMMENT
Kraus et al., 1995	MMN documentation of plasticity in processing associated with training.
Schulte-Körne et al., 1998	MMN measured for tonal and speech-sound stimuli; evidence of a phonological basis for dyslexia.
Schulte-Körne, Deimel, Bartling, & Remschmidt, 1999	MMN responses for temporal order differences for tonal signals smaller in dyslexic subjects than in control subjects.
Baldeweg et al., 1999	Smaller MMN response amplitude in dyslexic population for frequency (pitch) differences between standard and deviant stimuli, but not in a duration condition. Evidence of an auditory processing deficit.
Kujala et al., 2000	MMN differences between dyslexic and control subjects for stimuli consisting of tonal patterns; possible masking of sound processing by previous or surrounding sounds.
Kujala & Näätänen, 2001	Review article; the MMN literature provides evidence in dyslexia of abnormalities in processing of nonspeech and speech sounds.
Kujala, Kallis, Tervaniemi, & Näätänen, 2001	Training produced changes in auditory processing at the cortical level of the brain, as documented by the MMN response, that occurred concomitant with improved reading skills.
Leppanen et al., 2002	MMN response differences reported for infants at familial risk for dyslexia; possible left hemisphere site of dysfunction.
Kujala, Belitz, Tervaniemi, & Näätänen, 2003	Evidence presented for a backward masking mechanism in MMN response abnormalities in dyslexic adult subjects.
Renvall & Hari, 2003	Diminished magnetic MMN fields in the left hemisphere of adult dyslexic subjects for tonal stimuli.
Maurer et al., 2003b	MMN response deficits and scalp distribution differences were found for kindergarten children at familial risk for dyslexia in comparison to a control group using frequency and phoneme stimulus conditions.

of four identical tones, and poorer than normal performance for a corresponding behavioral task. The specific finding of this study and follow-up research by the same researchers (Kujala et al., 2001a,b; Kujala & Näätänen, 2001), an abnormal MMN response when an additional sound closely followed (10 ms) a tone pattern that had been shown when the third tone was not presented to elicit a response, suggests the possibility of a temporal deficit in auditory processing, and potential value of backward masking paradigms in the study of dyslexia. The very early detection with the MMN response of children at risk for such common and academically handicapping disorders as dyslexia (e.g., Guttorm, Leppänen, Tolvanen, & Lyytinen, 2003; Leppänen et al., 2002; Maurer et al., 2003a,b) opens up remarkable opportunities for early intervention and, essentially, preventive management. In addition, an increase in MMN response amplitude elicited by tone patterns from baseline measures to follow-up measures after intervention (auditory training) for dyslexia and language impairment provides neurophysiologic documentation of the benefit of therapy (e.g., Kujala et al., 2001a,b). Importantly, changes in the MMN response were related to improvement in reading performance.

LANGUAGE IMPAIRMENT. | Abnormal MMN response findings have been documented in children with specific language impairment (SLI), a deficit in oral language in children with normal hearing and intelligence who have enjoyed a typical learning environment (see Leppänen & Lyytinen, 1997 for review). The literature on MMN in SLI overlaps with papers on the MMN in dyslexia (also reviewed in this section). Friedrich, Weber, and Friederici (2004) also found delayed latency of the MMN response elicited by speech stimuli (long and short /ba/ syllables in the German language) in 8-week-old infants at risk for SLI due to family history, that is, SLI in parents or older siblings. The authors reported the presence of an MMN response in awakened infants and in sleep. Response latency was unchanged by state of arousal, whereas MMN response amplitude was larger when subjects were sleeping than in the awakened state.

In a series of reports, Kraus and colleagues (e.g., Cunningham et al., 2001; Kraus et al., 1996) describe for a group of children with learning disabilities, including apparently some with language impairment, age-adjusted abnormalities in late auditory responses, among them the MMN response elicited with speech sound stimuli. Differences in the MMN response between normal and learning impaired children were related to deficits in speech discrimination documented with behavioral tests.

Neuropsychiatric Disorders and Diseases

ALCOHOLISM. | The abnormal MMN pattern with long ISIs, described above for advancing age, is accentuated in persons with chronic alcohol abuse (Ahveninen et al., 2001; Polo, Escera, Gual, & Grau, 1999). It is unclear whether the MMN response can serve as a marker for vulnerability or risk of alcoholism, as findings vary considerably among studies (e.g., Sanchez-Turet & Serra-Grabulosa, 2002).

ALZHEIMER'S DISEASE. | The possible link between the MMN response and Alzheimer's disease is apparent, namely, a characteristic feature of Alzheimer's disease is loss of memory, and the MMN response is dependent on short-term sensory memory. Predictably, a number of investigators have applied the MMN response in persons with Alzheimer's disease (e.g., Gaeta, Friedman, Ritter, & Chen, 1999; Kazmerski, Friedman, & Ritter, 1997; Pekkonen, 2000; Pekkonen et al., 1994; Verleger et al., 1992; Yokoyama et al., 1995). The reader will recall that the majority of the authors of papers on the MMN response in Alzheimer's disease also have published information on the effects of aging on the MMN response. The effect of ISI on the MMN response is an important factor in studies of Alzheimer's disease. With relatively short ISIs, e.g., 1 to 1.5 seconds, the MMN response is typically normal in Alzheimer's disease (Gaeta et al., 1999; Kazmerski et al., 1997; Verlegere et al., 1992; Yokoyama et al., 1995), whereas significant reductions for MMN amplitude are found for longer ISIs, e.g., 3 or more seconds (Pekkonen et al., 1994). Riekkinen et al. (1997), in a study of the effect of a cholinesterase inhibitor tetrahydroaminoacridine (THA), a common medical therapy for cognitive dysfunction in Alzheimer's disease, on the MMN response found a paradoxical reduction of MMN amplitude with short ISIs (stimulus rate was 1/second).

BRAIN INJURY AND COMA. | MMN responses have been investigated in traumatic (closed) head injury as an index of underlying brain injury. Although findings among studies are not entirely consistent, there is evidence that the MMN can document during coma and with emergence from coma changes in attention (including reduced vigilance and distractibility), preattentive auditory processing, and other cognitive deficits, such as memory, information processing, and learning (Fischer et al., 1999; Fischer, Luaute, et al., 2004; Kaipio, Cheow, et al., 2000; Kaipio, Novitski, et al., 2001; Kane, Butler, & Simpson, 2000; Kane et al., 1993; Polo et al., 2002; Rugg et al., 1993). Amplitude of a MMN response elicited by tone stimuli is reduced in closed head injury. However, as noted by Fischer et al. (2004), "the presence of MMN is a predictor of awakening and pre-

cludes patients from moving to a permanent vegetative state" (p. 669).

In a study of seventy-nine patients with severe and diffuse brain injuries, including patients in a vegetative state, Kotchoubey et al. (2003) found MMN abnormalities for musical tones but not for simple pure-tone stimuli. The authors conclude that recording the MMN response with simple stimuli may, in clinical populations "lead to severe underestimation of the functional state of the patient's auditory system" (Kotchoubey et al., 2003, p. 129).

Application of the MMN response in coma secondary to brain injury was reviewed earlier in this chapter in the section on attention. Briefly, the appearance of the MMN to frequency differences between standard and deviant stimuli signified impending return to consciousness (Fischer et al., 1999; Kane et al., 1993; Kane et al., 1996), with specificity higher than sensitivity in the prediction of awakening.

PARKINSON'S DISEASE. | The MMN response evoked by frequency differences between the standard and deviant stimuli is smaller in amplitude for persons with Parkinson's disease than normal control subjects (Karayanidis et al., 1995; Pekkonen, 2000; Pekkonen et al., 1995). Inconsistencies in the details of findings among studies are likely the result of differences in methodology (attention versus passive conditions and dichotic versus monaural stimulus presentation), modest numbers of subjects (typically less than twenty), and a high degree of intersubject variation among subjects with Parkinson's disease. Based on the findings of studies published to date, including limitations in sensitivity and specificity, the MMN response cannot be relied upon for the diagnosis of Parkinson's disease or even the differentiation of patients with Parkinson's disease from normal elderly persons or patients with other neuropsychiatric diseases (e.g., Alzheimer's disease).

SCHIZOPHRENIA. | Using standard and deviant stimuli that differed in duration, Shelley and colleagues first described abnormal MMN response findings in schizophrenia back in 1991 (Shelley et al., 1991). Javitt et al. (1993) confirmed reduction in MMN response amplitude in schizophrenia with a stimuli differing in frequency. Reduced MMN response amplitude in schizophrenia was subsequently confirmed, and the pattern of findings expanded, by many other investigators (Alain et al., 1998; Catts et al., 1995; Gene-Cos, Ring, Pottinger, & Barrett, 1999; Hirayasu et al., 1998; Javitt, 2000; Javitt, Doneshka, Grochowski, & Ritter, 1995; Kasai et al., 1999; Kreitschmann-Andermahr et al., 1999; Michie et al., 2000; Oades, Dittman-Balcar, Zerbin, & Grzella, 1997; Shutara et al., 1996; Umbricht et al., 1998). In a review paper (German language), Rosburg, Kreitschmann-Andermahr, and Sauer (2004) summarize MMN findings in schizophrenia as reported in forty-three published studies. In general, at least in chronic (versus newly diagnosed patients), MMN amplitude reductions and latency prolongations for stimulus paradigms involving frequency and du-ration differences between standard and deviant stimuli were reported in schizophrenia. Some of the studies provided evidence of a relation between the degree of MMN ampli-tude reduction and severity of schizophrenia, as determined by selected symptoms. Medications (antipsychotic drugs) used in the management of schizophrenia do not appear to have an effect on the MMN response (Umbricht et al., 1998).

Diagnostic value and power for an auditory evoked re-sponse is greatly enhanced when a specific pattern of ab-normalities is characteristic of one disease or disorder and not others. Abnormal augmentation of the SP/AP ratio of the ECochG is, for example, a feature almost exclusively associated with the diagnosis of Ménière's disease. For neurodiagnostic ABR, a delay in the wave I to III latency interval rather conclusively points to unilateral (ipsilateral) retrocochlear auditory dysfunction in a limited anatomic region (eighth cranial nerve to caudal brainstem). There is evidence that manipulation of stimulus parameters in MMN measurement (e.g., the interval between deviant stimuli and probability of a deviant stimulus) yields changes in the MMN response that differentiate patients with schizophre-nia from not only normal subjects, but also aging adults and patients with other neuropsychiatric diseases, e.g., Alzheim-er's disease (e.g., Javitt, 2000). Specifically, with normal subjects and patients with schizophrenia, MMN amplitude changes inversely with probability of the deviant stimulus (decreased deviant stimulus probability produced a larger MMN response amplitude), but the effect was significantly less for schizophrenic patients than for age-matched control subjects. There was no difference between groups with ma-nipulations of the ISI for the deviant stimulus. In compari-son to schizophrenia, manipulation of the ISI for the deviant stimulus for patients with Alzheimer's disease, for example, produced significant changes in MMN response amplitude. Furthermore, there is the possibility that the MMN response can detect biological markers associated with the likelihood of being diagnosed with schizophrenia and with progression of the disease (Jessen et al., 2001; Michie, Innes-Brown, Todd, & Jablensky, 2002; Shinozaki et al., 2002). MMN ab-normalities in schizophrenia provide neurophysiologic evi-dence of a deficit in the formation of sensory memory and auditory perception, more pronounced for processes medi-ated in the frontal versus temporal lobes and perhaps related to disruption in the NMDA-receptor system (Javitt, 2000; Näätänen, 2003).

Other Disorders

SOCIALLY WITHDRAWN CHILDREN. | Citing literature on MMN response deficits in adult patient populations associ-ated with social withdrawal (e.g., schizophrenia and depres-sion) and the neuroanatomic regions involved in emotion, Bar-Haim et al. (2003) hypothesized that the MMN response would offer an electrophysiologic index of social withdrawal. The authors reported for a series of twenty-three socially withdrawn children abnormally prolonged MMN response latency and reduced amplitude, elicited by tonal stimuli (standard = 1000 Hz and deviant = 1100 Hz). Bar-Haim et al. (2003) speculate on a connection between frontal cortex dysfunction in socially withdrawn children and the MMN findings.

TINNITUS. | Weisz, Voss, Berg, and Elbert (2004) published what may be the first formal investigation of the MMN re-sponse in persons with bothersome tinnitus as their chief complaint. Using stimulus frequencies corresponding to the "lesion edge", i.e., the border of the frequency region for the patients' hearing loss, the authors found clear differences in the topographic distribution of the MMN response for fifteen persons with tinnitus in comparison to an equal number of control subjects.

CONCLUDING COMMENTS

As evident from the review in the present chapter, the MMN response is an objective and quantifiable index, or tool, for evaluating sensory representations in the central auditory nervous system, even for highly complex linguistic stimuli and before conscious attention. Among the auditory evoked responses, the MMN response is clearly in a class by itself in terms of the variety and potential complexity of stimuli that can be used in clinical measurement. Virtually any fea-ture of sound is effective as a difference between standard and deviant stimuli, including very small (fine) differences in frequency, intensity, duration, or some combination of features or temporal presentation of features. Speech stimuli are commonly applied in MMN measurement, ranging from acoustic cues within synthetic speech sound (phoneme) cat-egories (e.g., slight variations in speech-sound stimuli along the continuum from one phoneme to another) to linguisti-cally complex stimuli (e.g., words versus pseudowords). The feasibility of evoking the MMN response to complex speech stimuli is one of the main factors contributing to the value of the response in objectively evaluating auditory processing at the cortical level.

Recognition of the potential value of the MMN response for exploring high-level auditory information processing has led to a variety of clinical investigations in varied subject pop-ulations, from normal infants to diverse pediatric and adult patient populations, e.g., those with alcoholism, Alzheimer's disease, aphasia, auditory processing disorders (APD), autism, dyslexia, Parkinson's disease, and schizophrenia. Because the MMN response can be elicited with deviations in com-plex sounds, it is also well suited for the objective study—in subjects across the age spectrum from premature infants to elderly adults—of the perception, neural representation, and memory of many features of speech and nonspeech music, even rules associated with the perception of music and a specific language (or even multiple languages in the same subject). The MMN can also be applied in the investigation of the development and degeneration of these fundamental aspects of auditory processing and to document objectively (neuro-physiologically) the effects of training or therapy on auditory processing. Along with other cortical auditory evoked responses, the MMN is now a valuable research tool for probing the neurophysiologic underpinnings of auditory processing in normal persons and multiple patient populations.

15

CHAPTER

Electrically Evoked and Myogenic Responses

ELECTRICALLY EVOKED AUDITORY RESPONSES AND COCHLEAR IMPLANTS

Background

The primary clinical application of electrically evoked auditory evoked responses is with cochlear implant patients. Electrically evoked responses can be applied before, during, and after cochlear implantation. The major responses typically recorded with auditory stimulation—i.e., compound action potential (ECochG), ABR, AMLR, and ALR—can also be evoked with electrical stimulation. Latencies for electrically evoked auditory responses are, of course, shorter than for auditory evoked responses because the electrical stimulus directly activates neural pathways (spiral ganglion cells) and, therefore, is unaffected by time delays associated with acoustic travel time from an earphone to the tympanic membrane, transmission of mechanical energy through the middle ear and along the cochlear partition, excitation of hair cells, and synaptic transmission from hair cells to auditory nerve afferent fibers. Electrically evoked responses generated from the peripheral and central auditory system can be applied to assess neural survival and integrity as part of the determination of candidacy for cochlear implantation or to provide information needed for important clinical decisions, such as which ear will be implanted. Electrically evoked responses can also be recorded intraoperatively during cochlear implantation to verify adequate electrode placement and the integrity and function of cochlear implant components. After cochlear implantation, a variety of responses ranging from the electrical compound action potential (ECAP) to cortical responses (e.g., AMLR, P300, and MMN) can be evoked by either electrical stimulation directly within the cochlea via the device or by sound stimulation processed by the device. Importantly, there is no age restriction in the clinical application of electrically evoked auditory evoked responses. Clinical experience with these objective techniques has accumulated from patients ranging from infancy to advancing age.

The goal for some electrical measurements is postsurgical confirmation of the physical integrity and operating characteristics of the cochlear implant. The focus of the electrical measures is on the transmission to some type of recording device (i.e., a computer with a visual display) of detailed information on very specific internal and external components of the cochlear implant device. The term *telemetry* is often used to describe the quantification and transmission of the information from the cochlear implant for analysis by an audiologist or other person providing services to the patient. Common telemetric measures for cochlear implants are listed in Table 15.1. Cochlear implant telemetry is essential for initial and ongoing verification of hardware and technical integrity and, occasionally, for troubleshooting malfunction or failure of a cochlear implant. The topic, however, is outside of the scope of a discussion of electrically evoked auditory evoked responses. For details on specific methods for cochlear implant telemetry, the reader is referred to operation manuals prepared by the manufacturers of cochlear implants. The following review, therefore, is focused on

TABLE 15.1. Clinical Applications of Electrically Evoked Compound Action Potentials (ECAPs)

- Documentation of the integrity of the cochlear implant device.
- Estimation of detection thresholds and comfortable levels in infants, young children, and other patients who cannot be properly assessed with behavioral techniques.
- Reduced time required for mapping and initial programming of the cochlear implant in these patient populations.
- Measurement of interaction among electrode channels and elimination of channels that provide limited information and create undesirable interaction effects.
- Estimation of loudness and investigation of loudness mechanisms.
- Determination of most appropriate rates of stimulation.

---

electrophysiologic measurements of cochlear implant operation and patient response to sound processed with cochlear implants.

Electrically evoked auditory responses are applied in the evaluation of integrity of cranial (auditory) nerve and central auditory nervous system of patients with profound sensory (cochlear) hearing impairment when these patients are candidates for implantation of a cochlear prosthesis. The first publications describing characteristics and application of electrical evoked responses in the assessment of patient populations appeared in the 1970s, within a decade after the discovery of the ABR (Kileny, 1987; Simmons, Lusted, Meyers, & Shelton, 1984; Starr & Brackmann, 1979; Stypulkowski & van den Honert, 1984; Stypulkowski, van den Honert, & Kvistad, 1986; van den Honert & Stypulkowski, 1986). A brief review of electrically evoked auditory responses is presented here because the topic is now regularly reported in the literature, both as experimental and clinical procedures. Clinical investigators and practitioners around the world are recording electrical ABRs (EABRs) and AMLRs (EAMLRs) from pediatric and adult patients. As early as 1988, a panel of experts at the NIH Consensus Development Conference on Cochlear Implants recommended, "measurement of electrical auditory evoked potentials should be a basic component in candidate selection" (Volume 7, 2, May 4, 1988).

Dr. Paul Kileny, a clinical investigator who has for over twenty years published widely on the application of electrically evoked auditory responses before, during, and after cochlear implantation, edited a 2003 supplement to the *International Journal of Audiology* devoted to the topic. Dr. Kileny's comments in introduction of the journal issue are appropriate at the beginning of our discussion: "I believed then, as I believe now, that clinical neurophysiologic measures hold promise in practical applications such as the evaluation of candidacy in pediatric patients, and in under-

standing of fundamental neurophysiologic principles underling the auditory neural pathway-cochlear implant interface" (p. 32). The following discussion begins with an overview of principles important in the measurement of electrically evoked responses from the auditory system. A review of different electrically evoked responses follows. The clinical application of auditory (versus electrically) evoked responses in patients with cochlear implants is then reviewed.

ANATOMY. | Presumably, acoustical and electrical stimulation of the peripheral auditory system generates activity in equivalent regions of the auditory system, namely, the eighth nerve and auditory brainstem and cortex. This premise is essentially based on the similarity of surface recorded acoustically versus electrically evoked brainstem and middle latency responses, rather than any hard neurophysiologic evidence. Although similar anatomic regions underlie responses to both types of stimulation, different characteristic patterns of activity (e.g., discharge patterns) within these regions for electrical versus acoustic stimulation are likely (Kiang, 1965). As seen in Table 15.2, ABR and AMLR latency values are consistently shorter for electrical than acoustic stimulation. van den Honert and Stypulkowski (1986) provided a concise explanation for this distinction. ABR wave I latency is decreased with electrical stimulation because eighth-nerve fibers (primary auditory afferent neurons) are activated directly and with a high degree of synchrony. With acoustic stimulation, basilar membrane travel time precedes cochlear activation, and even with an abrupt (click) stimulus cochlear afferents are mostly activated in the basal region of the cochlea and all do not fire simultaneously. Cochlear physiology underlying ABR was described previously in Chapter 2. In contrast, with essentially direct electrical stimulation of the eighth nerve (via conduction from the promontory), basilar membrane travel time latency is eliminated, and af-

TABLE 15.2. Average Latency and Amplitude Values for Auditory Evoked Responses Evoked by Electrical versus Auditory Signals

COMPONENT	LATENCY (MS)		AMPLITUDE (µV)	
	Auditory	**Electrical**	**Auditory**	**Electrical**
ABR				
III	3.70	2.09	0.40	0.82
V	5.60	3.71	0.50	1.46
AMLR				
Na	15.0	15.4		
Pa	25.0	26.4		
Na-Pa			1.0	2.25
ALR				
N1	96	85.5		
P2	190	181.0		
N1-P2			10	5.65

Source: Data for electrical AERs adapted from Firszt, Chambers, Kraus, & Reeder, 2002.

ferents along a broad region of the cochlea (base to apex) fire synchronously. For these same reasons, latency of the electrical ABR shows little change as a function of stimulus intensity.

TEST PROTOCOLS. | *Stimuli* are typically biphasic square or rectangular electrical pulses. Pulse rate, duration (width), polarity, and amplitude vary from study to study. As an example of these parameters, van den Honert and Stypulkowski (1986) elicited EABRs in human subjects with a pulse rate of 20 to 25/sec, duration of 50 to 100 μsec (per phase), variable polarity and intensity in dB (usually 0 to 15 dB) referenced to perceptual threshold for the stimulus (dB SL). Kileny and colleagues (Kileny & Kemink, 1987; Kileny, Kemink, & Miller, 1989) described EAMLRs stimulated by with charge-balanced biphasic rectangular constant current pulses at a rate of 10 to 16/sec, with an on/off cycle of 2.5 or 5 ms, alternating polarity, and intensities in the range of 20 to 50 μA. Electrical stimuli may be delivered in two ways. Preoperatively (before the cochlear prosthesis is implanted), the electrical stimulus is delivered to the promontory via a needle electrode or, less often, to the round window. This technique is really an electrophysiologic alternative to the behavioral promontory test in assessing cochlear implant candidates. In the studies by Kileny and colleagues, electrical stimuli were presented, using a facial recess approach, to the round window with a Teflon-insulated tungsten electrode. The author uses a similar electrode type and a transtympanic promontory placement, as described in Chapter 4 for ECochG. Intra- or postoperatively, after cochlear prosthesis implantation, electrical pulses are presented via the power amplifier or external signal microprocessor component of the prosthesis coupled to the prosthesis electrodes within the cochlea. Successful measurement of evoked responses with electrical stimulation has been reported for single- and multiple-channel cochlear prostheses.

Stimulus artifact is a major problem in recording electrically evoked responses. Artifact is often far larger than the response, and artifact duration may extend beyond 5 ms and thus totally obscure early response components. Investigators reporting successful EABR measurement have minimized stimulus artifact duration with manipulations of pulse duration, and overall amount of artifact by reductions in intensity and alteration of the mode of presentation (bipolar versus monopolar electrodes). Because of the problem with contamination of EABR waveforms by stimulus artifact, some researchers have turned to EAMLR measurement for evaluation of cochlear implantation candidacy and intra- and postoperative performance.

In most respects, acquisition parameters are comparable for electrically versus acoustically evoked responses. For both EABR and EAMLR, the noninverting electrode is located on the vertex (Cz) or high forehead (Fz), and the inverting electrode is on the ipsilateral (for ABR or AMLR) or contralateral (for AMLR) mastoid or earlobe. The invert-

ing electrode is sometimes located contralateral to the side of stimulation in an attempt to minimize stimulus artifact. The ground electrode is usually placed on the forehead. For intraoperative applications of electrically evoked auditory responses, subdermal needle electrodes may be used instead of disc-type EEG electrodes. Filter settings should be as unrestrictive and filter slope as gradual as possible to reduce the likelihood of filter generated artifact components in the waveform. Band-pass filtering of 100 or even 300 to 3000 Hz is reported for ABR (e.g., van den Honert & Stypulkowski, 1986). With AMLR, high-pass filter cutoffs of 3 Hz and low-pass cutoffs of 1000 to 1500 Hz are used (Kileny et al., 1989). Notch filtering (at 60 Hz) is avoided. After averaging is complete, digital filtering can sometimes enhance the waveform for an electrically evoked auditory response. More than 1,000 stimulus repetitions are typically presented in averaging an EABR and EAMLR. It is important to note, in this regard, that apparent decay or adaptation has been associated with the repetitive stimulation necessary to average electrically evoked responses (van den Honert & Stypulkowski, 1986). No EABR could be detected in selected subjects who reported that stimulus "loudness" became inaudible during the course of testing.

Several other methodological issues add to the challenge of successfully recording and correctly interpreting electrically evoked auditory responses. One important concern is that reliably recorded activity following electrical stimulation does not necessarily arise from the auditory system. In the EABR waveform, components with latencies beyond 5 ms are more likely to be myogenic (generated by muscle or EMG) in nature, or generated within the vestibular system or by the facial nerve. Both vestibular and facial nerve elements are very close to the cochlea and may be stimulated electrically. Vestibular and myogenic responses may even occur within the initial 5 ms poststimulus period. EMG activity (e.g., vestibulo-ocular EMG) is distinguished from EABR by unusually large amplitude and longer latency. Both stimulus artifact and nonauditory evoked responses tend to be more serious problems with extracochlear (promontory) versus intracochlear (cochlear prosthesis) electrical stimulation. Failure to recognize nonauditory evoked responses is particularly serious in electrophysiologic evaluation of cochlear implant candidacy or performance because they can be recorded from patients with no perception of sound to electrical stimulation and, presumably, little or no eighth-nerve integrity.

An instrumentation problem must also be resolved before electrically evoked responses can be measured clinically. Since the acoustic stimulus delivering apparatus cannot be used in generating an electrical stimulus, some other device must be adapted to this function. Some clinical researchers have relied on the promontory stimulator provided by cochlear prosthesis manufacturers. The stimulator on the promontory must first be modified so that it simultaneously triggers the evoked response system to average in synch with stimulus presentation. Difficulty in triggering some evoked response systems externally and inflexibility in available stimulus parameters are limitations of this approach. Another alternative is to deliver the electrical pulse with the somatosensory stimulus portion of an evoked response system. This permits a wider range of stimulus options and eliminates the difficulties associated with interfacing an external device with the evoked response system. With most somatosensory stimulators, however, the smallest unit of current is 1 mA (1000 μA), and it is not possible to quantify stimulus current over the 0 to 1 mA range. Adequate stimulus accuracy, and a greater element of safety, can be obtained by inserting a current-limiting device between the stimulus generator and the patient.

Once the problems noted above (e.g., stimulus artifact, filter artifact, nonauditory waveform components, anesthesia) are solved, analysis of electrically evoked responses is essentially no different than for acoustically evoked responses. The main difference is that electrically evoked response latencies are shorter than those for acoustic stimulation, as displayed in Table 15.2.

ELECTRICAL VERSUS ACOUSTIC STIMULATION. | The preceding discussion focuses on the elicitation of auditory responses with electrical stimulation. The primary clinical purposes for electrically evoked auditory responses are to assess candidacy for cochlear implantation, to verify the integrity and performance of cochlear implant components, and to estimate communication benefit following cochlear implantation. Auditory evoked responses are generated when sounds presented via loudspeakers to the microphone of the cochlear implant are processed and converted to electrical signals. Auditory evoked responses in patients with cochlear implants are essentially an electrophysiological representation of the patient's behavioral response to sound. In other words, AERs recorded from patients with cochlear implants are really comparable to AERs recorded from any patient, except that sound is converted from an acoustical to an electrical signal by the cochlear implant rather than the ear. There are rather clear differences in the themes and findings for investigations of ECAP and EABR versus electrically evoked cortical responses. Electrically evoked responses arising from the auditory nerve and brainstem are applied most often in the definition of threshold for electrical stimulation and integrity of cochlear implant devices and auditory nerve survival. In contrast, cortical evoked responses are more often evoked clinically with acoustical stimulation after cochlear implantation to document performance, including speech perception, with the cochlear implant. Cortical auditory responses can be evoked by external electrical stimulation before cochlear implantation or with acoustic stimulation and internal electrical stimulation in cochlear implant users. The literature on the application of electrically evoked responses from the auditory cortex is expanding, particularly after cochlear implantation. One common theme in the literature is

the value of electrically evoked auditory cortical responses in documenting electrophysiologically the influence of auditory deprivation on auditory system development and, conversely, maturation and plasticity of central pathways with stimulation following cochlear implantation.

The application of electrically evoked auditory responses in patients with severe hearing loss, and also the measurement of auditory evoked responses following cochlear implantation, is now reviewed in anatomic sequence from the peripheral ECAP to cortical responses.

Electrically Evoked Compound Action Potentials (ECAP)

The foregoing review confirms that it is clinical feasible and useful to evoke auditory responses with electrical as well as acoustic signals. Electrically elicited auditory responses, e.g., electrical auditory brainstem or cortical responses, provide general information on the integrity of the auditory nerve prior to cochlear implantation. An electrical signal delivered via a needle electrode placed by a surgeon on the promontory (the medial wall of the middle ear) elicits compound action potentials (ensemble responses) from eighth-nerve fibers and pathways in the brainstem and higher auditory regions. Electrically elicited auditory responses are averaged for hundreds of signals and detected with a far-field technique, that is, with electrodes located at a distance from the cochlea. Figure 15.1 shows an example of an ECAP wave-

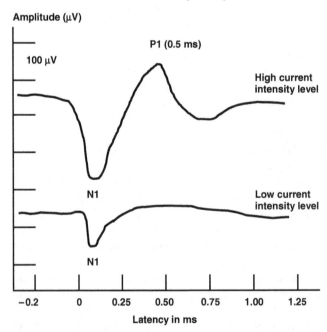

FIGURE 15.1. ECAP waveforms for a high and low level of electrical stimulation.

form for a high and low level of electrical stimulation. The technique, however, has at least three disadvantages in the evaluation of cochlear implants. First, the electrical stimulation simultaneously activates thousands of auditory nerve fibers. The waveforms recording recorded from the scalp reflect widespread electrophysiological activity, rather than spatially discrete excitation from selected neural channels. Second, response amplitude is small, rarely exceeding about 1.5 μV. Movement and muscle artifact often interfere with recordings. With pediatric patients, sedation is necessary to achieve an adequate signal-to-noise ratio for response detection. Finally, conventional electrically evoked auditory responses, only recorded before the cochlear implant surgery, reflect direct stimulation of the eighth cranial nerve fibers. The technique provides no information on performance of the cochlear implant.

Electrically evoked compound action potentials (ECAPs) are intracochlear evoked responses that offer a clinical tool for assessing the excitation of selected populations of neural fibers during stimulation with a multielectrode cochlear implant (Brown & Abbas, 1990; Brown, Abbas, Borland, & Bertschy, 1996), i.e., "the responsiveness of auditory neurons" (Rubinstein, 2004). Taking another complimentary perspective, ECAP measures can document channel interaction. As noted by Abbas, Hughes, Brown, and Miller (2004) "The lack of across-fiber independence in excitation is referred to as channel or spatial interaction and may impose significant limitations on performance in present cochlear implant designs" (p. 203). Simply put, it is desirable for one electrode to stimulate a very limited set of neural fibers and to reduce overlap or spread of stimulation from one electrode to nerve fibers that are stimulated also by another electrode. Measurement of the degree of overlap in the response to (spread of) electrical stimulation or, conversely, recordings that confirm the independence of individual electrodes and the absence of channel interaction appear to be related to performance of cochlear implants as determined with psychoacoustic measures.

Interest in ECAP as an objective measure of auditory nerve viability was generated largely from clinical reports in the mid-1980s of EABR recordings before, during, and after cochlear implantation (e.g., Simmons et al., 1984; Stypulkowski et al., 1986). EABR findings in cochlear implantation are reviewed in the next section. One early paper often cited now in publications on ECAP and EABR is the article by Robert Hall (1990) entitled "Estimation of Surviving Spiral Ganglion Cells in the Deaf Rat Using the Electrically Evoked Auditory Brainstem Response." In research conducted at the Auditory Prosthesis Research Laboratory at Massachusetts Eye and Ear Infirmary in Boston, Hall (1990), over a period of about 130 days from animals with normal cochlear function and other animals with total cochlear destruction caused by perfusion of the ototoxic drug neomycin, measured serially amplitude growth functions for major EABR peaks, including the P1 (i.e., the ECAP). Hall

(1990) states, "the measurements . . . presented here clearly confirm the theoretical prediction that the maximum amplitude of P1 is proportional to the number of excitable auditory nerve fibers" (p. 134). The author, however, goes on to point out the substantial amount of variability in findings for the amplitude growth functions that permit estimations of spiral ganglion cell integrity "only within rather large error bounds" (p. 134). Further qualifying the findings for clinical interpretation, Hall (1990) states, "additional experience in recording the rat's EABR will probably reduce that error, but even this kind of predictability may be difficult to achieve in humans. The variability in EABR amplitudes is likely to be greater than it is in the rat or other laboratory animals as a consequence of greater individual differences in subjects as well as greater variability in stimulating and recording conditions" (p. 134). Finally, the author reported "generally low correlations" for spiral ganglion cells counts and the amplitude of later EABR waves, thus providing an argument for the clinical application of ECAP versus EABR for estimating viability of the auditory nerve.

A detailed review of the literature describing techniques for determining with ECAP channel interaction and spread of neural excitation in cochlear implant users is beyond the scope of this discussion. Briefly, the amplitude of the response as recorded from different electrodes near or more distant from a fixed stimulating electrode can be calculated. Stimulus intensity level is, of course, an important factor in determining response amplitude. It is essential, therefore, for the level of stimulation to be consistent among electrodes. Equivalence in stimulus intensity among electrodes cannot always be verified. In addition, a robust neural response may be recorded via volume conduction from a rather distant stimulus electrode, rather than an adjacent or nearby electrode. [Note: The concept of volume conduction was reviewed in Chapter 2.] Another approach for determining electrode channel interaction for cochlear implants, and feasible with clinical cochlear implants, involves recording the ECAP with a probe electrical pulse presented to one electrode while a masker signal is presented to another electrode (e.g., Abbas et al., 2004; Cohen, Richardson, Saunders, & Cowan, 2003; Dees et al., 2005; Eisen & Franck, 2004; Miller, Arenberg, Middlebrooks, & Pfingst, 2003; van Weert, Stokroos, Rikers, & van Dijk, 2005). With this method, the extent of channel interaction can be calculated by measurement of the effect of the masker electrode location on ECAP amplitude for a given stimulus electrode. Generally, presentation of the masker signal precedes the probe stimulation by a brief time frame (e.g., 0.5 ms). The reader is referred for more details to original articles describing the "two-pulse forward masking paradigm" and other masker-probe methods.

The ECAP offers minimally two distinct clinical advantages in assessment of patients with cochlear implants. Psychoacoustic assessment is not be feasible for young children, yet ECAP can be recorded to provide physiologic information on cochlear implant performance. For older patients,

ECAP recordings often are less time consuming than psychoacoustic assessment. Furthermore, they complement and objectively verify behavioral findings.

Electrodes within the cochlear implant are numbered (e.g., 1, 2, . . . 15) sequentially in an apical to basal direction and separated by a space of about 1 mm. Briefly, an electrical signal is presented under computer control with one electrode among the 20-plus electrodes implanted in the cochlea. Neural recording is then made from another electrode located in the cochlear implant, close to the stimulating electrode. The primary function of multiple electrodes within a cochlear implant is to adequately code frequencies within complex sounds. The accuracy or "frequency resolution" of the coding process is largely dependent on the functional independence of individual electrodes. Conversely, cochlear implant performance is reduced, and subsequently speech recognition and perception performance, by "channel interaction" intracochlear recordings (e.g., Dorman, Smith, Smith, & Parkin, 1996; White, Mersnich, & Gardi, 1984). Ideally, cochlear implant electrodes can be located very close to the modiolar wall near the auditory afferent fibers and thus can activate auditory system with low levels of stimulation and, importantly, with a high degree of neuronal selectivity. That is, the electrode close to the modiolar wall should selectively stimulate a limited number of neurons and, at least theoretically, contribute to enhanced discrimination of acoustic signals, including speech sounds. Measurement of electrode interaction and related overlap in the stimulation of cochlear nerve fibers within the region of the electrodes is now possible with commercial instrumentation (Abbas et al., 2004; Cohen et al., 2003). Intracochlear stimulation and recording is illustrated schematically in Figure 15.2. One of the manufacturers of cochlear implant devices (Cochlear Corporation), developed a system for recording ECAPs consisting of computer software and multielectrode cochlear implant designs (CI24M and CI24R). With this device, the technique is referred to as Neural Response Telemetry, or NRT. Similar systems for measurement of ECAP available from at least two other cochlear implant manufacturers include Neural Response Imaging or NRI (Advanced Bionics Corp.) and Auditory Nerve Response Telemetry (MedEl).

In young and difficult-to-test children, ECAP measurements can contribute to decisions in cochlear implant fitting, such as selecting current levels for estimating subjective (psychophysical) detection threshold (T) and comfortable (C) settings (Brown et al., 2000; Franck & Norton, 2001). Children cannot describe the effect of changes in speech processor settings on their perception of sounds, but ECAP may offer in cochlear implant fitting an objective measure of individual electrode operation and channel interaction (Abbas et al., 2004). Factors that influence the isolation or, conversely, the overlap or spread in stimulation, of neurons with a multielectrode array in a cochlear implant include the intensity of the stimulus, the proportion of surviving and stimulable neurons, and the proximity of the electrode to the surviving,

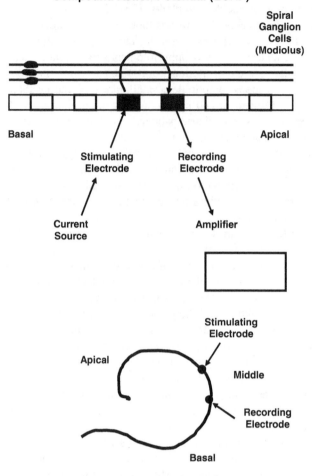

FIGURE 15.2. Schematic representation of intracochlear stimulus and recording electrodes in electrical compound action potential (ECAP).

i.e., "stimulable," neurons. Recent evidence suggests that parameters of auditory responses with intracochlear electrical stimulation, such as response threshold levels and amplitude, provide information on the extent of neural excitation and the closeness of the electrode to the nerve fibers (Abbas et al., 2004; Wackym et al., 2004). Concluding with the a statement by Rubinstein (2004), "The ECAP is not an empirical biological potential. It has precisely identifiable generators, and future applications may be far more useful than its current status as an indicator of electrical threshold" (p. S9).

ECAP TEST PROTOCOL. | Stimulus and acquisition parameters in ECAP measurement are summarized in Table 15.3. Options and values for some parameters are often unique to specific cochlear implant systems and manufacturers. Stimulus intensity, for example, is described by one manufacturer in "current unit levels" or CU that range from 1 up to over 200. The CUs roughly correspond to stimulus current of as

TABLE 15.3.   Guidelines for a Test Protocol for Electrically Evoked Compound Action Potential (ECAP)

Test parameters vary among manufacturers of cochlear implants with electrodes and software for recording ECAP.

PARAMETER	SELECTION
Stimulus	
Type	Biphasic constant current electrical pulse ("probe")
Masker	Biphasic electrical pulse
Stimulus (probe) duration	~25 to 50 µs
Masker duration	~25 to 50 µs
Masker probe interval	~500 µs
Site of stimulation	Selected intracochlear implant electrodes (intra- or postoperatively) from among up to 22 electrodes
Mode of stimulation	Bipolar (both electrodes within the cochlea) or monopolar (1 intracochlear and 1 extra-cochlear electrode, e.g., temporalis muscle)
Rate	~30 to 80/sec
Polarity	Alternating (bipolar); the first polarity change should be specified as either anodic (positive) or cathodic (negative)
Probe intensity	Variable in current units (CU)
Masker intensity	Higher than probe intensity (e.g., 10 CU)
Repetitions	~50 to 100 stimuli
Acquisition	
Electrode sites	Intracochlear implant electrodes (intra- or postoperatively) close to but several electrodes in the apical direction from the stimulus electrode
Analysis time	~5 ms
Analysis delay	>35 to 150 µs (between offset of stimulus and onset of signal averaging)
Filter settings	30 or 100 to 1500 Hz
Amplification (gain)	40 to 60 dB
Sweeps	~50 to >200 averages
Sampling rate	~20 Hz

low as about 10µA to a high of almost 200 mA (Abbas et al., 1999).

Stimulus artifact is a serious problem in recording the ECAP. With intracochlear ECAP measurement, the stimulating and recording electrodes are very close. Consequently, substantial stimulus artifact is detected with the recording electrode. The electrical artifact is usually larger in amplitude than the actual ECAP. Recall that the latency values of major ECAP components (N1 and P2) are short, e.g., 0.2 to 0.5 ms. Stimulus artifact within the initial portion of the waveform, therefore, may obscure detection of the ECAP. In addition, the large electrical artifact produces amplifier saturation. Electrophysiological activity can occur while the amplifier is recovering from saturation and, thus, the short latency ECAP components may go undetected. Electrical stimulus artifact must be diminished or in some way differentiated from the neural response to detect accurately the ECAP. Different solutions have been reported for minimizing stimulus artifact in ECAP measurement, including a masker-probe subtraction process, alternating stimulus polarity (or phase), artifact reduction pulse (ARP), and a technique of subtracting a template ("scaled template") of the stimulus artifact from the ECAP. Combinations of these techniques are available from some manufacturers of cochlear implants and reported in the literature (e.g., Battmer et al., 2004). Among these strategies for solving the problem of stimulus artifact in ECAP measurement, the masker-probe subtraction technique or algorithm, introduced by Charlet de Sauvage and colleagues (1983) is most often described in recent clinical papers due to its feasibility with commercial cochlear implant systems. The general technique is described with various terms, such as two-pulse subtraction, masked response extraction or MRE (e.g., Battmer et al., 2004), the masker-probe algorithm (e.g., Eisen & Franck, 2005), or simply the subtraction method (e.g., Abbas et al., 1999).

The masker-probe technique for reduction of electrical stimulus artifact in ECAP is illustrated schematically in Figure 15.3. Briefly, the ECAP is recorded in three different conditions. First, an ECAP is elicited only with an electrical stimulus (probe). Although the neural response (ECAP) may be present, it occurs within and cannot be distinguished from substantial electrical artifact. Electrical artifact is super-

Masker-Probe Subtraction Method in ECAP Measurement

A. Probe Only (neural response and probe artifact)

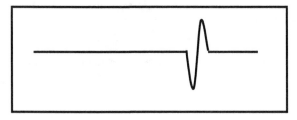

B. Masker and Probe (masker and probe artifact)

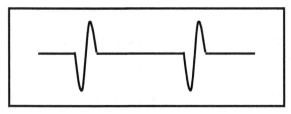

C. Masker Only (masker artifact)

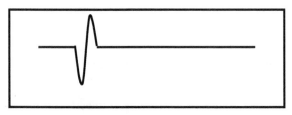

Subtraction Process to Derive Neural Response
A – (B – C)

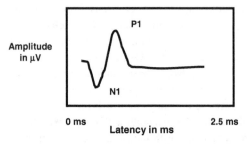

FIGURE 15.3. The masker-probe technique for reduction of electrical stimulus artifact and enhancement of the electrical compound action potential (ECAP).
Adapted from Dillier et al., 2002.

imposed on and contaminating the neural response. Next, the ECAP is recorded with a masker signal followed by the stimulus probe, described as the "masker-plus-probe condition" (Abbas et al., 1999). The time difference between the masker and the probe (the "masker advance") is typically on the order of 500 µs. The masker and probe signals are presented via the same intracochlear electrode and stimulate the same population of neurons. Because the probe stimulus is presented within the refractory period of the neurons, the masker effectively precludes the generation of a neural response by the probe stimulus. That is, the neurons are not yet ready to fire again within such as short time (500 µs) after being activated by the masker signal. With progressively longer masker-to-probe stimulus intervals, the masker signal generates a neural response and the probe also begins to generate a second neural response. With adequately long IPIs (several seconds), there would be two neural responses to two separate stimuli. Given the subsequent subtraction process, response amplitude decreases as the interpulse interval (IPI) increases and, conversely, ECAP amplitude increases as the IPI decreases. With the short (e.g., 500 µs) interval in the masker-probe condition used to record ECAP, there is no neural response to the probe stimulus. Finally, in the third recording condition, the masker signal alone is presented (refer again to Figure 15.3).

The ECAP is then derived, or resolved from the electrical artifact, by a multistep subtraction process. The waveform generated by the masker-probe combination is subtracted from the waveform produced in the probe alone condition, thus disentangling the neural response from the stimulus artifact. The resulting derived waveform, however, may contain residual electrical artifact associated with the masker signal and also neural activity generated by the masker signal. These unwanted sources of measurement "noise" are removed by further subtracting from the derived waveform the waveform recorded in the masker alone condition. Critical parameters affecting the quality of the ECAP include the stimulus and recording electrodes, including their location within the cochlea (basal, middle, apical) and their spatial relationship, the intensity level and the duration of the probe and masker pulses, and the delay between the masker and the probe signals. Each of these parameters is usually selected and varied with software supplied by the cochlear implant system manufacturer. Characteristics of the physiologic amplifier, such as linearity and resistance or susceptibility to saturation, also are important factors in successful ECAP measurement.

Common types of ECAP measurements include thresholds (T), amplitude growth functions (AGF), and recovery functions. Thresholds are, as expected, measured by recording ECAP at different stimulus intensity levels (in current units), including relatively low levels down to an intensity that produces no detectable response (see top portion of Figure 15.4). Amplitude growth functions are plots of ECAP amplitude (in µV) as a function of stimulus intensity level

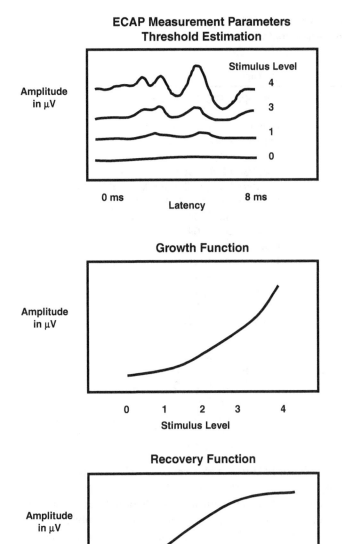

FIGURE 15.4. Illustration of common types of ECAP measurements including thresholds (T), amplitude growth functions (AGF), and recovery functions.

(in CU), as shown in the bottom portion of Figure 15.4. Of course, with an adequate number of stimulus intensity levels (e.g., in 5 CU increments), including minimal levels, ECAP thresholds can be calculated or interpolated from the low end of amplitude growth functions. Thresholds and amplitude growth functions are highly variable among subjects, with less variability within individual subjects. There is some evidence that ECAP thresholds decrease modestly for basal to apical electrode locations, although findings are not consistent among studies. Amplitude growth functions, in con-

trast, clearly decrease for apical to basal electrode locations. Recovery functions are measured with the masker-probe subtraction technique ("masked response subtraction") by manipulating the IPI. The interval between the masker and the probe pulses is also referred to as the masker probe interval, or the MPI (e.g., Battmer et al., 2004). With short IPIs, the neurons activated by masker are not recovered before the probe stimulus is presented, as described above. Therefore, no ECAP is generated. As the IPI is increased and approximates the end of the recovery period, the ECAP emerges. With further increases in the delay between the masker and probe, ECAP amplitude increases until, with an adequately long IPI, all neural fibers are activated maximally and amplitude reaches maximum (e.g., the amplitude saturates). The concept of ECAP recovery function was illustrated in Figure 15.4. The three ECAP response parameters are clearly not independent. The relation between ECAP threshold and AGF has already been noted. There is also evidence that recovery function vary with probe current level (Battmer et al., 2004).

CLINICAL APPLICATION OF ECAP. | Clinical measurement of the ECAP was introduced in 1996 (Brown et al., 1996). Since then, numerous investigators, some participating in multicenter trials, have reported intraoperative and postoperative ECAP recordings with Neural Response Telemetry (NRT), the system utilized in the Nucleus cochlear implant (Abbas et al., 1999; Brown, Abbas, & Gantz, 1998; Brown et al., 2000; Charasse, Chanal, Berger-Vachon, & Collet, 2004; Dillier et al., 2002; Franck & Norton, 2001; Gordon, Papsin, & Harrison, 2004; Hughes et al., 2000; Shallop, Facer, & Peterson, 1999; Smoorenburg, Willeboer, & van Dijk, 2002). During the same period, successful clinical measurement of ECAP was reported also for the Clarion cochlear implant device with the Neural Response Imaging (NRI) technique (e.g., Frijns, Briaire, & Grote, 2001). Findings confirmed the value of ECAP in programming cochlear implants, e.g., estimation of initial target settings, in young children. Studies also provided evidence of the contribution of ECAP data in decisions regarding the inclusion or exclusion of individual electrodes from the program in an attempt to maximize speech perception. The reader who is interested in the application of ECAP with a particular brand of cochlear implant is referred to the manufacturer and to articles describing research limited to a specific cochlear implant design, summarized in Table 15.4.

ECAP offers multiple advantages for clinical assessment of patients during or after cochlear implantation, as summarized in Table 15.5. Five distinct clinical applications of ECAP are reported in the literature. As noted below, the EABR can be applied clinically in essentially the same ways. One application of ECAP is assessment and documentation of auditory nerve integrity, i.e., the capacity of the afferent auditory neural fibers to respond when stimulated electrically. Functional integrity of auditory nerve fibers is,

TABLE 15.4. Selected Published Studies of Electrical Compound Action Potential (ECAP) Measurement with Cochlear Implants Available from Different Manufacturers

MANUFACTURER (ECAP TECHNIQUE)	DEVICE	SUBJECTS	STUDIES
Cochlear (NRT)	Nucleus 24M	14 adults; 14 children	Shallop, Facer, & Peterson, 1999
	Nucleus 24M	26 adults	Abbas et al., 1999
	Nucleus 24M	12 adults	Franck & Norton, 2001
	Nucleus 24M	60 children	Mason et al., 2001
	Nucleus 24M	23 children	Thai-Van et al., 2001
	Nucleus 24M	27 adults	Smoorenburg, Willeboer, & van Dijk, 2002
	Nucleus 24R	10 adults	Hay-McCutcheon et al., 2002
	Nucleus 24M	12 adults	Abbas et al., 2004
	Nucleus 24RCS	5 adults	Abbas et al., 2004
	Nucleus 24RCS	9 children	Wackym et al., 2004
	Nucleus 24M	6 adults	Charasse et al., 2004
	Nucleus 24M	2 children	Eisen & Franck, 2005
	Nucleus 24RCS	9 children	Eisen & Franck, 2005
	Nucleus 24M	147 adults	Dees et al., 2005
	Nucleus 24RCS	4 children; 10 adults	van Weert et al., 2005
Advanced Bionics (NRI)	Clarion HiFocus	16 children	Eisen & Franck, 2004
	Clarion HiFocus	8 children	Wackym et al., 2004
	Clarion CII	16 children	Eisen & Franck, 2005
	Clarion HiFocus	9 children; adults	Han et al., 2005

of course, a fundamental requirement for hearing and for success with a cochlear implant. With ECAP, documentation of functional integrity of the auditory fibers can be first made in the operating room within minutes after cochlear implantation. Since the technique is similar to ECAP measurement made in the weeks and months after cochlear implantation when the device is programmed, the intraoperative ECAP findings provide reasonable assurance that the patient will obtain benefit from cochlear implant, i.e., the patient will be able to hear. Conversely, absence of an ECAP when recorded intraoperatively does not necessarily mean that the cochlear implant has malfunctioned and the patient will not hear. Technical problems, such as excessive electrical artifact either in the recording environment or related to stimulation, may affect the quality, or even the detection, of the ECAP. Severe damage or dysfunction of the auditory nerve is an unlikely, but potential, explanation for the absence of an ECAP intraoperatively immediately after cochlear implantation. The likelihood of this explanation for the inability to detect an ECAP may be higher in selected patient populations, e.g., auditory neuropathy. A second, and related, application of ECAP is to confirm neural synchrony postoperatively (after cochlear implantation) in patients with the diagnosis of auditory neuropathy (Mason et al., 2003; Peterson et al., 2003; Shallop, Jin, Driscoll, & Tibesar, 2004; Shallop, Peterson, et al., 2001; Trautwein, Siniger, & Nelson, 2000).

Third, ECAP provides valuable information on the integrity of the cochlear implant device, including electrodes. Clinical experience confirms that abnormalities in intraoperative tests of cochlear implant function are not rare. For example, Mason (2004) reported detecting "anomalous findings" intraoperatively for about one-third of a consecutive series of twenty-nine children implanted with one brand and model of cochlear implant, with concerns about electrodes most common. Intraoperative electrophysiological findings (e.g., ECAP, EABR) can lead to an investigation of and, as needed, intervention for the problems, including reliance on a back-up device. As noted by Mason (2004) "Intraoperative electrophysiologic and objective measures play an important role in the management of children undergoing implant surgery . . ." (p. S37).

A fourth application of ECAP is to document postoperatively with serial measurements atypical and potentially serious variations in cochlear implant function in the weeks, months, and even years after cochlear implantation. Some changes in ECAP amplitude and threshold are expected among measurements made intraoperatively versus the initial months postoperatively. Malfunction of the cochlear implant can be detected with ECAP, even in young children who are unable to describe what they hear. Postoperative changes in the ECAP prompt troubleshooting to determine the cause of the problem, e.g., a breakdown in the internal receiver and stimulator, electrode failure, or other technical failures. Pe-

TABLE 15.5. Advantages and disadvantages among electrical auditory evoked response techniques*

RESPONSE	ADVANTAGES	DISADVANTAGES
ECAP	Large amplitude (up to 1500 µV) Not affected by muscle artifact Information specifically on neural function Information on cochlear implant integrity Independent of developmental status Closer relation to spiral ganglion cell viability Sedation not required Very quiet patient not necessary	Information limited to auditory nerve fibers No direct relation to speech perception with CI** Requires special manufacturer electrode and software Substantial electrical measurement artifact Poor relationship to speech perception
EABR	Doesn't require special manufacturer cochlear implant electrode and software Not affected by sedation or anesthesia Information on brainstem auditory function	Relatively small amplitude (1.5 µV or less) Poor relationship to speech perception Poorer relation to auditory nerve viability than ECAP
EAMLR	Information on auditory cortex Findings related to speech perception	Seriously affected by sedation and anesthesia
EALR	Information on auditory cortex Findings related to speech perception	Affected by sedation and anesthesia Affected by sleep
EP300	Information on auditory cortex Objective measure of speech perception	Affected by sedation and anesthesia Affected by sleep
EMMN	Information on auditory cortex Findings related to speech perception Not affected by sleep Can be recorded from infants	Affected by sedation and anesthesia

* ECAP = electrical compound action potential; EABR = electrical auditory brainstem response;
EAMLR = electrical auditory middle-latency response; EALR = electrical auditory late response;
EP300 = electrical P300 response; EMMN = electrical mismatch negativity response
** CI = cochlear implant

riodic ECAP measurement will also detect the development of unusual anatomic or physiologic abnormalities, including auditory nerve dysfunction secondary to pathology (e.g., tumors or viral infection).

Finally, the application of ECAP as an objective technique for programming cochlear implants has increased considerably with the reliance on cochlear implants as the treatment of choice for children with severe and profound hearing impairment at younger ages (less than 12 months). ECAP recorded intraoperatively or soon after cochlear implantation in young children is used to estimate and map objectively behavioral threshold (T) and comfort (C) levels and other stimulation parameters of cochlear implants (e.g., Cullington, 2000; Franck, 2002; Gantz, Brown, & Abbas, 1994; Hughes et al., 2000; Mason et al., 2001; Thai-Van et al., 2001). Application of ECAP in mapping and programming the speech processor of cochlear implants is the topic of ongoing investigation, as detailed by numerous articles in the literature. According to some investigators (e.g., Brown et al., 2000; Hughes et al., 2000; Smoorenburg et al., 2002), the relation between ECAP thresholds and subjective behaviorally estimated thresholds, and also maximum stimulation levels, is weak. In addition, Smoorenburg, Willeboer, and van Dijk (2002) found that "Prediction of the most critical factor in speech perception, the slope of the maximum stimulation curve, from ECAP thresholds is poor" (p. 335). However, Mason et al. (2001) reported in a series of sixty children implanted before 5 years of age that intraoperative ECAP thresholds were correlated significantly with initial threshold levels, as well as intraoperative EABR recordings. Similarly, Thai-Van and colleagues (2001) described a significant correlation between ECAP thresholds and behavioral levels, with the relationship remaining significant out to three to twelve months after implantation particularly for apical positioned electrodes.

Dees and no less than thirty-two co-authors from thirteen European countries (Dees et al., 2005) reported ECAP findings for 147 adults with cochlear implants. Subjects had multiple and generally imprecise etiologies for hearing loss, with the most common five described as progressive, meningitis, congenital, sudden/other, and unknown. Duration of hearing loss prior to implantation was also highly variable for the subject group, ranging from less than one year to over fifteen years. NRT measurements were made with the Nucleus 24® cochlear implant system (Cochlear Corp.). ECAP response parameters analyzed included test electrode location, morphology of the ECAP waveforms, electrophysiological and subjective threshold and loudness acceptance presentation levels, ECAP latency, and amplitude growth functions. Results of the study by Dees et al. (2005) may be summarized as follows:

- A clear ECAP was recorded in 96 percent of the subjects.
- An ECAP was also recorded from 96 percent of all electrodes that were tested in the group of subjects (e.g., 621 out of 647 electrodes).
- There was a relation between longer duration of deafness and lower tolerance levels for stimulation and the need for slower rates of stimulation for adequately high stimulation presentation level to produce a response.
- ECAP waveform morphology consisted of a single peak for 95 percent of the responses and a double peak for 7 percent.
- A double peak in the ECAP waveform was more common for responses recorded from apical electrode locations.
- ECAP amplitude varied widely among subjects, with the N1-P1 amplitude difference ranging from 12 to 633 μV.
- Also, within subjects, ECAP amplitude was highly variable for different electrode locations (e.g., 20 to 40 percent variability).
- The slope of the amplitude growth function for the ECAP was similarly variable among subjects, ranging from 1.2 μV/CU to 63.3 μV/CU. Slope was, to a lesser extent, variable among electrode locations within subjects. Typically, the slope for amplitude growth functions was between 5 and 20 μV/CU.
- At the loudest acceptable presentation level, ECAP latencies among electrode sites were on the average 0.32 to 0.34 ms for N1 (ranging from 0.22 to 0.62 ms) and 0.66 to 0.67 ms for P1 (ranging from 0.35 to 0.98 ms).
- Threshold of the ECAP was related to electrode location (threshold decreased gradually from electrode 20 to electrode 3).
- There was no clear correlation between ECAP threshold and two common subjective speech processor programming parameters, i.e., threshold or maximum comfortable loudness levels.

ECAP findings in patients with cochlear implants are characterized by large inter- and intrasubject variability (e.g., Dees et al., 2005). Current research is devoted largely to exploring factors contributing to the well-appreciated variability in electrophysiological and behavioral measures of cochlear implant performance. Among the possible factors are age of the patient, duration of deafness, etiology of hearing loss, the number of viable spiral ganglion cells, and location of the stimulating electrode within the cochlea and also in proximity to the modiolus (auditory nerve fibers). There is considerable current research interest in cochlear implant

designs and insertion techniques that minimize the distance between the electrodes and the auditory nerve fibers and the modiolus (e.g., Donaldson et al., 2001; Firszt et al., 2003; Pasanisi et al., 2002; Wackym et al., 2004). In theory, medial placement of the cochlear implant electrodes in close proximity to the auditory nerve fibers and spiral ganglion cells within the modiolus is optimal for cochlear implant performance. Related to this line of thinking is the suspicion that differences among individual electrodes in the distance between the electrode and the nerve fibers are a major factor in the variability in cochlear implant performance between patients, and even between electrodes for a single patient. Electrophysiological indices of enhanced cochlear implant performance include decreased (improved) thresholds and reduced channel interaction. In recent years, two devices or modifications in cochlear implant design have been introduced to achieve this goal.

One of the major cochlear implant manufacturers (Advanced Bionics) includes a positioner with the Clarion HiFocus II electrode that can be inserted immediately after implantation to push the electrodes toward the modiolus. Another manufacturer (Cochlear Corp.) offers a stylet for guiding and curling the Nucleus CI24R (CS) Contour electrode as it is inserted so the electrode is closer to the modiolus wall of the scala tympani. Eisen and Franck (2004) studied ECAP thresholds and amplitude growth functions (AGFs) with the Clarion HiFocus cochlear implant device in sixteen children. One purpose of the study was to evaluate the impact on cochlear implant performance of electrode location in patients implanted with versus without the use of a Silastic electrode positioning system. In theory, the positioner pushes the cochlear implant electrodes medially and closer to the auditory fibers (spiral ganglion cells), resulting in more effective stimulation with the cochlear implant. The benefits of smaller distance between the electrodes and auditory nerve fibers are intuitive. Less current is required to activate the neural fibers and stimulation is more specific to individual electrodes, i.e., there is less interaction between nearby electrodes (Fayad, Luxford, & Linthicum, 2000). Lower thresholds are desirable, for both subjective (behavioral) measures (e.g., Donaldson et al., 2001; Franck, Shah, Marsh, & Potsic, 2002; Mens, Boyle, & Mulder, 2003; Young & Grohne, 2001) and electrophysiological recordings (e.g., Cords et al., 2000; Firszt et al., 2003). Eisen and Franck (2004) found lower ECAP thresholds with the Silastic positioner, but only for the basal end of the implant. There was no difference in ECAP thresholds with versus without the positioner for apical electrodes. In this study, ECAP threshold was calculated by extrapolating from the linear portion of the amplitude growth function, rather than directly as the smallest detectable ECAP as stimulus intensity is decreased or increased. Lower thresholds are, of course, the reason for utilizing the device. However, the slopes of amplitude growth functions were not influenced by the positioner for any of the electrodes from the basal to the apical end of the cochlear implant. This was an unexpected outcome because, as Eisen and Franck (2004) point out, "If the distance between the electrode surface and the neural elements determined growth function slope, then we expect differences in slope between the presence and absence of the Silastic positioner. No gross differences appeared between these two groups" (p. 533).

Using a forward masking protocol, the same authors (Eisen & Franck, 2005) investigated in a group of twenty-seven children electrode interaction with either the Clarion II implant (Advanced Bionics) or the Nucleus 24 implant (Cochlear). While the probe electrode was held constant, a masker was moved from one electrode to another along the electrode array. Three probe electrode locations were assessed representing basal, medial, and apical sites. The authors reported increased electrode interaction as intensity of stimulation at the probe electrode increased. Electrode interaction was also related to location within the cochlea, with relatively smaller amounts of interaction in basal versus middle or apical probe sites. The relation of these findings to speech recognition or perception was not investigated. In another investigation of NRI with the Advance Bionic CII Bionic Ear system using HiResolution™ software, Han and colleagues in Beijing, China (Han et al., 2005), reported a correlation of NRI thresholds and most comfortable levels as determined behaviorally and used by patients in their "everyday HiResolution programs."

In an attempt to verify the benefits of positioning the cochlear implant closer to the modiolus (primary auditory nerves), Van Weert et al. (2005) recorded ECAP (NRT) intra-operatively in fourteen subjects implanted with the Nucleus C124R (CS) Contour implant before and after removal of a stylet designed to curl the electrode so that it would approximate the modiolus. The authors analyzed ECAP thresholds, amplitude growth functions, and electrode interaction (i.e., spread of excitation of auditory nerve fibers). The specificity of electrode stimulation was evaluated using the masker-and-probe technique, reported also by other authors with a different cochlear implant brand (e.g., Eisen & Franck, 2004). Citing other investigations (e.g., Cohen et al., 2003; Cords et al., 2000; Frijns, De Snoo, & Schoonhoven, 1995), Van Weert and colleagues (2005) state,

> Modiolar electrode placement has two possible advantages over conventional arrays. (i) Less power may be needed to stimulate the dentrites of the cochlear nerve fibers. This may result in reduced battery consumption, which is of obvious advantage to implant users. (ii) The implant may stimulate the auditory nerve more selectively, i.e., as each electrode is closer to the nerve, it is expected to stimulate a smaller (more localized) group of neurons. This reduced spread of excitation may result in larger perceived contrasts between sounds, which may contribute to improved speech discrimination. (p. 725)

The authors found no difference in the NRT thresholds or amplitude growth function before and immediately after

removal of the stylet for any electrode. As the authors note, it's possible that the electrode may in the weeks after surgery shift away from the modiolus. Analysis of electrode selectivity, or tuning curves, in NRT measurements showed narrower widths for electrodes at the basal and apical ends of the cochlear implant, but not for "mid-array" electrodes. Consistent with previous authors (e.g., Cohen et al., 2003), the findings reported by Van Weert et al. (2005) are "consistent with the hypothesis that modiolar placement of the electrode array improves stimulation selectivity" (p. 729). The effect was, however, small. And the authors further state: "Remarkably, we found no effect of modiolus hugging on the threshold of NRT responses" (p. 730).

Other research trends are also worthy of mention. Investigation of the application of ECAP (e.g., NRT) from the brainstem in programming auditory brainstem implants yielded disappointing findings (Otto, Waring, & Kuchta, 2005). Clinical studies are also underway to validate technological advances in cochlear implant hardware (e.g., amplifier noise floor and linearity) and software (e.g., artifact cancellation methods) with the goal of automating test protocols, decreasing ECAP measurement time, and enhance the accuracy and precision of ECAP recordings (e.g., Battmer et al., 2004).

Electrically Evoked Auditory Brainstem Response (EABR)

Reports describing measurement of the EABR date back to the 1980s—the first decade of clinical application of the acoustically evoked ABR (e.g., Black, Lilly, Fowler, & Stypulkowski, 1987; Pelizzone, Kasper, & Montandon, 1989; Shallop, Beiter, Goin, & Mischke, 1990; Smith & Simmons, 1983; van den Honert & Stypulkowski, 1986; Walsh & Leake-Jones, 1982). Historically, the main motivation for clinical application of EABR was to verify neural function of patients under consideration for cochlear implantation. Preoperatively, the EABR is stimulated with electrical signals delivered via a needle placed with a transtympanic technique on the promontory of the ear (medial wall of the middle ear space). However, can electrically evoked responses provide a means of quantifying eighth-nerve integrity (e.g., the percentage of surviving or functioning afferent fibers) before cochlear implantation, or of evaluating cochlear implant performance and patient communicative success with the implant (especially in children) following implantation? Much of the published research on EABR focuses on this question. An early use of EABR was identification of the ear (right versus left) that was most appropriate for cochlear implantation (Kileny, 1991). When the EABR was present with stimulation of one ear via a transtympanic technique, but not the other ear, the preoperative findings provided guidance for the laterality of cochlear implantation. Similarly, in combination with radiological findings, interear differences in the threshold of the EABR were applied in the estimation of neural survival and nerve stimulability and, therefore, decisions about which ear was implanted (e.g., Kileny, Zwolan, Zimmerman-Phillips, & Telian, 1994; Mason et al., 1997). In 1989, the National Institutes of Health Consensus Development Conference on Cochlear Implants recommended inclusion of preoperative EABR findings in decisions regarding cochlear implant candidacy. Based on analysis of data for a series of forty-three patients undergoing preoperative EABR measurement before cochlear implantation, Kileny et al. (1994) recommended for pediatric patients the application of electrophysiological measures (EABR) "to determine electrical excitability." However, subsequent studies suggest that the relation between preoperative EABR findings and postoperative cochlear implant performance is not clear-cut, a conclusion consistent with the cautious predictions made by Hall (1990) based on animal studies (detailed in the earlier discussion of ECAP). Nikolopoulos, Mason, O'Donaghue, and Gibbin (1999) described more identifiable EABRs, and significantly greater EABR amplitude values, for children with congenital deafness than for children with hearing loss following meningitis. The same British research group (Nikolopoulos, Mason, Gibbin, & O'Donaghue, 2000) found that EABR recorded preoperatively with promontory electrical stimulation from children did not predict speech perception and speech intelligibility with the cochlear implant. Indeed, cochlear implant performance for children with no detectable EABR with electrical stimulation at the promontory was comparable to performance for children with a clear preoperative response to promontory electrical stimulation.

The primary clinical purposes for electrically evoked auditory responses are to assess candidacy for cochlear implantation, to verify the integrity and performance of cochlear implant components, and to estimate communication benefit following cochlear implantation. Electrophysiological responses can also be evoked by auditory stimuli following cochlear implantation. Auditory evoked responses are generated when sounds presented via loudspeakers to the microphone of the cochlear implant are processed and converted to electrical signals. Auditory evoked responses in patients with cochlear implants are essentially an electrophysiological representation of the patient's behavioral response to sound. In other words, AERs recorded from patients with cochlear implants are really comparable to AERs recorded from any patient, except that sound is converted from an acoustical to an electrical signal by the cochlear implant rather than the ear.

EABR TEST PROTOCOL. | A test protocol for measurement of the EABR is displayed in Table 15.6. Similarities exist between the test protocols for acoustically versus electrically elicited ABRs. Naturally, stimulus parameters are substantially different for the electrically evoked response, in comparison to the conventional ABR.

As indicated above in the introduction to EABR, there are two general techniques for recording the EABR. Pre-

TABLE 15.6. Guidelines for a Test Protocol for Electrically Evoked Auditory Brainstem Response (EABR)

PARAMETER	SELECTION
Stimulus	
Type	Biphasic constant current electrical pulse
Mode of delivery	Needle electrode (preoperative) or cochlear implant electrode (intra- or postoperative)
Site of stimulation	Promontory (preoperative) or intracochlear (intra- or postoperative)
Rate	5 to >85 pulses/sec
Duration	~20 to 400 μsec per phase
Polarity	Alternating (bipolar)
Intensity	20 μA to 1 mA
Repetitions	≥1000
Acquisition	
Electrode sites	
Noninverting	Fz or Cz
Inverting	Noncephalic (nape of neck) or the contralateral ear (mastoid or earlobe)
Analysis time	10 ms, including a poststimulus delay of 1 to 1.5 ms in averaging to minimize electrical artifact
Filter settings	30 or 100 to 1500 Hz
Sweeps	≥1000

operatively, the EABR can be elicited with electrical stimuli generated by the evoked response system, delivered near the ear via a transtympanic needle placed on the promontory and recorded by the system as acoustically elicited ABRs are recorded. Recording ECochG with promontory electrodes was reviewed in Chapter 4. The technique for transtympanic placement of the needle electrode for electrical stimulation at the promontory is very similar. For adult patients, the tympanic membrane should be anesthetized locally and visualized with a microscope during electrode placement. General anesthesia is typically required for children undergoing promontory electrical stimulation. For direct electrical stimulation, the evoked response system must include the somatosensory option, permitting the generation of electrical pulses that can be manipulated in terms of duration, rate, intensity, and other parameters. Intensity levels, in particular, must be carefully controlled so that the auditory system is not overstimulated. Studies cited above clearly documented the clinical feasibility of eliciting EABRs with electrical stimulation delivered via a transtympanic needle placement on the promontory.

Alternatively, again preoperatively, electrical stimuli can be delivered to the patient with an external signal generator triggered by the evoked response system or with the evoked response system simultaneously triggered by the external signal generator to begin averaging with each stimulus presentation. The technique is described in detail in a series of papers published by Paul Kileny and colleagues during the 1990s (Kileny, 1991; Kileny, Zwolan, Zimmerman-Phillips, & Kemink, 1992; Kileny et al., 1994), and other authors (e.g., Mason et al., 1997; Nikopoulos et al., 1999). The external signal generator is often battery operated and capable of presenting constant current electrical pulses. Most clinical evoked response systems have an input for an external trigger signal, even though internal triggering is typically relied upon during clinical measurement of sensory evoked responses.

A recent paper by Kileny and Zwolan (2004) provides a good review of the transtympanic approach for evoking the EABR. EABRs were recorded from fifty-nine children in the operating room with the patient anesthetized immediately prior to cochlear implantation. Electrical stimuli were generated with a "custom-made stimulator" consistent of biphasic pulses, alternating in phase or polarity to minimize artifact, with a duration of 200 μs per phase and a maximum output of 999 μA. A "sync pulse" from the evoked response system triggered the stimulator. Stimuli were delivered to the promontory with a Teflon-insulated needle placed using the transtympanic technique. EABRs were recorded with electrodes (subdermal needles) on the forehead (noninverting) and contralateral ear (inverting) using physiologic filter settings of 10 or 30 Hz to 3000 Hz. Kileny and Zwolan (2004) report four criteria for determining which patients will be assessed with EABR: (1) temporal bone malformation, (2) inconclusive information about auditory thresholds due to young chronological or developmental age, (3) profound degree of hearing loss exceeding the maximum output of the audiometer, and (4) diagnosis of auditory neuropathy. EABR threshold was correlated with hearing loss, as indicated by the pure-tone average (PTA).

The second technique for recording EABR involves the cochlear implant. Postoperatively, that is, after the patient has undergone cochlear implantation, the EABR can be stimulated by the same intracochlear electrical signals, generated by the cochlear implant electrodes, that are used in recording the ECAP. With relatively minor modifications of the conventional ABR test protocol, the EABR is then recorded with the evoked response system. Once again, the evoked response system must be triggered by an external output of the cochlear implant system to average synchronously with the presentation of the intracochlear electrical signals.

One of the stimulus parameters modified from the conventional ABR for the EABR protocol is the location of the inverting electrode. Given the inevitable problem with excessive electrical stimulus artifact in EABR measurement, the inverting electrode is located at a distance from the site of stimulation, usually on either the contralateral ear or a noncephalic site (e.g., nape of the neck). It is desirable for the physiologic amplifier of the evoked response system to be recovery quickly from saturation due to high levels of electrical artifact. Other techniques for reducing stimulus-related electrical artifact include reducing amplifier sensitivity, reliance on a physiologic amplifier with a rapid recovery from saturation, using shorter electrode leads, alternating the stimulus polarity (biphasic pulses), delaying the onset of signal averaging until 1.5 to 2 ms (beyond most of the stimulus artifact).

As early as 1991, Abbas and Brown applied in EABR measurement the two-pulse (masker-probe) stimulus paradigm later commonly used in recording the ECAP. The goals of the study were to evaluate the refractory properties of the EABR and the effect of stimulus duration of the EABR, with the anticipation that findings might be related to performance on speech perception tasks. Neural recovery of the ABR, as evidenced by amplitude, increased directly with longer intervals between the masker signal and the probe, i.e., the inter-pulse interval (IPI). Recovery was generally complete when the probe followed the masker by 5 ms.

From the foregoing discussion, similarities are evident in clinical application and measurement of ECAP and EABR. The EABR, however, offers some distinct advantages in comparison to the ECAP, and also is characterized by some limitations, as summarized in Table 15.5. Clearly, one of the most important practical considerations in clinical measurement of electrophysiological responses is the state of the subject. A very quiet state of arousal is essential for EABR recordings, just as it is for acoustically elicited ABRs. Sedation of young children is, therefore, necessary for EABR assessment. As reviewed in the previous section, a quiet patient state is not required for ECAP measurement.

Thus, sedation is not needed for measurement of the ECAP, even in young and/or active children.

EABR ANALYSIS. | Differences between auditory and electrically evoked brainstem response waveforms are illustrated in Figure 15.5. Major components in the waveform of the EABR are sometimes designated with a lower case "e," e.g., wave eIII and wave eV. One obvious distinction is the sizable artifact produced by electrical stimulation, in comparison to acoustic stimulation (identified by the arrow in the figure), even when steps are taken in the test protocol to minimize the interference of stimulus artifact. Latency of waves is clearly shorter for responses elicited with electrical versus acoustic stimulation, as noted at the outset of this chapter. At a high stimulus–intensity level (i.e., close to maximum behavioral dynamic range), typical absolute latencies are, for example, about 1.30 ms for wave II, 2.10 ms for wave III, and 3.75 ms for wave V. Interwave latencies at the same high stimulus level are on the order of 0.80 ms for the II–III interval, 1.60 ms for the III–V interval, and 2.40 ms for the II–V interval (e.g., Firszt, Chambers, Kraus, & Reeder, 2002; Hervé, Truy, Durupt, & Collet, 1996; Pelizonne et al., 1989; Shallop et al., 1990). Wave V amplitude values at maximum intensity levels are between 1.00 and 1.46 μV, depending on the recording electrode along the cochlear implant array. Each of the response parameters for the EABR—latency, amplitude, and morphology—differs somewhat as a function of electrode position (i.e., from basal to apical). Wave V latency is, for example, longer for basal than apical electrodes (Abbas & Brown, 1991; Firszt et al., 2002). In comparison to waves for the ABR, morphology of brainstem response for electrical stimulation consists of all major waves except wave I and waves appear more rounded. In other respects, however, the ABR and EABR are similar. For example, increased stimulus intensity level (acoustic for ABR and electrical current for EABR) produces larger response amplitude and shorter latency. Similarly, during the first 24 months after birth, maturation of the auditory system and central nervous system affects both the acoustically and the electrically elicited ABR, although the age effect is less pronounced for EABR (Kileny & Zwolan, 2004). Developmental delays in maturation of the EABR secondary to auditory deprivation are, however, reported for children with severe-to-profound peripheral (sensory) hearing loss (Mason, 2003). Furthermore, EABR latency decreases and amplitude increases directly with ongoing cochlear implant use (Gordon, Papsin, & Harrison, 2003).

Dr. Steve Mason and British colleagues (e.g., Mason, Gibbin, Garnham, & O'Donaghue, 1996) described another wave occasionally observed within the time period of the EABR, but distinct from the conventional EABR wave I, wave III, and wave V. Referred to as the short latency component (SLC) by Mason et al. (1996), and the N3 component by Kato et al. (1998), the wave is elicited by high-intensity stimulation and appears as a negative peak with a latency of about 3 ms for acoustic stimuli and 2 ms for electrical stimuli, even in the absence of ABR or EABR wave V. The SLC is thought to be a response from the vestibular system, probably vestibular nuclei in the brainstem, rather than an auditory response (Mason, 2003; Mason et al., 1996). Another major nonauditory peak within the EABR analysis time is the compound muscle action potential sometimes observed in the 4 to 6 ms region after high-intensity electrical stimulation (Fifer & Novak, 1990; Kileny & Zwolan, 2004; Mason, 2003, 2004; van den Honert & Stypulkowski, 1986). Although the muscle response presumably reflects facial nerve rather than auditory system activation, it may interfere with confident analysis of the EABR wave V component.

CLINICAL APPLICATION OF EABR. | Clinical applications of EABR parallel those reviewed already for ECAP. One of the earliest applications of EABR, noted above, is assessment of the stimulability or integrity of the auditory nerve and, in addition, the auditory brainstem preoperatively using transtympanic promontory stimulation (e.g., Kileny, 1991; Kileny et al., 1992; Kileny et al., 1994; Mason et al., 1997). In the pediatric population, as described in a series of papers by Mason and colleagues (e.g., Mason, 2004; Mason, Dodd, Gibbin, & O'Donaghue, 2000; Mason et al., 1995; Mason et al., 1996) and others (e.g., Waring, 1992, 1995, 1996), measurement of the EABR intraoperatively at the time of cochlear implantation permits confirmation for the surgeon, audiologist, and the patient's parents of the functional integ-

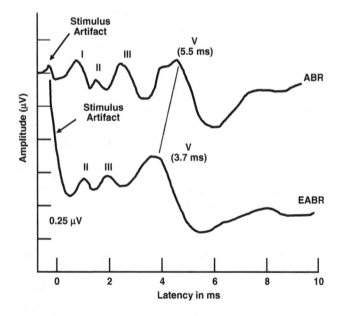

Auditory versus Electrically Evoked Brainstem Response

FIGURE 15.5. Examples of brainstem responses recorded by auditory stimulation (ABR) versus electrical stimulation (EABR).

rity of the cochlear implant device, including the electrode array. Another important and common pediatric application of EABR is estimation of physiologic threshold for electrical stimulation, a basic step in the process of programming a cochlear implant (e.g., Brown et al., 1994; Hodges, Ruth, Lambert, & Balkany, 1994; Shallop, Van Dyke, Goin, & Mischke, 1991; Truy et al., 1998). For adult patients with cochlear implants, threshold and comfortable levels for electrical stimulation can be confidently determined with behavioral test techniques. For infants and young children, however, behavioral techniques are not feasible. For programming cochlear implants in pediatric patient populations, EABR is a reliable alternative to behavioral techniques for estimating threshold and comfortable levels for electrical stimulation. The results of threshold estimation with EABR in patients with cochlear implants are not as accurate as the estimation of behavioral thresholds with conventional ABR in children with hearing impairment. One factor affecting accuracy of threshold estimation is electrode site within the cochlea. In general, the EABR has larger amplitudes and thresholds for lower stimulus intensity levels when evoked from apical electrode sites. Despite the imprecision in describing auditory function with electrical stimulation, EABR findings are a reasonable starting point for programming cochlear implants in children. In addition, the EABR is applied in estimations of the dynamic range for cochlear implant performance.

EABR parameters applied in programming cochlear implants include amplitude growth functions. Early animal investigations suggested that steep amplitude growth functions were correlated with survival of auditory neurons (e.g., Hall, 1990; Smith & Simmons, 1983; Walsh & Leake-Jones, 1982). Subsequent clinical experiences, however, were less positive. The relations between amplitude growth functions and most measures of cochlear implant performance are weak and not consistent among subjects (e.g., Abbas & Brown, 1991; Fifer & Novak, 1991), although research on the topic continues. The advantages for cochlear implant performance inherent in locating the electrode close to the afferent auditory nerve fibers in the modiolus were reviewed in the above ECAP discussion, namely, lower thresholds for stimulation, wider dynamic range for stimulation (between threshold and uncomfortable levels), less channel interaction, and reduced power (battery) consumption. There is some evidence that EABR thresholds are lower for cochlear implants designed to be in close proximity to the modiolus versus "straight array" electrodes (Cords et al., 2000).

Early attempts to find a strong correlation between EABR indices (e.g., thresholds, growth functions) with cochlear implant performance as defined by speech perception measures were generally disappointing (e.g., Abbas & Brown, 1991; Makhdoum, Groenen, Snik, & van den Broek, 1997). While some authors (e.g., Gallégo et al., 1998) reported statistically significant correlations between measures of EABR (absolute and interwave latencies) and speech per-

ception (correct identification of phonemes), more recent investigations have yielded somewhat negative findings (Firszt, Chambers, & Kraus, 2002; Kubo et al., 2001). In the words of Firszt et al. (2002), for example, "The parameters of the EABR (e.g., latency, maximum amplitude, normalized amplitude, and threshold of wave V) were not strongly associated with speech perception performance . . ." (p. 526). Nonetheless, the potential value of the EABR as an objective measure of cochlear implant function continues to be investigated. Electrically evoked cortical responses have more clinical value as prognostic indicators of cochlear implant performance, as reviewed in the next section.

Wackym and colleagues (2004) investigated in a series of seventeen young children (less than 3 years old) the impact of the Bionic Ear electrode positioning system and the Nucleus Contour device on the EABR parameters, including threshold, waveform morphology, latency, and amplitude. Although there was some evidence of a difference (improvement) in EABR threshold after insertion of the electrode positioner, it was not consistent among electrode sites but, rather, apparent only for selected electrodes and electrode positions. Cochlear implant brand was also a variable in the findings. As stated by Wackym et al. (2004), "Decreases in EABR wave V threshold and increases in supra-threshold wave V amplitude were significant for the tested basal electrode for the CII Bionic Ear and the tested apical electrode location for the Nucleus Contour device" (p. 71).

A handful of investigators have described findings for EABR versus ECAP for the same group of subjects (e.g., Brown et al., 2000; Hay-McCutcheon, Brown, Clay, & Seyle, 2002). Hay-McCutcheon et al. (2002) compared ECAP (i.e., NRT) and EABR measurements for a series of ten postlingually deafened adults (adults acquiring hearing loss after language development was complete) who were implanted with a precurved modiolus-hugging cochlear implant electrode design (Nucleus CI24R). The authors found a close correlation between thresholds measured with ECAP and EABR. Importantly, ECAP and EABR thresholds measured with the modiolus-hugging electrode design were equivalent to those reported earlier (Brown et al., 2000) for a conventional cochlear implant electrode design. That is, in agreement with the findings reported by other authors (e.g., Donaldson et al., 2001), electrophysiological recordings, specifically thresholds, failed to consistently verify enhanced stimulation of nerve fibers with the electrode designed to be closer to the modiolus. Results of the Hay-McCutcheon et al. (2002) study are, therefore, in agreement with those for the investigation reported by Wackym and colleagues (2004).

ELECTRICALLY EVOKED AUDITORY STEADY-STATE RESPONSE (ASSR). | In the era of universal newborn hearing screening, the ASSR has assumed an increasingly important role for frequency-specific estimation of auditory sensitivity in infants and young children. The ASSR is reviewed in Chapter 8. Menard and colleagues (2004) published what appears to be the first paper describing the application of ASSR as an objective measure of cochlear implant performance. Using the MASTER system (Bio-Logic Systems, Corp.), the ASSR was evoked with acoustic stimuli (80 Hz modulation frequency) presented to five adult cochlear implant (Digisonic, MXM Laboratories) subjects. Stimulus carrier frequencies and modulation rates of 600 Hz (80 Hz), 1000 Hz (77 Hz), 2000 Hz (83 Hz), and 3500 Hz (74 Hz) were presented to the implanted ear via an audiometer connected directly to the cochlear implant processor. Each carrier frequency was encoded and then delivered to a different individual electrode. Biphasic pulses generated by the cochlear implant were varied in duration and amplitude to manipulate the volume (intensity) of the stimulus level. ASSRs for various signal duration and amplitude values were compared to subjective measures of cochlear implant threshold and comfort levels. Well aware that electrical artifact could interfere with measurement of the ASSR, the authors carefully examined data for possible electrical artifact. Based on their analysis, Menard and colleagues (2004) conclude "that the recorded ASSR-like signals do not arise simply from electrical artifact generated by the electrodes of the implant, but contain components of a true physiologic response, suggesting the validity of the data for estimation of the auditory thresholds of an implanted subject" (p. S41). The authors found a "good correspondence" between the subjective behavioral threshold estimations and threshold durations of the electrically evoked ASSR and recommend further and more comprehensive investigation of the value of ASSR in fitting cochlear implants for very young or difficult-to-test children.

Electrically Evoked Cortical Auditory Evoked Responses

Electrically evoked cortical AERs described in the literature include the EAMLR, the EALR, the EP300, and the EMMN responses. Evidence is mounting that cortical electrical-evoked responses are an objective approach for predicting performance and even speech perception in pediatric cochlear implant patients. The insensitivity of the late responses to stimulus-related electrical artifact and the good relation between the late responses and perception of complex acoustic signals are in distinct contrast to the limited value of ECAP and EABR in estimating even basic parameters of cochlear implant performance. The divergence in prognostic value of responses arising from the cochlea versus the cortex is an excellent example of a fundamental auditory concept—we hear with our brain, not our ears. Cortical AERs also offer a clinical feasible objective measure of delayed maturation of the auditory system secondary to sensory deprivation experienced by children with severe-to-profound peripheral (sensory) hearing loss (Ponton, Moore, & Eggermont, 1999; Sharma, Dorman, & Spahr, 2002; Sharma et al., 2004) and, conversely, enhanced developmental trends reflecting the plasticity of the auditory cortex following stimulation with cochlear implantation.

ELECTRICAL AUDITORY MIDDLE-LATENCY RESPONSE (EAMLR). |
Investigation of the EAMLR in patients with cochlear implants dates back to 1989 (Kileny, Kemink, & Miller, 1989). In a study of electrical stimulation at the promontory following total destruction of the cochlear by labyrinthectomy, the same research group (Kemink, Kileny, Niparko, & Telian, 1991) documented EAMLR postoperatively for each of ten subjects. These authors (Rosenthal, Kileny, Boerst, & Telian, 1999) also described similar application of EAMLR recordings in patients with other rather unusual diseases associated with sensorineural hearing loss, such as MELAS (mitochrondrial encephalography lactic acidosis and stroke-like episodes) syndrome. The EAMLR offers at least three strengths as an electrophysiologic measure of auditory function in cochlear implant users. First, the relatively long latency wave components (e.g., Na and Pa) are far removed from the onset of stimulation and, therefore, not affected by electrical artifact. Second, the EAMLR is almost always detected in children about one year after cochlear implantation, although it is not typically recorded at the time of implantation. Third, with generators within the auditory cortex, the EAMLR is more closely related to "hearing" and communicative function than responses arising from the auditory nerve or brainstem.

A protocol for recording the EAMLR is summarized in Table 15.7. Stimulus parameters are similar to those used for EABR measurement, with the exception of those parameters that typically differ for ABR versus AMLR protocols, e.g., rate, physiologic filter settings, etc. Typical average latency values for EAMLR waves are approximately 14 to 19 ms for Na, 25 to 28 ms for the Pa, with Na-Pa amplitudes of 0.60 to 1.00 μV (Firszt et al., 2002). AMLR latency values with electrical stimulation tend to be somewhat shorter than latency values for acoustic stimulation. In a study of the AMLR Pb component (also referred to as P1), Curtis Ponton and colleagues (1996) found an average latency of 39.6 ms (standard deviation of 8.3 ms) for adults with cochlear implants versus that for normal-hearing adults (50.6 ms, standard deviation of 8.0 ms). The authors attribute the shorter latencies (about 2.5 to 3 ms) in cochlear implant patients to direct and perhaps more synchronous electrical stimulation of the auditory nerve fibers, i.e., "bypassing the auditory periphery (external auditory canal, middle ear, and cochlea)" (p. 62). The results of the study of Ponton et al. (1996) "provide strong evidence that plasticity of the auditory system is maintained in deaf children" (p. 64). In a study of twelve adult cochlear implant users and an equal number of age-matched control subjects, Kelly, Purdy, and Thorne (2005) found no difference between the composite acoustically elicited AMLR waveform recorded from normal hearers and the average EAMLR waveform recorded from subjects with cochlear implants. P1 amplitude values, however, differed for

TABLE 15.7. Guidelines for a Test Protocol for Electrically Evoked Auditory Middle-Latency Response (EAMLR)

PARAMETER	SELECTION
Stimulus	
Type	Biphasic constant current electrical pulse
Mode of delivery	Needle electrode (preoperative) or cochlear implant electrode (intra- or postoperative)
Site of stimulation	Promontory (preoperative) or intracochlear (intra- or postoperative)
Rate	<11 pulses/sec
Duration	~20 to 400 μsec per phase
Polarity	Alternating (bipolar)
Intensity	20 μA to 1 mA
Repetitions	≥500
Acquisition	
Electrode sites	
Noninverting	Fz or Cz
Inverting	Noncephalic (nape of neck) or the contralateral ear (mastoid or earlobe)
Analysis time	10 ms, including a poststimulus delay of 1 to 1.5 ms in averaging to minimize electrical artifact
Filter settings	10 to 1500 or 3000 Hz
Sampling rate	20,000 Hz
Sweeps	≥500

the two groups at some stimulus frequencies, but were equivalent at other frequencies. EAMLR latencies do not appear to differ as a function of cochlear implant electrode location, and amplitude of the EAMLR is directly related to electrical stimulus–intensity level (Firszt et al., 2002; Gordon, Papsin, & Harrison, 2005). Two important factors contributing to the likelihood that EAMLR components are detected in a patient with a cochlear implant are electrical stimulus intensity level and electrode position. A small proportion of patients with cochlear implants do not produce an EAMLR under optimal measurement conditions, e.g., maximum intensity levels and for any electrode within the array (Firszt et al., 2002).

Changes in the EAMLR latency and amplitude after cochlear implantation reflect the impact of deafness on auditory deprivation prior to cochlear implantation and also plasticity in central auditory function following cochlear implantation (Firszt et al., 2002; Kelly, Purdy, & Thorne, 2005; Ponton & Eggermont, 2001; Ponton et al., 1996; Shallop et al., 1990; Sharma et al., 2002; Sharma et al., 2004). In a longitudinal study of the EAMLR Pb component (described as the P1 component), Ponton et al. (1996) showed that maturation as defined by "age-dependent latency changes" was similar for children with normal hearing versus those following cochlear implantation. The P1 component is attributed to two auditory evoked responses—the AMLR and the ALR. Occurring normally with a latency of about 50 ms,

the component is labeled variously by different authors as "Pb," "P50," and "P1." Because the latency of the Pb (P50 or P1) wave is within the time frame typically associated with the auditory middle latency response, articles describing the P1 wave elicited by electrical stimuli or by speech signals in cochlear implant patients are included in this review of EAMLR literature, rather than in the subsequent section on the EALR. Measurement of the AMLR Pb (P50 or P1) component is reviewed in Chapter 11, while anatomic origins of the Pb (P1) are described in Chapter 2.

Kelly, Purdy, and Thorne (2005) reported smaller amplitudes for the EAMLR Na component as a function of the duration of deafness. Gordon, Papsin, and Harrison (2005) described longitudinal EAMLR findings in a series of fifty children with varied etiologies for hearing impairment (mostly prelingual) recorded during the first year of cochlear implant use and cross-sectional EAMLR findings for thirty-one children with over five years of cochlear implant experience. Subjects were awake during EAMLR measurement, except for data collected during surgery. The EAMLR was elicited with either biphasic pulses, usually with a duration of 205 μs, or monopolar pulses (duration of 25 to 150 μs), depending on which cochlear implant device was used by the subjects. Stimuli were presented via an electrode at the basal end of the cochlear implant electrode array. The EAMLR became more consistently detectable within the year after cochlear implantation and, by five years after cochlear implantation, all subjects yielded an EAMLR. Progressively shorter EAMLR latencies and larger amplitudes were associated with ongoing use of the cochlear implant. According to Gordon, Papsin, and Harrison (2005), this finding "suggests that the thalamo-cortical pathways of the auditory system remain plastic following a period of auditory deprivation and change in response to auditory input from the cochlear implant" (p. 86). Consistent with the cortical origin of the EAMLR, Firszt, Chambers, and Kraus (2002) found in their study of eleven adult cochlear implant patients that "normalized" amplitude of the response was correlated with behavioral measures of speech perception. However, consistent with previously reported findings (e.g., Makhdoum et al., 1997), other commonly analyzed EAMLR parameters (e.g., maximum amplitude and latency) were not closely related to speech perception scores.

Sharma and colleagues (2004) applied speech-evoked EALRs in an exploration of central auditory system maturation in two children with cochlear implants. Both children were implanted at 13 months of age. The stimulus was a synthetic speech sound (/ba/) presented to the implanted side of the subject's head in a sound booth via a loudspeaker. Children used their cochlear implant processors at customary settings while they viewed a cartoon or movie on a TV monitor. Stimulus and acquisition parameters were typical for a cortical evoked response protocol, including a noninverting electrode on Cz and an inverting electrode on the nonimplanted ear, a long analysis time (600 ms, with a 100 ms prestimulus time), and low physiologic filter settings (0.1 to 100 Hz). Within the initial three months after cochlear implantation, latency of the P1 component decreased rather dramatically, beginning far outside of the age-corrected normal region and at three months falling within the normal range. During the same time period, both children also evidenced rapid acquisition of speech skills. In a follow-up longitudinal investigation with twenty-one children with unilateral cochlear implants and two children with bilateral cochlear implants, Sharma, Dorman, and Kral (2005) confirmed their earlier findings. In addition, using the same speech signal (/ba/), the authors showed that changes in the EALR were more rapid for children implanted before 3.5 years versus those implanted after age 7 years. Remarkably, within just one week of the beginning of cochlear implant use, latency in the early-implanted children decreased by about 100 ms and fell within an age-corrected normal region. As Sharma, Dorman, and Kral (2005) point out, "Late-implanted children showed aberrant waveform morphology and significantly slower decreases in P1 latency postimplantation" (p. 134).

ELECTRICALLY EVOKED LATE LATENCY AUDITORY RESPONSE (EALR). | With the exception of the interpositioning of the cochlear implant components between the stimulus transducer and the auditory nerve, the technique and protocol for recording the EALR is very similar to the protocol for the conventional ALR (see Table 12.2 in Chapter 12). The auditory late response evoked by tonal or speech stimuli can be reliable recorded from most children and adults following cochlear implantation (e.g., Firszt et al., 2002; Groenen, Snik, & van den Broek, 1996; Makhdoum, Snik, & van den Broek, 1997; Maurer et al., 2002; Roman et al., 2005). Typical latency values for major EALR components, about 86 ms for N1 and 181 ms for P2, tend to be slightly shorter that those for the ALR evoked by acoustic stimuli, although differences are not generally significant (e.g., Brix & Gedlicka, 1991; Groenen et al., 1996; Makhdoum et al., 1997; Micco et al., 1995). Average amplitude for the N1-P2 difference for electrical stimulation ranges from 3.5 to 5.5 µV, depending the on the intensity level relative to the behavioral dynamic range (e.g., 100 percent BDR is maximum). Consistent with trends for the acoustically elicited ALR, latency of EALR decreases and amplitude increases as electrical stimulus intensity is increased. Minimum detection (threshold) levels for the EALR vary as a function of the cochlear implant electrode location. For example, Firszt et al. (2002) reported significant EALR threshold differences among electrodes, with the lowest average threshold for electrode 1 and the highest for electrode 7. In contrast, latencies for the EALR components (N1 and P2) were not related to electrode site. Groenen et al. (1996) found in ten adult cochlear implant users prolonged latencies, reduced amplitudes, and more variability for the N1 component in comparison to values for a control group of normal-hearing subjects. Although the pattern of findings was similar for the P2 component for tonal stimuli (500 and 1000 Hz), differences between groups were not significant for all speech stimuli (e.g., /ba/, /da/). Okusa, Shiraishi, Kubo, and Nageishi (1999), in an investigation of the P300 response in eight adult cochlear implant users, found no difference in the latency of the N1 and P2 components as a function of the difficulty of an oddball task for tonal stimuli (e.g., and easy task of 1000 versus 2000 Hz and a difficult task of 1000 versus 1100 Hz).

In the study of twelve adult postlingual cochlear implant users and an equal number of age-matched control subjects, cited above in the discussion of EAMLR papers, Kelly, Purdy, and Thorne (2005) reported considerably greater amplitude for the N1 component for subjects with normal hearing versus those with cochlear implants. In agreement with a report by Makhdoum et al. (1998), these authors also found a correlation between latency of the P2 component and speech recognition. When the ALR is elicited with acoustic stimuli, N1 latencies are slightly shorter for adult patients with cochlear implants than for age-matched control, whereas N1 amplitude values and the spatial scalp distributions of the N1 are equivalent for the two groups of subjects (Roman et al., 2005). According to Roman et al. (2005), "it appears that P2 latency is much too variable to be used for discriminating among CI [cochlear implant] users or even relative to normal-hearing persons" (p. 18).

Considering the well-recognized cortical origin of the EALR, one would expect response parameters to be predictive of cochlear implant performance, particularly speech perception. Indeed, confirming data reported in earlier studies (e.g., Makhdoum et al., 1997), Firszt, Chambers, and Kraus (2002) found that latency and amplitude measures of EALRs evoked by biphasic electrical pulses (produced by cochlear implants) "were strongly associated with speech perception abilities" (p. 527). Hoppe, Rosanowski, Iro, & Eysholdt (2001) found in eight adult cochlear implant patients a correlation between the EALR evoked by electric pulse trains (300 ms duration) and a behavioral measure of loudness perception.

ELECTRICALLY EVOKED P300 AUDITORY RESPONSE. | The statement opening the previous section on electrical evoked late response is appropriate also for the P300 response. That is, with the exception of the interpositioning of the cochlear implant components between the stimulus transducer and the auditory nerve, the technique and protocol for recording the electrically evoked P300 response is equivalent to the protocol for the conventional P300 (see Table 12.2 in Chapter 12). Findings for a growing number of papers on the P300 in cochlear implant users are quite encouraging (Beynon & Snik, 2004; Beynon, Snik, Stegman, & van den Broek, 2005; Groenen et al., 1996; Jordan et al., 1997; Kaga, Kodera, Hirota, & Tsuzulea, 1991; Kileny, 1991; Kileny, Boerst, & Zwolan, 1997; Micco et al., 1995; Oviatt & Kileny, 1991). Oviatt and Kileny (1991) reported in cochlear implant users delayed latency for the P3 component elicited by tonal differences between frequent and rare stimuli (500 versus 1000 Hz, and 500 versus 2000 Hz). In a follow-up study, Kileny et al. (1997) found that P300 responses for tonal signals (1500 versus 3000 Hz) recorded from children with cochlear implants were correlated with speech perception performance. In an investigation of speech sounds as stimuli for the P300 response in cochlear implant patients, Micco and colleagues (1995) found that responses with the cochlear implant approximated normal expectations.

Groenen et al. (1996) reported delayed P300 latency in adult cochlear implant users versus a normal-hearing control subjects. Interesting, a P3 peak was detected in most (eight out of nine) cochlear implant patients for some speech stimulus contrasts (e.g., /ba/ versus /da/) yet fewer cochlear implant patients (four out of nine) for other speech stimulus contrasts (e.g., /ba/ versus /pa/). Amplitude of the P300 response was typically smaller, and variability of latency and amplitude higher, for the cochlear implant group than for control subjects. The authors found significant positive relations between P300 amplitude and speech recognition performance, but not for P300 latency measures. The same Dutch research group (Beynon & Snik, 2004; Beynon et al., 2005) described for children and adults with cochlear implants patterns for the P300 response evoked by tonal (500 versus 1000 Hz) and speech stimuli, including a vowel contrast (/i/ versus /a/), and two phoneme contrasts involving consonants and place of articulation (/ba/ versus /da/) and voicing (/ba/ versus /pa/). P300 latencies were delayed and amplitudes reduced for patients with cochlear implants versus a control group. The P300 was "readily" and consistently evoked in persons with cochlear implants. Beynon and Snik (2004) conclude, based on their findings, "the P300 measurements are a valid tool to study speech processing in CI users. Furthermore, P300 measurements were sensitive enough to discriminate between strategies" (p. S46). That is, for an individual cochlear implant patient, speech-coding strategies could be differentiated on the basis of P300 response latency and amplitude values. Kelly, Purdy, and Thorne (2005) reported in adult cochlear implant users larger amplitude and shorter latency for the passively recorded P3a component as a function of the duration of cochlear implant use.

Okusa and colleagues (1999) from Osaka University in Japan described longer latencies and reaction times for the P300 response in cochlear implant users versus normal expectations as the discrimination difficulty increased for two tonal stimuli (as detailed above in the discussion of EALR findings for the article). The same research group, Kubo et al. (2001), reported longer latencies for the P300 response for adult patients with cochlear implants than for an age-matched normal-hearing control group. Also, among cochlear implant patients, P300 latency values were correlated with speech perception performance (consonant recognition scores, or CRS). Specifically, the average acoustically elicited P300 latency was 317 ms in the control group, whereas the electrically elicited P300 latency was 326 ms for patients with "good" speech recognition ability ($\geq$70 percent CRS) and 374 ms for patients with "fair" speech recognition ability (<70 percent CRS). Furthermore, based on serial measurements over a period of two years postimplantation, Kubo et al. (2001) reported "latency of P300 is closely related to speech reception ability over a long period after cochlear implantation" (p. 259).

ELECTRICALLY EVOKED MMN RESPONSE. | The MMN is not applied in clinical assessment patients with cochlear implants, just as the MMN is not incorporated into the clinical test battery for other patient populations. However, reports of studies of the MMN following cochlear implantation date back to the early 1990s (e.g., Groenen et al., 1996; Kileny et al., 1997; Kraus et al., 1993b; Ponton & Don, 1995) and are occasionally reported since then (e.g., Roman et al., 2005). Initial findings (Kraus et al., 1993b) suggested that MMN responses were similar for normal hearers and cochlear implant users. Groenen et al. (1996) subsequently reported a normal-appearing MMN response elicited by speech signals for cochlear implant subjects with good speech perception, whereas a clear MMN could not be detected from cochlear implant subjects with poorer speech recognition performance (as evaluated by the *Hearing in Noise Test (HINT)*. In the study of twelve adult cochlear implant users and an equal number of age-matched control subjects, noted above in the EAMLR and the EALR discussions, Kelly, Purdy, and Thorne (2005) recorded the MMN response less often in patients with cochlear implants than in normal subjects. The MMN showed some predictive value for identification of cochlear implant subjects with poorer versus better speech recognition scores. Roman and French colleagues (2005) investigated in eight adult cochlear implant patients and an age-matched control group the MMN response elicited by tone-burst stimuli (standard stimulus of 1000 Hz and a deviant stimulus of either 1500 Hz or 2000 Hz) presented via loudspeakers in the free-field. In general, MMN response parameters (e.g., latency, peak amplitude, and area) were not significantly different for cochlear implant users versus control subjects.

Music is a complex nonspeech acoustic signal investigated as the stimulus in some of the early studies of auditory evoked responses in persons with cochlear implants, even simple single electrode devices (e.g., Eddington et al., 1978; Fujita & Ito, 1999; Gfeller & Lansing, 1991; Pijl & Schwartz, 1995). In a clever investigation of music perception in cochlear implant users, and a follow-up to previous papers by the authors (Koelsch, Gunter, Friederici, & Schroeger, 2000; Koelsch, Schmidt, & Kansok, 2002), Koelsch and colleagues (2004) elicited the MMN response with musical chord sequences. A MMN wave was recorded with irregular chord stimulation from cochlear implant subjects, but amplitude values were smaller than for a normal-hearing control group. The findings "suggest that, despite the limited amount of sensory information provided by a CI, postlingually deafened CI users process musical information . . . with the same neural mechanisms as normal hearing controls" (Koelsch et al., 2004, p. 971).

VESTIBULAR EVOKED MYOGENIC POTENTIAL (VEMP)

Colebatch and colleagues in Sydney, Australia, first reported systematic clinical investigation of "myogenic potentials generated by click-evoked vestibulocollic reflex," also referred to by the authors as "vestibular evoked potentials" (Colebatch & Halmagyi, 1992; Colebatch, Halmagyi, & Skuse, 1994; Halmagyi & Colebatch, 1995). Robertson and Ireland in 1995 apparently coined the specific term "vestibular evoked myogenic potential," abbreviated VEMP. VEMP has, since then, assumed an important position in the test battery of clinics and medical centers worldwide offering services for patients with balance and vestibular disorders. The literature on VEMP has grown, especially since 2000. An Internet search with the keyword "VEMP" leads to the websites of numerous clinical facilities and hearing health care practices announcing the availability of vestibular evoked myogenic potentials along with other conventional vestibular procedures, such elecronystagmography (ENG), rotary

vestibular tests, and platform posturography. VEMP reflects vestibular system activity that is elicited by high-intensity sounds and detected as a change in muscle potentials within the neck. In the words of Ferber-Viart and French colleagues Dubreuil and Dubclaux (1999), "The human vestibule has preserved an ancestral sound sensitivity and it has been suggested that a reflex could originate from this property, thus indicating cervical muscle microcontractions secondary to strong acoustic stimulations" (p. 6). Specifically, a vestibular evoked myogenic potential is recorded as a change in activity within the sternocleidomastoid (SCM) muscle secondary to stimulation of the vestibular system with acoustic signals at intensity levels of about 90 dB HL and higher. As described by Zapala and Brey (2004), the "VEMP reflects a vestibulocollic reflex, that is, a quick reflexive change in muscle tone (flexor or extensor, depending on the muscle group) that occurs to stabilize the head following an unexpected translation." The vestibulocollic reflex (VCR) is one of three clinically recorded vestibular responses, the other two being the vestibulo-ocular (VOR) and vestibulospinal reflexes.

VEMPs are sometimes referred to as "sono-motor responses or reflexes," similar to the acoustic stapedial reflex and the postauricular muscle (PAM) response. The VEMP can be differentiated from these "sono-motor" responses in several ways. The VEMP is a unilateral response detected on the sternocleidomastoid (SCM) muscle on the side ipsilateral to the stimulated ear, whereas the acoustic reflex and PAM response are detected bilaterally with stimulation of one ear. In addition, the acoustic reflex and PAM response require some cochlear integrity, but the VEMP can be recorded in persons with profound hearing loss, i.e., deafness (e.g., Colebatch, Rothwell, Bronstein, & Hudman, 1994). VEMP is distinguished from the acoustic startle response by its shorter latency and its consistency with repeated stimulation. The acoustic startle response, in contrast, shows rapid habituation with repeated stimulation. High-intensity abrupt sounds, e.g., clicks or short tone bursts, activate the saccule, an otolith organ within the vestibular apparatus in the inner ear. The other otolith organ is the utricle. Stimulation of the saccule generates a response from corresponding vestibular afferent fibers (saccular nerve). The afferent fibers travel via the inferior vestibular nerve to the vestibular nucleus, with projections then to the spinal cord and then innervation of the SCM muscle, an anterior (strap) neck muscle. VEMPs do not reflect contraction of the SCM muscle but, rather, an alteration in tonic status of the muscle. Early investigations of patients with total unilateral dysfunction of the vestibular nerves secondary to surgical severing who showed no evidence of VEMP further confirmed the vestibular origin of the response (e.g., Colebatch, Halmagyi, & Skuse, 1994; Halmagyi & Colebatch, 1995).

The VEMP appears as a biphasic (positive and negative) response in the latency region of 10 to 25 ms. A VEMP waveform recorded from a young normal subject is illustrated in Figure 15.6. The response is actually a reflection

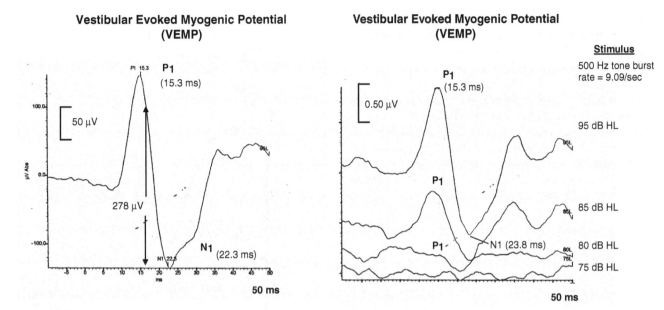

FIGURE 15.6. A vestibular evoked myogenic potential (VEMP) recording from a young female subject.

of transient inhibition (reduction) in SCM muscle activity secondary to acoustic stimulation of the saccule. Literature on VEMP is characterized by inconsistencies in how the two VEMP components are labeled. That is, some authors label the two components with a number (e.g., P1) and others utilize a latency designation (e.g., P13). There are also differences among publications in whether the waves are assigned positive or negative polarity (e.g., P13 versus N13). The literature even reveals discrepancies between upper and lowercase alphabetic labels for VEMP components (e.g., N13 versus n13). Explanations for some of these inconsistencies, and guidelines for analysis of VEMP waveforms, are offered in the following discussion of test parameters and waveform analysis.

Townsend and Cody (1971) introduced the concept of acoustic stimulation of the saccule in the early 1970s. However, years earlier Tullio (1929) described in patients vestibular symptoms generated by loud sounds, a clinical finding confirmed more recently by investigators of the VEMP (e.g., Colebatch et al., 1994). A few years after Tullio's observations, the famous Georg von Békésy recorded vestibular responses evoked by very high intensity sounds (>125 dB) as early as 1935 (von Békésy, 1935). Also, in the 1960s, Reginald Bickford and colleagues (Bickford, Jacobson, & Cody, 1964) reported a vestibular evoked myogenic response to high intensity sounds—the "inion response"—that was recorded from posterior neck muscles. Bickford's studies of myogenic responses during the same time period were noted in the historical review of the AMLR in Chapter 1. Subsequent studies in animals confirmed that loud sounds stimulate the otolith organs (e.g., Didier, Cazals, & Aurousseau, 1987; Young, Fernandez, & Goldberg, 1977). In addition to the ex-

perimental findings, beginning in the early 1990s numerous investigators provided ample evidence that the VEMP can be consistently recorded clinically (e.g., Colebatch & Halmagyi, 1992; Ferber-Viart et al., 1999; McCue & Guinan, 1994; Murofushi et al., 1995), and is indeed a vestibular response, rather than an auditory response (Murofushi, Matsuzaki, & Wu, 1999). For example, the VEMP can be recorded from persons with profound hearing impairment, so long as vestibular function is intact. In addition, VEMP can be recorded when auditory perception of the stimulus is masked by bone-conduction noise. Conversely, the VEMP disappears in severe vestibular dysfunction and when the vestibular nerves are sectioned surgically (e.g., Colebatch & Halmagyi, 1992; Murofushi, Matsuzaki, & Wu, 1999). Although the VEMP is clearly not an auditory evoked response, its measurement clinically is now falling within the purview of those professionals and practitioners who have the equipment for and expertise in recording auditory evoked responses. VEMP can be recorded with a conventional auditory evoked response system designed for ABR recordings, without any special software option or additional equipment or supplies. Since the late 1990s, audiologists, otolaryngologists, neurologists, and other health care professionals have assumed the responsibility for clinical measurement of vestibular function with VEMP much as they did about ten years earlier for measurement of facial electroneuronography (ENoG). Measurement, analysis, and clinical application of ENoG is reviewed in the next section of the chapter. The following overview is meant to introduce the reader to the principles and practices important for understanding the clinical application of VEMP. The information presented herein should, of course, be supplemented with intensive study of vestibular system anatomy and physiology, and practical experience with VEMP recording in normal persons and patients with balance and vestibular dysfunction of varying etiologies. Websites for academic departments of otolaryngology at medical schools (with residency programs) are a handy source of information on vestibular neuroscience and functional anatomy. Consistent with the test battery approach that is relied upon for clinical assessment of auditory and vestibular disorders, VEMP findings should not be analyzed and interpreted in isolation but, rather, within the context of the results for other procedures with proven test performance in this diagnostically challenging patient population.

Anatomy and Physiology

Although an understanding of vestibular system anatomy and physiology is essential for clinical application of the VEMP, adequate review of the topic is beyond the scope of this book. The reader is advised to rely on one or more of the numerous published books, book chapters, articles, or websites devoted to the vestibular system. One portion of the inner ear (about two-thirds) is important for auditory function and another (about a third) for vestibular function. The main structures within the vestibular part of the inner ear are the three semicircular canals (anterior, posterior, and horizontal or lateral), and the utricle, an otolith structure containing a region called the macula with otoliths (crystals of calcium carbonate within a gelatinous substance). The semicircular canals terminate in the utricle. One end of each semicircular canal is enlarged and forms the ampulla containing an epithelial structure, the ampullary crest covered by the cupula, and specialized receptor cells, e.g., vestibular hair cells. The term "pars superior" is sometimes used to describe the collection of vestibular structures that form the superior part of the inner ear. The other part of the inner ear—referred to sometimes as the "pars inferior"—consists of the cochlea and the saccule. The saccule, receptor of linear acceleration in mammals, is similar in anatomy to the utricle and is connected to the cochlea via the cochlear duct (ductus reuniens). In general, the semicircular canals are involved in dynamic functional response, i.e., detection and coding of rotation movements of the head in space and coordinating reflexive control of eye movements. In contrast, the utricle and saccule respond to static forces, i.e., maintaining posture and absolute position in space. The evolution of the two portions of the inner ear is interesting. In fish and primitive vertebrates, the pars superior is very easily distinguished from the pars inferior. The saccule within the pars inferior of primitive vertebrates functions not as a component in the vestibular system but, rather, along with another structure, the lagena, as a hearing organ (e.g., Lowenstein & Roberts, 1951; Popper, Platt, & Saidal, 1982). In humans and most vertebrates, the saccule remains sensitive to acoustic stimulation even though it is involved only in vestibular function, and not hearing.

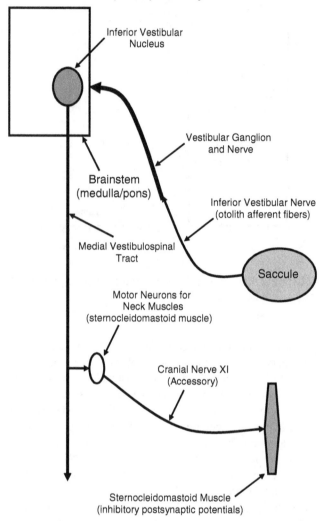

Vestibular Evoked Myogenic Potential (VEMP) Pathways

Inferior Vestibular Nucleus

Vestibular Ganglion and Nerve

Brainstem (medulla/pons)

Inferior Vestibular Nerve (otolith afferent fibers)

Medial Vestibulospinal Tract

Saccule

Motor Neurons for Neck Muscles (sternocleidomastoid muscle)

Cranial Nerve XI (Accessory)

Sternocleidomastoid Muscle (inhibitory postsynaptic potentials)

FIGURE 15.7. Schematic illustration of the anatomic structures and pathways underlying the vestibular evoked myogenic potential (VEMP).

Output from the peripheral vestibular structures is conveyed to the central nervous system via the vestibular nerves (see Figure 15.7). Animal (cat) investigations show that fibers within the vestibular nerve activated by acoustic stimulation of the saccule have spontaneous discharge rates within the range of 200 to 1000 Hz (McCue & Guinan, 1995; Todd, Cody, & Banks, 2000). The selective responsiveness of the saccular sensory system to a specific frequency region will be noted again in the following discussion of stimulus parameters for the VEMP test protocol. Stimulation of the saccule generates inhibitory postsynaptic potentials in motor neurons of the neck muscle (e.g., Todd, Cody, & Banks, 2000; Uchino et al., 1997). That is, following the presentation of a high-intensity sound, there is a temporary reduction in muscle activity, recorded as the positive wave in the

VEMP. Cell bodies for vestibular nerve fibers are in the vestibular ganglion (Scarpa's ganglion). Myelinated bipolar nerve cells extend from the innervation of the vestibular hair cells at their distal end to the termination of axons in the brainstem (the proximal end). There are superior and inferior components or divisions within the vestibular ganglion. With respect to VEMP anatomy, the superior division innervates the anterior portion of the macula within the saccule, whereas the inferior division innervates the posterior portion. Although the saccule is served by both the superior and inferior vestibular nerves, clinical findings in patients with various pathologies provide evidence that the VEMP is dependent on the integrity of the inferior vestibular portion of the auditory nerve. In contrast, the superior branch of the vestibular nerve innervates other peripheral vestibular structures (ampulla of anterior and horizontal canals and utricle). All vestibular nerve fibers run within the internal auditory meatus parallel to the cochlear nerve and the facial nerve on their way to the four vestibular nuclei (lateral, medial, superior, and inferior) in the caudal portion of the brainstem (the medulla/pons region). Early studies of the VEMP suggested that fibers from the saccule terminate in the medial vestibular nucleus, but findings were based on experiments with small animal models, such as guinea pig (Didier, Cazals, & Aurousseau, 1987). In mammals, however, fibers from the saccule, along with some from the semicircular canals and utricle, enter the inferior vestibular nucleus.

From the inferior vestibular nucleus the pathways underlying the VEMP traverse downward, primarily along the lateral vestibulospinal tract to the motor neurons within the eleventh (accessory) cranial nerve that innervate selected muscles in the neck (e.g., Todd, Cody, & Banks, 2000). The possibility of medial vestibulospinal tract involvement cannot be ruled out, particularly when there is bilateral activation of neck muscles with unilateral (monaural) stimulation. Vestibulospinal tracts descend within the brainstem, including the medulla and the cervical region of the spinal cord. Along the descending pathway, fibers from the vestibulospinal tract connect with neurons in the motor nucleus of cranial nerve XI (the accessory nerve). The SCM muscle is innervated mostly by the accessory cranial nerve (Fitzgerald, Comerford, & Tuffrey, 1982). From the motor nucleus of cranial nerve XI, nerve fibers take a rather indirect route from the medulla, through a cranial opening (jugular foramen) and then to neck muscles (SCM and trapezius muscles).

The VEMP is commonly recorded from an electrode placed on the sternocleidomastoid (SCM). However, sound-evoked myogenic potentials or changes in muscle tension, referred to sometimes as the "inion response" and also reflecting vestibular system function, can be detected from the posterior extensor muscles, including the trapezius muscle and the splenius capitis muscle (e.g., Ferber-Viart et al., 1998; Sakakura et al., 2005; Wu, Young, & Murofushi, 1999). The pathways involved in stimulating and recording the VEMP are ipsilateral (e.g., Halmagyi & Curthoys, 1999). In other words, stimulation of the right saccule by a high-intensity sound to the right ear produces a change in the contraction of the SCM muscle on the right side of the neck, and vice versa. Experiments in animals and humans involving single-unit techniques provide evidence of inhibition in activity of motor neurons innervating the SCM muscle following stimulation of the saccule (Colebatch & Rothewell, 1993; Kushiro et al., 1999). Masking sound presented at relatively high levels (>75 dB HL) to the nonstimulus ear, however, may result in attenuation of VEMP amplitude (e.g., Takegoshi & Murofushi, 2003), perhaps due to stapedius muscle contraction bilaterally. The rather short latency before the onset of the VEMP response (about 8 ms) suggests that few synapses—probably only two—are present in the neural pathways from the saccule to the SCM.

The rapid increase in clinical application of the VEMP is no doubt due in part to the rather unique information the procedure provides for diagnosis of vestibular disorders. With the VEMP, it's possible to evaluate integrity of the saccule and inferior vestibular nerve and, of course, dysfunction of these important structures. In contrast, other traditional techniques, such as electronystagmography (ENG) or the more recently introduced videonystagmography (VNG), primarily assess function of the superior semicircular canal and not the saccular and related pathways.

Measurement Protocols and Procedures

Colebatch et al. (1994) were among the first to systematically document the clinical feasibility of VEMP measurement and to suggest clinical applications of the new technique. Parameters of the VEMP (latency and amplitude) are highly dependent on stimulus parameters and, in addition, activity of the SCM muscle. Among the stimulus factors influencing VEMP are the type of stimulus (click versus tone burst), the frequency content of the stimulus (low- versus high-frequency tone bursts) and, of course, the intensity level of the stimulus. In general, tone bursts are more effective than clicks for elicitation of VEMP and, among tone-burst stimuli, low frequency more effective than high frequency. Within published papers, the most commonly used stimulus for clinical measurement of VEMP is a 500 Hz tone burst.

For successful measurement of the VEMP, the sternocleidomastoid muscle (SCM) must be maintained in tonic contraction (Bickford et al., 1964; Colebatch et al., 1994). That is, the VEMP is not produced by the contraction of a muscle but rather "the VEMP arises from modulation of background EMG activity and differs from neural potentials in that it requires tonic contraction of the muscle" (Welgampola & Colebatch, 2005).

STIMULUS PARAMETERS. | A protocol for VEMP measurement is summarized in Table 15.8. Stimuli for evoking VEMP are abrupt and very high intensity sounds, either clicks or tone bursts. Published evidence consistently confirms that tone bursts are more effective for elicitation of VEMP than click stimuli, and low-frequency tone bursts (≤1000 Hz) are more effective stimuli than higher frequency tone bursts (Akin & Murnane, 2001; Akin, Murnane & Proffitt, 2003; Murofushi, Matsuzaki, & Wu, 1999; Su, Huang, Young, & Chen, 2004; Todd, Cody, & Banks, 2000; Welgampola & Colebatch, 2001; Wu, Young, & Murofushi, 1999; Zapala & Brey, 2001). Animal investigations in the 1970s using single-unit recording techniques showed that among acoustic stimuli low-frequency tones are most effective for activating afferent fibers from the saccule, perhaps due to a phase-locking neural mechanism (Young, Fernandez, & Goldberg, 1977) and/or tuning of the sacculus portion of the otolith system (Schellart & Wubbels, 1998). Subsequent experimental findings in the early years of clinical VEMP measurement provided additional evidence of the particular responsiveness of vestibular nerve fibers to tonal stimuli within the region of 200 to 1000 Hz (McCue & Guinan, 1994). Todd, Cody, and Banks (2000) confirmed in human subjects frequency-specific tuning of the VEMP, with maximum amplitude in the region of 200 to 400 Hz. Although intersubject variability in VEMP amplitude was substantial, the tuning feature of the VEMP was remarkably well defined, frequency specific, and symmetrical for acoustic stimulation of the SCM muscles on the right and left side. As with AER measurement, durations for tone-burst stimuli in VEMP measurement are brief, on the order of several milliseconds. Also, consistent with expectations for AERs, such as the ABR, latencies of the VEMP components (P1 and N1) in normal adult subjects (e.g., Akin & Murnane, 2001; Basta, Todt, & Ernst, 2005) are shortest for click stimuli (about 11 ms for P1 and 18 ms for N1) and, among tone-burst stimuli, longer for lower frequencies (P1 and N1 latencies of about 18 ms and 25 ms respectively for 250 Hz) than higher frequencies (P1 and N1 latencies of about 12 ms and 17 ms respectively for 250 Hz). Welgampola and Colebatch (2001a) conducted a systematic investigation in twelve healthy young adult subjects of the effects on VEMP of stimulus frequency (for tone bursts), duration, and rate of presentation (interstimulus interval). VEMP amplitude increased as duration increased up to 7 ms, and then amplitude change reversed with decreasing amplitude for stimulus rates up to 20 ms. Welgampola and Colebatch (2001a) speculate that activation of the acoustic reflex with longer stimulus durations attenuates the VEMP. Similarly, these researchers found increased VEMP amplitude for longer interstimulus intervals up to 30 ms, but then progressively decreased amplitude for intervals of 50 ms and then 100 ms. Relatively slow rates of stimulus presentation (<6/sec) are need for generating optimal VEMP amplitudes. Increasing stimulus rate is associated with markedly decreased VEMP amplitude and greater likelihood that a VEMP will not be detected, even in normal subjects (Brantberg & Fransson, 2001; Wu, Young, & Murofushi, 1999). Latency, in contrast, is not significantly prolonged as stimulus rate increases (Brantberg & Fransson, 2001). VEMP findings in patients

TABLE 15.8. Guidelines for a Vestibular Evoked Myogenic Potentials (VEMPs) Test Protocol

PARAMETERS	RATIONALE/SELECTION
Stimulus	
Transducer	Insert earphones
Type	Click or tone burst (low frequency is optimal)
Duration	0.1 ms click or 2–0–2 cycle tone burst
Intensity	≥95 dB nHL
Polarity	Rarefaction
Rate	3 to 5/second
Acquisition	
Analysis time	
Prestimulus	10 to 20 ms
Poststimulus	50 to 100 ms
Electrode type	Large electrode on SCM muscle
Electrode location	
Noninverting	Midpoint of sternocleido-mastoid muscle
Inverting	Sternoclavicular junction or other sites, e.g., hand
Ground (common)	Forehead
Filter settings	
High-pass	1 to 30 Hz
Low-pass	250 to 1500 Hz
Notch	None
Amplification	× 50 to × 5000
Sweeps	45 to 250

with vestibular diseases are generally the same for click and tone-burst stimuli, that is, both types of stimuli yield either a normal response, a response with decreased amplitude, or an absent response. Approximately 10 percent of patients have divergent VEMP results for click versus tone-burst stimuli (Murofushi, Matsuzaki, & Wu, 1999).

To evoke a VEMP, acoustic stimuli delivered via air conduction must approach the maximum output limit of the signal generator for an evoked response system, i.e., >90 dB nHL or >120 dB SPL. Although clinically the VEMP is typically evoked with monaural stimulation, the response can be recorded simultaneously with binaural air-conduction stimulation (e.g., Murofushi, Iwasaki, Takai, & Takegoshi, 2005; Wang & Young, 2003). Based on an analysis of VEMP findings for twenty-eight patients with assorted otologic diseases, Murofushi et al. (2005) reported that 93 percent yielded the same results for binaural stimulation as for unilateral stimulation. The authors suggest the application of binaurally evoked VEMP as a clinical screening procedure for vestibulo-cochlear disorders. The VEMP can also be evoked with bone-conduction stimuli presented via a bone oscillator to the mastoid region (Sheykholeslami, Habiby, & Kaga, 2001; Sheykholeslami et al., 2000; Welgampola, Rosengren, Halmagyi, & Colebatch, 2003), but at output limits exceeding those typically available with evoked response systems and used for recording bone-conduction AERs. Bone-conduction stimuli for the VEMP, however, are delivered with the same type of oscillator (e.g., B71) used in measurement of the bone-conduction ABR (see Chapter 3 for details). For bone-conduction VEMPs, low-frequency tone-burst stimuli are preferable to clicks. Stimulation of one mastoid activates a bilateral saccular response and, with an appropriate two-channel electrode arrangement, the VEMP can be recorded simultaneously from each side. With calibration of high-intensity tone-burst (500 Hz) stimuli, VEMP latency values appear to be comparable for bone-and air-conduction stimulation (Basta, Todt, & Ernst, 2005). Sheykholeslami et al. (2001) confirmed that VEMPs evoked by tone-burst stimuli delivered via bone conduction show the same frequency tuning as VEMPs stimulated by air conduction, i.e., maximum amplitudes for tone-burst frequencies in the region of 200 to 400 Hz. These authors also demonstrated that the decrease in VEMP amplitude with increasing stimulus rate above 10/sec, described previously for air conduction, applies as well to stimuli delivered by bone conduction. Sheykholeslami et al. (2001) recommend clinical use of a stimulus rate of 10/sec, rather than commonly used slower rates (e.g., 5.1/sec) to reduce test time and patient discomfort, while preserving VEMP waveform morphology. There are reports documenting the elicitation of VEMP with nonacoustic stimuli, including electrical currents delivered in the mastoid region—galvanic-evoked myogenic potentials (Iwasaki et al., 2005; Murofushi, Takegoshi, Ohki, & Ozeki, 2002; Watson & Colebatch, 1998)—and also by uncalibrated taps delivered to the forehead, usually with a tendon hammer (Brantberg & Tribukait, 2002; Halmagyi, Yavor, & Colebatch, 1995). However, nonacoustic stimuli are not applied clinical measurement of the VEMP.

ACQUISITION PARAMETERS. | One of the most obvious distinctions in the protocol for measurement of VEMP versus auditory evoked responses is the role of muscle activity in the former. With AER measurement, minimizing or eliminating muscle activity and interference is always desirable to enhance waveform morphology and improve the accuracy of waveform analysis. Every attempt is made to keep the patient quiet with skeletal muscles in a relaxed state. For infants and young children, sedation or light anesthesia is typically required to achieve the necessary minimal state of arousal. In contrast, specific efforts are made in VEMP measurement to

increase muscle activity and to produce contraction of the muscles of interest, usually the sternocleidomastoid (SCM) muscle. Activation of the SCM muscles for VEMP measurement in adult patients is produced by manipulations of the head and neck, usually following detailed instructions by the tester and often with the assistance of the tester. At least three techniques are reported for producing and maintaining contraction of the SCM muscles. As shown in Figure 15.8, activation of the SCM muscle on one side of the neck can be generated by rotation of the subject's head to the opposite side, usually against some resistance, while he or she is sitting upright or lying supine (e.g., Murofushi et al., 1999). The VEMP must, of course, be recorded only from the SCM muscle that is activated, not the relaxed SCM muscle on the opposite site. Contraction of SCM muscles bilaterally can be produced by instructing the patient to lift his or her head slightly while lying either supine (on the back) or with the back elevated and head lifted (e.g., Brantberg & Fransson, 2001; Robertson & Ireland, 1995). The subject's head can then be rotated to one side for measurement of the VEMP on the opposite site—for example, rotated to the left to produce a easily identified contraction of the right SCM muscle.

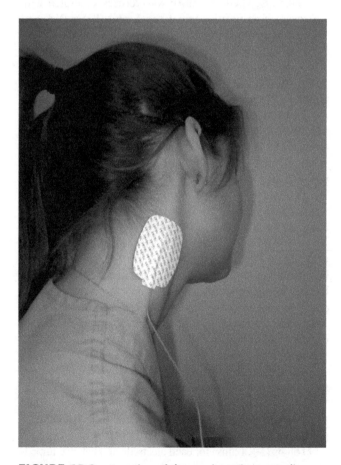

FIGURE 15.8. Location of the noninverting recording electrode on the sternocleidomastoid (SCH) muscle in VEMP measurement.

Another technique for activating bilateral SCM muscle activation requires the patient to press the forehead against a soft surface (e.g., padded wall or bar) while in a sitting position (Colebatch et al., 1994). The resistance to forward movement of the head generates contraction of SCM muscles on both sides of the neck. A goal with each of these manipulations is to maintain a reasonably consistent degree of tonic neck muscle activation.

Electrode locations used in recording the convention VEMP vary considerably among published reports, with related differences among studies in the polarity of VEMP waveforms. Confusion in the literature regarding polarity of VEMP waveforms is summarized below in a discussion of waveform analysis. Clearly, one electrode must be attached to the skin over the SCM muscle (see Figure 15.8). There is no apparent consensus or convention for electrode placement in VEMP measurement. A monopolar recording method is most often used, with a recording electrode (either noninverting or inverting) located on the surface of the SCM muscle, and the other recording electrode (either noninverting or inverting) located at another (non-SCM muscle) site, such as the nape of the neck or sternum. When the inverting electrode is located on the SCM muscle and the noninverting electrode is located elsewhere, a VEMP waveform is generated with a upward-going positive initial component (P1 or P13) and with a downward-going negative second component (N1 or N23). Reversing the sites for the noninverting and inverting electrodes results, of course, in a polarity inversion of the waveform (N13 and P23), but doesn't affect latency or amplitude of the components. The literature on VEMP contains numerous articles describing each type of electrode array, i.e., inverting versus noninverting electrode on the SCM muscle. VEMP activity is best detected with a relatively large electrode located near the midpoint (the middle third) or the upper third of the SCM muscle (e.g., Murofushi et al., 1999; Welgampola & Colebatch, 2005). Importantly, the site of the electrode on the SCM muscle must be symmetrical for the right and left side. That is, if the inverting electrode is affixed to the middle third of the SCM muscle on one side of the neck, then the inverting electrode on the opposite side should be placed in the same location on the muscle. The specific location of the other (usually inverting) recording electrode does not appear to be critical in VEMP measurement, as a wide variety of noncephalic sites are described in clinical papers (e.g., various points on the sternum, the sterno-clavicular junction, nape of neck, forehead, and even the hand). Although there is no convention for the ground (common) electrode site, the forehead is a popular choice clinically.

As with any evoked response test protocol, in VEMP measurement the skin should be prepared prior to electrode placement to produce interelectrode impedance of less than 5000 ohms (5 K ohms) for each electrode and balance impedance among electrodes (optimally within 2 K ohms). Electrode sites on the SCM muscle should be prepared on both sides (right and left) during preparation for VEMP measure-

ment. Detection of the VEMP with a large electrode on the SCM muscle is advisable for several related reasons. Zapala and Brey (2004) cite reasons for a large electrode, including the resulting greater surface area, the advantage of an enhanced signal-to-noise ratio and, consequently, higher response reliability and reduced demand for signal averaging and shorter test time. In addition, with a large electrode covering a rather expansive surface area, the precise location of the electrode exerts minimal influence on VEMP outcome. The authors recommend the use of a 2×3-inch disposable electrode for the inverting site (see Figure 15.8). Electrode options, including disposable electrode designs, were shown in Chapter 3 (Figure 3.9).

The electrode array for the inverting and noninverting electrode pair on each side constitutes a channel for two-channel evoked response systems. All electrodes can be plugged into the physiologic amplifier before the start of data collection. A VEMP will be recorded with the channel ipsilateral to the side of stimulation, with little or no VEMP activity detected from the contralateral electrode array. SCM muscle activity is sometimes observed on both sides with monaural acoustic stimulation, although amplitude is very small when recorded from the muscle contralateral to stimulation (Colebatch, Halmagyi, & Skuse, 1994). When the side of stimulation is reversed, the VEMP will be recorded in the opposite channel. With a one-channel evoked-response system, the electrodes for one side (usually the uninvolved side) are plugged in first, i.e., the electrode on the SCM muscle on the uninvolved side and the second recording electrode. Then, the electrode attached to the SCM muscle on the recorded side is removed from the physiologic amplifier and replaced by the electrode over the SCM muscle on the other side. As with ENoG measurement, the same test protocol is followed when assessing VEMP on each side (stimulating each ear). The general technique for skin preparation and electrode placement in evoked response measurement was described in Chapter 3.

In addition to the conventional sternocleidomastoid location for the recording electrode in VEMP measurement, the response can be detected with electrodes on posterior neck muscles, particularly the trapezius muscle and splenius capitis muscle (e.g., Ferber-Viart et al., 1998; Sakakura et al., 2005; Wu, Young, & Murofushi, 1999). Indeed, some of the earliest studies of VEMP focused on the "inion response" recorded from the posterior neck muscles (e.g., Bickford, Jacobson, & Cody, 1964). An inverting (reference) electrode is placed inferiorly at the nape of the neck (i.e., on the skin over the spinous portion of C7). Sakakura et al. (2005) defined the VEMP recorded from neck extensor muscles at the inion as follows:

- The threshold of the VEMP was higher than the threshold for hearing (over 60 dB). The authors also recorded a neck extensor muscle VEMP from patients who were deaf.

- Muscle tension was required for generation of the response.
- The response was abnormally small in amplitude or absent for patients with vestibular nerve dysfunction (e.g., acoustic tumors).
- Latency of the initial negative wave for the VEMP recorded from neck extensor muscles was equivalent to latency for the SCM muscle response.

According to Sakakura et al. (2005), the alternative electrode locations are better suited for VEMP measurement in elderly patients who are likely to lack muscle strength. With these posterior electrode locations, VEMP recordings can be performed with a patient seated comfortably in a chair or lying in a prone position on a bed, with no demand for tension of neck muscles (e.g., Todd, Cody, & Banks, 2000). In fact, subjects in the study reported by Sakakura et al. (2005) "were instructed to relax their bodies, and they were not required to contract their neck muscles." (p. 1769). These authors found that the VEMP recorded with from posterior muscles (neck extensor muscles) was comparable in latency, but considerably opposite in polarity (negative wave) than the VEMP recorded from the SCM muscle (positive wave). Absolute amplitude of the component was smaller for the neck extensor muscle response versus the SCM muscle response. In general, the proportion of young subjects generating a VEMP was higher for an electrode site on the SCM muscle (92%), rather than the neck extensor muscle site (74%). Among older subjects (over 70 years), only about 45 percent yielded a detectable VEMP for either electrode location. The lack of a detectable response in more than half of a group of normal subjects is clearly a disadvantage for clinical application of the neck extensor muscle VEMP technique. In addition, among the extensor muscles, the VEMP was smaller in amplitude when recorded from the bilateral splenius capitis muscle than from the median neck extensor muscle.

A time period of 50 to100 ms after stimulus presentation is used in VEMP measurement. Since the latest component in the VEMP waveform appears at about 23 ms, an analysis time of 50 ms is adequate. The VEMP protocol typically includes a prestimulus baseline time of 10 to 20 ms, or about 20 percent of the entire analysis time. Amplitude of the myogenic VEMP is considerably greater than the amplitude for any neurogenic response, for example, an auditory evoked response. A tenfold difference between the amplitude of the VEMP and the amplitude of AERs is typical. The amplitude excursion from trough to peak of the two VEMP components (P1 to N1 or n13 to p23) may exceed 200 µV. Because the response is robust, the amplifier setting for detection of the VEMP is only X5000, or often much less (e.g., ×50). In contrast, physiologic amplifier gain of X50000 to 100000 is required for AER recordings. Also, given the sizable amplitude of the VEMP, only modest signal averaging is required to confidently detect the presence of a response. A typical number of stimulus presentations, or sweeps, is 50 to 250. Physiologic filter settings for VEMP measurement must be selected to include the relatively low frequency content of the myogenic activity. The high-pass filter cutoff is usually within the region of 1 to 30 Hz, whereas a low-pass filter cutoff of 250 to 2500 Hz is typically utilized.

Analysis and Interpretation

VEMP WAVEFORM ANALYSIS. | With appropriate measurement parameters and conditions, a reliable VEMP with a positive peak and a negative peak is invariably recorded from normal young (<60 years) adults. A few more comments about waveform polarity are in order at the outset of the discussion of VEMP analysis. In published studies, there are inconsistencies in the polarity of the two components within the VEMP waveform. The differences in waveform polarity are associated with location of the noninverting and inverting electrodes relative to the SCM muscle, as noted in the preceding review of acquisition parameters. With an inverting electrode over the SCM muscle and the noninverting electrode at a remote location e.g., sternum or nape of the neck) away from the SCM muscle, the VEMP waveform consists of an up-going positive peak in the region of 10 to 18 ms followed by a down-going peak (negative trough) in the latency region of 17 to 26 ms (see Figure 15.9). The polarity of the VEMP components is reversed when the noninverting electrode is located on the SCM muscle and the inverting electrode, serving as a true reference, is located elsewhere on the body. As explained by Todd, Cody, and Banks (2000),

> . . . If one considers how such an arrangement [non-inverting electrode rostral on muscle to inverting electrode] would respond to a single action potential, then the polarity of the initial wave will depend on where the motor neuronal axons synapse with the muscle, i.e., the so-called motor point. If the motor point is closer to the negative electrode, then the polarity of the initial wave will be positive, since an action potential manifests itself as an increase in negativity on the surface of a muscle fibre." (p. 186).

The authors go on to emphasize the relation between excitatory and inhibitory modulation of SCM muscle contraction and polarity of the waveform. Given that the VEMP reflects an inhibitory response (decreased synchronization of motor unit action potentials), "in the case of a single action potential, the surface of the muscle will become relatively more negative for an 'excitatory pulse'. However, for an 'inhibitory pulse' the surface will become relatively less negative (Di Lazzaro, 1995)" (Todd, Cody, & Banks, 2000, p. 186).

In studies utilizing an electrode array with the noninverting electrode on the SCM muscle and the inverting at another location, the VEMP waves are described as n13 and p23, since the first component in the region of 13 ms has negative polarity and is plotted downward whereas the second component has a latency of about 23 ms, is positive

**Vestibular Evoked Myogenic Potential (VEMP)
Waveform Morphology and Analysis**

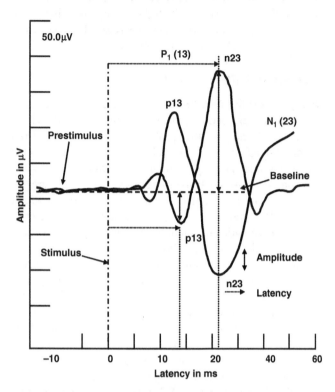

FIGURE 15.9. Analysis of the vestibular evoked myogenic potential (VEMP). The major component in the latency region of 23 ms may appear positive-going or negative-going depending on which electrode (noninverting or inverting electrode) is located on the sternocleidomastoid muscle.

in polarity, and is plotted upward. Adding to inconsistencies among published studies is the convention of the majority of VEMP investigators, particularly neurologists, of plotting positive peaks downward, and negative peaks upward (e.g., Colebatch et al., 1994; Welgampola & Colebatch, 2005). Latency and amplitude values for the two VEMP components (P1 and N2) are unaffected by the location of the noninverting and inverting electrodes, as long as one of them is on the SCM muscle. Exact latencies of VEMP components, of course, depend on stimulus parameters (e.g., type, frequency, and intensity) as reviewed above. In this chapter, the VEMP waveform will be described with a positive first peak (P1) and a negative second peak, or trough (N1), as recorded with the noninverting ("active") electrode located over the midpoint of the SCM muscle (see Figure 15.9).

The waveform of the VEMP recorded from the SCM muscle (with parameters shown in Table 15.8) consists of an onset of deviation from the baseline at 8 ms, a positive peak in the 13 ms latency region (P1 or p13), and then a negative trough at about 23 ms (N1 or n23). In most of the early papers on VEMP, components were labeled according to their

typical latency region (e.g., p13). Note that the alphabetic labels for VEMP components are sometimes in lower case, in contrast to the labels used for auditory evoked responses. In 1969, years before the first reports of VEMP, Yoshie and Okudaira (1969) suggested labeling peaks of muscle responses with lowercase letters to differentiate the myogenic peaks from those for responses arising from the sensory nervous system, such as AERs. More recently, however, Akin and Murnane (2001) introduced a alphabetical-numerical label system based on the sequence of peaks with uppercase letters to designated the peaks, e.g., P1 for the first positive peak and N1 for the first negative peak. Confusion might be generated by this alphabetical-numerical label system, since the same convention is also followed with cortical auditory evoked responses. Sometimes in VEMP recordings other waves are apparent at longer latencies. There is now, however, ample evidence that waves after the p13 (P1) and n23 (N1) do not originate from the vestibular system and are not components of the VEMP. On rare occasions, contralateral muscle activity (on the opposite side from the stimulus ear) is detected during VEMP measurement. Possibly a reflection of "vestibular hypersensitivity to sound" (Welgampola & Colebatch, 2005), the contralateral response is smaller in amplitude and opposite in polarity in comparison to the ipsilateral VEMP waveform (Colebatch et al., 1998).

Consistent with response characteristics for other electrophysiologic measures, VEMP latency is quite consistent among subjects, but intersubject VEMP amplitude is highly variable, with the trough-to-peak difference ranging from only 25 μV to well over 200 μV. Amplitude measures, however, are more sensitive to unilateral vestibular dysfunction (Brantberg & Fransson, 2001). Asymmetry in VEMP amplitude is a characteristic feature of the VEMP, even in normal subjects. For example, Brantberg and Fransson (2001) reported amplitude asymmetry in normal young adult subjects, as defined by the difference in amplitude between sides expressed as the range from the 25th to 75th quartile, 0.08 to 0.36 μV. Their data led to the conclusion "among the normals in the present study there was a rather large tendency to asymmetry in the VEMP amplitudes" (p. 195). VEMP amplitudes are, however, far more asymmetric for patients with vestibular dysfunction on one side. Although the variation in responses from one person to the next is probably a product of multiple factors, the level of tonic contraction of the SCM muscle—background EMG activity—plays a major role. In this respect, analysis of the vestibular-evoked muscle potential (VEMP) has features in common with analysis of the facial nerve myogenic response—electroneuronograpy (ENoG). Due to the wide variation in the size of VEMPs recorded in normal subjects, absolute amplitude is not a viable response parameter. The overall goal of VEMP analysis is to assess symmetry of vestibular, specifically saccular, function by comparing responses from the right versus left sides (Brantberg & Fransson, 2001). Abnormal asymmetry in VEMP amplitude is the distinctive clinical finding associated with unilateral vestibular dysfunction (Halmagyi, Colebatch, & Curthoys, 1994). A simple mathematical approach for calculating relative VEMP amplitude is now applied in clinical practice. Briefly, peak-to-trough amplitude of the major VEMP component (i.e., from the low point of the 13 ms negative wave to the peak of the 23 ms wave) is determined for right and left sides and then divided by the sum of the two amplitude measures. The interside amplitude calculation or difference or IAD (e.g., Wang & Young, 2004; Young & Kuo, 2004) is commonly expressed as an amplitude ratio for each side (A_L and A_R), or an "asymmetry ratio" by the following equation (Welgampola & Colebatch, 2005; Young, Wu, & Wu, 2002):

$$\text{Amplitude ratio (\%)} = \frac{(A_L - A_R)}{(A_L + A_R)}$$

where A = amplitude of the VEMP, and L and R refer to stimulation of the left and right sides. Reference to the comparison of responses from the right and left sides can, of course, be used with normal subjects or patients with suspected unilateral vestibular dysfunction. A minor variation of the interside amplitude approach is also utilized for VEMP analysis exclusively with patients having unilateral vestibular dysfunction, with a comparison of the VEMP for the involved or affected ("A") side versus the uninvolved or unaffected ("U") side (e.g., Murofushi, Matsuzaki, & Wu, 1999), as follows:

$$\text{Amplitude ratio (\%)} = \frac{(A_U - A_A)}{(A_U + A_A)}$$

The resulting ratio is analyzed in relation to normal expectations for VEMP amplitude symmetry. An inspection of the equation shows that smaller differences in the VEMP amplitude between the two sides produce a smaller amplitude ratio (in percent), whereas a discrepancy in amplitudes between sides (i.e., large amplitude from the normal side and depressed amplitude for the side of vestibular dysfunction), results in a higher value for the amplitude ratio (AR). Put another way, relatively lower VEMP amplitude on one side is a sign of vestibular abnormality. Investigation of VEMP amplitude data for right- versus left-side stimulation in groups of normal young adult subjects shows no significant difference, although in a given subject the VEMP may sometimes be larger for one side or the other (e.g., Young & Kuo, 2004). As expected, side-to-side differences are more often observed for VEMP amplitude than latency measures (Young & Kuo, 2004). Clinical investigations provide evidence that, for adult subjects less than 60 years old, an AR of ≤0.34 or 0.35 is considered normal, and an AR >0.34 or 0.35 is consistent with saccular dysfunction (e.g., Gans & Roberts, 2005; Murofushi, Matsuzaki, & Wu, 1999; Welgampola & Colebatch, 2001b, 2005; Young, Wu, & Wu, 2002). These values for analysis of VEMP amplitude ratios are based on published findings for normal young adult subjects.

In addition to the two major VEMP components just reviewed (P1 and N1), another wave possibly arising from the vestibular system, referred to as the "N3," is occasionally described in the literature (Kato et al., 1998; Murofushi et al., 2005; Nong et al., 2002; Ochi & Ohashi, 2001; Shiraishi et al., 1997). The nomenclature for the wave is somewhat confusing because the N3 is not the third of a sequence of negative waves in the VEMP waveform but, rather, a peak (trough) that appears at a poststimulus latency of approximately 3 ms. Indeed, the N3 wave is not a myogenic vestibular response like the VEMP. Rather, it appears to be an electrophysiological response, perhaps arising from the vestibular nucleus within the brainstem. The N3, therefore, might be described as a vestibular brainstem response (e.g., VBR), or a vestibular counterpart to the ABR. The N3 is, as the label implies, a negative polarity wave, sometimes found in the ABR that is evoked with high-intensity stimuli from persons with profound sensory hearing loss (e.g., Shiraishi et al., 1997). Because the N3 can be recorded in deafness, some authors speculated on a vestibular and, particularly, saccular origin (e.g., Kato et al., 1998; Nong et al., 2002; Ochi & Ohashi, 2001; Shiraishi et al., 1997). In the words of Kato et al. (1998), "the N3 potential is most likely not an auditory evoked response from the cochlea or a response from a semicircular canal, because it has a 3-ms latency, a sharp waveform, and is unassociated with vertigo. The results suggest that the N3 potential may be a saccular acoustic response" (p. 253). Using high intensity (95 dB nHL or 130 dB SPL) 1000 Hz tone-burst stimuli presented in the presence of ipsilateral white noise masking (100 dB SPL), Murofushi and colleagues (2005) also recorded what was described as the N3 wave in twenty-three of twenty-four normal-hearing young adult subjects. According to the authors (Murofushi et al., 2005), the likelihood of recording a vestibular response in their study was enhanced by the use of a high-intensity tone burst, and the likelihood of recording an auditory response was minimized by the use of a tone burst and also ipsilateral masking noise. Further confirming the vestibular nature of the N3 wave, Murofushi and colleagues (2005) demonstrated that findings for the N3 wave and the conventional VEMP recordings were in agreement, and the N3 wave was abnormal when measured in patients with known vestibular dysfunction.

NONPATHOLOGIC FACTORS: AGE IN CHILDREN. | Sheykholesami, Kaga, Megerian, and Arnold (2005) demonstrated that it was clinically feasible to record the VEMP from infants ranging in age from 1 to 12 months (average of 2.3 months). The VEMP was consistently detected in a series of twelve normal infants and another twelve infants with craniofacial anomalies, including bilateral aural atresia and Treacher-Collins syndrome. Stimuli were tone bursts of 500 Hz with rise/fall times of 1 ms and a plateau of 2 ms delivered via air conduction with supra-aural earphones and bone conduction with mastoid placement. Bone-conduction stimulation is, of course, more efficient than air-conduction stimulation for subjects with severe conductive hearing loss (e.g., aural atresia). During VEMP measurement, infants were lying "in a supine position on a parent's lap with their heads rotated as far as possible to the side contralateral to the stimulated ear. SCM muscles were kept contracted by using the routing reflex in the younger subjects. In older subjects, the contraction was maintained by hanging their head down and turned to the contralateral side . . ." (Sheykholesami et al., 2005, p. 1441). Latency of the N23 peak of the VEMP was shorter for the infants in comparison to adult expectations. The authors acknowledged that in infants it was difficult to maintain consistent muscle tension (EMG activity level) and, thus, VEMP amplitudes were more variable than those for VEMPs recorded from adults. Also, VEMP measurement in infants required two persons (one to operate the evoked response system and another to position the infant's head and maintain the proper level of muscle contraction). Nonetheless, the study suggests that it is possible to apply the VEMP in the identification of vestibular dysfunction in young children.

NONPATHOLOGIC FACTORS: ADVANCING AGE. | Age plays an important role in VEMP analysis. There are in the vestibular system age-related changes (Merchant et al., 2000; Tang, Lopez, & Baloh, 2001; Velasquez-Villasensor et al., 2000), similar to those occurring in the auditory system, including dysfunction of sensory structures (vestibular hair cells), neural components (Scarpa's ganglion cells), and changes in the central nervous system (cells within the vestibular nuclei in the brainstem). Evoking the VEMP with a 250 Hz tone-burst stimulus, Zapala and Brey (2004) describe a clear decrease in VEMP amplitude with advancing age over the range of 30 to 83 years and a trend toward increased VEMP latency with aging. An age-related change in latency of the VEMP, however, is not consistently reported. For example, Su et al. (2004) reported no age-related latency changes for VEMPs evoked with clicks for sixty subjects over the age range of 7 to 60 years. The authors did note a trend toward increased latency for a group of twenty subjects >60 years and a clear decrease in amplitude and the likelihood of detecting a VEMP for the subjects older than 60 years. Also, Basta, Todt, and Ernst (2005) described for three age groups (20 to 40 years, 41 to 60 years, and >60 years) equivalent latencies for the P1 and N1 components evoked by 500 Hz tone-burst stimuli. In a normal population (i.e., no diagnosis of vestibular disorder), VEMP amplitude declines with aging (Basta, Todt, & Ernst, 2005; Ochi & Ohashi, 2003; Su et al., 2004; Zapala & Brey, 2004) and the proportion of subjects producing a reliable VEMP decreases significantly after age 60 years (Welgampola & Colebatch, 2001b). Ochi and Ohashi (2003) further demonstrated an age-related increase in the threshold of acoustic stimulation of the VEMP, but no correlation between age and left-to-right differences in VEMP amplitude or threshold. Su et al. (2004) also confirmed no

age-related asymmetry in VEMP parameters (latency or amplitude).

The relation between age and VEMP amplitude is independent of a possible age-related decrease in tonic activity of the SCM muscle (e.g., Ochi & Ohashi, 2003). Clinically, the absence of a click-evoked VEMP for a patient over the age of 60 years may be entirely age related and not a sign of vestibular dysfunction. Other changes in VEMP with advancing age include increased thresholds for detection of a response, i.e., greater stimulus intensity levels are required to evoke the response and smaller intensity levels even at maximum stimulus intensity levels (Sakakura et al., 2005; Welgampola & Colebatch, 2001b). Whether interside differences are affected by age is unclear, as some investigators describe greater interaural asymmetry among older subjects (e.g., Welgampola & Colebatch, 2001b) and others find no age-related difference (e.g., Basta, Todt, & Ernst, 2005).

NONPATHOLOGIC FACTORS: GENDER. | In comparison to the multiple studies of aging on the VEMP, there are few published references on possible gender effects. The explanation for the paucity of data on VEMP and gender may be due to an appreciation of the absence of a relationship. Using 500 Hz tone-burst stimuli to evoke the VEMP, Basta, Todt, and Ernst (2005) found no differences between young adult males versus females for absolute latencies of the P1 and N1 waves or interside latency differences for the two components. Similarly, Akin, Murnane, and Proffitt (2003) reported no gender effect for latency and amplitude of VEMPs evoked with click stimuli.

PATHOLOGIC FACTORS. | One pathologic factor that has a major impact on measurement of the VEMP is conductive hearing loss. Because the VEMP is evoked with acoustic stimuli at intensity levels that are close to the maximum output limits of evoked response systems (e.g., >90 dB nHL), even a mild and perhaps clinically insignificant conductive hearing loss component may preclude VEMP measurement via air conduction (Bath, Harris, McEwan, & Yardley, 1999; Colebatch, Halmagyi, & Skuse, 1994; Halmagyi, Colebatch, & Curthoys, 1994; Yang & Young, 2003). That is, the attenuation of the effective stimulation of the saccule by a modest conductive hearing loss (e.g., 10 to 20 dB) is more than enough to obliterate the VEMP, just as using an acoustic stimulus intensity level of only 80 or 85 dB nHL would be inadequate. The impact of conductive hearing loss on the probability of detecting a VEMP leads to an important implication for clinical protocol. A basic audiologic assessment should be carried out before VEMP measurement. Tympanometry is sensitive to even slight middle ear dysfunction. In patients with clinical indications of middle ear disease, e.g., by history, otoscopic examination, absence of OAEs, and/or an abnormal tympanogram, pure-tone audiometry with air- and bone-conduction stimuli will document the degree of conductive hearing loss component. If a very slight conductive hearing loss component is present, it is reasonable to attempt VEMP measurement with air-conduction stimuli at a very high intensity level. If no VEMP activity is detected, or if the conductive hearing loss component is more than 5 dB and hearing sensitivity by bone-conduction stimulation is normal, then bone-conduction stimulation is in order. Patients with mixed hearing loss, i.e., a conductive hearing loss component is present but bone-conduction hearing is not normal, valid VEMP recording may not be possible.

Clinical Applications and Populations

Clinical reports describing VEMP findings for a variety of disease entities first appeared in the late 1990s (e.g., Brantberg et al., 1999; Halmagyi & Curthoys, 1999; Heide et al., 1999; Murofushi, Halmagyi, Yavor, & Colebatch, 1996; Murofushi, Matsuzaki, & Mizuno, 1998; Murofushi, Matsuzaki, & Wu, 1999). Studies and findings are summarized in Table 15.9. The majority of the pathologies, of course, affect the peripheral vestibular apparatus, sometimes in combination with auditory dysfunction or the neural pathways in the vestibular system. As a noninvasive measure of saccular function, VEMP plays an important, and rather unique, role in the vestibular test battery. In contrast, other clinical vestibular procedures, such as those within the ENG test battery, provide no information on the sacculus. Precise and comprehensive data on the sensitivity and specificity of the VEMP procedure for different vestibular diseases are now accumulating. Zapala and Brey (2004) reported for a series of sixty-four patients with various vestibular disorders VEMP sensitivity of 0.52 and specificity of 0.93, values similar to those for caloric procedures. Analysis of caloric and VEMP findings in combination yielded an increase in sensitivity to 0.81, although specificity showed a modest decrease to 0.89 (Zapala & Brey, 2004). Test specificity for VEMP, therefore, is generally considered high, up to 100 percent, for the VEMP technique (Heide, 1999), whereas sensitivity rates are reported to be within the range of 60 to 80 percent (e.g., Heide et al., 1999; Murofushi, Matsuzaki, & Mizuno, 1998). That is, false negative errors (normal findings in patients with confirmed vestibular dysfunction), as defined by normal amplitude ratios, are more commonly reported for VEMP than false positive errors (Murofushi, Matsuzaki, & Wu, 1999). Still, as noted by Zapala and Brey (2004), "Methods to improve the VEMP false-positive rate (possible the use of a 500 or 1000 Hz stimulus) would be helpful in improving test performance" (p. 213). VEMP findings, whether normal or abnormal, tend to be correlated with those for other vestibular tests, including the clinical vestibular examination (e.g., VOR), the ENG test battery, and computerized dynamic posturography, or CDP (Iwasaki et al., 2005; Robertson & Ireland, 1995; Zapala and Brey, 2004). Discrepancies between the VEMP and other measures of vestibular function are, of course, expected given the well-appreciated diversity of vestibular disorders. In addition, whether the VEMP is abnormal for an individual patient depends on the site of the vestibular pathology, specifically whether it affects function of the saccule. Differences in the outcome of VEMP and other clinical vestibular procedure are, in some cases, entirely logical due to the difference in anatomy of the responses. For example, the VEMP assesses function of the saccule and inferior vestibular nerve, whereas caloric measures within the ENG test battery assess function of the lateral semicircular canal and superior vestibular nerve. In an analysis of data for a series of 811 patients "with balance problems," Iwasaki et al. (2005) found that 40 (5 percent) had abnormal VEMPs, yet normal caloric test results. This group included twelve patients with the diagnosis of Ménière's disease, eight with an acoustic neuroma (tumor), six with sudden hearing loss with vertigo, and six with miscellaneous other diseases (e.g., cerebellar-pontine angle tumor, multiple sclerosis). In a follow-up study, Iwasaki et al. (2005) recorded abnormal VEMP findings more often than abnormal caloric test results in a series of twenty-two patients with sudden hearing loss with vertigo. The study illustrated the value of recording VEMP, in addition to conventional caloric tests, to extend the range of vestibular diagnosis to the saccule and inferior vestibular nerve in disorders, such as sudden hearing loss with vertigo, that are likely to affect these structures. Best agreement among vestibular procedures, including VEMP, occurs with total dysfunction of the peripheral vestibular apparatus (end organs). Limited published clinical investigation suggests that the VEMP is sensitive to vestibular deficits arising from lesions of the cranial nerves and central nervous system (Murofushi, Matsuzaki, & Takegoshi, 2001; Zapala & Brey, 2004). Such pathologies include vestibular schwannomas (acoustic tumors) and various neuropathologies in the medulla and pontine region of the brainstem (e.g., tumors, strokes).

Clinical reports on VEMP are reviewed herein for the most common vestibular disorders. The characteristic VEMP pattern in peripheral pathologies is absence of the response, although delayed latencies for VEMP components are recorded in some diseases (e.g., multiple sclerosis). Superior canal dehiscence syndrome (SCDS) is a distinct exception to these VEMP patterns. Vestibular sensitivity is enhanced in SCDS, as evidenced by larger than expected VEMP amplitudes and enhanced thresholds (e.g., 60 to 70 dB nHL versus $\geq$95 dB nHL). As already noted, basic audiologic assessment provides information valuable for interpretation of VEMP is patients with suspected conductive hearing loss. Clinical assessment of vestibular function is conducted with a battery of tests, each providing complementary information on integrity of vestibular structures. Examples of vestibular procedures include electronystagmography (ENG), platform posturography, and rotatory vestibular tests. Although VEMP is a valuable procedure for evaluating integrity of the saccule, it must be applied along with other procedures for adequate assessment of the vestibular system and, of course, for diagnosis of vestibular pathologies.

TABLE 15.9. Summary of Vestibular Evoked Myogenic Potential (VEMP) Findings in Selected Clinical Populations, Arranged Alphabetically

CLINICAL ENTITY	STUDIES	SUMMARY OF FINDINGS
Acoustic tumor (neuroma) (see Vestibular schwannoma)	Murofushi et al., 2001 Murofushi et al., 1998 Murofushi et al., 1996 Murofushi et al., 1999 Ushio, Matsuzaki, Takegoshi, & Murofushi, 2001 Tsutsumi et al., 2001 Zapala & Brey, 2004 Murofushi et al., 2005 Sakakura et al., 2005 Welgampola & Colebatch, 2005	Absent VEMP in ≥75% of patients.
Acute vertigo	Heide et al., 1999	
Auditory neuropathy	Sheykholeslami et al., 2000	
Aural atresia	Sheykholesami et al., 2005	
Benign paroxymal positional vertigo (BPPV)	Sakakura et al., 2005 Heide et al., 1999 Murofushi et al., 1999 Murofushi et al., 2005	Normal VEMP findings.
Cerebellar disease	Takegoshi & Murofushi, 2000 Murofushi et al., 2005	Normal VEMP findings.
Congenital malformation	Sheykholeslami, Habiby, & Kaga, 2001	
Endolymphatic hydrops	Murofushi, Matsuzaki, & Wu, 1999	Enhanced VEMP amplitudes.
Hearing loss (deafness)	Ackley, Tamaki, Oliszewski, & Inverso, 2004	
Herpes zoster otiticus	Welgampola & Colebatch, 2005	
Hunt syndrome	Sakakura et al., 2005	
Idiopathic sudden deafness	Sakakura et al., 2005 Iwasaki et al., 2005 Murofushi et al., 2005	Up to 75% with abnormal VEMP, with less than 50% with abnormal caloric test findings.
Idiopathic vestibulopathy	Matsuzaki & Murofushi, 2001	Absence of VEMP a characteristic finding.
Large vestibular aqueduct	Sheykholeslami et al., 2004	Lower than normal VEMP thresholds and higher amplitudes.
Machado-Joseph disease	Takegoshi & Murofushi, 2000	Most patients have abnormal VEMP findings.
Ménière's disease	de Waele et al., 1999 Heide et al., 1999 Seo, Node, Yukimasa, & Sakagami, 2003 Murofushi et al., 1999 Murofushi et al., 2001 Young, Wu, & Wu, 2003 Zapala & Brey, 2004 Murofushi et al., 2005 Sakakura et al., 2005 Welgampola & Colebatch, 2005	VEMP absent in 35 to 55% of patients, but possibly larger VEMP amplitudes in selected patients.
Migraine (basilar artery)	Liao & Young, 2004	VEMP may be delayed in latency or absent.
Multiple sclerosis	Shimizu, Murofushi, Sakurai, & Halmagyi, 2000 Murofushi et al., 2001	Prolonged VEMP latency values, or absent in some patients (<50%).

TABLE 15.9.   (continued)

CLINICAL ENTITY	STUDIES	SUMMARY OF FINDINGS
Neurofibromatosis 2	Wang et al., 2005	VEMP findings are typically normal.
Ramsay Hunt syndrome	Murofushi et al., 1999 Murofushi et al., 2005	Majority of patients have absent VEMP with vertigo.
Spinocerebellar degeneration		Delayed in latency or absent.
Stroke (brainstem)	Itoh et al., 2001 Chen & Young, 2003 Zapala & Brey, 2004	VEMP delayed in latency or absent.
Superior canal dehiscence	Brantberg et al., 1999 Watson et al., 2000 Brantberg et al., 2004 Welgampola & Colebatch, 2005	Enhanced VEMP thresholds and larger amplitudes.
Temporal bone fracture	Zapala & Brey, 2004	
Treacher-Collins Syndrome	Sheykholesami et al., 2005	
Tumor (brainstem)	Sakakura et al., 2005	
Vestibular neurectomy	Welgampola & Colebatch, 2001a,b	Absent VEMPs.
Vestibular neuritis	Murofushi et al., 1996 Murofushi et al., 1999 Ochi et al., 2003 Zapala & Brey, 2004 Monobe & Murofushi, 2004 Sakakura et al., 2005 Welgampola & Colebatch, 2005	Small amplitude; absent VEMP in 10 to 40% of patients.
Vestibular neuropathy (acute)	Heide et al., 1999 Zapala & Brey, 2004	High test specificity for VEMP in acute vertigo.
Wallenberg syndrome	Itoh et al., 2001	Abnormal VEMP with lower brainstem involvement.

* CPA = cerebello-pontine angle; CNS = central nervous system

ACOUSTIC TUMOR (NEUROMA). | VEMP findings tend to be abnormal in patients with acoustic tumors (vestibular schwannomas). Murofushi, Matsuzaki, and Mizuno, a group in the Department of Otolarynology at the University of Tokyo, have published numerous clinical studies of the VEMP. The authors reported abnormal VEMP findings in 80 percent of a patients with acoustic tumors, most often an absent response (Murofushi, Matsuzaki, & Mizuno, 1998; Murofushi et al., 2001). In a nondiagnostic application of VEMP recording in acoustic tumors (vestibular schwannomas), Magliulo et al. (2003) monitored vestibular nerve status with VEMP before and after surgery from removal of a 1.3 cm vestibular schwannoma. The VEMP was also normal, confirming that the tumor arose from the superior vestibular nerve and also that the inferior vestibular nerve remained intact post-operatively.

MÉNIÈRE'S DISEASE. | The literature includes a number of studies of VEMP in Ménière's disease (see listing in Table 15.9). Divergent VEMP findings characterize Ménière's disease, suggesting the possibility of more than one pathophysiologic process or mechanism underlying the disease. Interestingly, patients with Ménière's disease also show distinctively different patterns of findings for distortion product otoacoustic emissions (DPOAE). In patients with Ménière's disease, VEMPs may have reduced amplitude, they may be absent, or, paradoxically, amplitude of the VEMP may be abnormally large. Investigators commonly report abnormally reduced VEMP amplitudes or absence of the response in patients with Ménière's disease (e.g., de Waele et al., 1999; Iwasaki et al., 2005). However, Young, Wu, and Wu (2002) described "augmentation of vestibular responses" in patients with Ménière's disease and distended saccular hydrops, a finding confirmed also by others (e.g., Gans & Roberts, 2005). The diversity of VEMP findings in Ménière's disease may reflect variable sites of lesions, e.g., hair cells in the horizontal semicircular canal versus the saccule (de Waele et al., 1999), and pathophysiologic mechanisms. In general, the likelihood of VEMP abnormalities, including the absence of a response, in Ménière's disease increases directly with the degree of hearing loss, caloric weakness in electronystagmography (ENG), and for patients with deficits on the vestibular portions of a platform posturography test battery (e.g., de Waele et al., 1999; Robertson & Ireland, 1995). Murofushi et al. (2001) reported VEMP abnormalities (decreased amplitude or absence of the response) in 51 percent of forty-three patients with the diagnosis of Ménière's disease, even though latency was rarely prolonged when the VEMP was abnormal.

In another study by the same group of researchers, Murofushi, Matsuzaki, and Takegoshi (2001) documented with a series of seventeen patients with unilateral Ménière's disease that VEMP amplitude may increase following ingestion of glycerol, suggesting that VEMP abnormalities are sensitive to endolymphatic hydrops, and pathophysiology can involve the saccule. Magliulo et al. (2004) also investigated the effect of glycerol on VEMP, and also findings for pure-tone audiometry and DPOAEs. Data for a series of twenty-nine patients with an early diagnosis of endolymphatic hydrops confirmed the contribution of both DPOAEs and VEMP to the diagnosis, beyond information obtained from pure-tone audiometry. Close analysis of findings for VEMP and DPOAE, specifically the responsiveness of each measure to changes with glycerol administration, permits early diagnosis of endolymphatic hydrops and the categorization of patients into subgroups based on involvement of anterior versus posterior regions of the labyrinth.

Seo, Node, Yukimasa, and Sakagami (2003) conducted a similar study of VEMP in Ménière's disease using furosemide, a loop diuretic drug. The VEMP was detected in three out of seven patients after furosemide loading, even though it was not apparent before administration of the diuretic. For seven of the eighteen patients who yielded a clear VEMP before administration of the diuretic, the drug was associated with increased amplitude of the P1/N1 wave complex. The authors conclude that VEMP has value in the diagnosis of endolymphatic hydrops involving the saccule and for differentiating dysfunction of the saccule versus the cochlea. Overall, 40 percent of the patients with Ménière's disease yielded larger VEMP amplitudes following the administration of furosemide, even though audiometric status was unchanged. Also, for 24 percent of the twenty-five patients with apparently unilateral Ménière's disease, a change in the VEMP with furosemide was noted in the contralateral ear, suggesting the possible value of VEMP in detecting unsuspected bilateral Ménière's disease.

SUPERIOR CANAL DEHISCENCE SYNDROME (SCDS). | Contrary to the pattern of smaller VEMP amplitudes or absence of the VEMP associated with most peripheral diseases processes affecting the vestibular system, enlarged VEMPs are found in patients with the diagnosis of superior canal dehiscence syndrome (Brantberg et al., 1999; Watson, Halmagyi, & Colebatch, 2000). SCDS is most often unilateral, although bilateral pathology is also possible (Mikulec et al., 2004).

The pattern of hypersensitivity to sound stimulation reflected by VEMP findings in SCDS is consistent with the clinical sign known as Tullio's phenomenon, namely the generation of vestibular symptoms during exposure to high-intensity sounds (Colebatch et al., 1998; Colebatch et al., 1994; Watson, Halmagyi, & Colebatch, 2000). Tullio phenomenon has for over 100 years been recognized as a finding in different otologic pathologies in addition to SCDS, including syphilis and, occasionally, perilymphatic fistula, Ménière's disease, Lyme disease, and otitis media. Audiologic findings in SCDS invariably include a characteristic "conductive hyperacusis," i.e., better-than-normal hearing thresholds for bone conduction in combination with a clear air-bone gap (up to 60 dB) in patients with sensory (versus conductive) hearing loss, with normal acoustic reflexes and word recognition performance (Mikulec et al., 2004). Surgical management of SCDS, when indicated, consists of either repairing the surface of the superior semicircular canal or plugging the canal, with typically good postoperative status (total resolution or marked reduction of symptoms).

The VEMP is always recorded in patients with SCDS and is typically evoked with stimulus intensity levels down to 70 or 75 dB nHL, rather than the usual intensity levels exceeding 90 dB nHL. In addition, in SCDS at high-stimulus intensity levels VEMP amplitude values are consistently greater than expected (Colebatch et al., 1998; Colebatch et al., 1994; Mikulec et al., 2004; Watson, Halmagyi, & Colebatch, 2000). In fact, Gans and Roberts (2005) report a case study of SCDS with a reliable VEMP evoked by an acoustic stimulus as low as 62 dB nHL. Bone conduction stimulation also produces larger than normal VEMP amplitude in SCDS (Brantberg, Löfqvist, & Fransson, 2004). Bone-conduction stimulation to one mastoid generates a bilateral VEMP. For all four patients with unilateral SCDS, bone-conduction stimulation to one mastoid produced a normal VEMP from the uninvolved side and an abnormally large VEMP from the side with SCDS. In another group of three patients who had undergone unilateral labyrinthectomy, bone-conduction stimulation to either mastoid generated a normal VEMP from the normal ear and no VEMP from the operated ear. As an aside, the authors also confirmed that interaural (transcranial) attenuation was less for the 250 versus 500 Hz toneburst stimulus. Based on these findings, Brantberg, Löfqvist, and Fransson (2004) conclude that "patients with SCD syndrome have a vestibular hypersensitivity for bone conducted sounds" (p. 180), consistent with the Tullio phenomenon.

OTHER DISEASES AND DISORDERS. | Following vestibular neurectomy (surgical severing of the vestibular nerves typically in management of Ménière's disease), the VEMP is invariably absent (Welgampola & Colebatch, 2001a). Murofushi et al. (1996) described abnormal VEMP findings, often the absent of a response, for about one-third of a series of forty-seven patients with the diagnosis of vestibular neurolabyrinthitis. Some patients with vestibular neurolabyrinthitis later develop benign paroxysmal positional vertigo (BPPV). Interestingly, the authors provide evidence suggesting that patients with vestibular neurolabyrinthitis and absent VEMP are less likely to subsequently be diagnosed with BPPV and vice versa, i.e., vestibular neurolabyrinthitis patients with normal VEMP findings are at risk for development of BPPV. In another publication, Murofushi et al. (2001) describe an abnormal (decreased amplitude or absent) VEMP for 39 percent of sixty-two patients with vestibular neuritis and 25 percent of patients with multiple sclerosis. Monobe and Murofushi (2004) demonstrated the diagnostic value of eliciting the VEMP with bone conduction stimulation in a 3-year-old child with vestibular neuritis who also had bilateral otitis media with effusion and associated conductive hearing loss.

Application of VEMP in combination with the ABR enhances identification of brainstem lesions. Itoh et al. (2001) investigated both techniques in thirteen patients with brainstem lesions documented by MRI, include multiple sclerosis (N = 5), Wallenberg's syndrome (N = 4), brainstem hemorrhage (N = 3), and one patient with a pons-medulla infarction. Patients with lesions affecting the upper brainstem had abnormal ABRs but normal VEMP findings, whereas patients with lower brainstem (pons) involvement yielded abnormal findings for both ABR and VEMP.

The VEMP has also been recorded in the investigation of auditory and vestibular function in auditory neuropathy. Sheykholeslami et al. (2000) followed three patients with auditory neuropathy as defined by normal OAEs and cochlear microphonic potentials, mild-to-moderate hearing loss, poor word recognition scores, and absent ABRs. Sheykholeslami, Habiby, and Kaga (2001a,b) demonstrated the feasibility of recording VEMPs with bone conduction stimulation (clicks and tone bursts) in fifteen patients with severe conductive hearing loss secondary to bilateral aural atresia. Robust VEMPs were recorded from most patients, but responses evoked by tone-burst stimuli had larger amplitude and better morphology than those evoked by click stimuli.

The VEMP may contribute to documentation of the site of lesion in a variety of pathologies affecting the auditory and vestibular sensory and neural systems. Wang, Hsu, & Young (2005) describe normal VEMP findings in six out of seven adult patients with neurofibromatosis 2 (NF2), concluding that "neurofibromatosis 2 originates from the superior vestibular nerve more often than from the inferior nerve" (p. 72).

In a prospective study of twenty patients with basilar artery migraine, Liao and Young (2004) found delayed VEMP latency values in two patients and absence of the VEMP in seven patients, and one patient with an absent response on one side and a delayed response on the other side. Overall, one-half of the group yielded normal VEMP findings, whereas caloric responses were abnormal in 45 percent of the subject group. In the words of the authors, "Some patients with basilar artery migraine present absent or delayed vestibular evoked myogenic potentials, presumably because the descending pathway from the saccule through the brainstem to cranial nerve XI is interrupted, which is attributed to hypoperfusion in the territory of the basilar artery" (p. 1308).

Chen and Young (2003) describe VEMP findings for seven adult patients with MRI evidence of brainstem stroke including five with an infarction and two with hemorrhage. Vestibular abnormalities were found in all patients, with caloric deficits in 71 percent. VEMP results were normal in three ears and abnormal in eleven ears (absent in eight and delayed latencies in three). The authors conclude that "both caloric testing and VEMP tests should be performed" in brainstem stroke, as "caloric testing assesses the vestibulo-ocular reflex which passes upward through the upper brainstem, whereas VEMP test evaluates the sacculocollic reflex which travels downward through the lower brainstem" (p. 993).

Sheykholeslami, Schmerber, Kermany, and Kaga (2004) described, for the first time, VEMP findings for patients with large vestibular aqueduct syndrome, among the most common congenital inner ear abnormalies. Large vestibular aqueduct syndrome, confirmed by CT imaging, is associated with progressive, usually bilateral, sensorineural hearing loss and vestibular symptoms (e.g., vertigo) in childhood. The endolymphatic duct, and a vein and an artery, course through the vestibular aqueduct in the temporal bone. The three patients reported by Sheykholeslami and colleagues (2004) had lower VEMP thresholds (75 to 85 dB nHL) and considerably higher amplitudes than normal subjects, consistent with vestibular hypersensitivity to acoustic stimulation.

ELECTRONEURONOGRAPHY (ENoG)
Historical Overview and Clinical Rationale

Since about 1980, measurement of facial muscle activity evoked by stimulation of the facial nerve has become a common clinical procedure (Adour, Sheldon, & Kahn, 1980; Fisch, 1980; Gantz, Gmur, Holliday, & Fisch, 1984; May, Blumenthal, Klein, 1983; Niparko et al., 1989). Early on, the term *electroneuronography* (ENoG) was coined to refer to this response (Fisch, 1980). ENoG is also sometimes described as a facial nerve evoked response. These terms imply direct measurement of nerve activity following electrical stimulation. With ENoG, however, facial muscle activity secondary to facial nerve activity is actually being recorded. Therefore, facial electromyographic (EMG) evoked response is a more accurate term than ENoG. The logic behind this apparently semantic distinction will become clearer when the procedure is explained below. The term ENoG is, nonetheless, in general usage and consequently will be used in the following discussion. ENoG is within the scope of practice of audiologists based on both the American Academy of Audiology (AAA) and the American Speech-Language-Hearing Association (ASHA) Scope of

Practice statements. Audiologists have been evaluating facial nerve function for many decades, beginning with measurement of the acoustic reflex within the aural immittance test battery.

At first glance, ENoG would seem to be a rather simple procedure to perform. The test setup is straightforward, the patient need not be sedated and state of arousal doesn't influence results, and recordings are made with a single channel (only three recording electrodes). Also, little or no averaging is required since amplitude of the response is very high (often 1000 μV or more) in comparison to most other sensory evoked responses. Analysis also, on the surface, is rather simple, as it is based on response symmetry (i.e., comparison of response amplitude for the involved versus uninvolved side of the face). While ENoG is characterized by each of these features, reliability and validity of recordings depend to a large extent on the experience and technique of the tester, more so perhaps than for any other type of evoked response. The timing of the test after the onset of facial nerve dysfunction is an important factor in the outcome, as is the method of stimulation and certain subject characteristics, such as amount of body fat. Finally, the consequences of misinterpretation of findings may be very serious. At the extreme, a patient might undergo unnecessary potentially life-threatening surgery or, conversely, might mistakenly not be considered a candidate for surgery that would have restored facial nerve function.

The studies listed above have confirmed the value of ENoG in evaluation of facial nerve status in varied types of patients at risk for dysfunction, including those with congenital abnormalities, traumatic injury (temporal bone fracture), tumors in the area of the nerve and Bell's palsy. Ongoing assessment of facial nerve status intraoperatively is also now a common clinical practice (Delgado, Buchnett, Rosenholtz, & Chrissian, 1979; Gantz, 1985; Gantz, Gmur, & Fisch, 1982; Kileny & Niparko, 1988; Møller & Jannetta, 1984; Niparko et al., 1989), and there are devices specifically designed for this purpose. Applications of ENoG in the clinic are reviewed below later in this chapter.

Alternative Tests of Facial Nerve Function

Many other tests of facial nerve function have been or, for some procedures, continue to be applied in the assessment of facial nerve function. These include the Hilger test, electromyography, acoustic reflex testing, evoked accelerometry, antidromic nerve potentials, MRI and CT radiologic evaluations, maximal nerve stimulation tests, minimal nerve stimulation tests, transcranial magnetic stimulation, blink reflex tests, and others. The most commonly used facial nerve grading scale is the House-Brackmann (HB) scale. (see Table 15.10) The HB scale is used to approximate the quantity of volitional motion the patient has based on their clinical presentation. Although the HB scale is based on clinical observation, and variation among observers exists,

TABLE 15.10. House-Brackmann Clinical Grading System for Facial Nerve Function

ENoG is typically indicated for patients with grade VI paralysis.

GRADE	DESCRIPTION	FEATURES
I	Normal	Normal function of entire face
II	Mild dysfunction	Slight weakness Normal tone and symmetry at rest Eye closure Slight mouth asymmetry
III	Moderate dysfunction	Obvious difference between sides Normal symmetry at rest Eye closure with effort Weak mouth with maximum effort
IV	Moderately severe dysfunction	Obvious weakness and disfiguring asymmetry Normal symmetry and tone at rest Incomplete eye closure
V	Severe dysfunction	Barely perceptible motion Asymmetry at rest Incomplete eye closure
VI	Total paralysis	No movement

Adapted from House, J. W., & Brackmann, D. E. (1985). Facial nerve grading system. *Otolaryngology—Head and Neck Surgery 93,* 146–147.

the HB scale allows the clinician to grossly describe the characteristics and degree of facial nerve motion. In general, patients present with grade I through grade V. The HB scale has six grades. Each grade is reported as a fraction (i.e., 1/6 = grade I). A grade I presentation is perfectly normal. Grade II is a slight or mild weakness. Grade III is a moderate weakness with good (or normal) eye closure. Grade IV is a moderate weakness with no volitional eye closure. Grade V is a severe weakness. Grade VI is a total facial paralysis.

Facial Nerve Anatomy and Physiology

There are twelve pairs of cranial nerves. ENoG measurement pertains only to the seventh (VII) or facial cranial nerve. Each facial nerve has some 10,000 fibers. About two-thirds of the fibers are motor fibers, and the remaining one-third are sensory. The sensory portion of the facial nerve is referred to as the nervous intermedius. Only about half of the nerve fibers need be intact and functioning for essentially normal facial nerve function. As the facial nerve exits the brainstem, it traverses the cerebellopontine angle (CPA) to the medial end of the internal auditory canal (i.e., the porus acousticus). Progressing distally to the stylomastoid foramen, the facial nerve includes the labyrinthine segment, the tympanic segment, the pyramidal bend, the mastoid portion, and finally the stylomastoid foramen. The facial nerve exits the skull at the stylomastoid foramen. The vast majority of traumatic injuries (greater than 90 percent) are reported to be within the labyrinthine segment of the facial nerve.

COURSE OF THE FACIAL NERVE. | Selected schematic views of facial nerve anatomy are shown in Figure 15.10. The reader is urged to consult a basic otology, otolaryngology, or neuroanatomy text or recent review papers for a more detailed review of this complex topic. The sensory portion of the facial nerve is known as the nervous intermedius. Facial nerve anatomy can be divided into four general regions: the central pathways, an intracranial portion, a temporal bone portion, and branching of the nerve to parts of the face. Each of these major regions of facial nerve anatomy in turn has numerous components.

The first region is the central nervous system pathway. The most rostral portion of facial nerve anatomy is in the inferior portion of the pre-central gyrus of the motor strip, in the cortex of the frontal lobe of the brain. Fibers travel, initially via the internal capsule and then the pyramidal tracts, down to pons in the brainstem. Most, but not all, fibers cross from one side to the other (decussate) in the pons. The practical implication of this observation is that lesions

above the level of decussation will produce facial muscle dysfunction on the opposite side of the face. The brainstem center is the facial motor nucleus, a highly complex structure located in tegmentum (roof or dorsal portion) of the caudal (lower) pons and consisting of four major neuron groups. The facial nerve has different parts or roots and sensory as well as motor components. The facial nerve is therefore a mixed nerve. Some of the roots provide sensory innervation of regions of the body other than the face (e.g., skin, tongue, lacrimal glands, mucosa of nose and palate, external auditory canal). Efferent (motor) fibers of the facial nerve do not take a direct route when they leave the nucleus. Instead, fibers pass through the brainstem and course around the nucleus of the abducens (sixth) cranial nerve (the internal genu or knee of the facial nerve) before exiting the ventral and lateral portion of the pons.

The intracranial portion of the facial nerve, after it exits the brainstem, is within the cerebellopontine angle. Here the facial and auditory (eighth cranial) nerves come near each other. The anterior inferior cerebellar artery (AICA) is also nearby and may loop around either of the nerves. Both facial and auditory nerves travel together laterally and enter the internal auditory canal (IAC) within the temporal bone. In the IAC, the facial nerve takes a position anterior and superior to the auditory nerve. A branch of the AICA, the labyrinthine artery that supplies blood to the cochlea, wraps around and between the nerves within the IAC. Since the facial nerve is within the IAC meatus, this portion of its course is sometimes referred to the meatal segment. At the lateral (distal) end of the IAC the eighth and facial nerves part ways, with the former going on to the cochlear and vestibular labyrinth and the latter entering the fallopian canal still within the temporal bone.

The facial nerve route through the temporal bone is within the facial canal and has three main segments: the labyrinthine segment, the tympanic (or horizontal) segment, and the mastoid segment (see Figure 15.10). There are several notable features of this pathway. The canal is smallest in diameter at the meatus, where the nerve first enters. The labyrinthine portion is in the direction of the length (axis) of the temporal bone. Then, there is a genu (sharp, knee-shaped turn) just above the lowest part of the cochlea. This may be referred to as the external genu, in distinction to the internal (brainstem) genu mentioned above. The geniculate ganglion, a collection of facial neurons (cell bodies), is found at the external genu. At the genu, the facial nerve turns in a more lateral and posterior direction. In the next, tympanic or horizontal, segment, the nerve passes near the middle ear space. The facial nerve canal is found slightly above the oval window (the stapes footplate) and below the semicircular canal. At this point, the canal actually forms a bulge (prominence) in the medial middle ear wall, and it may be very thin or little more than mucosa.

The facial nerve travels from front to back through the middle ear space and then turns downward on its way to the

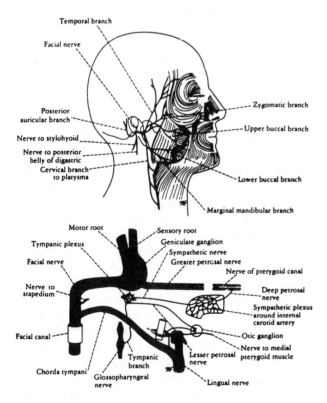

FIGURE 15.10. Simple diagram of different aspects of facial nerve anatomy.

mastoid. It is at the turn that the nerve gives off the stapedius branch, which innervates the stapedius muscle. The facial canal continues on vertically (the pyramidal segment) before ending at the stylomastoid foramen in the mastoid bone. Along the vertical route, the chorda tympani, another major branch of the facial nerve, arises and passes forward to the tongue and salivary glands. The facial nerve leaves the skull at the stylomastoid foramen (foramen means hole). This structure is located just behind the lower part of the external ear, and medial to the mastoid tip, which serves as protection. From the stylomastoid foramen, the nerve then goes forward and medial, passing under the lower part of external ear, across the ramus (upper portion) of the mandible, often through the parotid gland and then on to innervate the face. Along this route, numerous small branches leave for the ear, neck muscles, and other nearby structures. There are many normal variations in the relationship of the facial nerve to the parotid gland and in the exact patterns of branching of the nerve to the face. Five major branches are often identified that innervate the extent of the face. There is a temporal frontal portion going to the temple and forehead above the eyes, a zygomatic branch serving a region extending to below the eyes, a buchal branch above the mouth, and, finally, several lower branches traveling downward along the mandible. The region around the mouth (the orbicularis oris muscle) is richly innervated by the facial nerve. Three of these branches connect distally via anastomoses. The mandibular and frontal branches are anatomical exceptions. Facial paralysis is, therefore, unlikely when one of these three branches is injured.

TYPES OF FACIAL NERVE INJURY. | Dr. Ugo Fisch used three terms to describe the three primary types of facial nerve injury: neuropraxia, neurotmesis, and axonotmesis. It's not possible with ENoG recordings to differentiate between neurotmesis and axonotmesis. Neuropraxia is the most common finding associated with BP. In this situation, the patient experiences paralysis without peripheral nerve degeneration. The ENoG demonstrates a normal or reduced response. The nerve fibers and the sheath are anatomically intact, but the patient cannot move his or her facial muscles voluntarily (e.g., upon command to smile, close the eyes, etc). Facial nerve dysfunction associated with neuropraxia will usually reverse spontaneously over time. Axonotmesis is disruption of inner nerve fibers despite an intact outer casing (epineurium). ENoG measurement will yield no detectable response (i.e., a flat line). Neurotmesis is the most serious facial nerve outcome representing a total anatomic separation of the nerve. The ENoG waveform is essentially a flat line, and prognosis for return of function is very poor.

WALLERIAN DEGENERATION. | When BP and other facial nerve injuries occur, it takes some 72 hours or so for Wallerian degeneration (WD) to occur. WD is the process of denervation of the neural fibers, and it is a relatively slow process. WD occurs from proximal to distal anatomy. If a patient with an HB grade VI facial presentation is assessed one hour after the onset of BP, a normal ENoG is likely. That is, facial nerve fibers are physiologically intact, although nonfunctional volitionally. The resultant ENoG would be a false negative if the test was performed prior to complete WD. Therefore, it is important to wait approximately 72 hours before performing the first ENoG to allow the nerve to undergo complete WD. Results obtained prior to that time do not contribute to diagnosis as they may measure the status of the nerve before the damage is maximal.

ENoG Test Protocol

To be used in recording ENoG, an evoked response system must include capacity for generation of an electrical stimulus. The somatosensory evoked response (SSER) package or option for most instruments provides the necessary stimulus components and software for recording ENoG. In fact, many of the technical concerns in recording ENoG apply as well for SSERs. Measurement parameters for ENoG are summarized in Table 15.11, and the general stimulating and recording electrode sites are illustrated in Figure 15.11. Although most patients willingly undergo an ENoG procedure, anticipating that the findings will contribute to a resolution of their facial nerve dysfunction, simple instructions are important to enhance relaxation. Before the procedure begins, the patient should be informed that some wires will be taped to his or her face near the nose and mouth. Then, stimulation will be applied just behind the ear in order to test the facial nerve. The patient will feel a quick tapping sensation, but after a few minutes, the tapping feeling will decrease. The patient should sit comfortably, and tell the tester if he or she experiences excessive discomfort at any time during the procedure.

STIMULUS. | The stimulus is an electrical pulse, actually a small shock. Naturally, this description of the stimulus is not used with patients. Clinicians are advised to either perform the ENoG procedure on themselves or have a colleague record an ENoG to better appreciate patient's sensation of this stimulation and to develop the stimulus presentation technique. The electrical stimulation (again, the term "shock" is best avoided in the presence of patients) feels somewhat like a tapping sensation. Over most of the typical intensity range used clinically, this stimulus varies from just noticeable to moderately uncomfortable. Stimulus duration is usually 0.1 or 0.2 ms (100 or 200 μsec). The rate for continuous stimulation is slow (1 or 2/sec), and manual presentation of a single stimulus is optional for most evoked response systems. The slow stimulus rate increases the likelihood of a maximum response and, because few stimuli are required to observe a response, does not extend test time. In fact, most clinical evoked response systems do not permit rapid (greater than even 7 or 8/sec) electrical stimulus presentation. This is a

TABLE 15.11. Measurement parameters for recording ENoG in the clinic versus recording facial nerve integrity in the operating room.

PARAMETER	CLINICAL ENOG	INTRAOPERATIVE MONITORING
Stimulus		
Transducer	Pair of disc type electrode or prong	Subdermal needles
Type of stimulation	Electrical	Facial muscle activity monitored continuously to detect unintentional activation of nerve intraoperatively by surgical manipulations
Stimulus site	Stylomastoid foramen	Direct stimulation of facial nerve in internal auditory canal or posterior fossa
Orientation	Horizontal with cathode (negative) posterior	Monopolar cathode electrode on presumed nerve with anode located at remote location (e.g., shoulder)
Mode	Continuous	Gated (only during averaging)
Duration	0.2 ms (200 μs)	0.2 ms (200 μs)
Rate	1 stimulus/sec	1 stimulus/sec
Laterality	Unilateral; involved side first	Only on side of surgery
Stimulus intensity	15 to 40 mA	0.05 to 1 Ma (stimulation directly on facial nerve)
Acquisition		
Electrodes sites	Nasolabial fold	Corner of mouth and corner of eyes
Positive (noninverting)	Mouth	Corner of mouth and corner of eyes
Negative (inverting)	Alar region of nose	Corner of mouth and corner of eyes
Amplification	$\times$ 5000 or less	$< \times$ 5000
Filter settings	3 to 5000 Hz	3 to 5000 Hz
Analysis time	20 ms	20 ms
Prestimulus baseline	1 ms	1 ms
Number of sweeps	<20	<5
Response analysis	Side-to-side amplitude comparison	Acoustic events related to facial nerve activation; amplitude of response
Anesthesia	Not relevant	No neuromuscular blocker (no muscle paralyzing agent)

safety feature to prevent excessive stimulation (continuous high stimulus intensity at a fast rate). Electrical stimulus intensity for ENoG (also SSERs and electrically elicited AERs) is usually defined in milliamperes (mA), although some electrical pulse generators quantify stimulus–intensity in volts. The mA is a unit of current. Unlike AER measurement, a fixed stimulus intensity level is not employed with ENoG but, rather, stimulus intensity is gradually increased, typically in the range of 0 to 20 mA. Most commercially available systems require the clinician to set an upper limit for stimulus intensity (in mA) before testing begins. In any event, such a stimulus intensity limit is recommended for clinical facial nerve evaluations. Electrical stimulus intensity is increased (over the acceptable range) until a supra-maximal level is obtained. A supra-maximal stimulus intensity produces the largest possible facial muscle response on

the side of the face stimulated for the patient. That is, the stimulus intensity exceeds the level producing maximum response, and there is no further increase in response amplitude at greater stimulus intensity levels. Theoretically, at the supra-maximal stimulus intensity level the nerve is fully activated.

For routine clinical applications, the electrical pulse stimulus is delivered to the stylomastoid area. This location was defined above in the review of facial nerve anatomy. Bipolar stimulation is typically used. The two stimulating electrodes are placed so they straddle the earlobe, and then repeatedly relocated until the maximum response is obtained (refer to Figure 15.11). The positive electrode (anode) is positioned anteriorly, whereas the negative electrode (cathode) is positioned posteriorly. A mnemonic for recalling that the anode is positive is "A plus." Remember also that "black is

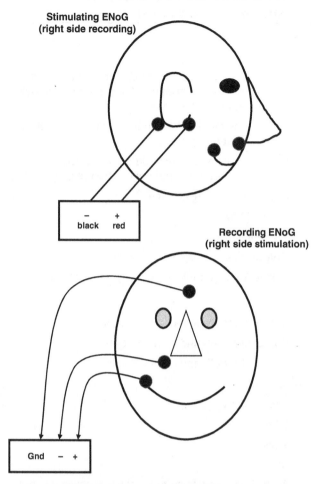

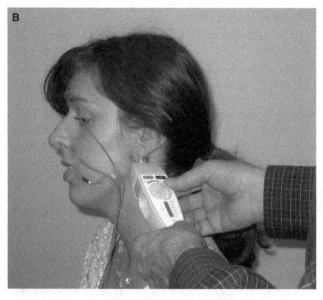

FIGURE 15.11. Stimulating and recording electrodes typically employed in electroneuronography (ENoG) measurement shown schematically (A) and in a photograph of a subject (B).

back." Vertical movement of the stimulus electrodes is useful in determining the optimal site, but movement of the electrodes anteriorly (forward toward the face) is poor technique. Placement of stimulating electrodes on the face in front of the ear may appear to produce a more distinct response. The nerve is more superficial in this location, which is near the stylomastoid foramen. The anterior electrode site, however, is more likely to stimulate one of the branches of the facial nerve, rather than the main trunk and, in addition, may be more likely to elicit masseter muscle activity. Continuous stimulation during testing is preferable to intermittent stimulation (only during averaging), both for patient comfort and for technical reasons (overcoming skin capacitance, as explained below).

Different stimulating electrode configurations are used in ENoG. Most evoked response systems with the option for electrical stimulation include an assembly that consists of a device for varying the percentage of maximum stimulus presented and along with two metal prongs (one anode and one cathode) and two corresponding jacks for plugging in electrode leads. A hand-held prong or electrode bar is preferable to the usual fixed electrode placement because it is easily relocated in attempts to find the optimum stimulus site. The skin surface in the area of stimulus electrode placement should be prepared by scrubbing vigorously with alcohol or an abrasive solution. Surface electrodes are almost always employed for clinical ENoG stimulation. Intraoperatively, facial muscle activity is often evoked with direct stimulation of the surgically exposed facial nerve.

ACQUISITION. | Acquisition parameters are displayed in Table 15.11. ENoG can be recorded with a single channel. Noninverting and inverting electrodes are typically located at the base of the nose and the corner of the mouth (nasolabial fold) on the stimulated side, as shown in Figure 15.11. [General electrode terminology and concepts are explained in Chapter 2.] In the interest of consistency in recording protocol, always place the noninverting (active) electrode of the pair at the corner of the mouth. The mnemonic "active mouth" helps to recall this protocol. Other recording electrode sites on the face are also acceptable. For example, some clinicians place an electrode at the base of the nose on each side. One of these electrodes is noninverting and the other is inverting. A ground (common) electrode can be located anywhere. A forehead site (Fpz) for the ground electrode is convenient and has the added advantage of being appropriate as a ground for AER measurement.

ENoG recording electrodes can either be affixed to the skin or movable. Fixed recording electrodes are applied in the same manner as other surface evoked-response electrodes. The skin is prepared by scrubbing with an abrasive solution. Conducting gel or paste is dabbed on the electrode and then the electrode is secured to the face with short pieces of tape. There are two clinical advantages of the standard fixed-electrode technique. One is consistency in electrode placement from one side to the other for a single patient and from one patient to the next. Also, fixing electrodes frees up one of the tester's hands. Disadvantages are inflexibility in location and relatively little pressure exerted by the electrodes. This latter feature is not really a serious limitation if interelectrode impedance is adequate. Interelectrode impedance should be less than 5000 ohms whenever possible, even though more vigorous preparation of skin at the nasiolabial fold may be necessary to meet this impedance criterion.

Amplification of X5000 is generally adequate because the response is large. Restrictive filtering should be avoided in order to eliminate the possibility of filter-related artifacts in the ENoG waveform. A filter setting of 3 or 10 to 10,000 Hz is recommended, even though the response spectrum is much more limited. The response usually occurs within the first 5 ms after stimulation, but an extended analysis time of 15 to 20 ms permits definition of a stable post stimulus baseline. Since the emphasis in ENoG analysis is amplitude, not latency, poorer latency resolution associated with a longer time period is not a concern. A pre-stimulus baseline period permits a clear view of stimulus artifact characteristics. However, stimulus artifact may be excessive because the stimulus electrodes are relatively close to the recording electrodes. The artifact is especially troublesome with evoked response equipment that automatically adjusts gain. The portion of the ENoG waveform of interest (i.e., the actual response) may be sized down so as to be undetectable. There are several solutions to the artifact problem. One is to manually set the gain, if possible, to comfortably encompass a response of normal amplitude on the display screen. This is actually a good technique for all evoked response recording. It permits online estimations of relative response amplitude for different stimulus intensity levels and between sides (or ears). Another approach is to set a poststimulus delay so that the entire artifact has subsided before averaging begins.

There is no correct number of stimulus repetitions (sweeps) for ENoG. The response is normally large enough to be recorded clearly with a single stimulus presentation. However, averaging over a modest number of stimulus presentations (e.g., 5 to 20) often produces a more stable and well-formed waveform. To achieve the most accurate and representative response, it is preferable to first stimulate for approximately 30 seconds with a given stimulus–intensity level and stimulus electrode site. This serves to maintain constant electrical capacitance across the skin. Replicated responses (two runs) are then averaged for a series of 5 to 20 stimuli each. The data are stored, the stimulus electrodes are relocated, and the process is repeated.

PROCEDURE. | Patients undergoing ENoG may be anxious in general and, in particular, apprehensive about the test procedure. Some patients may have already experienced discomfort or pain because of the disease process or during prior assessment of facial nerve status with the Hilger procedure. Posttrauma patients are often in pain and may have lacerations or contusions where the stimulus or recording electrodes are to be placed. The first step in successful ENoG evaluation is good bedside manner. As noted already, for conscious patients it is important to take time to completely explain the procedure. Sometimes briefly demonstrating the procedure on yourself or a colleague will effectively reduce the patient's concerns. Make it clear to the patient that he or she can stop the test if it becomes too uncomfortable, although this is not anticipated. With proper patient preparation, ENoG can be carried out with children as well as adults.

Following placement of recording electrodes bilaterally, as described above, and similar preparation of the skin at stimulus sites (scrubbing with an abrasive substance), the pair of stimulus electrodes is pressed gently but firmly against the skin in the region of the stylomastoid foramen (see Figure 15.11) on the presumably uninvolved (normal) side. Conducting gel or paste can be applied to each stimulus electrode, but this is not necessary. If used, the conducting material should never form a bridge connecting the two electrodes. Documentation of which side is normal versus abnormal is very important with ENoG because response analysis depends on asymmetry in amplitude. In many cases, differentiation of uninvolved versus involved sides is a matter of simply reviewing the patient's medical record, particularly the report of physical examination (PE) or neuroradiology, in search of a reference to a unilateral lesion. Another practical approach to the question is to ask the patient to smile in order to identify the stronger versus weaker side of the face. The referring physician can also indicate which side is considered at risk. Problems associated with differentiation of normal versus abnormal facial nerve function are discussed further below.

Once the stimulating electrodes are placed over the stylomastoid foramen region, stimulus intensity is gradually increased, typically by turning a knob on the stimulus assembly device. Intensity is slowly increased up to about 10 mA. In addition to reading stimulus intensity on the display screen of the evoked response equipment, the patient's face is monitored for signs of facial muscle activity, such as twitching movements around the mouth. Evidence of muscle twitching assures effective stimulation and provides a rough estimate of stimulus intensity. It is also a good practice to query the patient on the sensation. At at moderate intensity level, e.g., 10 mA, at least two replicated waveforms are recorded and stored and the intensity is increased in search of the supramaximal level. The maximum stimulus intensity necessary for a given patient depends on various factors, ranging from integrity of the nerve to the amount of adipose tissue (fat) between the nerve and stimulating electrode, as noted below. Often, replicated runs at several electrode sites for moderate (10 mA) and then at higher stimulus intensity levels, such as 15 mA or greater, are adequate in defining supra-maximal stimulation. This process is then repeated with stimulation of the involved (pathologic) side. Care is taken to achieve supra-maximal stimulation and, whenever possible, to duplicate the recording conditions on the "bad" versus "good" sides. If a normal response is not clearly observed on the involved side, the clinician is obligated to manipulate stimulus and recording parameters in search of a better response. Waveform analysis will now be described.

Waveform Analysis

NORMAL WAVEFORM PATTERNS. | As shown in Figure 15.12, normal ENoG waveform morphology may vary. The characteristic response is a biphasic waveform occurring within the first 5 to 7 ms after the electrical stimulus. There is, in sequence, a relatively small downward deflection, a prominent upward wave and then another downward component. The postresponse baseline may not be stable until 7 to 10 ms after stimulation. The prominent positive peak should be at least approximately 4 ms after the stimulus, even at high intensity levels. Normal variants are clear upward-going waves, which may be preceded but not followed by a negative wave, or vice versa (Figure 15.12). In ENoG, unlike AERs such as the ABR, there are no widely accepted conventions for waveform analysis.

While there is general agreement that response amplitude should be compared for the involved versus uninvolved side, specific guidelines for calculation of amplitude are lacking. The main issue is how to define the baseline for calculation of amplitude for the prominent upward-going peak.

Four choices are voltage difference from the positive peak to (1) preceding trough, (2) following trough, (3) a measure of prestimulus baseline, and (4) a measure of post response baseline. These different methods can yield highly divergent ENoG amplitude calculations. Clearly, a single method should be consistently used in a laboratory. However, waveform analysis becomes rather complicated when morphology differs from one patient to the next, from one test to the next for a given patient, from one side to the other within a patient, or even from one run to another on the same side of a patient in a single test session. Variability in findings due to waveform morphology and the method of analysis highlights the importance of recording a series of ENoG responses prior to test interpretation.

The most accepted abnormal ENoG criterion is documentation of amplitude for a response on the involved side that is less than 10 percent of the amplitude for the response on the uninvolved side. That is, ENoG analysis is typically based on a comparison of the amplitude of the facial nerve

Electroneuronography (ENoG) Analysis (At supra-maximal stimulation in mA)

$$\% \text{ Degeneration} = 100 - \frac{200\ \mu V}{1800\ \mu V} \times 100 = 92\%$$

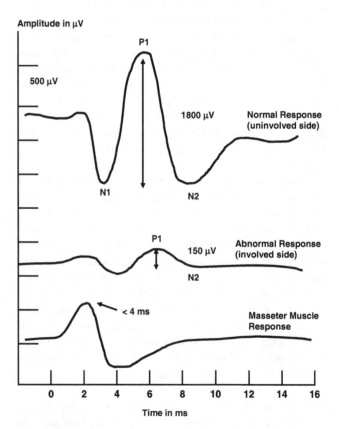

Electroneuronography (ENoG)

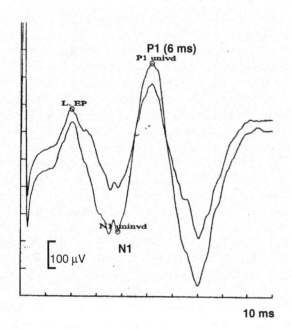

FIGURE 15.12. Example of normal and abnormal ENoG waveforms.

FIGURE 15.13. Strategies for analysis of the ENoG waveform.

response for the uninvolved ("good") side of the face versus the involved (paralyzed) side of the face. This analysis strategy is inappropriate, however, in patients with, or at at risk for, bilateral facial palsy, including those with Guillain-Barre syndrome, herpes zoster oticus, Stevens-Johns syndrome, polyneuritis, neurofibromatosis II, and bilateral temporal bone fractures. Supra-maximal stimulation of both sides is assumed. That is, stimulus intensity (in mA) is increased on each side (with corresponding calculation of response amplitude) until a further increase in stimulus intensity fails to produce greater amplitude. To be classified as significantly degenerated by these criteria, a facial nerve response must show greater than 90 percent degeneration in comparison to the presumably normal contralateral side (illustrated in Figure 15.13). Amplitude for the involved side is divided by amplitude for the uninvolved side, and then multiplied by 100 to yield a percentage value, as follows:

$$\text{Percent degeneration} = $$
$$100 - \frac{\text{amplitude } (\mu V) \text{ on involved side}}{\text{amplitude } (\mu V) \text{ on uninvolved side}} \times 100$$

In addition to being made with supra-maximal stimulus intensity levels, these calculations are consistently made with a single amplitude estimation method (see Figure 15.13). Other criteria for a significant interside difference in ENoG amplitude have been reported. For example, Kartush and colleagues (Kartush, Graham, & Kemink, 1986) describe as significant an amplitude decrease of 20 percent. With the 20 percent criterion, they report ENoG abnormalities (reduced response amplitude) for over a third of patients with acoustic tumors, even though facial function appeared normal as assessed clinically. These authors interpret this finding as consistent with subclinical degeneration or demyelination (Kartush, Graham, & Kemink, 1986).

The importance of applying supra-maximal stimulation, rather than a fixed intensity level for each side (e.g. 10 or 15 mA), cannot be overstated. For example, just increasing stimulus intensity from 15 to 20 mA may markedly increase response amplitude on the uninvolved or involved side and profoundly influence test interpretation.

ABNORMAL WAVEFORM PATTERNS. | Distance between stimulus and recording electrodes affects the latency of the response, but is not an important factor in ENoG amplitude. In fact, latency is frequently within normal expectations even though amplitude is abnormally reduced. This pattern implies that most of the nerve fibers are not functioning properly, but a small number of fibers, perhaps selected myelinated fibers, remain intact and are conducting a neural impulse without delay. The converse pattern, prolonged latency yet normal amplitude, is observed less often. There are several likely explanations for this ENoG finding. One is that most nerve fibers are functional, but they are not firing with the normal degree of synchrony. Desynchrony would also affect ampli-

tude to some extent. Demyelination of the distal portion of the facial nerve is probably the major factor in the finding of increased latency yet intact amplitude. While this is clearly not a normal pattern, its clinical significance is questionable. Marked reduction in amplitude, with or without concomitant latency prolongation, is invariably the ENoG finding that is relied on clinically. Again, an involved/uninvolved amplitude ratio of less than 10 percent is considered significantly abnormal.

Several important questions remain unanswered at this point. For example, what pathophysiologic processes underlie ENoG findings? At what point during the course of the facial nerve disease should ENoG be done? Finally, what are the clinical implications of a normal versus abnormal ENoG pattern? ENoG reflects distal facial nerve function. From the review of anatomy above, it was clear that there are extensive facial nerve pathways within the central nervous system and a complicated peripheral course through the cerebellopontine angle and temporal bone. In routine clinical ENoG, stimulation is presented to distal portion of the facial nerve only after it has exited the temporal bone, and the response is detected even more distal to the site of stimulation. This is referred to as *orthodromic* (*ortho* means "straight" and *dromo* means "running") nerve conduction. Another technique is based on *antidromic* conduction. Antidromic responses are produced by stimulation of distal portions of the facial nerve, e.g., on the face anterior to the ear, and recorded with electrodes placed more proximally (on the tympanic membrane, within the middle ear or intracranially). In the case of most facial nerve disorders, then, conduction is toward the site of lesion. Antidromic facial nerve responses also may offer additional and site specific information on nerve dysfunction (Kartush, Garcia, & Telian, 1987; Zealear, Hergon, & Korff, 1988; Zealear & Kurago, 1985). At this time, however, antidromic facial nerve conduction is not applied with regularity. One other type of nerve activity is ephaptic transmission. There may be abnormal connections between nerves, actually synapses where they do not normally occur. By means of these synapses, or ephapses, stimulation of and conduction along one division of the nerve leads to conduction along another division of the nerve.

The objective in routine clinical ENoG testing, therefore, is to evaluate the extent of neural degeneration in the distal portion of the nerve. Damage to one of the temporal bone segments of the facial nerve for example may, over two or three days or more, lead to degeneration of more distal portions of the nerve. The degeneration, known as Wallerian degeneration, proceeds outward (or downward) along the axon of the nerve, ultimately involving the axon of the nerve leading from the stylomastoid foramen to the face. The lesion may cause a total disruption in conduction through the nerve, as when the nerve is transected (severed) traumatically in a temporal bone fracture. More often, however, the disease process (e.g., edema, vascular, head trauma, surgical trauma, tumor) initially compromises but does not eliminate nerve function. There are then at least two possible courses for the disease. An almost immediate degeneration may progress from this site of lesion in a peripheral (distalward) direction, eventually reaching the face. The patient's facial movements, as in smiling or closing the eyes, may be impaired from the start because of damage somewhere between central pathways and the face, but early on the distal nerve has not degenerated and therefore ENoG confirms integrity. Another possibility is that the nerve is initially completely intact, both clinically and by ENoG. Dysfunction is delayed in onset, occurring presumably due to subsequent development of edema or constriction of the nerve.

In any event, ENoG measures the extent of facial nerve degeneration, not the extent of injury at the site of lesion. Overall functional status of the nerve from central pathways to the face is reflected by the patient's clinical status, i.e., his or her ability to activate facial muscles. It is, therefore, not uncommon to record a normal appearing ENoG from patients with apparently total facial paralysis. Sometimes, however, these patients will show facial muscle twitching during ENoG stimulation. An ENoG finding within the normal range (less than 90 percent degeneration) can also be obtained from patients showing no apparent facial muscle activity during stimulation. Finally, there are accounts of an abnormal ENoG among patients with normal clinical function (symmetrical smile, eyelids closed). As noted above, this is thought to reflect distal nerve demyelination or a reduction in the synchrony of neural activity.

From the foregoing discussion, it is apparent that the timing of ENoG after onset of facial nerve disease is an important factor. In general, the initial ENoG should be carried out within the first week post-insult. The date of injury is unambiguous when the etiology is trauma, but can be difficult to precisely determine for gradual onset facial nerve dysfunction. The initial ENoG provides a baseline measure of facial nerve status. Although ENoG within the first 24 hours after insult is not contraindicated, it is not necessary and for comatose head-injured patients may be complicated by medical therapy (chemical paralysis of facial muscles with neuroblockers). Serial ENoG assessments over the first two weeks post-insult are valuable to document the development of nerve degeneration. Surgery for correction of facial nerve disorder is much more likely to be effective if intervention occurs within twenty-one days (three weeks) post-insult. Surgery may begin with exploration of the nerve, but the primary goal in most cases is to release the nerve from excessive compression (decompression) at the site of lesion. The compression may be due to external pressure exerted by a structure (e.g., a growing tumor or a fractured bone) on the nerve, or to swelling of the nerve and surrounding blood vessels somewhere within the facial nerve canal. With vascular insult (an infarction), surgery is also directed toward removing fibrous tissue that may constrict nerve fibers.

Timing the ENoG Test

As noted above, Wallerian degeneration impacts the earliest reasonable test time. Typically, testing is delayed until 72 hours post-onset of paralysis. However, at the other end of the timing window is the twenty-one-day maximum. Specifically, if ENoG and subsequent surgical intervention are delayed past a twenty-one-day post-onset window, the test and possible surgical intervention are of questionable value. In essence, the ENoG should be performed for the first time at about 72 hours post-onset and again at three- to five-day intervals until a trend and confirmation can be obtained. If the trend and confirmation are determined prior to twenty-one days post-onset, surgical intervention may be an option. If the ENoG is not obtained prior to twenty-one days post-onset, it too is of little clinical use. Specifically, an ENoG obtained eight weeks after onset of facial paralysis is difficult, if not impossible, to interpret.

Recording Problems and Solutions

Some recording problems encountered in clinical ENoG are summarized in Table 15.12, along with possible solutions. Most of these difficulties can be overcome with common sense. Among the list, perhaps the two most frustrating and unsolvable test problems are found in those patients who are obese or at risk for bilateral dysfunction. In the obese patient, excessive adipose tissue (fat) in the neck around the region of the stylomastoid foramen serves to insulate the facial nerve from the stimulus. The characteristic ENoG finding is a very small response amplitude even on the uninvolved side. Obviously, there is no short-term solution to this big problem. A more effective stimulus is sometimes delivered by pressing the stimulus electrode prongs very firmly at the usual site. Another alternative, best taken with medical supervision, is insertion of stainless steel subdermal needle electrodes (see Chapters 2 and 4) vertically into the tissue. The remote danger of this approach, of course, is trauma to the nerve. A related type of measurement problem is presented by the patient with trauma-related edema and/or tenderness around the ear and neck in the region of the stylomastoid foramen. The two possible solutions just suggested for obese patients are usually inappropriate because they introduce an unacceptable amount of discomfort or even pain. A pain reliever or sedative might be useful in some patients, but deferring the test is probably the best overall solution. With both types of problems, if testing is completed and there is concern about stimulus effectiveness, this concern should be clearly stated in any report of the testing, and the findings qualified.

The majority of patients undergoing ENoG are suspected of unilateral facial nerve dysfunction, regardless of the etiology. Guidelines for determining the side at risk were noted above (e.g., chart review, clinical inspection of facial function, asking the patient's physician). One must keep in mind that these sources of information are not infallible. For example, patients with unilateral evidence of temporal bone

TABLE 15.12. Common ENoG Recording Problems and Solutions

SYMPTOM	PROBLEM(S)	SOLUTION(S)
Poor response bilaterally	Ineffective stimulus	Use needle electrodes
	Obesity	
	Bilateral dysfunction	Compare results to normal findings
	Edema at stimulus site	Relieve pain
	Tenderness limits proper stimulus electrode pressure	Defer pain
No response bilaterally	Chemical paralysis (in ICU or OR)	Reverse neuromuscular blocking agent medically
	Improper electrode placement	Verify correct electrode placement and usage
Poor response bilaterally	Inappropriate electrode site	Relocate stimulating electrodes
		Increase stimulus intensity to supra-maximal level
Short latency response	Masseter muscle response	Move stimulating electrodes posteriorly
Excessive artifact rejection	Stimulus artifact	Increase distance between stimulus and recording electrodes
		Avoid crossing stimulus and electrode wires
		Use poststimulus time
Delay	Very large response	Decrease amplification (gain) and/or increase sensitivity limits

fracture by computerized tomography (CT) may have contralateral facial nerve abnormalties. Any patient with clinical or historical evidence of facial nerve dysfunction on one side may have related or unrelated dysfunction on the opposite side as well.

Clinical Populations

Facial nerve paralysis is a debilitating condition. Patients with facial nerve disorders are often devastated due to the emotional and psychological impact of facial disfiguration and the subsequent physical limitations and difficulties associated with speaking, drinking, eating, and facial expression secondary to facial nerve disorders. Socialization and community participation is extraordinarily limited and difficult for many of these patients. The evaluation of facial nerve viability is a critically important part of management of facial nerve disorders. Depending on the outcome of the ENoG evaluation, the physicians involved may choose to "watch and wait," or they may elect to recommend surgical intervention. Surgical intervention is by no means trivial, and its utility is directly determined based on the ENoG evaluation. As summarized in Table 15.13, patients with facial nerve disorders have a variety of etiologies including Bell's palsy (BP), iatrogenic (surgically induced) injury, trauma to the temporal bone secondary to motor vehicle accidents (MVA), otitis media, herpes zoster oticus, multiple sclerosis, Melkersson-Rosenthal syndrome, mastoiditis, mumps, chicken pox, Gilllain-Barre syndrome, central nervous system disor-

ders (i.e., stroke), glomus jugulare, meningioma, facial nerve neuroma, and others. As noted previously, the House-Brackmann scale, summarized in Table 15.10, is one of the most common clinical approaches for categorizing facial nerve dysfunction. ENoG, however, has the feature of objectivity and provides quantification of facial nerve function or dysfunction.

BELL'S PALSY. | Bell's palsy (BP) is probably the single most common etiology of facial nerve disorders. Features of BP are summarized in Table 15.14. The incidence of BP in the

TABLE 15.13. Pathologies in the Differential Diagnosis of Facial Nerve Paralysis

- Idiopathic Bell's palsy
- Head (temporal bone) injury
- Herpes zoster oticus (Ramsay-Hunt syndrome)
- Otitis media with or without cholesteatoma
- Acute and chronic tympanomastoiditis
- Neoplasia (tumor), such as schwannomas or metastatic neoplasms
- Congenital facial paralysis (e.g., Treacher-Collins syndrome)
- Central nervous system disorder (e.g., stroke)
- Guillain-Barre syndrome
- Melkersson-Rosenthal syndrome
- Multiple sclerosis

TABLE 15.14. Features of Bell's Palsy

- Incidence is 13 to 18 per 100,000 depending on geographic location.
- There is a familial tendency for onset of Bell's palsy.
- Site of lesion most often is at narrowest region of fallopian canal ("meatal foramen").
- Onset of unilateral paralysis develops within 24 to 48 hours.
- Wallerian degeneration occurs within the 48- to 72-hour period after onset.
- Recovery is complete for about 75 to 80 percent of patients, beginning within three weeks after onset of paralysis.
- Approximately 15 percent of patients have some residual weakness, and 5 percent have severe or total paralysis.
- Bell's palsy may recur in about 7 to 10 percent of patients.

general population is about fifteen cases per 100,000 persons in the general population (0.00015 percent). BP has a familial tendency, although it is certainly not predictable across families or generations. BP will recur in 5 to 10 percent of patients. The time from onset of BP to total, unilateral facial paralysis is usually about 24 to 48 hours. Spontaneous recovery is common and usually occurs for some 75 to 80 percent of all patients in about three to four weeks. Of all BP patients, some 15 to 20 percent maintain a lifelong residual weakness following resolution of the BP, and about 5 percent of all patients have permanent weakness worse than HB grade 4/6. The etiology of BP is unknown. Various treatment options are available for the BP patient including surgical intervention, wait-and-watch approaches, acyclovir treatment, and other medical treatments.

NEUROPHYSIOLOGICAL MONITORING OF FACIAL NERVE FUNCTION. | A review of the principles, protocols, and procedures for intraoperative monitoring of facial nerve function is far beyond the scope of the present discussion of clinical assessment of facial nerve function with ENoG. The concepts reviewed herein, however, are directly applicable to the ongoing assessment of facial nerve function during surgeries that put the nerve at risk, such as surgical removal of an acoustic tumor. A few major distinctions between clinical ENoG assessment and intraoperative facial nerve monitoring warrant mention. During surgical procedures that pose risk to the facial nerve, it's possible for the surgeon to stimulate the nerve directly as it exits the brainstem (usually proximal to the region of greatest concern, e.g., a tumor) or at some more distal point along the nerve (e.g., within the internal auditory canal). In contrast, with clinical ENoG measurement, the facial nerve trunk is stimulated rather remotely, after it has exited the skull. The intensity level of direct nerve stimulation is, of course, a fraction of the stimulus–intensity levels used in ENoG measurement. Recording electrodes are located in similar locations for both clinical ENoG measurement and intraoperative monitoring. In the operating room with the patient anesthetized, however, subdermal needle electrodes are usually the recording technique of choice. During intraoperative monitoring, surgery-induced changes in facial nerve activity are inferred from an acoustic representation of stimulation (see Table 15.15), either inadvertent (e.g., stretching the nerve during tumor removal) or purposeful (e.g., electrical stimulation with a monopolar probe to verify identification of the facial nerve).

TABLE 15.15. Intraoperative Facial Nerve EMG and Acoustic Representation of Surgical Signals

STIMULUS	EMG	ACOUSTIC REPRESENTATION
Electrical	Precisely timed responses	Machine gun sound
Mechanical	Single polyphasic response (burst)	Synchronous clicking sound
Traction	Multiple asynchronous responses (train)	Popping corn, possibly delayed
Thermal	Initially: widened baseline	Initially: silent
	Later: multiple asynchronous responses	Later: popping corn

APPENDIX

Normative Data

Selected normative data for auditory evoked responses are summarized within this appendix. Manufacturers of auditory evoked response devices often provide normative data for specific auditory evoked responses, e.g., ABR, in either hard copy format (e.g., in the manual) or stored in electronic format on the device.

Two features of current evoked response devices are the options for adjusting stimulus–intensity levels for a particular clinical setting and for compiling normative data collected in the user's clinic. Normative behavioral threshold data can be collected within a clinic for each of the major types of stimulus, e.g., air-conduction click, bone-conduction click, and air-conduction tone bursts. The behavioral thresholds should be measured from young adult subjects with documented normal-hearing sensitivity (pure-tone thresholds of ≤15 dB HL). Once the average behavioral threshold is calculated for a small group (e.g., N = 10) of subjects, then that value is referred to as 0 dB nHL. The "dial" or "screen" intensity levels for the device can then be adjusted to correspond to the new behavioral data. If, for example, the average behavioral threshold for a 1000 Hz tone is 20 dB on the dial or screen, then that number really should be 0 dB nHL. Within an earphone calibration screen on the evoked response system, the user adjusts the intensity level for the 1000 Hz tone burst to 0 dB nHL, that is, intensity for the 1000 Hz stimulus is referenced to 0 dB nHL. Details on the steps of the stimulus calibration process for specific auditory evoked response devices are provided in the user manual. Stimuli used to elicit any auditory evoked response can, and should, be periodically calibrated using a sound level meter with reference to dB SPL. Insert earphones are calibrated with a 2 cc coupler or cavity (e.g, HA-2 or 711), supra-aural TDH earphones with a 6 cc coupler (NBS 9A), and the bone oscillator with an artificial mastoid (B & K 4930).

For example, the Audera device (GSI) includes a *Reference Data* option for depositing auditory evoked response latency and amplitude data for normal subjects of various ages and collected with different clinical protocols. Test parameters that must be documented and taken into account in collecting normative data include those summarized in an ABR test protocol (see Table 6.3), plus demographic subject data. A typical listing of critical subject data and test factors include:

- Number of subjects
- Age and gender of normal subjects
- Physical position of subjects during AER assessment (e.g., sitting versus supine)
- Subject state of arousal (e.g., awake, asleep, sedated)
- Type of transducer (e.g., ER-3A insert earphones, supra-aural TDH-39 earphones, B-70A bone oscillator)
- Stimulus type (e.g., air-conduction click, bone-conduction click, air-conduction tone burst)
- Stimulus polarity
- Rate of stimulus presentation
- Type and intensity level of masking (if any)
- Electrode locations
- The frequency of high- and low-pass filter settings, the slope of rolloffs for filters, and the types of filters (e.g., Butterworth)
- Number of sweeps

Once the local normative data are entered, the latency for auditory evoked responses (e.g., the ABR) recorded from individual patients with equivalent test protocols can be compared to normative latency–intensity functions.

A word about normative data for frequency-specific ABR measurement (tone-burst ABRs) is appropriate here. There are no published normative data for the latencies of ABRs evoked with tone-burst stimuli. Fortunately, the precise latency values of specific waves (e.g., wave V) for ABRs elicited by tone burst stimuli are not critical for their clinical application. The main objective in recording tone-burst ABRs from infants and young children is estimation of auditory threshold, rather than neurodiagnosis. Analysis of the tone burst ABR is mostly based the detection of a reliable wave V as stimulus intensity is progressively decreased. The exact latency of the wave V is not important. General expectations for the appropriate region for wave V latency with different tone-burst stimuli can be gained by first analyzing latency values for the ABR elicited with click stimuli. The latency of ABR wave V for high-frequency tone-burst stimuli (e.g., 4000 Hz) will approximate the wave V latency for a click-evoked ABR. ABR wave V latency values gradually increase for lower frequency tone-burst stimuli, even at high intensity levels. Of course, for each type of stimulus (click or tone burst), latency increases also as stimulus intensity is decreased.

TABLE A.1. Normal Cutoff Values for the ECochG Summating Potential to Action Potential (SP/AP) Ratio

ELECTRODE LOCATION (TYPE)	NORMAL	ABNORMAL
Ear canal (TIPtrode™)	0 to 50%	>50%
Tympanic membrane	0 to 35%	>35%
Promontory (transtympanic needle)	0 to 30%	>30%

TABLE A.2. Normative Data (Mean Values and One Standard Deviation, SD) for Auditory Brainstem Response (ABR) in Infants at Different Estimated Gestational Age (EGA) Categories. ABR test parameters are cited below.

EGA (WEEKS)	WAVE I LATENCY (65 dB nHL)	WAVE V LATENCY (65 dB nHL)	I–V INTERVAL (65 dB nHL)	WAVE V LATENCY (25 dB nHL)
33–34				
mean	3.50 ms	8.90 ms	5.37 ms	10.65 ms
(SD)	(0.38)	(0.63)	(0.50)	(0.66)
35–37				
mean	3.05 ms	8.26 ms	5.08 ms	9.76 ms
(SD)	(0.34)	(0.33)	(0.40)	(0.48)
38–40				
mean	3.12 ms	8.16 ms	5.01 ms	9.66 ms
(SD)	(0.34)	(0.42)	(0.31)	(0.70)
41+				
mean	2.95 ms	7.90 ms	4.94 ms	9.55 ms
(SD)	(0.35)	(0.38)	(0.24)	(0.64)

Transducer = insert earphones; Stimuli = clicks; Duration = 0.1 ms; Polarity = alternating; Presentation rate = 31.1/sec; Electrodes: noninverting = midline high forehead; inverting = ipsilateral mastoid; common = contralateral mastoid; Filter settings: high-pass = 30 Hz; low-pass = 3000 Hz; Replications = 2; Number of sweeps = >1000 (usually 2000 to 3000)

Criterion for pass with ABR screening = Presence of wave V at 25 dB nHL

From Van Riper & Kileny, 2002.

TABLE A.3.   Auditory Brainstem Response (ABR) Normative Data for Infants Including Absolute and Interwave Latency Values

Data in table are age-dependent correction factors, in milliseconds, for absolute ABR waves and for interpeak latencies. *Correction factors are added to the base value for adult normative data (see lowest line of the table).* The click stimulus intensity level was 70 dB nHL. The test protocol is summarized below.

	I	III	V	I–III	III–V	I–V
Part 1 preterm						
Gestational age (weeks)						
32	0.86	1.63	2.52	0.83	1.10	1.64
33	0.77	1.54	2.35	0.81	0.88	1.57
34	0.69	1.45	2.19	0.78	0.73	1.50
35	0.62	1.37	2.05	0.76	0.63	1.44
36	0.56	1.30	1.92	0.74	0.56	1.38
37	0.51	1.24	1.81	0.72	0.51	1.32
38	0.46	1.17	1.71	0.70	0.48	1.27
39	0.42	1.12	1.61	0.68	0.45	1.22
40	0.39	1.07	1.53	0.66	0.43	1.18
41	0.36	1.02	1.45	0.64	0.42	1.13
42	0.34	0.98	1.38	0.62	0.41	1.09
SD	0.24	0.29	0.29	0.32	0.26	0.33
High limit	2.13	4.24	6.09	2.59	2.34	4.42
Part 2 young postterm						
Age (weeks)						
1	0.36	1.02	1.45	0.64	0.42	1.13
2	0.34	0.98	1.38	0.62	0.41	1.09
3	0.32	0.94	1.32	0.61	0.40	1.06
4	0.30	0.90	1.27	0.59	0.39	1.02
6	0.27	0.83	1.17	0.56	0.38	0.95
8	0.25	0.78	1.09	0.53	0.37	0.90
10	0.23	0.73	1.02	0.51	0.36	0.85
12	0.22	0.69	0.97	0.49	0.35	0.80
16	0.20	0.63	0.89	0.45	0.33	0.72
20	0.19	0.58	0.83	0.41	0.32	0.66
24	0.18	0.54	0.78	0.38	0.30	0.62
Age (months)						
6	0.18	0.51	0.75	0.36	0.29	0.58
7	0.17	0.49	0.72	0.34	0.27	0.55
8	0.17	0.47	0.70	0.32	0.26	0.52
10	0.16	0.45	0.66	0.29	0.23	0.48
12	0.15	0.43	0.64	0.27	0.21	0.45
16	0.14	0.40	0.58	0.24	0.17	0.41
20	0.13	0.37	0.53	0.22	0.14	0.38
24	0.12	0.35	0.49	0.21	0.11	0.36
28	0.11	0.32	0.45	0.20	0.09	0.34
32	0.10	0.30	0.41	0.19	0.07	0.32
36	0.09	0.28	0.38	0.18	0.06	0.30
48	0.07	0.23	0.29	0.16	0.03	0.25
60	0.05	0.19	0.23	0.14	0.02	0.21
72	0.04	0.16	0.17	0.12	0.01	0.17
SD	0.24	0.25	0.24	0.26	0.23	0.27
High limit	2.06	4.17	6.02	2.52	2.27	4.35

(continued)

TABLE A.3. (continued)

	I	III	V	I–III	III–V	I–V
Part 3 old postterm						
Age (years)						
7	0.03	0.15	0.16	0.12	0.01	0.17
8	0.03	0.12	0.13	0.10	0.00	0.14
9	0.02	0.10	0.10	0.09	0.00	0.12
10	0.01	0.08	0.08	0.08	0.00	0.10
SD	0.17	0.17	0.21	0.15	0.14	0.22
High limit	1.94	4.05	5.90	2.40	2.15	4.23
Base (adult norm)	1.65	3.76	5.61	2.11	1.86	3.94

N = ears

Transducer = TDH-39 supra-aural earphones; Stimuli = clicks; Intensity = 70 dB nHL; Duration = 0.1 ms; Polarity = alternating; Presentation rate = 20/sec; Electrodes: noninverting = vertex or forehead; inverting = ipsilateral mastoid; common = contralateral mastoid; Filter settings: high pass = 100 Hz; low pass = 3000 Hz; Analysis time = 20 ms; Replications = 2; Number of sweeps = 2048.

From Issa & Ross, 1995.

TABLE A.4. Normative Data for Auditory Brainstem Response (ABR) in 189 Adult Subjects with Mean Age of 48 Years

ABR PARAMETER	NORMAL RANGE OF LATENCY (MS)
Wave I–III interval	1.23 to 2.85
Wave I–V Interval	
Males	3.57 to 4.56
Females	3.42 to 4.56
Interaural latency difference for wave V	−0.59 to 0.42
Rate-latency shift for wave V (11/sec to 88/sec)	0.12 to 1.32

Adapted from Lightfoot, G. R. (1992). ABR screening for acoustic neuromata: the role of rate-induced latency shift measurements. *British Journal of Audiology, 26,* 217–227.

TABLE A.5. Nontumor (Normative) Statistics for Auditory Brainstem Response (ABR) Wave Component Latency Parameters Used in Differentiation of Cochlear versus Eighth-Nerve Pathology in Adults

ABR LATENCY MEASURE (MS)	GROUP					
	Normal hearing (N = 786)			**Cochlear impairment (N = 1944)**		
	Mean	*(SD)*	*99%ile*	*Mean*	*(SD)*	*99%ile*
Absolute						
I	1.65	(0.14)	1.97	1.80	(0.23)	2.34
III	3.80	(0.18)	4.22	3.98	(0.24)	4.54
V	5.64	(0.23)	6.18	5.82	(0.27)	6.44
Interwave						
I–III	2.15	(0.14)	2.49	2.17	(0.18)	2.59
III–V	1.84	(0.14)	2.16	1.84	(0.16)	2.21
I–V	3.99	(0.20)	4.45	4.02	(0.24)	4.58
Interaural wave						
I	−0.02	(0.08)	0.21	−0.01	(0.25)	0.65
III	−0.03	(0.10)	0.26	−0.03	(0.23)	0.59
V	0.00	(0.11)	0.29	−0.03	(0.20)	0.52
Interaural interwave						
I–III	−0.01	(0.10)	0.25	−0.02	(0.16)	0.41
III–V	0.00	(0.10)	0.25	0.01	(0.14)	0.37
I–V	0.00	(0.11)	0.28	−0.02	(0.18)	0.46

Adapted from Joseph, West, Thornton, & Hermann, 1987.

TABLE A.6. A Simple Guideline for Remembering Important Response Parameters in Clinical Analysis of the ABR

The number five (5) is a critical clue (see bold font).

At a high click stimulus intensity, such as 8**5** dB nHL . . .

- Wave **V** latency is normally about **5.5** ms
- Wave V amplitude is about 0.**5** μV (microvolts)
- Upper end of the adult normal region for the wave I–**V** latency interval is 4.**50** ms
- Upper end of the term neonate normal region for the wave I–**V** latency interval is **5.**00 ms

TABLE A.7. Normative Latency and Amplitude Values for Auditory Late Response Components in Infants (N = 10) and Adults (N = 10) Reported in a Paper Describing the Passive P300 Response

	INFANTS		ADULTS	
ALR COMPONENT	**Mean**	**(SD)**	**Mean**	**(SD)**
Latency (ms)				
N1	205	(32.5)	96.0	(3.2)
P2	322	(33.7)	190	(10.9)
N2	454	(31.1)	235	(15.2)
Amplitude (μV)**				
N1	−6.8	(2.2)	−12.7	(4.0)
P2	8.1	(2.2)	11.0	(3.4)
N2	−7.2	(1.7)	4.8	(2.8)

* Measurement Parameters:
Signals in tones (standard = 1000 Hz; target = 2000 Hz); ISI = 2 seconds; Transducer = speaker 1.5 meters in front of subject; Rise/fall time = 9.9 ms; Plateau = 50 ms; Signal intensity = not specified; Noninverting electrode = Cz; Band-pass filter settings = 0.01 to 30 Hz; Analysis time = 1100 ms (prestimulus time = 110 ms)

** Amplitude was calculated with reference to the prestimulus baseline.

Adapted from McIsaac & Polich, 1992.*

TABLE A.8. Normative Latency and Amplitude Values for the Auditory Late Response Components and the P300 Response in Children and Adolescents (N = 80; age 8 to 18 years)

	FEMALE		MALE		COMBINED	
P300 COMPONENT	**Mean**	**(SD)**	**Mean**	**(SD)**	**Mean**	**(SD)**
Latency (ms)						
N1	95.9	(13.2)	96.1	(14.6)	96.0	(13.9)
P2	164.6	(17.8)	163.4	(24.0)	164.0	(20.9)
N2	222.1	(17.7)	214.4	(18.4)	218.3	(18.1)
P3	310.5	(19.2)	312.9	(15.6)	311.7	(17.4)
Amplitude (μV)**						
N1-P2	10.6	(3.8)	10.5	(4.8)	10.6	(4.0)
P2-N2	8.2	(2.4)	6.1	(4.2)	7.2	(3.3)
P2-P3	13.5	(3.5)	12.8	(3.3)	13.2	(3.4)

* Measurement Parameters:
Signals in tones (standard = 1000 Hz; target = 2000 Hz; target probability = 20%); ISI = 2 seconds; Mode of presentation = binaural; Transducer = "headphones"; Rise/fall time = 10 ms; Plateau = 30 ms; Signal intensity = 50 dB SL; Noninverting electrode = Pz; Band-pass filter settings = 0.01 to 70 Hz; Analysis time = not specified (prestimulus time = not specified)

** Amplitude was calculated with from trough-to-peak

Adapted from Zgorzalewicz, Galas-Zgorzalewicz, & Nowak, 2001.*

TABLE A.9. Average Latency and Amplitude Values for the P300 Response in Young and Older Adults (N = 72)

AGE GROUP	LATENCY (MS)	AMPLITUDE (μV)**
20 to 34 years (N = 19)	323	14.6
35 to 49 years (N = 9)	333	8.1
50 to 64 years (N = 12)	360	10.8
65 to 79 years (N = 15)	373	7.8
80 to 95 years (N = 17)	386	5.8

* Measurement Parameters:

Signals in tones (standard = 750 Hz; target = 1200 Hz; target probability = 20%); ISI = 1.5 seconds; Mode of presentation = not specified whether right ear, left ear, or binaural; Transducer = insert earphones; Rise/fall time = 10 ms; Plateau = 60 ms; Signal intensity = 80 dB (reference not specified); Noninverting electrode = Cz (data in the study were collected from 14 scalp electrodes); Band-pass filter settings = 0.10 to 70 Hz; Analysis time = 800 ms (prestimulus time = 100 ms)

** Amplitude was calculated with from prestimulus baseline to the P300 peak.

Adapted from Fjell & Walhovd, 2001.*

TABLE A.10. Normative Latency Values for the Vestibular Evoked Myogenic Potential (VEMP) in Normal Young Adult Subjects

Parameters for VEMP measurements in each study are summarized below.

STUDY/STIMULUS	LATENCY OF VEMP COMPONENTS (MS)			
	P1 (13 ms)		N1 (23 ms)	
	Absolute Mean (SD)	Between Sides Mean (SD)	Absolute Mean (SD)	Between Sides Mean (SD)
Robertson & Ireland, 1995	14.6 (2.0)	21.3 (1.6)		
Brantberg & Fransson, 2001	11.4 (range 10.62 to 11.59)		18.18 (range 17.34 to 19.20)	
Young & Kuo, 2004	13.7 (0.96)	NS*	20.2 (1.58)	NS*
Zapala & Brey, 2004	16.9 (1.43)	0.09 (1.35)	25.24 (1.63)	0.16 (1.42)
Sakakura et al., 2005	13.14 (0.85)		21.49 (2.74)	

* NS = Latency difference between sides not statistically significant (p > 0.05)

Measurement Parameters: Robertson & Ireland, 1995
Subjects: N = 7 (29 to 53 years); Stimulus = clicks; Polarity = rarefaction; Duration = 0.1 ms; Rate = 3/sec; Intensity level = 100 dB SL; Noninverting electrode = upper half of the SCM muscle; Inverting (reference) electrode = central sternum; Ground (common) electrode = not specified; Method for SCM muscle activation = supine with head elevated during data collection; Constant tonic activation = not specified; Filter settings = 20 to 10000 Hz; Analysis time = 80 ms; Prestimulus time = 20 ms; Stimulus repetitions (sweeps) = 512

Measurement Parameters: Brantberg & Fransson, 2001
Subjects: N = 23 (22 to 42 years); Stimulus = clicks; Polarity = rarefaction; Duration = 0.1 ms; Rate = 4/sec; Intensity level = 100 dB nHL; Noninverting electrode = "prominent part" of the SCM muscle; Inverting (reference) electrode = mid-point of sternum; Ground (common) electrode = upper part of sternum; Method for SCM muscle activation = supine with head elevated during data collection; Constant tonic activation = not specified; Filter settings = 20 - 2000 Hz; Analysis time = 50 ms; Prestimulus time = none; Stimulus repetitions (sweeps) = 128 X 2 = 256

Measurement Parameters: Young & Kuo, 2004
Subjects: N = 14 (22 to 26 years); Stimulus = binaural 500 Hz tone bursts; Ramp = 1 ms; Plateau = 2 ms; Duration = 4 ms; Rate = 5/sec; Intensity level = 95 dB HL; Noninverting electrode = upper half of the SCM muscle; Inverting (reference) electrode = lateral end of sternum; Ground (common) electrode = not specified; Method for SCM muscle activation = supine with head elevated during data collection; Constant tonic activation = 50 to 200 μV); Filter settings = 30 3000 Hz; Analysis time = 60 ms; Stimulus repetitions (sweeps) = 200

Measurement Parameters: Zapala & Brey, 2004
See Table A.11 for measurement parameters for Zapala & Brey, 2004.

Measurement Parameters: Sakakura et al., 2005
Subjects: N = 31 (20 to 39 years); Stimulus = 500 Hz tone burst; Rise/fall = 1 ms; Plateau = 2 ms; Duration = 4 ms; Rate = 5/sec; Intensity level = 105 dB (unit not specified); Noninverting electrode = upper half of the SCM muscle; Inverting (reference) electrode = upper middle end of sternum; Ground (common) electrode = not specified; Method for SCM muscle activation = seated in chair during data collection; Constant tonic activation = not specified; Filter settings = 20 to 2000 Hz; Analysis time = not specified; Prestimulus time = not specified; Stimulus repetitions (sweeps) = 200

From Robertson & Ireland, 1995; Young & Kuo, 2004.

TABLE A.11. Normative Amplitude Values for the Vestibular Evoked Myogenic Potential (VEMP) in Normal Young Adult Subjects.

Parameters for VEMP measurements in each study are summarized below.

	AMPLITUDE OF VEMP COMPONENTS (μV)			
	P1 (13 ms)		N1 (23 ms)	
STUDY/STIMULUS	Absolute Mean (SD)	Between Sides Mean (SD)	Absolute Mean (SD)	Between Sides Mean (SD)
Robertson & Ireland, 1995		P1/N1 = 65.3 (range 44.3 to 98.5)		
Brantberg & Fransson, 2001		P1/N1 = 10.2 (5.5)		
Young & Kuo, 2004		P1/N1 side difference = 0.89 (range 0.66 – 1.70)		
Zapala & Brey, 2004	P1/N1 = 180.71 (120.42)		P1/N1 side difference = 0.02 (0.19)	
Sakakura et al, 2005	58.62 (28.51)		61.72 (49.00)	

Measurement Parameters: Robertson & Ireland, 1995
Subjects: N = 7 (29 to 53 years); Stimulus = clicks; Polarity = rarefaction; Duration = 0.1 ms; Rate = 3/sec; Intensity level = 100 dB SL; Noninverting electrode = upper half of the SCM muscle; Inverting (reference) electrode = central sternum; Ground (common) electrode = not specified; Method for SCM muscle activation = supine with head elevated during data collection; Constant tonic activation = not specified; Filter settings = 20 to 10000 Hz; Analysis time = 80 ms; Prestimulus time = 20 ms; Stimulus repetitions (sweeps) = 512

Measurement Parameters: Brantberg & Fransson, 2001
N = 23 (22 to 42 years); Stimulus = 0.1 rarefaction clicks; Intensity level = 100 dB nHL; Rate = 4/sec; Noninverting electrode = prominent part of the sternoceidomastoid muscle; Inverting electrode = mid-portion of clavicle; Ground electrode = uppermost part of sternum; Method for SCM muscle activation = supine position with subject's head raised; Filter settings = 0.02 to 2000 Hz; Stimulus repetitions = 128; Analysis time = 50 ms

Measurement Parameters: Young & Kuo, 2004
Subjects: N = 14 (22 to 26 years); Stimulus = binaural 500 Hz tone bursts; Ramp = 1 ms; Plateau = 2 ms; Duration = 4 ms; Rate = 5/sec; Intensity level = 95 dB HL; Non-inverting electrode = upper half of the SCM muscle; Inverting (reference) electrode = lateral end of sternum; Ground (common) electrode = not specified; Method for SCM muscle activation = supine with head elevated during data collection; Constant tonic activation = 50 to 200 μV); Filter settings = 30 3000 Hz; Analysis time = 60 ms; Stimulus repetitions (sweeps) = 200

Measurement Parameters: Zapala & Brey, 2004
Subjects: N = 21 *presumed normal patients* (30 to 83 years); Stimulus = 250 Hz tone bursts; Rise/fall = 4 ms; Plateau = 0 ms; Duration = 8 ms; Rate = 5.1/sec; Intensity level = 90 dB HL (123 dB SPL); Non-inverting electrode = back of right hand; Inverting (reference) electrode = belly of SCM muscle; Ground (common) electrode = wrist; Method for SCM muscle activation = supine with 30° elevation of table with head elevated and rotated with test ear up during data collection; Constant tonic activation = not specified; Amplification = X5000; Filter settings = 1 to 250 Hz; Analysis time = 80 ms; Prestimulus time = 80 ms; Stimulus repetitions (sweeps) = 40 to 130

Measurement Parameters: Sakakura et al., 2005
Subjects: N = 31 (20 to 39 years); Stimulus = 500 Hz tone burst; Rise/fall = 1 ms; Plateau = 2 ms; Duration = 4 ms; Rate = 5/sec; Intensity level = 105 dB (unit not specified); Noninverting electrode = upper half of the SCM muscle; Inverting (reference) electrode = upper middle end of sternum; Ground (common) electrode = not specified; Method for SCM muscle activation = seated in chair during data collection; Constant tonic activation = not specified; Filter settings = 20 to 2000 Hz; Analysis time = not specified; Prestimulus time = not specified; Stimulus repetitions (sweeps) = 200

Source: Robertson & Ireland, 1995; Brantberg & Fransson, 2001; Young & Kuo, 2004; Zapala & Brey, 2004; Sakakura et al., 2005.

AABR: Automated auditory brainstem response.

A1, A2: 10–20 International system EEG electrode sites on the left (A1) and right (A2) earlobe. "A" refers to aural (from the Latin word *auris*).

ABG: Arterial blood gases (e.g., oxygen, carbon dioxide) Also, air-bone gap, the difference between hearing threshold levels for air-conducted pure-tone signals (presented with earphones) and bone-conducted pure-tone signals (presented with a bone oscillator).

acoustic: Related to sound or hearing.

acoustic (auditory) nerve: The eighth cranial nerve serving the senses of hearing (audition) and balance (vestibular function); the afferent pathway transmitting auditory information from the cochlea (inner ear) to the cochlear nuclei in the lower brainstem (pons).

acoustic (stapedial) reflex: A brainstem-mediated reflex in which the stimulus is a high-intensity (about 85 dB or more) sound, the afferent portion of the reflex arc is the eighth cranial nerve, the CNS portion consists of brainstem auditory centers and the efferent portion is the seventh cranial (facial) nerve innervating the stapedial muscle in the middle ear.

acoustic tumor: A neoplasm arising from the eighth cranial nerve, usually one of the vestibular portions (inferior or superior). Often referred to as acoustic neuroma, the proper term is "vestibular schwannoma."

action potential (AP): An electrical potential occurring over time and arising from the depolarization and repolarization of a cell or group of cells, such as neurons within the eighth cranial nerve.

active electrode: Usually refers to the noninverting electrode in AER measurements, e.g., the vertex electrode for ABR recordings. The term is usually not accurate because other electrodes in the electrode array also are actively detecting electrophysiologic activity from the ear, cranial nerves, or brain.

ad: Right ear (from the Latin *auris dextra*).

adaptive filtering: Filter characteristics are automatically altered to optimally filter a designated incoming electrical signal with the overall objective of improving the electrical signal-to-noise ratio.

ADHD: Attention-deficit/hyperactivity disorder.

afferent: Pertaining to a neural pathway leading from a sense organ (e.g., the ear) to the brain.

AIDS: Acquired immune deficiency syndrome; resulting from HIV (human immunodeficiency virus).

air-bone gap: A difference in dB between hearing thresholds for air- versus bone-conduction stimulation. Usually air-conduction thresholds are poorer than bone-conduction thresholds. The air-bone gap is an audiologic sign of conductive hearing impairment due to middle ear pathology.

air conduction: A mode for presenting auditory stimuli (sounds) via earphones placed over the ear or within the ear canal.

aliasing: Distortion in recording auditory evoked responses caused by insufficient sampling rate (too few data points) during the averaging process. Aliasing affects the latency and morphology (shape) of an auditory evoked response.

alpha rhythm: Electroencephalogram (EEG) activity within the 8 to 12 Hz frequency region, normally of high amplitude (greater than 50 µV); this EEG rhythm is sometimes associated with relaxation; the dominant EEG frequency of patients in alpha coma.

alternating stimulus polarity: Alternating presentation of rarefaction and condensation polarity stimuli, rather than stimuli of all one polarity.

AM: *See* amplitude modulation

AM²: Exponential amplitude modulation; a type of stimulus for elicitation of the auditory steady-state evoked response (ASSR).

AM3MF2: The abbreviation used for stimuli used in eliciting the auditory steady-state evoked response (ASSR) with modified or multiple carrier frequencies (e.g., 500, 1000, 2000, and 4000 Hz) and/or multiple modulation frequencies. *See* IAFM.

American Academy of Audiology (AAA): The major professional organization for audiologists in the United States of America, although audiologists from many other countries also hold membership status. The AAA website is www.audiology.org.

American National Standards Institute (ANSI): A government agency responsible for developing standards, including standards for design, construction, and performance of audiologic test equipment, e.g., earphones and audiometers.

American Speech-Language Hearing Association (ASHA): A professional organization for audiologists and (mostly) speech pathologists.

amplifier: An electronic device for increasing the magnitude (amount) of an electrical signal, i.e., increasing the gain.

Amplitrode™: A combination electrode and amplifier available from the manufacturer of evoked response systems (Vivosonic). The Amplitrode™ applies a high-pass 30 Hz filter, optimized for ABR measurement, and a low-pass RF filter prior to amplification.

amplitude: A measure of the size or magnitude of an auditory evoked response wave, usually made from either a peak to a preceding or following trough, or from the peak of a wave to some index of baseline; expressed in µvolts (microvolts). Calculation of the amplitude for wave V of the auditory brainstem response is often made from a shoulder on the wave to the following trough (low point)

amplitude modulation (AM): Change in the amplitude of a steady-state (sinusoidal or pure-tone) stimulus. Amplitude modulation in stimuli used to elicit the auditory steady-state response (ASSR) is often 100 percent and very rapid (> 60 times per second or > 60 Hz).

amyotrophic lateral sclerosis (ALS): A degenerative, terminal neuromuscular process known as Lou Gehrig's disease.

analog (analogue): A continuous varying signal over time (e.g., an evoked response), in contrast to a sequence of discrete values or a digital representation of the response.

analog-to-digital (A/D) converter: An electronic device that converts a continuously varying electrical signal (e.g., auditory evoked response) to a series of numeric values that can then be processed by a computer.

analysis: In auditory evoked response measurement the manual calculation of specific response parameters values, e.g., latency or amplitude, of wave components or the automated detection and confirmation statistically of an auditory evoked response.

analysis time: The time period after a stimulus is presented during which a response is averaged and analyzed (e.g., 15 ms for the auditory brainstem response).

anesthetic agent: A drug used to suppress consciousness before or during surgery, or perhaps for measurement of auditory evoked responses (e.g., the ABR) from young children who, without anesthesia, are too active physically to undergo assessment.

anode: The positive electrode of an electrode pair; often indicated by red (think "red hot").

APD: Auditory processing disorders (*see* auditory processing).

apex of cochlea: The upper portion of the cochlear (inner ear). Lower frequency sounds are represented in the apical region of the cochlea.

aphasia: Language dysfunction due to brain damage, often secondary to a cerebrovascular accident (stroke).

A/R: At risk.

array: A combination of electrodes used to record sensory evoked responses. The simplest electrode array used in recording the auditory brainstem response (ABR) consists of three electrodes (noninverting on forehead, inverting near or on the ear, and a common or ground electrode).

artifact (artefact): An unwanted electrical event or nonresponse activity in an auditory evoked response recording originating from a patient (e.g., neuromuscular electrical activity) or from external sources (e.g., airborne or power line electrical activity).

artifact rejection: A process during evoked response measurement for eliminating or reducing the unwanted contamination of the recording by artifact (nonresponse activity, e.g., muscle potentials).

as: Left ear (from Latin *auris sinistra*).

ASCII: The acronym for American Standard Code for Information Interchange (applies within the United States). The code consists of 128 characters (e.g., letters, numerals, punctuation marks) in a seven-bit binary format.

ASCVD: Arteriosclerotic cardiovascular disease.

ASSR: *See* auditory steady-state response.

at risk: For hearing loss, infants who are more likely than normal infants to have a hearing impairment according to specific risk indicators, e.g., low birth weight, craniofacial anomalies, perinatal infections, and others. The Joint Committee on Infant Hearing (*see* JCIH) defines risk indicators for neonatal, delayed onset, and progressive hearing loss in infants and young children.

attenuation: Reduction in the intensity of a stimulus or the amplitude of an evoked response.

audiogram: A graph of hearing sensitivity (hearing threshold levels in decibels or dB) for simple sinusoid (pure-tone) sounds as a function of their frequency (in cycles/second or Hertz, Hz). The audiogram is a common graph for defining the degree of hearing loss across a range of frequencies.

audiologist: A hearing health professional educated and trained to measure auditory system function and manage patients with auditory and communicative impairments with nonmedical and nonsurgical therapy. In the United States, minimum academic degree is the Doctor of Audiology degree (formerly the master's degree) and some audiologists hold the Ph.D. In some other countries, audiologists may practice with the bachelor's degree or other academic credentials.

audiology: The profession concerned with measurement of auditory system function and nonsurgical, nonmedical management of persons with auditory and communicative impairment. Clinical auditory neurophysiology is encompassed within the scope of practice for audiologists.

audiometry: Assessment of peripheral or central auditory function by means of behavioral and electrophysiological procedures.

auditory brainstem response (ABR): Electrical activity evoked (stimulated) by very brief sounds, originating from the eighth nerve or auditory portions of the brainstem and usually recorded from the surface of the scalp and external ear. Other terms or acronyms are brainstem evoked response (BSER), brainstem auditory evoked potential (BAEP), brainstem auditory evoked response (BAER).

auditory cortical radiations: Pathways within the brain leading from the upper regions of the brainstem and the thalamus to different portions of the auditory cortex.

auditory evoked response (AER): Electrical activity evoked (stimulated) by sounds arising from auditory portions of the peripheral or central nervous system and recorded with electrodes. AERs include but are not limited to the electrocochleogram, auditory brainstem response, auditory middle-latency response, 40 Hz response, auditory late response, and P300 response.

auditory late response (ALR): Electrical activity evoked by sound stimuli that originates from portions of the auditory cortex. The ALR is measured with electrodes placed on the scalp and occurs within a period of 100 to 300 ms after the sound is presented.

auditory middle-latency response (AMLR): Electrical activity evoked by sounds that originates from thalamocortical pathways, i.e., from the thalamus, fibers leading from the thalamus to the cortex, and the primary auditory cortex. The AMLR, measured with electrodes placed on the scalp over each cerebral hemisphere, occurs within a period of about 15 to 50 ms after a stimulus (sound) is presented.

auditory processing: The processing of auditory information (stimulus intensity, frequency, duration, and other temporal properties) anywhere within the auditory system from the cochlea (inner ear) rostrally through the nervous system.

auditory steady-state response (ASSR): A response arising from the auditory system (brainstem and/or cortical regions) elicited by sinusoidal (pure-tone or steady-state) stimuli that are modulated (changed) in amplitude or frequency, usually at a fast rate (e.g., > 60 Hz). The ASSR was formerly referred to as the steady-state evoked response (SSER) or steady-state evoked potential (SSEP).

auditory vertex response (AVR): A term formerly for referring to the auditory late response which occurs within a period of 100 to 300 ms after a stimulus is presented and is often recorded with an electrode placed on the vertex.

average (averaging): a process of summing the response to a repeated stimulus over a specific time period after the stimulus (e.g., 15 ms) and regularly dividing the summed response by the number of stimuli presented. Random electrical activity (noise) becomes smaller and electrical brain activity time-locked to the stimuli (signal) becomes larger with averaging.

band-pass (filter): A filter that allows energy within a certain range of frequencies to pass through (e.g., 30 to 1500 Hz) while frequencies below and above this range are rejected (filtered out).

base of cochlea: The lower portion (turns) of the cochlea (the inner ear). Higher frequency sounds are represented in the basal region of the cochlea.

basilar membrane: A very flexible partition or shelf of tissue running across the tube-like inner portion of the cochlea on which the actual sensory structures (the hair cells) are located (the organ of Corti).

Bereitschaftspotential: A direct current (DC) potential that precedes a motor reaction by the subject.

beta rhythm: Electroencephalogram (EEG) activity within the 13 to 30 Hz region, normally of low amplitude (less than 20 μVolts).

BF: Black female.

BID: Twice a day (from Latin *bis in die*).

bilateral: Both sides. A bilateral auditory response is generated from structures on each side of the central nervous system.

binaural: Both ears. A binaural stimulus is presented to both ears.

bipolar: A two-electrode recording array in which an electrode is located at each end or on each side of the dipole that is producing an auditory evoked response, i.e., both electrodes are "active" with respect to the electrical activity recorded.

bit: An abbreviation for binary digit. A bit is the smallest unit of data.

blink reflex: Brainstem reflex (the corneal response) that may be stimulated electrically in the supraorbital region or with tactile (touch) stimulation on the cornea. The afferent portion of the reflex arc is the fifth (trigeminal) cranial nerve. There are intermediate neurons in the lower brainstem. The efferent portion of the arc is the seventh cranial (facial) nerve that is involved in eye blinking.

BM: Black male.

bone conduction: Transmission of sound (mechanical vibrations) from the surface of the skull (e.g., at the mastoid or forehead) to the fluids of the cochlea. Sounds are then perceived in the usual way.

bone oscillator (vibrator): A small device (usually black plastic on the exterior with electronic components within, and about an inch square) that is used to present sounds (vibrations) to the skull in bone conduction auditory assessment. A Radioear B-70 or B-71 oscillator (vibrator) is recommended for AER stimulation.

BP: Blood pressure, recorded in mmHg (mercury).

brain electrical activity mapping (BEAM): Topographic display (color, shading, or numeric) of auditory evoked response amplitude recorded from multiple electrodes on the scalp (*see* Topographic evoked response mapping).

brainstem auditory evoked potential (BAEP): *See* auditory brainstem response (ABR).

brainstem auditory evoked response (BAER): *See* auditory brainstem response (ABR).

brainstem evoked response (BSER): *See* auditory brainstem response (ABR).

brainstem transmission time: A term sometimes used for the latency interval between components of the auditory brainstem response (ABR), e.g., the ABR wave I–V interval implying the time for conduction of neural impulses from the generator of one component to the other.

buffer: An electronic device either within a computer terminal or external (e.g., a printer buffer) that permits temporary storage of incoming data to allow the printer to keep pace with the computer or to free the computer up for other tasks while printing goes on.

bug: An error in a computer program or in the functioning of a computer.

byte: A coded group of binary bits that comprise a character (e.g., a letter, numeral, symbol, command).

c: With (from the Latin word *cum*).

C3, C4, C5, C6, C7, C8: International 10–20 system electrode locations in a coronal array on the left (odd numbers) and right (even numbers) of the head. The coronal (crown) array is identified as sites from the top and middle of the head (the vertex) down each side to the external auditory canal.

CA: Chronological age; cancer; or conceptional age.

calibration: Electronic or psychoacoustic determination that an electrical device (such as an amplifier) or an acoustic transducer (an earphone) is functioning according to defined characteristics. The term usually also implies correction of the device if necessary.

carrier frequency: In auditory steady-state response (ASSR) measurement, the stimulus is a sinusoid (carrier frequency) that is then modulated in amplitude or frequency to generate activity in the auditory system that can be detected with the evoked response system.

caudal: Toward the tail; inferior in position; for example, in the central nervous system the brainstem is caudal to the cerebrum.

CC: Chief complaint.

CCU: Coronary care unit.

central: Along the axis of the nervous system from the spinal cord upward through the brainstem to the cortex; *see* central nervous system.

central nervous system (CNS): The spinal cord, brainstem, cerebellum, and cerebrum; the axis or central core of the nervous system. Cranial nerves and other nerves and sensory structures (e.g., the inner ear) are part of the peripheral nervous system.

cerebellopontine angle (CPA): The angle formed or bordered by the cerebellum and lateral surface of the pons, located in the posterior fossa. The eighth (auditory) cranial nerve passes through the CPA. Some tumors (e.g., acoustic tumors and neurofibromas) may develop within or enter the CPA.

cerebral spinal fluid (CSF): The watery-appearing liquid in which the brain is bathed; it also fills the ventricles within the brain and the column within the spinal cord.

cerebrovascular accident (CVA): A stroke; brain damage resulting from interruption of blood supply to the brain.

channel: A single set of inputs into an evoked response system (e.g., from one pair of electrodes) or a single output from a stimulus generator (e.g., to the right earphone).

CHARGE syndrome: A collection of newborn defects. Letters in the acronym refer to the following disorders: **c**oloboma of the eye; **h**ead anomaly; **a**tresia (stenosis) of choana in the nose; **r**etardation of growth and/or development; **g**enital hypoplasia; and **e**ar anomalies and/or hearing impairment.

CHD: congenital heart disease.

chloral hydrate: A common medication for sedation for ABR measurement in children; in the hypnotic drug class; available as syrup, capsule, or suppository. Dosage of 50 or 75 mg of the drug per kg of body weight is commonly used.

click: A very brief-duration sound with almost instantaneous onset and duration and a wide range of frequencies, which is produced by a transient electrical pulse (usually 0.1 ms in duration).

CNS: Central nervous system (defined above).

cochlea: *See* inner ear. The word is from the Greek for snail.

cochlear microphonic (CM): An auditory electrical potential arising from the hair cells of the cochlea (mostly outer hair cells) that follows the polarity of a stimulus (i.e., like a microphone).

cochlear nuclei (CN): A collection of neuron cell bodies in the lower brainstem (pons) that synapse with fibers from the eighth (auditory) cranial nerve leading from the cochlea.

coma: An unconscious state in which a person has reduced responsiveness to external stimuli. *See* Glasgow Coma Scale.

command: A code that will cause a computer to perform a function.

common mode rejection (CMR): When the same (common) electrical signal is detected by two electrodes in an array or pair and is rejected or subtracted from itself (cancelled) by the differential amplifier. The common mode rejection ratio is a measure of how well the amplifier reduces common signals from signals that are different at each electrode (e.g., the response).

component: A peak in a response waveform; the wave I is a component of the auditory brainstem response. Some waves within later AERs (e.g., N1 in the auditory late response) may be made up of more than one component (e.g., N1a, N1b, N1c).

compound action potential (CAP): Simultaneously occurring action potentials from many nerve fibers.

computerized tomography: *See* CT.

conceptional age (CA): Age of a newborn infant based on dates of mother's last menstrual cycle versus a physical examination.

condensation (positive) stimulus polarity: Positive voltage electrical signal producing an outward movement of the transducer diaphragm with associated (compression) sound waves.

conductive (component or hearing loss): Hearing impairment due to an interruption of sound transmission through an abnormal middle ear. The abnormality often results from middle ear pathology, such as otitis media.

configuration: A term used to describe the shape or pattern of an audiogram, that is, how hearing loss varies as a function of test frequency. Three main configurations are sloping (high-frequency hearing loss), rising (low-frequency hearing loss) and flat.

contingent negative variation (CNV): A low-frequency, negative-voltage evoked response in the 300 to 500 ms region and associated with anticipation of a stimulus condition.

corpus callosum: A major collection of fibers connecting the two cerebral hemispheres; the largest and most rostral (superior in the nervous system) of multiple fiber tracts crossing (decussating) from one side to the other. The auditory pathways are within the posterior portion of the corpus collosum.

CPAP: Continuous positive airway pressure.

CPP: Cerebral perfusion pressure.

CPR: Cardiopulmonary resuscitation.

CPT: Current procedural terminology. CPT codes, listed in a comprehensive manual, are used by third-party payers (health insurance companies) in describing and classifying thousands of clinical procedures, including different auditory evoked response measures.

craniofacial: Involving the head and face. Craniofacial anomalies include preauricular (in front of the ear) tags and pits, and microtia (very small ears), and aural atresia (absence of external ears)

cross-correlation: A sophisticated mathematical procedure for assessing the variability of data points in a waveform that is useful in determining objectively and automatically the presence of an evoked response.

crossover (acoustic): Sound stimulus presented to one (test) ear travels around or across the head (via bone conduction) to stimulate the other (nontest) ear; *see* intraaural attenuation.

CSF: Cerebrospinal fluid.

CT: Computerized tomography, a neuroradiologic imaging technique; in lay terms, brain scan.

CVA: Cerebrovascular accident; a stroke. Brain injury (ischemia) related to an abnormal reduction of blood flow to brain tissue.

Cx: Cervical.

Cz: An electrode site in the International 10–20 system that is located on the vertex (top and center of head). "C" refers to coronal and "z" indicates the midline.

dB: *See* decibel.

dB nHL: Term used to describe and calibrate stimulus intensity level in auditory evoked response measurement. 0 dB nHL is the average behavioral threshold for a stimulus (e.g., a click or a tone burst) in a group of normal-hearing persons.

DC: Discontinue or discharge.

DD: Differential diagnosis.

dead ear: An audiologic/otologic slang term for a profound hearing impairment, i.e., an inner ear that is severely damaged and does not respond to sounds.

decay: Fatigue or decrease in response amplitude (rapid adaptation) with continued stimulation, e.g., acoustic stapedial reflex decay.

decibel (dB): A unit of sound intensity (loudness). A dB is the logarithm of the sound pressure of a sound to a reference sound pressure (usually 0.0002 dynes/cm). Clinically for adult patients, hearing threshold levels of 0 to 20 dB are considered to be within the normal range. Units for describing decibels include dB hearing level (HL), sound pressure level (SPL), sensation level (SL) and, for auditory evoked responses, dB normal hearing level (dB nHL).

deconvolution: Reducing a complex waveform with multiple frequencies into individual frequencies, as in spectral analysis.

decussation: A crossing of fibers from one side of the central nervous system to the other. A portion of the corpus callosum is a major decussation within the auditory system.

delta: Electroencephalogram (EEG) activity within the frequency band from 0 to 3 Hz, normally of low amplitude (less than 20 μvolts); delta, indicated by the symbol "Δ" also refers to any change in a quantity.

deviant: With measurement of the mismatch negativity (MMN) response, the rare or infrequent stimulus is referred to as the deviant stimulus, whereas the frequent stimulus is referred to as the standard. The MMN response is a reflection of the brain's unconscious detection of a difference (i.e., mismatch) between the standard and the deviant stimulus.

dichotic: Simultaneous presentation of a different sound (e.g., two different words) to each ear.

differential amplifier: An electrical device with two inputs that subtracts the voltage of one input from the other and then increases the amplitude (strength) of this voltage difference; *see* common mode rejection.

digital: In evoked response use, the process of assigning a number that quantifies response voltage at a specific time relative to the stimulus (e.g., before or after the stimulus).

diotic: presenting the same sound to both ears (*di* = two, *otic* = ears), but not necessarily simultaneously; *see* binaural.

dipole: An electrical source (as in the brain) with an axis that has a positive voltage charge at one end and a negative voltage charge at the other end. Dipoles are the final source of auditory evoked responses along the pathways within the auditory nervous system.

distal: Away (distant) from the center or medial (axes or axial) portion of a structure; for example, the cochlea is at the distal end of the eighth (auditory) cranial nerve; opposite of proximal.

DOB: Date of birth.

duration: The length of time (usually in ms in evoked response terminology) from the beginning to the end of a stimulus; includes the rise and fall times, and the plateau in between.

dwell time: The amount of time that an averaging computer requires for sampling electrical activity from the brain; shorter dwell times correspond to faster sampling and better time (latency) resolution.

dx: diagnosis.

earphone: A device for presenting a sound stimulus to the ear consisting of an acoustic transducer for converting an electrical signal to sound and a cushion that couples the transducer to the ear.

ECG (EKG): Electrocardiogram.

EEG: Electroencephalography (electroencephalogram).

efferent: Pertaining to transmission of neural information from the central nervous system out to a sensory receptor (e.g., the inner ear); descending (usually inhibitory) pathways; opposite of afferent.

eighth (auditory or acoustic) cranial nerve: The cranial nerve located within the temporal bone that transmits neural information from the cochlea (inner ear) to the brainstem; contains auditory and a vestibular portions.

electric response audiometry (ERA): An older, general term for auditory evoked responses. The term is not proper and most evoked responses do not assess hearing but, rather, electrical activity within a portion of the auditory nervous system.

electrocardiography (EKG): Electrophysiologic measurement of heart activity.

electrocochleography (ECochG, preferred, or ECoG): Evoked responses originating from the cochlea and eighth (auditory) cranial nerve, i.e., the summating potential (SP), the cochlear microphonic (CM), and the N1 component.

electrode: A device that makes contact with the body that conducts bioelectrical activity from the body via a wire lead to recording equipment in all sensory evoked responses. The electrode may be made up of metal in the shape of a cup, needle, or plate, or an adhesive material integrated with conducting gel. An electrode may also be used to deliver electrical stimulation to the body, e.g., in electroneuronography (ENoG) measurement of in somatosensory evoked response measurement.

electroencephalography (EEG): Ongoing electrical activity arising from the brain; background electrical activity during evoked response measurement. The conventional EEG frequency regions (delta, theta, alpha, beta) are within the region of 0 to about 30 Hz.

electromyography (EMG): Recording muscle activity electrophysiologically, usually with hook electrodes embedded in muscle.

electroneuronography (ENoG): Recording facial nerve/muscle activity electrophyiologically; technically electromyography of the facial muscles during stimulation of the facial nerve after it exits the skull. The facial nerve is usually stimulated at the stylomastoid foramen and activity is recorded with electrodes on the naso-labial fold.

electronystagmography (ENG): A test of vestibular (balance) functioning in which nystagmus (eyeball movements) are recorded electrophysiologically during stimulation of the vestibular system.

EMG: Electromyography (electromyogram).

envelope: The shape of the overall waveform of an acoustic stimulus that follows the rise, plateau and fall portions of the stimulus.

epoch: A time period, such as the analysis time in evoked response measurement. A typical epoch for the auditory brainstem response is 15 ms.

ER: Emergency room.

Erb's point: The region over the brachial plexus (the depression above the clavicle). This is an important electrode site in somatosensory evoked response measurement and the generator of the N9 component.

Event-related potential (ERP): The term used to describe certain evoked responses, such as the 40 Hz response or the P3 (P300) response, which are elicited with stimuli other than a simple sequence of brief-duration clicks or tones.

evoked: Elicited, stimulated, or activated. Sensory evoked responses are elicited, stimulated or activated by sensory (auditory, visual, somatosensory) stimuli (energy).

external auditory meatus: The opening of the outer ear leading to the external ear canal.

external ear: The portion of the ear that is normally visible. Major components of the external (or outer) ear include the pinna, concha, tragus, and external ear canal.

extratympanic: Lateral to (outside of) the tympanic membrane (eardrum). This term is often used to describe auditory evoked response electrodes located in the external ear canal.

fall time: The time (usually in milliseconds) from the maximum amplitude of a stimulus or the end of the plateau to some measure of baseline (zero voltage).

far-field response: A response recorded with electrodes relatively distant from the generator of the response. By definition, a slight change in electrode location has little or no effect on far-field response latency or amplitude. The auditory brainstem response is a far-field response.

fast Fourier transformation (FFT): A computerized technique, named after the French physicist and mathematician Baron Jean Baptiste Joseph Fourier (1768–1830), for separating a complex waveform consisting of multiple frequencies into individual frequency components.

FH: Family history.

filter: An electronic device for eliminating electrical energy in a specific frequency region while allowing other frequencies to pass on. Filters may be analog or digital. *See* high-pass, low-pass, and band-pass filters.

40 Hz (response): A periodic auditory evoked response to a stimulus repetition rate of approximately 40 per second that normally is of greater amplitude than the response to any single stimulus. Dr. Robert Galambos coined the term in the early 1980s.

Fpz: An electrode site (according to the 10–20 International electrode system) located in the midline on the lower portion of the forehead almost between the eyebrows.

frequency following response (FFR): An auditory evoked response to a continuous tone stimulus. The periodic waveform of the response is at the same frequency as the stimulus.

frequency modulation (FM): A change in the frequency of a stimulus used to elicit an auditory evoked response, such as the auditory steady-state response (ASSR). The warbled tone used in sound-field pure-tone audiometry is an example of a frequency-modulated stimulus.

frequency response: For acoustic transducers (e.g., earphones), the output of the transducer (usually in dB) across as a function of stimulus frequency. It is usually desirable for an earphone to have a wide, flat frequency response that produces equal amplitude output from very low to very high frequencies.

frequency specificity: The degree of precision in the spectrum of a stimulus. A pure-tone (a single sinusoid) stimulus has a very high degree of frequency specificity, whereas a click stimulus is associated with no frequency specificity (energy over a broad range of frequencies).

Fsp: The F-statistic for a single point; a statistical approach for confirming the likelihood that a response (e.g., auditory evoked response) is present and distinct from background electrical activity (noise). The Fsp is a common strategy for automated detection of the auditory brainstem response in newborn hearing screening.

FTND: Full-term normal delivery.

Fz: An electrode site (according to the 10–20 International electrode system) located in the midline on the forehead, approximately at the hairline (for persons without baldness).

gain: Increase in the amplitude or energy of an electrical signal with amplification. Gain is the difference between the input signal and the output signal.

gating (gate): The process in which an electrical signal is transmitted or stopped along an electrical pathway, often leading to a transducer (earphone). If the gate is open, the signal can pass on, but if the gate is closed, the signal does not pass on.

gestational age (GA): The age of a newborn infant determined by evaluation of physical, specifically, neurological maturity after birth and comparison to normative data for different ages after birth (usually in weeks).

Glasgow Coma Scale (GCS): A simple, clinical scale for grading neurological responsiveness and severity of brain injury based on eye opening, motor, and verbal responses. The GCS ranges from a low of 3 (totally unresponsive) to a high of 15 (totally responsive). A GCS of 8 or less indicates a severe brain injury.

gm: Gram = 1000 milligrams = 1/1000 kilograms = 15.43 grains.

ground: A connection from a piece of electronic equipment, or a person, to the actual ground or a relatively large metal structure. The ground electrode from a person is connected to the grounding circuit on an evoked response system. A good ground reduces electrical interference in evoked response recording.

hair cells: The initial sensory unit within in the auditory system, located in the cochlea (inner ear). Inner hair cells convert mechanical energy (movement) produced by sound stimulation to bioelectrical activity. Outer hair cells are capable of motility (movement). They are activated by sound stimulation to the ear. An important part of the cells, and the reason for their name, are clusters of tiny stereocilia (protein rods) resembling hairs on top of each cell.

haversine: One-half cycle of a sine wave (a pure tone). High-frequency haversines (e.g., for a 3000 Hz sine wave) are sometimes used as stimuli in evoked response measurement.

hearing loss (impairment): A problem with hearing that is characterized by decreased sensitivity to sound in comparison to normal hearing. *See* conductive, sensorineural, and mixed hearing loss.

hearing threshold level (HTL): The faintest intensity level (in dB hearing level) that a person can hear for a sound of a particular test frequency. A completely normal HTL is 0 dB HL (hearing level).

hemotympanum: Collection of blood in the middle ear space, behind the eardrum, usually resulting from head trauma in the region of the temporal bone.

Hertz (Hz): The unit of frequency of a sound, named after Heinrich Rudolf Hertz (1857–1894), a German physicist. One Hz = 1 cycle per second (cps).

Heschl's gyrus: The primary auditory cortex region of the brain, located on the superior gyrus of the temporal lobe.

high-pass (filter): A filter that passes electrical energy above a specific cutoff frequency and eliminates (filters out) energy below the frequency. A typical high-pass filter setting in auditory brainstem response measurement is 30 Hz. Some manufacturers of evoked response equipment refer to the high-pass filter cutoff at the "low-frequency filter."

H/O: History of.

hx: History.

IAFM: Independent amplitude and frequency modulation; a complex type of stimulus used to elicit the auditory steady-state response (ASSR).

ILD: See interear latency difference (ILD).

IM: Intramuscular. Injection of a drug into muscle tissue is usually in the upper arm or leg.

immittance (impedance) measurement: An electrophysiological procedure for evaluating middle ear function and the acoustic stapedial reflex based on measurement of impedance to (or admittance of) energy flow through the middle ear.

impedance (Z): Electrical; a measure of total opposition to energy (current) flow in an an electrical circuit. There are also mechanical and acoustic forms of impedance. Interelectrode impedance in evoked response measurement is the opposition to current flow between a pair of electrodes, reported as electrical resistance in ohms.

incus: An ossicle in the middle ear; the second (middle) of three tiny bones connecting the tympanic membrane to the cochlea (inner ear).

indifferent electrode: Usually the second electrode in an electrode pair in evoked response measurement. Also referred to as inactive, reference, or (properly) the inverting electrode. Unless this electrode is noncephalic, it is probably not actually "indifferent" or "inactive."

inferior colliculus: A large and complex nucleus within the midbrain (upper brainstem) region of the auditory system.

inion: The slight protuberance at the midline in the lower occipital region of the skull, on the back of the head just above the neck.

inner ear: Also called the cochlea. A snail-shaped structure located within the temporal bone containing the sensory organ for hearing. All acoustic stimulation must activate the inner ear to be perceived by as sound, therefore, all auditory evoked responses are dependent on integrity of the inner ear.

insert earphones: A type of earphone consisting of a transducer built into a small box and an acoustic tube for delivery of the sound stimulus to the ear. The tube is coupled to the ear by means of a small foam or rubber probe tip.

interaural attenuation: The isolation or attenuation produced by the head when sound is presented to one ear before it crosses over to the other (nontest ear). Interaural attenuation is greater for insert earphones than for supra-aural earphones. The latter are characterized by interaural attenuation of about the 40 to 50 dB.

interear latency difference (ILD): The difference in latency of an auditory evoked response component (usually auditory brainstem response [ABR wave V] for right versus left ear stimulation; a measure of the degree of auditory evoked response asymmetry, reported in milliseconds. An upper limit for normal ILD of 0.40 ms for the ABR wave is often used clinically.

internal auditory canal: The tubelike channel through the temporal bone leading from the inner ear to the middle cranial fossa of the skull; the eighth cranial nerve (auditory and vestibular portions) and the seventh (facial) cranial nerve course through the internal auditory canal, as well as blood vessels supplying the nerves and the inner ear.

International 10–20 Electrode System: Accepted nomenclature for designating electrode locations on the scalp, reported initially by Jasper in 1958.

interstimulus interval (ISI): The time interval (usually in milliseconds) between two successive stimuli. In general, interstimulus interval decreases as the rate of stimulation increases and vice versa.

interwave interval: The latency, or time, in milliseconds between any two waves (components) in an evoked response waveform. For example, the auditory brainstem response wave I to V interval is commonly measured clinically.

interwave latency difference (interval): A relative latency measure of the time between two waves in an auditory evoked response. The ABR wave I–V latency difference (interval) commonly calculated interwave latency difference.

intracranial pressure (ICP): Pressure (expressed in mmHg or sometimes cmH_2O) within the skull. Normal ICP is close to 0 mmHg and never greater than 20 mmHg. Abnormally elevated ICP secondary to brain edema and swelling is a major problem following severe brain injury.

intraoperative: During a surgical procedure, or operation.

intraventricular hemorrhage (IVH): Brain pathology consisting of discharge of large amounts of blood from cerebral vessels into the ventricular system of the brain; one of the more common brain pathologies in newborn infants.

invert: To reverse the polarity of a stimulus or a waveform, or turn it upside down. Waveforms can be inverted by reversing the electrodes in an electrode pair (i.e., the amplifier inputs) before evoked response recording or, with some evoked response systems, by a digital manipulation after the averaging process.

inverting versus noninverting (electrodes): Terms used to describe each electrode in a pair during evoked response recording. Electrical activity detected with the noninverting electrode does not change polarity during the amplification process, whereas the polarity of electrical activity detected with the inverting electrode is reversed (inverted) before the it is combined with the noninverting input and amplified.

IV: Intravenous. Injection or infusion of a substance, e.g., medication or fluid replacement, in a vein with a catheter (tube). Often done at the wrist or ankle.

JCIH: *See* Joint Committee on Infant Hearing.

Joint Committee on Infant Hearing: A multidisciplinary group with an interest in early identification and intervention for hearing loss in infants and young children with representation from audiology, pediatrics, otolaryngology, and other professions. The JCIH periodically prepares position statements.

kg: Kilogram = 1000 grams = 2.2 pounds (lb).

kilo (k): One thousand. For example, 1K Hz = 1000 Hz.

latency: A term used to describe the time at which an evoked response wave component occurs after a stimulus, or the time between two wave components; usually described in milliseconds (ms). The latency of auditory brainstem response wave V for a high-intensity stimulus is usually in the 5.0 to 6.0 ms region.

lateral lemniscus: The major ascending pathway in the auditory brainstem. The auditory brainstem response (ABR) wave V is generated by the lateral lemniscus.

LE: Lower extremity (leg).

logon: A form of stimulus sometimes used in auditory evoked response measurement defined by Davis (1976) as a sinusoid (pure tone) gating or shaped with a Gaussian envelope.

loudness: The psychological correlate to sound intensity. Increases in sound intensity are perceived as increased loudness. The relationship between intensity and loudness is not one-to-one but, rather, logarithmic.

low-pass (filter): A filter that passes electrical energy below a specific cutoff frequency and eliminates (filters out) energy above the frequency. A typical low pass filter setting in auditory brainstem response measurement is 3000 Hz. Some manufacturers of evoked response equipment refer to the low-pass filter cutoff at the "high-frequency filter."

M1, M2: The 10–20 International Electrode System labels for the left (1) and right (2) mastoid (M) sites.

MA: Mental age. A measure of age based on an evaluation neurological and/or cognitive functioning.

malleus: The first of the three tiny bones (ossicles) connecting the tympanic membrane to the inner ear. The umbo of the malleus rests against the inner surface of the tympanic membrane and can usually be seen with otoscopic examination of the ear.

MAP: Mean arterial blood pressure. A measure of blood pressure (BP) calculated as follows. MAP = systolic BP – diastolic BP/3 + diastolic BP.

mapping: Displaying the distribution or pattern of amplitudes for evoked response components (voltage distribution or topography) at a designated latency that are recorded simultaneously at numerous locations across the scalp. Mapping may be done continuously over a period of time.

masking (masker): Noise presented to the nontest ear in an audiometric procedure or auditory evoked response measurement. Common masking noises are either broadband or narrowband noise. Masking is used in an attempt to prevent a response from the nontest ear due to possible stimulus crossover from the test ear. Ipsilateral masking noise signals may be used in an attempt increase the frequency specificity of stimuli eliciting the auditory brainstem response (ABR).

MASTER: Multiple auditory steady-state response.

mastoid (bone): A portion of the temporal bone located behind the external ear. Bone-conduction stimulation is often applied to the mastoid bone.

medial geniculate body (MGB): A structure in the posterior region of the thalamus that contains major nuclei in the central auditory nervous system.

medulla: The lowest (most caudal) part of the brainstem, between the pons and the spinal cord. The initial auditory brainstem structures (e.g., cochlear nuclei) are in the pons-medulla border region.

Ménière's disease: Pathology affecting the cochlea and resulting in sensory (sensorineural) hearing impairment. Characteristic signs and symptoms are tinnitus, vertigo, sensation of ear fullness, and a fluctuating, often low-frequency, sensorineural hearing loss. Electrocochleography (ECochG) is useful in the diagnosis of Ménière's disease.

microphone: An electronic device for converting an acoustic signal (a sound) to an electrical signal.

microphonic: An electrical event within the cochlea. The cochlear microphonic (CM) is a cochlear response that reflects a tone stimulus much as a microphone produces an electrical signal that reflects an acoustic stimulus.

microsecond (μsec): One-millionth (1/1,000,000) of a second. 100 μsec equals 0.1 ms.

microvolt (μvolt or μV): One-millionth (1/1,000,000) of a volt. Amplitude of the ABR wave V is usually about 0.5 μV.

midbrain: Portion of the brainstem above the pons containing the inferior colliculus, an important center in the auditory nervous system.

middle ear: An opening within the temporal bone behind (medial to) the tympanic membrane and lateral to the cochlea containing the ossicles and middle ear muscles.

millisecond (ms): One-thousandth (1/1000) of a second. One ms equals 1000 microseconds. Latencies of auditory evoked response components are typically described in milliseconds or fractions of milliseconds. Latency of the ABR wave V at high stimulus intensity levels (e.g., 85 dB nHL) is normally about 5.5 to 6.0 ms.

mismatch negativity (MMN) response: The mismatch negativity (MMN) response is recorded with a rare or infrequent stimulus is referred to as the deviant stimulus and a frequent stimulus, referred to as the standard. The MMN response is a reflection of the brain's unconscious detection of a difference (i.e., mismatch) between the standard and the deviant stimulus. It appears as a negativity wave in the region of 100 to 200 ms after presentation of the stimuli.

mixed (hearing loss): Hearing loss with conductive (middle ear pathology) and a sensory (cochlear pathology) components. The audiogram shows a bone-conduction hearing deficit plus an air-bone gap.

modulation frequency: The rate (frequency) at which either amplitude or frequency of a stimulus (carrier tone) is changed in the stimulation of the auditory steady-state response (ASSR).

monaural: One ear. Monaural stimuli in auditory evoked response assessment are usually presented to first one ear (right or left) and then the other.

monitor: To continuously or to periodically measure status, such as central nervous system function. Auditory evoked responses are used as a monitoring technique in the operating room and in the intensive care unit.

monopolar: In evoked responses, monopolar refers to a recording electrode arrangement in which one electrode of a pair is detecting the response and the second electrode is "inactive," usually located distant from the response generator, and not detecting the response.

morphology: The shape, amplitude, clarity and general appearance of an evoked response waveform and its individual components.

ms: Millisecond = 1/1000 sec = 1000 microseconds.

multiple sclerosis (MS): A demyelinating disease of the nervous system. Evoked responses are often abnormal in patients with multiple sclerosis.

myogenic: Originating from muscle activity (versus neurogenic).

N1: A component in electrocochleography (ECochG) normally occurring approximately 1.5 to 2.0 ms after an acoustic stimulus and reflecting the compound action potential of the eighth cranial nerve ("N" stands for negative voltage and "1" indicates the first major wave of this response). The ECochG terms N1 and AP refer to the same component. Also, N1 is the first negative-voltage peak of the auditory late response normally occurring approximately 90 to 110 ms after an acoustic stimulus and, presumably, arising from auditory cortex.

N13: A somatosensory evoked response component with negative-voltage (as typically recorded) normally occurring at approximately 13 ms after an electrical pulse stimulus. A brainstem generator for N13 is suspected. Also, a VEMP component.

Na: The first major negative-voltage peak in the auditory middle latency response that precedes peak Pa and normally occurs approximately 13 to 15 ms after an acoustic stimulus. The generator of Na may be in the thalamus.

nanovolt (nv, nvolt): .001 µvolt.

nasion: A location on the scalp midline on the forehead, between the eyebrows. The ground electrode is often placed at the nasion in auditory evoked response measurement.

Nb: The second major negative-voltage (as typically recorded) peak in the auditory middle-latency response that follows peak Pa and normally occurs in the 30 to 40 ms region.

near-field response: A sensory evoked response recorded with an electrode close to or on the neural generator. Movement of the electrode a very small distance away from this site produces a marked reduction in response amplitude.

neonate: A newborn infant. As defined by the Joint Committee on Infant Hearing (JCIH), a neonate is an infant within the first month after term (40 weeks gestation), i.e., full-term, birth.

NL: Normal.

noise: In evoked response measurement noise is unwanted activity, either electrical or muscular, that interferes with detection of the response (the signal). A major objective in evoked response recording is maximizing the signal and minimizing the noise. Noise is also background sound (acoustic energy) that can interfere with (or mask) the stimulus in evoked response measurement. Types of acoustic noise are also used to mask out the nontest ear in audiologic and auditory evoked response measurement.

noncephalic: Not on the head. A noncephalic electrode is located off the head, e.g. on the nape of the neck (the bump where the neck meets the shoulders; approximately over the C7 vertebra.

noninverting electrode: A primary or "active" electrode in AER recording, usually leading to the positive voltage input of a differential amplifier. The vertex electrode in conventional ABR recordings.

normative data: Statistical information on normal characteristics of auditory evoked responses, such as latency or amplitude values or expected threshold intensity level for the response. Normative data is used to differentiate patients with peripheral or central auditory system dysfunction from patients without dysfunction.

notch, 60 Hz: A type of filter used in evoked response measurement designed to reduce interference from 60 Hz (cycle) electrical activity (power line noise). Notch filtering introduces filter distortion in responses and, unfortunately, rarely achieves the purpose of eliminating electrical artifact associated with 60 Hz interference.

NPO: Nothing by mouth (from Latin *non per os*).

NSFTD: Normal spontaneous full-term delivery.

nystagmus: Horizontal or, rarely, vertical movements of the eyeballs. Nystagmus may result from stimulation of the vestibular (balance) system. Recording nystagmus with electrodes placed around the eyes during stimulation of the vestibular system is electronystagmography (ENG).

O1, O2: International 10–20 Electrode System sites located on the scalp in the back of the head over the left (1) and right (2) occipital (O) regions of the brain.

OBS: Organic brain syndrome.

offline: In evoked responses, an offline activity is done when the machine is not being used during the measurement process. For example, offline data analysis takes place at some time after data acquisition is completed, either with or without the evoked response instrumentation.

ohm: A measure of electrical current resistance, named for a German physicist Georg Simon Ohm; the ohm is labeled sometimes with the symbol Ω. There is one ohm of resistance when one ampere of current is produced by one volt. Interelectrode impedance in evoked response measurement is optimally 5000 ohms or less, and balanced (difference of less than 2000 ohms between electrodes).

online: In evoked responses, an online analysis is done during data acquisition when the machine is involved in the auditory evoked response measurement process (*see* offline).

OP: Outpatient.

OR: Operating room.

organ of Corti: The sensory organ of hearing, located on the basilar membrane of the cochlea (inner ear) and containing inner and outer hair cells, as well as supporting cells. Mechanical energy is transduced to bioelectrical energy at the organ of Corti.

oscilloscope: An electronic device for visually displaying an electrical signal on a screen, permitting measurement of the signal's amplitude (e.g., in volts), frequency, or temporal characteristics.

otitis media: A general term for various forms of middle ear disease, such as serous otitis media, otitis media with effusion, purulent otitis media, and chronic otitis media. Otitis media is one of the most common childhood diseases and usually produces a conductive hearing loss (usually not permanent).

otoacoustic emissions (OAEs): Acoustic energy measured within the ear canal that is produced by the cochlea, specifically movement (motility) of outer hair cells. Evoked OAEs, including transient (TEOAEs) and distortion product (DPOAE) otoacoustic emissions are generated by acoustic stimulation of the ear.

otolaryngologist: An ear, nose, and throat (ENT) medical doctor. An otolaryngologist is a surgeon.

otologist: An otologist is an otolaryngologist (a surgeon) who specializes in diagnosis and treatment of ear and related (e.g., vestibular) problems.

otosclerosis: A bony degenerative disease process that can involve the stapes footplate and/or the cochlea; also called otospongeosus.

oval window: One of two openings into the inner ear (cochlea) from the middle ear space. Vibrations transmitted through the middle ear are send via the stapes footplate through the oval window into the inner ear (*see* round window).

P1: The first major positive-voltage (as typically recorded) peak in the auditory late response, normally occuring approximately 40 to 60 ms after an acoustic stimulus. The exact generator of P1 is not known, but auditory cortex contributions are confirmed.

P50: Another term used for the Pb wave of the auditory middle latency response, so named because the latency of the wave is approximately 50 ms.

P300 (P3): An auditory evoked response, sometimes called a cognitive or event-related response, occuring in the 300 ms region (with positive voltage, hence "P") after acoustic stimuli. The P300 is normally recorded when a person attends or listens for rare, oddball or target stimuli that are presented along with frequent stimuli.

Pa: The first major positive-voltage (as typically recorded) peak of the auditory middle-latency response, normally occurring approximately 25 to 30 ms after an acoustic stimulus. The generator of the Pa wave is thought to be mostly within the primary auditory cortex.

passive P3 response: A P300 response recorded without subject attention to the rare (infrequent) stimulus. The main component recorded in the passive P300 paradigm is the P3a.

Pb: The second major positive-voltage peak of the auditory middle latency response, occurring typically about 45 to 50 ms after the stimulus. Also, a P50 component.

PDD: Pervasive developmental disorder; a term used for various serious developmental and/or neurologic disorders, including, for example, autism, Asperger's disorder, and others.

PE: Physical examination.

peak: A component of an evoked response waveform, or the extreme amplitude for the component. With auditory evoked responses, the term peak is often used to describe a positive-voltage component and negative-voltage components are described simply as troughs, although potentially valuable response components may be overlooked with this approach.

peak equivalent sound pressure level (peSPL): A measure of sound intensity in which the maximum voltage of a transient stimulus, e.g., a click, is equated on an oscilloscope with the voltage of a tone stimulus of known intensity level in dB sound pressure level. The click intensity level is then defined in terms of a peak equivalent SPL.

PEEP: Positive end-expiratory pressure.

peripheral: In the nervous system, peripheral components lie outside of the central nervous system (the cerebrum, brainstem, cerebellum, and spinal cord) and include the cranial nerves (e.g., the eighth or auditory nerve).

PERLA: pupils equal, react to light, and accommodation.

phase: The zero voltage point at the beginning of the waveform of a stimulus or of a frequency component of a response waveform expressed in degrees or radians, such as 0 or 90 degrees. Phase of a response is related to latency.

phase coherence: The agreement or consistency in phase for multiple samples of response generated during measurement of an auditory evoked response, such as an auditory steady-state response (ASSR).

phonetically balanced (PB) word lists: A list of 25 or 50 single-syllable words in which speech sounds (phonemes) are represented with the occurrence expected in conversational or written speech.

PI: Present illness.

PICU: Pediatric intensive care unit.

pinna: The outer, most obvious portion of the ear, consisting of a cartilage framework. Parts of the pinna are the helix, the lobe, and the concha.

pitch: The perception of the frequency of sound. High pitches correspond to high frequency sounds and vice versa.

PKU: Phenylketonuria.

PO: By mouth (from Latin *per os*).

polarity: The voltage characteristics of a stimulus or response waveform. Stimuli are of negative (rarefaction), positive (condensation), or alternating polarity. Response polarity depends on the location relative to the neural generator of the electrode plugged into the positive input vs. the electrode plugged into the negative voltage inputs of the differential physiological amplifier.

pons: A low (caudal) portion of the brainstem just above the medulla and below the midbrain. Important auditory centers (e.g., cochlear nuclei, trapezoid body, superior colliculus, lateral lemniscus) and auditory brainstem response generators are located in the pons.

postauricular muscle (PAM): One of three muscles attaching the external ear (pinna) to the scalp. The PAM is located behind the ear. PAM activity in response to sound stimulation that interferes with auditory middle-latency response measurement is referred to as PAM artifact.

potential: A difference in electrical charge measured between two electrodes. In evoked response measurement, the source of electrical potentials is stimulus-evoked activity in sensory portions of the peripheral or central nervous system. The term potential is often used interchangeably with the term "response," as in referring to a type of response as a potential (e.g., brainstem auditory evoked potential).

PP: Post partum; after delivery of a newborn.

PPHD: Persistent pulmonary hypertension disease; a serious respiratory disorder affecting premature newborn infants.

PR: Per rectum (rectal site for recording temperature or administration of medication with suppository).

preamplifier: An electronic device that receives an electrical signal, such as an evoked response directly from the electrodes and increases the strength (amplitude) of the signal before it is sent on for further processing (amplification, filtering, averaging).

presbycusis: Decrease in hearing sensitivity associated with aging. Although hearing may first begin to show aging effects at 20 years, presbycusis usually does not cause speech perception difficulty and serious hearing impairment until age 60 or older.

prestimulus baseline: A period of time before the presentation of each stimulus during which bioelectric activity is collected. The prestimulus baseline provides an indication of the quality of measurement conditions during auditory evoked response measurement.

primary auditory cortex: The auditory cortical region, located on the superior plane and insula of the superior gyrus of the temporal lobe, which initially receives information from lower portions of the brain, such as the thalamus and brainstem. The primary auditory cortex is thought to contribute to the generation of components of the auditory middle latency response component, e.g, Pa.

PRN: As needed (from Latin *pro re nata*).

probe microphone: A tiny microphone, often located within a soft, small tube, placed within the external ear canal to measure sound intensity level near the eardrum. The probe microphone is connected to equipment for recording characteristics of sound.

probe stimulus: In P3 (P300) evoked response measurement, the oddball or rare stimulus that produces a large amplitude component at approximately 300 ms in the auditory late response.

promontory: A rounded bony projection on the inner (medial) wall of the middle ear that is the outer (lateral) wall of the first turn of the cochlea (inner ear). A site for electrode placement in electrocochleography (ECochG) using the transtympanic needle technique.

propofol: An anesthetic agent often used with children. Propofol is commonly administered during light anesthesia for ABR assessment of young children when muscle activity may interfere with recording.

proximal: Toward the center or medial part of a structure (e.g., the axial central nervous system); for example, the proximal end of the eighth (auditory) cranial nerve enters the brainstem; opposite of distal.

PT: Patient; physical therapy.

pure tone: A single frequency tonal sound, e.g., 1000 Hz; a sinusoid.

pure-tone average (PTA): The average of hearing threshold levels, in dB, usually at test frequencies of 500, 1000, and 2000 Hz. These frequencies are in the speech frequency region.

qd: Every day (from the Latin *quaque die*).

qh: Every hour (from the Latin *quaque hora*).

qid: Four times a day (from the Latin *quarter in die*).

ramp: The onset or rise portion of a stimulus, usually a tone, is shaped or modified in some way, rather than immediately rising to maximum (peak) amplitude within the first portion of the stimulus. Nonlinear ramping equations, e.g., Blackman, Gaussian, Cosine[2], are generally preferred for tonal stimuli used to elicit auditory evoked responses.

rarefaction (negative) stimulus polarity: The initial displacement of the stimulus is negative-polarity, produced by a negative-voltage electrical signal and inward movement of an acoustic transducer (e.g. earphone) diaphragm. Often incorrectly pronounced as "rarefraction."

rate (stimulus): The number of stimulus repetitions per unit of time, usually within one second. The stimulus rate is inversely related to the interstimulus interval (ISI). That is, ISIs are smaller for higher stimulus presentation rates. A stimulus rates in the range of 21.1/sec to 33.1/sec are often used in auditory brainstem response measurement.

RDS: Respiratory distress syndrome.

recovery time: The time period immediately after a neural unit is depolarized (fires) during which it is unable to be activated. Recovery times on the order of milliseconds are typical for cranial nerve and brainstem auditory responses, whereas dentritic postsynaptic excitatory responses underlying cortical auditory evoked responses have recovery times of greater than 5 seconds.

recruitment: A term referring to abnormally rapid growth of loudness. In some patients with cochlear hearing impairment, as the intensity level of a sound increases the perception of loudness increases, relatively greater than normal.

reference electrode: Usually the secondary electrode in an electrode pair. The term is often used improperly. Most reference electrodes located on the scalp are, in fact, active in detecting a response and are not a true reference, or neutral, electrode. The so-called reference electrode (best referred to as the inverting electrode) in auditory brainstem response measurement is usually on the earlobe or mastoid of the stimulated ear. An electrode located at a location off the head, e.g., the nape of the neck, is a true reference electrode.

reliability: In evoked response measurement, the amount of agreement or similarity between multiple sequential averaged waveforms; often used interchangeably with the terms repeatability and reproducibility. High reliability implies greater confidence that the waveform is indeed a representative response for a patient, and not noise.

REM: Rapid eye movement.

repetitions: The number of stimuli presented in recording or averaging a single auditory evoked response waveform. The terms repetitions and sweeps are synonymous. The number of stimulus repetitions required in auditory evoked response measurement is dependent on a variety of factors, especially the size of the response (the neural signal) and the magnitude of electrical noise encountered during recording. An adequate number of stimulus repetitions produce an adequate signal-to-noise ratio (SNR), usually a ratio of about 2:1.

resolution: In evoked responses, the accuracy or precision in calculating latency or amplitude values, that is, the smallest time or amplitude difference that can be measured for given measurement settings. As a rule, greater resolution is desirable. Resolution is dependent on the number of data sample points and the analysis time used in recording an evoked response.

reticular activating system (formation): A complex, multisynaptic pathway in the central nervous system (e.g., medial brainstem) involved in consciousness and arousal. The RAS (RAF) plays a role in the generation of cortical (longer latency) evoked responses, such as the auditory middle latency response.

retrocochlear: Referring to the eighth cranial nerve, or central auditory nervous system pathways. Retrocochlear auditory dysfunction often refers only to dysfunction involving the eighth (auditory) nerve.

rise time: The initial portion of a stimulus (usually described in ms) from its beginning at baseline to maximum or close-to-maximum amplitude. Rise time may include negative- and positive-polarity displacement in a tone stimulus. *See* ramp.

rising: An audiogram configuration or shape with poorer hearing in the low frequencies improving to better hearing in the high-frequency region. Often reflects a conductive hearing impairment (when bone-conduction hearing is normal).

R/O: Rule out; to determine that a patient does not have a particular disorder.

rollover: A somewhat paradoxical decrease in performance (percent correct) scores for a speech audiometry procedure at highest stimulus intensity level versus maximum scores at a lower intensity level. Rollover of greater than 20 percent is often considered a sign of retrocochlear auditory dysfunction.

root mean square (RMS): A calculation used in describing stimulus intensity level. RMS is the square root of the mean of the squared pressure and takes into account energy in the sound wave throughout the waveform, not just at the peak. For a pure tone, RMS sound pressure = $1/\sqrt{2}$.

rostral: Toward the head; superior; for example, the cerebrum is rostral to the brainstem in the central nervous system; opposite of caudal.

round window: One of two openings in the bony wall of the inner ear connecting the inner ear to the middle ear. The round window, which is covered with a thin membrane, acts as a pressure release valve permitting movement of inner ear fluids with movement of the stapes footplate (see oval window).

s: Without (from the Latin *sine*).

saccule: A sensory structure in the vestibular system that can be activated by high-intensity sounds. Adequate stimulation of the utricle is the first step in the generation of the vestibular evoked myogenic potential (VEMP).

saturation: When a neural unit, such as an eighth nerve fiber, reaches maximum firing rate. Also, a decrease in output at high stimulus inputs.

sedation: Drug-induced sleep. Conscious sedation with controlled substances (drugs), such as chloral hydrate, is sometimes needed in auditory brainstem response measurement to reduce interference of movement-related artifact that can obscure the small bioelectric activity underlying the response. Medical institutions require adherence to a protocol for monitoring by properly credentialed personnel physiologic status (e.g., heart rate, oxygen saturation, blood pressure) during conscious sedation.

sensation level (SL): A unit of intensity level for an acoustic stimulus; dB above some measure of an individual person's hearing threshold level. A stimulus intensity of 70 dB SL in evoked response measurement, for example, is 70 dB above the person's behavioral threshold for the click stimulus.

sensitivity: An amplifier setting that is defined by the positive and negative voltage limits for incoming electrical activity; closely related to physiologic amplification (greater sensitivity is more amplification). With some evoked response instruments, sensitivity is expressed in terms of ± microvolts (μV), e.g., +25 to –25 microvolts. Greater sensitivity means more stringent voltage limits.

sensorineural: Hearing loss due to cochlear (sensory) or eighth nerve (neural) auditory dysfunction. Most hearing impairments described as sensorineural are actually just sensory. The term "nerve deafness" is often used inappropriately to describe sensory hearing loss due to common etiologies, such as exposure to high-intensity noise and aging. Also sometimes referred to as neurosensory.

sensory evoked response (SER): A general term for a brain response produced by sensory stimulation, either auditory (e.g., clicking or brief tonal sounds delivered to the ear), somatosensory (e.g., small electrical pulses delivered to a peripheral nerve), or visual (e.g., flashes or patterns of light delivered to the eye).

sevofluorane: An anesthestic agent commonly used with children.

sign(s): The finding on a diagnostic procedure. For example, an increase in the auditory brainstem response (ABR) wave I to V latency interval, may be a sign of retrocochlear auditory dysfunction.

signal: A term sometimes used interchangeably with stimulus. With this use of the term, a signal can be light, sound, or tactile energy that may or may not be effective as a stimulus for a biologic response. Also, with reference to a signal-to-noise ratio (SNR), a signal is an event that is being measured, such as an evoked response, in contrast to extraneous activity, such as background electrical noise.

signal detection: A process for determining the presence of an event (a signal) which is usually embedded within background activity (noise). Signal detection is a function of the size of the signal and the size of the noise. It is often verified statistically with a method such as the Fsp.

signal-to-noise ratio (SNR): The ratio of an electrical signal (e.g., auditory evoked response) to background (nonresponse) electrical activity (noise). A SNR of 2:1 is usually required for confident clinical identification of an ABR.

slope: The portion of a wave component between the peak and some measure of baseline activity, or a trough (before or after the peak).

sloping: A term used in describing the configuration of a pure-tone audiogram, that is, how hearing loss varies as a function of test frequency. A sloping configuration shows progressively greater hearing loss for higher test frequencies. A common audiogram pattern, a sloping hearing loss is often associated with age-related cochlear dysfunction.

slow negative 10 ms (SN10): A relatively large, gradual negative voltage wave occurring in the 10 ms region in an auditory brainstem response recording. An analysis period of 13, about 13 ms or more, and a high-pass frequency filter setting of less than about 100 Hz are required to record an SN10 component. Structures within the inferior colliculus may contribute to generation of the SN10 wave.

smooth(ing): Digital manipulation of an evoked response waveform in which voltages for a sequence of three or more data points are added together. Smoothing may reduce the noisy appearance of waveforms containing excessive high-frequency electrical activity and facilitate identification of major wave components.

snow: A term used to describe diffuse scattering of waveform data points that may result from some types of excessive electrical artifact.

SOAP: Subjective, objective, assessment, and plans. A format for preparing the report of patient history and physical examination.

sound level meter: A device for measuring and quantifying sound intensity level in decibels (dB) sound pressure level (SPL).

sound pressure level (SPL): The amount or intensity of a sound, such as an acoustic stimulus for evoked responses, expressed in decibels (dB); an intensity level of 0 dB SPL is the smallest amount of displacement of air molecules caused by a sound that can be just be detected by the human ear at a given frequency; a physical scale for intensity level. The normal hearing SPL decibel (dB) reference is 20 µpascals, i.e., dB SPL = 20 log (Po/Pref), where Po is observed instantaneous pressure and Pref = 20 µpascals.

S/P: Status post; the event leading to the current illness, e.g., the patient is examined S/P head injury.

spectral content: The frequency composition of an electrical or acoustical signal. *See* frequency specificity.

spectral splatter: Energy at frequencies about and below the intended frequency of a stimulus. With tone-burst stimulation of the ABR, certain ramping equations (e.g., Blackman) produce stimuli with less spectral splatter (more frequency specificity).

spectrum (spectral): The amount of energy as a function of frequency, that is, the frequency composition, for an electrical (e.g., evoked response) or acoustical (e.g., stimulus) signal.

speech audiometry: Measurement of a person's threshold for a speech signal (i.e., the lowest intensity level for detection or understanding of speech) or speech understanding ability. Speech audiometry can be carried out with word or sentence materials.

speech frequencies: Frequencies within the 500 to 2000 or 3000 Hz region, which are important for the perception of speech.

spike: A very sharp increase in electrical or acoustical energy. Electrical potentials recording from single neurons (units) may appear as spikes, but a spike or spiking in an averaged evoked response waveform is usually due to electrical interference.

spiral ganglion: The collection of cell bodies of afferent auditory nerve fibers found within the modiolus of the cochlea. The spiral ganglion occurs after the fibers leave the hair cells of the cochlea but before the fibers form the eighth nerve.

SPL: *See* sound pressure level.

somatosensory evoked response (SSER): Electrical activity from the somatosensory nervous system (usually median or posterior tibial nerve, spinal cord, brainstem, and parietal cortex) elicited by electrical stimulation at the wrist or ankle.

staggered spondaic word (SSW) test: A clinical dichotic word test of central auditory nervous system functioning.

standard (stimulus): With measurement of the mismatch negativity (MMN) response, the frequent stimulus is referred to as the standard, whereas the rare or infrequent stimulus is referred to as the deviant stimulus. The MMN response is a reflection of the brain's unconscious detection of a difference (i.e., mismatch) between the standard and the deviant stimulus.

standard deviation: Statistical measure of variability.

stapedius muscle: The smallest muscle in the human body, attached to the posterior portion of the neck of the stapes and innervated by a branch of the seventh (facial) cranial nerve. The stapedius muscle contracts in response to high-intensity sounds (*see* acoustic stapedial reflex).

stapes: Pronounced *staypeez*; a tiny, stirrup-shaped bone (ossicle) within the medial portion of the middle ear space connecting another ossicle (the incus) to the oval window of the cochlea.

stat: At once (from the Latin *statim*).

static compliance: A measure of the flexibility (or stiffness) of the middle ear system at rest (i.e., at atmospheric pressure and without contraction of the stapedius muscle), often made during routine clinical acoustic impedance (immittance) measurement.

sternocleidomastoid (SCM) muscle: One of the so-called strap muscles in the neck. Running from the sternum in the chest up the lateral portion of the neck to the mastoid bone (behind the ear), the SCM muscle is the site for the electrode in measurement of the vestibular evoked myogenic potential (VEMP).

stimulus: A form of sound, light, tactile, or electrical energy that is presented to an organism (such as a human). An effective stimulus (e.g., an abrupt sound or click) produces activity, a response, in the peripheral and central nervous system (e.g., the auditory brainstem response).

stylomastoid foramen: An opening near the mastoid bone, behind and below the ear, from which the facial nerve exits before it courses toward the face. Site of stimulation for electroneuronography (ENoG).

summating potential (SP): A cochlear electrical response appearing as a shoulder on the initial portion of the N1 (action potential) component in electrocochleography. The SP potential is generated mostly by the inner hair cells.

superior olivary complex (SOC): A major collection of nuclei (cell bodies) in the lower portion of the brainstem (pons) in the auditory central nervous system. The SOC is the first place in the auditory nervous system where there is neural interaction secondary to stimulation of each ear (binaural stimulation). The SOC contributes to generation of the auditory brainstem response.

symptom: Usually defined as a subjective indication of change in bodily function by a patient. A headache or a decrease in hearing are examples of symptoms. *See also* signs.

synapse: The juncture between two nerves. The axon of one neuron approaches the cell body or dentrite of another neuron. Neural transmission in the central nervous system depends on biochemical communication between two nerves occurring at synapses.

syndrome: A collection of signs and symptoms that characterize a disease.

synthetic sentence identification (SSI): A speech audiometry measure in which the patient hears nonsense sentences, one at a time, in the presence of an ongoing meaningful background message (a story about Davy Crockett). The task is to identify which sentence among a list of ten is heard while ignoring the competing message. Scores are reported as percent correct responses. SSI is a sensitive measure of central auditory functioning.

Sx: Symptoms.

T3, T4, T5, T6, T7, T8: 10–20 International electrode system electrode sites located on the scalp over the temporal lobe region (odd numbers on the left side and even numbers on the right side).

temperature: Reported in degrees Centigrade (C) or Fahrenheit (F). To convert degrees F to degrees C: C = 5 (degrees F − 32)/9. To convert degrees C to degrees F: F = (degrees C × 9)/5 + 32. Normal temperature is 37 degrees C and 98.6 degrees F.

temporal bone: A very hard skull bone enclosing the external ear canal, the middle and inner ear, and, within the internal auditory canal, the eighth (auditory) cranial nerve.

thalamus: A subcortical oval-shaped structure on each side of the central nervous system that serves as a major relay station for sensory pathways (auditory, visual, somatosensory) between the brainstem and cortex. The medial geniculate body, an important auditory structure, is located on the posterior portion of thalamus.

theta: Electroencephalogram (EEG) activity in the 4 to 7 Hz region. Amplitude is usually described as moderate (20 to 50 µvolts).

tid: Three times a day (from the Latin *ter in die*).

time delay: A time interval between presentation of a stimulus for an evoked response and the initiation of response averaging.

tinnitus: The perception of a noise in the ear (e.g., ringing, cricket sound, roaring) even when there is no external sound; a phantom sound. Tinnitus is not a disease but, rather, a symptom associated with many disorders of the auditory system.

TM: Tympanic membrane.

tone burst: A brief (usually less than 1 second) tone stimulus with no specific duration characteristics. Tone-burst stimuli are effective in eliciting an auditory brainstem response.

tone pip: A brief tone stimulus sometimes defined as one complete cycle of the tone in the rise, plateau, and fall portions of the stimulus. A 1000 Hz tone pip, for example, would have rise, duration, and fall times of 1 ms each.

topographic: The recording and display of evoked response information with multiple electrodes distributed across the scalp. In early topographic studies, the waveforms were depicted at each electrode site. Evoked response amplitude at varying electrode sites is typically displayed in colors or shades and is analogous to a topographic relief map showing peaks and valleys as different shades or colors. Computerized evoked response topography has been referred to as brain mapping.

TORCH: A collection of perinatal medical problems that are often associated with hearing impairment. Abbreviations refer to: T = toxoplasmosis; O = ophthalmalogic disease; R = rubella; C = cytomegalovirus; H = herpes.

tragus: The small protrusion of tissue just anterior to the opening (meatus) of the external ear canal.

transducer: An electroacoustic device for converting energy from one form to another. An earphone is a transducer that converts electrical energy to acoustic energy (sound).

transient: A very brief duration (e.g., 0.1 ms) sound with almost instantaneous onset that is effective in eliciting short latency auditory evoked responses, e.g., the ABR.

transtympanic: An approach in electrocochleography (ECochG) for placement of a needle electrode on the promontory of the ear (bony medial wall of the middle ear space, i.e., the outer wall of the inner ear).

trapezoid body: An auditory brainstem pathway crossing from one side to the other. The first (most caudal) such decussation (crossing) in the auditory system, the trapezoid body is located in the pons.

trigger: An electrical signal (usually a pulse) that activates a device synchronously with another device. Evoked response systems are triggered to begin averaging with the presentation of a stimulus.

tympanogram: A measure of tympanic membrane mobility as a function of air pressure changes within the ear canal.

UE: Upper extremity.

unilateral: Pertaining to one side. A patient with a unilateral hearing loss has a hearing loss in one ear but not the other ear.

universal newborn hearing screening (UNHS): Hearing screening of all babies in a defined area (e.g., state, province, country).

validity (valid): How closely a measure actually reflects what is being measured. When a measurement produces the desired results. A valid auditory evoked response is one that accurately reflects underlying neurophysiologic status.

VD: Venereal disease.

VDRL: Venereal disease research laboratory; test for VD.

VEMP (vestibular evoked myogenic potential): A change in activity in the sternocleidomastoid muscle with high-intensity acoustic stimulation of saccule.

VER (visual evoked response): Activity in visual organs (e.g., retina), pathways (e.g. optic nerve and tracts), and centers of the brain (e.g., calcarine fissure in occipital lobe) that is elicited by photic (light) stimuli and recorded with electrodes, usually on the scalp. The typical VER occurs within a 250 ms period following stimulation.

versed: A conscious sedative sometimes used with children undergoing auditory brainstem response assessment.

vertex: A location on top of the head, in the center, defined as the intersection of lines constructed from one external ear canal to the other and from front to back along the midline (from nasion to inion). The vertex is a common electrode site in evoked response measurement.

vertigo: A balance (specifically vestibular) symptom. The patient experiences a spinning sensation or senses that the environment is spinning around him or her.

volume conduction: Instantaneous transmission or conduction of electrical activity from a neural generator through a medium (such as brain tissue and water) to a relatively distant point. For example, the auditory brainstem response is volume conducted from deep within the brainstem through the surrounding brain tissue, cranial bone and scalp to electrodes located on the outside of the head.

von Recklinghausen's disease: Another term for neurofibromatosis, a neuropathologic disease that is characterized by tumors within the central nervous system. The tumors may involve one or both eighth (auditory) cranial nerves and cause auditory evoked response abnormalities.

wave: A bump or deflection of voltage in an evoked response recording. A wave (component) is usually attributed to bioelectric activity (action potential or dentritic activity) of one or more neural generators.

wave I: Often the first component in an auditory brainstem response recording, normally occurring at about 1.5 ms for a high-intensity click stimulus and generated in the distal region of the eighth cranial nerve.

wave III: An auditory brainstem response component normally occurring at about 3.5 ms for a high-intensity click stimulus and generated within the lower (pons) portion of the auditory brainstem.

wave V: An auditory brainstem response component normally occurring at about 5.5 msec for a high-intensity click stimulus and generated within the upper (pons or midbrain) portion of the auditory brainstem.

waveform: An evoked response recording consisting of a series of waves or fluctuations in voltage. Each type of auditory evoked response has a characteristic normal waveform.

WF: White female.

WM: White male.

WNL: Within normal limits.

Z: Symbol in 10–20 International system for electrode nomenclature that is used for any electrode along the midline of the scalp.

Aaltonen, O., Eerola, O., Lang, A. H., Uusipaikka, E., & Tuomainen, J. (1994). Automatic discrimination of phonetically relevant and irrelevant vowel parameters as reflected by mismatch negativity. *Journal of the Acoustical Society of America, 96,* 1489–1493.

Aaltonen, O., Niemi, P., Nyrke, T., & Tuhkanen, M. (1987). Event-related brain potentials and the perception of phonetic continuum. *Biological Psychiatry, 24,* 197–207.

Aaltonen, O., Tuomainen, J., Laine, M., & Niemi, P. (1993). Cortical differences in tonal versus vowel processing as revealed by an ERP component called mismatch negativity (MMN). *Brain and Language, 44,* 139–152.

Abbas, P., & Brown, C. (1991a). Electrically evoked auditory brainstem response: Growth of response with current levels. *Hearing Research, 51,* 123–138.

Abbas, P., & Brown, C. (1991b). Electrically evoked auditory brainstem response: Refractory properties and strength-duration functions. *Hearing Research, 51,* 139–148.

Abbas, P., Brown, C., Shallop, J., Firszt, J., Hughes, M., Hong, S., & Staller, S. (1999). Summary of results using the Nucleus CI24M implant to record the electrically evoked compound action potential. *Ear and Hearing, 20,* 45–59.

Abbas, P., & Gorga, M. P. (1981). AP responses in forward-masking paradigms and their relationship to responses of auditory-nerve fibers. *Journal of the Acoustical Society of America, 69,* 492–499.

Abbas, P., Hughes, M., Brown, C., & Miller, C. (2004). Channel interaction in cochlear implant users evaluated using the electrically evoked compound action potential. *Audiology & Neuro-Otology, 9,* 203–213.

Abbate, C., Giorgianni, C., Munao, F., & Brecciaroli, R. (1993). Neurotoxicity induced by exposure to toluene. An electrophysiologic study. *International Archives of Occupational and Environmental Health, 64,* 389–392.

Abdala, C., & Folsom, R. (1995). Frequency contribution to the click-evoked auditory brain-stem response in human adults and infants. *Journal of the Acoustical Society of America, 97,* 2394–2404.

Abe, M. (1954). Electrical responses of the human brain to acoustic stimulus. *Tohoku Journal of Experimental Medicine, 60,* 47–58.

Abrahamian, H. A., Allison, T., Goff, W. R., & Rosner, B. S. (1963). Effects of thiopental on human cerebral evoked responses. *Anesthesiology, 24,* 650–657.

Abramovich, S. J., & Billings, R. (1981). Cochlear and brainstem auditory evoked potential recording in patients with unilateral sensorineural hearing loss. *Journal of Laryngology & Otology, 95,* 925–930.

Abramovich, S. J., Gregory, S., Slemick, M., & Stewart, A. (1979). Hearing loss in very low birthweight infants treated with neonatal intensive care. *Archives of Diseases in Children, 54,* 421–426.

Abramovich, S., & Prasher, D. K. (1986). Electrocochleography and brainstem potentials in Ramsay Hunt syndrome. *Archives of Otolaryngology—Head & Neck Surgery, 112,* 925–928.

Abramson, M., Stein, B. M., Pedley, T. A., Emerson, R. G., & Wazen, J. J. (1985). Intraoperative BAER monitoring and hearing preservation in the treatment of acoustic neuromas. *Laryngoscope, 95,* 1318–1321.

Abubakr, A., & Wambacq, I. (2003). The localizing value of auditory event-related potentials (P300) in patients with medically intractable temporal lobe epilepsy. *Epilepsy & Behavior, 4,* 692–701.

Acevedo, J. C., Sindou, M., Fischer, C., & Vial, C. (1997). Microvascular decompression for the treatment of hemifacial spasm. Retrospective study of a consecutive series of 75 operated patients—electrophysi-

ologic and anatomical surgical analysis. *Stereotactic and Functional Neurosurgery, 68,* 260–265

Achor, L. J., & Starr, A. (1980). Auditory brainstem responses in the cat: I. Intracranial and extracranial recordings. *Electroencephalography and Clinical Neurophysiology, 48,* 172–174.

Ackley, R., Tamaki, C., Oliszewski, C., & Inverso, D. (2004, September). Vestibular evoked myogenic potentials in deaf and hard of hearing subjects. *Insights in Practice: Clinical Topics in Otoneurology, 1–7.*

Adams, D., Watson, D. R., & McClelland, R. J. (1982). *The effects of diazepam on the auditory evoked brainstem potentials.* Paper presented at the Second International Symposium on Evoked Potentials, Cleveland, OH.

Adler, G., & Adler, J. (1989). Influence of stimulus intensity of AER components in the 80- to 200-millisecond latency range. *Audiology, 28,* 316–324.

Adler, L. E., Gerhardt, G. A., Franks, R., Baker, N., Nagamoto, H., Drebing, C., & Freeman, R. (1990). Sensory physiology and catecholamines in schizophrenia and mania. *Psychiatry Research, 31,* 297–309.

Adler, L. E., Olincy, A., Cawthra, E. M., McRae, K. A., Harris, J. G., Nagamoto, H. T., Waldo, M. C., Hall, M. H., Bowles, A., Woodward, L., Ross, R. G., & Freedman, R. (2004). Varied effects of atypical neuroleptics on P50 auditory gating in schizophrenia patients. *American Journal of Psychiatry, 161,* 1822–1828.

Adler, L. E., Olincy, A., Waldo, M., Harris, J. G., Griffith, J., Stevens, K., Flach, K., Nagamoto, H., Bickford, P., Leonard, S., & Freedman, R. (1998). Schizophrenia, sensory gating, and nicotinic receptors. *Schizophrenia Bulletin, 24,* 189–202.

Adler, L. E., Pachtman, E., Franks, R. D., Pecevich, M., Waldo, M. C., & Freedman, R. (1982). Neurophysiological evidence for a defect in neuronal mechanisms involved in sensory gating in schizophrenia. *Biological Psychiatry, 17,* 639–654.

Adour, K. K., Sheldon, M. I., & Kahn, Z. M. (1980). Maximal nerve excitability testing versus neuromyography: Prognostic value in patients with facial paralysis. *Laryngoscope, 90,* 1540–1547.

Adrian, E. D. (1930). The activity of the nervous system of the caterpillar. *Journal of Physiology, 30,* 34–36.

Agrawal, V., Shukla, R., Misra, P., Kapoor, R., & Malik, G. (1998). Brainstem auditory evoked response in newborns with hyperbilirubinemia. *Indian Pediatrics, 35,* 513–518.

Aguilar, E. A., Hall, J. W., III, & Mackey-Hargadine, J. R. (1986). Neurootologic evaluation of the acute severely head-injured patient: Correlation among physical findings, auditory evoked responses and computerized tomography. *Archives of Otolaryngology—Head & Neck Surgery, 94,* 211–219.

Aguirre, M., & Broughton, R. J. (1987). Complex event-related potentials (P300 and CNV) and MSLT in the assessment of excessive daytime sleepiness in narcolepsy-cataplexy. *Electroencephalography and Clinical Neurophysiology, 67,* 298–316.

Ahveninen, J., Jääskeläinen, I. P., Pekkonen, E., Hallberg, A., Hietanen, M., Näätänen, R., & Sillanaukee, P. (2001). Global field power of auditory N1 correlates with impaired verbal-memory performance in human alcoholics. *Neuroscience Letters, 285,* 131–134.

Ahveninen, J., Jääskeläinen, I. P., Pekkonen, E., Hallberg, A., Hietanen, M., Näätänen, R., & Sillanaukee, P. (1999). Post-withdrawal changes in middle-latency auditory evoked potentials in abstinent human alcoholics. *Neuroscience Letters, 268,* 57–60.

Ainslie, P. J., & Boston, J. R. (1980). Comparison of auditory evoked potentials for monaural and binaural stimuli. *Electroencephalography and Clinical Neurophysiology, 49,* 291–302.

Akaboshi, S., Tomita, Y., Suzuki, Y., Une, M., Sohma, O., Takashima, S., & Takeshita, K. (1997). Peroxisomal bifunctional enzyme deficiency: Serial neurophysiological examinations of a case. *Brain and Development, 19,* 295–299.

Akin, F., & Murnane, O. (2001). Vestibular evoked myogenic potentials: Preliminary report. *Journal of the American Academy of Audiology, 12,* 445–452.

Akin, F., Murnane, O., & Proffitt, T. (2003). The effects of click and toneburst stimulus parameters on the vestibular evoked myogenic potential (VEMP). *Journal of the American Academy of Audiology, 14,* 500–509.

Akiyama, Y., Schutze, F. J., Schultz, M. A., & Parmalee, A. H. (1969). Acoustically evoked responses in premature and full term newborn infants. *Electroencephalography and Clinical Neurophysiology, 26,* 371–380.

Alain, C., & Woods, D. L. (1997). Attention modulates auditory pattern memory as indexed by event-related brain potentials. *Psychophysiology, 34,* 534–546.

Alain, C., Woods, D. L., & Covarrubias, D. (1997). Activation of duration-sensitive auditory cortical fields in humans. *Electroencephalography and Clinical Neurophysiology, 104,* 531–539.

Alain, C., Woods, D. L., & Knight, R. T. (1998). A distributed cortical network for auditory sensory memory in humans. *Brain Research, 812,* 23–37.

Alain, C., Woods, D. L., & Ogawa, K. H. (1994). Brain indices of automatic pattern processing. *Neuroreport, 6,* 140–144.

Alexander, J., Bauer, L. O., Kuperman, S., Morzorati, S., O'Connor, S. J., Rohrbaugh, J., Porjesz, B., Begleiter, H., & Polich, J. (1996). Hemispheric differences for P300 amplitude from an auditory oddball task. *International Journal of Psychophysiology, 21,* 189–196.

Alexander, J., & Polich, J. (1997). Handedness and P300 from auditory stimuli. *Brain and Cognition, 35,* 259–270.

Alexander, J., Polich, J., Bloom, F., Bauer, L., Kuperman, S., Rohrbaugh, J., Morzorati, S., O'Connor, S., Porjesz, B., & Begleiter, H. (1994). P300 from an auditory oddball task: Inter-laboratory consistency. *International Journal of Psychophysiology, 17,* 35–46.

Alexander, M., Thomas, S., Mohan, P., & Narendranathan, M. (1995). Prolonged brainstem auditory evoked potential latencies in tropical pancreatic diabetics with normal hearing. *Electromyography and Clinical Neurophysiology, 35,* 95–98.

Alho, K., Paavilainen, P., Reinikainen, K., Sams, & Näätänen, R. (1986). Separability of different negative components of the event-related potential associated with auditory stimulus processing. *Psychophysiology, 23,* 613–623.

Alho, K., Sainio, K., Sajaniemi, N., Reinikainen, K., & Näätänen, R. (1990). Event-related brain potential of human newborns to pitch change of an acoustic stimulus. *Electroencephalography and Clinical Neurophysiology, 77,* 151–155.

Alho, K., Sams, M., Paavilainen, P., & Näätänen, R. (1986). Small pitch separation and the selective-attention effect on the ERP. *Psychophysiology, 23,* 189–197.

Alho, K., Tervaniemi, M., Huotilainen, M., Lavikainen, J., Tiitinen, H., Ilmoniemi, R. J., Knuutila, J., & Näätänen, R. (1996). Processing of complex sounds in the human auditory cortex as revealed by magnetic brain responses. *Psychophysiology 33,* 369–375.

Alho, K., Woods, D. L., Algazi, A., Knight, R. T., and Näätänen, R. (1994). Lesions of frontal cortex diminish the auditory mismatch negativity. *Electroencephalography & Clinical Neurophysiology, 91,* 353–362.

Alho, K., Woods, D. L., Algazi, A., & Näätänen, R. (1992). Intermodal selective attention: II. Effects of attentional load on processing auditory and visual stimuli in central space. *Electroencephalography and Clinical Neurophysiology, 82,* 356–368.

Allison, R. S., & Millar, J. H. D. (1954). Prevalence and familial incidence of disseminated sclerosis: A report to the Northern Hospitals Authority on the result of a three-year survey. *Ulster Medical Journal, 23,* 1–92.

Allison, T., Wood, C. C., & Goff, W. R. (1983). Brain stem auditory, pattern-reversal visual, and short-latency somatosensory evoked potentials: Latencies in relation to age, sex, and brain and body size. *Electroencephalography and Clinical Neurophysiology, 55,* 619–636.

Almadori, G., Ottaviani, F., Paludetti, G., Rosignoli, M., Gallucci, L., D'Alatri, L., & Vergoni, G. (1988). Auditory brainstem responses in noise-induced permanent hearing loss. *Audiology, 27,* 36–41.

Alonso-Prieto, E., Alvarez-Gonzalez, M. A., Fernandez-Concepcion, O., & Jimenez-Conde, A. (2002). [Usefulness of P300 as a tool for diagnosing alterations in sustained attention in ischemic cerebrovascular disease]. *Review of Neurology, 34,* 1105–1109.

Amadeo, M., & Shagass, C. (1973). Brief latency click evoked potentials during waking and sleep in man. *Psychophysiology 10,* 244–250.

Amantini, A., Rossi, L., de Scisciolo, G., & Bindi, A., et al. (1984). Auditory evoked potentials (early, middle, late components) and audiological tests in Friedreich's ataxia. *Electroencephalography and Clinical Neurophysiology, 58,* 37–47.

Amatuzzi, M. G., Northrop, C., Liberman, M. C., Thornton, A., Halpin, C., Herrmann, B., Pinto, L. E., Saenz, A., Carranza, A., & Eavey, R. D. (2001). Selective inner hair cell loss in premature infants and cochlea pathological patterns from neonatal intensive care unit autopsies. *Archives of Otolaryngology—Head & Neck Surgery, 127,* 629–636.

Ambrosini, A., De Pasqua, V., Afra, J., Sandor, P. S., & Schoenen, J. (2001). Reduced gating of middle-latency auditory evoked potentials (P50) in migraine patients: Another indication of abnormal sensory processing? *Neuroscience Letters, 306,* 132–134.

Amenedo, E., & Diaz, F. (1998). Effects of aging on middle-latency auditory evoked potentials: A cross-sectional study. *Biological Psychiatry, 43,* 210–219.

American Academy of Pediatrics Task Force on Newborn and Infant Hearing. (1999). Newborn and infant hearing loss: Detection and Intervention. *Pediatrics, 103,* 527–529.

American National Standards Institute (ANSI). (1960). *American national standard acoustical terminology (S1.1).* New York: Acoustical Society of America.

American Psychiatric Association. (1980). *Diagnostic and statistical manual of mental disorders (DSM III)* (3rd ed.). Arlington VA: American Psychiatric Publishing.

Amin, S. B., Orlando, M. S., Dalzell, L. E., Merle, K. S., & Guillet, R. (1999). Morphological changes in serial auditory brain stem responses in 24 to 32 weeks' gestational age infants during the first week of life. *Ear and Hearing, 20,* 410–418.

Anand, N., Gupta, A., & Raj, H. (1991). Auditory brainstem response in neonates with hypoxic-ischemic-encephalopathy following preinatal asphyxia. *Indian Pediatrics, 28,* 901–907.

Anderer, P., Semlitsch, H. V., & Saletu, B. (1996). Multichannel auditory event-related brain potentials: Effects of normal aging on the scalp distribution of N1, P2, N2 and P300 latencies and amplitudes. *Electroencephalography and Clinical Neurophysiology. 99,* 458–472.

Anderson, D. C., Bundlie, S., & Rockswold, G. L. (1984). Multimodality evoked potentials in closed head trauma. *Archives of Neurology, 41,* 369–374.

Anderson, D. J., Rose, J. E., Hind, J. E., & Brugge, J. F. (1971). Temporal position of discharges in single auditory nerve fibers within the cyle of a sine-wave stimulus: Frequency and intensity effects. *Journal of the Acoustical Society of America, 49,* 1131–1139.

Anderson, H., Barr, B., & Wedenberg, E. (1970). Early diagnosis of VIIIth-nerve tumours by acoustic reflex tests. *Acta Otolaryngologica (Supplement), 263,* 232–237.

Anft, D., Jamali, Y., Scholz, G., & Mrowinski, D. (2001). Electrocochleography and phase audiometry in diagnosis of Ménière's disease. *HNO, 49,* 102–108.

Annett, M. (1970). A classification of hand preference by association analysis. *British Journal of Psychology, 61,* 303–321.

Anteby, I., Hafner, H., Pratt, H., & Uri, N. (1986). Auditory brainstem evoked potentials in evaluating the central effects of middle ear effusion. *International Journal of Pediatrics, 12,* 1.

Antinoro, F., Skinner, P. H., & Jones, J. J. (1969). Relation between sound intensity and amplitude of the AER at different stimulus frequencies. *Journal of the Acoustical Society of America, 46,* 1433–1436.

Antonelli, A. R., Bellotto, R., & Grandori, F. (1987). Audiologic diagnosis of central versus eighth nerve and cochlear auditory impairment. *Audiology, 26,* 209–226.

Antonelli, A. R., Bonfioli, F., Cappiello, J., Peretti, G., Zanetti, D., & Capra, R. (1988). Auditory evoked potentials test battery related to magnetic resonance imaging for multiple sclerosis patients: Evaluation of test findings and assessment of diagnostic criteria. *Scandinavian Audiology (Supplement), 33,* 191–196.

Antonelli, A., & Grandori, F. (1984). Some aspects of the auditory nerve responses evoked by tone bursts. *British Journal of Audiology, 18,* 117–126.

Anyanwu, E., Campbell, A. W., & High, W. (2002). Brainstem auditory evoked response in adolescents with acoustic mycotic neuroma due to environmental exposure to toxic molds. *International Journal of Adolescent Medicine & Health, 14,* 67–76.

Aoyagi, M., Kim, Y., Yokoyama, J., Kiren, T., Suzuki, Y., & Koike, Y. (1990). Head size as a basis of gender difference in the latency of the brainstem auditory-evoked response. *Audiology, 29,* 107–112.

Aoyagi, M., Suzuki, Y., Yokota, M., Furuse, H., Watanabe, T., & Ito, T. (1999). Reliability of 80-Hz amplitude-modulation-following response detected by phase coherence. *Audiology & Neuro-Otology, 4,* 28–37.

Aoyagi, M., Yokota, M., Nakamura, T., Tojima, H., Kim, Y., Suzuki, Y., et al. (1994). Hearing preservation and improvement of auditory brainstem response findings after acoustic neuroma surgery. *Acta Otolaryngologica, 511,* 40–46.

Arakawa, K. (1998). Summating potential evoked by long-tone burst stimuli in Ménière's disease. *Nippon Jiblinkoka Gakkai Kaiho, 101,* 53–62.

Aran, J. M. (1971). The electro-cochleogram: Recent results in children and in some pathological cases. *Archives of Klinikum Experimental Ohren-, Nasen- und Kehlkopfheilkunde, 198,* 128–141.

Aran, J. M., & Charlet de Sauvage, R. (1976). Clinical value of cochlear microphonic recordings. In R. J. Ruben, C. Eberling, & G. Salomon (Eds.), *Electrocochleography* (pp. 55–65). Baltimore: University Park Press.

Aran, J. M., & LeBert, G. (1968). Les responses nerveuses cochleaires chez l'homme. Image du functionment de l'oreille et nouveau test d'audiometrie objective. *Revue de Laryngologie, 89,* 361.

Aran, J. M., Portmann, C., Delaunay, J., Pelerin, J., & Lenoir, J. (1969). L'electro-cochleogramme: Methodes et premiers resultas chez l'enfant. *Revue de Laryngologie, 90,* 615.

Arciniegas, D., Olincy, A., Topkoff, J., McRae, K., Cawthra, E., Filley, C. M., Reite, M., & Adler, L. E. (2000). Impaired auditory gating and P50 nonsuppression following traumatic brain injury. *Journal of Neuropsychiatry & Clinical Neuroscience, 12,* 77–85.

Arehole, S. (1995). A preliminary study of the relationship between long latency response and learning disorder. *British Journal of Audiology, 29,* 295–298.

Arenberg, I. K., Ackley, R. S., Ferraro, J., & Muchnik, C. (1988). EcoG results in perilymphatic fistula: Clinical and experimental studies. *Otolaryngology—Head & Neck Surgery, 99,* 435–443.

Arenberg, I. K., Gibson, W. P. R., Bohlen, H. K. H., & Best, L. (1989). An overview of diagnostic and intraoperative electrocochleography for inner ear disease. *Insights in Otolaryngology, 4,* 1–6.

Arenberg, I. K., Kobayashi, H., Obert, A. D., & Gibson, W. P. (1993). Intraoperative electrocochleography of endolymphatic hydrops surgery using clicks and tone bursts. *Acta Otolaryngologica Supplement, 504,* 58–67.

Arezzo, J., Pickoff, A., & Vaughan, H. G., Jr. (1975). The sources and intracerebral distribution of auditory evoked potentials in the alert rhesus monkey. *Brain Research, 90,* 57–73.

Arikan, M., Devrim, M., Oran, O., Inan, S., Elhih, M., & Demiralp, T. (1999). Music effects on event-related potentials of humans on the basis of cultural environment. *Neuroscience, 268,* 21–24.

Arinami, T., Kondo, I., Hamaguchi, H., Tamura, K., & Hirano, T. (1988). Auditory brainstem responses in the fragile X syndrome. *American Journal of Human Genetics, 43,* 46–51.

Arlinger, S. D. (1977). Auditory processing of frequency ramps. *Audiology, 16,* 480–486.

Arlinger, S. D. (1981). Technical aspects of stimulation, recording, and signal processing. *Scandinavian Audiology, 13,* 41–53.

Arlinger, S. D., & Kylen, P. (1977). Bone-conducted stimulation in electrocochleography. *Acta Otolaryngologica, 84,* 377–384.

Arriaga, M., Chen, D., & Fukushima, T. (1997). Individualizing hearing preservation in acoustic neuroma surgery. *Laryngoscope, 107,* 1043–1047.

Arsenault, M. D,. & Benitez, J. T. (1991). Electrocochleography: A method for making the Stypulkowski-Staller electrode and testing technique. *Ear and Hearing, 12,* 358–360.

Arslan, E., Prosser, S., & Michelini, S. (1981). The auditory brainstem response to binaural delayed stimuli in man. *Scandinavian Audiology, 13,* 75–81.

Asai, H., & Mori, N. (1989). Change in the summating potential and action potential during the fluctuating of hearing in Ménière's disease. *Scandinavian Audiology, 18,* 13–17.

Aso, S. (1990). [Clinical electrocochleography in Ménière's disease]. *Nippon Jibiinkoka Gakkai Kaiho, 93,* 1093–1105.

Aso, S., & Gibson, W. P. (1994). Electrocochleography in profoundly deaf children: Comparison of promontory and round window techniques. *American Journal of Otology, 15,* 376–379.

Aso, S., Watanabe, Y., & Mizukoshi, K. (1991). A clinical study of electrocochleography in Ménière's disease. *Acta Otolaryngologica, 111,* 44–52.

Atienza, M., & Cantero, J. L. (2001). Complex sound processing during human REM sleep by recovering information from long-term memory as revealed by the mismatch negativity (MMN). *Brain Research, 90,* 151–160.

Atienza, M., Cantero, J. L., & Dominguez-Marin, E. (2002). Mismatch negativity (MMN): An objective measure of sensory memory and long-lasting memories during sleep. *International Journal of Psychophysiology, 46,* 215–225.

Atienza, M., Cantero, J., & Escera, C. (2001). Auditory information processing during human sleep as revealed by event-related brain potentials. *Clinical Electroencephalography, 112,* 2031–2045.

Ayerbe, I., Ucelay, I., Portmann, D., Negrevergne, M., & Bovard, D. (1991). [Cochlea-vestibular syndrome disclosing dolicho-ectasis of the basilar trunk and vertebral artery.]. *Revue Laryngologie Otologie et Rhinologie (Bord), 112,* 165–168.

Azumi, T., Nakashima, K., & Takahashi, K. (1995). Aging effects on auditory middle latency responses. *Electromyography and Clinical Neurophysiology, 35,* 397–401.

Azzena, C. B., Conti, G., Santarelli, R., Ottaviani, F., Paludetti, G., & Maurizi, M. (1995). Generation of human auditory steady-state responses (SSRs). I: Stimulus rate effects. *Hearing Research, 83,* 1–8.

Babkoff, H., Pratt, H., & Kempinski, D. (1984). Auditory brainstem evoked potential latency-intensity functions: A corrective algorithm. *Hearing Research, 16,* 243–249.

Bacon, S. P., & Vermeister, N. F. (1985). Temporal modulation transfer function in normal-hearing and hearing-impaired listeners. *Audiology, 24,* 117–134.

Baiocco, F., Testa, D., d'Angelo, A., & Cocchini, F. (1984). Abnormal auditory evoked potentials in Dejerine-Sottas disease: Report of two cases with central acoustic and vestibular impairment. *Journal of Neurology, 231,* 46–49.

Baldeweg, T., Williams, J. D., & Gruzelier, J. H. (1999). Differential changes in frontal and sub-temporal components of mismatch negativity. *International Journal of Psychophysiology, 33,* 143–148.

Baldwin, R. L., & LeMaster, K. (1989). Neurofibromatosis-2 and bilateral acoustic neuromas: Distinctions from neurofibromatosis-1 (Von Recklinghausen's disease). *The American Journal of Otology, 10,* 439–442.

Baldy-Moulinier, M., Rondouin, G., Touchon, J., Billiard, M., Zinszner, J., & Cadihac, J. (1984). Brain-stem auditory evoked potentials in the assessment of the transient ischemic attacks of the arterial vertebrobasilar system. *Monograph of Neurological Science, 11,* 216–221.

Balfour, P., Pillion, J., & Gaskin, A. (1998). Distortion product otoacoustic emission and auditory brain stem response measures of pediatric sensorineural hearing loss with islands of normal sensitivity. *Ear and Hearing, 19,* 463–472.

Balkany, T. J., Downs, M. P., Jafek, B. W., & Krajicek, M. J. (1979). Hearing loss in Down's syndrome: A treatable handicap more common than generally recognized. *Clinical Pediatrics, 18,* 116–118.

Bancaud, J., Bloch, V., & Paillard, J. (1953). Contribution of E.E.G. a l'etude des potentiels evoques chez l'homme au niveau du vertex. *Revue Neurologie, 89,* 399–418.

Banerjee, A., Whyte, A. & Atlas, M. D. (2005). Superior canal dehiscence: Review of a new condition. *Clinical Otolaryngology, 30,* 9–15.

Bank, J. (1991). Brainstem auditory evoked potentials in migraine after Rausedyl provocation. *Cephalalgia, 11,* 277–279.

Bao, X., & Wong, V. (1998). Brainstem auditory-evoked potential evaluation in children with meningitis. *Pediatric Neurology, 19,* 109–112.

Barajas, J. J. (1985). Brainstem response auditory as subjective and objective test for neurological diagnosis. *Scandinavian Audiology, 14,* 57–62.

Barajas, J. J., Fernandez, R., & Bernal, M. R. (1988). Middle latency and 40 Hz auditory evoked responses in normal hearing children: 500 Hz thresholds. *Scandinavian Audiology (Supplement), 30,* 99–104.

Baran, J. A., Bothfeldt, R. W., & Musiek, F. E. (2004). Central auditory deficits associated with compromise of the primary auditory cortex. *Journal of the American Academy of Audiology, 15,* 106–116.

Baran, J. A., Catherwood, K. P., & Musiek, F. E. (1995). "Negative" ABR findings in an individual with a large brainstem tumor: Hit or miss? *Journal of the American Academy of Audiology, 6,* 211–216.

Baran, J. A., Musiek, F., Long, R. R., & Ommaya, A. (1988). Topographic mapping of brain electrical activity in the assessment of central auditory nervous system pathology. *American Journal of Otology, 9,* 72–76.

Baranak, C. C., Marsh, R. R., & Potsic, W. P. (1984). Sedation in brainstem response audiometry. *International Journal of Pediatric Otorhinolaryngology, 8,* 55–59.

Bar-Haim, Y., Marshall, P. J., Fox, N. A., Schorr, E. A., & Gordon-Salant, S. (2003). Mismatch negativity in socially withdrawn children. *Biological Psychiatry, 54,* 17–24.

Barkovich, A. J., Wippold, F. J., & Brammer, R. E. (1986). False-negative MR imaging of an acoustic neuroma. *American Journal of Neuroradiology, 7,* 363–364.

Barnet, A., & Goodwin, R. S. (1965). Averaged evoked electroencephalographic responses to sound. *Electroencephalography and Clinical Neurophysiology, 18,* 441–450.

Barnet, A., & Lodge, A. (1967). Diagnosis of hearing loss in infancy by means of EEG audiometry. *Clinical Proceedings of Children's Hospital in Washington, D.C., 23,* 1–18.

Barnet, A., Ohlrich, E. S., Weiss, I. P., & Shanks, B. (1975). Auditory evoked potentials during sleep in normal children from ten days to three years of age. *Electroencephalography and Clinical Neurophysiology, 39,* 29–41.

Barnett, S. B. (1980). The influence of ultrasound and temperature on the cochlear microphonic response following a round window irradiation. *Acta Otolaryngologica, 90,* 32–39.

Barratt, H. (1980). Investigations of the mastoid electrode contribution to brain stem auditory evoked response. *Scandinavian Audiology, 9,* 203–211.

Barrett, G., Nehshige, R., & Shibasaki, H. (1987). Human auditory and somatosensory event-related potentials: Effects of response condition and age. *Electroencephalography and Clinical Neurophysiology, 66,* 409–419.

Barrs, D., Brackmann, D., Olson, J. E., & House, W. F. (1985). Changing concepts of acoustic tumor diagnosis. *Archives of Otolaryngology, 111,* 17–21.

Barrs, D., Luxford, W., Becker, T. S., & Brackmann, D. (1984). Computed tomography with gas cisternography for detection of small acoustic tumors. *Archives of Otolaryngology, 110,* 535–537.

Barry, R. J., Johnstone, S. J., & Clarke, A. R. (2003). A review of electrophysiology in attention-deficit/hyperactivity disorder: II. Event-related potentials. *Clinical Neurophysiology, 114,* 184–198.

Bartel, D. R., Markand, O. N., & Kolar, O. J. (1983). The diagnosis and classification of multiple sclerosis: Evoked responses and spinal fluid electrophoresis. *Neurology, 33,* 611–617.

Barth, P., Wanders, R., Schutgens, R., Bleeker-Wagemakers, E., & van Heemstra, D. (1990). Peroxisomal oxidation defect with detectable peroxisomes: A case with neonatal onset and progressive course. *European Journal of Paediatrics, 149,* 722–726.

Bartnik, E. A., Blinowska, K. J., & Durka, P. J. (1992). Single evoked potential reconstruction by means of wavelet transform. *Biological Cybernetics, 67,* 175–181.

Basar, E., Gonder, A., & Ungan, P. (1976a). Important relation between EEG and brain evoked potentials: I. Resonance phenomena in subdural structures of the cat brain. *Biological Cybernetics, 25,* 27–40.

Basar, E., Gonder, A., & Ungan, P. (1976b). Important relation between EEG and brain evoked potentials: II. A systems analysis of electrical signals from the human brain. *Biological Cybernetics, 25,* 41–48.

Basta, D., Todt, I., & Ernst, A. (2005). Normative data for P1/N1-latencies of vestibular evoked myogenic potentials induced by air- or bone-conducted tone bursts. *Clinical Neurophysiology, 116,* 2216–2219.

Bastuji, H., & García-Larrea, L. (1999). Evoked potentials as a tool for the investigation of human sleep. *Sleep Medical Review, 3,* 23–45.

Bastuji, H., García-Larrea, L., Franc, C., & Mauguiere, F. (1995). Brain processing of stimulus deviance during slow-wave and paradoxical sleep: A study of human auditory evoked responses using the oddball paradigm. *Journal of Clinical Neurophysiology, 12,* 155–167.

Bastuji, H., Perrin, F., & García-Larrea, L. (2002). Semantic analysis of auditory input during sleep: Studies with event related potentials. *International Journal of Psychophysiology, 46,* 243–255.

Bath, A., Beynon, G. J., Moffat, D. A., & Baguley, D. M. (1998). Effective anaesthesia for transtympanic electrocochleography. *Auris Nasus Larynx, 25,* 137–141.

Bath, A., Harris, N., McEwan, J., & Yardley, M. (1999). Effect of conductive hearing loss on the vestibulo-colic reflex. *Clinical Otolaryngology, 24,* 181–183.

Batra, R., Kuwada, S., & Stanford, T. R. (1989). Temporal coding of envelopes and their interaural delays in the inferior colliculus of the unanesthetized rabbit. *Journal of Neurophysiology, 61,* 257–268.

Battista, R., Wiet, R., & Paauwe, L. (2000). Evaluation of three intraoperative auditory monitoring techniques in acoustic neuroma surgery. *American Journal of Otology, 21,* 244–248.

Battmer, R., Dillier, N., Lai, W., Weber, B., Brown, C., Gantz, B., Roland, J., Cohen, N., Shapiro, W., Pesch, J., Killian, M., & Lenarz, T. (2004). Evaluation of the Neural Response Telemetry (NRT) capabilities of the Nucleus Research Platform 8: Initial results from the NRT trial. *International Journal of Audiology, 43,* S10–S15.

Bauch, C. D., & Olsen, W. (1986). The effect of 2000–4000 Hz hearing sensitivity on ABR results. *Ear and Hearing, 7,* 314–317.

Bauch, C. D., & Olsen, W. (1989). Wave V interaural latency differences as a function of asymmetry in 2000–4000 Hz hearing sensitivity. *American Journal of Otology, 10,* 389–392.

Bauch, C. D., & Olsen, W. O. (1990). Comparison of ABR amplitudes with TIPtrode and mastoid electrodes. *Ear and Hearing, 11,* 463–467.

Bauch, C. D., Olsen, W. O., & Harner, S. G. (1983). Auditory brain-stem response and acoustic reflex test: Results for patients with and without tumor matched for hearing loss. *Archives of Otolaryngology, 109,* 522–525.

Bauch, C. D., Rose, D. E., & Harner, S. (1980). Brainstem responses to tone pip and click stimuli. *Ear and Hearing, 1,* 181–184.

Bauch, C. D., Rose, D. E., & Harner, S. (1981). Auditory brainstem responses in ears with hearing loss: Case studies. *Scandinavian Audiology, 10,* 247–254.

Bauch, C. D., Rose, D. E., & Harner, S. (1982). Auditory brainstem response results from 255 patients with supsected retrocochlear involvement. *Ear and Hearing, 3,* 83–86.

Bauch, C. D., Rose, D. E., & Harner, S. G. (1983). Auditory brain-stem response results for patients with suspected retrocochlear involvement. *Ear and Hearing, 3,* 83–86.

Beagley, H. A., & Knight, J. J. (1967). Changes in auditory evoked response with intensity. *Journal of Laryngology & Otology, 81,* 861–873.

Beagley, H. A., Sayers, B. M., & Ross, A. J. (1979). Fully objective ERA by phase spectral analysis. *Acta Otolaryngologica, 78,* 270–278.

Beagley, H. A., & Sheldrake, J. B. (1978). Differences in brainstem response latency with age and sex. *British Journal of Audiology, 12,* 69–77.

Beattie, R. C. (1988). Interaction of click polarity, stimulus level, and repetition rate on the auditory brainstem response. *Scandinavian Audiology, 17,* 99–109.

Beattie, R. C., & Boyd, R. (1984). Effects of click duration on the latency of the early evoked response. *Journal of Speech and Hearing Research, 27,* 70–76.

Beattie, R. C., Garcia, E., & Johnson, A. (1996). Frequency-specific auditory brainstem responses in adults with sensorineural hearing loss. *Audiology, 35,* 194–203.

Beattie, R. C., Moretti, M., & Warren, V. (1984). Effects of rise fall time, frequency, and intensity on the early/middle evoked response. *Journal of Speech and Hearing Disorders, 49,* 114–127.

Beattie, R. C., & Torre, P. (1997). Effects of rise-fall time and repetition rate on the auditory brainstem response to 0.5 and 1 kHz tone bursts using normal-hearing and hearing-impaired subjects. *Scandinavian Audiology, 26,* 23–32.

Beattie, R. C., Zipp J. A., Schaffer, C. A., & Silzel, K. L. (1992). Effects of sample size on the latency and amplitude of the auditory evoked response. *American Journal of Otology, 13,* 55–67.

Beauchaine, K. A., Kaminski, J. R., & Gorga, M. P. (1987). Comparison of Beyer DT48 and Etymotic insert earphones: Auditory brain stem response measurements. *Ear and Hearing, 8,* 292–297.

Beckerman, R., Meltzer, J., Sola, A., Dunn, D., & Wegmann, M. (1986). Brain-stem auditory response in Ondine's syndrome. *Archives of Neurology, 43,* 698–701.

Begleiter, H., Porjesz, B., Bihari, B., & Kissin, B. (1984). Event-related brain potentials in boys at risk for alcoholism. *Science, 225,* 1493–1496.

Begleiter, H., Porjesz, B., & Chou, C. L. (1981). Auditory brainstem potentials in chronic alcoholics. *Science, 211,* 1064–1066.

Begleiter, H., Porjesz, B., Chou, C. L., & Aunon, J. L. (1983). P3 and stimulus incentive value. *Psychophysiology, 20,* 95–101.

Beiser, M., Himmelfarb, M. Z., Gold, S., & Shanon, E. (1985). Maturation of auditory brainstem potentials in neonates and infants. *Journal of Pediatric Otorhinolaryngology, 9,* 69–76.

Beiter, R. C., & Hogan, D. D. (1973). Effects of variations in stimulus rise-decay time upon the early components of the auditory evoked response. *Electroencephalography and Clinical Neurophysiology, 34,* 203–206.

Békèsy, G. v. (1935). [Uber akustiche Reizung des Vestibularapparates.]. *Pflugers Archives, 236,* 59–76.

Békèsy, G. v. (1960). *Experiments in hearing.* New York: McGraw-Hill.

Bell, S. L., Allen, R., & Lutman, M. E. (2001). The feasibility of maximum length sequences to reduce acquisition time of the middle latency response. *Journal of the Acoustical Society of America, 109,* 1073–1081.

Bell, S. L., Smith, D.C., Allen, R., & Lutman, M. E. (2004). Recording the middle latency response of the auditory evoked potential as a measure of depth of anaesthesia. A technical note. *British Journal of Anaesthesia, 92,* 442–445.

Bellman, S., Barnard, S., & Beagley, H. A. (1984). A nine-year review of 841 children tested by transtympanic electrocochleography. *Journal of Laryngology & Otology, 98,* 1–9.

Benita, M., & Conde, H. (1972). Effects of local cooling upon conduction and synaptic transmission. *Brain Research, 14,* 133–151.

Benna, P., Gilli, M., Ferrero, P., & Bergamasco, B. (1982). Brain stem auditory evoked potentials in supratentorial tumours. *Electroencephalography and Clinical Neurophysiology, 54,* 8–9.

Bennett, M. J. (1980). Trials with the auditory response cradle II: The neonatal response to an auditory stimulus. *Audiology, 14,* 1–6.

Beresford, H. R. (1984). Legal aspects of terminating care. *Seminars in Neurology, 4,* 23–29.

Bergenius, J., Borg, E., & Hirsch, A. (1983). Stapedius reflex test, brainstem audiometry and opto-vestibular tests in diagnosis of acoustic neurinomas: A comparison of test sensitivity in patients with moderate hearing loss. *Scandinavian Audiology, 12,* 3–9.

Bergsmark, J., & Djupesland, G. (1968). Heredopathia atactica polyneuritiformis (Refsum's deseases). An audiological examination of two patients. *European Neurology, 1,* 122–130.

Berlad, I., & Pratt, H. (1995). P300 in response to the subject's own name. *Electroencephalography and Clinical Neurophysiology, 96,* 472–474.

Berlin, C. I. (1999). Auditory neuropathy: Using OAEs and ABRs from screening to management. *Seminars in Hearing, 20,* 307–315.

Berlin, C. I., Bordelon, J., St. John, P., Wilensky, D., Hurley, A., Kluka, E., & Hood, L. J. (1998). Reversing click polarity may uncover auditory neuropathy in infants. *Ear and Hearing,* 37–47.

Berlin, C. I., Cullen, J. K., Jr., Ellis, M. S., Lousteau, R. J., Yarbrough, W. M., & Lyons, G. D., Jr. (1974). Clinical application of recording human VIIIth nerve action potentials from the tympanic membrane. *Transactions of the American Academy of Ophthalmology and Otolaryngology, 78,* 401–410.

Berlin, C. I., Hood, L. J., Hurley, A., & Wen, H. (1994). Contralateral suppression of otoacoustic emissions: An index of the function of the medial olivocochlear system. *Archives of Otolaryngology—Head & Neck Surgery, 110,* 3–21.

Berlin, C. I., Hood, L., Morlet, T., Den, Z., Goforth, L., Tedesco, S., Li, L., Buchler, K., & Keats, B. (2000). The search for auditory neuropathy patients and connexin 26 patients in schools for the deaf. *Abstracts of the Association for Research in Otolaryngology, 23,* 23–24.

Berlin, C. I., Hood, L., Morlet, T., Rose, K., & Brashears, S. (2003). Auditory neuropathy/dys-synchrony: Diagnosis and management. *Mental Retardation and Developmental Disabilities Research Review, 9,* 225–231.

Berlin, C. I., Hood, L., & Rose, K. (2001). On renaming auditory neuropathy as auditory dys-synchrony: Implications for a clearer understanding of the underlying mechanisms and management options. *Audiology Today, 13,* 15–17.

Bernal, J., Harmony, T., Rodriguez, M., Reyes, A., Yanez, G., Fernandez, T., Galan, L., Silva, J., Bouzas, A., Rodriguez, H., Guerrero, V., & Marosi, E. (2000). Auditory event-related potentials in poor readers. *International Journal of Psychophysiology, 36,* 11–23.

Bernard, P. (1980). Alterations of auditory evoked potentials during the course of chloroquine treatment. *Acta Otolaryngologica (Stockholm), 99,* 387–392.

Bess, F. J., & Paradise, J. (1994). Universal newborn hearing screening: Not risk-free and not supported by the evidence. *Pediatrics, 93,* 330–334.

Bess, F. J., Peek, B. F., & Chapman, J. J. (1979). Further observations on noise levels in infant incubators. *Pediatrics, 63,* 100–106.

Beynon, A., & Snik, A. (2004). Use of the event-related P300 potential in cochlear implant subjects for the study of strategy-dependent speech processing. *International Journal of Audiology, 43,* S44–S47.

Beynon, A., Snik, A., Stegeman, D., & van den Broek, P. (2005). Discrimination of speech sound contrasts determined with behavioral tests and event-related potentials in cochlear implant recipients. *Journal of the American Academy of Audiology, 16,* 42–53.

Beynon, G. J., Clarke, N., & Baguley, D. M. (1995). Patient comfort in audiological testing. *British Journal of Audiology, 29,* 1–5.

Bhargava, V. K., & McKean, C. M. (1977). Role of 5-hydroxytryptamine in the modulation of acoustic brainstem (far-field) potentials. *Neuropharmacology, 16,* 447–449.

Bhargava, V. K., Salamy, A., & McKean, C. M. (1978). Effect of cholinergic drugs on the auditory evoked responses (far-field) in rats. *Neuroscience, 3,* 821–826.

Bickford, R. G. (1964). The interaction of averaged multisensory responses recorded at the inion. *Electroencephalography and Clinical Neurophysiology, 17,* 713.

Bickford, R. G., Galbraith, R. F., & Jacobson, J. L. (1963). The nature of averaged evoked potentials recorded from the human scalp. *Electroencephalography and Clinical Neurophysiology, 15,* 720.

Bickford, R. G., Jacobson, J. L., & Cody, D. T. R. (1964). Nature of average evoked potentials to sound and other stimuli in man. *Annals of the New York Academy of Sciences, 112,* 204–223.

Black, F., Lilly, D., Fowler, L., & Stypulkowski, P. (1987). Surgical evaluation of candidates for cochlear implants. *Annals of Otology, Rhinology and Laryngology, 96,* 96–99.

Black, F., Pesznecker, S., Allen, K., & Gianna, C. (2001). A vestibular phenotype for Waardenburg syndrome? *Otology and Neurotology, 22,* 188–194.

Black, J. A., Fariello, R. G., & Chun, R. W. (1979). Brainstem auditory evoked response in adrenoleukodystrophy. *Annals of Neurology, 6,* 269–270.

Blegvad, B. (1975). Binaural summation of surface-recorded electrocochleographic responses. *Scandinavian Audiology, 4,* 233–238.

Blegvad, B., Svane-Knudsen, V., & Borre, S. (1984). ABR in patients with congenital/early acquired sensorineural hearing loss, abnormal stapedius reflex thresholds and speech retardation. *Scandinavian Audiology, 13,* 41–46.

Bobbin, R. P., May, M., & Lemoine, R. L. (1979). Effects of pentobarbital and ketamine on brainstem auditory potentials. *Archives of Otolaryngology, 105,* 467–470.

Bock, G. R., & Saunders, J. C. (1977). A critical period of acoustic trauma in the hamster and its relation to cochlear development. *Science, 197,* 396–398.

Bockenheimer, S. T., Schmidt, C. L., & Zöllner, C. (1984). Neuro-otological findings in patients with small acoustic neuromas. *Archives of Otorhinolaryngology, 239,* 31–39.

Bodis-Wollner, I. (1985). Utility of evoked potentials. *Journal of the American Medical Association, 254,* 3490.

Boezeman, E. H. J. F., Kapteyn, T. S., Feenstra, L., & Snel, A. M. (1985). Verification of the air-bone gap using cancellation and evoked responses. *Audiology, 24,* 174–185.

Boezeman, E. H. J. F., Kapteyn, T. S., Visser, S. L., & Snel, A. M. (1983). Effect of contralateral and ipsilateral masking of acoustic stimulation on the latencies of auditory evoked potentials from cochlea and brain stem. *Electroencephalography and Clinical Neurophysiology, 55,* 710–713.

Bojrab, D. I., Bhansali, S. A., & Andreozzi, M. P. (1994). Intraoperative electrocochleography during endolymphatic sac surgery: Clinical results. *Otolaryngology—Head & Neck Surgery, 111,* 478–484.

Bolz, J., & Giedke, H. (1982). Brain stem auditory evoked responses in psychiatric patients and healthy controls. *Journal of Neural Transmission, 54,* 285–291.

Bomba, M., & Pang, E. (2004). Cortical evoked potentials in autism: A review. *International Journal of Psychophysiology, 53,* 161–169.

Bonafe, A., Manelfe, C., Clanet, M., Fraysse, B., Soulier, M. J., Kersaint-Gilly, A. D., et al. (1985). Electrophysiology: CT correlations in exploration for acoustic neurinoma. *Journal of Neuroradiology, 12,* 61–70.

Bonhomme, V., Plourde, G., Meuret, P., Fiset, P., & Backman, S. B. (2001). Auditory steady-state response and bispectral index for assessing level of consciousness during propofol sedation and hypnosis. *Anaesthesia & Analgesia, 91,* 1398–1403.

Booth, B. (1980). Ménière's disease: The selection and assessment of patients for surgery using electrocochleography. *Annals of the Royal College of Surgeons of England, 62,* 415–425.

Borg, E. (1981a). Brainstem responses to filtered sinewaves for frequency specific determination of auditory sensitivity in rats and rabbits. *Scandinavian Audiology (Supplement), 13,* 33–34.

Borg, E. (1981b). Physiological mechanisms in auditory brainstem-evoked response. *Scandinavian Audiology, 13,* 11–22.

Borg, E., & Löfqvist, L. (1982). Auditory brainstem response (ABR) to rarefaction and condensation clicks in normal and abnormal ears. *Scandinavian Audiology, 11,* 227–235.

Borg, E., Löfqvist, L., & Rosen, F. (1981). Brainstem response (ABR) in conductive hearing loss. *Scandinavian Audiology, 13,* 95–97.

Borsanyi, S., & Blanchard, C. L. (1964). Auditory evoked brain responses in man. *Archives of Otolaryngology, 80,* 149–154.

Borton, T., Eby, T., Ball, E., Nolen, B., & Bradley, E. (1992). Stimulus repetition rate effect on the auditory brainstem response in systemic lupus erythematosus. *Laryngoscope, 102,* 335–339.

Boshuizen, H., van der Lem, G., Kauffman-de Boer, M., van Zanten, G. A., Oudesluys-Murphy, A., & Verkerk, P. (2001). Costs of different strategies for neonatal hearing screening: A modeling approach. *Archives of Disease in Childhood, 85,* F177–F181.

Boston, J. R. (1981). Spectra of auditory brainstem responses and spontaneous EEG. *IEEE Transactions on Biomedical Engineering, 28,* 334–341.

Boston, J. R. (1989). Automated interpretation of brainstem auditory evoked potentials: A prototype system. *IEEE Transactions in Biomedical Engineering, 36,* 528–532.

Boston, J. R., & Ainslie, P. J. (1980). Effects of analogue and digital filtering on brainstem auditory evoked potentials. *Electroencephalography and Clinical Neurophysiology, 48,* 361–364.

Böttcher-Gandor, C., & Ullsperger, P. (1992). Mismatch negativity in event-related potentials to auditory stimuli as a function of varying interstimulus interval. *Psychophysiology, 29,* 546–550.

Bouchard, K. R., & Bojrab, D. (1988). *Electrocochleography: Intra-operative SP/AP ratios.* Rockville, MD: American Speech-Language-Hearing Association.

Boutros, N. N., & Belger, A. (1999). Midlatency evoked potentials attenuation and augmentation reflect different aspects of sensory gating. *Biological Psychiatry, 45,* 917–922.

Boutros, N. N., Campbell, D., Petrakis, I., Krystal, J., Caporale, M., & Kosten, T. (2000). Cocaine use and the mid-latency auditory evoked responses. *Psychiatry Research, 96,* 117–126.

Boutros, N. N., Overall, J., & Zouridakis, G. (1991). Test-retest reliability of the P50 mid-latency auditory evoked response. *Psychiatry Research, 39,* 181–192.

Boutros, N. N., Torello, M. W., Barker, B. A., Tueting, P. A., Wu, S. C., & Nasrallah, H. A. (1995). The P50 evoked potential component and mismatch detection in normal volunteers: Implications for the study of sensory gating. *Psychiatry Research, 57,* 83–88.

Brackmann, D. (1984). A review of acoustic tumors. *American Journal of Otology, 5,* 233–244.

Brackmann, D., & Bartels, L. J. (1980). Rare tumors of the cerebellopontine angle. *Archives of Otolaryngology—Head & Neck Surgery, 88,* 555–559.

Brackmann, D., Owens, R., Friedman, R., Hitselberger, W., De la Cruz, A., House, J., Nelson, R., Luxford, W., Slattery, W., III. & Fayad, J. (2000). Prognostic factors for hearing preservation in vestibular schwannoma surgery. *American Journal of Otology, 2,* 417–424.

Brackmann, D., & Selters, W. A. (1976). Electrocochleography in Ménière's disease and acoustic neuromas. In R. J. Ruben, C. Elberling & G. Salo-

mon (Eds.), *Electrocochleography* (pp. 315–329). Baltimore: University Park Press.

Braff, D. L., & Geyer, M. A. (1990). Sensorimotor gating and schizophrenia. Human and animal model studies. *Archives of General Psychiatry, 47,* 181–188.

Bramon, E., Rabe-Hesketh, S., Sham, P., Murray, R. M., & Frangou, S. (2004). Meta-analysis of the P300 and P50 waveforms in schizophrenia. *Schizophrenia Research, 70,* 315–329.

Brantberg, K. (1996). Easily applied ear canal electrodes improve the diagnostic potential of auditory brainstem response. *Scandinavian Audiology, 25,* 147–152.

Brantberg, K., & Fransson, P. (2001). Symmetry measures of vestibular evoked myogenic potentials using objective detection criteria. *Scandinavian Audiology, 30,* 189–196.

Brantberg, K., Fransson, P., Hansson, H., & Rosenhall, U. (1999). Measures of the binaural interaction component in human auditory brainstem response using objective detection criteria. *Scandinavian Audiology, 28,* 15–26.

Brantberg, K., Löfqvist, L., & Fransson, P. (2004). Large vestibular evoked myogenic potentials in response to bone-conducted sounds in patients with superior canal dehiscence syndrome. *Audiology & Neuro-Otology, 9,* 173–182.

Brantberg, K., & Tribukait, A. (2002). Vestibular evoked myogenic potentials in response to laterally directed skull taps. *Journal of Vestibular Research, 12,* 35–45.

Brattico, E., Tervaniemi, M., Valimaki, V., Van Zuijen, T., & Peretz, I. (2003). Cortical correlates of acquired deafness to dissonance. *Annals of the New York Academy of Science, 999,* 158–160.

Brecher, M., & Begleiter, H. (1983). Event-related brain potentials to high-incentive stimuli in unmedicated schizophrenic patients. *Biological Psychiatry, 18,* 661–674.

Brett, B., Di, S., Watkins, L., & Barth, D. S. (1994). A horseradish peroxidase study of parallel thalamocortical projections responsible for the generation of mid-latency auditory-evoked potentials. *Brain Research, 647,* 65–75.

Bridger, M. W., & Graham, J. M. (1985). The influence of raised body temperature on auditory evoked brainstem responses. *Clinical Otolaryngology & Allied Sciences, 10,* 195–199.

Brinkmann, R. D., & Scherg, M. (1979). Human auditory on and off potentials of the brainstem. *Scandinavian Audiology, 8,* 27–32.

Britt, R. H., Lyons, B. E., Pounds, D. W., & Prionas, S. D. (1983). Feasibility of ultrasound hyperthermia in the treatment of malignant brain tumors. *Medical Instrumentation, 17,* 172–177.

Brix, R., & Gedlicka, W. (1991). Late cortical auditory potentials evoked by electrostimulation in deaf and cochlear implant patients. *European Archives of Otorhinolaryngology, 248,* 442–444.

Brookhauser, P. E., Gorga, M. P., & Kelly, W. J. (1990). Auditory brainstem response results as predictors of behavioral auditory thresholds in severe and profound hearing impairment. *Laryngoscope, 100,* 803–810.

Brown, C. J., & Abbas, P. J. (1990). Electrically evoked whole-nerve action potentials. II. Parametric data from the cat. *Journal of the Acoustical Society of America, 88,* 2205–2210.

Brown, C. J., Abbas, P. J., Borland, J., & Bertschy, M. R. (1996). Electrically evoked whole nerve action potentials in Ineraid cochlear implant users: Responses to different stimulating electrode configurations and comparison to psychophysical responses. *Journal of Speech & Hearing Research, 39,* 453–467.

Brown, C., Abbas, P., Fryauf-Bertschy, H., Kelsay, D., & Gantz, B. (1994). Intra-operative and post-operative electrically evoked auditory brainstem responses in Nucleus cochlear implant users: Implications for the fitting process. *Ear and Hearing, 15,* 168–176.

Brown, C. J., Abbas, P. J., & Gantz, B. J. (1998). Preliminary experience with neural response telemetry in the Nucleus CI24M cochlear implant. *American Journal of Otology, 19,* 320–327.

Brown, C., Hughes, M., Luk, B., Abbas, P., Wolaver, A., & Gervais, J. (2000). The relationship between EAP and EABR thresholds and levels used to program the Nucleus 24 speech processor: Data from adults. *Ear and Hearing, 21,* 151–163.

Brown, F. R., Shimizu, H., McDonald, J. M., Moser, A. B., Marquis, P., Chen, W. W., et al. (1981). Auditory evoked brainstem response and high-performance liquid chromatography sulfatide assay as early indices of metachromatic leukodystrophy. *Neurology, 31,* 980–985.

Brown, R. M., Crane, A. M., & Goldman, P. S. (1979). Regional distribution of monoamines in the cerebral cortex and subcortical structures of the rhesus monkey: Concentrations and in vivo synthesis rates. *Brain Research, 168,* 133–150.

Brown, W. S., Marsh, J. T., & LaRue, A. (1982). Event-related potentials in psychiatry: Differentiating depression and dementia in the elderly. *Bulletin of the Los Angeles Neurological Society, 47,* 91–107.

Brown, W. S., Marsh, J. T., & LaRue, A. (1983). Exponential electrophysiological aging: P3 latency. *Electroencephalography & Clinical Neurophysiology, 55,* 277–285.

Brown, W. S., Marsh, J. T., & Smith, J. C. (1973). Contextual meaning effects on speech-evoked potentials. *Behavioral Biology, 9,* 755–761.

Brown, W. S., Marsh, W. T., & Smith, J. C. (1976). Evoked potential waveform differences produced by the perception of different meanings of an ambiguous phrase. *Electroencephalography and Clinical Neurophysiology, 41,* 113–123.

Browning, S., Mohr, G., Dufour, J. J., Rapaport, J. M., Zeitoumi, A., Provencal, C., Hernandes, Y., Surkis, S., Druker, S., & Davis, N. L. (2001). Hearing preservation in acoustic neuroma surgery. *Journal of Otolaryngology, 30,* 307–315.

Brualla, J., Romero, M. F., Serrano, M., & Valdizan, J. R. (1998). Auditory event-related potentials to semantic priming during sleep. *Electroencephalography and Clinical Neurophysiology, 108,* 283–290.

Bruce, D. A., Shut, L., Bruno, L. A., Wood, J. H., & Sutton, L. N. (1978). Outcome following severe head injuries in children. *Journal of Neurosurgery, 48,* 679–688.

Bruder, G. E., Tenke, C. E., Stewart, J. W., Towey, J. P., Leite, P., Voglmaier, M., & Quitkin, F. M. (1995). Brain event-related potentials to complex tones in depressed patients: Relations to perceptual asymmetry and clinical features. *Psychophysiology, 32,* 373–381.

Bruder, G. E., Towey, J. P., Stewart, J. W., Friedman, D., Tenke, C., & Quitkin, F. M. (1991). Event-related potentials in depression: Influence of task, stimulus hemifield and clinical features on P3 latency. *Biological Psychiatry, 30,* 233–246.

Brugge, J., Anderson, D., Hind, J., & Rose, J. (1969). Time structure of discharges in single auditory nerve fibers of the squirrel monkey in response to complex periodic sound. *Journal of Neurophysiology, 32,* 386–401.

Bruneau, N., Roux, S., Adrien, J. L., & Barthelemy, C. (1999). Auditory associative cortex dysfunction in children with autism: Evidence from late auditory evoked potentials (N1 wave-T complex). *Clinical Neurophysiology, 110,* 1927–1934.

Bruneau, N., Roux, S., Guerin, P., Barthelemy, C., & Lelord, G. (1997). Temporal prominence of auditory evoked potentials (N1 wave) in 4- to 8-year-old children. *Psychophysiology, 34,* 32–38.

Buchsbaum, M. S. (1977). The middle evoked response components and schizophrenia. *Schizophrenia Bulletin, 3,* 93–104.

Buchwald, J. S., Erwin, R. J., Read, S., Van Lancker, D., & Cummings, J. L. (1989). Midlatency auditory evoked responses: Differential abnormality of P1 in Alzheimer's disease. *Electroencephalography and Clinical Neurophysiology, 74,* 378–384.

Buchwald, J. S., Erwin, R., Van Lancker, D., Guthrie, D., Schwafel, J., & Tanguay, P. (1992). Midlatency auditory evoked responses: P1 abnormalities in adult autistic subjects. *Electroencephalography and Clinical Neurophysiology, 84,* 164–171.

Buchwald, J. S., & Huang, C. M. (1975). Far-field acoustic response: Origins in the cat. *Science, 189,* 382–384.

Buchwald, J. S., Rubinstein, E. H., Schwafel, J., & Strandburg, R. J. (1991). Midlatency auditory evoked responses: Differential effects of a cholinergic agonist and antagonist. *Electroencephalography and Clinical Neurophysiology, 80,* 303–309.

Budd, T. W., Barry, R. J., Gordon, E., Rennie, C., & Michie, P. T. (1998). Decrement of the N1 auditory event-related potential with stimulus repetition: Habituation vs. refractoriness. *International Journal of Psychophysiology, 31,* 51–68.

Buettner, U. W., Stohr, M., & Koletzki, E. (1983). Brainstem auditory evoked potential abnormalities in vascular formations of the posterior fossa. *Journal of Neurology, 229,* 247–254.

Buller, N., Shivili, Y., Laurian, N., Laurian, L., & Zohar, Y. (1988). Delayed brainstem auditory evoked responses in diabetic patients. *Journal of Laryngology & Otology, 102,* 857–860.

Burkard, R. (1984). Sound pressure level measurement and spectral analysis of brief acoustic transients. *Electroencephalography and Clinical Neurophysiology, 57,* 83–91.

Burkard, R., & Hecox, K. (1983). The effect of broadband noise on the human brainstem auditory evoked response: I. Rate and intensity effects. *Journal of the Acoustical Society of America, 74,* 1204–1223.

Burkard, R., & Hecox, K. E. (1987). The effect of broadband noise on the human brain-stem auditory evoked response. IV. Additivity of forward-masking and rate-induced wave V latency shifts. *Journal of the Acoustical Society of America, 81,* 1064–1072.

Burkard, R., Shi, Y., & Hecox, K. (1990a). A comparison of maximum length and Legendre sequences for the derivation of brain-stem auditory-evoked responses at rapid rates of stimulation. *Journal of the Acoustical Society of America, 87,* 1656–1664.

Burkard, R., Shi, Y., & Hecox, K. (1990b). Brain-stem auditory evoked responses elicited by maximum length sequences: Effect of simultaneous masking noise. *Journal of the Acoustical Society of America, 87,* 1665–1672.

Burkard, R., & Voight, H. F. (1989). Stimulus dependencies of the gerbil brain-stem auditory evoked response (BAER): II. Effects of broadband noise level and high-pass masker cutoff frequency across click polarity. *Journal of the Acoustical Society of America, 85,* 2526–2535.

Burkey, J., Rizer, F., Schuring, A., Fucci, M., & Lippy, W. (1996). Acoustic reflexes, auditory brainstem response, and MRI in the evaluation of acoustic neuromas. *Laryngoscope, 106,* 839–841.

Burrows, D. L., & Barry, S. J. (1990). Electrophysiological evidence for the critical band in humans: Middle-latency responses. *Journal of the Acoustical Society of America, 88,* 180–184.

Butinar, D., Zidar, J., Leonardis, L., et al. (1999). Hereditary auditory, vestibular, motor, and sensory neuropathy in a Slovenian Roma (Gypsy) kindred. *Annals of Neurology, 46,* 36–44.

Butler, R. A. (1968). The effect of changes in stimulus frequency and intensity on habituation of the human vertex potential. *Journal of the Acoustical Society of America, 44,* 945–950.

Butler, R. A., Keidel, W. D., & Spreng, M. (1969). An investigation of the human cortical evoked potential under conditions of monaural and binaural stimulation. *Acta Otolaryngologica, 68,* 317–326.

Butler, R. A., Konishi, T., & Fernandez, C. (1960). Temperature coefficients of cochlear potentials. *American Journal of Physiology, 199,* 688–692.

Cacace, A. T., & McFarland, D. J. (2003). Quantifying signal-to-noise ratio of mismatch negativity in humans. *Neuroscience Letters, 341,* 251–255.

Cacace, A. T., Parnes, S., Lovely, T., & Kalathia, A. (1994). The disconnected ear: Phenomenological effects of a large acoustic tumor. *Ear and Hearing, 15,* 287–298.

Cacace, A. T., Satya-Murti, S., & Wolpaw, J. R. (1990). Human middle-latency auditory evoked potentials: Vertex and temporal components. *Electroencephalography and Clinical Neurophysiology, 77,* 6–18.

Cacace, A. T., Shy, M., & Satya-Murti, S. (1980). Brainstem auditory evoked potentials: A comparison of two high-frequency filter settings. *Neurology, 30,* 765–767.

Cagy, M., & Infantosi, A. F. (2002). Unconsciousness indication using time-domain parameters extracted from mid-latency auditory evoked potentials. *Journal of Clinical Monitoring and Computaton, 17,* 361–366.

Caird, D., Sondheimer, D., & Klinke, R. (1985). Intra- and extracranially recorded auditory evoked potentials in the cat. I. Source location and binaural interaction. *Electroencephalography and Clinical Neurophysiology, 61,* 50–60.

Callan, D., Lasky, R., & Fowler, C. (1999). Neural networks applied to retrocochlear diagnosis. *Journal of Speech, Language, and Hearing Research, 42,* 287–299.

Callaway, E. (1975). *Brain electrical potentials and individual psychological differences.* New York: Grune and Stratton.

Callaway, E., & Halliday, R. A. (1973). Evoked potential variability: Effects of age, amplitude, and methods of measurement. *Electroencephalography and Clinical Neurophysiology, 34,* 125–133.

Camilleri, A. E., & Howarth, K. L. (2001). Prognostic value of electrocochleography in patients with unilateral Ménière's disease undergoing saccus surgery. *Clinical Otolaryngology, 26,* 257–260.

Campanella, G., DeFalco, F. A., Santoro, V., Perretti, A., Cassandro, E., & Mosca, F. (1984). Specific impairment of BAERs in Friedreich's ataxia: Importance of auditory evoked responses in the clinical evaluation and differential diagnosis. *Journal of Neurological Science, 65,* 111–120.

Campbell, F., Atkinson, J., Francis, M., & Green, D. (1977). Estimation of auditory thresholds using evoked potentials. A clinical screening test. *Progress in Clinical Neurophysiology, 2,* 8–78.

Campbell, K. B., Bell, J., & Bastien, C. (1992). Evoked potential measures of information processing during natural sleep. In R. J. Broughton, & R. D. Ogilvie (Eds.), *Sleep, arousal and performance: A tribute to Bob Wilkinson* (pp. 88–116). Boston: Birkhauser.

Campbell, K. B., & Colrain, I. M. (2002). Event-related potential measures of the inhibition of information processing: II. The sleep onset period. *International Journal of Psychophysiology, 46,* 197–214.

Campbell, K. B., & de Lugt, D. R. (1995). Event-related potential measures of cognitive deficits following closed head injury. *Handbook of Neuropsychology, 10,* 269–297.

Campbell, K. B., Suffield, J. B., & Deacon, D. L. (1990). Electrophysiological assessment of cognitive disorder in closed head-injured outpatients. *Electroencephalography and Clinical Neurophysiology, Supplement, 41,* 202–215.

Campbell, K. C., Faloon, K. M., & Rybak, L. P. (1993). Noninvasive electrodes for electrocochleography in the chinchilla. *Archive of Otolaryngology—Head & Neck Surgery, 119,* 767–771.

Campbell, K. C., Harker, L. A., & Abbas, P. J. (1992). Interpretation of electrocochleography in Ménière's disease and normal subjects. *Annals of Otology, Rhinology & Laryngology, 101,* 496–500.

Campbell, M. J., Lewis, D. A., Foote, S. L., & Morrison, J. H. (1987). Distribution of choline acetyltransferase-, serotonin-, dopamine-beta-hydroxylase-, tyrosine hydroxylase-immunoreactive fibers in monkey primary auditory cortex. *Journal of Comparative Neurology, 8,* 209–220.

Campbell, P., Harris, C., Hendricks, S., & Sirimanna, T. (2004). Bone conduction auditory brainstem responses in infants. *Journal of Laryngology & Otology, 118,* 117–122.

Campbell, P., Harris, C., Sirimanna, T., & Vellodi, A. (2003). A model of neuronopathic Gaucher disease. *Journal of Inherited Metabolic Disorders, 26,* 629–639.

Campbell, P., Harris, C., & Vellodi, A. (2004). Deterioration of the auditory brainstem response in children with type 3 Gaucher disease. *Neurology, 63,* 385–387.

Cane, M., O'Donoghue, G., & Lutman, M. (1992). The feasability of using oto-acoustic emissions to monitor cochlear function during acoustic neuroma surgery. *Scandinavian Audiology, 21,* 173–176.

Caravaglios, G., Natale, E., Ferraro, G., Fierro, B., Raspanti, G., & Daniele, O. (2001). Auditory event-related potentials (P300) in epileptic patients. *Clinical Neurophysiology, 31,* 121–129.

Cardenas, A. T., McCallin, K., Hopkins, R., & Fein, G. (1997). A comparison of the repetitive click and conditioning-testing P50 paradigms. *Electroencephalography and Clinical Neurophysiology, 104,* 157–164.

Carlin, L., Roach, E. S., Riela, A., Spudis, E., & McLean, W. T. (1983). Juvenile metachromatic leukodystrophy: Evoked potentials and computerized tomography. *Annals of Neurology, 13,* 105–106.

Carlton, E. H., & Katz, S. (1980). Is Weiner filtering an effective method of improving evoked potential estimation? *IEEE Transactions on Biomedical Engineering, BME-27,* 187–192.

Carrillo-de-la-Pena, M. T., & Cadaveira, F. (2000). The effect of motivational instructions on P300 amplitude. *Clinical Neurophysiology, 30,* 232–239.

Carrillo-de-la-Pena, M. T., & García-Larrea, L. (1999). On the validity of interblock averaging of P300 in clinical settings. *International Journal of Psychophysiology, 34,* 103–112.

Cashman, M. Z., & Rossman, R. N. (1983). Diagnostic features of the brainstem response in identifying cerebellopointine angle tumours. *Scandinavian Audiology, 12,* 35–41.

Cashman, M. Z., Stanton, S. G., Sagle, C., & Barber, H. O. (1993). The effect of hearing loss on ABR interpretation: Use of a correction factor. *Scandinavian Audiology, 22,* 153–158.

Cassandro, E., Mosca, F., Sequino, L., DeFalco, F. A., & Campanella, G. (1986). Otoneurological findings in Friedrich's ataxia and other inherited neuropathies. *Audiology, 5,* 84–91.

Catts, S. V., Shelley, A. M., Ward, P. B., Liebert, B., McConaghy, N., Andrews, S., & Michie, P. T. (1995). Brain potential evidence for an auditory sensory memory deficit in schizophrenia. *American Journal of Psychiatry, 152,* 213–219.

Cebulla, M., Stürzebecher, E., & Wernecke, K. (2000). Objective detection of auditory brainstem potentials. *Scandinavian Audiology, 29,* 44–51.

Celebisoy, N., Aydogdu, I., Ekmekci, O., & Akurekli, O. (1996). Middle latency auditory evoked potentials (MLAEPs) in multiple sclerosis (MS). *Acta Neurologica Scandinavia, 93,* 318–321.

Celesia, G. G. (1976). Organization of auditory cortical areas in man. *Brain, 99,* 403–414.

Celesia, G. G., Broughton, R., Rasmussen, T., & Branch, C. (1968). Auditory evoked responses from the exposed human cortex. *Electroencephalography and Clinical Neurophysiology, 24,* 458–466.

Čeponiene, R., Alku, P., Westerfield, M., Torki, M., & Townsend, J. (2005). ERPs differentiate syllable and nonphonetic sound processing in children and adults. *Psychophysiology, 42,* 391–406.

Čeponiene, R., Lepisto, T., Shestakova, A., Vanhala, R., Alku, P., Näätänen, R., & Yaguchi, K. (2003). Speech-sound-selective auditory impairment in children with autism: They can perceive but do not attend. *Proceedings of the National Academy of Sciences of the United States of America 100,* 5567–5572.

Čeponiene, R., Rinne, T., & Näätänen, R. (2002). Maturation of cortical sound processing as indexed by event-related potentials. *Clinical Neurophysiology, 113,* 870–882.

Čeponiene, R., Shestakova, A., Balan, P., Alku, P., Yiaguchi, K., & Näätänen, R. (2001). Children's auditory event-related potentials index sound complexity and "speechness." *International Journal of Neuroscience, 109,* 245–260.

Cevette, M. (1984). Auditory brainstem response testing in the intensive care unit. *Seminars in Hearing, 5,* 57–69.

Chaimoff, M., Nageris, B., Sulkes, J., Spitzer, T., & Kalmanowitz, M. (1999). Sudden hearing loss as a presenting symptom of acoustic neuroma. *American Journal of Otology, 20,* 157–160.

Chambers, R. D. (1992). Differential age effects for components of the adult auditory middle latency response. *Hearing Research, 58,* 121–131.

Chambers, R. D., Rowan, L. E., Matthies, M. L., & Novak, M. A. (1989). Auditory brain-stem responses in children with previous otitis media. *Archives of Otolaryngology—Head & Neck Surgery, 115,* 452–457.

Chan, F., Lam, F., Poon, P., & Qiu, W. (1995). Detection of brainstem auditory evoked potential by adaptive filtering. *Medical Biology, Engineering & Computing, 33,* 69–75.

Chan, Y. W., Woo, E. K. W., Hammond, S. R., Yiannikas, C., & McLeod, J. G. (1988). The interaction between sex and click polarity in brainstem auditory potentials evoked from control subjects of Oriental and Caucasian origin. *Electroencephalography and Clinical Neurophysiology, 71,* 77–80.

Chandler, D., & Grantham, D. (1992). Minimal audible movement angle in the horizontal plane as a function of stimulus frequency and bandwidth, source azimuth, and velocity. *Journal of the Acoustical Society of America, 91,* 1624–1636.

Chandrasekhar, S., Brackmann, D., & Devgan, K. (1995). Utility of auditory brainstem response audiometry in diagnosis of acoustic neuromas. *American Journal of Otology, 16,* 63–67.

Chang, B., & Morariu, M. A. (1979). Transient traumatic "locked-in" syndrome. *European Neurology, 18,* 391–394.

Chang, Y. C., Yeh, C. Y., & Wang, J. D. (1995). Subclinical neurotoxicity of mercury vapor revealed by a multimodality evoked potential study of chloralkali workers. *American Journal of Industrial Medicine, 27,* 271–279.

Charachon, R., & Dumas, G. (1980). Value of early auditory evoked potentials in non-traumatic diseases of the brain stem. *Journal Francais Oto-Rhino-Laryngologie, Audiophonologie, Chirurgie Maxillo-Faciale, 29,* 569–588.

Charasse, B., Chanal, J., Berger-Vachon, C., & Collet, L. (2004). Influence of stimulus frequency on NRT recordings. *International Journal of Audiology, 43,* 236–244.

Charlet de Sauvage, R. (1983). [Evoked auditory potentials using electric stimulation of the ear. Experimental study]. *Review de Laryngologie, Otologie & Rhinologie (Bordeaux), 104,* 157–165.

Charuvanji, A., Visudhiphan, P., Chiemchanya, S., & Tawin, C. (1990). Sensorineural hearing loss in children recovering from purulent meningitis: A study in Thai children at Ramathibodi Hospital. *Journal of the Medical Association of Thailand, 73,* 253–257.

Chassard, D., Joubaud, A., Colson, A., Guiraid, M., Dubreuil, C., & Bansillon, V. (1989). Auditory evoked potentials during propofol anaesthesia in man. *British Journal of Anaesthesia, 62,* 522–526.

Chatrian, G. E., Petersen, M. C., & Lazarte, J. A. (1960). Responses to clicks from the human brain: Some depth electrographic observations. *Electroencephalography and Clinical Neurophysiology, 12,* 479–489.

Chatrian, G. E., Wirch, A. L., Edwards, K. H., Lettich, E., & Snyder, J. M. (1984). Cochlear summating potential recorded from the external auditory meatus of normal humans: Amplitude-intensity functions and relationship to auditory nerve action potential. *Electroencephalography and Clinical Neurophysiology, 59,* 396–410.

Chatrian, G. E., Wirch, A. L., Edwards, K. H., Lettich, E., & Snyder, J. M. (1985). Cochlear summating potentials to broadband clicks detected from the human external auditory meatus: A study of subjects with normal hearing for age. *Ear and Hearing, 6,* 130–138.

Chayasirisobhon, S., Green, V., Mason, K., & Berchou, R. (1984). The brainstem auditory evoked potential in phenytoin intoxication. In R. H. Nodar & C. Barber (Eds.), *Evoked Potentials II: The Second International Evoked Potentials Symposium* (pp. 506–509). Boston: Butterworth.

Chayasirisobhon, S., Yu, L., Griggs, L., Westmoreland, S., & Leu, N. (1996). Recording of brainstem evoked potentials and their association with gentamicin in neonates. *Pediatric Neurology, 14,* 277–280.

Chen, C. S., & Wong, Y. C. (1993). Transtympanic electrocochleography in Ménière's disease. *Chung Hua I. Hsueh Tsa Chih (Taipei), 52,* 319–324.

Chen, C. S., & Young, Y. (2003). Vestibular evoked myogenic potentials in brainstem stroke. *Laryngoscope, 113,* 990–993.

Chen, S., Yang, E., Kwan, M., Chang, P., Shiao, A., & Lien, C. (1996). Infant hearing screening with an automated auditory brainstem response screener and the auditory brainstem response. *Acta Paediatrica, 85,* 14–18.

Chen, T., & Chen, S. (1993). Effects of aircraft noise on hearing and auditory pathway function of school-age children. *International Archives of Occupational and Environmental Health, 65,* 107–111.

Chen, Y., Chow, J., & Lee, I. (2001). Comparison the cognitive effect of anti-epileptic drugs in seizure-free children with epilepsy before and after drug withdrawal. *Epilepsy Research, 44,* 65–70.

Chen, Y., & Ding, Y. (1999). Relationship between hypertension and hearing disorders in the elderly. *East African Medical Journal, 76,* 344–347.

Chen, Y. J., & Hsu, C. C. (1994). Effects of prenatal exposure to PCBs on the neurological function of children: A neuropsychological and neurophysiological study. *Developmental Medicine & Child Neurology, 36,* 312–320.

Cheour, M., Alho, K., Čeponiene, R., Reinikainen, K., Sainio, K., Pohjavuori, M., Aaltonen, O., & Näätänen, R. (1998a). Maturation of mismatch negativity in infants. *International Journal of Psychophysiology, 29,* 217–226.

Cheour, M., Čeponiene, R., Leppanen, P., Alho, K., Kujala, T., Renlund, M., Fellman, V., & Näätänen, R. (2002). The auditory sensory memory trace decays rapidly in newborns. *Scandinavian Journal of Psychology, 43,* 33–39.

Cheour, M., Haapanen, M. L., Čeponiene, R., Hukki, J., Ranta, R., & Näätänen, R. (1998). Mismatch negativity (MMN) as an index of auditory sensory memory deficit in cleft-palate and CATCH syndrome children. *Neuroreport, 9,* 2709–2712.

Cheour, M., Kushnerenko, E., Čeponiene, R., Fellman, V., & Näätänen, R. (2002). Electric brain responses obtained from newborn infants to changes in duration in complex harmonic tones. *Developmental Neuropsychology, 22,* 471–479.

Cheour-Luhtanen, M., Alho, K., Sainio, K., Rinne, T., Reinikainen, K., Pohjavuori, M., Renlund, M., Aaltonen, O., Eerola, O., & Näätänen, R. (1996). The ontogenetically earliest discriminative response of the human brain. *Psychophysiology, 33,* 478–481.

Cheour-Luhtanen, M., Haapanen, M. L., Hukki, J., Čeponiene, R., Kurjenluoma, S., Alho, K., Tervaniemi, M., Ranta, R., & Näätänen, R. (1997). The first neurophysiological evidence for cognitive brain dysfunctions in children with CATCH. *Neuroreport, 8,* 1785–1787.

Cherian, B., Singh, T., Chacko, B., & Abraham, A. (2002). Sensorineural hearing loss following acute bacterial meningitis in non-neonates. *Indian Journal of Pediatrics, 69,* 951–955.

Chermak, G., & Musiek, F. E. (1997). *Central auditory processing disorders.* San Diego: Singular Publishing Group.

Chiappa, K. H. (1980). Pattern shift visual, brainstem auditory, and short-latency somatosensory evoked potentials in multiple sclerosis. *Neurology, 30,* 110–123.

Chiappa, K. H. (1983). *Evoked potentials in clinical medicine.* New York: Raven Press.

Chiappa, K. (1997). Brainstem auditory evoked potentials: Interpretation. In K. Chiappa (Ed.), *Evoked potentials in clinical medicine* (pp 199–268). Philadelphia: Lippincott-Raven.

Chiappa, K. H., Gladstone, K. J., & Young, R. R. (1979). Brainstem auditory evoked responses: Studies of waveform variations in 50 normal human subjects. *Archives of Neurology, 36,* 81–87.

Chiappa, K. H., Harrison, J. L., Brooks, E. B., & Young, R. R. (1980). Brainstem auditory evoked responses in 200 patients with multiple sclerosis. *Annals of Neurology, 7,* 135–143.

Chiappa, K. H., & Norwood, A. E. (1977). A comparison of the clinical utility of pattern-shift visual evoked responses and brainstem auditory evoked responses in multiple sclerosis. *Neurology, 27,* 297.

Chiappa, K. H., & Ropper, A. H. (1982). Evoked potentials in clinical medicine. *New England Journal of Medicine, 306,* 1140–1150.

Chiappa, K. H., & Young, R. R. (1985). Evoked responses: Overused, underused, or misused? *Archives of Neurology, 42,* 76–77.

Chiarenza, G. A., D'Ambrosio, G. M., & Cazzullo, A. G. (1988). Sex and ear differences of brain-stem acoustic evoked potentials in a sample of normal full-term newborns: Normative study. *Electroencephalography and Clinical Neurophysiology, 71,* 357–366.

Chiba, S., Motoi, Y., Noro, H., Asakura, K., & Matsumoto, H. (1990). [A case of pure trigeminal motor neuropathy.]. *Rinsho Shinkeigaku, 30,* 883–887.

Chisin, M., Gafni, M., & Sohmer, H. (1983). Patterns of auditory nerve and brainstem evoked responses to different types of peripheral hearing loss. *Archives of Otorhinolaryngology, 237,* 165–173.

Chisin, R., Perlman, M., & Sohmer, H. (1979). Hearing loss following neonatal hyperbilirubinemia. *Annals of Otorhinolaryngology, 88,* 352–357.

Chokroverty, S., Duvoisin, R. C., Lepore, F., & Nicklas, W. (1984). Brainstem auditory and pattern-reversal visual evoked potential study in olivopontocerebellar degeneration. In R. H. Nodar & C. Barber (Eds.), *Evoked Potentials II: The Second International Evoked Potentials Symposium* (pp. 637–642). Boston: Butterworth.

Chu, N. S., & Squires, K. C. (1980). Auditory brainstem response study of alcoholic patients. *Pharmacology and Biochemical Behavior, 1,* 241–244.

Chu, N. S., Squires, K. C., & Starr, A. (1978). Auditory brainstem potentials in chronic alcohol intoxication and alcohol withdrawal. *Archives of Neurology, 35,* 596–602.

Chu, N. S., Squires, K. C., & Starr, A. (1982). Auditory brainstem responses in chronic alcoholic patients. *Electroencephalography and Clinical Neurophysiology, 54,* 418–425.

Chu, N. S., & Yang, S. S. (1987). Brain-stem auditory evoked potentials in different types of hepatic diseases. *Electroencephalography and Clinical Neurophysiology, 67,* 337–339.

Chu, N. S., Yang, S. S., & Cheng, C. L. (1985). Somatosensory evoked potentials: Monitoring cerebral functions following liver transplantation. *Clinical Encephalography, 16,* 192–194.

Chung, W. H., Cho, D. Y., Choi, J. Y., & Hong, S. H. (2004). Clinical usefulness of extratympanic electrocochleography in the diagnosis of Ménière's disease. *Otology & Neurotology, 25,* 144–149.

Church, M., Eldis, F., Blakley, B., & Bawle, E. (1997). Hearing, language, speech, vestibular, and dentofacial disorders in fetal alcohol syndrome. *Alcoholism: Clinical and Experimental Research, 21,* 227–237.

Church, M., & Kaltenbach, J. (1997). Hearing, speech, language, and vestibular disorders in the fetal alcohol syndrome: A literature review. *Alcoholism: Clinical and Experimental Research, 21,* 495–512.

Church, M. W., & Williams, H. L. (1982). Dose- and time-dependent effects of ethanol on brain stem auditory evoked responses in young adult males. *Electroencephalography Clinical Neurophysiology, 54,* 161–174.

Ciesielski, K. T., Courchesne, E., & Elmasian, R. (1990). Effects of focused selected attention tasks on event related potentials in autistic and normal individuals. *Electroencephalography and Clinical Neurophysiology, 75,* 207–220.

Clayton, L. G., & Rose, D. E. (1970). Auditorily evoked cortical responses in normal and recruiting ears. *Journal of Auditory Research, 10,* 79–81.

Clementz, B. A., Geyer, M. A., & Braff, D. L. (1997). P50 suppression among schizophrenia and normal comparison subjects: A methodological analysis. *Biological Psychiatry, 41,* 1035–1044.

Clemis, J. D. (1984). Hearing conservation in acoustic tumor surgery: Pros and cons. *Archives of Otolaryngology—Head & Neck Surgery, 92,* 156–161.

Clemis, J. D., & McGee, T. (1979). Brainstem electric response audiometry in the differential diagnosis of acoustic tumors. *Laryngoscope, 89,* 31–42.

Clemis, J. D., & Mitchell, C. (1977). Electroencephalography and brainstem responses used in the differential diagnosis of acoustic tumors. *Laryngoscope, 89,* 31–42.

Clifford-Jones, R. E., Clarke, G. P., & Mayles, P. (1979). Crossed acoustic response combined with visual and somatosensory evoked responses in the diagnosis of multiple sclerosis. *Journal of Neurology, Neurosurgery, & Psychiatry, 42,* 749–752.

Coats, A. C. (1965). Temperature effects on the peripheral auditory apparatus. *Science, 150,* 1481–1483.

Coats, A. C. (1974). On electrocochleographic electrode design. *Journal of the Acoustical Society of America, 56,* 708–711.

Coats, A. C. (1978). Human auditory nerve action potentials in brainstem evoked responses: Latency intensity functions in detection of cochlear and retrocochlear abnormality. *Archives of Otolaryngology, 104,* 709–717.

Coats, A. C. (1981). The summating potential and Ménière's disease: I. Summating potential amplitude in Ménière's and non Ménière's ears. *Archives of Otolaryngology, 107,* 199–208.

Coats, A. C. (1984). Instrumentation. In E. J. Moore (Ed.), *Bases of auditory brain-stem evoked responses.* New York: Grune & Stratton.

Coats, A. C. (1986). The normal summating potential recorded from external ear canal. *Archives of Otolaryngology, 112,* 759–768.

Coats, A. C., & Alford, B. R. (1981). Ménière's disease and the summating potential: III. Effect of glycerol administration. *Archives of Otolaryngology, 107,* 469–473.

Coats, A. C., & Dickey, J. R. (1970). Nonsurgical recording of human auditory nerve action potentials and cochlear microphonics. *Journal of the Acoustical Society of America, 79,* 844–852.

Coats, A. C., Jenkins, H., & Monroe, B. (1984). Auditory evoked potentials: The cochlear summating potential in detection of endolymphatic hydrops. *American Journal of Otology, 5,* 443–446.

Coats, A. C., & Kidder, H. R. (1980). Earspeaker coupling effects on auditory action potential and brainstem responses. *Archives of Otolaryngology, 106,* 339–344.

Coats, A. C., & Martin, J. L. (1977). Human auditory nerve action potentials and brainstem evoked responses: Effect of audiogram shape and lesion location. *Archives of Otolaryngology, 103,* 605–622.

Coats, A. C., Martin, J. L., & Kidder, H. R. (1979). Normal short-latency electrophysiological filtered click responses recorded from vertex and external auditory meatus. *Journal of the Acoustical Society of America, 65,* 747–758.

Cody, D. T. R., & Bickford, R. G. (1965). Cortical audiometry: An objective method of evaluating auditory acuity in man. *Mayo Clinic Proceedings, 40,* 273–287.

Cody, D. T. R., & Bickford, R. G. (1969). Averaged evoked myogenic responses in normal man. *Laryngoscope, 79,* 400–416.

Cody, D. T. R., Jacobson, J. L., Walker, J. C., & Bickford, R. G. (1964). Averaged evoked myogenic and cortical potentials to sound in man. *Annals of Otology, Rhinology, & Laryngology, 73,* 763–777.

Cody, D. T. R., & Klass, D. W. (1968). Cortical audiometry: Potential pitfalls in testing. *Archives of Otolaryngology, 88,* 396–406.

Cody, D. T. R., Klass, D. W., & Bickford, R. G. (1967). Cortical audiometry: An objective method of evaluating auditory function in awake and sleeping man. *Transactions of the American Academy of Ophthalmology and Otolaryngology, 19,* 81–91.

Cohen, L., Richardson, L., Saunders, E., & Cowan, R. (2003). Spatial spread of neural exitation in cochlear implant recipients: Comparison of improved ECAP method and psychophysical forward masking. *Hearing Research, 179,* 72–87.

Cohen, L., Rickards, F., & Clark, G. (1991). A comparison of steady-state evoked potentials to modulated tones in awake and sleeping humans. *Journal of the Acoustical Society of America, 90,* 2467–2479.

Cohen, M. M. (1982). Coronal topography of the middle latency auditory evoked potentials (MLAEPs) in man. *Electroencephalography and Clinical Neurophysiology, 53,* 231–236.

Cohen, M. S., & Britt, R. H. (1982). Effects of sodium pentobarbital, ketamine, halothane, and chloralose on brainstem auditory evoked responses. *Anaesthesia and Analgesia, 61,* 338–343.

Cohen, N., Lewis, W., & Ransohoff, J. (1993). Hearing preservation in cerebellopontine angle tumor surgery: the NYU experience 1974–1991. *American Journal of Otology, 14,* 423–433.

Cohn, A. I., LeLiever, W. C., Hokanson, J. A., & Quinn, F. B. (1986). Acoustic neurinoma diagnostic model evaluation using decision support systems. *Archives of Otolaryngology—Head & Neck Surgery, 112,* 830–835.

Cohn, E., Kelley, P., Fowler, T., Gorga, M., Lefkowitz, D., Kuehn, H., Schaefer, B., Gobar, L., Hahn, F., Harris, D., & Kimberling, W. (1999). Clinical studies of families with hearing loss attributable to mutations in the connexin 26 gene (GJB2/DFNB1). *Pediatrics, 103,* 546–550.

Colebatch, J., Day, B., Bronstein, A., et al. (1998). Vestibular hypersensitivity to clicks is characteristic of the Tullio phenomenon. *Journal of Neurology, Neurosurgery, & Psychiatry, 65,* 670–678.

Colebatch, J., & Hamalgyi, G. (1992). Vestibular evoked myogenic potentials in human neck muscles before and after unilateral vestibular de-afferentiation. *Neurology, 42,* 1635–1636.

Colebatch, J., Halmagyi, G., & Skuse, N. (1994). Myogenic potentials generated by a click evoked vestibulocollic reflex. *Journal of Neurology, Neurosurgery, & Psychiatry, 57,* 190–197.

Colebatch, J., & Rothwell, J. (1993). Vestibular-evoked EMG responses in human neck muscles. *Journal of Physiology, 47,* 34–91.

Colebatch, J., Rothwell, J., Bronstein, A., & Hudman, H. (1994). Click-evoked vestibular activation in the Tullio phenomenon. *Journal of Neurology, Neurosurgery, & Psychiatry, 57,* 1538–1540.

Colletti, V., & Fiorino, F. G. (1994). Vulnerability of auditory function during acoustic neuroma surgery. *Acta Otolaryngologica (Stockholm), 116,* 264–270.

Colletti, V., Fiorino, F. G., Carner, M., & Tonoli, G. (1997a). Mechanisms of auditory impairment during acoustic neuroma surgery. *Otolaryngology—Head & Neck Surgery, 117,* 596–605.

Colletti, V., Fiorino, F. G., Mocella, S., et al. (1997b). ECoG, CNAP, and ABR monitoring during acoustic neuroma surgery. *Audiology, 37,* 27–37.

Colrain, I. M., DiParsia, P., & Gora, J. (2000). The impact of prestimulus EEG frequency on auditory evoked potentials during sleep onset. *Canadian Journal of Experimental Psychology, 54,* 243–254.

Comi, G. (1997). Evoked potentials in diabetes mellitus. *Clinical Neuroscience, 4,* 74–379.

Committee on Hearing and Equilibrium. (1995). Committee on Hearing and Equilibrium guidelines for the evaluation of hearing preservation in acoustic neuroma (vestibular schwannoma). *Archives of Otolaryngology—Head & Neck Surgery, 113,* 179–180.

Concu, A., Carcassi, A. M., Piras, M. B., Blanco, S., & Argiolas, A. (1978). Evidence for a correlation between the latency of an early component of auditory evoked potentials and the brain levels of serotonin in albino rats. *Experienientia, 34,* 375–377.

Cone-Wesson, B., Parker, J., Swiderski, N., & Rickards, F. (2002). The auditory steady-state response: Full term and premature neonates. *Journal of the American Academy of Audiology, 13,* 260–269.

Cone-Wesson, B., & Ramirez, G. (1997). Hearing sensitivity in newborns estimated from ABRs to bone-conducted sounds. *Journal of the American Academy of Audiology, 8,* 299–307.

Cone-Wesson, B., Rickards, F., Poulis, C., Parker, J., Tan, L., & Pollard, J. (2002). The auditory steady-state response: Clinical observations and applications in infants and children. *Journal of the American Academy of Audiology, 13,* 270–282.

Cone-Wesson, B., Rickards, F., Swiderski, N., & Parker, J. (2002). The auditory steady-state response: full-term and premature neonates. *Journal of the American Academy of Audiology, 13,* 260–269.

Cone-Wesson, B., Vohr, B. R., Sininger, Y. S., Widen, J. E., Folsom, R. C., Gorga, M. P., & Norton, S. J. (2000). Identification of neonatal hearing impairment: Infants with hearing impairment. *Ear and Hearing, 21,* 488–507.

Conijn, E. A. J. G., Brocaar, M. P., & van Zanten, G. A. (1990). Monaural versus binaural auditory brainstem response thresholds to clicks masked by high-pass noise in normal-hearing subjects. *Audiology, 29,* 29–35.

Conijn, E. A. J. G., Brocaar, M. P., & van Zanten, G. A. (1993). Frequency-specific aspects of the auditory brainstem response threshold elicited by 1000-Hz filtered clicks in subjects with sloping cochlear hearing losses. *Audiology, 32,* 1–11.

Conijn, E. A. J.G, van der Drift, J. F. C., Brocaar, M. P., & van Zanten, G. A. (1989). Conductive hearing loss assessment in children with otitis media with effusion. A comparison of pure tone and BERA results. *Clinical Otolaryngology, 14,* 115–120.

Conlon, B. J., & Gibson, W. P. (1999). Ménière's disease: The incidence of hydrops in the contralateral asymptomatic ear. *Laryngoscope, 109,* 1800–1802.

Conlon, B. J., & Gibson, W. P. (2000). Electrocochleography in the diagnosis of Ménière's disease. *Acta Otolaryngologica, 120,* 480–483.

Connolly, P. K., Stout, G. G., Williams, S. T., Jorgensen, S., & Smith, R. J. H. (1990). Oral habilitation of the child with no response on brainstem audiometry. *Pediatrics, 86,* 217–220.

Conti, G., Arslan, E., Camurri, L., et al. (1984). Electrocochleography and ABR in pediatric audiology: Comparison of results in threshold detection. *Acta Otorhinolaryngologica Italia, 4,* 655–666.

Conti, G., Modica, V., Castrataro, A., Fileni, A., & Colosimo, C., Jr. (1988). Latency of the auditory brainstem response (ABR) and head size: Evidence of the relationship by means of radiographic data. *Scandinavian Audiology (Supplement), 30,* 219–223.

Coons, H., Klorman, R., & Borgstedt, A. (1987). Effects of methylphenidate on adolescents with a childhood history of attention deficit disorder. II. Information processing. *Journal of the American Academy of Child and Adolescent Psychiatry, 26,* 368–374.

Cordone, A., Bavazzano, M., Sismondini, A., Mora, R., D'Angelo, M., Cordone, G., & Salami, A. (1999). Studio dei potenziali evocati uditivi a media latenza nella malattia di Alzheimer: valutazione delle onde P1 e P3. [Mid-latency auditory evoked responses in Alzheimer's disease: Evaluation of P1 and P3 waves]. *Acta Otorhinolaryngologica Italia, 19,* 64–69.

Cords, S., Reuter, G., Issing, P., Sommer, A., Kuzma, J., & Lenarz, T. (2000). A silastic positioner for a modiolus-hugging position of intracochlear electrodes: Electrophysiologic effects. *American Journal of Otology, 21,* 212–217.

Corley, V. M., & Crabbe, L. S. (1999). Auditory neuropathy and a mitochondrial disorder in a child: Case study. *Journal of the American Academy of Audiology, 10,* 484–488.

Cornacchia, L., Martini, A., & Morra, B. (1983). Air and bone conduction brain stem responses in adults and infants. *Audiology, 22,* 430–437.

Costa Neto, T., Ito, Y., Fukuda, Y., Gananca, M., & Caovilla, H. (1991). Effects of gender and head size on the auditory brainstem response. *Revue Laryngologie, Otologie, & Rhinologie (Bordeaux), 112,* 17–19.

Cote, C. J., Karl, H. W., Notterman, D. A., Weinberg, J. A., & McCloskey, C. (2000). Adverse sedation events in pediatrics: Analysis of medications used for sedation. *Pediatrics,106,* 633–644.

Cote, K. (2002). Probing awareness during sleep with the auditory odd-ball paradigm. *International Journal of Psychophysiology, 46,* 227–241.

Cottrell, G., & Gans, D. (1995). Auditory-evoked response morphology in profoundly-involved multi-handicapped children: Comparisons with normal infants and children. *Audiology, 34,* 189–206.

Counter, S. A., & Buchanan, L. H. (2002). Neuro-ototoxicity in Andean adults with chronic lead and noise exposure. *Journal of Occupational & Environmental Medicine, 44,* 30–38.

Counter, S. A., Buchanan, L., Ortega, F., & Laurell, G. (1997). Normal auditory brainstem and cochlear function in extreme pediatric plumbism. *Journal of Neurological Sciences, 152,* 85–92.

Courchesne, E. (1978a). Changes in P3 waves with event repetition: Long-term effects on scalp distribution and amplitude. *Electroencephalography and Clinical Neurophysiology, 45,* 745–766.

Courchesne, E. (1978b). Neurophysiological correlates of cognitive development: Changes in long-latency event-related potentials from childhood to adulthood. *Electroencephalography and Clinical Neurophysiology, 45,* 468–482.

Courchesne, E., Hillyard, S. A., & Galambos, R. (1975). Stimulus novelty, task relevance and the visual evoked potential in man. *Electroencephalograpy and Clinical Neurophysiolology, 39,* 131–143.

Courchesne, E., Kilman, B., Galambos, R., & Lincoln, A. (1984). Autism: Processing of novel auditory information assessed by event-related brain potentials. *Electroencephalography and Clinical Neurophysiology, 59,* 238–248.

Courchesne, E., Lincoln, A., Kilman, B., & Galambos, R. (1985). Event-related brain potential correlates of the processing of novel visual and auditory information in autism. *Journal of Autism and Developmental Disorders, 15,* 55–76.

Courchesne, E., Lincoln, A. J., Yeung-Courchesne, R., Elmasian, R., & Grillon, C. (1989). Pathophysiologic findings in nonretarded autism and receptive developmental language disorder. *Journal of Autism and Developmental Disorders, 19,* 1–17.

Coutinho, M., Rocha, V., & Santos, M. (2002). Auditory brainstem response in two children with autism. *International Journal of Pediatric Otorhinolaryngology, 66,* 81–85.

Cowan, N. (1984). On short and long auditory stores. *Psychology Bulletin, 96,* 341–370.

Cowell, P. E., Turetsky, B. I., Gur, R. C., Grossman, R. I., Shtasel, D. L., & Gur, R. E. (1994). Sex differences in aging of the human frontal and temporal lobes. *Journal of Neuroscience, 14,* 4748–4755.

Cox, L. C. (1985). Infant assessment: Developmental and age-related considerations. In J. T. Jacobson (Ed.), *The auditory brainstem response* (pp. 297–316). San Diego: College-Hill Press.

Cox, L. C., Hack, M., & Metz, D. A. (1981). Brainstem evoked response audiometry in the premature infant population. *International Journal of Pediatric Otorhinolaryngology, 3,* 213–224.

Cox, R. M. (1986). NBS-9A coupler-to-eardrum transformation: TDH-39 and TDH-49. *Journal of the Acoustical Society of America, 79,* 120–123.

Cracco, R. Q. (1985). Utility of evoked potentials. *Journal of the American Medical Association, 254,* 3490.

Crain, M. R., & Dolan, K. D. (1990). Internal auditory canal enlargement in Paget's disease appearing as bilateral acoustic neuromas. *Annals of Otology, Rhinology & Laryngology, 99,* 833–834.

Cranford, J. L., Rothermel, A. K., Walker, L., Stuart, A., & Elangovan, S. (2004). Effects of discrimination task difficulty on N1 and P2 components of late auditory evoked potential. *Journal of the American Academy of Audiology, 15,* 456–461.

Creasey, H., & Rapoport, S. I. (1985). The aging human brain. *Annals of Neurology, 17,* 2–10.

Creel, D. J., Kivlin, J. D., & Wolfey, D. E. (1984). Auditory brain-stem responses in Marcus Gunn ptosis. *Electroencephalography and Clinical Neurophysiology, 59,* 341–344.

Creutzfeldt, O. D., Arnold, P. M., Becker, D., Langestein, S., Tirsch, W., Wilhelm, H., & Wuttke, W. (1976). EEG changes during spontaneous and controlled menstrual cycles and their correlation with psychological performance. *Electroencephalography and Clinical Neurophysiology, 40,* 113–131.

Creutzfeldt, O. D, Hellweg, F. C., & Schreiner, C. (1980). Thalamocortical transformation of responses to complex auditory stimuli. *Experimental Brain Research, 39,* 87–104.

Crottaz-Herbette, S., & Ragot, R. (2000). Perception of complex sounds: N1 latency codes pitch and topography codes spectra. *Clinical Neurophysiology, 111,* 1759–1766.

Crowley, K. E., & Colrain, I. M. (2004). A review of the evidence for P2 being an independent component process: Age, sleep & modality. *Clinical Neurophysiology, 115,* 732–744.

Crowley, K. E., Trinder, J., & Colrain, I. M. (2002). An examination of evoked-K-complex amplitude and frequency of occurrence in the elderly. *Journal of Sleep Research, 11,* 129–140.

Csépe, V. (1995). On the origin and development of the mismatch negativity. *Ear and Hearing, 16,* 91–104.

Csépe, V., Osman-Sagi, J., Molnar, M., & Gosy, M. (2001). Impaired speech perception in aphasic patients: Event-related potential and neuropsychological assessment. *Neuropsychologia, 39,* 1194–1208.

Csépe, V., Pantev, C., Hoke, M., Hampson, S., & Ross, B. (1992). Evoked magnetic responses of the human auditory cortex to minor pitch changes: Localization of the mismatch field. *Electroencephalography and Clinical Neurophysiology, 84,* 538–548.

Cueva, R. (2004). Auditory brainstem response versus magnetic resonance imaging for the evaluation of asymmetric sensorineural hearing loss. *Laryngoscope, 114,* 1686–1692.

Cueva, R. A., Morris, G. F., & Prioleau, G. R. (1998). Direct cochlear nerve monitoring: First report on a new atraumatic, self-retaining electrode. *American Journal of Otology, 19,* 203–207.

Cullen, J., Ellis, M., Berlin, C. I., & Lousteau, R. J. (1972). Human acoustic nerve action potential recordings from the tympanic membrane without Anaesthesia. *Acta Otolaryngologica, 74,* 15–22.

Cullington, H. (2000). Preliminary neural response telemetry results. *British Journal of Audiology, 34,* 131–140.

Cunningham, J., Nicol, T., Zecker, S. G., & Kraus, N. (2000). Speech-evoked neurophysiologic responses in children with learning problems: Development and behavioral correlates of perception. *Ear and Hearing, 21,* 554–568.

Cunningham, J., Nicol, T., Zecker, S. G., & Kraus, N. (2001). Neurobiologic responses to speech in noise in children with learning problems: Deficits and strategies for improvement. *Clinical Neurophysiology, 112,* 758–767.

Curry, S. (1980). Event-related potentials as indicators of structural and functional damage in closed head injury. In H. Kornhuber & L. Deeke, (Eds.), *Motivation, motor and sensory processes of the brain: Electrical potentials, behaviour, and clinical use* (pp. 507–515). Amsterdam: Elsevier.

Cutler, J. R., Aminoff, M. J., & Brant-Zawadzki, M. B. (1986). Evaluation of patients with multiple sclerosis by evoked potentials and magnetic resonance imaging: A comparative study. *Annals of Neurology, 20,* 645–648.

Czigler, I., Csibra, G., & Csontos, A. (1992). Age and inter-stimulus interval effects on event-related potentials to frequent and infrequent auditory stimuli. *Biological Psychology, 33,* 195–206.

Dafny, N., & Rigor, B. M. (1978). Neurophysiological approach as a tool to study effects of drugs on the central nervous system: Dose-effect of ketamine. *Experimental Neurology, 59,* 275–285.

Dalebout, S. D., & Fox, L. G. (2000). Identification of the mismatch negativity in the responses of individual listeners. *Journal of the American Academy of Audiology, 11,* 12–22.

Dalebout, S. D., & Fox, L. G. (2001). Reliability of the mismatch negativity in the responses of individual listeners. *Journal of the American Academy of Audiology, 12,* 245–253.

Dalebout, S. D., & Robey, R. (1997). Comparison of the intersubject and intrasubject variability of exogenous and endogenous auditory evoked potentials. *Journal of the American Academy of Audiology, 8,* 342–354.

Dalebout, S. D., & Stack, J. W. (1999). Mismatch negativity to acoustic differences not differentiated behaviorally. *Journal of the American Academy of Audiology, 10,* 388–399.

Dallos, P. (1973). *The auditory periphery.* New York: Academic Press.

Dallos, P. (1975). Electrical correlates of mechanical events in the cochlea. *Audiology, 14,* 408–418.

Dallos, P., & Cheatham, M. A. (1976). Compound action potential (AP) tuning curves. *Journal of the Acoustical Society of America, 59,* 591–597.

Dallos, P., & Olsen, W. (1964). Integration of energy at threshold with gradual rise-fall tone pips. *Journal of the Acoustical Society of America, 36,* 743.

Dallos, P., Schoeny, Z., & Cheatham, M. (1972). Cochlear summating potentials: Descriptive aspects. *Acta Otolaryngologica (Supplement), 302,* 1–46.

Daly, D., Roeser, R. J., Aung, M. H., & Daly, D. D. (1977). Early evoked potentials in patients with acoustic neuroma. *Electroencephalography and Clinical Neurophysiology, 43,* 151–159.

Daniels, D. L., Millen, S. J., Meyer, G. A., Pojunas, K. W., Kilgore, D. P., Shaffer, K. A., et al. (1987). MR detection of tumor in the internal auditory canal. *American Journal of Neuroradiology, 8,* 249–252.

Danner, C., Mastrodimos, B., & Cueva, R. A. (2004). A comparison of direct eighth nerve monitoring and auditory brainstem response in hearing preservation surgery for vestibular schwannoma. *Otology and Neurotology, 25,* 826–832.

Danos, P., Kasper, S., Scholl, H. P., Kaiser, J., Ruhrmann, S., Hoflich, G., & Moller, H. J. (1994). Clinical response to sleep deprivation and auditory-evoked potentials—preliminary results. *Pharmacopsychiatry, 27,* 70–71.

D'Arcy, R. C. N., & Connolly, J. F. (1999). An event-related brain potential study of receptive speech comprehension using a modified Token Test. *Neuropsychologia, 37,* 1477–1489.

D'Arcy, R. C. N., Connolly, J. F., Service, E., Hawco, C. S., & Houlihan, M. E. (2004). Separating phonological and semantic processing in auditory sentence processing: A high-resolution event-related brain potential study. *Human Brain Mapping, 22,* 40–51.

Darling, R. M., & Price, L. L. (1990). Loudness and auditory brain stem evoked response. *Ear and Hearing, 11,* 289–295.

Daruna, J., Nelson, A., & Green, J. (1989). Unilateral temporal lobe lesions alter P300 scalp topography. *International Journal of Neuroscience, 46,* 243–247.

Daspit, C. P., Raudzens, P. A., & Shetter, A. G. (1982). Monitoring of intraoperative auditory brain stem responses. *Archives of Otolaryngology—Head & Neck Surgery, 90,* 108–116.

Dau, T., Wagner, O., Mellert, V., & Kollmeier, B. (2000). Auditory brainstem responses with optimized chirp signals compensating basilar-membrane dispersion. *Journal of the Acoustical Society of America, 107,* 1530–1540.

Dauman, R. (1991). Electrocochleography: Applications and limitations in young children. *Acta Otolaryngologica (Stockholm), Supplement, 482,* 14–26.

Dauman, R., Aran, J. M., Charlet de Sauvage, R., & Portmann, M. (1988). Clinical significance of the summating potential in Ménière's disease. *American Journal of Otology, 9,* 31–38.

Dauman, R., Aran, J. M., & Portmann, M. (1986). Summating potential and water balance in Ménière's disease. *Annals of Otology, Rhinology & Laryngology, 95,* 389–395.

Dauman, R., & Charlet de Sauvage, R. (1984). Continuous monitoring of SP and CAP during glycerol test in Ménière's disease. *Revue de Laryngologie, Otologie, Rhinologie, 105,* 219–221.

Dauman, R., Szyfter, W., Charlet de Sauvage, R., & Cazals, Y. (1984). Low frequency thresholds assessed with 40 Hz MLR in adults with impaired hearing. *Archives of Otorhinolaryngology, 240,* 85–89.

Davies, M., Kane, R., & Valentine, J. (1984). Impaired hearing in X-linked hypophosphataemic (vitamin-D-resistant) osteomalacia. *Annals of Internal Medicine, 100,* 230–232.

Davis, H. (1958). A mechano-electrical theory of cochlear action. *Annals of Otology, Rhinology & Laryngology, 67,* 789–801.

Davis, H. (1964). Enhancement of evoked cortical potentials in humans related to a task requiring a decision. *Science, 145,* 182–183.

Davis, H. (1965). Slow cortical responses evoked by acoustic stimuli. *Acta Otolaryngologica (Supplement), 59,* 179–185.

Davis, H. (1973). Sedation of young children for electric response audiometry. *Audiology, 12,* 55–57.

Davis, H. (1976a). Brain stem and other response audiometry. *Annals of Otology, Rhinology & Laryngology, 85,* 3–14.

Davis, H. (1976b). Principles of electric response audiometry. *Annals of Otology, Rhinology & Laryngology, 85,* 1–96.

Davis, H. (1979). United States–Japan seminar on auditory responses from the brainstem. *Laryngoscope, 39,* 1336–1339.

Davis, H., Bowers, C., & Hirsh, S. K. (1968). Relations of the human vertex potential to acoustic input: Loudness and masking. *Journal of the Acoustical Society of America, 43,* 431–438.

Davis, H., Davis, P. A., Loomis, A. L., Harvey, E. N., & Hobart, G. (1939). Electrical reactions of the human brain to auditory stimulation during sleep. *Journal of Neurophysiology, 2,* 500–514.

Davis, H., Deatherage, B. H., Eldredge, D. H., & Smith, C. A. (1958). Summating potentials of the cochlea. *American Journal of Physiology, 195,* 251–261.

Davis, H., & Hirsh, S. K. (1979). A slow brain stem response for low-frequency audiometry. *Audiology, 18,* 445–461.

Davis, H., Hirsh, S. K., Popelka, G. R., & Formby, C. (1984). Frequency sensitivity and thresholds of brief stimuli suitable for electric response audiometry. *Audiology, 23,* 59–74.

Davis, H., Hirsh, S. K., & Turpin, L. L. (1983). Possible utility of middle latency responses in electric response audiometry. *Advances in Otorhinolaryngology, 31,* 208–216.

Davis, H., Hirsh, S. K., Turpin, L. L., & Peacock, M. E. (1985). Threshold sensitivity and frequency specificity in auditory brainstem response audiometry. *Audiology, 24,* 54–70.

Davis, H., Mast, T., Yoshie, N., & Zerlin, S. (1966). The slow response of the human cortex to auditory stimuli: Recovery process. *Electroencephalography and Clinical Neurophysiology, 21,* 105–113.

Davis, H., & Onishi, S. (1969). Maturation of auditory evoked potentials. *International Audiology, 8,* 24–33.

Davis, H., & Zerlin, S. (1966). Acoustic relations of the human vertex potential. *Journal of the Acoustical Society of America, 39,* 109–116.

Davis, P. A. (1939). Effects of acoustic stimuli on the waking human brain. *Journal of Neurophysiology, 2,* 494–499.

Davis, R. L., & Robertson, D. M. (Eds.). (1991). *Textbook of neuropathy* (2nd ed.). Baltimore, MD: Williams & Wilkins.

Davis, S. L., Aminoff, M. J., & Berg, B. O. (1985). Brainstem auditory evoked potentials in children with brainstem or cerebellar dysfunction. *Archives of Neurology, 42,* 156–160.

Davis-Gunter, M., Lowenheim, H., Gopal, K., & Moore, E. (2001). The I' potential of the human auditory brainstem response to paired click stimuli. *Scandinavian Audiology, 30,* 50–60.

Dawson, G. D. (1951). A summation technique for detecting small signals in a large irregular background. *Journal of Physiology, 115,* 2.

Dawson, G. D., Finley, C., Phillips, S., Galpert, L., & Lewy, A. (1988). Reduced P3 amplitude of the event-related brain potential: Its relationship to language ability in autism. *Journal of Autism and Developmental Disorders, 18,* 493–504.

Dawson, W. W., & Doddington, H. W. (1973). Phase distortion of biological signals: Extraction of signals from noise without phase error. *Electroencephalography and Clinical Neurophysiology, 34,* 207–211.

Deacon, D., Nousak, J. M., Pilotti, M., Ritter, W., & Yang, C. M. (1998). Automatic change detection: Does the auditory system use representations of individual stimulus features or gestalts? *Psychophysiology, 35,* 413–419.

Deans, J. A., Birchall, J. P., & Mendelow, A. D. (1990). Acoustic neuroma and the contralateral ear: Recovery of auditory brainstem response abnormalities after surgery. *The Journal of Laryngology, 104,* 565–569.

Deans, J. A., Hill, J., Birchall, J. P., Davison, T., Fitzgerald, J. E., & Elliott, C. (1996). The effect of electrode position in electrocochleography. *Clinical Otolaryngology, 21,* 317–323.

DeBrey, H. B., & Eggermont, J. J. (1978). The influence of cochlear temperature on the electrical travelling wave pattern in the guinea pig cochlea. *Acta Otolaryngologica, 85,* 363–371.

Debruyne, D. F. (1984). Binaural interaction in early, middle, and late auditory evoked responses. *Scandinavian Audiology, 13,* 293–296.

Debruyne, D. F., Hombergen, G., & Hoekstra, M. (1980). Normale waarden in de brainstem electric response audiometry (BERA). *Acta Oto-Rhino-Laryngology Belgium, 34,* 238–296.

DeCasper, A. J., & Fifer, W. P (1980). Of human bonding: Newborns prefer their mothers' voices. *Science, 208,* 1174–1176.

De Chicchis, A. R., Carpenter, M., Cranford, J. L., & Hymel, M. R. (2002). Electrophysiologic correlates of attention versus distraction in young and elderly listeners. *Journal of the American Academy of Audiology, 13,* 383–391.

Decker, T. N., & Howe, S. W. (1981). Auditory tract asymmetry in brainstem electrical responses during binaural stimulation. *Journal of the Acoustical Society of America, 69,* 1084–1090.

Dees, D., Dillier, N., Lai, W., von Wallenberg, E., Van Dijk, J., Akdas, F., Aksit, M., Batman, C., Beynon, A., Burdo, S., Chanal, J., Collet, L., Conway, M., Coudert, C., Craddock, L., Cullington, H., Deggouj, N., Fraysse, B., Grabel, S., Kiefer, J., Kiss, J., Lenarz, T., Mair, A., Maune, S., Muller-Deile, J., Piron, J., Razza, S., Tasche, C., Thai-Van, H., Toth, F., Truy, E., Uziel, A., & Smoorenburg, G. (2005). Normative findings of electrically evoked compound action potential measurements using the neural response telemetry of the Nucleus CI24M cochlear implant system. *Audiology & Neuro-Otology, 10,* 105–116.

Dehaene-Lambertz, G., & Dehaene, S. (1994). Speed and cerebral correlates of syllable discrimination in infants. *Nature, 370,* 292–295.

Dehan, C., & Jerger, J. (1990). Analysis of gender differences in the auditory brainstem response. *Laryngoscope, 100,* 18–24.

deJesus, P. V., Hausmanowa-Petrusewicz, I., & Barch, R. L. (1973). The effect of cold on nerve conduction of human slow and fast nerve fibers. *Neurology, 23,* 1182–1189.

Dejong, R. (1982). Central nervous system manifestations of DM. *Postgraduate Medicine, 71,* 50–67.

Deka, R. C., Kacker, S. K., & Tandon, P. N. (1987). Auditory brain-stem evoked responses in cerebellopontine angle tumors. *Archives of Otolaryngology—Head & Neck Surgery, 113,* 647–650.

Deldin, P. J., Duncan, C. C., & Miller, G. A. (1994). Season, gender, and P300. *Biological Psychology, 39,* 15–28.

Delgado, R., & Özdamar, O. (1994, April/May). Automated auditory brainstem response interpretation. *IEEE EMB,* 227–237.

Delgado, T. E., Bucheit, W. A., Rosenholtz, H. R., & Chrissian, S. (1979). Intra-operative monitoring of facial muscle evoked responses obtained by intracranial stimulation of the facial nerve: A more accurate technique for facial nerve dissection. *Neurosurgery, 4,* 418–421.

Deltenre, P., Mansbach, A. L., Bozet, C., Clercx, A., & Hecox, K. E. (1997). Temporal distortion products (kernel slices) evoked by maximum-length sequences in auditory neuropathy: Evidence for a cochlear pre-synaptic origin. *Electroencephalography and Clinical Neurophysiology, 104,* 10–16.

Deltenre, P., Van Nechel, C., Strul, S., & Ketelaer, P. (1984). A five-year prospective study on the value of multimodal evoked potentials and blink reflex, as an aid to the diagnosis of suspected multiple sclerosis. In R. H. Nodar & C. Barber (Eds.), *Evoked Potentials II: The Second International Evoked Potentials Symposium* (pp. 603–608). Boston: Butterworth.

Deltenre, P., Vercruyzze, A., Van Nechel, C., Ketelaer, P., Capon, A., Colin, F., et al. (1979). Early diagnosis of multiple sclerosis by combined multimodal evoked potentials: Results and practical considerations. *Journal of Biomedical Engineering, 1,* 17–21.

deLugt, D. R., Loewy, D. H., & Campbell, K. B. (1996). The effect of sleep onset on event related potentials with rapid rates of stimulus presentation. *Electroencephalograpy and Clinical Neurophysiology, 98,* 484–492.

Demiralp, T., Ademoglu, A., Schurmann, M., Basar-Eroglu, C., & Başar, E. (1999). Detection of P300 waves in single trials by the wavelet transform (WT). *Brain and Language, 66,* 108–128.

Dempsey, J. J., Censoprano, E., & Mazor, M. (1986). Relationship between head size and latency of the auditory brainstem response. *Audiology, 25,* 258–262.

Dennenberg, V., Kertesz, A., & Cowell, P. (1991). A factor analysis of the human's corpus callosum. *Brain Research, 548,* 126–132.

Dennis, J. M., & Earley, D. A. (1988). Monitoring surgical procedures with the auditory brainstem response. *Seminars in Hearing, 9,* 113–125.

Densert, B., Arlinger, S., Sass, K., & Hergils, L. (1994). Reproducibility of the electric response components in clinical electrocochleography. *Audiology, 33,* 254–263.

Deol, M. S. (1981). The inner ear in Bronx waltzer mice. *Acta Otolaryngologica, 92,* 331–336.

Deouell, L. Y., Bentin, S., & Giard, M. H. (1998). Mismatch negativity in dichotic listening: Evidence for interhemispheric differences and multiple generators. *Psychophysiology, 35,* 355–365.

Derbyshire, A. J., & Davis, H. (1935). The action potentials of the auditory nerve. *American Journal of Physiology, 113,* 476–504.

deRegnier, R. A., Nelson, C. A., Thomas, K. M., Wewerka, S., & Georgieff, M. K. (2001). Neurophysiologic evaluation of auditory recognition memory in healthy newborn infants and infants of diabetic mothers. *Journal of Pediatrics, 137,* 777–784.

Desaulty, A., Lansiaux, V., Moreau, L., & Vandorpe, C. (1992). [Retrocochlear deafness, acoustic neurinoma and early evoked auditory potentials—apropos of a series of 113 patients.]. *Acta Otorhinolaryngologica Belgium, 46,* 77–83.

Despland, P. A., & Galambos, R. (1980). The auditory brainstem response (ABR) is a useful diagnostic tool in the intensive care nursery. *Pediatric Research, 14,* 154–158.

De Waele, C., Tran Ba Huy, P., Diard, J., Freyss, G., & Vidal, P. (1999). Saccular dysfunction in Ménière's patients. A vestibular-evoked myogenic potential study. *Annals of the New York Academy of Sciences, 871,* 392–397.

de Weerd, J. P. C. (1981). A posteriori time-varying filtering of averaged evoked potentials: I. Introduction and conceptual basis. *Biological Cybernetics, 41,* 211–222

de Weerd, J. P. C., & Kap, J. I. (1981). Spectro-temporal representations and time-varying spectra of evoked potentials. *Biological Cybernetics, 41,* 101–117.

Diaz, F., Cadaveira, F., & Grau, C. (1990). Short- and middle-latency auditory evoked potentials in abstinent chronic alcoholics: Preliminary findings. *Electroencephalography and Clinical Neurophysiology, 77,* 145–150.

Diaz, F., & Zurron, M. (1995). Auditory evoked potentials in Down's syndrome. *Electroencephalography and Clinical Neurophysiology, 96,* 526–537.

Didier, A., Cazals, Y., & Aurousseau, C. (1987). Brainstem connections of the anterior and posterior parts of the saccule of the guinea pig. *Acta Otolaryngologica, 104,* 385–391.

Dierks, T., Linden, D. E., Jandl, M., Formisano, E., Goebel, R., Lanfermann, H., & Singer, W. (1999). Activation of Heschl's gyrus during auditory hallucinations. *Neuron, 22,* 615–621.

Dillier, N., Lai, W., Almqvist, B., Frohne, C., Muller-Deile, J., Stecker, M., & von Wallenberg, E. (2002). Measurement of the electrically evoked compound action potential via a neural response telemetry system. *Annals of Otology, Rhinology & Laryngology, 111*, 414.

DiLorenzo, L., Foggia, L., Panza, N., Calabrese, M., Motta, G., Orio, F. J., & Lombardi, G. (1995). Auditory brainstem responses in thyroid diseases before and after therapy. *Hormone Research, 43*, 200–205.

Dimitrijevic, A., John, M. S., & Picton, T. W. (2004). Auditory steady-state responses and word recognition scores in normal-hearing and hearing-impaired adults. *Ear and Hearing, 25*, 68–84.

Dimitrijevic, A., John, M., Van Roon, P., & Picton, T. (2001). Human auditory steady-state responses to tones independently modulated in both frequency and amplitude. *Ear and Hearing, 22*, 100–111.

Dimitrijevic, A., John, M., Van Roon, P., Purcell, D., Adamonis, J., Ostroff, J., et al. (2002). Estimating the audiogram using multiple auditory steady-state responses. *Journal of the American Academy of Audiology, 13*, 205–224.

Dimpfel, W., Todorova, A., & Vonderheid-Guth, B. (1999). Pharmacodynamic properties of St. John's wort: A single blind neurophysiological study in healthy subjects comparing two commercial preparations. *European Journal of Medical Research, 4*, 303–312.

Diner, B. C., Holcomb, P. J., & Dykman, R. A. (1985). P300 in major depressive disorder. *Psychiatry Research, 15*, 175–184.

DiPaolo, B., DiMarco, T., Cappelli, P., et al. (1988). Electrophysiological aspects of nervous conduction in uremia. *Clinical Nephrology, 32*, 242–248.

Dittmann-Balcar, A., Thienel, R., & Schall, U. (1999). Attention-dependent allocation of auditory processing resources as measured by mismatch negativity. *Neuroreport, 10*, 3749–3753.

Djupesland, G., Flottorp, G., Modalsli, B., Tevete, O., & Sortland, O. (1981). Acoustic brainstem resposne in diagnosis of acoustic neuroma. *Scandinavian Audiology (Supplement), 13*, 109–112.

Dobie, R. A., & Norton, S. J. (1980). Binaural interaction in human auditory evoked potentials. *Electroencephalography and Clinical Neurophysiology, 49*, 303–313.

Dobie, R. A., & Wilson, M. J. (1989). Analysis of auditory evoked potentials by magnitude-squared coherence. *Ear and Hearing, 10*, 2–13.

Döller, C. F., Opitz, B., Mecklinger, A., Krick, C., Reith, W., & Schroger, E. (2003). Prefrontal cortex involvement in preattentive auditory deviance detection: Neuroimaging and electrophysiological evidence. *NeuroImage, 20*, 1270–1282.

Dolphin, W. (1997). The envelope following response to multiple tone pair stimuli. *Hearing Research, 110*, 1–14.

Dolphin, W. F., & Mountain, D. C. (1992). The envelope following response: Scalp potentials elicited in the Mongolian gerbil using sinusoidally AM acoustic signals. *Hearing Research, 58*, 70–78.

Domico, W. D., & Kavanaugh, K. T. (1986). Analog and zero phase-shift digital filtering of the auditory brainstem resonse of the waveform. *Ear and Hearing, 7*, 377–382.

Don, M. (2002). Auditory brainstem response testing in acoustic neuroma diagnosis. *Current Opinions in Archives of Otolaryngology—Head & Neck Surgery, 10*, 376–381.

Don, M., Allen, A. R., & Starr, A. (1977). Effect of click rate on the latency of auditory brainstem responses in humans. *Annals of Otology, Rhinology & Laryngology, 86*, 186–195.

Don, M., & Eggermont, J. J. (1978). Analysis of the click-evoked brainstem potentials in man using high-pass noise masking. *Journal of the Acoustical Society of America, 63*, 1084–1092.

Don, M., Eggermont, J. J., & Brackmann, D. (1979). Reconstruction of the audiogram using brain stem responses and high-pass noise masking. *Annals of Otology, Rhinology & Laryngology (Supplement), 57*, 1–20.

Don, M., Elberling, C., & Waring, M. (1984). Objective detection of averaged auditory brainstem response. *Scandinavian Audiology, 13*, 1–36.

Don, M., & Kwong, B. (2002). Differential diagnosis. In J. Katz (Ed.). *Handbook of clinical audiology* (pp. 274–297). Baltimore: Lippincott Williams & Wilkins.

Don, M., Kwong, B., Tanaka, C., Brackmann, D., & Nelson, R. (2005). The stacked ABR: A sensitive and specific screening tool for detecting small acoustic tumors. *Audiology & Neuro-Otology, 10*, 274–290.

Don, M., Masuda, A., Nelson, R., & Brackmann, D. (1997). Successful detection of small acoustic tumors using the stacked derived band ABR method. *American Journal of Otolaryngology, 18*, 608–621.

Don, M., Ponton, C., Eggermont, J., & Masuda, A. (1993). Gender differences in cochlear response time: An explanation for gender amplitude differences in the unmasked auditory brainstem response. *Journal of the Acoustical Society of America, 94*, 2135–2148.

Don, M., Ponton, C., Eggermont, J., & Masuda, A. (1994). Auditory brainstem response (ABR) peak amplitude variability reflects individual differences in cochlear response times. *Journal of the Acoustical Society of America, 96*, 3476–3491.

Don, M., Vermiglio, A., Ponton, C., & Eggermont, J. (1996). Variable effects of click polarity on auditory brain-stem response latencies: Analyses of narrow-band ABRs suggest possible explanation. *Journal of the Acoustical Society of America, 100*, 458–466.

Donald, M., Bird, C., Lawson, J., Letemendia, F., Monga, T., Surridge, D. H. C., et al. (1981). Delayed auditory brainstem responses in diabetes mellitus. *Journal of Neurology, Neurosurgery, & Psychiatry, 44*, 641–644.

Donaldson, G., Peters, M., Ellis, M., Friedman, B., Levine, S., & Rimell, F. (2001). Effects of the Clarion Electrode Positioning System on auditory thresholds and comfortable loudness levels in pediatric patients with cochlear implants. *Archives of Otolaryngology—Head & Neck Surgery, 127*, 956–960.

Donaldson, G., & Ruth, R. (1993). Derived band auditory brainstem response estimates of traveling wave velocity in humans. I. Normal-hearing subjects. *Journal of the Acoustical Society of America, 93*, 940–951.

Donchin, E. (1966). A multivariate approach to the analysis of average evoked potentials. *IEEE Transactions on Biomedical Engineering, 13*, 131–139.

Donchin, E. (1969). Data analysis techniques in evoked potential research. In E. Donchin & D. B. Lindsley (Eds.), *Averaged evoked potentials: Methods, results, evaluation.* Washington, DC: Government Printing Office.

Donchin, E., & Coles, M. G. H. (1988). Is the P300 component a manifestation of context updating? *Behavioral and Brain Science, 11*, 357–374.

Donchin, E., & Heffley, E. F. (1978). Multivariate analysis of event-related potentials data: A tutorial review. *Multidisciplinary Perspectives in Event-Related Brain Potential Research, 9*, 553–572.

Donchin, E., Ritter, W., & McCallum, W. C. (1978). Cognitive psychophysiology: The endogenous components of the ERP. In E. Callaway, P. Tueting, & S. H. Koslow (Eds.), *Event-related brain potentials in man* (pp. 349–411). New York: Academic Press.

Doring, W. H., & Daub, D. (1980). Acoustically evoked responses under sedation with diazepam. *Archives of Otorhinolaryngology, 227*, 522–525.

Dorman, M., Smith, L., Smith, M., & Parkin, J. (1996). Frequency discrimination and speech recognition by patients who use the Ineraid and continuous interleaved sampling cochlear-implant signal processors. *Journal of the Acoustical Society of America, 99*, 1174–1184.

Dornhoffer, J. L. (1998). Diagnosis of cochlear Ménière's disease with electrocochleography. *ORL: Journal for Otorhinolaryngolaryngology and its Related Specialities, 60*, 301–305.

Dornhoffer, J. L., & Arenberg, I. K. (1993). Diagnosis of vestibular Ménière's disease with electrocochleography. *American Journal of Otology, 14*, 161–164.

Dornhoffer, J., Helms, J., & Hoehmann, D. (1995). Hearing preservation in acoustic tumor surgery: Results and prognostic factors. *Laryngoscope, 105*, 184–187.

Doty, R. L., Hall, J. W. I., Flickinger, G. L., & Sondheimer, S. J. (1982). Cyclical changes in olfactory and auditory sensitivity during the menstrual cycle: No attentuation by oral contraceptive medication. In W. E. Breiphol (Ed.), *Olfaction and endocrine regulation* (pp. 35–42). London: IRL Press.

Douek, E., Gibson, W., & Humphries, K. (1973). The crossed acoustic response. *Journal of Laryngology & Otology, 87*, 711–726.

Downs, M. P., & Sterritt, G. M. (1967). A guide to newborn and infant hearing screening programs. *Archives of Otolaryngology, 85*, 37–44.

Doyle, D. J. (1975). Some comments on the use of Weiner filtering for estimation of evoked potentials. *Electroencephalography and Clinical Neurophysiology, 38*, 533–534.

Doyle, D. J., & Hyde, M. L. (1981a). Analogue and digital filtering of auditory brainstem responses. *Scandinavian Audiology, 10*, 81–89.

Doyle, D. J., & Hyde, M. L. (1981b). Digital inverse filtering of distorted auditory brainstem response. *Scandinavian Audiology, 10*, 261–263.

Doyle, K. J., Sininger, Y., & Starr, A. (1998). Auditory neuropathy in childhood. *Laryngoscope, 108*, 1374–1377.

Drake, M. E., Jr., Huber, S. J., Pakalnis, A., & Phillips, B. B. (1993). Neuropsychological and event-related potential correlates of nonepileptic seizures. *Journal of Neuropsychiatry & Clinical Neuroscience, 5,* 102–104.

Drake, M. E., Weate, S. J., & Newell, S. A. (1996). Auditory evoked potentials in postconcussive syndrome. *Electromyography and Clinical Neurophysiology, 36,* 457–462.

Drake, M. J., Burgess, R., Gelety, T., Ford, C., & Brown, M. (1986). Long-latency auditory event-related potentials in epilepsy. *Clinical Electroencephalography, 17,* 10–13.

Dreyer, M., Rudiger, H., Bujara, K., et al. (1982). The syndrome of diabetes insipidus, diabetes mellitus, optic atrophy, deafness, and other abnormalities (DIDMOAD syndrome). *Wiener Klinische Wochenschrift (Klin Wochenschr), 60,* 471–475.

Drummond, J. C., Todd, M. M., & Sang, H. (1985). The effect of high dose sodium thiopental on brain stem auditory and median nerve somatosensory evoked responses in humans. *Anesthesiology, 63,* 249–254.

Dubois, M., Coppola, R., Buchsbaum, M. S., & Lees, D. E. (1981). Somatosensory evoked potentials during whole body hyperthermia in humans. *Electroencephalography and Clinical Neurophysiology, 52,* 157–162.

Dubois, M., Sato, S., Chassy, J., & MacNamara, T. (1982). Effect of enflurane on brain stem auditory evoked response (BAER). *Electroencephalography and Clinical Neurophysiology, 53,* 36P.

Dubowitz, L. N. S., Dubowitz, W., & Goldberg, C. (1970). Clinical assessment of gestational age. *Journal of Pediatrics, 77,* 1–10.

Duffy, F. H. (1982). Topographic display of evoked potentials: Clinical applications of brain electrical activity mapping (BEAM). In I. B. Wollner (Ed.), *Evoked potentials* (pp. 183–196). Annals of the New York Academy of Science, New York.

Duffy, F. H., Burchfield, J. D., & Lombroso, C. T. (1979). Brain electrical activity mapping (BEAM): A new method for extending the clinical utility of EEG and evoked potential data. *Annals of Neurology, 5,* 309–321.

Duncan, C. C., Kosmidis, M. H., & Mirsky, A. F. (2005). Closed head injury-related information processing deficits: an event-related potential analysis. *International Journal of Psychophysiology, 58,* 133–157.

Duncan, C. C., Rumsey, J. M., Wilkniss, S. M., Denckla, M. B., Hamburger, S. D., & Odou-Potkin, M. (1994). Developmental dyslexia and attention dysfunction in adults: Brain potential indices of information processing. *Psychophysiology, 31,* 386–401.

Duncan, R. G., Sanders, R. A., & McCullough, D. W. (1979). Preservation of auditory-evoked brainstem responses in anaesthetized children. *Canadian Anaesthesiology Society Journal, 26,* 492–495.

Duncan-Johnson, C. C., & Donchin, E. (1977). On quantifying surprise: The variation of event-related potentials with subjective probability. *Psychophysiology, 14,* 456–467.

Duquette, P., Murray, T. J., Pleines, J., Ebers, G. C., Sadovnick, D., Weldon, P., Warren, S., & Paty, D. W. (1987). Multiple sclerosis in childhood: Clinical profile in 125 patients. *Journal of Pediatrics, 111,* 359–363.

Durieux-Smith, A., Picton, T., Edwards, C., Goodman, J. T., & MacMurray, B. (1985). The Crib-O-Gram in the NICU: An evaluation based on brain stem electric response audiometry. *Ear and Hearing, 6,* 20–24.

Durmus, C., Yetiser, S., & Durmus, O. (2004). Auditory brainstem evoked potentials in insulin-dependent (ID) and non-insulin-dependent (NID) diabetic subjects with normal hearing. *International Journal of Audiology, 43,* 29–33.

Durrant, J. D. (1990). Extratympanic electrode support via vented earmold. *Ear and Hearing, 11,* 468–469.

Durrant, J. D., Burns, A., & Ronis, R. (1977). Electrocochleographic studies in animals. *Advances in Otorhinolaryngology, 22,* 14–23.

Durrant J. D., & Ferraro J. A. (1991). Analog model of human click-elicited SP and effects of high-pass filtering. *Ear and Hearing, 12,* 144–148.

Durrant, J. D., Wang, J., Ding, D. L., & Salvi, R. J. (1998). Are inner or outer hair cells the source of summating potentials recorded from the round window? *Journal of the Acoustical Society of America, 104,* 370–377.

Dus, V., & Wilson, S. J. (1975). The click-evoked post-auricular myogenic response in normal subjects. *Electroencephalography and Clinical Neurophysiology, 39,* 523–525.

Dustman, R. E., & Callner, D. A. (1979). Cortical evoked responses and response decrement in nonretarded and Down's syndrome individuals. *American Journal of Mental Deficiency, 83,* 391–397.

Dustman, R. E., Emmerson, R., & Shearer, D. (1994). Physical activity, age, and cognitive-neuropsychological function. *Journal of Aging and Physical Activity, 2,* 143–181.

Dutton, R. C., Smith, W. D., Rampil, I. J., Chortkoff, B. S., & Eger, E. I. (1999). Forty-hertz midlatency auditory evoked potential activity predicts wakeful response during desflurane and propofol anaesthesia in volunteers. *Anesthesiology, 91,* 1209–1220.

Ebner, A., Haas, J. C., Lucking, C. H., Schily, M., Wallesch, C. W., & Zimmermann, P. (1986). Event-related brain potentials (P300) and neuropsychological deficit in patients with focal brain lesions. *Neuroscience Letters, 64,* 330–334.

Eccard, K. D., & Weber, B. A. (1983). Influence of electrode impedance on auditory brain stem response recordings in the intensive care nursery. *Ear and Hearing, 4,* 104–105.

Eddington, D., Dobelle, W., Brackmann, D., Mladejovsky, M., & Parkin, J. (1978). Place and periodicity pitch by stimulation of multiple scala tympani electrodes in deaf volunteers. *Transcripts of the American Society of Artificial Internal Organs, 24,* 1–5.

Eddins, A. C., & Peterson, J. R. (1999). Time-intensity trading in the late auditory evoked potential. *Journal of Speech, Language and Hearing Research, 42,* 516–525.

Edwards, B., Kileny, P., & Van Riper, L. (2002). CHARGE syndrome: A window of opportunity for audiologic intervention. *Pediatrics, 110,* 119–126.

Edwards, C., Durieux-Smith, A., & Picton, T. (1985). Auditory brainstem response audiometry in neonatal hydrocephalus. *Journal of Otolaryngology (Supplement), 14,* 40–46.

Edwards, R. M., Buchwald, J. S., Tanguay, P. E., & Schwafel, J. A. (1982). Sources of variability in auditory brain stem evoked potential measures over time. *Electroencephalography and Clinical Neurophysiology, 53,* 125–132.

Edwards, R. M., Squires, N., Buchwald, J. S., & Tanguay, P. E. (1983). Central transmission time differences in the auditory brainstem responses as a function of sex, age, and ear of stimulation. *International Journal of Neuroscience, 18,* 59–66.

Eggermont, J. J. (1974). Basic principles for electrocochleography. *Acta Otolaryngologica (Supplement), 316,* 7–16.

Eggermont, J. J. (1976a). Electrocochleography. In W. D. Keidel & W. D. Neff (Eds.), *Handbook of sensory physiology: Auditory system, clinical and special topics* (pp. 85–104). New York: Springer-Verlag.

Eggermont, J. J. (1976b). Summating potentials in electrocochleography: Relation to hearing disorders. In R. J. Ruben, C. Elberling, & G. Salomon (Eds.), *Electrocochleography* (pp. 67–87). Baltimore: University Park Press.

Eggermont, J. J. (1977). Compound action potential tuning curves in normal and pathological human ears. *Journal of the Acoustical Society of America, 62,* 1247–1251.

Eggermont, J. J. (1979). Summating potentials in Ménière's disease. *Archives of Otorhinolaryngology, 222,* 65–75.

Eggermont, J. J. (1983). Physiology of the developing auditory system. In S. Trehub & B. Schneider (Eds.), *Auditory development in infancy.* New York: Plenum Press.

Eggermont, J. J. (1985a). To BER or not to BER: That is the question. In S. Trehub & B. Schneider (Eds.), *Auditory development in infancy* (pp. 177–180). New York: Plenum Press.

Eggermont, J. J. (1985b). Evoked potentials as indicators of auditory maturation. *Acta Otolaryngologica (Supplement), 421,* 41–47.

Eggermont, J. J., Brown, D., Ponton, C., & Kimberley, B. (1996). Comparison of distortion product otoacoustic emission (DPOAE) and auditory brain stem response (ABR) traveling wave delay measurements suggest frequency-specific synapse maturation. *Ear and Hearing, 17,* 386–394.

Eggermont, J. J., & Don, M. (1980). Analysis of the click-evoked brainstem potentials in humans using high-pass noise masking: II. Effects of click intensity. *Journal of the Acoustical Society of America, 68,* 1671–1675.

Eggermont, J. J., Don, M., & Brackmann, D. (1980). Electrocochleography and auditory brainstem electric responses in patients with pontine angle tumors. *Annals of Otology, Rhinology & Laryngology, 89,* 1–19.

Eggermont, J. J., & Odenthal, D. W. (1974a). Methods in electrocochleography. Electrocochleography: Basic principles and clinical application. *Acta Otolaryngologica (Supplement), 316,* 17–23.

Eggermont, J. J., & Odenthal, D. W. (1974b). Action potentials and summating potentials in the normal human cochlea. In Electrocochleography: Basic principles and clinical application. *Acta Otolaryngologica (Supplement), 316,* 39–61.

Eggermont, J. J., Odenthal, D. W., Schmidt, P. H., & Spoor, A. (1974). Electrocochleography: Basic principles and clinical application. *Acta Otolaryngologica (Supplement), 316,* 5–84.

Eggermont, J. J., & Salamy, A. (1988). Development of ABR parameters in a preterm and a term born population. *Ear and Hearing, 9,* 283–289.

Ehle, A. L., Steward, R. M., Lellelid, N. A., & Leventhal, N. A. (1984). Evoked potentials in Huntington's disease: A comparative and longitudinal study. *Archives of Neurology, 41,* 379–382.

Eichlin, F. A. (1965). Spasm of basilar and vertebral arteries caused by experiemental subarachnoid hemorrhage. *Journal of Neurosurgery, 23,* 1–11.

Eisen, A., & Cracco, R. Q. (1983). Overuse of evoked potentials: Caution. *Neurology, 33,* 618–621.

Eisen, M., & Franck, K. (2004). Electrically evoked compound action potential amplitude growth functions and HiResolution programming levels in pediatric CII implant subjects. *Ear and Hearing, 25,* 528–538.

Eisen, M., & Franck, K. (2005). Electrode insertion in pediatric cochlear implant subjects. *Journal of the Association for Research in Otolaryngology, 6,* 160–170.

Elberling, C. (1974). Action potentials along the cochlear partition recorded from the ear canal in man. *Scandinavian Audiology, 3,* 13–19.

Elberling, C. (1976). Stimulation of cochlear action potentials recorded from the ear canal in man. In R. J. Ruben, C. Elberling, & G. Salomon (Eds.), *Electrocochleography* (pp. 151–168). Baltimore: University Park Press.

Elberling, C. (1978). Compound impulse response for the brain stem derived through combinations of cochlear and brain stem recordings. *Scandinavian Audiology, 7,* 147–157.

Elberling, C. (1979). Auditory electrophysiology: Spectral analysis of cochlear and brain stem evoked potentials. *Scandinavian Audiology, 8,* 57–64.

Elberling, C., & Don, M. (1984). Quality estimation of averaged auditory brainstem response. *Scandinavian Audiology, 13,* 187–197.

Elberling, C., & Don, M. (1987). Threshold characteristics of the human auditory brain stem response. *Journal of the Acoustical Society of America, 81,* 115–121.

Elberling, C., & Parbo, J. (1987). Reference data for ABRs in retrocochlear diagnosis. *Scandinavian Audiology, 16,* 49–55.

Elberling, C., & Salomon, G. (1973). Cochlear microphonics recorded from the ear canal in man. *Acta Otolaryngologica, 75,* 489–495.

Elberling, C., & Wahlgreen, O. (1985). Estimation of auditory brainstem response, ABR, by means of Bayesian inference. *Scandinavian Audiology, 14,* 89–96.

Eldredge, D. H. (1974). Inner ear cochlear mechanics and cochlear potential. In W. D. Keidel & W. D. Neff (Eds.), *Handbook of sensory physiology.* New York: Springer-Verlag.

Elidan, J., Sohmer, H., Gafni, M., & Kahana, E. (1982). Contribution of changes in click rate and intensity on diagnosis of multiple sclerosis by brainstem auditory evoked potentials. *Acta Neurologica Scandinavian, 65,* 570–585.

El-Kashlan, H., Eisenmann, D., & Kileny, P. (2000). Auditory brainstem response in small acoustic neuromas. *Ear and Hearing, 21,* 257–262.

Elkind-Hirsch, K., Stoner, W., Stach, B., & Jerger, J. (1992b). Estrogen influences auditory brainstem responses during the normal menstrual cycle. *Hearing Research, 60,* 143–148.

Elkind-Hirsch, K., Wallace, E., Malinak, L., & Jerger, J. (1994). Sex hormones regulate ABR latency. *Archives of Otolaryngology—Head & Neck Surgery, 110,* 46–52.

Elkind-Hirsch, K., Wallace, E., Stach, B., & Jerger, J. (1992a). Cyclic steroid replacement alters auditory brainstem responses in young women with premature ovarian failure. *Hearing Research, 64,* 93–98.

Elliott, F. A., & McKissock, W. (1954). Acoustic neuroma early diagnosis. *Lancet, 267,* 1189–1191.

Elting, J. W., van der Naalt, J., van Weerden, T. W., De Keyser, J., & Maurtitis, N. M. (2005). P300 after head injury: Pseudodelay caused by reduced P3A amplitude. *Clinical Neurophysiology, 116,* 2606–2612.

Elwany, S., & Kamel, T. (1988). Sensorineural hearing loss in sickle cell crisis. *Laryngoscope, 98,* 386–389.

Emerson, R. G., Brooks, E. B., Parker, S. W., & Chiappa, K. H. (1982). Effects of click polarity on brainstem auditory evoked potentials in normal subjects and patients: Unexpected sensitivity of wave V. *Annals of the New York Academy of Science, 388,* 710–721.

Enoki, H. (1990). P300 of auditory event-related potentials: The effects of development and aging in humans. *Japanese Journal of EEG & EMG, 18,* 60–67.

Epstein, C. M., Stappenbeck, R., & Karp, H. R. (1980). Brainstem auditory evoked responses in palatal myoclonus. *Annals of Neurology, 7,* 592.

Erwin, R. J., & Buchwald, J. S. (1986). Midlatency auditory evoked responses: Differential recovery cycle characteristics. *Electroencephalography and Clinical Neurophysiology, 64,* 417–423.

Erwin, R. J., Mawhinney-Hee, M., Gur, R. C., & Gur, R. E. (1991). Midlatency auditory evoked responses in schizophrenia. *Biological Psychiatry, 30,* 430–442.

Escera, C., Alho, K., Schroger, E., & Winkler, I. (2000). Involuntary attention and distractibility as evaluated with event-related brain potentials. *Audiology & Neuro-Otology, 5,* 151–166.

Euler, M., & Kiessling, J. (1983). Far-field cochlear microphonics in man and their relation to cochlear integrity. *Electroencephalography and Clinical Neurophysiology, 56,* 86–89.

Eysholdt, V., & Schreiner, C. (1982). Maximum length sequences: A fast method for measuring brainstem-evoked responses. *Audiology, 21,* 242–250.

Fabiani, M., Sohmer, H., Tait, C., Gafni, M., & Kinart, R. (1979). A functional measure of brain activity. *Electroencephalography and Clinical Neurophysiology, 47,* 483–491.

Fabry, L. (1998). Case study—identification and management of auditory neuropathy. A sound foundation through early amplification. In *Proceedings of an International Conference* (pp. 237–245). www.phonak.com

Factor, S. A., & Dentinger, M. P. (1987). Early brain-stem auditory evoked responses in vertebrobasilar transient ischemic attacks. *Archives of Neurology, 44,* 544–547.

Faingold, C. L., & Stittsworth, J. D., Jr. (1981). Phenytoin: Plasma levels and behavioral changes associated with supression of auditory evoked potentials in the cat. *Neuropharmacology, 20,* 445–449.

Fan, Y., Jiang, J., & Qian, T. (1994). [Significance of brainstem auditory evoked potential determination in chronic renal failure and maintenance hemodialysis patients.]. *Zhongguo Zhong Xi Yi Jie He Za Zhi, 14,* 220–221.

Faught, E., & Oh, S. J. (1984). Clinical correlations with brainstem auditory evoked responses in brainstem infarction. In R. H. Nadar & C. Barber (Eds.), *Proceedings of the Second International Symposium on Evoked Potentials* (pp. 285–312). Boston: Butterworth.

Fayad, J., Luxford, W., & Linthicum, F. (2000). The Clarion electrode positioner: Temporal bone studies. *American Journal of Otology, 21,* 226–229.

Feblot, P. D., & Uziel, A. (1982). Detection of acoustic neuromas with brainstem auditory evoked potentials: Comparison between cochlear and retrocochlear abnormalities. In J. Coujon, F. Mauguiere, & M. Revol (Eds.), *Clinical applications of evoked potentials in neurology* (pp. 169–176). New York: Raven Press.

Fedele, D., Martini, A., Cardone, C., Comacchio, F., Bellavere, F., Molinari, G., et al. (1984). Impaired auditory brainstem-evoked responses in insulin-dependent diabetic subjects. *Diabetes, 33,* 1085–1089.

Fein, G., Biggins, C., & MacKay, S. (1996). Source origin of a 50-msec latency auditory evoked field component in young schizophrenic men. *Biological Psychiatry, 24,* 495–506.

Fein, G., & Turetsky, B. (1989). P300 latency variability in normal elderly: Effects of paradigm and measurement technique. *Electroencephalography and Clinical Neurophysiology, 72,* 384–394.

Fellman, V., Kushnerenko, E., Mikkola, K., Čeponiene, R., Leipala, J., & Näätänen, R. (2004). Atypical auditory event-related potentials in preterm infants during the first year of life: A possible sign of cognitive dysfunction? *Pediatric Research, 5,* 291–297.

Ferber-Viart, C., Colleaux, B., Laoust, L., Dubreuil, C., & Duclaux, R. (1998). Is the presence of transient evoked otoacoustic emissions in ears with acoustic neuroma significant? *Laryngoscope, 108,* 605–609.

Ferber-Viart, C., Dubreuil, C., & Duclaux, R. (1999). Vestibular evoked myogenic potentials in humans: A review. *Acta Otolaryngologica, 119*, 6–15.

Ferguson, M., Smith, P., Lutman, M., Mason, S., Coles, R., & Gibbin, K. (1996). Efficiency of tests used to screen for cerebellopontine angle tumours: A prospective study. *British Journal of Audiology, 30*, 159–176.

Ferraro, J. A., Arenberg, I. K., & Hassanein, R. (1985). Electrocochleography and symptoms of inner ear dysfunction. *Archives of Otolaryngology, 111*, 71–74.

Ferraro, J. A., Blackwell, W. L., Mediavilla, S. J., & Thedinger, B. S. (1994). Normal summating potential to tone bursts recorded from the tympanic membrane in humans. *Journal of the American Academy of Audiology, 5*, 17–23.

Ferraro, J. A., & Durrant, J. (1989). *Effects of high-pass filtering on the human electrocochleogram.* Rockville, MD: American Speech-Language-Hearing Association.

Ferraro, J. A., & Ferguson, R. (1989). Tympanic ECochG and conventional ABR: A combined approach for the identification of wave I and the I-V interwave interval. *Ear and Hearing, 10*, 161–166.

Ferraro, J. A., Murphy, G., & Ruth, R. (1986). A comparative study of primary electrodes used in extratympanic electrocochleography. *Seminars in Hearing*, 279–287.

Ferraro, J. A., & Tibbils, R. P. (1999). SP/AP area ratio in the diagnosis of Ménière's disease. *American Journal of Audiology, 8*, 21–28.

Ferree, T. C., Luu, P. L., Russell, G. S., & Tucker, D. M. (2001). Scalp electrode impedance infection risk and EEG data quality. *Clinical Neurophysiology, 112*, 536–544.

Ferri, R., Elia, M., Agarwal, N., Lanuzza, B., Musumeci, S. A., & Pennisi, G. (2003). The mismatch negativity and the P3a components of the auditory event-related potentials in autistic low-functioning subjects. *Clinical Neurophysiology, 114*, 1671–1680.

Ferron, P., Ouellet, Y., Rouillard, R., & Desgange, R. (1983). Electrocochleography in the child: 300 case study. *Journal of Otolaryngology, 12*, 235–237.

Fifer, R. C. (1985). *The MLR and SSEP in neonates.* Houston, TX: Baylor College of Medicine.

Fifer, R. C., & Novak, M. A. (1990). Myogenic influences on the electrical auditory brainstem response (EABR) in humans. *Laryngoscope, 100*, 1180–1184.

Fifer, R. C., & Novak, M. (1991). Prediction of auditory nerve survival in humans using the electrical auditory brainstem response. *American Journal of Otology, 12*, 350–356.

Fifer, R. C., & Sierra-Irizarry, B. (1988). Clinical applications of the auditory middle latency response. *American Journal of Otology, 9*, 47–56.

Filipo, R., Cordier, A., Barbara, M., & Bertoli, G. A. (1997). Electrocochleographic findings: Ménière's disease versus sudden sensorineural hearing loss. *Acta Otolaryngologica Supplement, 526*, 21–23.

Fine, E. J., & Hallett, M. (1980). Neurophysiological study of subacute combined degeneration. *Journal of Neurological Science, 45*, 331–336.

Finitzo, T., & Freeman, F. (1989). Spasmodic dysphonia, whether and where: Results of seven years of research. *Journal of Speech and Hearing Research, 32*, 541–555.

Finitzo, T., & Pool, K. D. (1987). Brain electrical activity mapping. *Asha, 29*, 21–25.

Finitzo-Hieber, T., Hecox, K., & Kone, B. (1979). Brainstem auditory potentials in patients with congenital atresia. *Laryngoscope, 89*, 1151–1158.

Finitzo-Hieber, T., Simhadri, R., & Hieber, J. P. (1981). Abnormalities of the auditory brainstem response in post-meningitic infants and children. *International Journal of Pediatric Otorhinolaryngology, 3*, 275–286.

Finley, W., Faux, S., Hutcheson, J., & Amstutz, L. (1985). Long-latency event-related potentials in the evaluation of cognitive function in children. *Neurology, 35*, 323–327.

Firszt, J., Chambers, R., & Kraus, N. (2002). Neurophysiology of cochlear impant users II: Comparison among speech perception, dynamic range, and physiologic measures. *Ear and Hearing, 23*, 516–531.

Firszt, J., Chambers, R., Kraus, N., & Reeder, R. (2002). Neurophysiology of cochlear implant users I: Effects of stimulus current level and electrode site on the electrical ABR, MLR, and N1-P2 response. *Ear and Hearing, 23*, 502–515.

Firszt, J., Gaggl, W., Runge-Samuelson, C., Burg, L., & Wackym, P. (2004). Auditory sensitivity in children using the auditory steady-state response. *Archives of Otolaryngology—Head & Neck Surgery, 130*, 536–540.

Firszt, J., Wackym, P., Gaggl, W., Burg, L., & Reeder, R. (2003). Electrically evoked auditory brainstem responses for lateral and medial placement of the Clarion HiFocus electrode. *Ear and Hearing, 24*, 184–190.

Fisch, U. (1980). Maximal nerve excitability testing versus electroneuronography. *Archives of Otolaryngology, 106*, 352–357.

Fischer, C., Bognar, L., Turjman, F., & Lapras, C. (1995). Auditory evoked potentials in a patient with a unilateral lesion of the inferior colliculus and medial geniculate body. *Electroencephalography and Clinical Neurophysiology, 96*, 261–267.

Fischer, C., Bognar, L., Turjman, F., Villanyi, E., & Lapras, C. (1994). Auditory early- and middle-latency evoked potentials in patients with quadrigeminal plate tumors. *Neurosurgery, 35*, 45–51.

Fischer, C., Luaute, J., Adeleine, P., & Morlet, D. (2004). Predictive value of sensory and cognitive evoked potentials for awakening from coma. *Neurology, 63*, 69–673.

Fischer, C., Mauguiere, F., Echallier, J. F., & Coujon, J. (1982). Contribution of brainstem auditory evoked potentials to diagnosis of tumors and vascular diseases. In J. Courjin, F. Mauguiere, & M. Revol (Eds.), *Clinical applications of evoked potentials in neurology* (pp. 177–185). New York: Raven Press.

Fischer, C., Mauguiere, F., Ibanez, V., Confavreux, C., & Chazot, G. (1985). The acute deafness of definite multiple sclerosis: BAEP patterns. *Electroencephalography and Clinical Neurophysiology, 61*, 7–15.

Fischer, C., Morlet, D., & Giard, M. (2000). Mismatch negativity and N100 in comatose patients. *Audiology & Neuro-Otology, 5*, 192–197.

Fischer, C., Morlet, D., Bouchet, P., Luaute, J., Jourdan, C., & Salord, F. (1999). Mismatch negativity and late auditory evoked potentials in comatose patients. *Clinical Neurophysiology. 110*, 1601–1610.

Fischer, G., Constantini, J. L., & Mercier, P. (1980). Improvement of hearing after microsurgical removal of acoustic neurinoma. *Neurosurgery, 7*, 154–159.

Fischer, G., Fischer, C., & Remond, J. (1992). Hearing preservation in acoustic neurinoma surgery. *Journal of Neurosurgery, 76*, 910–917.

Fisher, A. L., Hymel, M. R., Cranford, J. L., & DeChicchis, A. R. (2000). Electrophysiologic signs of auditory distraction in elderly listeners. *Journal of the American Academy of Audiology, 11*, 36–45.

Fitzgerald, M., Comerford, P., & Tuffrey, A. (1982). Sources of innervation of the neuromuscular spindles in sternomastoid and trapezius. *Journal of Anatomy, 134*, 471–490.

Fjell, A. M., & Walhovd, K. B. (2001). P300 and neuropsychological tests as measures of aging: Scalp topography and cognitive changes. *Brain Topography, 14*, 25–40.

Fjermedal, O., & Laukli, E. (1989a). Pediatric auditory brainstem response and pure-tone audiometry: Threshold comparisons. *Scandinavian Audiology, 18*, 105–111.

Fjermedal, O., & Laukli, E. (1989b). Low-level 0.5 and 1 KHz auditory brainstem responses. *Scandinavian Audiology, 18*, 177–183.

Fletcher, H. (1940). Auditory patterns. *Review of Modern Physics, 12*, 47–65.

Fobel, O., & Dau, T. (2004). Searching for the optimal stimulus eliciting auditory brainstem responses in humans. *Journal of the Acoustical Society of America, 116*, 2213–2222.

Folsom, R. C. (1984). Frequency specificity of human auditory brainstem responses as revealed by pure-tone masking profiles. *Journal of the Acoustical Society of America, 75*, 919–924.

Folsom, R. C., Weber, B., & Thompson, G. (1983). Auditory brainstem responses in children with recurrent middle ear disease. *Annals of Otology, Rhinology & Laryngology, 92*, 249–253.

Folsom, R. C., Widen, J. E., & Wilson, W. R. (1983). Auditory brainstem responses in infants with Down's syndrome. *Archives of Otolaryngology, 109*, 607–610.

Folsom, R. C., & Wynne, M. K. (1987). Auditory brain stem responses from human adults and infants: Wave V tuning curves. *Journal of the Acoustical Society of America, 81*, 412–417.

Ford, J. M. (1999). Schizophrenia: The broken P300 and beyond. *Biological Psychiatry, 36*, 667–682.

Ford, J. M., Mathalon, D. H., Marsh, L., Faustman, W., Harris, D., Hoff, A., Beal, M., & Pfeifferbaum, A. (1999). P300 amplitude is related to clinical state in severely and moderately ill patients with schizophrenia. *Biological Psychiatry, 46*, 94–101.

Ford, J. M., Mathalon, D. H., Kalba, S., Marsh, L., & Pfefferbaum, A. (2001). N1 and P300 abnormalities in patients with schizophrenia, epilepsy, and epilepsy with schizophrenialike features. *Biological Psychiatry, 49,* 848–860.

Ford, J. M., Mathalon, D. H., Kalba, S., Whitfield, S., Faustman, W. O., & Roth, W. T. (2001). Cortical responsiveness during inner speech in schizophrenia: An event-related potential study. *American Journal of Psychiatry, 158,* 1914–1916.

Ford, J. M., Mathalon, D. H., Marsh, L., Faustman, W. O., Harris, D., Hoff, A. L., Beal, M., & Pfefferbaum, A. (1999). P300 amplitude is related to clinical state in severely and moderately ill patients with schizophrenia. *Biological Psychiatry, 46,* 94–101.

Ford, J. M, Roth, W. T., & Kopell, B. S. (1976). Auditory evoked potentials to unpredictable shifts in pitch. *Psychophysiology, 13,* 32–39.

Ford, J. M., Roth, W. T., Mohs, R., Hopkins, W., & Kopell, B. S. (1979). Event-related potentials recorded from young and old adults during a memory retrieval task. *Electroencephalography and Clinical Neurophysiology, 47,* 450–459.

Formby, C. (1987). Modulation threshold functions for chronologically impaired Ménière's patients. *Audiology, 26,* 89–102.

Forss, N., Mäkelä, J. P., McEvoy, L., & Hari, R. (1993). Temporal integration and oscillatory responses of the human auditory cortex revealed by evoked magnetic fields to click trains. *Hearing Research, 68,* 89–96.

Fowler, B., & Lindeis, A. E. (1992). The effects of hypoxia on auditory reaction time and P300 latency. *Aviation, Space & Environmental Medicine, 63,* 976–981

Fowler, C. (1992). Effects of stimulus phase on the normal auditory brainstem response. *Journal of Speech and Hearing Research, 35,* 167–174.

Fowler, C., & Broadard, R. S. (1988). Low-frequency activity in the binaural interaction component of the auditory brain stem response. *Ear and Hearing, 9,* 65–69.

Fowler, C., & Leonards, J. S. (1985). Frequency dependence of the binaural interaction component of the auditory brainstem response. *Audiology, 24,* 420–429.

Fowler, C., & Noffsinger, D. (1983). Effects of stimulus repetition rate and frequency on the auditory brainstem response in normal, cochlear-impaired, and VIII nerve/brainstem-impaired subjects. *Journal of Speech and Hearing Research, 26,* 560–567.

Fowler, C., & Swanson, M. R. (1989). The 40-Hz potential and SN10 as measures of low-frequency thresholds. *Scandinavian Audiology, 18,* 27–33.

Fox, L. G., & Dalebout, S. D. (2002). Use of the median method to enhance the detection of the mismatch negativity in the responses of individual listeners. *Journal of the American Academy of Audiology, 13,* 83–92.

Foxe, J., & Stapells, D. (1993). Normal infant and adult auditory brainstem responses to bone conduction tones. *Audiology, 32,* 95–109.

Fradis, M., Podoshin, L., Ben-David, J., et al. (1989). Brainstem auditory evoked potentials with increased stimulus rate in patients suffering from systemic lupus erythamatosus. *Laryngoscope, 99,* 325–329.

Franck, K. H. (2002). A model of a nucleus 24 cochlear implant fitting protocol based on the electrically evoked whole nerve action potential. *Ear and Hearing, 23,* 67S–71S.

Franck, K. H., & Norton, S. (2001). Estimation of psychophysical levels using the electrically evoked compound action potential measured with neural response telemetry capabilities of Cochlear Corporation's CI24M Device. *Ear and Hearing, 22,* 289–299.

Franck, K. H., Shah, U. K., Marsh, R. R., & Potsic, W. (2002). Effects of Clarion electrode design on mapping levels in children. *Annals of Otology, Rhinology & Laryngology, 111,* 1128–1132.

Frank, T., & Crandell, C. C. (1986). Acoustic radiation produced by B-71, B-72, and KH 70 bone vibrators. *Ear and Hearing, 7,* 344–347.

Frank, Y., Seiden, J., & Napolitano, B. (1994). Event-related potentials to an 'oddball' auditory paradigm in children with learning disabilities with or without attention deficit hyperactivity disorder. *Clinical Electroencephalography, 25,* 136–141.

Frank, Y., Vishnubhakat, S., & Pahwa, S. (1992). Brainstem auditory evoked responses in infants and children with AIDS. *Pediatric Neurology, 8,* 262–266.

Freedman, R., Adler, L. E., Myles-Worsley, M., Nagamoto, H. T., Miller, C., Kisley, M., McRae, K., Cawthra, E., & Waldo, M. (1996). Inhibitory gating of an evoked response to repeated auditory stimuli in schizophrenic and normal subjects. Human recordings, computer simulation, and an animal model. *Archives of General Psychiatry, 19,* 1114–1121.

Freedman, R., Adler, L. E., Waldo, M. C., Pachtman, E., & Franks, R. D. (1983). Neurophysiological evidence for a defect in inhibitory pathways in schizophrenia: Comparison of medicated and drug-free patients. *Biological Psychiatry, 18,* 537–551.

Freedman, R., Olincy, A., Ross, R. G., Waldo, M. C., Stevens, K. E., Adler, L. E., & Leonard, S. (2003). The genetics of sensory gating deficits in schizophrenia. *Current Psychiatry Report, 5,* 155–161.

Freedman, R., Waldo, M., Bickford-Winner, P., & Nagamoto, H. (1991). Elementary neuronal dysfunction in schizophrenia. *Schizophrenia Research, 4,* 233–243.

Fria, T. J., & Doyle, W. J. (1984). Maturation of the auditory brain stem response (ABR): Additional perspectives. *Ear and Hearing, 5,* 361–365.

Fria, T. J., & Sabo, D. L. (1979, March). The use of brainstem auditory electric responses in children: Practical considerations. *Hearing Aid Journal,* 20–23.

Fria, T. J., & Sabo, D. L. (1980). Auditory brainstem responses in children with otitis media with effusion. *Annals of Otology, Rhinology & Laryngology, 89,* 200–206.

Fridman, J., John, E. R., Bergelson, M., Kaiser, J. B., & Baird, H. W. (1982). Application of digital filtering and automatic peak detection of brain stem auditory evoked potentials. *Electroencephalography and Clinical Neurophysiology, 53,* 405–416.

Fridman, J., Zappalla, R., Bergelson, M., Greenblatt, E., Malis, L., Morrell, F., Hoeppner, T. (1984). Applications of phase spectral analysis for brain stem auditory evoked potential detection in normal subjects and patients with posterior fossa tumors. *Audiology, 23,* 99–113.

Friedman, W. A., Kaplan, B. J., Gravenstein, D., & Rhoton, A. L. (1985). Intraoperative brain-stem auditory evoked potentials during posterior fossa microvascular decompression. *Journal of Neurosurgery, 62,* 552–557.

Friedrich, M., Weber, C., & Friederici A. D. (2004). Electrophysiological evidence for delayed mismatch response in infants at-risk for specific language impairment. *Psychophysiology, 41,* 772–782.

Frijns, J. H. M., Briaire, J. J., & Grote, J. J. (2001). The importance of human cochlear anatomy for the results with modiolus hugging multichannel cochlear implants. *Otology and Neuro-Otology, 22,* 340–349.

Frijns, J., DeSnoo, S., & Schoohoven, R. (1995). Potential distributions and neural excitation patterns in a rotationally symmetric model of the electrically stimulated cochlea. *Hearing Research, 87,* 170–186.

Froding, C. A. (1960). Acoustic investigation of newborn infants. *Acta Otolaryngologica, 52,* 31–41.

Frodl, T., Hampel, H., Juckel, G., Burger, K., Padberg, F., Engel, R., Møller, H., & Hegerl, U. (2002). Value of event-related P300 subcomponents in the clinical diagnosis of mild cognitive impairment and Alzheimer's disease. *Psychophysiology, 39,* 175–181.

Frodl, T., Meisenzahl, E. M., Gallinat, J., Hegerl, U., & Møller, H. J. (1998). Markers from event-related potential subcomponents and reaction time for information processing dysfunction in schizophrenia. *European Archives of Psychiatry and Clinical Neuroscience, 248,* 307–313.

Frodl-Bauch, T., Bottlender, R., & Hegerl, U. (1999). Neurochemical substrates and neuroanatomical generators of the event-related P300. *Neuropsychobiology, 40,* 86–94.

Frodl-Bauch, T., Kathmann, N., Møller, H. J., & Hegerl, U. (1997). Dipole localization and test-retest reliability of frequency and duration mismatch negativity generator processes. *Brain Topography, 10,* 3–8.

Fromm, B., Nylen, C. O., & Zotterman, Y. (1935). Studies in the mechanism of the Wever and Bray effect. *Acta Otolaryngologica, 22,* 477–486.

Fruhstorfer, H. (1971). Habituation and dishabituation of the human vertex response. *Electroencephalography and Clinical Neurophysiology, 30,* 306–312.

Fruhstorfer, H., Soveri, P., & Jarvilehto, T. (1970). Short-term habituation of the auditory evoked response in man. *Electroencephalography and Clinical Neurophysiology, 28,* 153–161.

Fujikawa, S. M., & Weber, B. A. (1977). Effects of increased stimulus rate on brainstem electric response (BER) audiometry as a function of age. *Journal of the American Auditory Society, 3,* 147–150.

Fujioka, T., Trainor, L. J., Ross, B., Kakigi, R., & Pantev, C. (2004). Musical training enhances automatic encoding of melodic contour and interval structure. *Journal of Cognitive Neuroscience, 16,* 1010–1021.

Fujita, M., Hosoki, M., & Miyazaki, M. (1981). Brainstem auditory evoked responses in spinocerebellar degeneration and Wilson disease. *Annals of Neurology, 9,* 42–47.

Fujita, S., & Ito, J. (1999). Ability of nucleus cochlear implantees to recognize music. *Annals of Otology, Rhinology & Laryngology, 108,* 634–640.

Fukai, M., Motomura, N., Kobayashi, S., Asaba, H., & Sakai, T. (1990). Event-related potential (P300) in epilepsy. *Acta Neurologica Scandinavia, 82,* 197–202.

Fullerton, B. C., & Hosford, H. L. (1979). Effects of midline brain stem lesions on the short-latency auditory evoked response. *Society of Neurosciences, 5,* 20.

Fulton, R., & Lloyd, L. (1968). Hearing impairment in a population of children with Down's syndrome. *American Journal of Mental Deficiency, 73,* 298–302.

Funakawa, I., Ogoshi, M., Shibazaki, K., Koga, M., & Yuki, N. (1999). [A case of Bickerstaff's brainstem encephalitis during pregnancy.]. *Rinsho Shinkeigaku, 39,* 1045–1048.

Funasaka, S., & Ito, S. (1986). Stimulus duration and waves of auditory brainstem response. *Audiology, 25,* 176–183.

Furst, M., Levine, R. A., & McGaffigan, P. M. (1985). Click lateralization is related to the B component of the dichotic brainstem auditory evoked potentials of human subjects. *Journal of the Acoustical Society of America, 78,* 1644–1651.

Gabor, D. (1947). Acoustical quanta and the theory of hearing. *Nature, 159,* 591–594.

Gaeta, H., Friedman, D., Ritter, W., & Cheng, J. (1999). Changes in sensitivity to stimulus deviance in Alzheimer's disease: An ERP perspective. *Neuroreport, 10,* 281–287.

Gaetz, M., & Bernstein, D. M. (2001). The current status of electrophysiologic procedures for the assessment of mild traumatic brain injury. *Journal of Head Trauma Rehabilitation, 16,* 386–405.

Gaetz, M., & Weinberg, H. (2000). Electrophysiological indices of persistent post-concussion symptoms. *Brain Injury, 14,* 815–832.

Gafni, M., Sohmer, H., Weizman, Z., & Robinson, M. J. (1980). Analysis of auditory nerve-brainstem responses (ABR) in neonates and very young infants. *Archives of Otorhinolaryngology, 229,* 167–174.

Galambos, R. (1956). Suppression of auditory nerve activity by stimulation of efferent fibers to cochlea. *Journal of Neurophysiology, 19,* 424–437.

Galambos, R. (1976). *Hearing and Davis: Essays honoring Hallowell Davis.* St. Louis: Washington University Press.

Galambos, R., & Hecox, K. (1978). Clinical applications of the auditory brainstem response. *Otolaryngology Clinics of North America, 11,* 709–722.

Galambos, R., Hicks, G. E., & Wilson, M. J. (1984). The auditory brain stem response reliably predicts hearing loss in graduates of a tertiary intensive care nursery. *Ear and Hearing, 5,* 254–260.

Galambos, R., Makeig, S., & Talmachoff, P. J. (1981). A 40-Hz auditory potential recorded from the human scalp. *Proceedings of the National Academy of Science USA, 78,* 2643–2647.

Galambos, R., & Wilson, M. (1994). Newborn hearing thresholds measured by both insert and earphone methods. *Journal of the American Academy of Audiology, 5,* 141–145.

Galbraith, G. C. (2001). Enhanced brainstem and cortical evoked response amplitudes: single-trial covariance analysis. *Perceptual Motor Skills, 92,* 659–672.

Galbraith, G. C., & Arroyo, C. (1993). Selective attention and brainstem frequency-following responses. *Biological Psychology, 37,* 3–22.

Gallégo, S., Frachet, B., Micheyl, C., Truy, E., & Collet, L. (1998). Cochlear implant performance and electrically-evoked auditory brain-stem response characteristics. *Electroencephalography and Clinical Neurophysiology, 108,* 521–525.

Gallinat, J., Bottlender, R., Juckel, G., Munke-Puchner, A., Stotz, G., Kuss, H. J., Mavrogiorgou, P., & Hegerl, U. (2000). The loudness dependency of the auditory evoked N1/P2-component as a predictor of the acute SSRI response in depression. *Psychopharmacology (Berl), 148,* 404–411.

Gamble, B. A., Meyerhoff, W. L., Shoup, A. G., & Schwade, N. D. (1999). Salt-load electrocochleography. *American Journal of Otology, 20,* 325–330.

Gans, R., & Roberts, R. (2005). Vestibular evoked myogenic potential: A tutorial. *Audiology Today, 17,* 23–25.

Gantz, B. (1985). Intraoperative facial nerve monitoring. *The American Journal of Otology (Supplement), 6,* 58–61.

Gantz, B., Brown, C., & Abbas, P. (1994). Intraoperative measures of electrically evoked auditory nerve compound action potential. *American Journal of Otology, 15,* 1–8.

Gantz, B., Gmur, A., & Fisch, U. (1982). Intraoperative electromyography in Bell's palsy. *American Journal of Otolaryngology, 3,* 273–278.

Gantz, B., Gmur, A., Holliday, M., & Fisch, U. (1984). Electroneurographic evaluation of the facial nerve: Method and technical problems. *Annals of Otology, Rhinology & Laryngology, 93,* 394–398.

Gantz, B., Harker, L., Parnes, L., et al. (1986). Middle cranial fossa acoustic neuroma excision: Results and complications. *Annals of Otology, Rhinology & Laryngology, 95,* 454–459.

Gardi, J. N., & Berlin, C. I. (1981). Binaural interaction components: Their possible origins in guinea pig auditory brainstem response. *Archives of Otolaryngology, 107,* 164–168.

Gardi, J. N., & Bledsoe, S. C., Jr. (1981). The use of kainic acid for studying the origins of scalp-recorded auditory brainstem response in the guinea pig. *Neuroscience Letters, 26,* 143–149.

Gardi, J. N., Martin, W., & Jewett, D. L. (1980). Planar-curve analysis of auditory brain stem responses: Preliminary observations. *Journal of the Acoustical Society of America, 68,* S19.

Garg, B. P., Markand, O. N., & Bustion, P. F. (1982). Brainstem auditory evoked responses in hereditary motor-sensory neuropathy: Site of origin of wave II. *Neurology, 32,* 1017–1019.

Garg, B. P., Markand, O. N., DeMyer, W. E., & Warren, C. (1983). Evoked response studies in patients with adrenoleukodystrophy and heterozygous relatives. *Archives of Neurology, 40,* 356–359.

Gawel, M. J., Das, P., Vincent, S., & Rose, F. C. (1981). Visual and auditory evoked responses in patients with Parkinson's disease. *Journal of Neurology, Neurosurgery, and Psychiatry, 44,* 227–232.

Ge, N. N., Shea, J. J., Jr., & Orchik, D. J. (1997). Cochlear microphonics in Ménière's disease. *American Journal of Otology, 18,* 58–66.

Ge, X., & Shea, J. J., Jr. (2002). Transtympanic electrocochleography: A 10-year experience. *Otology and Neuro-Otology, 23,* 799–805.

Geisler, C. D. (1960). Average response to clicks in man recorded by scalp electrodes. *MIT Technical Report, 380,* 1–158.

Geisler, C. D., Frishkopf, L. S., & Rosenblith, W. A. (1958). Extracranial responses to acoustic clicks in man. *Science, 128,* 1210–1211.

Geisler, G. D. (1964). Discussion of "Nature of average evoked potentials to sound and other stimuli in man." *Annals of the New York Academy of Sciences, 112,* 218.

Geisler, M. W., & Polich, J. (1990). P300 and time of day: Circadian rhythms, food intake, and body temperature. *Biological Psychology, 31,* 117–136.

Geisler, M. W., & Polich, J. (1992). P300 and individual differences: Morning/evening activity preference, food, and time-of-day. *Psychophysiology, 29,* 86–94.

Gene-Cos, N., Ring, H. A., Pottinger, R. C., & Barrett, G. (1999). Possible roles for mismatch negativity in neuropsychiatry. *Neuropsychiatry, Neuropsychology & Behavioral Neurology, 12,* 17–27.

Gentili, F., Lougheed, W., Yasashiro, K., & Corrado, C. (1985). Monitoring of sensory evoked potentials during surgery of skull base tumors. *Canadian Journal of Neurological Science, 12,* 336–340.

Geraud, G., Coll, J., Anre-Bes, M. C., Arbus, L., Locamme, Y., & Bes, A. (1982). Brainstem auditory evoked potentials in multiple sclerosis: Influence of body temperature increase. In J. Coujon, F. Mauguiere, & M. Revol (Eds.), *Clinical applications of evoked potentials in neurology* (pp. 501–505). New York: Raven Press.

Gerhardt, H. J., Wagner, H., & Werbs, M. (1985). Electrocochleography (ECochG) and brain stem evoked response recordings (BSER) in the diagnosis of acoustic neuromas. *Acta Otolaryngologica, 99,* 384–386.

Gerling, I. J. (1989). Interaction of stimulus parameters on the auditory brain stem response: A normal variant. *Ear and Hearing, 10,* 117–123.

Gerull, G., Giesen, M., Knupling, R., & Mrowinski, D. (1981). Medium-latency acoustically evoked brain potentials used for examination of the auditory pathway. *Laryngology and Rhinology, 60,* 135–138.

Gerull, G., & Mrowinski, D. (1984). Brain stem potentials evoked by binaural click stimuli with differences in interaural time and intensity. *Audiology, 23,* 265–276.

Gerull, G., Mrowinski, D., Janssen, T., & Anft, D. (1985). Brainstem and cochlea potentials evoked by rarefaction and condensation single-slope stimuli. *Scandinavian Audiology, 14,* 141–150.

Gfeller, K., & Lansing, C. (1991). Melodic, rhythmic and timbral perception of adult cochlear implant users. *Journal of Speech and Hearing Research, 34,* 916–920.

Ghisolfi, E. S., Maegawa, G. H., Becker, J., Zanardo, A. P., Strimitzer, I. M. Jr., Prokopiuk, A. S., Pereira, M. L., Carvalho, T., Jardim, L. B., & Lara, D. R. (2004b). Impaired P50 sensory gating in Machado-Joseph disease. *Clinical Neurophysiology, 115,* 2231–2235.

Ghisolfi, E. S., Margis, R., Becker, J., Zanardo, A. P., Strimitzer, I. M., & Lara, D. R. (2004a). Impaired P50 sensory gating in post-traumatic stress disorder secondary to urban violence. *International Journal of Psychophysiology, 51,* 209–214.

Ghisolfi, E. S., Prokopiuk, A. S., Becker, J., Ehlers, J. A., Belmonte-de-Abreu, P., Souza, D. O., & Lara, D. R. (2002). The adenosine antagonist theophylline impairs P50 auditory sensory gating in normal subjects. *Neuropsychopharmacology, 27,* 629–637.

Ghorayeb, B. Y., Yeakley, J. W., Hall, J. W. III, & Jones, E. B. (1987). Unusual complications of temporal bone fractures. *Archives of Otolaryngology—Head and Neck Surgery, 113,* 749–753.

Ghosh, S., Gupta, A. K., & Mann, S. S. (2002). Can electrocochleography in Ménière's disease be noninvasive? *Journal of Otolaryngology, 31,* 371–375.

Giard, M. H., Perrin, F., Pernier, J., & Bouchet, P. (1990). Brain generators implicated in the processing of auditory stimulus deviance: A topographic event-related potential study. *Psychophysiology, 27,* 627–640.

Giard, M. H., Perrin, F., & Peronnet, F. (1988). Several attention-related wave forms in auditory areas: A topographic study. *Electroencephalography and Clinical Neurophysiology, 69,* 371–384.

Gibson, W. P. R. (1975). The crossed acoustic response—A post-aural myogenic response. Thesis, Doctor of Medicine, University of London, London.

Gibson, W. P. R. (1978). *Essentials of clinical electric response audiometry.* New York: Churchill Livingstone.

Gibson, W. P. R. (1982). Electrocochleography. In A. M. Halliday (Ed.), *Evoked potentials in clinical testing* (pp. 283–311). Edinburgh: Churchill Livingstone.

Gibson, W. P. R. (1991). The use of intraoperative electrocochleography in Ménière's surgery. *Acta Otolaryngologica Supplement, 485,* 65–73.

Gibson, W. P. R. (1992). Electrocochleography in the diagnosis of perilymphatic fistula: Intraoperative observations and assessment of a new diagnostic office procedure. *American Journal of Otology, 13,* 146–151.

Gibson, W. P. R., & Beagley, H. A. (1976a). Electrocochleography in the diagnosis of acoustic neuroma. *Journal of Laryngology and Otology, 90,* 127–137. Ref ID: 627

Gibson, W. P. R., & Beagley, H. A. (1976b). Transtympanic electrocochleography in the investigation of retrolabyrinthine disorders. *Revue de Laryngologie, Otologie, Rhinologie, 97,* 507–510.

Gibson, W. P. R., Moffat, D. A., & Ramsden, R. T. (1977). Clinical electrocochleography in the diagnosis and management of Ménière's disorder. *Audiology, 16,* 389–401.

Gibson, W. P. R., Prasher, D. K., & Kilkenny, G. (1983). Diagnostic significance of transtympanic electrocochleography in Ménière's disease. *Annals of Otology, Rhinology, & Laryngology, 92,* 155–159.

Giesser, B. S., Kurtzberg, D., Vaughan, H. G., Jr., Arezzo, J., Aisen, M. L., Smith, C. R., et al. (1987). Trimodal evoked potentials compared with magnetic resonance imaging in the diagnosis of multiple sclerosis. *Archives of Neurology, 44,* 281–284.

Gillberg, C., Rosenhall, U., & Johansson, E. (1983). Auditory brainstem responses in childhood psychosis. *Journal of Autism and Developmental Disorders, 13,* 181.

Gillberg, C., Wahltrom, J., Johansson, R., Tornblom, M., & Albertsson-Wikland, K. (1986). Folic acid as an adjunct in the treatment of children with the autism fragile-X syndrome (AFRAX). *Developmental Medicine and Child Neurology, 28,* 624–627.

Gilroy, J., & Lynn, G. E. (1978). Computerized tomography and auditory-evoked potentials: Use in the diagnosis of olivopontocerebellar degeneration. *Archives of Neurology, 35,* 143–147.

Gilroy, J., Lynn, G. E., & Pellerin, R. J. (1977). Auditory evoked brain stem potentials in a case of "locked-in" syndrome. *Archives of Neurology, 34,* 492–495.

Gilroy, J., Lynn, G. E., Ristow, G. E., & Pellerin, R. J. (1977). Auditory evoked brain stem potentials in a case of "locked-in" syndrome. *Archives of Neurology, 34,* 492–495.

Glaser, E. M., & Ruchkin, D. (1976). *Principles of neurobiological signal analysis.* New York: Academic Press.

Glasscock, M. I., Dickens, J. R., & Wiet, R. (1979). Preservation of hearing in acoustic tumor surgery: Middle fossa approach. In H. Silverstein & H. Norrell (Eds.), *Neurological surgery of the ear* (pp. 284–286). Birmingham: Aesculapius Publishers.

Glasscock, M. I., Hays, J. W., Miller, G. W., Drake, F. D., & Kanok, M. M. (1978). Preservation of hearing in tumors of the internal auditory canal and cerebellopontine angle. *Laryngoscope, 88,* 43–55.

Gleich, L., Urbina, M., & Pincus, R. (1994). Asymptomatic congenital syphilis and auditory brainstem response. *International Journal of Pediatric Otorhinolaryngology, 30,* 11–13.

Godey, B., Morandi, X., Beust, L., Brassier, G., & Bourdiniere, J. (1998). Sensitivity of auditory brainstem response in acoustic neuroma screening. *Acta Otolaryngologica, 118,* 501–504.

Godey, B., Schwartz, D., de Graaf, J. B., Chauvel, P., & Liegeois-Chauvel, C. (2001). Neuromagnetic source localization of auditory evoked fields and intracerebral evoked potentials: A comparison of data in the same patients. *Clinical Neurophysiolology, 112,* 1850–1859.

Goff, G. D., Matsumiya, Y., Allison, T., & Goff, W. R. (1977). The scalp topography of human somatosensory and auditory evoked potentials. *Electroencephalography and Clinical Neurophysiology, 42,* 57–76.

Goff, W. R., Allison, T., & Vaughan, H. G., Jr. (1978). The functional neuroanatomy of event-related potentials. In E. Callaway, E. Tueting, & S. H. Koslow (Eds.), *Event-related potentials in man* (pp. 1–79). New York: Academic Press.

Goin, D., Staller, S., Asher, D., & Mischke, R. E. (1982). Summating potential in Ménière's disease. *Laryngoscope, 92,* 1383–1389.

Goitein, K., Fainmesser, P., & Sohmer, H. (1983). Cerebral perfusion pressure and auditory brain-stem responses in childhood CNS disease. *American Journal of Diseases in Children, 137,* 777–781.

Gold, S., Cahani, M., Sohmer, H., Horowitz, M., & Shahar, A. (1985). Effects of body temperature elevation of auditory nerve-brainstem evoked responses and EEGs in rats. *Electroencephalography and Clinical Neurophysiology, 60,* 146–153.

Goldberg, J. M., & Moore, R. Y. (1967). Ascending projections of the lateral lemniscus in the cat and monkey. *Journal of Comparative Neurology, 129,* 143–156.

Goldie, W. D., Chiappa, K. H., & Young, R. R. (1981). Brainstem auditory and short-latency somatosensory evoked responses in brain death. *Neurology, 31,* 248–256.

Goldie, W. D., van Eyes, J., & Baram, T. Z. (1987). Brain stem auditory evoked potentials as a tool in the clinical assessment of children with posterior fossa tumors. *Journal of Child Neurology, 2,* 272–275.

Goldsher, M., Pratt, H., Hassan, A., Shenhav, R., Eliachar, I., & Kanter, Y. (1986). Auditory brainstem evoked potentials in insulin-dependent diabetics with and without peripheral neuropathy. *Acta Otolaryngologica, 102,* 204–208.

Goldstein, A., Spencer, K. M., & Donchin, E. (2002). The influence of stimulus deviance and novelty on the P300 and novelty P3. *Psychophysiology, 39,* 781–790.

Goldstein, M. H., Jr., & Kiang, N. Y. S. (1958). Synchrony of neural activity in electric responses evoked by transient acoustic stimuli. *Journal of the Acoustical Society of America, 30,* 107–114.

Goldstein, P. J., Krumholz, A., Felix, J. K., Shannon, D., & Carr, R. F. (1979). Brainstem evoked responses in neonates. *American Journal of Obstetrics and Gynecology, 135,* 622–631.

Goldstein, R. (1984). Editorial: Dimensions of the averaged electroencephalic response (AER). *Ear and Hearing, 5,* 185–186.

Goldstein, R., & Rodman, L. B. (1967). Early components of averaged evoked responses in rapidly repeated auditory stimuli. *Journal of Speech and Hearing Research, 10,* 697–705.

Goldstein, R., Rodman, L. B., & Karlovich, R. S. (1972). Effects of stimulus rate and number on the early components of the averaged electroencephalic response. *Journal of Speech and Hearing Research, 15,* 559–566.

Gomot, M., Giard, M. H., Adrien, J. L., Barthelemy, C., & Bruneau, N. (2002). Hypersensitivity to acoustic change in children with autism: Electrophysiological evidence of left frontal cortex dysfunctioning. *Psychophysiology, 39,* 577–584.

Gomot, M., Giard, M. H., Roux, S., Barthelemy, C., & Bruneau, N. (2000). Maturation of frontal and temporal components of mismatch negativity (MMN) in children. *Neuroreport, 11,* 3109–3112.

Gonsalvez, C. J., Gordon, E., Anderson, J., Pettigrew, G., Barry, R. J., Rennie, C., & Meares, R. (1995). Numbers of preceding nontargets differentially affect responses to targets in normal volunteers and patients with schizophrenia: A study of event-related potentials. *Psychiatry Research, 58,* 69–75.

Goodin, D. S., & Aminoff, M. (1987). Electrophysiological differences between demented and non-demented patients with Parkinson's disease. *Annals of Neurology, 21,* 90–94.

Goodin, D. S., Desmedt, J., Maurer, K., & Nuwer, M. (1994). IFCN recommended standards for long-latency auditory event-related potentials. Report of an IFCN committee. *Electroencephalography and Clinical Neurophysiology, 91,* 18–20.

Goodin, D. S., Squires, K., Henderson, B., & Starr, A. (1978a). Age-related variations in evoked potentials to auditory stimuli in normal human subjects. *Electroencephalography and Clinical Neurophysiology, 44,* 447–458.

Goodin, D. S., Squires, K., Henderson, B., & Starr, A. (1978b). An early event-related cortical potential. *Psychophysiology, 15,* 360–365.

Goodin, D. S., Squires, K. C., & Starr, A. (1978). Long latency event-related components of the auditory evoked potentials in dementia. *Brain, 101,* 635–648.

Goodin, D. S., Squires, K. C., & Starr, A. (1983). Variations in early and late event-related components of the auditory evoked potential with task difficulty. *Electroencephalography and Clinical Neurophysiology, 66,* 680–686.

Goodman, J. M., & Heck, L. L. (1977). Confirmation of brain death at bedside by isotope angiography. *Journal of the American Medical Association, 238,* 966–968.

Goodman, J. M., Heck, L. L., & Moore, B. D. (1985). Confirmation of brain death with portable isotope angiography: A review of 204 cases. *Neurosurgery, 16,* 492–497.

Goodman, W. S., Appleby, S. V., Scott, J. W., & Ireland, P. E. (1964). Audiometry in newborn children by electroencephalography. *Laryngoscope, 74,* 1316–1328.

Gopal, K. V., Bishop, C. E., & Carney, L. (2004). Auditory measures in clinically depressed individuals. II. Auditory evoked potentials and behavioral speech tests. *International Journal of Audiology, 43,* 499–505.

Gopal, K., Daly, D., Daniloff, R., & Pennartz, L. (2000). Effects of selective serotonin reuptake inhibitors on auditory processing: Case study. *Journal of the American Academy of Audiology, 11,* 454–463.

Gordon, K. A., Papsin, B. C., & Harrison, R. V. (2003). Activity-dependent developmental plasticity of the auditory brain stem in children who use cochlear implants. *Ear and Hearing, 24,* 485–500.

Gordon, K., Papsin, B., & Harrison, R. (2004). Programming cochlear implant stimulation levels in infants and children with a combination of objective measures. *International Journal of Audiology, 43,* S28–S32.

Gordon, M., & Cohen, N. (1995). Efficacy of auditory brainstem response as a screening test for small acoustic neuromas. *American Journal of Otology, 16,* 136–139.

Gorga, M. P., & Abbas, P. J. (1981). Forward-masking AP tuning curves in normal and in acoustically traumatized ears. *Journal of the Acoustical Society of America, 70,* 1322–1330.

Gorga, M. P., Beauchaine, K. A., Reiland, J. K., Worthington, D. W., & Javel, E. (1984). Effects of stimulus duration on ABR thresholds and on behavioral thresholds. *Journal of the Acoustical Society of America, 76,* 616–619.

Gorga, M. P., Kaminski, J. R., & Beauchaine, K. A. (1988). Auditory brainstem responses from graduates of an intensive care nursery using an insert earphone. *Ear and Hearing, 9,* 144–147.

Gorga, M., Kaminski, J., & Beauchaine, K., (1991). Effects of stimulus phase on the latency of the auditory brainstem response. *Journal of the American Academy of Audiology, 2,* 1–6.

Gorga, M., Kaminski, J., Beauchaine, K, & Bergman, B. (1993). A comparison of auditory brainstem response thresholds and latencies elicited by air- and bone-conducted stimuli. *Ear and Hearing, 14,* 85–94.

Gorga, M. P., Kaminski, J. R., Beauchaine, K. A., & Jesteadt, W. (1988). Auditory brainstem responses to tone bursts in normally hearing subjects. *Journal of Speech and Hearing Research, 31,* 87–97.

Gorga, M. P., Kaminski, J. R., & Carr, R. F. (1987). Auditory brain stem responses to high-frequency tone bursts in normal-hearing subjects. *Ear and Hearing, 8,* 222–226.

Gorga, M., Neely, S., Hoover, B., Dierking, D., Beauchaine, K., & Manning, C. (2004). Determining the upper limits of stimulation for auditory steady-state response measurements. *Ear and Hearing, 25,* 302–307.

Gorga, M. P., Preissler, K., Simmons, J., Walker, L., & Hoover, B. (2001). Some issues relevant to establishing a universal newborn hearing screening program. *Journal of the American Academy of Audiology, 12,* 101–112.

Gorga, M. P., Reiland, J. K., & Beauchaine, K. A. (1985). Auditory brainstem responses in a case of high-frequency hearing loss. *Journal of Speech and Hearing Disorders, 50,* 346–350.

Gorga, M. P., Reiland, J. K., Beauchaine, K. A., Worthington, D. W., & Jesteadt, W. (1987). Auditory brainstem responses from graduates of an intensive care nursery: Normal patterns of response. *Journal of Speech and Hearing Research, 30,* 311–318.

Gorga, M. P., & Thornton, A. R. (1989). The choice of stimuli for ABR measurements. *Ear and Hearing, 10,* 217–230.

Gorga, M. P., Worthington, D. W., Reiland, J. K., Beauchaine, K. A., & Goldgar, D. E. (1985). Some comparisons between auditory brainstem response threshold, latencies, and the pure-tone audiogram. *Ear and Hearing, 6,* 105–112.

Gosepath, K., Maurer, J., & Mann, W. (1995). [Diagnostic intra-meatal acoustic neurinoma—the role of acoustically evoked brain stem potentials and other otoneurologic studies]. *Laryngorhinootologie, 74,* 728–732.

Gothgen, S., Jacobs, L., & Newman, R. P. (1981). Brainstem auditory evoked responses and palatal myoclonus. *Annals of Neurology, 9,* 309.

Gott, P. S., & Hughes, E. C. (1989). Effect of noise masking on the brainstem and middle-latency auditory evoked potentials. *Electroencephalography and Clinical Neurophysiology, 74,* 131–138.

Graham, J., Greenwood, R., & Lecky, B. (1980). Cortical deafness: A case report and review of the literature. *Journal of Neurological Science, 48,* 35–49.

Graham, S. J., Scaife, J. C., Balboa Verduzco, A. M., Langley, R. W., Bradshaw, C. M., & Szabadi, E. (2004). Effects of quetiapine and haloperidol on prepulse inhibition of the acoustic startle (eyeblink) response and the N1/P2 auditory evoked response in man. *Journal of Psychopharmacology, 18,* 173–180.

Grandjean, P., Weihe, P., Burse, V., Needham, L., Storr-Hansen, E., Heinzow, B., et al. (2001). Neurobehavioral deficits associated with PCB in 7-year-old children potentially exposed to seafood neurotoxins. *Neurotoxicology and Teratology, 23,* 305–317.

Grandori, F. (1979). Interpretation of the whole-nerve action potential off-effect in response to tone bursts. *Audiology, 18,* 109–188.

Grandori, F. (1986). Field analysis of auditory evoked brainstem potentials. *Hearing Research, 21,* 51–58.

Grantham, D. (1986). Detection and discrimination of simulated motion of auditory targets in the horizontal plane. *Journal of the Acoustical Society of America, 79,* 1939–1949.

Gravendeel, D. W., & Plomp, R. (1960). Perceptive bass deafness. *Acta Otolaryngologica, 51,* 548.

Green, J. B., Burba, A., Freed D. M., Elder, W. W., & Xu, W. (1997). The P1 component of the middle latency auditory potential may differentiate a brainstem subgroup of Alzheimer disease. *Alzheimer Disease and Associated Disorders, 11,* 153–157.

Green, J. B., Flagg, L., Freed, D. M., & Schwankhaus, J. D. (1992). The middle latency auditory evoked potential may be abnormal in dementia. *Neurology, 42,* 1034–1036.

Green, J. B., Walcoff, M., & Lucke, J. F. (1982). Phenytoin prolongs far-field somatosensory and auditory evoked potential interpeak latencies. *Neurology, 32,* 85–88.

Greenberg, H. J., & Metting, P. J. (1974). Averaged encephalic response of aphasics to linguistic and nonlinguistic auditory stimuli. *Journal of Speech and Hearing Research, 17,* 113–124.

Greenberg, R. P., & Becker, D. P. (1976). Clinical applications and results of evoked potentials in patients with severe head injury. *Surgical Forum, 26,* 484–486.

Greenberg, R. P., Becker, D. P., Miller, J. D., & Mayer, D. J. (1977). Evaluation of brain function in severe head trauma with multimodality evoked potentials: II. Localization of brain dysfunction in correlation with post-traumatic neurologic conditions. *Journal of Neurosurgery, 47,* 163–177.

Griffiths, S., & Chambers, R. (1991). The amplitude modulation-following response as an audiometric tool. *Ear and Hearing, 12,* 235–241.

Grillon, C., Ameli, R., & Braff, D. L. (1991). Middle latency auditory evoked potentials (MAEPs) in chronic schizophrenics. *Schizophrenia Research, 5,* 61–66.

Grillon, C., Courchesne, E., & Akshoomoff, N. A. (1989). Brainstem auditory evoked potentials and middle latency responses in non-retarded subjects with infantile autism and receptive developmental language disorders. *Journal of Autism and Developmental Disorders, 19,* 255–269.

Grimes, A. M., Elks, M. L., Grunberger, G., & Pikus, A. M. (1983). Auditory brain-stem responses in adrenomyeloneuropathy. *Archives of Neurology, 40,* 574–576.

Grimes, A. M., Grady, C., & Pikus, A. (1987). Auditory evoked potentials in patients with dementia of the Alzheimer type. *Ear and Hearing, 8,* 157–161.

Grimm, M., Czerny, M., Baumer, H., Kilo, J., Madl, C., Kramer, L., Rajek, A., & Wolner, E. (2001). Normothermic cardiopulmonary bypass is beneficial for cognitive brain function after coronary artery bypass grafting—a prospective randomized trial. *European Journal of Cardiothoracic Surgery, 18,* 270–275.

Groenen, P., Snik, A., & van den Broek, P. (1996). On the clinical relevance of mismatch negativity: Results from subjects with normal hearing and cochlear implant users. *Audiology & Neuro-Otology, 1,* 112–124.

Grönfors, T. (1993a). Identification of auditory brainstem responses. *International Journal of Biomedical Computation, 32,* 171–179.

Grönfors, T. (1993b). Peak identification of auditory brainstem responses with multi-filters and attributed automation. *Computer Methods and Programs in Biomedicine, 40,* 83–87.

Gross, M. M., Begleiter, H., Tobin, M., & Kissin, B. (1965). Auditory evoked response comparison during counting clicks and reading. *Electroencephalography and Clinical Neurophysiology, 18,* 451–454.

Gross, M. M., Begleiter, H., Tobin, M., & Kissin, B. (1966). Changes in auditory evoked response induced by alcohol. *Journal of Nervous and Mental Diseases, 143,* 152–156.

Grosse-Aldenhovel, H., Gallencamp, U., & Sulemana, C. (1991). Juvenile onset diabetes mellitus, central diabetes insipidus and optic atrophy (Wolfram syndrome), neurological findings and prognostic implications. *Neuropediatrics, 22,* 103.

Grundy, B. L. (1983). Intraoperative monitoring of sensory-evoked potentials. *Anesthesiology, 58,* 72–87.

Grundy, B. L., Jannetta, P. J., Procopio, P. T., Lina, A., Boston, J. R., & Doyle, E. (1982). Intraoperative monitoring of brain-stem auditory evoked potentials. *Journal of Neurosurgery 57,* 674–681.

Grundy, B. L., Lina, A., Procopio, P. T., & Jannetta, P. J. (1981). Reversible evoked potential changes with retraction of the eighth cranial nerve. *Anaesthesia and Analgesia, 60,* 835–838.

Gstoettner, W., Neuwirth-Reidl, K., Swoboda, H., Mostbeck, W., & Burian, M. (1992). Specificity of auditory brainstem response audiometry criteria in acoustic neuroma screening as a function of deviations of reference values in patients with cochlear hearing loss. *European Archives of Otorhinolaryngology, 249,* 253–256.

Guerit, J. M. (1991). [Brain stem auditory evoked potentials. Anatomophysiological basis. Neurological applications] *Acta Otorhinolaryngologic Belgium, 45,* 171–203.

Guerit, J. M. (1992). Evoked potentials: A safe brain-death confirmatory tool? *European Journal of Medicine, 1,* 233–243.

Guerit, J. M., Verougstraete, D., de Tourtchaninoff, M., Debatisse, D., & Witdoeckt, C. (1999). ERPs obtained with the auditory oddball paradigm in coma and altered states of consciousness: Clinical relationships, prognostic value, and origin of components. *Clinical Neurophysiology, 110,* 1260–1269.

Guidelines. (1981). Guidelines for the determination of death: Report to the medical consultants on the diagnosis of death to the President's Commission for the Study of Ethical Problems in Medicine and Biomedical and Behavioral Research. *Journal of the American Medical Association, 246,* 2184–2186.

Guinan, J. J., & Peake, W. T. (1967). Middle-ear characteristics of anesthetized cats. *Journal of the Acoustical Society of America, 41,* 1237–1261.

Gummow, L., Dustman, R., & Keaney, R. (1986). Cerebrovascular accident alters P300 event-related potential characteristics. *Electroencephalography and Clinical Neurophysiology, 63,* 128–137.

Gunn, T., & Belmonte, M. (1977). Juvenile diabetes mellitus, optic atrophy, sensory nerve deafness, and diabetes insipidus—a syndrome. *Journal of Pediatrics, 90,* 856–857.

Gupta, P. R., Guilleminault, C., & Dorfman, L. J. (1981). Brainstem auditory evoked potentials in near-miss sudden infant death syndrome. *Journal of Pediatrics, 98,* 791–795.

Guthkelch, A. N., Sclabassi, R. J., & Vries, J. K. (1982). Changes in the visual evoked potentials of hydrocephalic children. *Neurosurgery, 11,* 599–602.

Guttorm, T. K., Leppänen, P. H. T., Tolvanen, A., & Lyytinen, H. (2003). Event-related potentials in newborns with and without familial risk for dyslexia: Principal component analysis reveals differences between the groups. *Journal of Neural Transmission, 110,* 1059–1074.

Haapaniemi, J. J., Laurikainen, E. T., Johansson, R., Rinne, T., & Varpula, M. (2000). Audiovestibular findings and location of an acoustic neuroma. *European Archives of Otorhinolaryngology, 257,* 237–241.

Haberman, R. S., II, & Kramer, M. B. (1989). False positive MRI and CT findings of an acoustic neuroma. *The American Journal of Otology, 10,* 301–303.

Habib, M. (2000). Mechanisms of dyslexia. *Brain, 123,* 2373–2399.

Hagan, C., Malkmus, D., & Durham, P. (1979). *Measures of cognitive functioning in the rehabilitation facility.* Downey, CA: Professional Staff Association, Rancho Los Amigos Hospital, Inc.

Hagberg, B., Aicardi, J., Dias, K., & Ramos, O. (1983). A progressive syndrome of autism, dementia, ataxia, and loss of purposeful hand use in girls: Rhett's syndrome: Report of 35 cases. *Annals of Neurology, 14,* 471–479.

Haglund, Y., & Persson, H. E. (1990). Does Swedish amateur boxing lead to chronic brain damage? 3. A retrospective clinical neurophysiological study. *Acta Neurologica Scandinavia, 82,* 353–360.

Hahn, M., Lamprecht-Dinnesen, A., Heinecke, A., Hartmann, S., Bulbul, S., Schroder, G., Steinhard, J., Louwen, F., & Seifert, E. (1999). Hearing screening in healthy newborns: Feasibility of different methods with regard to test time. *International Journal of Pediatric Otorhinolaryngology, 51,* 83–89.

Haig, A. R., Gordon, E., Rogers, G., & Anderson, J. (1995). Classification of single-trial ERP sub-types: Application of globally optimal vector quantization using simulated annealing. *Electroencephalography and Clinical Neurophysiology, 94,* 288–297.

Halford, J. J. (2003). Neurophysiologic correlates of psychiatric disorders and potential applications in epilepsy. *Epilepsy and Behavior, 4,* 375–385.

Halgren, E., Baudena, P., Clarke, J. M., Heit, G., Liegeois, C., Chauvel, P., & Musolino, A. (1995). Intracerebral potentials to rare target and distractor auditory and visual stimuli. I. Superior temporal plane and parietal lobe. *Electroencephalography and Clinical Neurophysiology, 94,* 191–220.

Halgren, E., Marinkovic, K., & Chauvel, P. (1998). Generators of the late cognitive potentials in auditory and visual oddball tasks. *Electroencephalography and Clinical Neurophysiology, 106,* 156–164.

Halgren, E., Squires, N. K., Wilson, C. L., Rohrbaugh, J. W., Babb, T. L., & Crandall, P. H. (1980). Endogenous potentials generated in the human hippocampal formation and amygdala by infrequent events. *Science, 210,* 803–805.

Halgren, E., Stapleton, J. M., Smith, M., & Altafullah, I. (1986). Generators of the human scalp P3(s). In R. Q. Cracco & I. Bodis-Wollner (Eds.), *Evoked potentials.* New York: Liss.

Hall, J. I., & Denneny, J. I. (1993). Audiologic and otolaryngologic findings in progeria: Case report. *Journal of the American Academy of Audiology, 4,* 116–121.

Hall, J. L. (1965). Binaural interaction in the accessory superior-olivary nucleus of the cat. *Journal of the Acoustical Society of America, 37,* 814–823.

Hall, J. W., III. (1981). Central auditory function in spastic dysphonia. *American Journal of Otolaryngology, 2,* 188–198.

Hall, J. W., III. (1985). The acoustic reflex in central auditory dysfunction. In M. L. Pinheiro & F. E. Musiek (Eds.), *Assessment of Auditory dysfunction: Foundations and clinical correlates* (pp. 103–130). Baltimore: Williams & Wilkins.

Hall, J. W., III. (1985). Effects of high-dose barbiturates on the acoustic reflex and auditory evoked responses: Two case reports. *Acta Otolaryngologica, 100,* 387–398.

Hall, J. W., III. (1986). Auditory brainstem response spectral content in comatose head-injured patients. *Ear and Hearing, 7,* 383–387.

Hall, J. W., III. (1988). Auditory evoked responses in the management of acutely brain-injured children and adults. *American Journal of Otology, 9,* 36–46.

Hall, J. W., III. (1991). The classic site-of-lesion test battery: Foundation of diagnostic audiology. In W. Rintelmann (Ed.), *Hearing assessment* (2nd ed., pp. 653–677). Austin TX: Pro-Ed.

Hall, J. W., III. (1992). *Handbook of auditory evoked responses.* Boston: Allyn and Bacon.

Hall, J. W., III. (1994). Bone conduction ABR: Clinically useful and clinically feasible. *The Hearing Journal 47,* 10–14, 1994.

Hall, J. W., III. (2000). Screening for and assessment of infant hearing impairment. *Journal of Perinatology, 20,* S113-S121.

Hall, J. W., III. (2000a). *Handbook of otoacoustic emissions.* San Diego: Singular Publishing Group.

Hall, J. W., III. (2003). *Clinical experience with the auditory steady state response.* Paper presented at the Annual Convention of the American Academy of Audiology, San Antonio, Texas.

Hall, J. W., III. (2004). The clinical challenges of bone conduction measurement: Some old and new solutions. *The Hearing Journal, 57,* 10–14.

Hall, J. W., III, Brown, D. P., & Mackey-Hargadine, J. (1985). Pediatric applications of serial auditory brainstem and middle late measurements. *International Journal of Pediatric Otorhinolaryngology, 9,* 201–218.

Hall, J. W., III, Bull, J., & Cronau, L. (1988). The effect of hypo- versus hyperthermia on auditory brainstem response: Two case reports. *Ear and Hearing, 9,* 137–143.

Hall, J. W., III, Gray, L. C., Brown, D. P., & Tompkins, S. M. (1986). Clinical applications of new concepts in auditory brainstem response measurement. *Hearing Instruments, 37,* 11–21.

Hall, J. W., III, Hargadine, J. R., & Allen, S. J. (1985). Monitoring neurologic status of comatose patients in the intensive care unit. In J. T. Jacobson (Ed.), *The auditory brainstem response* (pp. 253–283). San Diego: College-Hill Press.

Hall, J. W., III, Huangfu, M., & Gennarrelli, T. A. (1982). Auditory function in acute head injury. *Laryngoscope, 93,* 383–390.

Hall, J. W., III, & Jonas, A. (1988*). Auditory function in rickets.* Paper presented at the annual meeting of the American Auditory Society, Chicago.

Hall, J. W., III, Kileny, P. R., & Ruth, R. A. (1987). *Clinical trials for the ALGO-1 newborn hearing screening device.* Tenth biennial meeting of the International Electric Response Study Group, Charlottesville VA.

Hall, J. W., III, Kileny, P., Ruth, R., & Peters Kripal, J. (1987). Newborn auditory screening with ALGO-1 vs. conventional auditory brainstem response. American Speech-Language-Hearing Association Meeting, New Orleans, LA.

Hall, J. W., III, Mackey-Hargadine, J., & Kim, E. E. (1985). Auditory brainstem response (ABR) in determination of brain death. *Archives of Otolaryngology, 111,* 613–620.

Hall, J. W., III, Morgan, S. H., Mackey-Hargadine, J., Aguilar, E. A. III, & Jahrdoerfer, R. A. (1984). Neuro-otologic applications of simultaneous multi-channel auditory evoked response recordings. *Laryngoscope, 94,* 883–889.

Hall, J. W., III, & Mueller, H. G., III. (1997). *Audiologists' desk reference. Volume, I.* San Diego: Singular Publishing Group.

Hall, J. W., III, & Rupp, K. A. (1997). Auditory brainstem response: Recent developments in recording and analysis. *Advances in Otorhinolaryngology, 53,* 21–45.

Hall, J. W., III, Smith, S. D., & Popelka, G. R. (2004). Newborn hearing screening with combined otoacoustic emissions and auditory brainstem responses. *Journal of the American Academy of Audiology, 15,* 414–425.

Hall, J. W., III, & Tucker, D. A. (1985). Auditory evoked responses in traumatic head injury. *The Hearing Journal, 38,* 23–29.

Hall, J. W., III, & Tucker, D. A. (1986). Sensory evoked responses in the intensive care unit. *Ear and Hearing, 7,* 220–232.

Hall, J. W., III, Tucker, D. A., Fletcher, S. J., & Habersang, R. (1988). Auditory evoked responses in the management of head-injured children. In M. E. Miner & K. E. Wagner (Eds.), *Neurotrauma: Treatment, rehabilitation, and related issues* (2nd ed.). Boston: Butterworth.

Hall, J. W., III, Winkler, J. B., Herndon, D. N., & Gary, L. B. (1986). Auditory brainstem response in young burn wound patients treated with ototoxic drugs. *International Journal of Pediatric Otorhinolaryngology, 12,* 187–203.

Hall, R. (1990). Estimation of surviving spiral ganglion cells in the deaf rat using the electrically evoked auditory brainstem response. *Hearing Research, 45,* 123–136.

Halliday, A. M., & Mason, A. A. (1964). The effect of hypnotic aneasthesia on cortical responses. *Journal of Neurology Neurosurgery, and Psychiatry, 27,* 300–312.

Hallpike, C. S., Harriman, D. G., & Wells, C. E. (1980). A case of afferent neuropathy and deafness. *Journal of Laryngology & Otology, 8,* 945–64.

Halmagyi, G. M., & Colebatch, J. G. (1995). Vestibular evoked myogenic potentials in the sternomastoid are not of lateral canal origin. *Acta Otolaryngologica, 520,* 1–3.

Halmagyi, G. M., Colebatch, J. G., & Curthoys, I. S. (1994). New tests of vestibular function. *Baillieres Clinical Neurology, 3,* 485–500.

Halmagyi, G., & Curthoys, I. (1999). Clinical testing of otolith function. *Annals of the New York Academy of Sciences, 871,* 195–204.

Halmagyi, G., Yavor, R., & Colebatch, J. (1995). Tapping the head activates the vestibular system: A new use for the clinical reflex hammer. *Neurology, 45,* 1927–1929.

Hamada, R., Yoshida, Y., Kuwano, A., Mishima, I., & Igata, A. (1982). [Auditory brainstem responses in fetal organic mercury poisoning.]. *Shinkei-Naika, 16,* 282–285.

Hamaguchi, H., Hashimoto, T., Mori, K., Tayama, M., Fukuda, K., Endo, S., et al. (1993). Moebius syndrome: Continuous tachypnea verified by a polygraphic study. *Neuropediatrics, 24,* 319–323.

Hamill, T., Hussing, R., & Sammeth, C. (1991). Rapid threshold estimation using the "chained stimuli" technique for auditory brainstem response measurement. *Ear and Hearing, 12,* 229–234.

Hammerschlag, P. E., Berg, H. M., Prichep, L. S., John, E. R., Cohen, N. L., & Ransohoff, J. (1986). Real-time monitoring of brainstem auditory evoked response (BAER) during cerebellopontine angle (CPA) surgery. *Otolaryngology—Head & Neck Surgery, 95,* 538–542.

Hammond, E. J., & Wilder, B. J. (1983). Evoked potentials in olivopontocerebellar atrophy. *Archives of Neurology, 40,* 366–369.

Hammond, S. R., & Yiannikas, C. (1987). The relevance of contralateral recordings and patient disability to assessment of brain-stem auditory evoked potential abnormalities in multiple sclerosis. *Archives of Neurology, 44,* 382–387.

Han, D., Chen, X., Zhao, X., Kong, Y., Li, Y., Liu, S., Liu, B., & Mo, L. (2005). Comparisons between neural response imaging thresholds, electrically evoked auditory reflex thresholds and most comfortable loudness levels in CII Bionic Ear users with HiResolution™ sound processing strategies. *Acta Otolaryngologica, 125,* 732–735.

Hanner, P., Rosenhall, U., Karlsson, B., Badr, G., Anderson, O., Frisen, L., & Edstrom, S. (1985). Clinical evaluation of central auditory lesions in patients with Bell's palsy. *Audiology Italie, 2,* 30–35.

Hannley, M., Jerger, J., & Rivera, V. (1983). Relationships among auditory brainstem responses, masking level differences and the acoustic reflex in multiple sclerosis. *Audiology, 22,* 20–33.

Hansch, E. C., Syndulko, K., Cohen, S., Goldberg, Z., Potvin, A., & Tourellotte, W. (1982). Cognition in Parkinson disease: An event-related potential perspective. *Annals of Neurology, 11,* 599–607.

Hansen, C. C., & Reske-Nielsen, E. (1965). Pathological studies in presbycusis. *Archives of Otolaryngology, 82,* 115–132.

Hansen, J. C., & Hillyard, S. A. (1980). Endogenous brain potentials associated with selective auditory attention. *Electroencephalography and Clinical Neurophysiology, 49,* 277–290.

Hansen, J. C., & Hillyard, S. A. (1984). Effects of stimulation rate and attribute cuing on event-related potentials during selective auditory attention. *Psychophysiology, 21,* 394–405.

Harbin, T. J., Marsh, G. R., & Harvey, M. T. (1984). Differences in the late components of the event-related potential due to age and to semantic and non-semantic tasks. *Electroencephalography and Clinical Neurophysiology, 59,* 489–496.

Harder, H., & Arlinger, S. (1981). Ear canal compared to mastoid electrode placement in ABR. *Scandinavian Audiology (Supplement), 13,* 55–57.

Harder, H., Arlinger, S., & Kylen, P. (1983). Electrocochleography with bone-conducted stimulation: A comparative study of different methods of stimulation. *Acta Otolaryngologica (Stockholm), 95,* 35–45.

Hardy, R. W., Kinney, S. E., Lueders, H., & Lesser, R. P. (1982). Preservation of cochlear nerve function with the aid of brain stem auditory evoked potentials. *Neurosurgery, 11,* 16–19.

Hare, T. A., Wood, J. H., Manyam, B. V., Gerner, R. H., Ballenger, J. C., & Post, R. M. (1982). Central nervous system: Aminobutyric acid activity in man. *Archives of Neurology, 39,* 247–249.

Hari, R., Aittoniemi, K., Jarvinen, M. L., Katila, T., & Varpula, T. (1980). Auditory evoked transient and sustained magnetic fields of the human brain. Localization of neural generators. *Experimental Brain Research, 40,* 237–240.

Hari, R., Kaila, K., Katila, T., Tuomisto, T., & Varpula, T. (1982). Inter-stimulus interval dependence of the auditory vertex response and its magnetic counterpart: Implications for their neural generation. *Electro-encephalography and Clinical Neurophysiology, 54,* 561–569.

Hari, R., Pelizzone, M., Mäkelä, J. P., Hallstrom, J., Leinonen, L., & Lounasmaa, O. V. (1987). Neuromagnetic responses of the human auditory cortex to on- and offsets of noise bursts. *Audiology, 26,* 31–43.

Hari, R., Sams, M., & Jarvilehto, T. (1979). Auditory evoked transient and sustained potentials in the human EEG: I. Effects of expectation of stimuli. *Psychiatric Research, 1,* 297–306.

Hari, R., Sukava, R., & Haltia, M. (1982). Brainstem auditory evoked responses and alpha-pattern coma. *Annals of Neurology, 11,* 187–189.

Harker, L. A., Hosick, E., Voots, R. J., & Mendel, M. I. (1977). Influence of succinylchooline on middle component auditory evoked potentials. *Archives of Otolaryngology, 103,* 133–137.

Harkins, S. W. (1981a). Effects of age and interstimulus level on the brainstem auditory evoked potential. *International Journal of Neuroscience, 15,* 107–118.

Harkins, S. W. (1981b). Effects of presenile dementia of the Alzheimer's type on brainstem transmission time. *International Journal of Neuroscience, 15,* 165–170.

Harkins, S. W., Gardner, D. F., & Anderson, R. A. (1985). Auditory and somatosensory far-field evoked potentials in diabetes mellitus. *International Journal of Neuroscience, 28,* 41–47.

Harkrider, A. W., & Champlin, C. A. (2001a). Acute effect of nicotine on non-smokers: II. MLRs and 40-Hz responses. *Hearing Research, 160,* 89–98.

Harkrider, A. W., & Champlin, C. A. (2001b). Acute effect of nicotine on non-smokers: III. LLRs and EEGs. *Hearing Research, 160,* 99–110.

Harkrider, A. W., Champlin, C. A., & McFadden, D. (2001). Acute effect of nicotine on non-smokers: I. OAEs and ABRs. *Hearing Research, 160,* 73–88.

Harner, S. G., Harper, C., Beatty, C., Litchy, W., & Ebersold, M. (1996). Far-field auditory brainstem response in neurotologic surgery. *American Journal of Otology, 17,* 150–153.

Harner, S. G., & Laws, E. R., Jr. (1981). Diagnosis of acoustic neurinoma. *Neurosurgery, 9,* 373–379.

Harper, C. M., Harner, S. G., Slavit, D. H., Litchy, W. J., Daube, J. R., Beatty, C. W., & Ebersold, M. J. (1992). Effect of BAEP monitoring on hearing preservation during acoustic neuroma resection. *Neurology, 42,* 1551–1553.

Harris, D. P., & Hall, J. W., III. (1990). Feasibility of auditory event-related potential measurement in brain injury rehabilitation. *Ear and Hearing, 11,* 340–350.

Harris, F. J. (1978). On the use of windows for harmonic analysis with the discrete Fourier transform. *IEEE Transactions in Acoustics, Speech, and Signal Processing, 66,* 51–83.

Harris, S., Broms, P., & Mollerstrom, B. (1981). ABR in the mentally retarded child. *Scandinavian Audiology (Supplement), 13,* 149–150.

Harrison, R. V. (1998). An animal model of auditory neuropathy. *Ear and Hearing, 19,* 355–361.

Hart, C. W., Cokely, C. G., Schupbach, J., Dal Canto, M. C., & Coppleson, L. W. (1989). Neurotologic findings of a patient with acquired immune deficiency syndrome. *Ear and Hearing, 10,* 69–76.

Hart, R. G., & Davenport, J. (1981). Diagnosis of acoustic neuroma. *Neurosurgery, 9,* 450–463.

Hart, R. G., Gardner, D. P., & Howieson, J. (1983). Acoustic tumors: Atypical features and recent diagnostic tests. *Neurology, 33,* 211–221.

Hart, R. G., & Sherman, D. G. (1982). The diagnosis of multiple sclerosis. *Journal of the American Medical Association, 247,* 498–503.

Hashimoto, I. (1982). Auditory evoked potentials from the human midbrain: Slow brain stem responses. *Electroencephalography and Clinical Neurophysiology, 53,* 652–657.

Hashimoto, I., Ishiyama, Y., & Tozuka, G. (1979). Bilaterally recorded brainstem auditory evoked responses: Their asymmetric abnormalities and lesions of the brainstem. *Archives of Neurology, 36,* 161–167.

Hashimoto, I., Ishiyama, Y., Tozuka, G., & Mitzutani, H. (1980). Monitoring brainstem function during posterior fossa surgery with brainstem auditory evoked potentials. In C. Barber (Ed.), *Proceedings of an international evoked potentials meeting held in Nottingham, England* (pp. 377–390). Lancaster: MTP Press.

Hashimoto, I., Ishiyama, Y., Yoshimoto, R., & Nemoto, S. (1981). Brainstem auditory evoked potentials recorded directly from human brainstem and thalamus. *Brain, 104,* 841–859.

Hatanaka, T., Takedatsu, M., Yasuhara, A., & Kobayashi, Y. (1992). Serial electrophysiological study on two infants with acute facial palsy. *Electromyography and Clinical Neurophysiology, 32,* 155–159.

Hatanaka, T., Yasuhara, A., Hori, A., & Kobayashi, Y. (1990). Auditory brain stem response in newborn infants: Masking effect on ipsi- and contralateral recording. *Ear and Hearing, 11,* 233–236.

Haug, G. (1977). Age and sex dependence of the size of normal ventricles on computed tomography. *Neuroradiology, 14,* 201–204.

Haung, C.-M., & Buchwald, J. S. (1978). Factors that affect the amplitudes of vertex short-latency acoustic responses in the cat. *Electroencephalography and Clinical Neurophysiology, 44,* 179–186.

Hausler, R., & Levine, R. A. (1980). Brainstem auditory evoked potentials are related to interaural time discrimination in patients with multiple sclerosis. *Brain Research, 191,* 589–594.

Hausler, S. L., Bresman, M. J., Reinherz, E. L., & Weiner, H. L. (1982). Childhood multiple sclerosis: Clinical features and demonstration of changes in T cell subsets with disease activity. *Annals of Neurology, 11,* 463–468.

Hawes, M. D., & Greenberg, H. J. (1981). Slow brain-stem responses (SN10) to tone pips in normally hearing newborns and adults. *Audiology, 20,* 113–122.

Hayes, D. (1994). Hearing loss in infants with craniofacial anomalies. *Archives of Otolaryngology—Head & Neck Surgery,11,* 39–45.

Hayes, D., & Jerger, J. (1982). Auditory brainstem response (ABR) to tonepips: Results in normal and hearing-impaired subjects. *Scandinavian Audiology, 11,* 133–142.

Hayes, E., Warrier, C. M., Nicol, T., Zecker, S. G., & Kraus, N. (2003). Neural plasticity following auditory training in children with learning problems. *Clinical Neurophysiology, 114,* 673–684.

Hay-McCutcheon, M., Brown, C., Clay, K., & Seyle, K. (2002). Comparison of electrically evoked whole-nerve action potential and electrically evoked auditory brainstem response thresholds in Nucleus CI24R cochlear implant recipients. *Journal of the American Academy of Audiology, 13,* 416–427.

Hecht, C., Honrubia, V., Wiet, R., et al. (1997). Hearing preservation after acoustic neuroma resection with tumor size used as a clinical prognosticator. *Laryngoscope, 107,* 1122–1126.

Hecox, K. (1975). Electrophysiological correlates of human auditory development, In L. B. Cohen & P. Salaptex (Eds.), *Infant perception: From sensation to cognition.* New York: Academic Press.

Hecox, K. (1983). Role of auditory brain stem response in the selection of hearing aids. *Ear and Hearing, 4,* 51–55.

Hecox, K., & Burkard, R. (1982). Developmental dependencies of the human brainstem auditory evoked response. *Annals of the New York Academy of Sciences, 388,* 538–556.

Hecox, K., & Cone, B. (1981). Prognostic importance of brainstem evoked potentials after asphyxia. *Neurology, 31,* 1429–1433.

Hecox, K., Cone, B., & Blaw, M. (1981). Brainstem auditory evoked response in the diagnosis of pediatric neurologic diseases. *Neurology, 31,* 832–840.

Hecox, K., & Galambos, R. (1974). Brain stem auditory evoked responses in human infants and adults. *Archives of Otolaryngology, 99,* 30–33.

Hecox, K., Patterson, J., & Birman, M. (1989). Effect of broadband noise on the human brain stem auditory evoked responses. *Ear and Hearing, 10,* 346–353.

Hecox, K., Squires, N., & Galambos, R. (1976). Brainstem evoked response in man: I. Effect of stimulus rise-fall time and duration. *Journal of the Acoustical Society of America, 60,* 1187–1192.

Hegerl, U., Bottlender, R., Gallinat, J., Kuss, H. J., Ackenheil, M., & Moller, H. J. (1998). The serotonin syndrome scale: First results on validity. *European Archives of Psychiatry and Clinical Neuroscience, 248,* 96–103.

Hegerl, U., & Juckel, G. (1994). Auditory evoked dipole source activity: Indicator of central serotonergic dysfunction in psychiatric patients? *Pharmacopsychiatry, 27,* 75–78.

Hegerl, U., Wulff, H., & Muller-Oerlinghausen, B. (1992). Intensity dependence of auditory evoked potentials and clinical response to prophylactic lithium medication: A replication study. *Psychiatry Research, 44,* 181–190.

Heide, G., Freitag, S., Wollenberg, I., Iro, H., Schimrigk, K., & Dillmann, U. (1999). Click evoked myogenic potentials in the differential diagnosis of acute vertigo. *Journal of Neurology, Neurosurgery and Psychiatry, 66,* 787–790.

Heinke, W., Kenntner, R., Gunter, T. C., Sammler, D., Olthoff, D., & Koelsch, S. (2004). Sequential effects of increasing propofol sedation on frontal and temporal cortices as indexed by auditory event-related potentials. *Anesthesiology, 100,* 617–625.

Hellekson, C. A., Allen, A., Greely, H., Emergy, S., & Reeves, A. (1979). Comparison of interwave latencies of brainstem auditory evoked responses in narcoleptics, primary insomniacs and normal controls. *Electroencephalography and Clinical Neurophysiology, 47,* 742–744.

Henry, J., Fausti, S., Kempton, J., Trune, D., & Mitchell, C. (2000). Twenty-stimulus train for rapid acquisition of auditory brainstem responses in humans. *Journal of the American Academy of Audiology, 11,* 103–113.

Herdman, A. T., Lins, O., Van Roon, P., Stapells, D., Scherg, M., & Picton, T. (2002). Intracerebral sources of human auditory steady-state responses. *Brain Topography, 15,* 69–86.

Herdman, A. T., Picton, T. W., & Stapells, D. R. (2002). Place specificity of multiple auditory steady-state responses. *Journal of the Acoustical Society of America, 112,* 1569–1582.

Herdman, A. T., & Stapells, D. R. (2001). Thresholds determined using the monotic and dichotic multiple auditory steady-state response technique in normal-hearing subjects. *Scandinavian Audiology, 30,* 41–49.

Herdman, A. T., & Stapells, D. (2003). Auditory steady-state response thresholds of adults with sensorineural hearing impairments. *International Journal of Audiology, 42,* 237–248.

Herman, C. J., & Bignall, K. E. (1967). Effects of diphenylhydantoin on spontaneous and evoked activity in cat under chloralose anaesthesia. *Electroencephalography and Clinical Neurophysiology, 23,* 351–359.

Herrmann, B., Thornton, A., & Joseph, J. (1995). Automated infant hearing screening using the ABR: Development and validation. *American Journal of Audiology, 4,* 6–14.

Hervé, T., Truy, E., Durupt, I., & Collet, L. (1996). A new stimulation strategy for recording electrical auditory evoked potentials in cochlear implant patients. *Electroencephalography and Clinical Neurophysiology, 100,* 472–478.

Hicks, G. E. (1980). Auditory brainstem response: Sensory assessment by bone conduction masking. *Archives of Otolaryngology, 106,* 392–395.

Higashi, K. (1991). Otologic findings of Didmoad syndrome. *American Journal of Otology, 12,* 57–60.

Hildesheimer, M., Muchnik, C., & Rubenstein, M. (1985). Problems in interpretation of brainstem-evoked response audiometry. *Audiology, 24,* 374–379.

Hillyard, S. A. (1984). Cognitive functions and event-related potentials. In R. H. Nodar & C. Barber (Eds.), *Evoked potentials II. The Second International Evoked Potentials Symposium* (pp. 51–62). Boston: Butterworth.

Hillyard, S. A., Hink, R. F., Schwent, V. L., & Picton, T. (1973). Electrical signs of selective attention in the human brain. *Science, 182,* 177–180.

Hillyard, S. A., & Kutas, M. (1983). Electrophysiology of cognitive processing. *Annual Review of Psychology, 34,* 33–61.

Hillyard, S. A., & Picton, T. W. (1978). On and off components in the auditory evoked potential. *Perception and Psychophysics, 24,* 391–398.

Hillyard, S. A., Picton, T. W., & Regan, D. (1978). Sensation, perception, and attention: Analysis using ERPs. In P. Tueting & S. H. Koslow (Eds.), *Event-related potentials in man.* New York: Academic Press.

Hilz, M., Litscher, G., Weis, M., Claus, D., Druschky, K., Pfurtscheller, G., et al. (1991). Continuous multivariable monitoring in neurological intensive care patients—preliminary reports on four cases. *Intensive Care Medicine, 17,* 87–93.

Hink, R. F., & Hillyard, S. A. (1976). Auditory evoked potentials during selectively listening to dichotic speech messages. *Perception and Psychophysics, 20,* 236–242.

Hink, R. F., & Hillyard, S. A. (1978). Electrophysiological measures of attentional processes in man as related to the study of schizophrenia. *Journal of Psychiatric Research, 14,* 155–165.

Hirata, M., & Kosaka, H. (1993). Effects of lead exposure on neurophysiological parameters. *Environmental Research, 63,* 60–69.

Hirata, M., Ogawa, Y., Okayama, A., & Goto, S. (1992). Changes in auditory brainstem response in rats chronically exposed to carbon disulfide. *Archives of Toxicology, 66,* 334–338.

Hirayasu, Y., Potts, G. F., O'Donnell, B. F., Kwon, J. S., Arakaki, H., Akdag, S. J., Levitt, J. J., Shenton, M. E., & McCarley, R. W. (1998). Auditory mismatch negativity in schizophrenia: Topographic evaluation with a high-density recording montage. *American Journal of Psychiatry, 155,* 1281–1284.

Hirsch, A., & Anderson, H. (1980). Audiological test results in 96 patients with tumors affecting the eighth nerve. *Acta Otolaryngologica (Supplement), 369,* 1–26.

Hirsch, B., Durrant, J., Yetiser, S., Kamerer, D., & Martin, W. (1996). Localizing retrocochlear hearing loss. *American Journal of Otology, 17,* 537–546.

Ho, K. J., Kileny, P. R., Paccioretti, D., & McLean, D. R. (1987). Neurologic, audiologic, and electrophysiologic sequelae of bilateral temporal lobe lesions. *Archives of Neurology, 44,* 982–987.

Hodges, A., Ruth, R., Lambert, P., & Balkany, T. (1994). Electric auditory brain-stem responses in Nucleus multichannel cochlear implant users. *Archives of Otolaryngology—Head & Neck Surgery, 120,* 1093–1099.

Hoffer, M. E., Kopke, R. D., Weisskopf, P., Gottshall, K., Allen, K., & Wester, D. (2001). Microdose gentamicin administration via the round window microcatheter: Results in patients with Ménière's disease. *Annals of the New York Academic Science, 942,* 46–51.

Hofmann, G., & Flach, M. (1981). Brainstem evoked resonse audiometry via air- and bone-conducted stimulation. *Laryngology Rhinology Otology, 60,* 254–267. (German).

Hohmann, D. (1992). [Intraoperative monitoring with transtympanic electrocochleography]. *HNO, 40,* 133–139.

Hohmann, D., Kahaly, G., & Warzelhan, J. (1990). The effect of hyperlipidemia and hypothyroidism on auditory evoked brainstem responses. *HNO, 38,* 446–450.

Hoke, M. (1976). Cochlear mircophonics in man and its probable importance in objective audiometry. In R. Ruben, C. Elberling, & G. Salomon (Eds.), *Electrocochleography* (pp. 41–54). Baltimore: University Park Press.

Hoke, M., Lutkenhoner, B., & Bappert, E. (1980). Brainstem evoked resonses specific to low-frequency region. *Scandinavian Audiology (Supplement), 11,* 105–115.

Hoke, M., Wickesberg, R. E. & Lutkenhoner, B. (1984). Time- and intensity-dependent low-pass filtering of auditory brain stem responses. *Audiology, 23,* 195–205.

Holcomb, P., Ackerman, P., & Dykman, R. (1986). Auditory event-related potentials in attention and reading disabled boys. *International Journal of Psychophysiology, 3,* 263–273.

Holliday, P. O., Pillsbury, D., Kelly, D. L., & Dillard, R. (1985). Brain stem auditory evoked potentials in Arnold-Chiari malformation: Possible prognostic value and change with surgical decompression. *Neurosurgery, 16,* 48–53.

Holt, L. E., Raine, A., Pa, G., Schneider, L. S. Henderson, V. W., & Pollock, V. E. (1995). P300 topography in Alzheimer's disease. *Psychophysiology, 32,* 257–265.

Hömberg, V., Grünewald, G., & Grünewald-Zuberbier, E. (1981). The variation of P300 amplitude in a money-winning paradigm in children. *Psychophysiology, 18,* 258–262.

Hömberg, V., Hefter, H., Granseyer, G., Strauss, W., Lange, H., & Hennerici, M. (1986). Event-related potentials inpatients with Huntington's disease and relatives at risk in relation to detailed psychometry. *Electroencephalography and Clinical Neurophysiology, 63,* 552–569.

Honrubia, V., & Ward, P. H. (1969). Dependence of the cochlear microphonics and summating potential on the endocochlear potential. *Journal of the Acoustical Society of America, 46,* 388–392.

Hood, L. J., & Berlin, C. I. (1987). Comparison of guinea pig toneburst versus derived action potential sinusoidal recordings. *Association for Research in Otolaryngology* (Abstract), 1–8.

Hood, L. J., Martin, D. A., & Berlin, C. I. (1990). Auditory evoked potentials differ at 50 milliseconds in right- and left-handed listeners. *Hearing Research, 45,* 115–122.

Hooks, R. G., & Weber, B. A. (1984). Auditory brain stem responses of premature infants to bone-conducted stimuli: A feasibility study. *Ear and Hearing, 5,* 42–46.

Hoppe, U., Rosanowski, F., Iro, H., & Eysholdt, U. (2001). Loudness perception and late auditory evoked potentials in adult cochlear implant users. *Scandinavian Audiology, 30,* 119–125.

Horikawa, M., Ohtaki, E., Urabe, F., Kawano, Y., Amamoto, M., & Matsuishi, T. (1993). Long-term observation of the changing brainstem auditory evoked potentials in a case of infantile opsoclonus-polymyclonia syndrome. *Brain Development, 15,* 308–310.

Horner, K. C., & Cazals, Y. (1988). Independent fluctuations of the round-window summating potential and compound action potential following the surgical induction of endolymphatic hydrops in the guinea pig. *Audiology, 27,* 147–155.

Horovitz, S. G., Skudlarski, P., & Gore, J. C. (2002). Correlations and dissociations between BOLD signal and P300 amplitude in an auditory oddball task: A parametric approach to combining fMRI and ERP. *Magnetic Resonance Imaging, 20,* 319–325.

Hosford-Dunn, H., Mendelson, T., & Salamy, A. (1981). Binaural interactions in the short-latency evoked potentials of neonates. *Audiology, 20,* 394–408.

Hosick, E. C., & Mendel, M.- I. (1975). Effects of secobarbital on the late components of the auditory evoked potentials. *Revue de Larygologie Otologie Rhinologie (Bordeaux), 96,* 185–191.

Hosono, S., Ohno, T., Kimoto, H., Nagoshi, R., Shimizu, M., Nozawa, M., et al. (2002). Follow-up study of auditory brainstem responses in infants with high unbound bilirubin levels treated with albumin infusion therapy. *Pediatric International, 44,* 488–492.

Hoth, S. (1986). Reliability of latency and amplitude on values of auditory-evoked potentials. *Audiology, 25,* 248–257.

Hotz, M. A., Allum, J. H., Kaufmann, G., Follath, F., & Pfaltz, C. R. (1990). Shifts in auditory brainstem response latencies following plasma-level-controlled aminoglycoside therapy. *European Archives of Otorhinolaryngology, 247,* 202–205.

Hoult, C. (1985). Inverting click polarity: Some effects on the morphology of the brainstem auditory evoked response. *Australian Journal of Audiology, 7,* 33–42.

House, W. F. (1979). *Acoustic tumor.* Baltimore: University Park Press.

Howard, L., & Polich, J. (1985). P300 latency and memory span development. *Developmental Psychology, 21,* 283–289.

Hsu, J., Lui, T., Yu, C., Chen, Y., Chang, C., & Tan, P. (1992). The simultaneous use of electrocochleogram, brainstem auditory evoked potential and facial muscle EMG in cerebellopontine angle tumor removal. *Journal of Formosa Medical Association, 91,* 580–584.

Huang, C.-M., & Buchwald, J. S. (1978). Factors that affect the amplitudes of vertex short-latency acoustic responses in the cat. *Electroencephalography and Clinical Neurophysiology, 44,* 179–186.

Huang, T., Chang, Y., Lee, S., Chen, F., & Chopra, I. (1989). Visual, brainstem auditory and somatosensory evoked potential abnormalities in thyroid disease. *Thyroidology, 1,* 137–142.

Hughes, G., Josey, A., Glasscock, M. E., III, Jackson, C., Ray, W., & Sismanis, A. (1981). Clinical electroneuronography: Statistical analysis of controlled measurements in 22 normal subjects. *Laryngoscope, 91,* 1834–1846.

Hughes, J. R., & Fino, J. (1980). Usefulness of piezoelectric earphones in recording brain stem auditory evoked potentials: A new early deflection. *Electroencephalography and Clinical Neurophysiology, 48,* 357–360.

Hughes, J. R., & Fino, J. J. (1984). Neurophysiological studies on conjoined twins. *Neuropediatrics, 15,* 220–225.

Hughes, J. R., Fino, J., & Gagnon, L. (1981). The importance of phase stimulus and the reference recording electrode in brain stem auditory evoked potentials. *Electroencephalography and Clinical Neurophysiology, 51,* 611–623.

Hughes, M., Brown, C., Abbas, P., Wolaver, A., & Gervais, J. (2000). Comparison of EAP thresholds with MAP levels in the Nucleus 24 cochlear implant: Data from children. *Ear and Hearing, 21,* 164–174.

Humes, L. E., & Ochs, M. G. (1982). Use of contralateral masking in the measurement of the auditory brainstem response. *Journal of Speech & Hearing Research, 25,* 528–535.

Humphries, K. N., Ashcroft, P. B., & Douek, E. E. (1977). Extra-tympanic electrocochleography. *Acta Otolaryngologica (Stockholm), 83,* 303–309.

Humphries, K. N., Gibson, W. P. R., & Douek, E. E. (1976). Objective methods of hearing assessment: A system for recording the crossed acoustic response. *Medical Biology and Engineering, 14,* 1–7.

Huotilainen, M., Tiitinen, H., Lavikainen, J., Ilmoniemi, R. J., Pekkonen, E., Sinkkonen, J., Laine, P., & Näätänen, R. (1995). Sustained fields of tones and glides reflect tonotopy of the auditory cortex. *Neuroreport, 6,* 841–844.

Hutchinson, M., Blandford, S., & Glynn, D. (1984). Clinical correlates of abnormal brain-stem auditory evoked responses in multiple sclerosis. *Acta Neurologica Scandinavia, 69,* 90–95.

Hyde, M. L. (1985). Frequency-specific BERA in infants. *Journal of Otolaryngology (Toronto Supplement), 14,* 19–27.

Hyde. M. L., & Blair, R. L. (1981). The auditory brainstem response in neuro-otology: Prospective and problems. *Journal of Otolaryngology, 10,* 117–125.

Hyde, M. L., Stephens, S. D. G., & Thornton, A. R. D. (1976). Stimulus repetition rate and early brainstem responses. *British Journal of Audiology, 10,* 41–50.

Hymel, M. R., Cranford, J. L., & Stuart, A. (1998). Effects of contralateral speech competition on auditory event-related potentials recorded from elderly listeners: Brain map study. *Journal of the American Academy of Audiology, 9,* 385–397.

Ibanez, V., Deiber, P., & Fischer, C. (1989). Middle latency auditory evoked potentials in cortical lesions: Criteria of interhemispheric asymmetry. *Archives of Neurology, 46,* 1325–1332.

Igarashi, M., Neely, J. G., & Anthony, P. F. (1976). Cochlear nerve degeneration in adrenocerebroleukodystrophy. *Archives of Otolaryngology, 102,* 722–726.

Iijima, M., Osawa, M., Iwata, M., Miyazaki, A., & Tei, H. (2000). Topographic mapping of P300 and frontal cognitive function in Parkinson's disease. *Behavioral Neurology, 12,* 143–148.

Ikner, C., & Hassen, A. (1990). The effects of tinnitus on ABR latencies. *Ear and Hearing, 11,* 16–20.

Iley, K., & Addis, R. (2000). Impact of technology choice on service provision for universal newborn hearing screening within a busy district hospital. *Journal of Perinatology, 20,* S122–S127.

Ilvonen, T., Kujala, T., Kozou, H., Kiesilainen, A., Salonen, O., Alku, P., & Näätänen, R. (2004). The processing of speech and non-speech sounds in aphasic patients as reflected by the mismatch negativity (MMN). *Neuroscience Letters, 366,* 235–240.

Inagaki, M., Kaga, M., Nihei, K., Naitoh, H., Takayama, S., & Sugai, K. (1999). The value of serial auditory brainstem response in patients with subacute sclerosing panencephalitis. *Journal of Child Neurology, 14,* 422–427.

Inayoshi, S., Okajima, T., Sannomiya, K., & Tsuda, T. (1993). [Brainstem and middle auditory evoked potentials in Minimata disease.]. *Clinical Encephalography, 35,* 588–592.

Ino, T., & Mizoi, K. (1980). Vector analysis of auditory brainstem response (BSR) in human beings. *Archives of Otorhinolaryngology, 226,* 55–62.

Inoue, K., Tanaka, H., Scaglia, F., Araki, A., Shaffer L. G., & Lupski, J. R. (2001). Compensating for central nervous system dysmyelination: Females with a proteolipid protein gene duplication and sustained clinical improvement. *Annals of Neurology, 50,* 747–754.

Inoue, T., Kawasaki, H., Shiraishi, S., & Takasaki, M. (1992). Effects of high-dose fentanyl anaesthesia on auditory brain stem responses. *Masui, 41,* 1414–1418.

Irving, R., Jackler, R., & Pitts, L. (1998). Hearing preservation in patients undergoing vestibular schwannoma surgery: Comparison of middle fossa and retrosigmoid approaches. *Journal of Neurosurgery 88,* 840–845.

Iselin-Chaves, I. A., El Moalem, H. E., Gan, T. J., Ginsberg, B., & Glass, P. S. (2000). Changes in the auditory evoked potentials and the bispectral index following propofol or propofol and alfentanil. *Anesthesiology, 92,* 1300–1310.

Islam, M., Asano, K., Tabata, H., Ohkuma, H., & Suzuki, S. (2002). Pineal region tumor manifesting initially as hearing impairment. *Neurologia Medico-Chirugica (Tokyo), 42,* 301–304.

Issa, A., & Ross, H. F. (1995). An improved procedure for assessing ABR latency in young subjects based on a new normative data set. *International Journal of Pediatric Otorhinolaryngology, 32,* 35–47.

Ito, H. (1984). Auditory brainstem response in NICU infants. *International Journal of Pediatric Otorhinolaryngology, 8,* 155–162.

Itoh, A., Kim, Y. S., Yoshioka, K., Kanaya, M., Enomoto, H., Hiraiwa, F., & Mizuno, M. (2001). Clinical study of vestibular-evoked myogenic potentials and auditory brainstem responses in patients with brainstem lesions. *Acta Otolaryngologica Supplement, 545,* 116–119.

Itoh, K., Kawai, S., Nishino, M., Lee, Y., Negishi, H., & Itoh, H. (1992). [The clinical and pathological features of siblings with infantile neuro-axonal dystrophy—early neurological, radiological, neuroelectrophysi-ological and neuropathological characteristics.] *No To Hattatsu, 24,* 283–288.

Ivey, R. G., & Schmidt, H. B. (1993). P300 response: Habituation. *Journal of the American Academy of Audiology, 4,* 182–188.

Iwanami, A., Kamijima, K., & Yoshizawa, J. (1996). P300 component of event-related potentials in passive tasks. *International Journal of Neuroscience, 84,* 121–126.

Iwasaki, S., Takai, Y., Ozeki, H., Ito, K., Karino, S., & Murofushi, T. (2005). Extent of lesions in idiopathic sudden hearing loss with vertigo: Study using click and galvanic vestibular evoked myogenic potentials. *Archives of Otolaryngology—Head & Neck Surgery, 131,* 857–862.

Izuma, S. (1980). The effects of rejection slope and passband of input filter on MLR. *Audiology (Japan), 23,* 184–203.

Jääskeläinen, I. P., Ahveninen, J., Bonmassar, G., Dale, A. M., Ilmoniemi, R. J., Levanen, S., Lin, F. H., May, P., Melcher, J., Stufflebeam, S., Ti-itinen, H., & Belliveau, J. W. (2004). Human posterior auditory cortex gates novel sounds to consciousness. *Proceedings of the National Academy of Sciences of the United States of America, 101,* 6809–6814.

Jääskeläinen, I. P., Hautamaki, M., Näätänen, R., & Ilmoniemi, R. J. (1999). Temporal span of human echoic memory and mismatch negativity: Revisited. *Neuroreport, 10,* 1305–1308.

Jabbari, B., Schwartz, D., Chikarmane, A., & Fadden, D. (1982). Somato-sensory and brain stem auditory evoked response abnormalities in a family with Friedreich's ataxia. *Electroencephalography and Clinical Neurophysiology, 53,* 24–25P.

Jackler, R. K., Shapiro, M. S., Dillon, W. P., Pitts, L., & Lanser, M. J. (1990). Gadolinium-DTPA enhanced magnetic resonance imaging in acoustic neuroma diagnosis and management. *Archives of Otolaryngology—Head & Neck Surgery, 102,* 670–677.

Jackson, L. E., & Roberson, J. B., Jr. (2000). Acoustic neuroma surgery: Use of cochlear nerve action potential monitoring for hearing preservation. *American Journal of Otology, 21,* 249–259.

Jacobs, B., & Schneider, S. (2003). Analysis of lexical-semantic processing and extensive neurological, electrophysiological, speech perception, and language evaluation following a unilateral left hemisphere lesion: Pure word deafness? *Aphasiology, 17,* 23–141.

Jacobson, G. P. (1990, Winter). False-negative outcomes in evoked potential monitoring: A review. *American Society of Evoked Potential Monitoring Newsletter,* 5–8.

Jacobson, G. P., Lombardi, M. A., Gibbens, N. D., Ahmad, M. D., & New-man, C. W. (1992). The effects of stimulus frequency and recording site on the amplitude and latency of multichannel cortical auditory evoked potential (CAEP) component N1. *Ear and Hearing, 13,* 300–306.

Jacobson, G. P., Means, E. D., & Dhib-Jalbut, S. (1986). Delay in the absolute latency of auditory brainstem response (ABR) component P1 in acute inflammatory demyelinating disease. *Scandinavian Audiology, 15,* 121–124.

Jacobson, G. P., & Newman, C. W. (1989). Absence of rate-dependent BAEP P5 latency changed in patients with definite multiple sclerosis: Possible physiological mechanisms. *Electroencephalography and Clinical Neurophysiology, 74,* 19–23.

Jacobson, G. P., Newman, C., Monsell, E., & Wharton, J. (1993). False negative auditory brainstem response findings in vestibular schwannoma: case reports. *Journal of the American Academy of Audiology, 4,* 355–359.

Jacobson, G. P., Newman, C. W., Privitera, M., & Grayson, A. S. (1991). Differences in superficial and deep source contributions to middle latency auditory evoked potential Pa component in normal subjects and patients with neurologic disease. *Journal of the American Academy of Audiology, 2,* 7–17.

Jacobson, G. P., & Tew, J. M., Jr. (1987). Intraoperative evoked potential monitoring. *Journal of Clinical Neurophysiology, 4,* 145–176.

Jacobson, J. T. (1983). Effects of rise time and noise masking on tone pip auditory brainstem responses. *Seminars in Hearing, 4,* 363–373.

Jacobson, J. T. (Ed.). (1985). *The auditory brainstem response.* San Diego: College-Hill Press.

Jacobson, J. T., & Jacobson, C. A. (1994). The effects of noise in transient EOAE newborn hearing screening. *International Journal of Pediatric Otorhinolaryngology, 29,* 235–248.

Jacobson, J. T., Jacobson, C., & Spahr, R. (1990). Automated and conventional ABR screening techniques in high-risk infants. *Journal of the American Academy of Audiology, 1,* 187–195.

Jacobson, J. T., Morehouse, C. R., & Johnson, M. J. (1982). Strategies for infant auditory brainstem response assessment. *Ear and Hearing, 3,* 263–270.

Jacobson, J. T., Murray, T. J., & Deppe, U. (1987). The effects of ABR stimulus repetition rate in multiple sclerosis. *Ear and Hearing, 8,* 115–120.

Jahrsdoerfer, R. A., & Hall, J. W., III. (1986). Congenital malformation of the ear. *American Journal of Otology, 7,* 267–269.

Jahrsdoerfer, R. A., Hall, J. W., III, & Gray, L. C. (1988). A review of syndromes that deafen. In F. H. Bess (Ed.), *Hearing impairment in children* (pp. 57–64). Parkton, MD: York Press.

Jahrsdoerfer, R. A., Yeakley, J. W., Hall, J. W., III, Robbins, K. T., & Gray, L. C. (1985). High resolution CT scaning and ABR in congenital aural atresia-patient selection and surgical correlation. *Archives of Otolaryngology—Head & Neck Surgery, 93,* 292–298.

Jain, S., & Maheshwari, M. C. (1984). Brainstem auditory evoked responses in coma due to meningoencephalitis. *Acta Neurologica Scandinavia, 69,* 163–167.

Jannetta, P. J. (1981). Hemifacial spasm. In J. Samii (Ed.), *The cranial nerves* (pp. 484–493). New York: Springer.

Jannetta, P. J., Møller, A. R., & Møller, M. B. (1984). Technique of hearing preservation in small acoustic neuromas. *Annals of Surgery, 200,* 513–523.

Jansson-Verkasalo, E., Čeponiene, R., Kielinen, M., Suominen, K., Jantti, V., Linna, S. L., Moilanen, I., & Näätänen, R. (1993). Deficient auditory processing in children with Asperger Syndrome, as indexed by event-related potentials. *Neuroscience Letters, 338,* 197–200.

Jansson-Verkasalo, E., Čeponiene, R., Valkama, M., Vainionpaa, L., Laita-kari, K., Alku, P., Suominen, K., & Näätänen, R. (2003). Deficient speech-sound processing, as shown by the electrophysiologic brain mismatch negativity response, and naming ability in prematurely born children. *Neuroscience Letters, 348,* 5–8.

Jansson-Verkasalo, E., Korpilahti, P., Jantti, V., Valkama, M., Vainionpaa, L., Alku, P., Suominen, K., & Näätänen, R. (2004). Neurophysiologic correlates of deficient phonological representations and object naming in prematurely born children. *Clinical Neurophysiology, 115,* 179–187.

Jaramillo, M., Paavilainen, P., & Näätänen, R. (2000). Mismatch negativity and behavioural discrimination in humans as a function of the magnitude of change in sound duration. *Neuroscience Letters, 290,* 101–104.

Jasper, H. H. (1958). The ten twenty electrode system of the international federation. *Electroencephalography and Clinical Neurophysiology, 10,* 371–375.

Jastreboff, P. J., Gray, W. C., & Gold, S. L. (1996). Neurophysiological approach to tinnitus patients. *American Journal of Otology, 17,* 236–240.

Javel, E., Mouney, D. F., McGee, J., & Walsh, E. J. (1982). Auditory brainstem responses during systemic infusion of lidocaine. *Archives of Otolaryngology, 108,* 71–76.

Javitt, D. C. (2000). Intracortical mechanisms of mismatch negativity dysfunction in schizophrenia. *Audiology & Neuro-Otology, 5,* 207–215.

Javitt, D. C., Doneshka, P., Grochowski, S., & Ritter, W. (1995). Impaired mismatch negativity generation reflects widespread dysfunction of working memory in schizophrenia. *Archives of General Psychiatry, 52,* 550–558.

Javitt, D. C., Doneshka, P., Zylberman, I., Ritter, W., & Vaughan, H. G., Jr. (1993). Impairment of early cortical processing in schizophrenia: an event-related potential confirmation study. *Biological Psychiatry, 33,* 513–519.

Javitt, D. C., Grochowski, S., Shelley, A. M., & Ritter, W. (1998). Impaired mismatch negativity (MMN) generation in schizophrenia as a function of stimulus deviance, probability, and interstimulus/interdeviant interval. *Electroencephalography and Clinical Neurophysiology, 108,* 143–153.

Javitt, D. C., Schroeder, C. E., Steinschneider, M., Arezzo, J. C., & Vaughan, H. G., Jr. (1992). Demonstration of mismatch negativity in the monkey. *Electroencephalography and Clinical Neurophysiology, 83,* 87–90.

Jeng, F., Brown, C., Johnson, T., & Vander Werff, K. (2004). Estimating air-bone gaps using auditory steady-state responses. *Journal of the American Academy of Audiology, 15,* 67–78.

Jennett, B., & Teasdale, G. (1981). *Management of head injuries.* Philadelphia: F. A. Davis.

Jensen, E. W., Lindholm, P., & Henneberg, S. W. (1996). Autoregressive modeling with exogenous input of middle-latency auditory-evoked potentials to measure rapid changes in depth of anaesthesia. *Methods of Information in Medicine, 35,* 256–260.

Jensen, E. W., Nygaard, M., & Henneberg, S. W. (1998). On-line analysis of middle latency auditory evoked potentials (MLAEP) for monitoring depth of anaesthesia in laboratory rats. *Medical Engineering & Physics, 20,* 722–728.

Jeon, Y., & Polich, J. (2001). P300 asmmetry in schizophrenia: A meta-analysis. *Psychiatric Research, 104,* 61–74.

Jerger, J. (1987). Diagnostic audiology: Historical perspective. *Ear and Hearing (Supplement), 8,* 7–12.

Jerger, J., Chmiel, R., Frost, J. D., Jr., & Coker, N. (1986). Effect of sleep on the auditory steady state evoked potential. *Ear and Hearing, 7,* 240–245.

Jerger, J., Chmiel, R., Glaze, D., & Frost, J. D., Jr. (1987). Rate and filter dependence of the middle-latency response in infants. *Audiology, 26,* 269–283.

Jerger, J., & Estes, R. (2002). Asymmetry in event-related potentials to simulated auditory motion in children, young adults, and seniors. *Journal of the American Academy of Audiology, 13,* 1–13.

Jerger, J., & Hall, J. W., III. (1980). Effects of age and sex on auditory brainstem response (ABR). *Archives of Otolaryngology, 106,* 387–391.

Jerger, J., & Hayes, D. (1976). The cross-check principle in pediatric audiometry. *Archives of Otolaryngology, 102,* 614–420.

Jerger, J., Hayes, D., & Jordan, C. (1980). Clinical experience with auditory brainstem response in pediatric assessment. *Ear and Hearing, 1,* 19–25.

Jerger, J., & Johnson, K. (1988). Interactions of age, gender, and sensorineural hearing loss on ABR latency. *Ear and Hearing, 9,* 168–176.

Jerger, J., Martin, J., & McColl, R. (2004). Interaural cross correlation of event-related potentials and diffusion tensor imaging in the evaluation of auditory processing disorder: A case study. *Journal of the American Academy of Audiology, 15,* 79–87.

Jerger, J., & Mauldin, L. (1978/1979). Prediction of sensorineural hearing level from the brainstem evoked response. *Archives of Otolaryngology, 104,* 456–461.

Jerger, J., & Musiek, F. (2000). Report of the consensus conference on the diagnosis of auditory processing disorders in school-aged children. Consensus Development Conference. *Journal of the American Academy of Audiology, 11,* 467–474.

Jerger, J., & Musiek, F. (2002). On the diagnosis of auditory processing disorder: A reply to "Clinical and research concerns regarding the 2000 APD consensus report and recommendations." *Audiology Today, 14,* 19–21.

Jerger, J., Oliver, T. A., Chmiel, R. A., & Rivera, V. M. (1986). Patterns of auditory abnormality in multiple sclerosis. *Audiology, 25,* 193–209.

Jerger, J., & Tillman, T. (1960). A new method for the clinic determination of sensori-neural acuity level (SAL). *Archives of Otolaryngology, 71,* 948–955.

Jerger, J., Weikers, N. J., Sharbrough, F. W., III, & Jerger, S. (1969). Bilateral lesions of the temporal lobe: A case study. *Acta Otolaryngologica (Supplement), 258,* 5–51.

Jerger, K., Biggins, C., & Fein, G. (1992). P50 suppression is not affected by attentional manipulations. *Biological Psychiatry, 15,* 365–377.

Jerger, S., & Jerger, J. (1983). Evaluation of diagnostic audiometric tests. *Audiology, 22,* 144–161.

Jerger, S., & Jerger, J. (1985). Audiologic applications of early, middle, and late auditory evoked potentials. *The Hearing Journal, 38,* 31–36.

Jerger, S., Jerger, J., & Loiselle, L. (1989). Pediatric central auditory dysfunction: Comparison of children with confirmed lesions versus suspected processing disorders. *American Journal of Otology, 9,* 63–71.

Jessen, F., Fries, T., Kucharski, C., Nishimura, T., Hoenig, K., Maier, W., Falkai, P., & Heun, R. (2001). Amplitude reduction of the mismatch negativity in first-degree relatives of patients with schizophrenia. *Neuroscience Letters, 309,* 185–188.

Jewett, D. L. (1970). Volume-conducted potentials in response to auditory stimuli as detected by averaging in the cat. *Electroencephalography and Clinical Neurophysiology, 28,* 609–618.

Jewett, D. L., Romano, M. N., & Williston, J. S. (1970). Human auditory evoked potentials: Possible brainstem components detected on the scalp. *Science, 167,* 1517–1518.

Jewett, D. L., & Williston, J. S. (1971). Auditory evoked far fields averaged from the scalp of humans. *Brain, 4,* 681–696.

Jiang, Z. (1995). Maturation of the auditory brainstem in low risk-preterm infants: A comparison with age-matched full term infants up to six years. *Early Human Development, 42,* 49–65.

Jiang, Z., & Tierney, T. (1996). Binaural interaction in human neonatal auditory brainstem. *Pediatric Research, 39,* 708–714.

Jiang, Z., Brosi, D., & Wilkinson, A. (1998). Immaturity of electrophysiological response of the neonatal auditory brainstem to high repetition rates of click stimulation. *Early Human Development, 52,* 133–143.

Jirsa, R. E., & Clontz, K. B. (1990). Long latency auditory event-related potentials from children with auditory processing disorders. *Ear and Hearing, 11,* 222–232.

Johannsen, H. S., & Lehn. T. (1984). The dependence of early acoustically evoked potentials on age. *Archives of Otorhinolaryngology, 240,* 153–158.

Johansson, R. K., Haapaniemi, J. J., & Laurikainen, E. A. (1997). Transtympanic electrocochleography in evaluation of cochleovestibular disorders. *Acta Otolaryngologica (Stockholm), Supplement, 529,* 63–65.

John, M. S., Brown, D., Muir, P., & Picton, T. (2004). Recording auditory steady-state responses in young infants. *Ear and Hearing, 25,* 539–553.

John, M. S., Dimitrijevic, A., & Picton, T. (2003a). Auditory steady-state responses to exponential modulation envelopes. *Ear and Hearing, 23,* 106–117.

John, M. S., Dimitrijevic, A., & Picton, T. (2003b). Efficient stimuli for evoking auditory steady-state responses. *Ear and Hearing, 24,* 406–423.

John, M. S., Dimitrijevic, A., Van Roon, P., & Picton, T. W. (2001). Multiple auditory steady-state responses to AM and FM stimuli. *Audiology & Neuro-Otology, 6,* 12–27.

John, M. S., Lins, O., Boucher, B., & Picton, T. (1998). Multiple auditory steady-state responses (MASTER): Stimulus and recording parameters. *Audiology, 37,* 59–82.

John, M. S., & Picton, T. W. (2000). Human auditory steady-state responses to amplitude-modulated tones: Phase and latency measurements. *Hearing Research, 141,* 57–79.

John, M. S., & Picton, T. (2000). MASTER: A Windows program for recording multiple auditory steady-state responses. *Computer Methods for Programming in Biomedicine , 61,* 25–150.

John, M. S., Purcell, D., Dimitrijevic, A., & Picton, T. (2002). Advantages and caveats when recording steady-state responses to multiple simultaneous stimuli. *Journal of the American Academy of Audiology, 13,* 246–259.

Johnson, B. W., Weinberg, H., Ribary, U., Cheyene, D. O., & Ancill, R. (1988). Topographic distribution of the 40 Hz auditory evoked-related potential in normal and aged subjects. *Brain Tomography, 1*(2), 117–121.

Johnson, M. R., & Adler, L. E. (1993). Transient impairment in P50 auditory sensory gating induced by a cold-pressor test. *Biological Psychiatry, 33,* 380–387.

Johnson, R. (1986). A triarch model of P300 amplitude. *Psychophysiology, 23,* 367–384.

Johnson, R. (1988). The amplitude of the P300 component of the event-related potential: review and synthesis. *Advances in Psychophysiology, 3,* 69–137.

Johnson, R. (1989). Developmental evidence for modality-dependent P300 generations: A normative study. *Psychophysiology, 26,* 651–666.

Johnson, R., Fitzpatrick, J., & Hahn, D. (1993). Calcinosis cutis following electromyographic examination. *Cutis, 52,* 161–164.

Johnston, V. S., Miller, D. R., & Burleson, M. H. (1986). Multiple P3s to emotional stimuli and their theoretical significance. *Psychophysiology, 23,* 684–694.

Johnstone, S., & Barry, R. (1996). Auditory event-related potentials to a two-tone discrimination paradigm in attention deficit hyperactivity disorder. *Psychiatric Research, 64,* 179–192.

Joint Committee on Infant Hearing. (1982). Joint Committee on Infant Hearing 1982 position statement. *Pediatrics, 70,* 496–497.

Joint Committee on Infant Hearing. (2000a). *Position Statement 2000.* Retrieved from American Academy of Audiology website (www.audiology.org).

Joint Committee on Infant Hearing. (2000b). Year 2000 position statement: Principles and guidelines for early hearing detection and intervention programs. Joint Committee on Infant Hearing, American Academy of Audiology, American Academy of Pediatrics, American Speech-

Language-Hearing Association, and Directors of Speech and Hearing Programs in State Health and Welfare Agencies. *Pediatrics, 106,* 798–817.

Joint Committee on Infant Hearing. (2000c). Year 2000 position statement: principles and guidelines for early hearing detection and intervention programs. *American Journal of Audiology, 9,* 9–29.

Jones, S., & Van der Poel, J. (1990). Binaural interaction in the brain-stem auditory evoked potential: Evidence for a delay line coincidence detection mechanism. *Electroencephalography and Clinical Neurophysiology, 77,* 214–224.

Jongsma, M. L. A., Desain, P., & Honing, H. (2004). Rhythmic context influences the auditory evoked potentials of musicians and nonmusicians. *Biological Psychology, 66,* 29–152.

Jonkman, L., Kemner, C., Verbaten, M., Koelega, H., Camfferman, G., van der Gaag, R., Buitelaar, J., & van Engeland, H. (1997). Event-related potentials and performance of attention-deficit hyperactivity disorder: Children and normal controls in auditory and visual selective attention tasks. *Biological Psychiatry, 41,* 595–611.

Jordan, K. (1993). Continuous EEG and evoked potential monitoring in the neuroscience intensive care unit. *Journal of Clinical Neuroscience, 10,* 445–475.

Jordan, K., Schmidt, A., Plotz, K., Von Specht, H., Begall, K., et al. (1997). Auditory event-related potentials in post- and prelingually deaf cochlear implant recipients. *American Journal of Otology, 18,* 116–117.

Joseph, J. M., West, C. A., Thornton, A. R., & Herrmann, B. S. (1987). *Improved decision criteria for evaluation of clinical ABR's.* Paper presented at the biennial meeting of the International Electric Response Audiometry Study Group, Charlottesville, VA.

Josey, A. F., Glasscock, M. E., II, & Musiek, F. E. (1988). Correlation of ABR and medical imaging in patients with cerebellopontine angle tumors. *American Journal of Otology, 9,* 12–16.

Joutsiniemi, S. L., Ilvonen, T., Sinkkonen, J., Huotilainen, M., Tervaniemi, M., Lehtokoski, A., Rinne, T., & Näätänen, R. (1998). The mismatch negativity for duration decrement of auditory stimuli in healthy subjects. *Electroencephalography and Clinical Neurophysiology, 108,* 154–159.

Juckel, G., Molnar, M., Hegerl, U., Csépe, V., & Karmos, G. (1997). Auditory-evoked potentials as indicator of brain serotonergic activity—first evidence in behaving cats. *Biological Psychiatry, 15,* 1181–1195.

Judd, L. L., McAdams, L., Budnick, B., & Braff, D. L. (1992). Sensory gating deficits in schizophrenia: New results. *American Journal of Psychiatry, 49,* 488–493.

Jutras, B., Russell, L., Hurteau, A., & Chapdelaine, M. (2003). Auditory neuropathy in siblings with Waardenburg's syndrome. *International Journal of Pediatric Otorhinolaryngology, 67,* 1133–1142.

Kadner, A., Viirre, E., Wester, D.C., Walsh, S. F., Hestenes, J., Vankov, A., & Pineda, J. A. (2002). Lateral inhibition in the auditory cortex: An EEG index of tinnitus? *Neuroreport, 13,* 443–446.

Kadobayashi, I., Kira, Y., Toyoshima, A., & Nishijima, H. (1984). A study of auditory middle latency responses in relation to electrode combinations and stimulus conditions. *Audiology, 23,* 509–519.

Kadobayashi, I., & Toyoshima, A. (1984). Effects of attention on auditory evoked middle latency potentials. *Folia Psychiatrica Neurology Japan, 38,* 459–463.

Kaga, K., Hink, R. F., Shinoda, Y., & Suzuki, J. (1980). Evidence for a primary cortical origin of a middle latency auditory evoked potential in cats. *Electroencephalography and Clinical Neurophysiology, 50,* 254–266.

Kaga, K., Ichimura, K., Kitazumi, E., Kodama, K., & Tamai, F. (1996). Auditory brainstem responses in infants and children with anoxic brain damage due to near-suffocation or near-drowning. *International Journal of Pediatric Otorhinolaryngology, 36,* 231–239.

Kaga, K., Iwasaki, S., Tamura, A., Suzuki, J., & Haebara, H. (1997). Temporal bone pathology of acoustic neuroma correlating with presence of electrocochleography and absence of auditory brainstem response. *Journal of Laryngology & Otology, 111,* 967–972.

Kaga, K., Kodera, K., Hirota, E., & Tsuzuka, T. (1991). P300 response to tones and speech sounds after cochlear implant: A case report. *Laryngoscope, 101,* 905–907.

Kaga, K., Kurauchi, T., Yumoto, M., & Uno, A. (2004). Middle-latency auditory-evoked magnetic fields in patients with auditory cortex lesions. *Acta Otolaryngologica, 124,* 376–380.

Kaga, K., & Marsh, R. R. (1986). Auditory brainstem responses in young children with Down's syndrome. *International Journal of Pediatric Otorhinolaryngology, 11,* 29–38.

Kaga, K., Marsh, R., & Fukuyama, Y. (1982). Auditory brain stem responses in infantile spasms. *International Journal of Pediatric Otorhinolaryngology, 4,* 57–67.

Kaga, K., Ono, M., Yakumaru, K., Owada, M., & Mizutani, T. (1998). Brainstem pathology of infantile Gaucher's disease with only wave I and II of auditory brainstem response. *Journal of Laryngology & Otology, 112,* 1069–1073.

Kaga, K., Setou, M. & Nakamura, M. (2001). Bone-conducted sound lateralization of interaural time difference and interaural intensity difference in children and a young adult with bilateral microtia and atresia of the ears. *Acta Otolaryngologica, 121,* 274–277.

Kaga, K., Shindo, M., Gotoh, O., & Tamura, A. (1990). Speech perception and auditory P300 potentials after section of the posterior half of the truncus of the corpus callosum. *Brain Topography, 3,* 175–181.

Kaga, K., Tamai, F., Kitazumi, E., & Kodama, K. (1995). Auditory brainstem responses in children with Cornelia de Lange syndrome. *International Journal of Pediatric Otorhinolaryngology, 31,* 137–146.

Kaga, K., Tanaka, Y., & Fukuyama, Y. (1981). Behavioral responses to sounds and auditory brain stem responses of infants with infantile spasms. *Brain Development, 13,* 517–525.

Kaga, K., Yokochi, K., Kodama, K., Kitazumi, E., & Marsh, R. (1986). Absence of later auditory brain stem response components, congenital horizontal nystagmus, and hypotonia in male infants. *Annals of Otology, Rhinology, & Laryngology, 95,* 203–206.

Kaga, M., Azuma, C., Imamura, T., & Murakami, T. (1982). Auditory brainstem response (ABR) in infantile Gaucher's disease. *Neuropediatrics, 13,* 207–210.

Kaga, M., Naitoh, H., & Nihei, K. (1987). Auditory brainstem response in Leigh's syndrome. *Acta Paediatrica Japan, 29,* 254–260.

Kahana, L., Rosenblith, W. A., & Galambos, R. (1950). Effect of temperature change on round-window response in the hamster. *American Journal of Physiology, 163,* 213–223.

Kahkonen, S., Ahveninen, J., Jaaskelainen, I. P., Kaakkola, S., Näätänen, R., Huttunen, J., & Pekkonen, E. (2001). Effects of haloperidol on selective attention: A combined whole-head MEG and high-resolution EEG study. *Neuropsychopharmacology, 25,* 498–504.

Kahkonen, S., Ahveninen, J., Pekkonen, E., Kaakkola, S., Huttunen, J., Ilmoniemi, R. J., & Jaaskelainen, I. P. (2002). Dopamine modulates involuntary attention shifting and reorienting: An electromagnetic study. *Clinical Neurophysiology, 113,* 1894–1902.

Kaipio, M. L., Cheour, M., Ceponiene, R., Ohman, J., Alku, P., & Näätänen, R. (2000). Increased distractibility in closed head injury as revealed by event-related potentials. *Neuroreport, 11,* 1463–1468.

Kaipio, M. L., Novitski, N., Tervaniemi, M., Alho, K., Ohman, J., Salonen, O., & Näätänen, R. (2001). Fast vigilance decrement in closed head injury patients as reflected by the mismatch negativity (MMN). *Neuroreport, 12,* 1517–1522.

Kalayam, B., Alexopoulos, G., Kindermann, S., Kakuma, T., Brown, G., & Young, R. (1998). P300 latency in geriatric depression. *American Journal of Psychiatry, 155,* 425–427.

Kalayam, B., Alexopoulos, G., Musiek, F., Kakuma, T., Toro, A., Silbersweig, D., & Young, R. (1997). Brainstem evoked response abnormalities in late-life depression with vascular disease. *American Journal of Psychiatry, 154,* 970–975.

Kalaydijieva, L., Nikolova, A. Turnev, I., Petrova, J., Hristova, A., & Ishpekova, R. (1998). Hereditary motor and sensory neuropathy—Lom, a novel demyelinating neuropathy associated with deafness in gypsies. Clinical, electrophysiological and nerve biopsy findings. *Brain, 121,* 399–408.

Kaldestad, R., Wingaard, L., & Hansen, T. (2002). [Screening for congenital hearing loss—a pilot project.]. *Tiddskrift for den Norske Laegeforening, 122,* 2190–2193.

Kalita, J., & Misra, U. (1999). Brainstem auditory evoked potential in Japanese encephalitis. *Journal of the Neurological Sciences, 165,* 24–27.

Kalita, J., & Misra, U. (2001). Brainstem auditory evoked potentials in tubercular meningitis and their correlation with radiological findings. *Neurology of India, 49,* 51–54.

Kalmanchev, R., Avila, A., & Symon, L. (1986). The use of brainstem auditory evoked potentials during posterior fossa surgery as a monitor of brainstem function. *Acta Neurochirurgica, 82,* 128–136.

Kaminer, M., & Pratt, H. (1987). Three-channel Lissajous' trajectory of auditory brainstem potentials evoked by specific frequency bands (derived responses). *Electroencephalography and Clinical Neurophysiology, 66,* 167–174.

Kamuro, K., Inagaki, M., & Tomita, Y. (1992). [Correlation between morphological abnormalities of Chiari malformation and evoked potentials]. *No To Hattatsu, 24,* 554–558.

Kane, N. M., Butler, S. R., & Simpson, T. (2000). Coma outcome prediction using event-related potentials: P$_3$ and mismatch negativity. *Audiology & Neuro-Otology, 5,* 186–191.

Kane, N. M., Curry, S. H., Butler, S. R., & Cummins, B. H. (1993). Electrophysiological indicator of awaking from coma. *Lancet, 341,* 688.

Kane, N. M., Curry, S. H., Rowlands, C. A., Manara, A. R., Lewis, T., Moss, T., Cummins, B. H., & Butler, S. R. (1996). Event-related potentials—neurophysiological tools for predicting emergence and early outcome from traumatic coma. *Intensive Care Medicine, 22,* 39–46.

Kankkunen, A., & Rosenhall, U. (1985). Comparison between thresholds obtained with pure-tone audiometry and the 40-Hz middle latency response. *Scandinavian Audiology, 14,* 99–104.

Kanzaki, J., Ogawa, K., Shiobara, R., & Toya, S. (1989). Hearing preservation in acoustic neuroma surgery and postoperative audiologic findings. *Acta Otolaryngologica, 107,* 474–478.

Kanzaki, J., Oushi, T., Yokobori, H., & Ino, T. (1982). Electrocochleographic study of summating potentials in Ménière's disease. *Audiology, 21,* 409–424.

Kapoor, R., Makharia, A., Shukla, R., Misra, P., & Sharma, B. (1997). Brainstem auditory evoked response in tuberculous meningitis. *Indian Journal of Pediatrics, 64,* 399–407.

Karaaslan, F., Gonul, A. S., Oguz, A., Erdinc, E., & Esel, E. (2003). P300 changes in major depressive disorders with and without psychotic features. *Journal of Affective Disorders, 73,* 283–287.

Karayanidis, F., Andrews, S., Ward, P. B., & Michie, P. T. (1995). ERP indices of auditory selective attention in aging and Parkinson's disease. *Psychophysiology, 32,* 335–350.

Karhu, J., Herrgard, E., Paakkonen, A., Luoma, L., Airaksinen, E., & Partanen, J. (1997). Dual cerebral processing of elementary auditory input in children. *Neuroreport, 8,* 1327–1330.

Karnaze, D., Gott, P., Mitchell, F., & Loftin, J. (1984). Brainstem auditory evoked potentials are normal in idiopathic sleep apnea. *Annals of Neurology, 15,* 406.

Karnaze, D. S., Marshall, L. F., McCarthy, C. S., Klauber, M. R., & Bickford, R. G. (1982). Localizing and prognostic value of auditory evoked responses in coma after closed head injury. *Neurology, 32,* 299–302.

Karp, B., & Laureno, R. (1993). Pontine and extrapontine myelinolysis: A neurologic disorder following rapid correction of hyponatremia. *Medicine (Baltimore), 72,* 359–373.

Kartush, J., Garcia, P., & Telian, S. A. (1987). The source of far-field antidromic facial nerve potentials. *American Journal of Otology, 8,* 199–204.

Kartush, J., Graham, M. D., & Kemink, J. L. (1986). Electroneuronography: Preoperative facial nerve assessment in acoustic neuroma surgery. *American Journal of Otology, 7,* 322–325.

Kasaba, T., Kosaka, Y., & Itoga, S. (1991). Effects of intravenous lidocaine administration on auditory brainstem response. *Masui, 40,* 931–935.

Kasaba, T., Nonoue, T., Yanagidani, T., Maeda, M., Aoki, S., Sakaguchi, T., et al. (1991). Effect of lumbar epidural anaesthesia on brainstem auditory response. *Masui, 40,* 16–20.

Kasai, K., Nakagome, K., Itoh, K., Koshida, I., Hata, A., Iwanami, A., Fukuda, M., Hiramatsu, K. I., & Kato, N. (1999). Multiple generators in the auditory automatic discrimination process in humans. *Neuroreport, 10,* 2267–227.

Kaseda, Y., Tobimatsu, S., Morioka, T., & Kato, M. (1991). Auditory middle-latency responses in patients with localized and non-localized lesions of the central nervous system. *Journal of Neurology, 238,* 427–432.

Katayama, J., & Polich, J. (1996). P300, probability, and the three-tone paradigm. *Electroencephalography and Clinical Neurophysiology, 100,* 555–562.

Katayama, J., & Polich, J. (1998). Stimulus context determines P3a and P3b. *Psychophysiology, 35,* 23–33.

Katbamma, B., Metz, D., Adelman, C., & Thodi, C. (1993). Auditory-evoked responses in chronic alcohol and drug abusers. *Biological Psychiatry, 33,* 750–752.

Kathmann, N., Frodl-Bauch, T., & Hegerl, U. (1999). Stability of the mismatch negativity under different stimulus and attention conditions. *Clinical Neurophysiology, 110,* 317–323.

Kato, T., Shiriashi, K., Eura, Y., Shibata, K., Sakata, T., Morizono, T., & Soda, T. (1998). A neural response with 3-ms latency evoked by loud sound in profoundly deaf patients. *Audiology & Neuro-Otology, 3,* 253–264.

Kaukoranta, E., Hari, R., & Lounasmaa, O. V. (1987). Responses of the human auditory cortex to vowel onset after fricative consonants. *Experimental Brain Research, 69,* 19–23.

Kaustio, O., Partanen, J., Valkonen-Korhonen, M., Viinamaki, H., & Lehtonen, J. (2002). Affective and psychotic symptoms relate to different types of P300 alteration in depressive disorder. *Journal of Affective Disorders, 71,* 43–50.

Kavanagh, K. T., & Beardsley, J. V. (1979). Brainstem auditory evoked responses. *Annals of Otology, Rhinology & Laryngology (Supplement), 88, 58,* 1–28.

Kavanagh, K. T., & Domico, W. D. (1986). High-pass digital filtration of the 40 Hz response and its relationship to the spectral content of the middle latency and 40 Hz responses. *Ear and Hearing, 7,* 93–99.

Kavanagh, K. T., Domico, W. D., Franks, R., & Han, J. C. (1988). Digital filtering and spectral analysis of the low intensity ABR. *Ear and Hearing, 9,* 43–47.

Kavanagh, K. T., Gould, H., McCormick, G., & Franks, R. (1989). Comparison of the identifiability of the low intensity ABR and MLR in the mentally handicapped patient. *Ear and Hearing, 10,* 124–130.

Kavanagh, K. T., Harker, L. A., & Tyler, R. S. (1984). Auditory brainstem and middle latency responses: I. Effects of response filtering and waveform identification; II. Threshold responses to a 500-Hz tone pip. *Acta Otolaryngologica (Stockholm), 108,* 1–12.

Kazmerski, V. A., Friedman, D., & Ritter, W. (1997). Mismatch negativity during attend and ignore conditions in Alzheimer's disease. *Biological Psychiatry, 42,* 382–402.

Keating, L. W., & Ruhm, H. B. (1971). Some observations on the effects of attention to stimuli on the amplitude of the acoustically evoked response. *Audiology, 10,* 177–184.

Keidel, W. D., & Spreng, M. (1965). Neurophysiological evidence for the Steven's power function in man. *Journal of the Acoustical Society of America, 38,* 191–195.

Keith, W. J., & Greville, K. A. (1987). Effects of audiometric configuration on the auditory brainstem response. *Ear and Hearing, 8(1),* 49–55.

Kellényi, L., Thuroczy, G., Faludy, B., & Lenard, L. (1999). Effects of mobile GSM radiotelephone exposure on the auditory brainstem response (ABR). *Neurobiology, 7,* 79–81.

Kelly, A., Purdy, S., & Thorne, P. (2005). Electrophysiological and speech perception measures of auditory processing in experienced adult cochlear implant users. *Clinical Neurophysiology, 116,* 1235–1246.

Kelly-Ballweber, D., & Dobie, R. A. (1984). Binaural interaction measured behaviorally and electrophysiologically in young and old adults. *Audiology, 23,* 181–194.

Kemink, J. L., Kileny, P. R., Niparko, J. K., & Telian, S. A. (1991). Electrical stimulation of the auditory system after labyrinthectomy. *American Journal of Otology, 12,* 7–10.

Kemink, J., LaRouere, M., Kileny, P., et al. (1990). Hearing preservation following suboccipital removal of acoustic neuromas. *Laryngoscope, 100,* 597–602.

Kemner, C., Oranje, B., Verbaten, M. N., van Engeland, H. (2002). Normal P50 gating in children with autism. *Journal of Clinical Psychiatry, 63,* 214–217.

Kemner, C., Verbaten, M. N., Cuperus, J. M., Camfferman, G., & van Engeland, H. (1995). Auditory event-related brain potentials in autistic children and three different control groups. *Biological Psychiatry, 38,* 150–165.

Kemner, C., Verbaten, M. N., Koelega, H. S., Buitelaar, J. K., van der Gaag, R. J., Camfferman, G., & van Engeland, H. (1996). Event-related brain potentials in children with attention-deficit and hyperactivity disorder: Effects of stimulus deviancy and task relevance in the visual and auditory modality. *Biological Psychiatry, 40,* 522–534.

Kenemans, J. L., Verbaten, M. N., Roelofs, J. W., & Slangen, J. L. (1989). "Initial-" and "change-orienting" reactions, trial event-related potentials. *Biological Psychology, 28,* 199–226.

Kennedy, C. (1999). Controlled trial of universal neonatal screening for early identification of permanent childhood hearing impairment: Coverage, positive predictive value, effect on mothers and incremental yield. *Acta Paediatrica, 88,* 73–75.

Kevanishvili, Z., & Aphonchenko, V. (1979). Frequency composition of brainstem auditory evoked potentials. *Scandinavian Audiology, 8,* 51–55.

Kevanishvili, Z., & Aphonchenko, V. (1981). Click polarity inversion effects upon the human brainstem auditory evoked potential. *Scandinavian Audiology, 10,* 141–147.

Kevanishvili, Z., & Lagidze, Z. (1987). Masking level difference: An electrophysiological approach. *Scandinavian Audiology, 16,* 3–11.

Khardori, R., Soler, N. G., Good, D.C., Develesc-Howard, A. B., Broughton, D., & Walbert, J. (1986). Brainstem auditory and visual evoked potentials in Type 1 (insulin-dependent) diabetic patients. *Diabetologia, 29,* 362–365.

Khecheniashvili, S. N., & Kevanishvili, Z. S. (1974). Experiences in computer audiometry (EcoG and ERA). *Audiology, 13,* 391–402.

Khedr, E., El Toony, L., & Tarkhan, M. (2000). Peripheral and central nervous system alterations in hypothyroidism: Electrophysiological findings. *Neuropsychobiology, 41,* 88–94.

Khosbin, S., & Hallett, M. (1981). Multimodality evoked potentials and blink reflex in multiple sclerosis. *Neurology, 31,* 138–144.

Kiang, N. Y.-S. (1965). *Discharge patterns of single nerve fibers in the cat's auditory nerve.* Cambridge, MA: MIT Press.

Kiang, N. Y.-S. (1975). Stimulus representation in discharged patterns of auditory neurons. In E. L. Eagles (Ed.), *The nervous system: Human communication and its disorder* (vol. 3). New York: Raven Press.

Kiang, N. Y.-S., Crist, A. H., French, M. A., & Edwards, A. G. (1963). Postauricular electric response to acoustic stimuli in humans. *Quarterly Progress Report, MIT, 2,* 218–225.

Kidd, G., Burkard, R., & Mason, C. (1993). Auditory detection of the human brainstem auditory evoked response. *Journal of Speech and Hearing Research, 36,* 442–447.

Kileny, P. R. (1981). The frequency specificity of tone-pips evoked auditory brain stem responses. *Ear and Hearing, 2,* 127–270.

Kileny, P. R. (1983). Auditory evoked middle latency responses: Current issues. *Seminars in Hearing, 4,* 403–413.

Kileny, P. R. (1984). Comments on auditory brainstem responses to middle- and low-frequency tone pips. *Audiology, 23,* 75–84.

Kileny, P. R. (1985). Middle latency (MLR) and late vertex auditory evoked responses (LVAER) in central auditory dysfunction. In M. L. Pinheiro & F. E. Musiek (Eds.), *Assessment of central auditory dysfunction: Foundations and clinical correlates* (pp. 87–102). Baltimore: Williams & Wilkins.

Kileny, P. R. (1987). Algo-1 automated infant hearing screener: Preliminary results. *Seminars in Hearing, 8,* 125–131.

Kileny, P. R. (1988). New insights on ABR infant hearing screening. *Scandinavian Audiology (Supplement), 30,* 81–88.

Kileny, P. R. (1991). Use of electrophysiologic measures in the management of children with cochlear implants: Brainstem, middle latency, and cognitive (P300) responses. *American Journal of Otology, 12,* 37–42.

Kileny, P. R., & Berry, D. A. (1983). Selective impairment of late vertex and middle latency auditory evoked responses in multiply handicapped infants and children. In G. Mencher & S. Gerber (Eds.), *The multiply handicapped hearing impaired child* (pp. 233–258). New York: Grune & Stratton.

Kileny, P. R., Boerst, A., & Zwolan, T. (1997). Cognitive evoked potentials to speech and tonal stimuli in children with implants. *Archives of Otolaryngology—Head & Neck Surgery, 117,* 161–169.

Kileny, P. R., Dodson, D., & Gelfand, E. (1983). Middle-latency auditory evoked responses during open-heart surgery with hypothermia. *Electroencephalography and Clinical Neurophysiology, 55,* 268–276.

Kileny, P. R., Edwards, B., Disher, M., & Telian, S. (1998). Hearing improvement after resection of cerebellopontine angle meningioma: Case study of the preoperative role of transient evoked otoacoustic emissions. *Journal of the American Academy of Audiology, 9,* 251–256.

Kileny, P. R., & Kemink, J. L. (1987). Electrically evoked middle-latency auditory potentials in cochlear implant candidates. *Archives of Otolaryngology—Head & Neck Surgery, 113,* 1072–1077.

Kileny, P. R., Kemink, J., & Miller, J. (1989). An intrasubject comparison of electric and acoustic middle latency responses. *American Journal of Otology, 10,* 23–27.

Kileny, P. R., & Kripal, J. P. (1987). Test-retest variability of auditory event-related potentials. *Ear and Hearing, 8,* 110–114.

Kileny, P. R., & Magathan, M. G. (1987). Predictive value of ABR in infants and children with moderate to profound hearing impairment. *Ear and Hearing, 8*(4), 217–221.

Kileny, P. R., Miller, J. M., Ruth, R. A., Berlin, C. I., Miyamoto, R. T., Stypulkowski, P. H., Don, M., Thornton, A. R., Abbis, P. J., & Shepherd, R. K. (1988). *Evoked responses to electrical stimulation of the auditory system.* Session presented at the American Speech-Language Hearing Association Convention, Boston, November 20.

Kileny, P. R., & Niparko, J. K. (1988). Intraoperative monitoring of auditory and facial nerve functions in neurotologic surgery. *Advances in Otolaryngology Head and Neck Surgery, 2,* 55–88.

Kileny, P. R., Paccioretti, D., & Wilson, A. F. (1987). Effects of cortical lesions on middle-latency auditory evoked responses (MLR). *Electroencephalography and Clinical Neurophysiology, 66,* 108–120.

Kileny, P. R., & Shea, S. L. (1986). Middle-latency and 40 Hz auditory evoked responses in normal-hearing subjects: Click and 500 Hz thresholds. *Journal of Speech and Hearing Research, 29,* 20–28.

Kileny, P. R., & Zwolan, T. (2004). Pre-perioperative transtympanic electrically evoked auditory brainstem response in children. *International Journal of Audiology, 43,* S16–S21.

Kileny, P. R., Zwolan, T., Zimmerman-Phillips, S., & Kemink, J. (1992). A comparison of round-window and transtympanic promontory electrical stimulation in cochlear implant candidates. *Ear and Hearing, 13,* 294–299.

Kileny, P. R., Zwolan, T., Zimmerman-Phillips, S., & Telian, S. (1994). Electrically evoked auditory brain-stem response in pediatric patients with cochlear implants. *Archives of Otolaryngology—Head & Neck Surgery, 120,* 1083–1090.

Killion, M. (1984). New insert earphones for audiometry. *Hearing Instruments, 35,* 28–29.

Killion, M., Wilbur, L., & Gudmundsen, G. (1985). Insert earphones for more interaural attenuation. *Hearing Instruments, 36,* 34–36.

Kimura, D. (1961). Cerebral dominance and the perception of verbal stimuli. *Canadian Journal of Psychology, 15,* 166–171.

Kimura, H., Aso, S., & Watanabe, Y. (2003). Prediction of progression from atypical to definite *Ménière's* disease using electrocochleography and glycerol and furosemide tests. *Acta Otolaryngologica, 123,* 388–395.

Kimura, J. (1985). Abuse and misuse of evoked potentials as a diagnostic tool. *Archives of Neurology, 42,* 78–80.

Kinarti, R., & Sohmer, H. (1982). Analysis of auditory brain stem response sources along the basilar membrane to low-frequency filtered clicks. *Israel Journal of Medical Sciences, 18,* 93–98.

King, C., Nicol, T., McGee, T., & Kraus, N. (1999). Thalamic asymmetry is related to acoustic signal complexity. *Neuroscience Letters,* 89–92.

King, C., Warrier, C. M., Hayes, E., & Kraus, N. (2002). Deficits in auditory brainstem pathway encoding of speech sounds in children with learning problems. *Neuroscience Letters, 319*(2), 111–115.

Kinoshita, S., Maeda, H., Nakamura, J., Kodama, E., & Morita, K. (1995). Reliability of the probability effect on event-related potentials during repeated testing. *Kurume Medical Journal, 42,* 199–210.

Kinoshita, Y., Tanaka, Y., Yasuhara, A., Matsuzaki, S., Kuriki, H., & Kobayashi, Y. (1992). A case of deletion of the short arm of chromosome 10 with severe hearing loss and brainstem dysfunction. *American Journal of Perinatology, 9,* 299–301.

Kiren, T., Aoyagi, M., Furuse, H., & Koike, Y. (1994). An experimental study on the generator of amplitude-modulation following response. *Acta Otolaryngologica Supplement, 511,* 28–33.

Kisley, M. A., Olincy, A., Robbins, E., Polk, S. D., Adler, L. E., Waldo, M. C., & Freedman, R. (2003a). Sensory gating impairment associated with schizophrenia persists into REM sleep. *Psychophysiology, 40,* 29–38.

Kisley, M. A., Polk, S. D., Ross, R. G., Levisohn, P. M., & Freedman, R. (2003b). Early postnatal development of sensory gating. *Neuroreport, 14,* 693–697.

Kitahara, M., Takada, T., Yazawa, Y., & Matsubara, H. (1981). Electrocochleography in the diagnosis of Ménière's disease. In K. H. Vosteen, H. Schuknecht, & C. R. Pfalz (Eds.), *Ménière's disease: Pathogenesis, diagnosis and treatment* (pp. 163–169). Stuttgart: Thieme.

Kitahara, Y., Fukatsu, O., & Koizumi, Y. (1995). Effect of sevoflurane and nitrous oxide *Anaesthesia* on auditory brainstem responses in children. *Masui, 44,* 805–809.

Kitaoku, Y. (1994). Extratympanic electrocochleography during glycerol dehydration test in unilateral Ménière's disease. *Nippon Jiblinkoka Gakkai Kaiho, 97,* 1281–1290.

Kitaoku, Y., Nario, K., & Matsunaga, T. (1993). Extratympanic electrocochleography during glycerol dehydration test in control subjects with normal hearing. *Nippon Jiblinkoka Gakkai Kaiho, 96,* 2032–2038.

Kitchin, C., Counts, L., & Gerstenhaber, M. (2003, November 13). Input filter prevents instrumentation-amp RF-rectification errors. *EDN,* 101–102.

Kjaer, M. (1979). Evaluation and gradation of brain stem auditory evoked potentials in patients with neurological diseases. *Acta Neurologica Scandinavia, 60,* 231–242.

Kjaer, M. (1980). Recognizability of brain stem auditory evoked potential components. *Acta Neurologica Scandinavia, 60,* 20–33 (d).

Kjaer, M. (1983). Evoked potentials. With special reference to the diagnostic value in multiple sclerosis. *Acta Neurologica Scandinavia, 67,* 67–89.

Klein, A. J. (1983). Properties of the brain-stem response slow-wave component: II. Frequency specificity. *Archives of Otolaryngology, 109,* 74–78.

Klein, A. J. (1984). Frequency and age-dependent auditory evoked thresholds in infants. *Hearing Research, 16,* 291–297.

Klein, A. J., & Mills, J. H. (1981). Physiological (waves I and V) and psychological tuning curves in human subjects. *Journal of the Acoustical Society of America, 69,* 760–768.

Klein, A. J., & Teas, D.C. (1978). Acoustically dependent latency shifts of BSER (wave V) in man. *Journal of the Acoustical Society of America, 63,* 1887–1895.

Klin, A. (1993). Auditory brainstem responses in autism: brainstem dysfunction or peripheral hearing loss? *Journal of Autism and Developmental Disorders, 23,* 15–35.

Klorman, R., Brumaghim, J., Fitzpatrick, P., & Borgstedt, A. (1991). Methylphenidate speeds evaluation processes of attention deficit disorder adolescents during a continuous performance test. *Journal of Abnormal Child Psychology, 19,* 236–283.

Klorman, R., Brumaghim, J. T., Fitzpatrick, P. A., & Borgstedt, A. D. (1992). Methylphenidate reduces abnormalities of stimulus classification in adolescents with attention deficit disorder. *Journal of Abnormal Psychology, 101,* 130–138.

Klorman, R., Salzman, L., Bauer, L., Coons, H., Borgstedt, A., & Halpern, W. (1983). Effects of two doses of methylphenidate on cross-situational and borderline hyperactive children's evoked potentials. *Electroencephalography and Clinical Neurophysiology, 56,* 169–185.

Knight, R. T. (1984). Decreased response to novel stimuli after prefrontal lesions in man. *Electroencephalography and Clinical Neurophysiology, 59,* 9–20.

Knight, R. T. (1996). Contribution of human hippocampal region to novelty detection. *Nature, 383,* 256–259.

Knight, R. T., & Brailowsky, S. (1990). Auditory evoked potentials from the primary auditory cortex of the cat: topographic and pharmacological studies. *Electroencephalography and Clinical Neurophysiology, 77,* 225–232.

Knight, R. T., Hillyard, S. A., Woods, D. L., & Neville, H. J. (1980). The effects of frontal and temporal-parietal lesions on the auditory evoked potential in man. *Electroencephalography and Clinical Neurophysiology, 50,* 112–124.

Knight, R. T., Scabini, D., Woods, D., & Clayworth, C. (1989). Contributions of temporal-parietal junction to the human auditory P300. *Brain Research, 502,* 109–116.

Knoll, O., Harbort, U., Schulte, K., & Zimpel, F. (1982). Quantitative survey of uremic brain dysfunction by auditory evoked potentials. In J. Courjon, F. Mauguiere, & M. Revol (Eds.), *Clinical applications of evoked potentials in neurology* (pp. 227–232). New York: Raven Press.

Kobayashi, H., Arenberg, I. K., Ferraro, J. A., & VanderArk, G. D. (1993). Delayed endolymphatic hydrops following acoustic tumor removal with intraoperative and postoperative auditory brainstem response improvements. *Acta Otolaryngologica Supplement, 504,* 74–78

Kobylarz, E. J., & Schiff, N. D. (2004). Functional imaging of severely brain-injured patients: Progress, challenges, and limitations. *Archives of Neurology, 61,* 1357–1360.

Kochanek, K., Tacikowska, G., Pierchala, K., Olczak, J., Dobrzynski, P., & Stelmaszek, K. (1998). [Auditory brainstem responses in the diagnosis of retrocochlear hearing loss: Selected case reports.]. *Otolaryngology Poland, 52,* 69–76.

Kodera, H., Yamane, H., Yamada, O., & Suzuki, J.-I. (1977). The effects of onset, offset and rise-decay times of tone bursts on brain stem responses. *Scandinavian Audiology, 6,* 205–210.

Kodera, K., Yamada, O., Yamane, H., & Suzuki, J. I. (1978). Effects of number and interstimulus interval of tone pips on fast responses. *Audiology, 17,* 500–510.

Koeda, T., & Kohno, Y. (1992). [Non-verbal auditory agnosia with EEG abnormalities and epilepsy: An unusual case of Landau-Kleffner syndrome.]. *No To Hattatsu, 24,* 262–267.

Koelsch, S., Gunter, T., Friederici, A., & Schroger, E. (2000). Brain indices of music processing: 'Non-musicians' are musical. *Journal of Cognitive Neuroscience, 12,* 520–541.

Koelsch, S., Maess, B., Grossmann, T., & Friederici, A. D. (2003). Electric brain responses reveal gender differences in music processing. *Neuroreport, 14,* 09–713.

Koelsch, S., Schmidt, B., & Kansok, J. (2002). Influences of musical expertise on the ERAN: An ERP study. *Psychophysiology, 39,* 657–663.

Koelsch, S., Schroger, E., & Tervaniemi, M. (1999). Superior pre-attentive auditory processing in musicians. *Neuroreport, 10,* 1309–1313.

Koelsch, S., Wittfoth, M., Wolf, A., Muller, J., & Hahne, A. (2004). Music perception in cochlear implant users: An event-related potential study. *Clinical Neurophysiology, 115,* 966–972.

Koenig, S., Gendelman, H. E., Orenstein, J. M., Dal Canto, M. C., Pezeshkpour, G. H., Yungbluth, M., Janotta, F., & Askamit, A. (1986). Detection of AIDS virus in macrophages in brain tissue from AIDs patients with encephalography. *Science, 5,* 1089–1094.

Kohelet, D., Arbel, E., Goldberg, M., & Arlazoroff, A. (2000). Brainstem auditory evoked response in newborns and infants. *Journal of Child Neurology, 15,* 33–35.

Kohelet, D., Usher, M., Arbel, E., Arlasoroff, A., & Goldberg, M. (1990). Effect of gentamycin on the auditory brainstem evoked response in term infants: A preliminary report. *Pediatric Research, 28,* 232–234.

Komsuoglu, S. S., Jones, L. A., & Harding, G. F. (1981). Visual and auditory evoked potentials in a case of Marchiafava Bignami Disease. *Clinical Electroencephalography, 12,* 72–78.

Kondo, H., Harayama, H., Shinozawa, K., Yuasa, T., & Miyatake, T. (1990). [Auditory brainstem response and somatosensory evoked potential in Machado-Joseph disease in Japanese families.] *Rinsho Shinkeigaku, 30,* 723–727.

Konradsson, K. S., Carlborg, B., Grenner, J., & Tjernstrom, O. (1999). Electrocochleographic and audiometric evaluation of hypobaric effect in Ménière's disease. *Laryngoscope, 109,* 59–64.

Kooi, K. A., Tipton, A. C., & Marshall, R. E. (1971). Polarities and field configurations of the vertex components of the human auditory evoked response: A reinterpretation. *Electroencephalography and Clinical Neurophysiology, 31,* 166–169.

Kopell, B. S., Roth, W. T., & Tinklenberg, J. R. (1978). Time-course effects of marijuana and ethanol on event-related potentials. *Psychopharmacology, 56,* 15–20.

Korczak, P. A., Kurtzberg, D., & Stapells, D. R. (2005). Effects of sensorineural hearing loss and personal hearing AIDS on cortical event-related potential and behavioral measures of speech-sound processing. *Ear and Hearing, 26,* 165–185.

Korein, J. (1980). Brain death. In J. E. Kottrel & H. Turndorf (Eds.), *Anaestesiology in neurosurgery* (pp. 282–331). St. Louis: CV Mosby.

Korpelainen, J., Kauhanen, M., Mononen, H., Hiltunen, P., Sotaniemi, K., Suominen, K., & Myllyla, V. (2000). Auditory P300 event related potential in minor ischemic stroke. *Acta Neurologica Scandinavia, 101,* 202–208.

Korpilahti, P., Krause, C. M., Holopainen, I., & Lang, A. H. (2001). Early and late mismatch negativity elicited by words and speech-like stimuli in children. *Brain and Language, 76,* 332–339.

Korpilahti, P., & Lang, H. A. (1994). Auditory ERP components and mismatch negativity in dysphasic children. *Electroencephalography and Clinical Neurophysiology, 91,* 256–264.

Koshino, Y., Nishio, M., Murata, T., Omori, M., Murata, I., Sakamoto, M., & Isaki, K. (1993). The influence of light drowsiness on the latency and amplitude of P300. *Clinical Electroencelphography, 24,* 110–113.

Kotchoubey, B., & Lang, S. (2001). Event-related potentials in an auditory semantic oddball task in humans. *Neuroscience Letters, 310,* 93–96.

Kotchoubey, B., & Lang, S. (2002). Auditory mismatch: Not every mismatch-related negativity is a mismatch negativity. *Journal of Psychophysiology, 16,* 243.

Kotchoubey, B., Lang, S., Baales, R., Herb, E., Maurer, P., Mezger, G., Schmalohr, D., Bostanov, V., & Birbaumer, N. (2001). Brain potentials in human patients with extremely severe diffuse brain damage. *Neuroscience Letters, 301,* 37–40.

Kotchoubey, B., Lang, S., Herb, E., Maurer, P., Schmalohr, D., Bostanov, V., & Birbaumer, N. (2003). Stimulus complexity enhances auditory discrimination in patients with extremely severe brain injuries. *Neuroscience Letters, 352,* 129–132.

Kotlarz, J. P., Eby, T. L., & Borton, T. E. (1992). Analysis of the efficiency of retrocochlear screening. *Laryngoscope, 102,* 1108–1112.

Kovach, M., Campbell, K., Herman, K., et al. (2002). Anticipation in a unique family with Charcot-Marie-Tooth syndrome and deafness: Delineation of the clinical features and review of the literature. *American Journal of Medical Genetics, 108,* 295–303.

Koyama, S., Kuroda, K., Aizawa, H., Kikuchi, K., & Kusunoki, S. (1998). [Bickerstaff's brainstem encephalitis with one-and-a-half syndrome.] *Rinsho Shinkeigaku, 38,* 849–852.

Koyuncu, M., Mason, S. M., & Saunders, M. W. (1994). Electrocochleography in endolymphatic hydrops using tone-pip and click stimuli. *Clinical Otolaryngology, 19,* 73–78.

Kraiuhin, C., Gordon, E., Coyle, S., Sara, G., Rennie, C., Howson, A., Landau, P., & Meares, R. (1990). Normal latency of the P300 event-related potential in mild-to-moderate Alzheimer's disease and depression. *Biological Psychiatry, 28,* 372–386.

Kramer, S., & Teas, D. (1982). Forward masking of the auditory nerve (N1) and brainstem (wave V) responses in humans. *Journal of the Acoustical Society of America, 72,* 795–803.

Kraus, N. (1999). Speech sound perception, neurophysiology, and plasticity. *International Journal of Pediatric Otorhinolaryngology, 47,* 123–129.

Kraus, N. (2001). Auditory pathway encoding and neural plasticity in children with learning problems. *Audiology & Neuro-Otology, 6,* 221–227.

Kraus, N., Bradlow, A. R., Cheatham, M. A., Cunningham, J., King, C. D., Koch, D. B., Nicol, T. G., McGee, T. J., Stein, L. K., & Wright, B. A. (2000). Consequences of neural asynchrony: a case of auditory neuropathy. *Journal of the Association for Research in Otolaryngology, 1,* 33–45.

Kraus, N., & Cheour, M. (2000). Speech sound representation in the brain. *Audiology & Neuro-Otology, 5,* 140–150.

Kraus, N., Kileny, P., & McGee, T. (1994). Middle latency auditory evoked potentials. In J. Katz, (Ed.), *Handbook of Clinical Audiology* (4th ed., pp. 378–405). Baltimore: Williams & Wilkins.

Kraus, N., Koch, D. B., McGee, T. J., Nicol, T. G., & Cunningham, J. (1999). Speech-sound discrimination in school-age children: psychophysical and neurophysiologic measures. *Journal of Speech, Language and Hearing Research, 42,* 1042–1060.

Kraus, N., & McGee, T. (1988). Color imaging of the human middle latency response. *Ear and Hearing, 9,* 159–167.

Kraus, N., & McGee, T. (1990). Clinical applications of the middle latency response. *Journal of the American Academy of Audiology, 1,* 130–133.

Kraus, N., & McGee, T. (1993). Clinical implications of primary and nonprimary pathway contributions to the middle latency response generating system. *Ear and Hearing, 14,* 36–48.

Kraus, N., & McGee, T. (1995). The middle latency response generating system. *Electroencephalography and Clinical Neurophysiology, Supplement, 44,* 93–101.

Kraus, N., McGee, T., Carrell, T., King, C., Littman, T., & Nicol, T. (1994). Discrimination of speech-like contrasts in the auditory thalamus and cortex. *Journal of the Acoustical Society of America, 96,* 2758–2768.

Kraus, N., McGee, T., Carrell, T. D., & Sharma, A. (1995). Neurophysiologic bases of speech discrimination. *Ear and Hearing, 16,* 19–37.

Kraus, N., McGee, T., Carrell, T., Sharma, A., Micco, A., & Nicol, T. (1993a). Speech-evoked cortical potentials in children. *Journal of the American Academy of Audiology, 4,* 238–248.

Kraus, N., McGee, T. J., Carrell, T. D., Zecker, S. G., Nicol, T. G., & Koch, D. B. (1996). Auditory neurophysiologic responses and discrimination deficits in children with learning problems. *Science, 273,* 971–973.

Kraus, N., McGee, T., & Comperatore, C. (1989). MLRs in children are consistently present during wakefulness, stage 1, and REM sleep. *Ear and Hearing, 10,* 339–345.

Kraus, N., McGee, T., Ferre, J., Hoeppner, J. A., Carrell, T., Sharma, A., & Nicol, T. (1993b). Mismatch negativity in the neurophysiologic/behavioral evaluation of auditory processing deficits: A case study. *Ear and Hearing, 14,* 223–234.

Kraus, N., McGee, T. J., & Koch, D. B. (1998a). Speech sound perception and learning: biologic bases. *Scandinavian Audiology Supplement, 49,* 7–17.

Kraus, N., McGee, T. J., & Koch, D. B. (1998b). Speech sound representation, perception, and plasticity: a neurophysiologic perceptive. *Audiology & Neuro-Otology, 3,* 168–182.

Kraus, N., McGee, T., Littman, T., & Nicol, T. (1992). Reticular formation influences on primary and non-primary auditory pathways as reflected by the middle latency response. *Brain Research, 587,* 186–194.

Kraus, N., McGee, T., Littman, T., Nicol, T., & King, C. (1994). Nonprimary auditory thalamic representation of acoustic change. *Journal of Neurophysiology, 72,* 1270–1277.

Kraus, N., McGee, T., Micco, A., Sharma, A., Carrell, T., & Nicol, T. (1993). Mismatch negativity in school-age children to speech stimuli that are just perceptibly different. *Electroencephalography and Clinical Neurophysiology, 88,* 123–130.

Kraus, N., McGee, T., Sharma, A., Carrell, T., & Nicol, T. (1992). Mismatch negativity event-related potential elicited by speech stimuli. *Ear and Hearing, 13,* 158–164.

Kraus, N., Micco, A., Koch, D., McGee, T., Carrell, T., Sharma, A., Wiet, R., & Weingarten, C. (1993c). The mismatch negativity cortical evoked potential elicited by speech in cochlear-implant users. *Hearing Research, 65,* 118–124.

Kraus, N., & Nicol, T. (2003). Aggregate neural responses to speech sounds in the central auditory system. *Speech Communication, 41,* 35–47.

Kraus, N., Özdamar, O., Heydemann, P. T., Stein, L., & Reed, N. L. (1984). Auditory brainstem responses in hydrocephalic patients. *Electroencephalography and Clinical Neurophysiology, 59,* 310–331.

Kraus, N., Özdamar, O., Hier, D., & Stein, L. (1982). Auditory middle latency responses (MLRs) in patients with cortical lesions. *Electroencephalography and Clinical Neurophysiology, 54,* 275–287.

Kraus, N., Özdamar, O., Stein, L., & Reed, N. (1984). Absent auditory brain stem response: Peripheral hearing loss or brain stem dysfunction? *Laryngoscope, 94,* 400–406.

Kraus, N., Reed, N., Smith, D. I., Stein, L., & Cartee, C. (1987). High-pass filter setting affect the detectability of MLRs in humans. *Electroencephalography and Clinical Neurophysiology, 68,* 234–236.

Kraus, N., Smith, D. I., & McGee, T. (1988). Midline and temporal lobe MLRs in the guinea pig originate from different generator systems: A conceptual framework for new and existing data. *Electroencephalography and Clinical Neurophysiology, 70,* 1–18.

Kraus, N., Smith, D., Reed, N. L., Stein, L. K., & Cartee, C. (1985). Auditory middle latency responses in children: Effects of age and diagnostic category. *Electromyography and Clinical Neurophysiology, 62,* 343–351.

Kreitschmann-Andermahr, I., Rosburg, T., Demme, U., Gaser, E., Nowak H., & Sauer, H. (2001). Effect of ketamine on the neuromagnetic mismatch field in healthy humans. *Brain Research & Cognitive Brain Research, 12,* 109–116.

Kreitschmann-Andermahr, I., Rosburg, T., Meier, T., Volz, H. P., Nowak, H., & Sauer, H. (1999). Impaired sensory processing in male patients with schizophrenia: A magnetoencephalographic study of auditory mismatch detection. *Schizophrenia Research, 35,* 121–129.

Krishnan, A. (1999). Human frequency-following responses to two-tone approximations of steady-state vowels. *Audiology & Neuro-Otology, 4,* 95–103.

Krishnan, A., & McDaniel, S. (1998). Binaural interaction in the human frequency-following response: Effects of interaural intensity difference. *Audiology & Neuro-Otology, 3,* 291–299.

Kriss, A., Prasher, D. K., & Pratt, R. T. C. (1984). Brainstem evoked potentials followed methohexitone *Anaesthesia* and unilateral ect. In R. H. Nodar & C. Barber (Eds.), *Evoked Potentials II: The Second International Evoked Potentials Symposium.* Boston: Butterworth.

Krough, H. J., Khan, M. A., & Fosuig, L. (1977). N1 to P2 component of the auditory evoked potential during alcohol intoxication and interaction of pyrithioxine in healthy adults. *Electroencephalography and Clinical Neurophysiology, 44,* 1–7.

Krueger, W. W., & Storper, I. S. (1997). Electrocochleography in retrosigmoid vestibular nerve section for intractable vertigo caused by Ménière's disease. *Otolaryngology—Head & Neck Surgery, 116,* 593–596.

Krueger, W. W., & Wagner, A. P. (1997). Needle placement with transtympanic electrocochleography. *Laryngoscope, 107,* 1671–1673.

Krumholz, A., Singer, H. S., Niedermeyer, E., Burnite, R., & Harris, K. (1983). Electrophysiological studies in Tourette's syndrome. *Annals of Neurology, 14,* 638–641.

Krumholz, A., Weiss, H. D., Goldstein, P. J., & Harris, K. C. (1981). Evoked responses in vitamin B12 deficiency. *Annals of Neurology, 9,* 407–409.

Krumm, M., & Cranford, J. L. (1989). Effects of contralateral speech competition on the late auditory evoked potential in children. *Journal of the American Academy of Audiology, 5,* 127–132.

Kubo, T., Yamamoto, K., Iwaki, T., Matsukawa, M., Doi, K., & Tamura, M. (2001). Significance of auditory evoked responses (EABR and P300) in cochlear implant subjects. *Acta Otolaryngologica, 121,* 257–261.

Kugelman, A., Hadad, B., Ben David, J., Podoshin, L., Borochowitz, Z., & Bader, D. (1997). Preauricular tags and pits in the newborn: The role of hearing tests. *Acta Paediatrica, 86,* 170–172.

Kugler, C., Taghavy, A., & Platt, D. (1993). The event-related P300 potential analysis of cognitive human brain aging: A review. *Gerontology, 39,* 280–303.

Kujala, T., Belitz, S., Tervaniemi, M., & Näätänen, R. (2003). Auditory sensory memory disorder in dyslexic adults as indexed by the mismatch negativity. *European Journal of Neuroscienc, 17,* 1323–1327.

Kujala, T., Kallio, J., Tervaniemi, M., & Näätänen, R. (2001). The mismatch negativity as an index of temporal processing in audition. *Clinical Neurophysiology, 112,* 1712–1719.

Kujala, T., Karma, K., Čeponiene, R., Belitz, S., Turkkila, P., Tervaniemi, M., & Näätänen, R. (2001). Plastic neural changes and reading improvement caused by audiovisual training in reading-impaired children. *Proceedings of the National Academy of Science (U.S.A.), 98,* 10509–10514.

Kujala, T., Myllyviita, K., Tervaniemi, M., Alho, K., Kallio, J., & Näätänen, R. (2000). Basic auditory dysfunction in dyslexia as demonstrated by brain activity measurements. *Psychophysiology, 37,* 262–266.

Kujala, T., & Näätänen, R. (2001). The mismatch negativity in evaluating central auditory dysfunction in dyslexia. *Neuroscience and Bio-Behavior Review, 25,* 535–543.

Kulynych, J. J., Vladar, K., Jones, D. W., & Weinberger, D. R. (1993). Gender differences in the normal lateralization of the supratemporal cortex: MRI surface-rendering morphometry of Heschl's gyrus and the planum temporale. *Cerebral Cortex, 4,* 107–118.

Kumagami, H., Nishida, H., & Baba, M. (1982). Electrocochleographic study of Ménière's disease. *Archives of Otolaryngology, 108,* 284–288.

Kumar, V., & Tandon, O. (1997). Neurotoxic effects of rubber factory environment. An auditory evoked potential study. *Electromyography and Clinical Neurophysiology, 37,* 469–473.

Kupperman, G. L., & Mendel, M. I. (1974). Threshold of the early components of the averaged electroencephalic response determined with tone pips and clicks during drug-induced sleep. *Audiology, 13,* 379–390.

Kurauchi, T., Kaga, K., & Shindo, M. (1996). Abnormalities of ABR and auditory perception test findings in acquired palatal myoclonus. *International Journal of Neuroscience, 85,* 273–283.

Kurtz, I., & Sokolov, Y. (2005, February). Novel method of reducing the effect of electric and magnetic fields on auditory evoked potentials. *Abstracts of the 28th Annual Midwinter Research Meeting, Association for Research in Otolaryngology, 506,* 178.

Kurtzberg, D. (1989). Cortical event-related potential assessment of auditory system function. *Seminars in Hearing, 10*(3), 252–261.

Kurtzberg, D., Hilpert, P., Kreuzer, J. A., Stone, C. L., & Vaughan, H. G., Jr. (1986). Topographic analysis of auditory evoked potentials to speech sounds in infants. In W. C. McCallum, R. Zappoli, & F. Denoth (Eds.), *Cerebral psychophysiology: Studies in event-related potentials* (pp. 326–328). New York: Elsevier Science Publishers.

Kurtzberg, D., Hilpert, P. L., Kreuzer, J. A., & Vaughan, H. G., Jr. (1984). Differential maturation of cortical auditory evoked potentials to speech sounds in normal fullterm and very low-birthweight infants. *Developmental Medicine—Child Neurology, 26,* 466–475.

Kurtzberg, D., Stone, C. L., & Vaughan, H. G. (1986). Cortical responses to speech sounds in the infant. In R. Q. Cracco & I. Bodis-Wollner (Eds.), *Evoked potentials* (pp. 513–520). New York: Liss.

Kurtzberg, D., Vaughan, H. G., Jr., Courchesne, E., Friedman, D., Harter, M. R., & Putnam, L. E. (1984). Developmental aspects of event-related potentials. *Annals of the New York Academy of Science, 425,* 300–318.

Kurtzberg, D., Vaughan, H. G., Jr., Kreuzer, J. A., & Fliegler, K. Z. (1995). Developmental studies and clinical application of mismatch negativity: Problems and prospects. *Ear and Hearing, 16,* 105–117.

Kurtzke, J. G. (1970). Clinical manifestations of multiple sclerosis. In P. J. Vinken & G. W. Bruyn (Eds.), *Handbook of clinical neurology* (pp. 161–216). Amsterdam: North-Holland Publishing.

Kusakari, J., Okitsu, R., Kobayashi, T., Rokugo, M., Tomioka, S., Arakawa, E., Oyama, K., & Hashimoto, S. (1981). ABR audiometry in the diagnosis of cerebellopontine angle tumors. *Otorhinolaryngology, 43,* 336–344.

Kushiro, K., Zakir, M., Ogawa, Y., Sato, H., & Uchino, Y. (1999). Saccular and utricular inputs to sternocleidomastoid motoneurons of decerebrate cats. *Experimental Brain Research, 126,* 410–416.

Kushnerenko, E., Čeponiene, R., Balan, P., Fellman, V., & Näätänen, R. (2002). Maturation of the auditory change detection response in infants: A longitudinal ERP study. *Neuroreport, 13,* 1843–1848.

Kushnerenko, E., Cheour, M., Čeponiene, R., Fellman, V., Renlund, M., Soininen, K., Alku, P., Koskinen, M., Sainio, K., & Näätänen, R. (2001). Central auditory processing of durational changes in complex speech patterns by newborns: An event-related brain potential study. *Developmental Neuropsychology, 19,* 83–97.

Kutas, M., & Hillyard, S. A. (1980). Reading senseless sentences: Brain potentials reflect semantic incongruity. *Science, 207,* 203–205.

Kutas, M., & Hillyard, S. A. (1982). The lateral distribution of event-related potentials during sentence processing. *Neuropsychologia, 20,* 589–590.

Kutas, M., & Hillyard, S. A. (1983). Event-related brain potentials to grammatical errors and semantic anomalies. *Memory and Cognition, 11,* 539–550.

Kutas, M., & Hillyard, S. A. (1984). Brain potentials during reading reflect word expectancy and semantic association. *Nature, 307,* 161–163.

Kutas, M., Neville, H. J., & Holcomb, P. J. (1987). A preliminary comparison of the N400 response to semantic anomalies during reading, listening and signing. *Electroencephalography and Clinical Neurophysiology, Supplement, 39,* 325–330.

Kutas, M., Van Petten, C., & Besson, M. (1988). Event-related potential asymmetries during the reading of sentences. *Electroencephalograpy and Clinical Neurophysiology, 69,* 218–233.

Kuwada, S., Anderson, J., Batra, R., Fitzpatrick, D., Teissier, N., & D'Angelo, W. (2002). Sources of the scalp-recorded amplitude-modulation following response. *Journal of the American Academy of Audiology, 13,* 188–204.

Kuwada, S., & Batra, R. (1999). Coding of sound envelopes by inhibitory rebound of the superior olivary complex in the unanesthetized rabbit. *Journal of Neuroscience, 19,* 2273–2287.

Kuwada, S., Batra, R., & Maher, V. L. (1986). Scalp potentials of normal and hearing-impaired subjects in response to sinusoidally amplitude-modulated tones. *Hearing Research, 21,* 179–192.

Kylen, P., Harder, H., Jervall, L., & Arlinger, S. (1982). Reliability of bone-conducted electrocochleography: A clinical study. *Scandinavian Audiology, 11,* 223–226.

Lacey, D., & Terplan, K. (1984). Correlating auditory evoked and brainstem histological abnormalities in infantile Gaucher's disease. *Neurology, 34,* 539–541.

Lader, M. (1977). Effects of psychotropic drugs on auditory evoked potentials in man. In J. E. Desmedt (Ed.), *Auditory evoked potentials in man: Psychopharmacology correlates of evoked potentials* (pp. 142–159). Basel, Switzerland: Karger.

Lai, C., Tai, C., Liu, R., & Howng, S. (1997). A longitudinal study of central and peripheral nerve conduction in hypothyroid rats. *Journal of Neurological Science, 148,* 139–145.

Lajtman, Z., Marinovic, F., Krpan, D., & Gasparovic, S. (1993). Summating potentials in the differential diagnosis of cochlear pathology. *Lijec. Vjesn., 115,* 238–240.

Lambert, P., & Ruth, R. A. (1988). Simultaneous recording of noninvasive EcoG and ABR for use in intraoperative monitoring. *Archives of Otolaryngology—Head & Neck Surgery, 98,* 575–580.

Lammers, W. J., & Badia, P. (1989). Habituation of P300 to target stimuli. *Physiology & Behavior, 45,* 595–601.

Lane, R. H., Kupperman, G. L., & Goldstein, R. (1971). Early components of the averaged electroencephalic response in relation to rise-decay time and duration of pure tones. *Journal of Speech and Hearing Research, 14,* 408–415.

Lane, R. H., Mendel, M. I., Kupperman, G. L., Vivion, M. C., Buchanan, L. H., & Goldstein, R. (1974). Phase distortion of averaged electroencephalic response. *Archives of Otolaryngology, 99,* 428–432.

Lang, A. H., Eerola, O., Korpilahti, P., Holopainen, I., Salo, S., & Aaltonen, O. (1995). Practical issues in the clinical application of mismatch negativity. *Ear and Hearing, 16,* 118–130.

Lang, A. H., Happonen, J., & Salmivalli, A. (1981). An improved technique for the noninvasive recording of auditory brainstem responses with a specially constructed metal electrode. *Scandinavian Audiology, Supplement, 13,* 59–62.

Lang, A. H., Jantti, V., Nyrke, T., & Happonen, J. M. (1981). The application of FFT and inverse FFT in the analysis of ABR waveform variation. *Scandinavian Audiology (Supplement), 13,* 65–67.

Lang, S. F., Nelson, C. A., & Collins, P. F. (1990). Event-related potentials to emotional and neutral stimuli. *Journal of Clinical and Experimental Neuropsychology, 12,* 946–958.

Lanser, M. J., Sussman, S. A., & Frazer, K. (1992). Epidemiology, pathogenesis, and genetics of acoustic tumors. *Otolaryngology Clinics of North America, 25,* 499–520.

Lary, S., Briassoulis, G., de Vries, L., Dubowitz, L. M. S., & Dubowitz, V. (1985). Hearing threshold in preterm and term infants by auditory brainstem response. *Journal of Pediatrics, 107,* 593–599.

Lasky, R. E. (1984). A developmental study on the effect of stimulus rate on the auditory evoked brain-stem response. *Electroencephalography and Clinical Neurophysiology, 59,* 411–419.

Lasky, R. E., & Rupert, A. (1982). Temporal masking of auditory evoked brainstem responses in human newborns and adults. *Hearing Research, 6,* 315–334.

Lasky, R. E., Rupert, A., & Walker, M. (1987). Reproducibility of auditory brainstem responses as a function of the stimulus, scorer, and subject. *Electroencephalography and Clinical Neurophysiology, 68,* 45–57.

Laukli, E., & Mair, I. W. S. (1981). Early auditory-evoked responses: Spectral content. *Audiology, 20,* 453–464.

Laukli, E., & Mair, I. W. S. (1985). Auditory brainstem responses of the cat: On- and off-responses. *Audiology, 24,* 217–226.

Laukli, E., & Mair, I. W. S. (1985). Low-frequency sensorineural hearing loss. *Scandinavian Audiology, 14,* 133–139.

Laureano, A. N., McGrady, M. D., & Campbell, K. C. (1995). Comparison of tympanic membrane-recorded electrocochleography and the auditory brainstem response in threshold determination. *American Journal of Otology, 16,* 209–215.

Lauter, J., Oyler, R., & Lord-Maes, J. (1993). Amplitude stability of auditory brainstem responses in two groups in two groups of children compared with adults. *British Journal of Audiology, 27,* 263–271.

Lavikainen, J., Tiitinen, H., May, P., & Näätänen, R. (1997). Binaural interaction in the human brain can be non-invasively accessed with long-latency event-related potentials. *Neuroscience Letters, 222,* 37–40.

Lazorthes, G., LaComme, Y., Ganbert, J., & Planel, H. (1961). La constitution du nerf auditif. *Presse Medicine, 69,* 1067–1068.

Lazzaro, H., Anderson, J., Gordon, E., Clarke, S., Leong, J., & Meares, R. (1997). Single trial variability within the P300 (250–500 ms) processing window in adolescents with attention deficit hyperactivity disorder. *Psychiatric Research, 73,* 91–101.

Lee, B., & Newberg, A. (2005). Neuroimaging in traumatic brain imaging. *NeuroRx, 2,* 372–383.

Lee, Y. S., Lueders, H., Dinner, D. S., Lesser, R. P., Hahn, J., & Klemm, G. (1984). Recording of auditory evoked potentials in man using chronic subdural electrodes. *Brain, 107,* 115–131.

Legatt, A. D. (2002). Mechanisms of intraoperative brainstem auditory evoked potential changes. *Journal of Clinical Neurophysiology, 19,* 396–408.

Legatt, A. D., Pedley, T. A., Emreson, R. G., Stein, B. M., & Abramson, M. (1988). Normal brain-stem auditory evoked potentials with abnormal latency-instensity studies in patient with acoustic neuromas. *Archives of Neurology, 45,* 1326–1330.

Lehnhardt, M. L. (1971). Effects of frequency modulation on auditory evoked response. *Audiology, 10,* 18–22.

Lehnhardt, M. L. (1981). Childhood central auditory processing disorder with brainstem auditory evoked response verification. *Archives of Otolaryngology, 107,* 623–625.

Lehnhardt, M. L. (1982). Wave V latency and chirp (linear frequency ramp): Repetition rate. *Audiology, 21,* 425–432.

Lehtonen, J. B. (1973). Functional differentiation between late components of visual evoked potentials recorded at occiput and vertex: Effect of stimulus interval and contour. *Electroencephalography and Clinical Neurophysiology, 35,* 75–82.

Lehtonen, J. B., & Koivikko, M. J. (1971). The use of a non-cephalic reference electrode in recording cerebral evoked potentials in man. *Electroencephalography and Clinical Neurophysiology, 31,* 154–156.

Lemons, J., Fanaroff, A., Stewart, E., Bantkover, J., Murray, G., & Diefendorf, A. (2002). Newborn hearing screening: Cost of establishing a program. *Journal of Perinatology, 22,* 120–124.

Lempert, J., Wever, E., & Lawrence, M. (1947). The cochleogram and its clinical applications: A preliminary report. *Archives of Otolaryngology, 45,* 61–67.

Lenarz, T., & Ernst, A. (1992). Intraoperative monitoring by transtympanic electrocochleography and brainstem electrical response audiometry in acoustic neuroma surgery. *European Archives of Otorhinolaryngology, 249,* 257–262.

Lenarz, T., & Sachsenheimer, W. (1985). Prognostic factors for postsurgical hearing and facial nerve function in cases of cerebellopontine angle tumors: The meaning of brain stem evoked response audiometry (BERA). *Acta Neurochirurgica, 78,* 21–27.

Lenn, N., Olsho, L., & Turk, W. (1986). Auditory processing deficits in a patient with Rett syndrome. *American Journal of Medical Genetics, 24,* 153–156.

Lenzi, A., Chiarelli, G., & Sambataro, G. (1989). Comparative study of middle-latency responses and auditory brainstem responses in elderly subjects. *Audiology, 28,* 144–151.

Leonardis, L., Zidar, J., Popovic, M., et al. (2000). Hereditary motor and sensory neuropathy associated with auditory neuropathy in a Gypsy family. *Pfluger Archives of the European Journal of Physiology, 439,* R208–R210.

Leppanen, P. H., & Lyytinen, H. (1997). Auditory event-related potentials in the study of developmental language-related disorders. *Audiology & Neuro-Otology, 2,* 308–340.

Leppanen, P. H., Richardson, U., Pihko, E., Eklund, K. M., Guttorm, T. K., Aro, M., & Lyytinen, H. (2002). Brain responses to changes in speech sound durations differ between infants with and without familial risk for dyslexia. *Developmental Neuropsychology, 22,* 407–422.

Lesperence, M., Grundfast, K., & Rosenbaum, K. (1998). Otologic manifestations of Wolf-Hirschorn syndrome. *Archives of Otolaryngology—Head & Neck Surgery, 124,* 193–196.

Lev, A., & Sohmer, H. (1972). Sources of averaged neural responses recorded in animal and human subjects during cochlear audiometry. *Archives of Klinische and Experimentale Ohren, Nasen Kehlkopfheilkunde, 201,* 79–90.

Levänen, S., Ahonen, A., Hari, R., McEvoy, L., & Sams, M. (1996). Deviant auditory stimuli activate human left and right auditory cortex differently. *Cerebral Cortex, 6,* 288–296.

Levänen, S., Hari, R., McEvoy, L., & Sams, M. (1993). Responses of the human auditory cortex to changes in one versus two stimulus features. *Experimental Brain Research, 97,* 177–183.

Levi, E., Folsom, R., & Dobie, R. (1993). Amplitude-modulation following response (AMFR): Effects of modulation rate, carrier frequency, age and state. *Hearing Research, 68,* 42–52.

Levine, R. A. (1981). Binaural interaction in brainstem potentials of human subjects. *Annals of Neurology, 9,* 384–393.

Levine, R. A, & Davis, P. (1991). Origin of the click-evoked binaural interaction potential, beta, of humans. *Hearing Research, 57,* 121–128.

Levine, R. A., & McGaffigan, P. M. (1983). Right-left asymmetries in the human brain stem: Auditory evoked potentials. *Electroencephalography and Clinical Neurophysiology, 55,* 532–537.

Levine, R. A., Ojemann, R. G., Montogomery, W. W., & McGaffigan, P. M. (1984). Monitoring auditory evoked potentials during acoustic neuroma surgery: Insights in the mechanism of the hearing loss. *Annals of Otology, Rhinology & Laryngology, 93,* 116–123.

Levine, S. C., Antonelli, P., Le, C., & Haines, S. (1991). Relative value of diagnostic tests for small acoustic neuromas. *American Journal of Otology, 12,* 41–346.

Levine, S. C., Margolis, R. H., Fournier E. M., & Winzenburg, S. M. (1992). Tympanic electrocochleography for evaluation of endolymphatic hydrops. *Laryngoscope, 102,* 614–622.

Levit, R. A., Sutton, S., & Zubin, J. (1973). Evoked potential correlates of information processing in psychiatric patients. *Psychological Medicine, 3,* 487–494.

Lew, G. S., & Polich, J. (1993). P300, habituation, and response mode. *Physiological Behavior, 53,* 111–117.

Lew, H., Lee, E., Miyoshi, Y., Chang, D., Date, E., & Jerger, J. (2004). Brainstem auditory-evoked potentials as an objective tool for evaluating hearing dysfunction in traumatic brain injury. *American Journal of Physical Medicine and Rehabilitation, 83*, 210–215.

Li, X., Sokolov, Y., & Kunov, H. (2002). *System and method for processing low signal-to-noise ratio signals.* U.S. Patent 6,463,411. Issued October 8, 2002. US Class: 704/226; 381/71.6; 381/317, Intl. Class: H04B 015/00; G10L 021/02; H04R 025/00. Filed: May 7, 2001, Application No. 849451.

Liang, J., Lee, W., Young, C., Peng, S., & Shen, Y. (2002). Agyria-pachygyria: Clinical, neuroimaging, and neurophysiologic correlations. *Pediatric Neurology, 27*, 171–176.

Liao, L., & Young, Y. (2004). Vestibular evoked myogenic potentials in basilar artery migraine. *Laryngoscope, 114*, 1305–1309.

Liao, T. J., Nakanishi, H., & Nishikawa, H. (1993). The effect of acupuncture stimulation of the middle latency auditory evoked potential. *Tohoku Journal of Experimental Medicine, 170*, 103–112.

Liasis, A., Bamiou, D. E., Campbell, P., Sirimanna, T., Boyd, S., & Towell, A. (2003). Auditory event-related potentials in the assessment of auditory processing disorders: A pilot study. *Neuropediatrics, 34*, 23–29.

Liberson, W. T. (1966). The study of evoked potentials in aphasics. *American Journal of Physical Medicine, 45*, 135–142.

Liebenthal, E., Ellingson, M. L., Spanaki, M. V., Prieto, T. E., Ropella, K. M., & Binder, J. R. (2003). Simultaneous ERP and fMRI of the auditory cortex in a passive oddball paradigm. *NeuroImage, 19*, 1395–1404.

Liegeois-Chauvel, C., Musolino, A., Badier, J. M., Marquis, P., & Chauvel, P. (1994). Evoked potentials recorded from the auditory cortex in man: Evaluation and topography of the middle latency components. *Electroencephalography and Clinical Neurophysiology, 92*, 204–214.

Lightfoot, G. (1992). ABR screening for acoustic neuromata: The role of rate-induced latency shift measurements. *British Journal of Audiology, 26*, 217–227.

Lightfoot, G. (1993). Correcting for factors affecting ABR wave V latency. *British Journal of Audiology, 27*, 211–220.

Likosky, W., & Elmore, R. S. (1982). Exacerbation detection in multiple sclerosis by clinical and evoked potential techniques: a preliminary report. *Advances in Neurology, 32*, 535–540.

Lincoln, A. J., Courchesne, E., Harms, L., & Allen, M. (1993). Contextual probability evaluation in autistic, receptive developmental language disorder and control children: Event-related brain potential evidence. *Journal of Autism and Developmental Disorders, 23*, 37–58.

Linden, D. E., Prvulovic, D., Formisano, E., Vollinger, M., Zanella, F. E., Goebel, R., & Dierks, T. (1999). The functional neuroanatomy of target detection: an fMRI study of visual and auditory oddball tasks. *Cerebral Cortex, 9*, 815–823.

Linden, R. D., Campbell, K., Hamel, G., & Picton, T. (1985). Human auditory steady-state evoked potentials during sleep. *Ear and Hearing, 6*, 167–174.

Linden, R. D., Picton, T. W., Hamel, G., & Campbell, K. B. (1987). Human auditory steady-state potentials during selective attention. *Electroencephalography and Clinical Neurophysiology, 66*, 145–159.

Ling, D., Ling, A. H., & Doehring, D. G. (1970). Stimulus, response and observed variables in the auditory screening of newborn infants. *Journal of Speech and Hearing Research, 13*, 9–18.

Linker, S., Ruckenstein, M., Acker, J., & Gardner, G. (1997). An accurate, cost-effective approach for diagnosing retrocochlear lesions utilizing the T2-weighted, fast-spin echo magnetic resonance imaging scan. *Laryngoscope, 107*, 1525–1529.

Lins, O., Picton, P., Picton, T., Champagne, S., & Durieux-Smith, A. (1995). Auditory steady-state responses to tones amplitude-modulated at 80–110 Hz. *Journal of the Acoustical Society of America, 97*, 3051–3063.

Lins, O., & Picton, T. (1995). Auditory steady-state responses to multiple simultaneous stimuli. *Electroencephalography and Clinical Neurophysiology, 96*, 420–432.

Lins, O., Picton, T., Boucher, B., Durieux-Smith, A., Champagne, S., Moran, L., et al. (1996). Frequency-specific audiometry using steady-state responses. *Ear and Hearing, 17*, 81–96.

Linsay, K. W., Carlin, J., Kennedy, I., Fry, J., McInnes, A., & Teasdale, G. M. (1981). Evoked potentials in severe head injury: Analysis and relation to outcome. *Journal of Neurology, Neurosurgery, and Psychiatry, 44*, 796–802.

Lippe, W., & Rubel, E. W. (1983). Development of place principle: Tonotopic organization. *Science, 219*, 514–516.

Lisowska, G., Namylowski, G., Morawski, K., & Strojek, K. (2001). Early identification of hearing impairments in patients with type-I diabetes mellitus. *Otology and Neurotology, 22*, 316–320.

Litscher, G. (1995). Continuous auditory evoked potential monitoring during nocturnal sleep. *International Journal of Neuroscience, 82*, 135–142.

Litscher, G., Schwartz, G., & Reimann, R. (1996). Abnormal brainstem auditory evoked potentials in a girl with the central alveolar hypoventilation syndrome. *International Journal of Neuroscience, 87*, 113–117.

Little, J. R., Lesser, R. P., Lueders, H., & Furlan, A. J. (1983). Brain stem auditory evoked potentials in posterior circulation surgery. *Neurosurgery, 12*, 496–502.

Littman, T., Kraus, N., McGee, T., & Nicol, T. (1992). Binaural stimulation reveals functional differences between midline and temporal components of the middle latency response in guinea pigs. *Electroencephalography and Clinical Neurophysiology, 84*, 362–372.

Litvan, H., Jensen, E. W., Revuelta, M., Henneberg, S. W., Paniagua, P., Campos, J. M., Martinez, P., Caminal, P., & Villar Landeira, J. M. (2002). Comparison of auditory evoked potentials and the A-line ARX Index for monitoring the hypnotic level during sevoflurane and propofol induction. *Acta Anaesthesiologica Scandinavia, 46*, 245–251.

Liu, C., Lin, S., & Chang, Y. (2001). Cochlear vertebral entrapment syndrome: A case report. *European Journal of Radiology, 40*, 147–150.

Lloyd, L., & Reid, M. (1967). The incidence of hearing impairment in an institutionalized mentally retarded population. *American Journal of Mental Deficiency, 71*, 746–763.

Lockwood, A., Berlin, C., Hood, L., Burkard, R., & Salvi, R. (1999). PET studies of auditory pathways in patients with auditory neuropathy. *Annals of Neurology, 46*, 460.

Loewy, D. H., Campbell, K. B., & Bastien, C. (1996). The mismatch negativity to frequency deviant stimuli during natural sleep. *Electroencephalography and Clinical Neurophysiology, 98*, 493–501.

Loftus, B., & Wazen, J. J. (1990). A false-positive gadolinium-enhanced MRI: Acoustic neuroma versus cochleovestibular neuritis. *Otolaryngology—Head & Neck Surgery, 103*, 299.

Loiselle, D. L., Stamm, J. S., Matininsky, S., & Whipple, S. C. (1980). Evoked potential and behavioral signs of attentional dysfunction in hyperactive boys. *Psychophysiology, 17*, 193–201.

Long, J. K., & Allen, N. (1984). Abnormal brainstem auditory evoked potentials following Ondine's curse. *Archives of Neurology, 41*, 1104–1110.

Lonsdale, D., Nodar, R. H., & Orlowski, J. P. (1979). The effects of thiamine on abnormal brainstem auditory evoked potentials. *Cleveland Clinic Quarterly, 46*, 83–88.

Lopez, L., Jurgens, R., Diekmann, V., Becker, W., Ried, S., Grozinger, B., & Erne, S. N. (2003). Musicians versus nonmusicians—A neurophysiological approach. *Neurosciences and Music, 999*, 124–130.

Lopez-Diaz-de-Leon, E., Silva-Rojas, A., Ysunza, A., Amavisca, R., & Rivera, R. (2003). Auditory neuropathy in Friedreich ataxia: A report of two cases. *International Journal of Pediatric Otorhinolaryngology, 67*, 641–648.

Lopez-Escamez, J., Salguero, G., & Salinero, J. (1999). Age and sex differences in latencies of waves I, III and V in auditory brainstem response of normal hearing subjects. *Acta Otolaryngologica, 53*, 09–115.

Lopponen, H., Sorri, M., Serlo, W., & von Wendt, L. (1989). Audiological findings of shunt-treated hydrocephalus in children. *International Journal of Pediatric Otorhinolaryngology, 18*, 21–30.

Lorente de No, R. (1947). *A study of nerve physiology.* New York: Rockefeller University Press.

Lorenz, J., Brooke, S., Petersen, R., Torok, Z., & Wenzel, J. (1995). Brainstem auditory evoked potentials during a helium-oxygen saturation dive to 450 meters of seawater. *Undersea Hyperbaric Medicine, 22*, 229–240.

Louza, M. R., Maurer, K., & Neuhauser, B. (1992). Functional relationship between brain regions in schizophrenia evaluated with Pearson's correlation between event-related potentials. *Electromyography and Clinical Neurophysiology, 32*, 611–614.

Lowenstein, O., & Roberts, T. (1951). The localization and analysis of the responses to vibration from the isolated elasmobranch labyrinth: A contribution to the problem of the evolution of hearing in vertebrates. *Journal of Physiology, 114*, 471–489.

Lucertini, M., Ciniglio-Appiani, G., Antonini, R., & Urbani, L. (1993). Effects of hypobaric hypoxia on the middle-latency and steady-state auditory evoked potentials. *Audiology, 32,* 356–362.

Lumenta, C. B. (1984). Measurements of brain-stem auditory evoked potentials in patients with spontaneous intracerebral hemorrhage. *Journal of Neurosurgery, 60,* 548–552.

Lumenta, C. B., Kramer, M., & Bock, W. J. (1986). Monitoring of brain stem function by brain stem auditory evoked potentials (BAEP). In M. Samii (Ed.), *Surgery in and around the brain stem and the third ventricle: Anatomy, pathology neurophysiology, diagnosis and treatment* (pp. 168–180). New York: Springer-Verlag.

Luts, H., Desloovere, C., Kumar, A., Vandermeersch, E., & Wouters, J. (2004). Objective assessment of frequency-specific hearing thresholds in babies. *International Journal of Pediatric Otorhinolaryngology, 68,* 915–926.

Luts, H., & Wouters, J. (2005). Comparison of MASTER and AUDERA for measurement of auditory steady-state responses. *International Journal of Audiology, 44,* 244–253.

Lutschg, J., Meyer, E., Jeanneret-Iseli, C., & Kaiser, G. (1985). Brainstem auditory evoked potentials in meningomyelocele. *Neuropediatrics, 16,* 202–204.

Lutschg, J., Pfenninger, J., Ludin, H. P., & Fassela, F. (1983). Brain-stem auditory evoked potentials in neurointensively treated comatose children. *American Journal of Disease in Children, 137,* 421–426.

Lutzenberger, W., Elbert, T., Rockstroh, B., & Birbaumer, N. (1979). The effects of self-regulation of slow cortical potentials on performance in a signal detection task. *International Journal of Neuroscience, 9,* 175–183.

Lynn, G. E., Cullis, P. A., & Gilroy, J. (1983). Olivopontocerebellar degeneration: Effects on auditory brainstem responses. *Seminars in Hearing, 4,* 375–383.

Lynn, G. E., & Gilroy, J. (1984). Auditory evoked potentials in vertebrobasilar arterial occlusive disease. In R. Berguer & R. B. Bauer (Eds.), *Vertebrobasilar arterial occlusive disease* (pp. 85–94). New York: Raven Press.

Mabin, D., LeGuyader, J., & Le Mevel, J. C. (1985). Brainstem auditory evoked responses in chronic alcoholism. *Clinical Neurophysiology, 14,* 323–328.

Machado, C., Valdes, P., Garcia-Tigera, J., Virues, T., Biscay, R., Miranda, J., Coutin, P., Roman, J., & Garcia, O. (1991). Brain-stem auditory evoked potentials and brain death. *Electroencephalography and Clinical Neurophysiology, 80,* 392–389.

Mackersie, C., Down, K. E., & Stapells, D. R. (1993). Pure-tone masking profiles for human auditory brainstem and middle latency responses. *Hearing Research, 65,* 61–68.

Madden, C., Hilbert, L., Rutter, M., Greinwald, J., & Choo, D. (2002). Pediatric cochlear implantation in auditory neuropathy. *Otology and Neuro-Otology, 23,* 163–168.

Maddox, H. E., III. (1982). The lateral approach to acoustic tumors. *Annals of Otology, Rhinology & Laryngology, 91,* 240–245.

Madhavan, G. (1992). Minimal repetition evoked potentials by modified adaptive line enhancement. *IEEE Transactions in Biomedical Engineering, 39,* 760–764.

Madhavan, G., de Bruin, H., Upton, A., & Jernigan, M. (1986). Classification of brain-stem auditory evoked potentials by syntactic methods. *Electroencephalography and Clinical Neurophysiology, 65,* 289–296.

Maeshima, S., Itakura, T., Komai, N., Matsumoto, T., & Ueyoshi, A. (2002). Relationships between event-related potentials (P300) and activities of daily living in Parkinson's disease. *Brain Injury, 16,* 1–8.

Magdziarz, D., Wiet, R., Dinces, E., & Adamiec, L. (2000). Normal audiologic presentations in patients with acoustic neuroma: An evaluation using strict audiologic parameters. *Archives of Otolaryngology Head and Neck Surgery, 122,* 157–162.

Magliulo, G., Cianfrone, G., Gagliardi, M., Cuiuli, G., & D'Amico, R. (2004). Vestibular evoked myogenic potentials and distortion-product otoacoustic emissions combined with glycerol testing in endolymphatic hydrops: Their value in early diagnosis. *Annals of Otology Rhinology and Laryngology, 113,* 1000–1005.

Magliulo, G., Gagliardi, M., Appiani, G., & D'Amico, R. (2003). Preservation of the saccular nerve and of the vestibular evoked myogenic potential during vestibular schwannoma surgery. *Otology and Neurotology, 24,* 308–311.

Mair, I. W. S., & Laukli, E. (1985). Frequency specificity of the auditory brainstem responses in the cat. *Acta Otolaryngologica (Stockholm), 99,* 377–383.

Mair, I. W. S., Laukli, E., & Pedersen, E. K. (1980). Auditory brain-stem electric responses evoked with suprathreshold tone-bursts. *Scandinavian Audiology, 9,* 153–160.

Maiste, A. C., Wiens, A. S., Hunt, M. J., Scherg, M., & Picton, T. W. (1995). Event-related potentials and the categorical perception of speech sounds. *Ear and Hearing, 16,* 68–90.

Majkowski, J., Bochenek, Z., Bochenek, W., Knapil-Fajalowska, D., & Kopec, J. (1971). Latency of averaged evoked potentials to contralateral and ipsilateral stimuli. *Brain Research, 25,* 416–419.

Makashima, K., & Tanaka, K. (1971). Pathological changes of inner ear and central auditory pathways in diabetes. *Annals of Otology Rhinology and Laryngology, 80,* 218–228.

Mäkelä, A. M., Alku, P., May, P. J. Makinen, V., & Tiitinen, H. (2004). The auditory n100m response reflects changes in speech fundamental frequency. *Neurology and Clinical Neurophysiology, 30,* 49.

Mäkelä, A. M., Makinen, V., Nikkila, M., Ilmoniemi, R. J., & Tiitinen, H. (2001). Magnetoencephalographic (MEG) localization of the auditory N400m: Effects of stimulus duration. *Neuroreport, 12,* 49–53.

Mäkelä, J. P., Hämäläinen, M., Hari, R., & McEvoy, L. (1994). Whole head mapping of middle-latency auditory evoked magnetic fields. *Electroencephalography and Clinical Neurophysiology, 92,* 414–421.

Mäkelä, J. P., & Hari, R. (1987). Evidence for cortical origin of the 40 Hz auditory evoked response in man. *Electroencephalography and Clinical Neurophysiology, 66,* 539–546.

Makhdoum, M. J., Groenen, P., Snik, A., & van den Broek, P. (1998). Intra- and interindividual correlations between auditory evoked potentials and speech perception in cochlear implant users. *Scandinavian Audiology, 27,* 13–20.

Makhdoum, M. J., Snik, A. F., & van den Broek, P. (1997). Cochlear implantation: A review of the literature and the Nijmegen results. *Journal of Laryngology & Otology, 111,* 1008–1017.

Malinoff, R., & Spivak, L. (1990). Effects of stimulus parameters on auditory brainstem response spectral analysis. *Audiology, 29,* 21–28.

Mancuso, G., Tosti, A., Fanti, P., Berndondini, R., Mongiorgi, R., & Morandi, A. (1990). Cutaneous necrosis and calcinosis following electroencephalography. *Dermatologica, 181,* 324–326.

Mangham, C. (1991). Hearing threshold difference between ears at risk of acoustic tumor. *Archives of Otolaryngology—Head and Neck Surgery, 105,* 814–817.

Manley, J. A., & Johnstone, B. M. (1974). A comparison of cochlear summating potentials in the bat and guinea pig, including temperature effects. *Journal of Comparative Physiology, 88,* 43–66.

Manninen, P., Lam, A. M., & Nicholas, J. F. (1985). The effects of isoflurane-nitrous oxide anaesthesia on brainstem auditory evoked potentials in humans. *Anaesthesia and Analgesia, 64,* 43–47.

Mantzaridis, H., & Kenny, G. N. (1997). Auditory evoked potential index: A quantitative measure of changes in auditory evoked potentials during general anaesthesia. *Anaesthesia, 52,* 1030–1036.

Marangos, N. (1992). Diagnostic value of transtympanic electrocochleography: Case reports. *Otolaryngol. Pol,. 46,* 402–405.

Marangos, N., Maier, W., Merz, R., & Laszig, R. (2001). Brainstem response to cerebellopontine angle tumors. *Otology and Neurotology, 22,* 95–99.

Marangos, N., Schipper, J., & Richter, B. (1999). [Objective auditory brainstem response threshold deficits in patients with cerebellopontine angle tumors.]. *HNO, 47,* 804–808.

Margolis, R. H., Levine, S. C., Fournier, E. M., Hunter, L. L., Smith, S. L., & Lilly, D. J. (1992). Tympanic electrocochleography: normal and abnormal patterns of response. *Audiology, 31,* 8–24.

Margolis, R. H., Rieks, D., Fournier, E. M., & Levine, S. E. (1995). Tympanic electrocochleography for diagnosis of Ménière's disease. *Archives of Otolaryngology—Head & Neck Surgery, 121,* 44–55.

Markand, O. N., Garg, B. P. & Brandt, J. K. (1982). Non-ketotic hyperglycinemia: Electroencephalographic and evoked potential abnormalities. *Neurology, 32,* 151–156.

Markand, O. N., DeMyer, W. E., Worth, R. M., & Warren, C. (1982). Multimodality evoked responses in leukodystrophies. In J. Courjon, R. Mauguiere, & M. Revol (Eds.), *Clinical applications of evoked potentials in neurology* (pp. 409–416). New York: Raven Press.

Marsh, J. T., Brown, W. S., & Smith, J. C. (1974). Differential brainstem pathways for the conduction of auditory frequency-following responses. *Electroencephalography and Clinical Neurophysiology, 36,* 415–242.

Marsh, R. R. (1988). Digital filtering of auditory evoked potentials. *Ear and Hearing, 9,* 101–107.

Marsh, R. R., Frewen, T. C., Sutton, L. N., & Potsic, W. P. (1984). Resistance of the auditory brain stem response to high barbiturate levels. *Archives of Otolaryngology—Head & Neck Surgery, 92,* 685–688.

Marshall, L. F., Smith, R. W., & Shapiro, H. M. (1979). The outcome with aggressive treatment in severe head injuries: I. The significance of intracranial pressure monitoring. *Journal of Neurosurgery, 50,* 20–25.

Marshall, N. K., & Donchin, E. (1981). Circadian variations in the latency of brainstem responses and its relation to body temperature. *Science, 212,* 356–358.

Martin, B. A., & Boothroyd, A. (1999). Cortical, auditory, event-related potentials in response to periodic and aperiodic stimuli with the same spectral envelope. *Ear and Hearing, 20,* 33–44.

Martin, B. A., Kurtzberg, D., & Stapells, D. R. (1999). The effects of decreased audibility produced by high-pass noise masking on N1 and the mismatch negativity to speech sounds /ba/and /da. *Journal of Speech, Language and Hearing Research, 42,* 271–286.

Martin, B. A., Shafer, V. L., Morr, M. L., Kreuzer, J. A., & Kurtzberg, D. (2003). Maturation of mismatch negativity: A scalp current density analysis. *Ear and Hearing, 24,* 463–471.

Martin, B. A., & Stapells, D. R. (2005). Effects of low-pass noise masking on auditory event-related potentials to speech. *Ear and Hearing, 26,* 195–213.

Martin, D., & Cranford, J. L. (1991). Age-related changes in binaural processing. I. Evoked potential findings. *American Journal of Otology, 12,* 357–364.

Martin, L. J., Barajas, J. J., & Fernandez, R. (1989). Auditory P3 development in childhood. *Scandinavian Audiology (Suppl), 30,* 105–109.

Martin, L., Barajas, J. J., Fernandez, R., & Torres, E. (1988). Auditory event-related potentials in well-characterized groups of children. *Electroencephalography and Clinical Neurophysiology, 71,* 375–381.

Martin, M. E., & Moore, E. J. (1977). Scalp distribution of early (0 to 10 msec) auditory evoked responses. *Archives of Otolaryngology, 103,* 326–328.

Martini, A., Comacchia, F., Fedele, D., Crepaldi, G., & Sala, O. (1987). Auditory brainstem evoked response in the clinical evaluation and follow-up of insulin dependent diabetic subjects. *Acta Otolaryngologica, 103,* 620–627.

Martini, A., Comacchio, F., & Magnavita, V. (1991). Auditory brainstem and middle latency evoked responses in the clinical evaluation of diabetes. *Diabetic Medicine, 8.* Spec No:S74–7.

Marvel, J. B., Jerger, J. F., & Lew, H. L. (1992). Asymmetries in topographic brain maps of auditory evoked potentials in the elderly. *Journal of the American Academy of Audiology, 3,* 361–368.

Maslan, M. J., Latack, J. T., Kemink, J. L., & Graham, M. D. (1986). Magnetic resonance imaging of temporal bone and cerebellopontine angle lesions. *Archives of Otolarngology—Head & Neck Surgery, 112,* 410–415.

Mason, J. A., DeMichele, A., Stevens, C., Ruth, R., Hashisaki, G., et al. (2003). Cochlear implantation in patients with auditory neuropathy of various etiologies. *Laryngoscope, 113,* 45–49.

Mason, J. A., & Hermann, K. R. (1998). Universal newborn hearing screening by automated auditory brainstem response measurement. *Pediatrics, 101,* 221–227.

Mason, J. A., Mason, S., & Gibbin, K. (1995). Raised ABR threshold after suction aspiration of glue from the middle ear: Three case studies. *Journal of Laryngology and Otology, 109,* 726–728.

Mason, S. (1988). On-line computer scoring of the auditory brainstem response for estimation of hearing threshold. *Audiology, 23,* 277–296.

Mason, S. (2003). The electrically evoked auditory brainstem response. In H. Cullington (Ed.), *Cochlear implants: Objective measures.* (pp. 130–159). London: Whurr.

Mason, S. (2004). Electrophysiologic and objective monitoring of the cochlear implant during surgery: implementation, audit and outcomes. *International Journal of Audiology, 43,* S33-S38.

Mason, S., Cope, Y., Garnham, J., O'Donoghue, G. M., & Gibbin, K. P. (2001). Intra-operative recordings of electrically evoked auditory nerve action potentials in young children by use of neural response telemetry with the nucleus C124M cochlear implant. *Brititsh Journal of Audiology, 35,* 225–235.

Mason, S., Davis, A., Wood, S., & Farnsworth A. (1998). Field sensitivity of targeted neonatal hearing screening using the Nottingham ABR Screener. *Ear and Hearing, 19,* 91–102.

Mason, S., Dodd, M., Gibbin, K., & O'Donaghue, G. (2000). Assessment of the functioning of peripheral auditory pathways after cochlear re-implantation in young children using intra-operative objective measures. *British Journal of Audiology, 34,* 179–186.

Mason, S., Garnham, C., Sheppard, S., O'Donaghue, G., & Gibbin, K. (1995). An intraoperative test protocol for objective assessment of the Nucleus 22-Channel cochlear implant. *Advances in Otorhinolaryngology, 50,* 38–44.

Mason, S., Gibbin, K., Garnham, C., & O'Donaghue, G. (1996). Intraoperative electrophysiological and objective tests after cochlear re-implantation in a young child. *British Journal of Audiology, 30,* 67–70.

Mason, S., & Mellor, D. H. (1984). Brain-stem, middle latency and late cortical evoked potentials in children with speech and language disorders. *Electroencephalography and Clinical Neurophysiology, 59,* 297–309.

Mason, S., O'Donaghue, G., Gibbin, K., Garnham, C., & Jowett, C. (1997). Perioperative electrical auditory brain stem response in candidates for pediatric cochlear implantation. *American Journal of Otology, 18,* 466–471.

Mast, T. E. (1965). Short latency human evoked reponses to clicks. *Journal of Applied Physiology, 20,* 725–730.

Mathalon, D. H., Ford, J. M., Rosenbloom, M., & Pfefferbaum, A. (2000). P300 reduction and prolongation with illness duration in schizophrenia. *Biological Psychiatry, 47,* 413–427.

Matheson, J. K., Harrington, H., & Hallet, M. (1983). Abnormalities of somatosensory, visual, and brainstem evoked potentials in amyotrophic lateral sclerosis. *Muscle Nerve, 6,* 529.

Mathiak, K., Rapp, A., Kircher, T. T., Grodd, W., Hertrich, I., Weiskopf, N., Lutzenberger, W., & Ackermann, H. (2002). Mismatch responses to randomized gradient switching noise as reflected by fMRI and whole-head magnetoencephalography. *Human Brain Mapping, 16,* 190–195.

Matsuura, K., Tono, T., Hara, Y., Ueki, Y., Ushisako, Y., & Morimitsu, T. (1996). [Tympanic electrocochleography with disposable electrode]. *Nippon Jibiinkoka Gakkai Kaiho, 99,* 1016–1025.

Matsuyama, Z., Katayama, S., & Nakamura, S. (1993). [A case of sodium bromate intoxication with cerebral lesion.]. *Rinsho Shinkeigaku, 33,* 535–540.

Matsuzaki, M., & Murofushi, T. (2001). Vestibular evoked myogenic potentials in patients with idiopathic bilateral vestibulopathy: Report of three cases. *ORL: Journal of Otorhinolaryngology and its Related Specialties, 63,* 349–352.

Matsuzawa, T., Hashimoto, M., Nara, H., Yoshida, M., Tamura, S., & Igarashi, T. (1997). Current status of conducting function tests in repeated dose toxicity studies in Japan. *Journal of Toxicological Science, 22,* 375–382.

Matthews, W. B., Read, D. J., & Poutney, E. (1979). Effect of raising body temperature on visual and somatosensory evoked potentials in patients with multiple sclerosis. *Journal of Neurology, Neurosurgery, and Psychiatry, 42,* 250–255.

Matthews, W. B., & Small, D. G. (1979). Serial recording of visual and somatosensory evoked potentials in multiple sclerosis. *Journal of Neurological Sciences, 40,* 11–21.

Matthews, W. B., Wattam-Bell, J. R. B., & Poutney, E. (1982). Evoked potentials in the diagnosis of multiple sclerosis: A follow up study. *Journal of Neurology, Neurosurgery, and Psychiatry, 45,* 202–307.

Matthies, C., & Samii, M. (1997). Direct brainstem recording of auditory evoked potentials during vestibular schwannoma resection: Nuclear BAEP recording. *Journal of Neurosurgery, 86,* 1057–1062.

Mauldin, L., & Jerger, J. (1979). Auditory brainstem evoked responses to bone-conducted signals. *Archives of Otolaryngology, 105,* 656–661.

Maurer, J., Collet, L., Pelster, H., Truy, E., & Gallego, S. (2002). Auditory late cortical response and speech recognition in Digisonic cochlear implant users. *Laryngoscope, 112,* 2220–2224.

Maurer, K., Schafer, E., & Leitner, H. (1980). The effects of varying stimulus polarity (rarefaction vs. condensation) on early auditory evoked potentials (EAEPs). *Electroencephalography and Clinical Neurophysiology, 50,* 332–334.

Maurer, K., Strumpel, D., & Wende, S., (1982). Acoustic tumor detection with early auditory evoked potentials and neuroradiological methods. *Journal of Neurology, 227,* 117–185.

Maurer, U., Bucher, K., Brem, S., & Brandeis, D. (2003a). Altered responses to tone and phoneme mismatch in kindergartners at familial dyslexia risk. *Neuroreport, 14,* 2245–2250.

Maurer, U., Bucher, K., Brem, S., & Brandeis, D. (2003b). Development of the automatic mismatch response: from frontal positivity in kindergarten children to the mismatch negativity. *Clinical Neurophysiology, 114,* 808–817.

Maurizi, M., Altissimi, G., Ottaviani, F., Paludetti, G., & Bambini, M. (1982). Auditory brainstem responses (ABR) in the aged. *Scandinavian Audiology, 11,* 213–221.

Maurizi, M., Ottaviani, F., Alamdori, G., Falchi, M., & Paludetti, G. (1987). Auditory brainstem and middle-latency responses in Bell's palsy. *Audiology, 26,* 111–116.

Maurizi, M., Ottaviani, F., Paludetti, G., et al. (1985). Contribution to the differentiation of peripheral versus central tinnitus via auditory brainstem response evaluation. *Audiology, 24,* 207–216.

Maurizi, M., Ottaviani, F., Paludetti, G., & Lungarotti, S. (1985). Audiological findings in Down's children. *International Journal of Pediatric Otorhinolaryngology, 9,* 227–232.

Maurizi, M., Ottaviani, F., Paludetti, G., Alamodir, G., & Tassoni, A. (1985). Contribution to the differentiation of peripheral versus central tinnitus via auditory brain stem response evaluation. *Audiology, 24,* 207–216.

Maurizi, M., Paludetti, G., Ottaviani, F., & Rosignoli, M. (1984). Auditory brainstem responses to middle- and low-frequency tone pips. *Audiology, 23,* 75–84.

Maurizi, M., Paludetti, G., Ottaviani, F., & Rosignoli, M. (1986). Effects of high-pass filtering on the waveform and threshold of auditory brainstem responses to tone pips. *Audiology, 25,* 124–128.

May, M., Blumenthal, F., & Klein, S. (1983). Acute Bell's palsy: Prognostic value of evoked electromyography, maximal stimulation, and other electrical tests. *American Journal of Otology, 4,* 350–361.

May, P., Tiitinen, H., Ilmoniemi, R. J., Nyman, G., Taylor, J. G., & Näätänen, R. (1999). Frequency change detection in human auditory cortex. *Journal of Computers and Neuroscience, 6,* 99–120.

Maybeck, P. S. (1979). *Stochastic models, estimation and control.* New York: Academic Press.

Mazzini, L., Zaccala, M., Gareri, F., Giordano, A., & Angelino, E. (2001). Long-latency auditory-evoked potentials in severe traumatic brain injury. *Archives of Physical and Medical Rehabilitation, 82,* 57–65.

McAlpine, D., Lumsden, C. E., & Acheson, E. D. (1972). *Multiple sclerosis: A reappraisal.* Edinburgh: Churchill Livingstone.

McArthur, G. M., Bishop, D. V. M., & Proudfoot, M. (2003). Do video sounds interfere with auditory event-related potentials? *Behavior Research Methods—Instruments and Computers, 35,* 329–333.

McCall, S., Chertoff, M., & Ferraro, J. (1998). Effects of in-situ calibration of click-stimuli on the auditory brainstem response. *Journal of the American Academy of Audiology, 9,* 127–133.

McCallum, W. C., & Curry, S. H. (1981). The form and distribution of auditory evoked potentials and CNVs when stimuli and responses are lateralized. *Progressive Brain Research, 54,* 767–775.

McCallum, W. C., Farmer, S. F., & Pocock, P. V. (1984). The effects of physical and semantic incongruities on auditory event-related potentials. *Electroencephalography and Clinical Neurophysiology, 59,* 477–488.

McCandless, G. A., & Best, L. (1964). Evoked responses to auditory stimuli in man using a summing computer. *Journal of Speech and Hearing Research, 7,* 193–202.

McCandless, G. A., & Rose, D. E. (1970). Evoked cortical responses to stimulus change. *Journal of Speech and Hearing Research, 13,* 624–634.

McCarley, R. W., Wible, C. G., Frumin, M., Hirayasu, Y., Levitt, J. J., Fischer, I. A., & Shenton, M. E. (1999). MRI anatomy of schizophrenia. *Biological Psychiatry, 45,* 1099–1119.

McCarthy, G. (1992). *Intracranial recordings in humans.* In Twelfth Annual Carmel Conference, Carmel, CA.

McCarthy, G., Luby, M., Gore, J., & Goldman-Rakic, P. (1997). Infrequent events transiently activate human prefrontal and parietal cortex as measured by functional MRI. *Journal of Neurophysiology, 77,* 1630–1634.

McClelland, R. J., & McCrae, R. S. (1979). Intersubject variability of the auditory-evoked brain-stem potentials. *Audiology, 18,* 462–471.

McClelland, R. J., Eyre, D. G., Watson, D., Calvert, G. J., & Sherrard, E. (1992). Central conduction time in childhood autism. *British Journal of Psychiatry, 160,* 659–663.

McCue, M., & Guinan, J. J. (1994). Acoustically responsive fibers in the vestibular nerve of the cat. *Journal of Neuroscience, 14,* 6058–6070.

McCue, M. P., & Guinan, J. J., Jr. (1995). Spontaneous activity and frequency selectivity of acoustically responsive vestibular afferents in the cat. *Journal of Neurophysiology, 74,* 1563–1572.

McDonald, J. M., & Shimizu, H. (1981). Frequency specificity of the auditory brain stem response. *American Journal of Otolaryngology, 2,* 36–42.

McDonald, W. I., & Sears, T. A. (1970). The effects of experimental demyelination of conduction in the central nervous system. *Brain, 93,* 583–598.

McDonald, W. L., & Halliday, A. M. (1977). Diagnosis and classification of multiple sclerosis. *British Medical Bulletin, 33,* 4–8.

McDonnell, D. E., Jabbari, B., Spinella, G., Mueller, H. G., & Klara, P. M. (1990). Delayed hearing loss after neurovascular decompression. *Neurosurgery, 27,* 997–1003.

McFadden, D. (2002). Masculinization effects in the auditory system. *Archives of Sexual Behavior, 31,* 93–105.

McFarland, W. H., Vivion, M. C., & Goldstein, R. (1977). Middle components of the AER to tone-pips in normal-hearing and hearing-impaired subjects. *Journal of Speech & Hearing Research, 20,* 781–798.

McFarland, W. H., Vivion, M. C., Wolf, K. E., & Goldstein, R. (1975). Reexamination of effects of stimulus rate and number on the middle components of the averaged electroencephalic response. *Audiology, 14,* 456–465.

McFarlane, A. C., Weber, D. L., & Clark, C. R. (1993). Abnormal stimulus processing in posttraumatic stress disorder. *Biological Psychiatry, 34,* 311–320.

McGee, T. J., & Clemis, J. D. (1982). Effects of conductive hearing loss on auditory brainstem response. *Annals of Otology, Rhinology, and Laryngology, 91,* 304–309.

McGee, T., & Kraus, N. (1996). Auditory development reflected by middle latency response. *Ear and Hearing, 17,* 419–429.

McGee, T., Kraus, N., Comperatore, C., & Nicol, T. (1991). Subcortical and cortical components of the MLR generating system. *Brain Research, 544,* 211–220.

McGee, T., Kraus, N., Killion, M., Rosenberg, R., & King, C. (1993). Improving the reliability of the auditory middle latency response by monitoring EEG delta activity. *Ear and Hearing, 14,* 76–84.

McGee, T., Kraus, N., & Manfredi, C. (1988). Toward a strategy for analyzing the auditory middle-latency response waveform. *Audiology, 27,* 119–130.

McGee, T., Kraus, N., & Nicol, T. (1997). Is it really a mismatch negativity? An assessment of methods for determining response validity in individual subjects. *Electroencephalography and Clinical Neurophysiology, 104,* 359–368.

McGee, T., Wolters, C., Stein, L., Kraus, N., Johnson, D., Boyer, K., et al. (1992). Absence of sensorineural hearing loss in treated infants and children with congenital toxoplasmosis. *Archives of Otolaryngology—Head & Neck Surgery, 106,* 75–80.

McIsaac, H., & Polich, J. (1992). Comparison of infant and adult P300 from auditory stimuli. *Journal of Experimental Child Psychology, 53,* 115–128.

McLeod, B., & Boheimer, N. (1985). Propofol ('Dipaivan') infusion as main agent for day case surgery. *Postgraduate Medical Journal, 61,* 105–107.

McPherson, D. L., Amlie, R., & Foltz, E. (1985). Auditory brainstem responses in infant hydrocephalus. *Child's Nervous System, 1,* 70–76.

McPherson, D. L., Hirasugi, R., & Starr, A. (1985). Auditory brain stem potentials recorded at different scalp locations in neonates and adults. *Annals of Otology, Rhinology, and Laryngology, 94,* 236–243.

McPherson, D. L., & Salamat, M. R. (2004). Interactions among variables in the P300 response to a continuous performance task in normal and ADHD adults. *Journal of the American Academy of Audiology, 15,* 666–677.

McPherson, D. L., & Starr, A. (1993). Binaural interaction in auditory evoked potentials: Brainstem, middle- and long-latency components. *Hearing Research, 66,* 91–98.

McPherson, D., & Starr, A. (1995). Auditory time-intensity cues in the binaural interaction component of the auditory evoked potentials. *Hearing Research, 89,* 162–171.

McRandle, C. C., & Goldstein, R. (1973). Effects of alcohol on the averaged electroencephalic response to clicks. *Journal of Speech and Hearing Research, 16,* 353–359.

McRandle, C. C., Smith, M. A., & Goldstein, R. (1974). Early average electroencephalic responses to clicks in neonates. *Annals of Otology, Rhinology and Laryngology, 83,* 695–702.

McSherry, J. W., Walter, C. I., & Horber, J. D. (1982). Acute visual evoked potential changes in hydrocephalus. *Electroencephalography and Clinical Neurophysiology, 53,* 331–333.

Meador, K., Loring, D., King, D., Gallagher, B., Rogers, O., Smith, J., & Flanigin, H. (1988). Spectral power of human limbic evoked potentials: Relationship to seizure onset. *Annals of Neurology, 23,* 145–151.

Meador, K., Loring, D., King, D., & Nichols, F. (1988). The P3 evoked potential transient global amnesia. *Archives of Neurology, 45,* 465–467.

Megala, A. L., & Teyler, T. J. (1979). Habituation and the human evoked potential. *Journal of Comparative Physiology & Psychology, 93,* 175–183.

Meier, S., Narabayashi, O., Probst, R., & Schmuziger, N. (2004). Comparison of currently available devices designed for newborn hearing screening using automated auditory brainstem and/or otoacoustic emission measurements. *International Journal of Pediatric Otorhinolaryngology, 68,* 927–934.

Meister, M., Johnson, A., Popelka, G. R., Kim, G. S., & Whyte, M. P. (1986). Audiologic findings in young patients with hypophosphatemic bone disease. *Annals of Otology, Rhinology, and Laryngology, 95,* 415–420.

Menard, M., Gallego, S., Berger-Vachon, C., Durrant, J., & Collet, L. (2004). Auditory steady-state response evaluation of auditory thresholds in cochlear implant patients. *International Journal of Audiology, 43,* S39–S43.

Mendel, M. I., Adkinson, C. D., & Harker, L. A. (1977). Middle components of the auditory evoked potentials in infants. *Annals of Otology, Rhinology, and Laryngology, 86,* 293–299.

Mendel, M. I., & Goldstein, R. (1969). Stability of the early components of the averaged electroencephalic response. *Journal of Speech and Hearing Research, 12,* 351–361.

Mendel, M. I., & Goldstein, R. (1971). Early components of the averaged electroencephalic response to constant level clicks during all-night sleep. *Journal of Speech & Hearing Research, 14,* 829–840.

Mendel, M. I., & Hosick, E. C. (1975). Effects of secobarbital on the early components of the auditory evoked potentials. *Revue Laryngologie, Otologie, Rhinologie, 96,* 180–184.

Mendel, M. I., Hosick, E. C., Windman, T., Davis, H., Hirsh, S. K., & Dinges, D. F. (1975). Audiometric comparison of the middle and late components of the adult auditory evoked potentials awake and asleep. *Electroencephalography and Clinical Neurophysiology, 38,* 27–33.

Mendelson, T., & Salamy, A. (1981). Maturational effects on the middle components of the averaged encephalic response. *Journal of Speech and Hearing Research, 24,* 140–144.

Mendelson, T., Salamy, A., Lenoir, M., & McKean, C. M. (1979). Brainstem evoked potential findings in children with otitis media. *Archives of Otolaryngology, 105,* 17–20.

Mens, L., Boyle, P., & Mulder, J. (2003). The Clarion electrode positioner: Approximation to the medial wall and current focussing? *Audiology and Neurootology, 8,* 166–175.

Merchant, S., Velasquez-Villasenor, L., Tsuji, K., Glynn, R., Wall, C. I., & Rauch, S. (2000). Temporal bone studies of the human peripheral vestibular system. Normative vestibular hair cell data. *Annals of Otology, Rhinology,& Laryngology, 181,* 3–13.

Messick, J. M., Newberg, L. A., Nugent, M., & Fanst, R. J. (1985). Principles of neuroanesthesia for the neurosurgical patient with CNS pathophysiology. *Anesthesia and Analgesics, 64,* 143–174.

Messner, A., Price, M., Kwast, K., Gallagher, K., & Forte, J. (2001). Volunteer-based universal newborn hearing screening program. *International Journal of Pediatric Otorhinolaryngology, 60,* 123–130.

Metrick, S. A., & Brenner, R. P. (1982). Abnormal brainstem auditory evoked potentials in chronic paint sniffers. *Annals of Neurology, 12,* 553–556.

Metting Van Rijn, A. C., Kuiper, A. P., Dankers, T. E., & Grimbergen, C. A. (1996). Low-cost active electrode improves the resolution in biopoten-tial recordings, *Proceedings of the 18th Annual International Conference of the IEEE, 31,* 101–102.

Metzger, L. J., Carson, M. A., Paulus, L. A., Lasko, N. B., Paige, S. R., Pitman, R. K., & Orr, S. P. (2002). Event-related potentials to auditory stimuli in female Vietnam nurse veterans with posttraumatic stress disorder. *Psychophysiology, 39,* 49–63.

Meurer, J., Malloy, M., Kolb, M., Subichin, S., & Fleischfresser, S. (2000). Newborn hearing testing at Wisconsin hospitals: A review of the need for universal screening. *Wisconsin Medical Journal, 99,* 43–46.

Meyer, C., Witte, J., Hildmann, A., Hennecke, K. H., Schunck, K. U., Maul, K., Franke, U., Fahnenstich, H., Rabe, H., Rossi, R., Hartmann, S., & Gortner, L. (1999). Neonatal screening for hearing disorders in infants at risk: Incidence, risk factors, and follow-up. *Pediatrics, 104,* 900–904.

Meyerhoff, W. L., & Yellin, M. W. (1990). Summating potential/action potential ratio in perilymph fistula. *Archives of Otolaryngology—Head & Neck Surgery, 102,* 678–682.

Micco, A., Kraus, N., Koch, D., McGee, T., Carrell, T., et al. (1995). Speech-evoked cognitive P300 potentials in cochlear implant recipients. *American Journal of Otology, 16,* 514–520.

Michael, R., Klorman, R., Salzman, L., Borgstedt, A., & Dainer, K. (1981). Normalizing effects of methylphenidate on hyperactive children's vigilance performance and evoked potentials. *Psychophysiology, 18,* 665–677.

Michalewski, H. J., Thompson, L. W., Patterson, J. V., Bowman, T. E., & Litzelman, D. (1980). Sex differences in the amplitudes and latencies of the human auditory brainstem potential. *Electroencephalography and Clinical Neurophysiology, 48,* 351–356.

Michie, P. T. (2001). What has MMN revealed about the auditory system in schizophrenia? *International Journal of Psychophysiology, 42,* 177–194.

Michie, P. T., Budd, T. W., Todd, J., Rock, D., Wichmann, H., Box, J., & Jablensky, A. V. (2000). Duration and frequency mismatch negativity in schizophrenia. *Clinical Neurophysiology, 111,* 1054–1065.

Michie, P. T., Innes-Brown, H., Todd, J., & Jablensky, A. V. (2002). Duration mismatch negativity in biological relatives of patients with schizophrenia spectrum disorders. *Biological Psychiatry, 52,* 749–758.

Michie, P. T., Solowij, N., Crawford, J. M., & Glue, L. C. (1993). The effects of between-source discriminability on attended and unattended auditory ERPs. *Psychophysiology, 30,* 205–220.

Middleton, M., Wilson, K., & Keith, R. (1997). Central auditory evaluation of patients with spasmodic dysphonia. *Ear Nose and Throat Journal, 76,* 710–715.

Miezejeski, C., Heaney, G., Belser, R., Brown, W., Jenkins, E., & Sersen, E. (1997). Longer brainstem auditory evoked response latencies of individuals with Fragile X syndrome related to sedation. *American Journal of Medical Genetics, 74,* 167–171.

Mikulec, A., McKenna, M., Ramsey, M., Rosowski, J., Herrmann, B., Rauch, S., Curtin, H., & Merchant, S. (2004). Superior semicircular canal dehiscence presenting as conductive hearing loss without vertigo. *Otology and Neurotology, 25,* 121–129.

Milford, C. A., & Birchall, J. P. (1988/1989). Steady-state auditory evoked potentials to amplitude-modulated tones in hearing-impaired subjects. *British Journal of Audiology, 23,* 137–142.

Milhorat, T. H. (1984). Hydrocephalus: Historical notes, etiology, and clinical diagnosis. In American Association of Neurological Surgeons, Inc. (Ed.), *Pediatric neurosurgery: Surgery of the developing nervous system* (pp. 197–210). New York: Grune and Stratton.

Miller, A. L., Arenberg, J. G., Middlebrooks, J. C., & Pfingst, B. E. (2001). Cochlear implant thresholds: Comparison of middle latency responses with psychophysical and cortical-spike-activity thresholds. *Hearing Research, 152,* 55–66.

Minami, T., Kurokawa, T., Inoue, T., Takaki, S., & Goya, N. (1984). Primary brainstem hemorrhage in a child: Usefulness of auditory brainstem response (ABR). *Neuropediatrics, 15,* 99–101.

Minoda, R., Uno, K., Toriya, T., Eura, M., Noguchi, S., & Masuyama, K. (1999). Neurologic and otologic findings in Fisher's syndrome. *Auris Nasus Larynx, 26,* 153–158.

Minoli, I., & Moro, G. (1985). Constraints of intensive care units and follow-up studies in prematures. *Acta Otolaryngologica, 421,* 62–67.

Minor, L., Solomon, D., Zinreich, J., & Zee, D. (1998). Sound- and/or pressure-induced vertigo due to bone dehiscence of the superior semicircular canal. *Archives of Otolaryngology—Head and Neck Surgery, 124,* 249–258.

Mitchell, C., Kempton, J., Creedon, T., & Trune, D. (1996). Rapid acquisition of auditory brainstem responses with multiple frequency and intensity tone-bursts. *Hearing Research, 99,* 38–46.

Mitchell, C., Kempton, J., Creedon, T., & Trune, D. (1999). The use of a 56-stimulus train for the rapid acquisition of auditory brainstem responses. *Audiology and Neuro-Otology, 4,* 80–87.

Miyamoto, R. T., Campbell, R. L., Fritsch, M., & Lochmueller, G. (1990). Preservation of hearing in neurofibromatosis 2. *Archives of Otolaryngology—Head & Neck Surgery, 103,* 619–624.

Miyao, M., Kudo, H., Chiku, Y., et al. (1983). Auditory brainstem evoked responses in degenerative disease in children. *No To Hattatsu, 15,* 402–409.

Mizrahi, E. M., Maulsby, R. L., & Frost, J. D. (1983). Improved wave V resolution by dual-channel brainstem auditory evoked potential recording. *Electroencephalography and Clinical Neurophysiology, 55,* 105–107.

Mizukoshi, K., Shojaku, H., Aso, S., Asai, M., & Watanabe, Y. (2001). Ménière's disease and delayed endolymphatic hydrops in children. *Acta Otolaryngology Supplement, 545,* 6–9.

Mizukoshi, K., Shojaku, H., Aso, S., & Watanabe, Y. (2000). Clinical study of elderly patients with Ménière's and related diseases. *Auris Nasus Larynx, 27,* 167–173.

Mochizuki, Y., Go, T., Ohkubo, H., Tatara, T., & Motomura, T. (1982). Developmental changes of brainstem auditory evoked potentials (BAEPs) in normal human subjects from infants to young adults. *Brain Development, 4,* 127–136.

Moffat, D. A., Baguley, D. M., Harries, M. L., Atlas, M., & Lynch, C. A. (1992). Bilateral electrocochleographic findings in unilateral Ménière's disease. *Otolaryngology—Head & Neck Surgery, 107,* 370–373.

Mogensen, F., & Kristensen, O. (1979). Auditory double click evoked potentials in multiple sclerosis. *Acta Neurologica Scandinavia, 59,* 96–107.

Mohamed, A. S., Iacono, R. P., & Yamada, S. (1996). Normalization of middle latency auditory P1 potential following posterior ansa-pallidotomy in idiopathic Parkinson's disease. *Neurology Research, 18,* 516–520.

Mokotoff, B., Schulman-Galambos, C., & Galambos, R. (1977). Brain stem auditory evoked responses in children. *Archives of Otolaryngology, 103,* 38–43.

Mokrusch, R. Schramm, J., & Fahlbusch, R. (1985). Repeatedly reversible alteration of acoustic-evoked brainstem responses with a cystic craniopharyngioma. *Surgical Neurology, 24,* 571–577.

Møller, A. R. (1981). Latency in the ascending auditory pathway determined using continuous sounds: Comparison between transient and envelope latency. *Brain Research, 207,* 184–188.

Møller, A. R. (1983a). Improving brainstem auditory evoked potential recordsing by digital filtering. *Ear and Hearing, 4,* 108–113.

Møller, A. R. (1983c). *Auditory physiology.* New York: Academic Press.

Møller, A. R. (1985). Origin of latency shift of cochlear nerve potentials with sound intensity. *Hearing Research, 17,* 177–189.

Møller, A. R. (1986). Effect of click spectrum and polarity on round window N1-N2 response in the rat. *Audiology, 25,* 29–43.

Møller, A. R. (1987a). Auditory evoked potentials to continuous amplitude-modulated sounds: Can they be described by linear methods? *Electroencephalography and Clinical Neurophysiology, 71,* 226–232.

Møller, A. R. (1987b). Auditory evoked potentials to continuous amplitude-modulated tones: Can they be described by linear methods? *Electroencephalography and Clinical Neurophysiology, 71,* 226–232.

Møller, A. R. (1996). Monitoring auditory function during operations to remove acoustic tumors. *American Journal of Otology, 17,* 452–460.

Møller, A. R., & Blegvad, B. (1976). Brainstem response in patients with sensorineural hearing loss. *Scandinavian Audiology, 5,* 115–127.

Møller, A. R., & Jannetta, P. J. (1981). Compound action potentials recorded intracranially from the auditory nerve in man. *Journal of Experimental Neurology, 74,* 862–874.

Møller, A. R., & Jannetta, P. J. (1982). Evoked potentials from the inferior colliculus in man. *Electroencephalography and Clinical Neurophysiology, 53,* 612–620

Møller, A. R., & Jannetta, P. J. (1983a). Auditory evoked potentials recorded from the cochlear nucleus and its vicinity in man. *Journal of Neurosurgery, 59,* 1013–1018.

Møller, A. R., & Jannetta, P. J. (1983b). Interpretation of brainstem auditory evoked potentials: Results from intracranial recordings in humans. *Scandinavian Audiology, 12,* 125–133.

Møller, A. R., & Jannetta, P. J. (1984). Monitoring auditory nerve potentials during operations in the cerebellopontine angle. *Otolaryngology, Head and Neck Surgery, 92,* 434–439.

Møller, A. R., Jannetta, P., & Møller, M. B. (1982). Intracranially recorded auditory nerve response in man. *Archives of Otolaryngology, 108,* 77–82.

Møller, A. R., & Jho, H. D. (1989). Responses from the exposed human auditory nerve to pseudorandom noise. *Hearing Research, 42,* 237–252.

Møller, A. R., Jho, H. D., Yokota, M., & Jannetta, P. J. (1995). Contribution from crossed and uncrossed brainstem structures to the brainstem auditory evoked potentials: A study in humans. *Laryngoscope, 105,* 596–605.

Møller, A. R., & Møller, M. (1983). Brainstem auditory evoked potentials in patients with cerebellopontine angle tumors. *Annals of Otology, Rhinology & Laryngology, 92,* 645–650.

Møller, A. R., Møller, M., & Jannetta, M. (1982). Brain stem auditory evoked potentials in patients with hemifacial spasm. *Laryngoscope, 92,* 848–852.

Møller, M. B., & Møller, A. R. (1985). Audiometric abnormalities in hemifacial spasm. *Audiology, 24,* 396–405.

Mongey, A. B., Glynn, D., Hutchinson, M., & Bresnihan, B. (1987). Clinical neurophysiology in the assessment of neurological symptoms in systemic lupus erythematosus. *International Rheumatology, 7,* 49–52.

Monobe, H., & Murofushi, T. (2004). Vestibular neuritis in a child with otitis media with effusion: Clinical application of vestibular evoked myogenic potential by bone-conducted sound. *International Journal of Pediatric Otorhinolaryngology, 68,* 1455–1458.

Mononen, L. J., & Seitz, M. R. (1977). An AER analysis of contralateral advantage in the transmission of auditory information. *Neuropsychologia, 15,* 165–173.

Montandon, P. B., Cao, M. H., Engel, R. T., & Grajew, T. (1979). Auditory nerve and brainstem responses in the newborn and in preschool children. *Acta Otolaryngologica, 87,* 279–286.

Montandon, P. B., Megill, N. D., Kahn, A. R., Peake, W. T., & Kiang, N. Y. S. (1975). Recording auditory-nerve potentials as an office procedure. *Annals of Otolaryngology, Rhinology, and Laryngology, 84,* 2–10.

Moore, E. J. (Ed.). (1983). *Bases of auditory brain-stem evoked responses.* New York: Grune and Stratton.

Moore, E., Semela, J., Rakerd, B., Robb, R., & Ananthanarayan, A. (1992). The I' potential of the brain-stem auditory-evoked potential. *Scandinavian Audiology, 21,* 153–156.

Moore, J. K. (1987a). The human auditory brainstem: A comparative view. *Hearing Research, 29,* 1–32.

Moore, J. K. (1987b). The human auditory brainstem as a generator of auditory evoked potentials. *Hearing Research, 29,* 33–43.

Moore, J. K., Ponton, C. P., Eggermont, J. J., Wu, B. J.-C., & Huang, J. Q. (1996). Perinatal maturation of the ABR: Changes in path length and conduction velocity. *Ear and Hearing, 17,* 411–418.

Moore, R. D., Smith, C. R., & Lietman, P. S. (1984). Risk factors for the development of auditory toxicity in patients receiving aminoglycosides. *Journal of Infectious Diseases, 149,* 23–30.

Mora, J. A., Exposito, M., Solis, C., & Barajas, J. J. (1990). Filter effects and low stimulation rate on the middle-latency response in newborns. *Audiology, 29,* 329–335.

Morawski, K., Namyslowski, G., Lisowska, G., Bazowski, P., Kwiek, S., & Telischi, F. F. (2004). Intraoperative monitoring of cochlear function using distortion product otoacoustic emissions (DPOAEs) in patients with cerebellopontine angle tumors. *Otology and Neuro-Otology, 25,* 818–825.

Morgan, D. E., Zimmerman, M. C., & Dubno, J. R. (1987). Auditory brain stem evoked response characteristics in the full-term newborn infant. *Annals of Otology, Rhinology, and Laryngology, 96,* 142–151.

Mori, K., Uchida, Y., Nishimura, T., & Eghwrudjakpor, P. (1988). Brainstem auditory evoked potentials in Chiari-II malformation. *Child's Nervous System, 4,* 154–157.

Mori, N., Asai, H., Doi, K., & Matsunaga, T. (1987). Diagnostic value of extratympanic electrocochleography in Ménière's disease. *Audiology, 26,* 103–110.

Mori, N., Asai, H., & Sakagami, M. (1990). Relationship between results of electrocochleography and caloric test in Ménière's disease. *ORL, 222,* 63–75.

Morita, Y., Morita, K., Yamamoto, M., Waseda, Y., & Maeda, H. (2001). Effects of facial affect recognition on the auditory P300 in healthy subjects. *Neuroscience Research, 41*, 89–95.

Morlet, T., Ferber-Viart, C., Putet, G., Sevin, F., & Duclaux, R. (1998). Auditory screening in high-risk pre-term and full-term neonates using transient evoked otoacoustic emissions and brainstem auditory evoked potentials. *International Journal of Pediatric Otorhinolaryngology, 45*, 31–40.

Morr, M. L., Shafer, V. L., Kreuzer, J. A., & Kurtzberg, D. (2002). Maturation of mismatch negativity in typically developing infants and preschool children. *Ear and Hearing, 23*, 118–136.

Morrison, A. W., Moffat, D. A., & O'Connor, A. F. (1980). Clinical usefulness of electrocochleography in Meniere's disease: An analysis of dehydrating agents. *Otolaryngology Clinics of North America, 13*, 703–721.

Mosko, S. S., Pierce, S., Holowach, J., & Sassim, J. (1981). Normal brainstem auditory evoked potentials recoded in sleep apneics during waking as a function of arterial oxygen saturation during sleep. *Electroencephalography and Clinical Neurophysiology, 51*, 477–482.

Mouney, D. F., Berlin, C. I., Cullen, J. K., & Hughes, L. F. (1978). Changes in human eighth nerve action potential as a function of stimulation rate. *Archives of Otolaryngology, 104*, 551–554.

Moushegian, G., Rupert, A. L., & Stillman, R. D. (1973). Scalp-recorded early responses in man to frequencies in the speech range. *Electroencephalography and Clinical Neurophysiology, 35*, 665–667.

Muchnik, C., Neeman, R. K., & Hildesheimer, M. (1995). Auditory brainstem response to bone-conducted clicks in adults and infants with normal hearing and conductive hearing loss. *Scandinavian Audiology, 24*, 185–191.

Muchnik, C., Rubel, Y., Zohar, Y., & Hildesheimer, M. (1995). Auditory brainstem response in obstructive sleep apnea patients. *Journal of Basic Clinical Physiology and Pharmacology, 6*, 139–148.

Mueller, H. G., III, & Hall, J. W., III. (1998). *Audiologists' desk reference: Volume II.* San Diego: Singular Publishing Group.

Mulert, C., Juckel, G., Augustin, H., & Hegerl, U. (2002). Comparison between the analysis of the loudness dependency of the auditory N1/P2 component with LORETA and dipole source analysis in the prediction of treatment response to the selective serotonin reuptake inhibitor citalopram in major depression. *Clinical Neurophysiology, 113*, 1566–1572.

Müller, V., Birbaumer, N., Preissl, H., Braun, C., & Lang, F. (2002). Effects of water on cortical excitability in humans. *European Journal of Neuroscience, 15*, 528–538.

Müller-Gass, A., & Campbell, K. (2002). Event-related potential measures of the inhibition of information processing: I. Selective attention in the waking state. *International Journal of Psychophysiology, 46*, 177–195.

Müller-Gass, A., Marcoux, A., Logan, J., & Campbell, K. B. (2001). The intensity of masking noise affects the mismatch negativity to speech sounds in human subjects. *Neuroscience Letters, 299*, 197–200.

Munte, T. F., Nager, W., Beiss, T., Schroeder, C., & Altenmuller, E. (2003). Specialization of the specialized: Electrophysiological investigations in professional musicians. *Neurosciences and Music, 999*, 131–139.

Murakami, T., Nakagome, K., Kamio, S., Kasai, K., Iwanami, A., Hiramatsu, K., Fukuda, M., Hata, A., Honda, M., Watanabe, A., & Kato, N. (2002). The effects of benzodiazepines on event-related potential indices of automatic and controlled processing in schizophrenia: a preliminary report. *Progress in Neuropsychopharmacology and Biological Psychiatry, 26*, 651–661.

Murata, K., Araki, A., & Aono, H. (1990). Central and peripheral nervous system effects of hand-arm vibrating tool operation: A study of brainstem auditory-evoked potential and peripheral nerve condition. *International Archives of Occupational and Environmental Health, 62*, 183–188.

Murata, K., Araki, S., Tanigawa, T., & Uchida, E. (1992). Acute effects of alcohol on cognitive function and central nervous system assessed by auditory event-related potentials. *Nippon Eiseigaku Zasshi, 47*, 958–964.

Murata, K., Araki, A., Yokoyama, K., Nomiyama, K., Nomiyama, H., Tao, Y., & Liu, S. (1995). Autonomic and central nervous system effects of lead in female glass workers in China. *American Journal of Industrial Medicine, 28*, 233–244.

Murata, K., Araki, S., Yokoyama, K., Okomura, T., Ishimatsu, S., Takasu, N., & et al. (1997). Asymptomatic sequelae to acute sarin poisoning in the central and autonomic nervous system 6 months after the Tokyo subway attack. *Journal of Neurology, 244*, 601–606.

Murata, K., Araki, A., Yokoyama, K., Uchida, E., & Fujimura, Y. (1993). Assessment of central, peripheral, and autonomic nervous system functions in lead workers: Neuroelectrophysiological studies. *Environmental Research, 61*, 323–336.

Murata, K., Weihe, P., Araki, S., Jorgensen, E., & Grandjean, P. (1999). Evoked potentials in Faroese children prenatally exposed to methylmercury. *Neurotoxicology and Teratology, 21*, 471–472.

Murata, K., Weihe, P., Budtz-Jorgensen, E., Jorgensen, P., & Grandjean, P. (2004). Delayed brainstem auditory evoked potential latencies in 14-year-old children exposed to methylmercury. *Journal of Pediatrics, 144*, 177–183.

Murata, K., Weihe, P., Renzoni, A., Debes, F., Vasconcelos, R., Zino, F., Araki, S., Jorgensen, P., White, R., & Grandjean, P. (1999). Delayed evoked potentials in children exposed to methylmercury from seafood. *Neurotoxicology and Teratology, 21*, 343–348.

Murofushi, T., Curthoys, I. S., Topple, A. N., Colebatch, J. G., & Halmagyi, G. M. (1995). Responses of guinea pig primary vestibular neurons to clicks. *Exploratory Brain Research, 103*, 174–178.

Murofushi, T., Halmagyi, G., Yavor, R., & Colebatch, J. (1996). Absent vestibular evoked myogenic potentials in vestibular neurolabyrinthitis. An indicator of inferior vestibular nerve involvement? *Archives of Otolaryngology—Head & Neck Surgery, 122*, 845–849.

Murofushi, T., Iwasaki, S., Takai, Y., & Takegoshi, H. (2005). Sound-evoked neurogenic responses with short latency of vestibular origin. *Clinical Neurophysiology, 116*, 401–405.

Murofushi, T., Matsuzaki, M., & Mizuno, M. (1998). Vestibular evoked myogenic potentials in patients with acoustic neuromas. *Archives of Otolaryngology—Head & Neck Surgery, 124*, 509–512.

Murofushi, T., Matsuzaki, M., & Takegoshi, H. (2001). Glycerol affects vestibular evoked myogenic potentials in Ménière's disease. *Auris Nasus Larynx, 28*, 205–208.

Murofushi, T., Matsuzaki, M., & Wu, C. (1999). Short tone burst-evoked myogenic potentials on the sternocleidomastoid muscle. *Archives of Otolaryngology—Head & Neck Surgery, 125*, 660–664.

Murofushi, T., Takegoshi, H., Ohki, M., & Ozeki, H. (2002). Galvanic-evoked myogenic responses in patients with an absence of click-evoked vestibulocollic reflexes. *Clinical Neurophysiology, 113*, 305–309.

Murphy, M., & Selesnick, S. (2002). Cost-effective diagnosis of acoustic neuromas: A philosophical, macroeconomic, and technological decision. *Archives of Otolaryngology—Head & Neck Surgery, 127*, 253–259.

Murray, G., Ormson, M., Loh, M., Ninan, B., Ninan, D., Dockery, L., & Fanaroff, A. (2004). Evaluation of Natus ALGO 3 newborn hearing screener. *Journal of Obstetric, Gynecologic, & Neonatal Nursing, 33*, 183–190.

Musiek, F. E. (1982). ABR in 8th-nerve and brain-stem disorders. *The American Journal of Otology, 3*, 243–248.

Musiek, F. E., & Baran, J. (1986). Neuroanatomy, neurophysiology, and central auditory assessment: I. Brain stem. *Ear and Hearing, 7*, 207–219.

Musiek, F. E., & Baran, J. A. (1990). Canal electrode electrocochleography in patients with absent wave I ABRs. *Archives of Otolaryngology—Head & Neck Surgery, 103*, 25–31.

Musiek, F. E., & Baran, J. A. (2004). Audiological correlates to a rupture of a pontine arteriovenous malformation. *Journal of the American Academy of Audiology, 15*, 161–171.

Musiek, F. E., Baran, J. A., & Shinn, J. (2004). Assessment and remediation of an auditory processing disorder associated with head trauma. *Journal of the American Academy of Audiology, 15*, 117–132.

Musiek, F. E., Charette, L., Kelly, T., Lee, W., & Musiek, E. (1999). Hit and false positive rates for middle latency response in patients with central nervous system involvement. *Journal of the American Academy of Audiology, 10*, 124–132.

Musiek, F. E., Charette, L., Morse, D., & Baran, J. A. (2004). Central deafness associated with a midbrain lesion. *Journal of the American Academy of Audiology, 15*, 133–151.

Musiek, F. E., & Geurkink, N. A. (1981). Auditory brainstem and middle latency evoked response sensitivity near threshold. *Annals of Otology, Rhinology & Laryngology, 90*, 236–240.

Musiek, F. E., & Geurkink, N. A. (1982). Auditory brainstem response and central auditory test findings for patients with brainstem lesions: A preliminary report. *Laryngoscope, 92*, 891–900.

Musiek, F. E., Geurkink, N. A., Weider, D. J., & Donnelly, K. (1984). Past, present, and future applications of the auditory middle latency response. *Laryngoscope, 94*(12), 1545–1552.

Musiek, F. E., Gollegly, K. M., Kibbe, K. S., & Reeves, A. G. (1989). Electrophysiologic and behavioral auditory findings in multiple sclerosis. *American Journal of Otology, 10*(5), 343–350.

Musiek, F. E., Gollegly, K. M., Kibbe, K. S., & Verkest, S. B. (1988). Current concepts on the use of ABR and auditory psychophysical tests in the evaluation of brain stem lesions. *The American Journal of Otology, 9,* 25–35.

Musiek, F. E., & Hanlon, D. (1999). Neuroaudiological effects in a case of fatal dimethylmercury poisoning. *Ear and Hearing, 20,* 271–275.

Musiek, F. E., Josey, A. F., & Glasscock, M. E., III. (1986). Auditory brainstem response in patients with acoustic neuromas: Wave presence and absence. *Archives of Otolaryngology, Head and Neck Surgery, 112,* 186–189.

Musiek, F. E., & Kibbe, K. (1986). Auditory brain stem response wave IV-V abnormalities from the ear opposite large cerebellopontine lesions. *American Journal of Otology, 7,* 253–257.

Musiek, F. E., Kibbe, K., Rackliffe, L., & Weider, D. J. (1984). The auditory brain stem response I-V amplitude ratio in normal, cochlear, and retrocochlear ears. *Ear and Hearing, 5,* 52–55.

Musiek, F. E., & Lee, W. (1995). The auditory brain stem response in patients with brain stem or cochlear pathology. *Ear and Hearing, 16,* 631–636.

Musiek, F. E., Verkest, S. B., & Gollegly, K. M. (1988). Effects of neuromaturation on auditory-evoked potentials. *Seminars in Hearing, 9,* 1–14.

Musiek, F. E., Weider, E. J., & Mueller, R. J. (1983). Reversible audiological results in a patient with an extra-axial brain stem tumor. *Ear and Hearing, 4,*

Mustillo, P. (1984). Auditory deficits in multiple sclerosis. A review. *Audiology, 23,* 145–164.

Muthane, U., Satishchandra, P., & Subhash, M. (1993). Visual and auditory evoked potentials in early onset Parkinson's disease and their relationship to cerebrospinal fluid monoamine metabolites. *Movement Disorders, 8,* 344–348.

Näätänen, R. (1975). Selective attention and evoked potentials in humans—a critical review. *Biological Psychology, 2,* 237–307.

Näätänen, R. (1982). Processing negativity: An evoked-potential reflection of selective attention. *Psychological Bulletin, 92,* 605–640.

Näätänen, R. (1990). The role of attention in auditory information processing as revealed by event-related potentials and other brain measures of cognitive function. *Behavioral and Brain Sciences, 13,* 201–288.

Näätänen, R. (1992). *Attention and brain function.* Hillsdale, NJ: Erlbaum.

Näätänen, R. (1995). The mismatch negativity: A powerful tool for cognitive neuroscience. *Ear and Hearing, 16,* 6–18.

Näätänen, R. (2000). Mismatch negativity (MMN). Perspectives for application. *International Journal of Psychophysiology, 37,* 3–10.

Näätänen, R. (2003). Mismatch negativity: Clinical research and possible applications. *International Journal of Psychophysiology, 48,* 179–188.

Näätänen, R., & Alho, K. (1997). Mismatch negativity—the measure for central sound representation accuracy. *Audiology & Neuro-Otology, 2,* 341–353.

Näätänen, R., & Escera, C. (2000). Mismatch negativity: Clinical and other applications. *Audiology & Neuro-Otology, 5,* 105–110.

Näätänen, R., Gaillard, A. W. K., & Mäntysalo, S. (1978). Early selective-attention effect on evoked potential reinterpretation. *Acta Psychologica, 42,* 313–329.

Näätänen, R., Jiang, D., Lavikainen, J., Reinikainen, K., & Paavilainen, P. (1993). Event-related potentials reveal a memory trace for temporal features. *Neuroreport, 5,* 310–312.

Näätänen, R., Lehtokoski, A., Lennes, M., Cheour, M., Huotilainen, M., Iivonen, A., Vainio, M., Alku, P., Ilmoniemi, R. J., Luuk, A., Allik, J., Sinkkonen, J., & Alho, K. (1997). Language-specific phoneme representations revealed by electric and magnetic brain responses. *Nature, 385,* 432–434.

Näätänen, R., & Michie, P. T. (1979). Early selective attention effects on the evoked potential: A critical review and reinterpretation. *Biological Psychology, 8,* 81–136.

Näätänen, R., Paavilainen, P., Alho, K., Reinikainen, K., & Sams, M. (1987). The mismatch negativity to intensity changes in an auditory stimulus sequence. *Electroencephalography and Clinical Neurophysiology, Supplement, 40,* 125–131.

Näätänen, R., Paavilainen, P., Tiitinen, H., Jiang, D., & Alho, K. (1993). Attention and mismatch negativity. *Psychophysiology, 30,* 436–450.

Näätänen, R., Pakarinen, S., Rinne, T., & Takegata, R. (2004). The mismatch negativity (MMN): Towards the optimal paradigm. *Clinical Neurophysiology, 115,* 140–144.

Näätänen, R., & Picton, T. W. (1987). The N1 wave of the human electric and magnetic response to sound: A review and an analysis of the component structure. *Psychophysiology, 24,* 375–425.

Näätänen, R., Sams, M., Alho, K., Paavilainen, P., Reinikainen, K., & Sokolov, E. N. (1998). Frequency and location specificity of the human vertex N1 wave. *Electroencephalography and Clinical Neurophysiology, 69,* 523–531.

Näätänen, R., Simpson, M., & Loveless, N. E. (1982). Stimulus deviance and evoked potentials. *Biological Psychiatry, 14,* 53–98.

Näätänen, R., Tervaniemi, M., Sussman, E., Paavilainen, P., & Winkler, I. (2001). "Primitive intelligence" in the auditory cortex. *Trends in Neuroscience, 24,* 283–288.

Näätänen, R., & Winkler, I. (1999). The concept of auditory stimulus representation in cognitive neuroscience. *Psychological Bulletin, 125,* 826–859.

Nadol, J., Chiong, C., Ojemann, R., et al. (1992). Preservation of hearing and facial nerve function in resection of acoustic neuroma. *Laryngoscope, 102,* 1153–1158.

Naessens, B., Gordts, F., Clement, P., & Buisseret, T. (1996). Re-evaluation of the ABR in the diagnosis of CPA tumors in the MRI-era. *Acta Otorhinolaryngologica Belgium, 50,* 99–102.

Naganuma, Y., Konishi, T., Murakami, M., Hongou, K., Yamatani, M., & Okada, T. (1991). [Age-related changes of auditory event-related potential (P300) in children]. *No To Hattatsu, 23,* 194–199.

Nagata, K., Tazawa, T., Mizukami, M., & Araki, G. (1984). Application of brainstem auditory evoked potentials to evaluation of cerebral herniation. In R. H. Nodar & C. Barber (Eds.), *Evoked Potentials II: The Second International Evoked Potentials Symposium* (pp. 183–193). Boston: Butterworth.

Nager, W., Kohlmetz, C., Altenmuller, E., Rodriguez-Fornells, A., & Munte, T. F. (2003a). The fate of sounds in conductors' brains: An ERP study. *Cognitive Brain Research, 17,* 83–93.

Nager, W., Kohlmetz, C., Joppich, G., Mobes, J., & Munte, T. F. (2003b). Tracking of multiple sound sources defined by interaural time differences: Brain potential evidence in humans. *Neuroscience Letters, 344,* 181–184.

Nager, W., Teder-Salejarvi, W., Kunze, S., & Munte, T. F. (2003c). Preattentive evaluation of multiple perceptual streams in human audition. *Neuroreport, 14,* 871–874.

Nagy, E., Potts, G. F., & Loveland, K. A. (2003). Sex-related ERP differences in deviance detection. *International Journal of Psychophysiology, 48,* 285–292.

Naito, R., Hayashida, T., Mochizuki, M., Kojima, H., & Kaga, K. (1999). Auditory brainstem response and neuropathology in a case of systemic T-cell lymphoma with intracranial metastasis. *ORL Journal for Otorhinolaryngology and its Related Specialties, 61,* 108–112.

Nakagawa, M., Yoshikawa, H., Ando, I. & Ichikawa, G. (1999). Equivalent dipoles for middle latency auditory evoked potentials using the dipole tracing method. *Auris Nasus Larynx, 26,* 245–256.

Nakano, S., Imamura, S., Tokunaga, K., Tsuji, S., & Hashimoto, I. (1997). Evoked potentials in patients with chronic respiratory insufficiency. *Internal Medicine, 36,* 270–275.

Narayan, R. K., Greenberg, R. P., Miller, J. D., & Becker, D. P. (1981). Improved confidence of outcome prediction in severe head injury. A comparative analysis of the clinical examination, multimodality evoked potentials, CT scanning and intracranial pressure. *Journal of Neurosurgery, 54,* 751–762.

Nash, C. L., Loring, A., Schatzinger, L. A., & Brown, R. H. (1977). Spinal cord monitoring during operative treatment of the spine. *Clinical Orthopedics and Related Research, 54,* 751–762.

Nashida, T., Yabe, H., Sato, Y., Hiruma, T., Sutoh, T., Shinozaki, N., & Kaneko, S. (2000). Automatic auditory information processing in sleep. *Sleep, 23,* 821–828.

National Institutes of Health. (1993, May 4). *Consensus conference statement. identification of hearing impairment in infants and young children.* Bethesda, MD: Author.

National Instruments. (2000). *LabVIEW measurements manual.* Austin, TX: Author.

Naunton, R. F., & Zerlin, S. (1976). Human whole-nerve response to clicks of various frequency. *Audiology, 15,* 1–9.

Navaratnarajah, M., Thornton, C., Heneghan, C. P. H., Bateman, E., & Jones, J. G. (1983). Effect of etomidate on the auditory evoked response in man. *British Journal of Anesthesia*, 1157P–1158P.

Negishi, H., Lee, Y., Nishino, M., Itoh, K., Kawai, S., Takada, S., et al. (1993). [Prognostic significance of auditory brainstem responses in full-term newborn infants with intracranial hemorrhages.]. *No To Hattatsu, 25*, 33–39.

Negri, M., Bacciu, A., Fava, G., Pasanisi, E., Piazza, F., & Bacciu, S. (1996). [Electrocochleography by extra- and transtympanic methods: the results in a group of normal subjects]. *Acta Bio-medica de L'Ateneo, 67*, 177–183.

Nelson, C., Collins, P., & Torres, F. (1991). P300 brain activity in seizure patients preceding temporal lobectomy. *Archives of Neurology, 48*, 141–147.

Nelson, D. A., & Lassman, F. M. (1968). Effects of intersignal interval on the human auditory evoked response. *Journal of the Acoustical Society of America, 44*, 1529–1532.

Nelson, M. D., Hall, J. W., III, & Jacobson, G. P. (1997). Factors influencing the auditory middle latency response Pb component (P1). *Journal of American Academy of Audiology, 8*, 89–99.

Neuloh, G., & Curio, G. (2004). Does familiarity facilitate the cortical processing of music sounds? *Neuroreport, 15*, 2471–2475.

Neville, H. J., Kutas, M., & Schmidt, A. (1982). Event-related potential studies of cerebral specialization during reading: I. Studies of normal adults. *Brain and Language, 16*, 300–315.

Newlon, P. G., Greenberg, R. P., Enas, F. F., & Becker, D. P. (1983). Effects of therapeutic pentobarbital coma on multimodality evoked potentials. *Journal of Neurosurgery, 12*, 613–619.

Newman, R. L., Connolly, J. F., Service, E., & Mcivor, K. (2003). Influence of phonological expectations during a phoneme deletion task: Evidence from event-related brain potentials. *Psychophysiology, 40*, 640–647.

Newton, M. R., Barrett, G., Callanan, M. M., & Towell, A. D. (1989). Cognitive event-related potentials in multiple sclerosis. *Brain, 112*, 1637–1660.

Neylan, T. C., Fletcher, D. J., Lenoci, M., McCallin, K., Weiss, D. S., Schoenfeld, F. B., Marmar, C. R., & Fein, G. (1999). Sensory gating in chronic posttraumatic stress disorder: reduced auditory P50 suppression in combat veterans. *Biological Psychiatry, 46*, 1656–1664.

Ng, M., Srireddy, S., Horlbeck, D. M., & Niparko, J. K. (2001). Safety and patient experience with transtympanic electrocochleography. *Laryngoscope, 111*, 792–795.

Niedzielska, G., & Katska, E. (1998). ABR disturbances in children with insulin dependant diabetes mellitus. *International Journal of Pediatric Otorhinolaryngology, 44*, 1–4.

Nielsen-Bohlman, L., Knight, R. T., Woods, D. L., & Woodward, K. (1991). Differential auditory processing continues during sleep. *Electroencephalography and Clinical Neurophysiology, 79*, 281–290.

Nighoghossian, N., Neuschwander, P., Sonnet, M., Audrat, P., Bouffard, Y., & Trouillas, P. (1991). [Neurological manifestations in the vertebro-basilar system suggesting pregnancy toxemia.] *Revue Française de Gynecologie et d'Obstetrique, 86*, 119–122.

Nikiforidis, G., Tsambaos, D., Karamitsos, D., Koutsojannis, C., & Georgiou, S. (1993). Abnormalities of the auditory brainstem response in vitiligo. *Scandinavian Audiology, 22*, 97–100.

Nikiforidis, G., Tsambaos, D., Karamitsos, D., Koutsojannis, C., & Georgiou, S. (1994). Effects of oral isotretinoin on human auditory brainstem response. *Dermatology, 189*, 62–64.

Nikolopoulos, T., Mason, S., Gibbin, K., & O'Donaghue, G. (2000). The prognostic value of promontory electric auditory brain stem response in pediatric cochlear implantation. *Ear and Hearing, 21*, 236–241.

Nikolopoulos, T., Mason, S., O'Donaghue, G., & Gibbin, K. (1999). Integrity of the auditory pathway in young children with congenital and postmeningitic deafness. *Annals of Otology Rhinology and Laryngology, 108*, 327–330.

Niparko, J. K., Kileny, P. R., Kemink, J. L., Lee, J. M. & Graham, M. D. (1989). Neurophysiologic intraoperative monitoring. II. Facial nerve function. *The American Journal of Otology, 10*, 55–61.

Niparko, J. K., Kileny, P. R., Kemink, J. L., Lee, J. M., & Graham, M. D. (1989). Neurophysiologic intraoperative monitoring. II. Facial nerve function. *The American Journal of Otology*, 55–61.

Nishida, H., Komatsuzaki, A., & Noguchi, Y. (1998). A new electrode (HN-5) for CM measurement in extratympanic electrocochleography. *Audiology, 37*, 7–16.

Nishida, H., Tanaka, Y., Okada, M., & Inoue, Y. (1995). Evoked otoacoustic emissions and electrocochleography in a patient with multiple sclerosis. *Annals of Otology, Rhinology & Laryngology, 104*, 456–462.

Nishida, S., Nakamura, M., Suwazono, S., Honda, M., & Shibasaki, H. (1997). Estimate of physiological variability of peak latency in single sweep P300. *Electroencephalography and Clinical Neurophysiology, 104*, 431–436.

Nishida, S., Nakamura, M., Suwazono, S., Honda, M., Nagamine, T., & Shibasaki, H. (1994). Automatic detection method for P300 waveform in the single sweep records by using a neural network. *Medical Engineering and Physics, 16*, 425–429.

Nishiyama, T., Matsukawa, T., & Hanaoka, K. (2004). A comparison of the clinical usefulness of three different electroencephalogram monitors: Bispectral index, processed electroencephalogram, and Alaris auditory evoked potentials. *Anaesthesia & Analgesia, 98*, 1341–1345.

Nodar, R. H., Hahn, J., & Levine, H. L. (1980). Brain stem auditory evoked potentials in determining site of lesion of brain stem gliomas in children. *Laryngoscope, 90*, 258–265.

Nodar, R. H., Lonsdale, D., & Orlowski, J. (1980). Abnormal brainstem auditory evoked potentials in infants with threatened sudden infant death syndrome. *Otolaryngology—Head & Neck Surgery, 88*, 619–621.

Noffsinger, D., Martinez, C. D., & Schaefer, A. B., (1982). Auditory brainstem responses and masking level difference from persons with brainstem lesions. *Scandinavian Audiology (Suppl), 15*, 157–165.

Noffsinger, D., Olsen, W. O., Carhart, R., Hart, C. W., & Sahgal, V. (1972). Auditory and vestibular aberrations in multiple sclerosis. *Acta Otolaryngologica (Suppl), 303*, 1–63.

Noguchi, Y., Komatsuzaki, A., & Nishida, H. (1999). Cochlear microphonics for hearing preservation in vestibular schwannoma surgery. *Laryngoscope, 109*, 1982–1987.

Nong, D. X., Ura, M., Kyuna, A., Owa, T., & Noda, Y. (2002). Saccular origin of acoustically evoked short latency negative response. *Otology and Neuro-Otology, 23*, 953–957.

Norcia, A. M., Sato, T., Shinn, P., & Mertus, J. (1986). Methods for the identification of evoked response components in the frequency and combined time/frequency domains. *Electroencephalography and Clinical Neurophysiology, 65*, 212–226.

Nordby, H. K., & Nesbakken, R. (1984). The effect of high dose barbiturate decompression after severe head injury: A controlled clinical trial. *Acta Neurochirugica, 72*, 157–166.

Norton, S. J., Gorga, M. P., Widen, J. E., Folsom, R. C., Sininger, Y., Cone-Wesson, B., Vohr, B. R., Mascher, K., & Fletcher, K. (2000). Identification of neonatal hearing impairment: Evaluation of transient evoked otoacoustic emission, distortion product otoacoustic emission, and auditory brain stem response test performance. *Ear and Hearing, 21*, 508–528.

Noseworthy, J. H., Miller, J., Murray, T. J., & Regan, D. (1981). Auditory brainstem responses in postconcussion syndrome. *Archives of Neurology, 38*, 275–278.

Nousak, J., & Stapells, D. (1992). Frequency specificity of the auditory brainstem responses to bone conducted tones. *Ear and Hearing, 13*, 87–95.

Nousak, J. M., & Stapells, D. (1999, November). *ABR/MR results for 1000-Hz tones in hearing-impaired subjects.* Paper presented at the Annual Convention of the American Speech-Language-Hearing Association, San Francisco.

Novick, B., Vaughan, H. G., Kurtzberg, D., & Simson, R. (1980). An electrophysiologic indication of auditory processing defects in autism. *Psychiatry Research, 3*, 107–114.

Nowosielski, J. E., Redhead, T. J., & Kattula, S. P. (1991). Extratympanic electrocochleography with a conductive fluid and flexible electrode. *British Journal of Audiology, 25*, 345–349.

Nuwer, M. R. (1986). *Evoked potential monitoring in the operating room.* New York: Raven Press.

Nuwer, M. R., Perlman, S. L., Packwood, J. W., & Kark, R. A. P. (1982). Evoked potential abnormalities in the various inherited ataxias. *Annals of Neurology, 13*, 20–27.

Oades, R. D., Dittman, B., Schepker, R., Eggers, C., & Zerbin, D. (1996). Auditory event-related potentials (ERPs) and mismatch negativity (MMN) in healthy children and those with attention-deficit or Tourette/tic symptoms. *Biological Psychiatry, 43*, 163–185.

Oades, R. D., Dittmann-Balcar, A., Zerbin, D., & Grzella, I. (1997). Impaired attention-dependent augmentation of MMN in nonparanoid vs paranoid schizophrenic patients: A comparison with obsessive-compulsive disorder and healthy subjects. *Biological Psychiatry, 41,* 1196–1210.

Oades, R. D., Walker, M. K., Geffen, L. B., & Stern, L. M. (1988). Event-related potentials in autistic and healthy children on an auditory choice reaction task. *International Journal of Psychophysiology, 6,* 25–37.

Oates, P. A., Kurtzberg, D., & Stapells, D. R. (2002). Effects of sensorineural hearing loss on cortical event-related potential and behavioral measures of speech-sound processing. *Ear and Hearing, 23,* 399–415.

Oates, P., & Purdy, S. C. (2001). Frequency specificity of the human auditory brainstem and middle latency responses using notched noise masking. *Journal of the Acoustical Society of America, 110,* 995–1009.

Oates, P., & Stapells, D. R. (1997). Frequency specificity of the human auditory brainstem and middle latency responses to brief tones. I. High pass noise masking. *Journal of the Acoustical Society of America, 102,* 3597–3608.

Ochi, K., & Ohashi, T. (2001). Sound-evoked myogenic potentials and responses with 3 ms latency in auditory brain-stem responses. *Laryngoscope, 111,* 1818–1821.

Ochi, K., & Ohashi, T. (2003). Age-related changes in the vestibular-evoked myogenic potentials. *Otolaryngology—Head & Neck Surgery, 129,* 655–659.

Ochi, K., Kinoshita, H., Kenmochi, M., Nishino, H., & Ohashi, T. (2003). Neurotological findings in a patient with narrow internal auditory canal: a case report. *Auris Nasus Larynx, Supplement, 30,* S93–S96.

Ochs, R., Markand, O. N., & DeMyer, W. E. (1979). Brainstem auditory evoked responses in leukodystrophies. *Neurology, 29,* 1089–1093.

Odenthal, D. W., & Eggermont, J. J. (1974). Clinical electrocochleography. *Acta Otolaryngologica (Stockholm, Suppl), 316,* 62–74.

Odenthal, D. W., & Eggermont, J. J. (1976). Electrocochleography study in Meniere's disease and pontine angle neurinoma. In R. J. Ruben, C. Elberling, & G. Salomon, (Eds.), *Electrocochleography* (pp. 331–352). Baltimore: University Park Press.

O'Donnell, B., Friedman, S., Squires, N., Maloon, A., Drachman, D., & Swearer, J. (1990). Active and passive P300 latency in dementia. *Neuropsychiatry Neurophysiology and Behavioral Neurology, 3,* 164–169.

O'Donnell, B., Squires, K., Martz, J., Chen, C., & Phay, A. (1987). Evoked potential changes and neuropsychological performance in Parkinson's disease. *Biological Psychiatry, 24,* 23–37.

O'Donovan, C. A., Beagley, H. A., & Shaw, M. (1980). Latency of brainstem response in children. *British Journal of Audiology, 14,* 23–29.

Oeken, J. (1996). [Assessment of cochlear function with distortion products of otoacoustic emissions in acoustic neuroma]. *HNO, 44,* 677–684.

Ogilvie, R. D., Simons, I. A., Kuderian, R. H., MacDonald, T., & Rustenburg, J. (1991). Behavioral, event-related potential, and EEG/FFT changes at sleep onset. *Psychophysiology, 28,* 54–64.

Ogleznev, K. Y., Zaretsky, A. A., & Shesterikov, S. A. (1983). Brain stem auditory evoked potentials: Reduction of evaluation errors. *Electroencephalography and Clinical Neurophysiology, 55,* 331–332.

Oh, S. J., Kuba, T., & Soya, A. (1981). Lateralization of brainstem lesions by brainstem auditory evoked potentials. *Neurology, 31,* 14–18.

Ohashi, T. (1983). Electrophysiological analysis of cochlear CD potential in man: Pathophysiology of electrocochleographic SP. *Practical Otolaryngology Kyoto* (Suppl), *6*(76), 2857–2895.

Ohashi, T., Akagi, M., Ochi, K., Kenmochi, M., Kinoshita, H., & Yoshino, K. (1996). Diagnostic significance of electrocochleogram and auditory evoked brainstem response in totally or subtotally deaf patients. *Acta Otolaryngologica, 522,* 11–16.

Ohashi, T., Ochi, K., Kinoshita, H., Kenmochi, M., Kikuchi, K., Nishino, H., & Taguchi, Y. (2001). Electrocochleogram after transection of vestibulo-cochlear nerve in a patient with a large acoustic neurinoma. *Hearing Research, 154,* 26–31.

Ohashi, T., Ochi, K., Okada, T., & Takeyama, I. (1991). Long-term follow-up of electrocochleogram in Ménière's disease. *ORL, 53,* 131–136.

Ohlrich, E. S., & Barnet, A. B. (1972). Auditory evoked responses during the first year of life. *Electroencephalography and Clinical Neurophysiology, 32,* 161–169.

Ohlrich, E. S., Barnet, A. B., Weiss, I. P., & Shanks, B. L. (1978). Auditory evoked potential development in early childhood: A longitudinal study. *Electroencephalograpy and Clinical Neurophysiology, 44,* 411–423.

Ojemann, R. G., Levine, R. A., Montgomery, W. M., & McGaffigan, P. (1984). Use of intraoperative auditory evoked potentials to preserve hearing in unilateral acoustic neuroma removal. *Journal of Neurosurgery, 61,* 938–948.

Okazaki, H. (1983). *Fundamentals of neuropathology.* New York: Igaku-Shoin.

Okita, T. (1979). Event-related potentials and selective attention to auditory stimuli varying pitch and localization. *Biological Psychology, 9,* 271–284.

Okita, T., & Ohtani, A. (1977). The effects of active attention switching between the ears on averaged evoked potentials. *Electroencephalography and Clinical Neurophysiology, 42,* 198–204.

Okitsu, R. Kusakari, J., Ito, K., & Tomioka, S. (1980). Study of simultaneous lobe-vertex recording technique in auditory brainstem response. *Otorhinolaryngology, 42,* 282–291.

Okitsu, T. (1984). Middle components of the auditory evoked response in young children. *Scandinavian Audiology, 13,* 83–86.

Oku, T., & Hasegewa, M. (1997). The influence of aging on auditory brainstem response and electrocochleography in the elderly. *ORL Journal for Otorhinolaryngology & its Related Specialties, 59,* 141–146.

Okusa, M., Shiraishi, T., Kubo, T., & Nageishi, Y. (1999). Effects of discrimination difficulty on cognitive event-related brain potentials in patients with cochlear implants. *Archives of Otolaryngological—Head & Neck Surgery, 121,* 610–615.

O'Mahoney, D., Rowan, M., Feely, J., Walsh, J., & Coakley, D. (1994). Primary auditory pathway and reticular activating system dysfunction in Alzheimer's disease. *Neurology, 44,* 2089–2094.

O'Malley, S. Ramsden, R. T., Latif, F., Kane, R., & Davies, M. (1985). Electrocochleographic changes in the hearing loss associated with X-linked hypophosphataemic osteomalacia. *Acta Otolaryngologica, 100,* 13–18.

Onishi, S., & Davis, H. (1968). Effects of duration and rise time of tone bursts on evoked V potentials. *Journal of the Acoustical Society of America, 44,* 582–591.

Onitsuka, T., Ninomiya, H., Sato, E., Yamamoto, T., & Tashiro, N. (2003). Differential characteristics of the middle latency auditory evoked magnetic responses to interstimulus intervals. *Clinical Neurophysiology, 114,* 1513–1520.

Onofrj, M., Curatola, L., Malatesta, G., et al. (1992). Delayed P3 event-related potentials (ERPs) in thalamic hemorrhage. *Electroencephalography and Clinical Neurophysiology, 83,* 52–61.

Onofrj, M., Thomas, A., Paci, C., Scesi, M., & Tombari, R. (1997). Event related potentials recorded in patients with locked-in syndrome. *Journal of Neuropsychiatry & Neurosurgical, & Psychiatry, 63,* 759–764.

Opitz, B., Mecklinger, A., Von Cramon, D. Y., & Kruggel, F. (1999). Combining electrophysiological and hemodynamic measures of the auditory oddball. *Psychophysiology, 36,* 142–147.

Oranje, B., van Berckel, B. N., Kemner, C., van Ree, J. M., Kahn, R. S., & Verbaten, M. N. (2000). The effects of a sub-anaesthetic dose of ketamine on human selective attention. *Neuropsychopharmacology, 22,* 293–302.

Orchik, D. J., Ge, N. N., & Shea, J. J., Jr. (1998). Action potential latency shift by rarefaction and condensation clicks in Meniere's disease. *Journal of the American Academy of Audiology, 9,* 121–126.

Orchik, D. J., Shea, J. J., Jr., & Ge, X. (1993). Transtympanic electrocochleography in Meniere's disease using clicks and tone-bursts. *American Journal of Otology, 14,* 290–294.

Ornitz, E. M., & Walter, D. O. (1975). The effect of sound pressure waveform on human brain stem auditory evoked responses. *Brain Research, 92,* 490–498.

Ornitz, E. M., Ritvo, E. R., Carr, E. M., Panman, L. M., & Walter, R. D. (1967). The variabililty of the auditory averaged evoked response during sleep and dreaming in children and adults. *Electroencephalograpy and Clinical Neurophysiology, 22,* 514–524.

Osman, K., Pawlas, K., Schutz, A., Gazdzik, M., Sokal, J., & Vahter, M. (1999). Lead exposure and hearing effects in children in Katowice, Poland. *Environmental Research, 80,* 1–8.

Osterhammel, P. (1981). The unsolved problems in analog filtering on the auditory brain stem responses. *Scandinavian Audiology, Supplement, 13,* 69–74.

Osterhammel, P. A., Shallop, J. K., & Terkildsen, K. (1985). The effect of sleep on the auditory brainstem response (ABR) and the middle latency response (MLR). *Scandinavian Audiology, 14,* 47–50.

Osterhammel, P. H., Davis, H., Wier, C. C., & Hirsh, S. K. (1973). Adult auditory evoked vertex potentials in sleep. *Audiology, 12,* 116–128.

Osterhout, L., Allen, M. D., McLaughlin, J., & Inoue, K. (2002). Brain potentials elicited by prose-embedded linguistic anomalies. *Memory and Cognition, 30,* 1304–1312.

Ostroff, J. M., Martin, B. A., & Boothroyd, A. (1998). Cortical evoked response to acoustic change within a syllable. *Ear and Hearing, 19,* 290–297.

Ostroff, J. M., McDonald, K. K., Schneider, B. A., & Alain, C. (2003). Aging and the processing of sound duration in human auditory cortex. *Hearing Research, 181,* 1–7.

Otto, D. A., & Fox, D. A. (1993). Auditory and visual dysfunction following lead exposure. *Neurotoxicology, 14,* 191–207.

Otto, S., Waring, M., & Kuchta, J. (2005). Neural response telemetry and auditory/nonauditory sensations in 15 recipients of auditory brainstem implants. *Journal of the American Academy of Audiology, 16,* 219–227.

Otto, W. C., & McCandless, G. A. (1982). Aging and the auditory brainstem response. *Audiology, 21,* 466–473.

Oudesluys-Murphy, A. M., & Harlaar, J. (1997). Neonatal hearing screening with an automated auditory brainstem response screener in the infant's home. *Acta Paediatrica, 86,* 651–655.

Oviatt, D., & Kileny, P. (1991). Auditory event-related potentials elicited from cochlear implant recipients and hearing subjects. *American Journal of Audiology, 1,* 48–55.

Owen, M., Morcross-Nechay, K., & Howie, V. (1993). Brain stem auditory evoked potentials in young children before and after tympanostomy tube placement. *International Journal of Pediatric Otorhinolaryngology, 25,* 105–117.

Oysu, C., Aslan, I., Basaran, B., & Baserer, N. (2001). The site of the hearing loss in Refsum's disease. *International Journal of Pediatric Otorhinolaryngology, 61,* 129–134.

Ozata, M., Ozkardes, A., Bulur, M., Beyhan, Z., Corakci, A., Yardim, M., & Gundogan, M. (1996). Central and peripheral neural responses in males with ideopathic hypogonadotrophic hypogonadism. *Journal of Endocrinology Investigations, 19,* 449–454.

Ozcan, C., Ozbek, E., Soylu, A., Yilmaz, U., Guzelipek, M., & Balbay, M. D. (2001). Auditory event-related potentials in patients with premature ejaculation. *Urology, 58,* 1025–1029.

Özdamar, O., & Dallos, P. (1976). Input-output functions of cochlear whole-nerve action potentials: Interpretation in terms of one population of neurons. *Journal of the Acoustical Society America, 59,* 43–147.

Özdamar, O., & Kalayci, T. (1999). Median averaging of auditory brain stem responses. *Ear and Hearing, 20,* 253–264.

Özdamar, O., & Kraus, N. (1983). Auditory middle-latency responses in humans. *Audiology, 22,* 34–49.

Özdamar, O., Kraus, N., & Curry, F. (1982). Auditory brain stem and middle latency responses in a patient with cortical deafness. *Electroencephalograpy and Clinical Neurophysiology, 53,* 224–230.

Özdamar, O., Kraus, N., & Grossmann, J. (1986). Binaural interaction in the auditory middle latency response of the guinea pig. *Electroencephalograpy and Clinical Neurophysiology, 63,* 224–230.

Özdamar, O., Kraus, N., & Stein, L. (1983). Auditory brainstem responses in infants recovering from bacterial meningitis. *Archives of Otolaryngology, 109,* 12–18.

Özdirim, E., Topcy, M., Ozon, A., & Cila, A. (1996). Cockayne syndrome: Review of 25 cases. *Pediatric Neurology, 15,* 312–316.

Paavilainen, P., Alho, K., Reinikainen, K., Sams, M., & Näätänen, R. (1991). Right hemisphere dominance of different mismatch negativities. *Electroencephalography and Clinical Neurophysiology, 78,* 466–479.

Paetau, R., Ahonen, A., Salonen, O., & Sams, M. (1995). Auditory evoked magnetic fields to tones and pseudowords in healthy children and adults. *Journal of Clinical Neurophysiology, 12,* 177–185.

Pakalnis, A., Drake, M. E., Jr., Dadmehr, N., & Weiss, K. (1987). Correlation of EEG, evoked potentials, and magnetic resonance imaging in evaluation of multiple sclerosis. *Electromyography and Clinical Neurophysiology, 27,* 489–492.

Pal, P. K., Jayakumar, P. N., Taly, A. B., Nagaraja, D., & Rao, S. (1999). Early onset cerebellar ataxia with retained tendon reflexes (EOCA) and olivopontocerebellar atrophy (OPCA): A computed tomographic study. *Neurology India, 47,* 276–281

Pal, P. K., Taly, A. B., Nagaraja, D., & Jayakumar, P. N. (1995). Early onset cerebellar ataxia with retained tendon reflexes: A clinical, electrophysiological and computed tomographic study. *Journal for the Association of Physicians, India, 43,* 608–613.

Palaskas, C. W., Wilson, M. J., & Dobie, R. A. (1989). Electrophysiologic assessment of low-frequency hearing: sedation effects. *Archives of Otolaryngology—Head & Neck Surgery, 101,* 434–441.

Palenga, R., Valigi, F., & Bicciolo, C. (1985). Use of brain-stem evoked responses in the ischemic pathology of the vertebrobasilar area. *Otorhinolarynogologia, 35*(5): 439–442.

Palludetti, G., Maurizi, M., & Ottaviani, F. (1983). Effects of stimulus repetition rate on the auditory brainstem response (ABR). *American Journal of Otology, 4,* 226–234.

Palludetti, G., Ottaviani, F., Gallai, V., Tassoni, A., & Maurizi, M. (1985). Auditory brainstem responses (ABR) in multiple sclerosis. *Scandinavian Audiology, 14,* 27–34.

Palva, T., Troupp, H., & Jauhianen, T. (1985). Hearing preservation in acoustic neurinoma surgery. *Acta Otolaryngologica, 99,* 1–7.

Pang, E. W., Edmonds, G. E., Desjardins, R., Khan, S. C., Trainor, L. J., & Taylor, M. J. (1998). Mismatch negativity to speech stimuli in 8-month-old infants and adults. *International Journal of Psychophysiology, 29,* 227–236.

Pang, E. W., & Taylor, M. J. (2000). Tracking the development of the N1 from age 3 to adulthood: An examination of speech and non-speech stimuli. *Clinical Neurophysiology, 111,* 388–397.

Pantev, C., Bertrand, O., Eulitz, C., Verkindt, C., Hampson, S., Schuierer, G., & Elbert, T. (1995). Specific tonotopic organizations of different areas of the human auditory cortex revealed by simultaneous magnetic and electric recordings. *Electroencephalograpy and Clinical Neurophysiology, 94,* 26–40.

Pantev, C., Lagidze, S., Pantev, M., & Kevanishvili, Z. (1985). Frequency-specific contributions to the auditory brain stem response derived by means of pure-tone masking. *Audiology, 24,* 275–287.

Pantev, C., & Pantev, M. (1982). Derived brain stem responses by means of pure-tone masking. *Scandinavian Audiology, 11,* 15–22.

Pantev, C., Ross, B., Fujioka, T., Trainor, L. J., Schulte, M., & Schulz, M. (2003). Music and learning-induced cortical plasticity. *Neurosciences and Music, 999,* 438–450.

Papanicolaou, A. C., Levin, H. S., & Eisenberg, H. M. (1984). Evoked potential correlates of recovery from aphasia after focal left hemisphere injury in adults. *Neurosurgery, 14,* 412–415.

Papanicolaou, A. C., Loring, D. W., & Eisenberg, H. M. (1985). Relationship between stimulus intensity and the P300. *Psychophysiology, 22,* 326–329.

Papanicolaou, A., Loring, D., & Eisenberg, H. (1985). Stimulus offset P3 and temporal resolution of uncertainty. *International Journal of Psychophysiology, 3,* 29–31.

Pappas, D. G., Pappas, D. G., Carmichael, L., Hyatt, D. P., & Toohey, L. M. (2000). Extratympanic electrocochleography: Diagnostic and predictive value. *American Journal of Otology, 21,* 81–87.

Parasuraman, R. (1978). Auditory evoked potentials and divided attention. *Psychophysiology, 15,* 460–465.

Parker, D. J., & Thornton, A. R. D. (1978). The validity of the derived cochlear Nerve and brainstem evoked responses of the human auditory system. *Scandinavian Audiology, 7,* 45–52.

Parsons, F. G., & Keene, L. (1919). Sexual differences in the skull. *Journal of Anatomy, 54,* 58–65.

Parthasarathy, T., Borgsmiller, P., & Cohlan, B. (1998). Effects of repetition rate, phase, and frequency on the auditory brainstem response in neonates and adults. *Journal of the American Academy of Audiology, 9,* 134–140.

Parthasarathy, T., & Moushegian, G. (1993). Rate, frequency, and intensity effects on early auditory evoked potentials and binaural interaction component in humans. *Journal of the American Academy of Audiology, 4,* 229–237.

Parving, A. (1984). Inherited low-frequency hearing loss: A new mixed conductive/sensorineural entity? *Scandinavian Audiology, 13,* 47–56.

Parving, A., Elberling, C., Balle, V., Parbo, J., Dejgaard, A., & Parving, H. (1990). Hearing disorders in patients with insulin dependent diabetes mellitus. *Audiology, 29,* 113–121.

Parving, A., Elberling, C., & Smith, T. (1981). Auditory electrophysiology: findings in multiple sclerosis. *Audiology, 20,* 123–142.

Parving, A., Salomon, G., Elberling, C., Larsen, B., & Lassen, N. A. (1980). Middle components of the auditory evoked response in bilateral temporal lobe lesions. *Scandinavian Audiology, 9,* 161–167.

Pasanisi, E., Vincenti, V., Bacciu, A., Guida, M., & Bacciu, S. (2002). The nucleus contour electrode array: An electrophysiological study. *Laryngoscope, 112,* 1653–1656.

Pasman, J. W., Rotteveel, J. J., de Graaf, R., Maassen, B., & Notermans, S. L. (1991). Detectability of auditory evoked response components in preterm infants. *Early Human Development, 26,* 129–141.

Pastores, G., Michels, V., & Jack, C. (1991). Early childhood diagnosis of acoustic neuromas in presymptomatic individuals at risk for neurofibromatosis 2. *American Journal of Medical Genetics, 41,* 325–329.

Patrick, G., Straumanis, J. J., Struve, F. A., Fitz-Gerald, M. J., & Manno, J. E. (1997). Early and middle latency evoked potentials in medically and psychiatrically normal daily marihuana users: A paucity of significant findings. *Clinical Electroencephalography, 28,* 26–31.

Patrick, G., Straumanis, J. J., Struve, F. A., Nixon, F., Fitz-Gerald, M. J., Manno, J. E., & Soucair, M. (1995). Auditory and visual P300 event related potentials are not altered in medically and psychiatrically normal chronic marihuana users. *Life Sciences, 56,* 2135–2140.

Patterson, J. V., Michalewski, H. J., & Starr, A. (1988). Latency variability of the components of auditory event-related potentials to infrequent stimuli in aging, Alzheimer-type dementia, and depression. *Electroencephalography and Clinical Neurophysiology, 71,* 450–460.

Patterson, J. V., Michalewski, H. J., Thompson, L. W., Bowman, T. E., & Litzelman, D. K. (1981). Age and sex differences in the human auditory system. *Journal of Gerontology, 36,* 455–462.

Patuzzi, R. B., & O'Beirne, G. A. (1999). A correlation method for detecting the sound-evoked post-auricular muscle response (PAMR). *Hearing Research, 138,* 147–162.

Pauwels, H.P., Vogeleer, M., Clement, P. A., Rousseeuw, P. J., & Kaufman, L. (1982). Brainstem electric response audiometry in newborns. *International Journal of Pediatric Otorhinolaryngology, 4,* 317–323.

Pazo-Alvarez, P., Cadaveira, F., & Amenedo, E. (2003). MMN in the visual modality: A review. *Biological Psychology, 63,* 199–236.

Peake, W. T., & Kiang, N. Y. S. (1962). Cochlear responses to condensation and rarefaction clicks. *Biophysical Journal, 2,* 23–34.

Pearce, J., Crowell, D., Tokioka, A., & Pacheco, G. (1989). Childhood developmental changes in the auditory P300. *Journal of Child Neurology, 4,* 100–106.

Peck, J. E. (1984). Hearing loss in Hunter's syndrome. II. Mucopolysaccaridosis. *Ear and Hearing, 5,* 243–246.

Pedersen, L., & Trojaborg, W. (1981). Visual, auditory and somatosensory pathway involvement in hereditary cerebellar ataxia, Friedreich's ataxia and familial spastic paraplegia. *Electroencephalography and Clinical Neurophysiology, 52,* 283–297.

Pekkonen, E. (2000). Mismatch negativity in aging and in Alzheimer's and Parkinson's diseases. *Audiology & Neuro-Otology, 5,* 216–224.

Pekkonen, E., Jousmaki, V., Kononen, M., Reinikainen, K., & Partanen, J. (1994). Auditory sensory memory impairment in Alzheimer's disease: An event-related potential study. *Neuroreport, 5,* 2537–2540.

Pekkonen, E., Katila, H., Ahveninen, J., Karhu, J., Huotilainen, M., & Tuhonen, J. (2002). Impaired temporal lobe processing of preattentive auditory discrimination in schizophrenia. *Schizophrenia Bulletin, 28,* 467–474.

Pekkonen, E., Rinne, T., & Näätänen, R. (1995). Variability and replicability of the mismatch negativity. *Electroencephalography and Clinical Neurophysiology, 96,* 546–554.

Pekkonen, E., Rinne, T., Reinikainen, K., Kujala, T., Alho, K., & Näätänen, R. (1996). Aging effects on auditory processing: an event-related potential study. *Experimental Aging Research, 22,* 171–184.

Peled, R., Pratt, H., Scharf, B., & Lavie, P. (1983). Auditory brainstem evoked potentials during sleep apnea. *Neurology, 33,* 419–423.

Pelizzone, M., Kasper, A., & Montandon, P. (1989). Electrically evoked responses in cochlear implant patients. *Audiology, 28,* 230–238.

Pelson, R. O., & Budden, S. S. (1987). Auditory brainstem response findings in Rhett syndrome. *Brain Development, 9,* 514–516.

Peltola, M., Jaaskelainen, S., Heinonen, O., Falck, B., Nanto-Salonen, K., Heinanen, K., et al. (2002). Peripheral nervous system in gyrate atrophy of the choroid and retina with hyperornithinemia. *Neurology, 59,* 735–740.

Perez, G., Rodrigo, C., Perolada Valmana, J., Ibanez, A., & Morera, P. (1997). [Cochleovestibular nerve compression syndrome. A case report.] *Acta Otorhinolaringologica Espana, 48,* 305–308.

Perez-Abalo, M., Savio, G., Torres, A., Martin, V., Rodriguez, E., & Galan, L. (2001). Steady state responses to multiple amplitide-modulated tones: An optimized method to test frequency-specific thresholds in hearing-impaired children and normal-hearing subjects. *Ear and Hearing, 22,* 200–211.

Perez-Abalo, M., Valdes-Sosa, M., Bobes, M., Galan, L., & Biscay, R. (1988). Different functional properties of on and off components in auditory brainstem response to tone bursts. *Audiology, 27,* 249–259.

Perlman, H., & Case, T. (1941). Electrical phenomena of the cochlea in man. *Archives of Otolaryngology, 34,* 710–718.

Perlman, H., Kimura, R., & Fernandez, C. (1959). Experiments on temporary obstruction of the internal auditory artery. *Laryngoscope, 69,* 591–613.

Perlman, M., Fainmesser, P., Sohmer, H., Tamari, H., Wax, Y., & Pevsmer, B. (1983). Auditory nerve-brainstem evoked responses in hyperbilirubinemic neonates. *Pediatrics, 72,* 658–664.

Peronnet, F., & Michal, F. (1977). The asymmetry of the auditory evoked potentials in normal man and in patients with brain lesions. In C. Barber (Ed.), *Evoked potentials* (pp. 317–324). Baltimore: University Park Press.

Peronnet, F., Michal, F., Echallier, J. F., & Girod, J. (1974). Coronal topography of human auditory evoked responses. *Electroencephalography and Clinical Neurophysiology, 37,* 225–230.

Perrault, N., & Picton, T. W. (1984). Event-related potentials recorded from the scalp and nasopharynx. II. N2, P3 and slow wave. *Electroencephalography and Clinical Neurophysiology, 59,* 261–278.

Perrin, F., Bastuji, H., & García-Larrea, L. (2002). Detection of verbal discordances during sleep. *Neuroreport, 19,* 1345–1349.

Perrin, F., Bastuji, H., Mauguiere, F., & García-Larrea, L. (2000). Functional dissociation of the early and late portions of human K-complexes. *Neuroreport, 11,* 1637–1640.

Perrin, F., García-Larrea, L., Mauguiere, F., & Bastuji, H. (1999). A differential brain response to the subject's own name persists during sleep. *Clinical Neurophysiology, 110,* 2153–2164.

Peters, J. F., & Mendel, M. I. (1974). Early components of the averaged electroencephalic response to monaural and binaural stimulation. *Audiology, 13,* 195–204.

Peterson, A., Shallop, J., Driscoll, C., Breneman, A., Babb, J., et al. (2003). Outcomes of cochlear implantation in children with auditory neuropathy. *Journal of the American Academy of Audiology, 14,* 188–201.

Pettigrew, A., & Hutchinson, I. (1985). Effects of alcohol on functional development of the auditory pathway in the brainstem of infants and chick embryo. In M. O'Connor, (Ed.), *Mechanisms of alcohol damage in utero.* (pp. 24–26). Ciba Foundation Symposium. London: Pitman.

Pettigrew, C. M., Murdoch, B. E., Kei, J., Chenery, H., Sockalingam, R., Ponton, C. W., Finnigan, S., & Alku, P. (2004a). Processing of English words with fine acoustic contrasts and simple tones: A mismatch negativity study. *Journal of the American Academy of Audiology, 15,* 47–66.

Pettigrew, C. M., Murdoch, B. E., Ponton, C. W., Finnigan, S., Alku, P., Kei, J., Sockalingam, R., & Chenery, H. J. (2004b). Automatic auditory processing of English words as indexed by the mismatch negativity, using a multiple deviant paradigm. *Ear and Hearing, 25,* 284–301.

Pettigrew, C. M., Murdoch, B., Ponton, C., Kei, J., Chenery, H., & Alku, P. (2004c). Subtitled videos and mismatch negativity (MMN) investigations of spoken word processing. *Journal of the American Academy of Audiology, 15,* 469–485.

Pfefferbaum, A., Buchsbaum, M., & Gips, J. (1971). Enhancement of the averaged evoked response to tone onset and cessation. *Psychophysiology, 8,* 332–339.

Pfefferbaum, A., Ford, J. M., & Kraemer, H. C. (1990). Clinical utility of long latency 'cognitive' event-related potentials (P3): The cons. *Electroencephalography and Clinical Neurophysiology, 76,* 6–12.

Pfefferbaum, A., Ford, J. M., Roth, W. T., & Kopell, B. S. (1980). Age-related changes in auditory event-related potentials. *Electroencephalography and Clinical Neurophysiology, 49,* 266–276.

Pfefferbaum, A., Ford, J. M., Weller, B. J., & Kopell, B. S. (1985). ERPs to response production and inhibition. *Electroencephalography and Clinical Neurophysiology, 60,* 423–434.

Pfefferbaum, A., Ford, J. M., Wenegrat, B. G., Roth, W. T., & Kopell, B. S. (1984). Clinical application of the P3 component of event-related potentials. I Normal Aging. *Electroencephalography and Clinical Neurophysiology, 59,* 85–103.

Pfefferbaum, A., Ford, J. M., White, P. M., & Roth, W. T. (1989). P3 in schizophrenia is affected by stimulus modality, response requirements, medication status, and negative symptoms. *Archives of General Psychiatry, 46,* 1035–1044.

Pfefferbaum, A., Horvath, T. B., Roth, W. T., & Kopell, B. (1979). Event-related potential changes in chronic alcoholics. *Electroencephalography and Clinical Neurophysiology, 46,* 637–647.

Pfefferbaum, A., Roth, W. T., Tinklenberg, J. R., Rosenbloom, J. J., & Kopell, B. S. (1979). The effects of ethanol and meperidine on auditory evoked potentials. *Drug and Alcohol Dependency, 4,* 371–380.

Pfefferbaum, A., Wenegrat, B. G., Ford, J. M., Roth, W. T., & Kopell, B. S. (1984). Clinical application of the P3 component of event-related potentials. II. Dementia, depression and schizophrenia. *Electroencephalography and Clinical Neurophysiology, 59,* 104–124.

Pfeiffer, R. R. (1974). Consideration of the acoustic stimulus. In W. D. Keidel & W. D. Neff (Eds.), *Handbook of sensory physiology: Auditory system. Anatomy and physiology.* New York: Springer-Verlag .

Pfeiffer, R. R., & Kim, D. O. (1972). Response patterns of single cochlear nerve fibers to click stimuli: Descriptions for cat. *Journal of Acoustical Society of America, 52,* 1669–1677.

Pfurtscheller, G. (1992). Event-related synchronization (ERS): An electrophysiological correlate of cortical areas at rest. *Electroencephalography and Clinical Neurophysiology, 83,* 62–69.

Philbert, B., Durrant, J., Ferber-Viart, C., Duclaux, R., Veuillet, E., & Collet, L. (2003). Stacked tone-burst-evoked auditory brainstem response (ABR): Preliminary findings. *International Journal of Audiology, 42,* 71–81.

Phillips, K. R., Potvin, A. R., Syndulko, K., Cohen, S. N., Tourtelotte, W. W., & Potvin, J. H. (1983). Multimodality evoked potentials and neurophysiological tests in multiple sclerosis: Effects of hyperthermia on test results. *Archives of Neurology, 40,* 159–164.

Phillips, N. A., Connolly, J. F., Mate-Kole, C. C., & Gray, J. (1997). Individual differences in auditory middle latency responses in elderly adults and patients with Alzheimer's disease. *International Journal of Psychophysiology, 27,* 125–136.

Piatt, J. H., Jr., & Schiff, S. J. (1984). High dose barbiturate therapy in neurosurgery and intensive care. *Neurosurgery, 15,* 427–444.

Piatt, J. H., Radtke, R. A., & Erwin, C. W. (1985). Limitations of brain stem auditory evoked potentials for intraoperative monitoring during a posterior fossa operation: Case report and technical note. *Neurosurgery, 16,* 818–821.

Pickles, J. O. (1988). *An introduction to the physiology of hearing.* New York: Academic Press.

Picton, T. W. (1995). The neurophysiological evaluation of auditory discrimination. *Ear and Hearing, 16,* 1–5.

Picton, T. W., Alain, C., Otten, L., Ritter, W., & Achim, A. (2000). Mismatch negativity: Different water in the same river. *Audiology & Neuro-Otology, 5,* 111–139.

Picton, T. W., Bentin, S., Berg, P., Donchin, E., Hillyard, S., Johnson, R., Jr., Miller, G., Ritter, W., Ruchkin, D., Rugg, M., & Taylor, M. (2000). Guidelines for using human event-related potentials to study cognition: Recording standards and publication criteria. *Psychophysiology, 37,* 127–152.

Picton, T. W., Dimitrijevic, A., John, M. S., & Van Roon, P. (2001). The use of phase in the detection of auditory steady-state responses. *Clinical Neurophysiology, 112,* 1698–1711.

Picton, T. W., Durieux-Smith, A., Champagne, S., Whittingham, J., Moran, L., Giguere, C., et al. (1998). Objective evaluation of aided thresholds using auditory steady-state responses. *Journal of the American Academy of Audiology, 9,* 315–331.

Picton, T. W., & Hillyard, S. A. (1974). Human auditory evoked potentials. II. Effects of attention. *Electroencephalography and Clinical Neurophysiology, 36,* 191–199.

Picton, T. W., Hillyard, S. A., & Galambos, R. (1971). Human auditory attention: A central or peripheral process? *Science, 173,* 351–353.

Picton, T. W., Hillyard, S. A., & Galambos, R. (1976). Habituation and attention in the auditory system. In W. Keidel & W. Neff (Eds.), *Handbook of sensory physiology: The auditory system.* (pp. 345–389). Berlin: Springer.

Picton, T. W., Hillyard, S. A., Krausz, H. I., & Galambos, R. (1974). Human auditory evoked potentials. I. Evaluation of the components. *Electroencephalography and Clinical Neurophysiology, 36,* 179–190.

Picton, T. W., & John, M. (2004). Avoiding electromagnetic artifacts when recording auditory steady-state responses. *Journal of the American Academy of Audiology, 15,* 541–554.

Picton, T. W., John, M., Dimitrijevic, A., & Purcell, D. (2003). Human auditory steady-state responses. *International Journal of Audiology, 42,* 177–219.

Picton, T. W., Ouelette, K., Hamel, G., & Smith, A. D. (1979). Brainstem evoked potential to tonepips in notched noise. *Journal of Otolaryngology, 8,* 289–314.

Picton, T. W., Skinner, C., Champagne, S., Kellett, A., & Maiste, A. (1987). Potentials evoked by the sinusoidal modulation of the amplitude or frequency of a tone. *Journal of the Acoustical Society of America, 82,* 165–178.

Picton, T. W., Stapells, D. R., & Campbell, K. B. (1981). Auditory evoked potentials from the human cochlea and brainstem. *Journal of Otolaryngology (Toronto), 10,* 1–14.

Picton, T. W., Stapells, D. R., Perrault, N., Baribeau-Braun, J., & Stuss, D. T. (1984). Human event-related potentials: Current perspectives. In R. H. Nodar & C. Barber (Eds.), *Evoked potentials II* (pp. 3–16). Boston: Butterworth.

Picton, T. W., Woods, D. L., & Proulx, G. B. (1978). Human auditory sustained potentials. II. Stimulus relationships. *Electroencephalography and Clinical Neurophysiology, 45,* 198–210.

Picton, T. W., Woods, D. L., Baribeau-Braun, J., & Healey, T. M. G. (1977). Evoked potential audiometry. *Journal of Otolaryngology (Toronto), 6,* 90–119.

Pietrowsky, R., Dentler, M., Fehm, H., & Born, J. (1992). Effects of calcitonin on human auditory and visual evoked brain potentials. *Psychopharmacology (Berlin), 107,* 50–54.

Pijl, S. (1987). Effects of click polarity on ABR peak latency and morphology in a clinical population. *Journal of Otolaryngology, 16,* 89–96.

Pijl, S., & Schwartz, D. (1995). Melody recognition and musical interval perception by deaf subjects stimulated with electrical pulse trains through single cochlear electrodes. *Journal of the Acoustical Society of America, 98,* 886–895.

Pikus, A. (1995). Pediatric audiologic profile in type 1 and type 2 neurofibromatosis. *Journal of the American Academy of Audiology, 6,* 54–62.

Pillion, J., & Naidu, S. (2000). Auditory brainstem repsonse findings in Rett syndrome: Stability over time. *Journal of Pediatrics, 137,* 393–396.

Pillion, J., Rawool, V., & Naidu, S. (2000). Auditory brainstem reponses in Rett syndrome: Effects of hyperventilation, seizures, and tympanometric variables. *Audiology, 39,* 80–87.

Plum, F., & Posner, J. B. (1980). *The diagnosis of stupor and coma.* Philadelphia: F. A. Davis.

Podoshin, L., Ben-David, Y., Pratt, H., Fradis, M., & Feiglin, H. (1986). Noninvasive recordings of cochlear evoked potentials in Ménière's disease. *Archives of Otolaryngology—Head & Neck Surgery, 112,* 827–829.

Podoshin, L., Ben-David, J., Pratt, H., Fradis, M., Sharf, B., Weller, B., et al. (987). Auditory brainstem and visual evoked potentials in patients with migraine. *Headache, 27,* 27–29.

Polich, J. (1986). Attention, probability, and task demands as determinants of P300 latency from auditory stimuli. *Electroencephalography and Clinical Neurophysiology, 63,* 251–259.

Polich, J. (1986). Normal variation of P300 from auditory stimuli. *Electroencephalography and Clinical Neurophysiology, 65,* 236–240.

Polich, J. (1986). P300 development from auditory stimuli. *Psychophysiology, 23,* 590–597.

Polich, J. (1987). Response mode and P300 from auditory stimuli. *Biological Psychology, 25,* 61–71.

Polich, J. (1989). P300 for a passive auditory paradigm. *Electroencephalography and Clinical Neurophysiology, 74,* 312–320.

Polich, J. (1996). Meta-analysis of P300 normative aging studies. *Psychophysiology, 33,* 334–353.

Polich, J. (1997). EEG and ERP assessment of normal aging. *Electroencephalography and Clinical Neurophysiology, 104,* 244–256.

Polich, J. (2004). Clinical application of the P300 event-related brain potential. *Physical Medicine and Rehabilitation Clinics of North America, 15,* 133–161.

Polich, J., Alexander, J., Bauer, L., Kuperman, S., Morzorati, S., O'Connor, S., Porjesz, B., Rohrbaugh, J., & Begleiter, H. (1997). P300 topography of amplitude/latency correlations. *Brain Topography, 9,* 275–282.

Polich, J., & Bloom, F. E. (1987). P300 from normals and adult children of alcoholics. *Alcohol, 4,* 301–305.

Polich, J., & Bondurant, T. (1997). P300 sequence effects, probability, and interstimulus interval. *Psychology and Behavior, 61,* 843–849.

Polich, J., Ehlers, C. E., Otis, S., Mandell, A. J., & Bloom, F. E. (1986). P300 reflects the degree of cognitive decline in dementing illness. *Electroencephalography and Clinical Neurophysiology, 63,* 138–144.

Polich, J., Eischen, S. E., & Collins, G. E. (1994). P300 from a single auditory stimulus. *Electroencephalography and Clinical Neurophysiology, 92,* 253–261.

Polich, J., & Herbst, K. (2000). P300 as a clinical assay: Rationale, evaluation, and findings. *International Journal of Psychophysiology, 38,* 3–19.

Polich, J., & Hoffman, L. (1998). P300 and handedness: On the possible contribution of corpus callosal size to ERPs. *Psychophysiology, 35,* 497–507.

Polich, J., Howard, L., & Starr, A. (1983). A P300 latency correlates with digit span. *Psychophysiology, 20,* 665–669.

Polich, J., Howard, L., & Starr, A. (1985). Stimulus frequency and masking as determinants of P300 latency in event-related potentials from auditory stimuli. *Biological Psychology, 21,* 309–318.

Polich, J., Ladish, C., & Burns, T. (1990). Normal variation of P300 in children: Age, memory span and head size. *International Journal of Psychophysiology, 3,* 237–248.

Polich, J., & Lardon, M. (1997). P300 and long-term physical exercise. *Electroencephalography and Clinical Neurophysiology, 103,* 493–498.

Polich, J., & McIsaac, H. K. (1994). Comparison of auditory P300 habituation from active and passive conditions. *International Journal of Psychophysiology, 17,* 25–34.

Polich, J., Moore, A. P., & Wiederhold, M. D. (1995). P300 assessment of chronic fatigue syndrome. *Journal of Clinical Neurophysiology, 12,* 186–191.

Polich, J., Pollock, V., & Bloom, F. (1994). Meta-analysis of P300 amplitude from males at risk for alcoholism. *Psychological Bulletin, 115,* 55–73.

Polich, J., Romine, J. S., Sipe, J. C., Aung, M., & Dalessio, D. J. (1992). P300 in multiple sclerosis: A preliminary report. *International Journal of Psychophysiology, 12,* 155–163.

Polich, J., & Squires, L. R. (1993). P300 from amnesic patients with bilateral hippocampal lesions. *Electroencephalography and Clinical Neurophysiology, 86,* 408–417.

Polizzi, A., Mauceri, L., & Ruggieri, M. (1999). Hypotonia, congenital nystagmus, ataxia, and abnormal auditory brainstem responses: A report on the first white patient. *Developmental Medicine and Child Neurology, 41,* 51–54.

Pollock, V. E., & Schneider, L. S. (1989). Effects of tone stimulus frequency on late positive component activity (P3) among normal elderly subjects. *International Journal of Neuroscience, 45,* 127–132.

Polo, M. D., Escera, C., Gual, A., & Grau, C. (1999). Mismatch negativity and auditory sensory memory in chronic alcoholics. *Alcohol Clinical and Experimental Research, 23,* 1744–1750.

Polo, M. D., Newton, P., Rogers, D., Escera, C., & Butler, S. (2002). ERPs and behavioural indices of long-term preattentive and attentive deficits after closed head injury. *Neuropsychologia, 40,* 2350–2359.

Polyakov, A., & Pratt, H. (1994). Three-channel Lissajous' trajectory of human middle latency auditory evoked potentials. *Ear and Hearing, 15,* 390–399.

Ponton, C. W., & Don, M. (1995). The mismatch negativity in cochlear implant users. *Ear and Hearing, 16,* 131–146.

Ponton, C. W., Don, M., Eggermont, J. J., & Kwong, B. (1997). Integrated mismatch negativity (MMNi): A noise-free representation of evoked responses allowing single-point distribution-free statistical tests. *Electroencephalography and Clinical Neurophysiology, 104,* 143–150.

Ponton, C. W., Don, M., Eggermont, J., Waring, M., Kwong, B., & Masuda, A. (1996). Auditory plasticity in children after long periods of complete deafness. *Neuroreport, 8,* 61–65.

Ponton, C. W., Don, M., Eggermont, J. J., Waring, M. D., & Masuda, A. (1996). Maturation of human cortical auditory function: Differences between normal-hearing children and children with cochlear implants. *Ear and Hearing, 17,* 430–437.

Ponton, C. W., & Eggermont, J. J. (2001). Of kittens and kids: Altered cochlear maturation following profound deafness and cochlear implant use. *Audiology & Neuro-Otology, 6,* 263–280.

Ponton, C. W., Eggermont, J. J., Don, M., Waring, M. D., Kwong, B., Cunningham, J., & Trautwein, P. (2000). Maturation of the mismatch negativity: effects of profound deafness and cochlear implant use. *Audiology & Neuro-Otology, 5,* 167–185.

Ponton, C. W., Moore, J. K., & Eggermont, J. J. (1996). Auditory brain stem response generation by parallel pathways: Differential maturation of axonal conduction time and synaptic transmission. *Ear and Hearing, 17,* 402–410.

Ponton, C. W., Moore, J. K., & Eggermont, J. J. (1999). Prolonged deafness limits auditory system developmental plasticity: evidence from an evoked potentials study in children with cochlear implants. *Scandinavian Audiology, 28 (Supplement 51),* 13–22.

Pool, K. D., Finitzo, T., Hong, C. T., Rogers, J., & Pickett, R. B. (1989). Infarction of the superior temporal gyrus: A description of auditory evoked potential latency and amplitude topology. *Ear and Hearing, 10,* 144–152.

Popescu, M., Papadimitriou, S., Karamitsos, D., & Bezerianos, A. (1999). Adaptive denoising and multiscale detection of the V wave in brainstem auditory evoked potentials. *Audiology & Neuro Otology, 4,* 38–50.

Popper, A., Platt, C., & Saidal, W. (1982). Acoustic functions in the fish ear. *Trends in Neuroscience, 5,* 276–280.

Porjesz, B., & Begleiter, H. (1981). Human evoked brain potentials and alcohol. *Alcoholism: Clinical and Experimental Research, 5,* 304–317.

Portmann, M., Dauman, R., Duriez, F., Portmann, D., & Dhillon, R. (1989). Modern diagnostic strategy for acoustic neuromas. *Archives of Otorhinolaryngology, 246,* 286–291.

Portnoy, R. K., Kurtzberg, D., Arezzo, J. C., Sands, G. H., Miller, A., & Vaughan, H. G., Jr. (1985). Return to alertness after brain-stem hemorrhage: A case with evoked potential and roentgenographic evidence of bilateral tegmental damage. *Archives of Neurology, 42,* 85–88.

Poth, E., Boettcher, F., Mills, J., & Dubno, J. (2001). Auditory brainstem responses in younger and older adults for broadband noises separated by a silent gap. *Hearing Research, 161,* 81–86.

Potter, D., & Barrett, K. (1999). Assessment of mild head injury with ERPs and neuropsychological tasks. *Journal of Psychophysiology, 13,* 200–206.

Potter, D., Bassett, M., Jory, S., & Barrett, K. (2001). Changes in event-related potentials in a three-stimulus auditory oddball task after mild head injury. *Neuropsychologia, 39,* 1464–1472.

Potter, D., Pickles, C., Roberts, R., & Rugg, M. (1992). The effects of scopolamine on event-related potentials in a continuous recognition memory task. *Psychophysiology, 29,* 29–37.

Pou, A. M., Hirsch, B. E., Durrant, J. D., Gold, S. R., & Kamerer, D. B. (1996). The efficacy of tympanic electrocochleography in the diagnosis of endolymphatic hydrops. *American Journal of Otology, 17,* 607–611.

Poungvarin, N. (1991). Multifocal brain damage due to lacquer sniffing: The first case report of Thailand. *Journal of the Medical Association of Thailand, 74,* 296–300.

Pradhan, S. N., & Galambos, R. (1963). Some effects of anesthetics on the evoked responses in the auditory cortex of cats. *Journal of Pharmacology and Experimental Therapy, 139,* 97–106.

Prasher, D. K., & Gibson, W. P. R. (1980a). Brain stem auditory evoked potential: Significant latency differences between ipsilateral and contralateral stimulation. *Electroencephalography and Clinical Neurophysiology, 50,* 240–246.

Prasher, D. K., & Gibson, W. P. R. (1980b). Brain stem auditory evoked potentials: A comparison study of monaural versus binaural stimularion in the detection of multiple sclerosis. *Electroencephalography and Clinical Neurophysiology, 50,* 247–253.

Prasher, D. K., & Gibson, W. P. R. (1984). Paradoxical reduction in AP amplitude on binaural stimulation. In R. H. Nodar & C. Barber (Eds.), *Evoked potentials II: The Second International Evoked Potentials Symposium,* pp. 157–181. Boston: Butterworth.

Prasher, D. K., Sainz, M., & Gibson, W. P. R. (1982). Binaural voltage summation of brainstem auditory evoked potentials: An adjunct to the diagnostic criteria for multiple sclerosis. *Annals of Neurology, 11,* 86–91.

Pratap-Chand, R., Sinniah, M., & Salem, F. (1988). Cognitive evoked potential (P300): A metric for cerebral concussion. *Acta Neurologica Scandinavica, 78,* 185–189.

Pratt, H., Ben-David, Y., Peled, R., Podoshin, L., & Scharf, B. (1981). Auditory brain stem potentials: Clinical promise of increasing stimulus rate. *Electroencephalography and Clinical Neurophysiology, 51,* 80–90.

Pratt, H., Berlad, I., & Lavie, P. (1999). "Oddball" event-related potentials and information processing during REM and non-REM sleep. *Clinical Neurophysiology, 110,* 53–61.

Pratt, H., & Bleich, N. (1982). Auditory brain stem potentials evoked by clicks in notch-filtered masking noise. *Electroencephalography and Clinical Neurophysiology, 53,* 417–426.

Pratt, H., Brodsky, G., Goldsher, M., et al. (1986). Auditory brainstem evoked potentials in patients undergoing dialysis. *Electroencephalography and Clinical Neurophysiology, 63,* 18–24.

Pratt, H., & Sohmer, H. (1976). Intensity and rate function of cochlear and brainstem evoked responses to click stimuli in man. *Archives of Otorhinolaryngology, 212,* 85–92.

Pratt, H., & Sohmer, H. (1977). Correlations between psychophysical magnitude estimates and simultaneously obtained auditory nerve, brain stem and cortical responses to click stimuli in man. *Electroencephalography and Clinical Neurophysiology, 43,* 802–812.

Pratt, H., & Sohmer, H. (1978). Comparison of hearing threshold determined by auditory pathway electric responses and by behavioral responses. *Audiology, 17,* 285–292.

Pratt, H., Urbach, D., & Bleich, N. (1989). Auditory brainstem evoked potentials peak identification by finite impulse response digital filters. *Audiology, 28,* 272–283.

Pratt, H., Yitzhak, E. B., & Attias, J. (1984). Auditory brain stem potentials evoked by clicks in notch-filtered masking noise. *Audiology, 23,* 380–387.

Pribram, K. H., Rosner, B. R., & Rosenblith, W. A. (1954). Electrical responses to acoustic clicks in monkey: Extent of neocortex activated. *Journal of Neurophysiology, 17,* 336–344.

Prieve, B. A., Gorga, M. P., & Neely, S. T. (1991). Otoacoustic emissions in an adult with severe hearing loss. *Journal of Speech and Hearing Research, 34,* 379–385.

Prijs, V. F. (1991). Evaluation of electrocochleographic audiogram determination in infants. *Acta Otolaryngologica Supplement, 482,* 27–33.

Pritchard, W. (1981). Psychophysiology of P300. *Psychological Bulletin, 89,* 506–540.

Prosser, S., & Arslan, E. (1985). Does general anaesthesia affect the child's auditory middle latency repsonse (MLR)?. *Scandinavian Audiology, 14,* 105–107.

Prosser, S., & Arslan, E. (1987). Prediction of auditory brainstem wave V latency as a diagnostic tool of sensorineural hearing loss. *Audiology, 26,* 179–187.

Prosser, S., Arslan, E., & Pastore, A. (1984). Auditory brain-stem response and hearing threshold in cerebellopontine angle tumours. *Archives of Otorhinolaryngology, 239,* 183–189.

Psatta, D. M., & Matei, M. (1988). Age-dependent amplitude variation of brain-stem auditory evoked potentials. *Electroencephalography and Clinical Neurophysiology, 71,* 27–32.

Ptok, M., Blachnik, P., & Schonweiler, R. (2004). NC-ERP in APD children with and without attention deficits. *HNO, 52,* 67–74.

Puce, A., Donnan, G. A., & Bladin, P. F. (1989b). Comparative effects of age on limbic and scalp P3. *Electroencephalography and Clinical Neurophysiology, 74,* 385–393.

Puce, A., Donnan, G. A., & Bladin, P. (1989a). Limbic P3 potentials, seizure location, and surgical pathology in temporal lobe epilepsy. *Annals of Neurology, 26,* 377–385.

Puente, A., Ysunza, A., Pamplona, M., Silva-Rojas, A., & Lara, C. (2002). Short latency and long latency auditory evoked responses in children with attention deficit disorder. *International Journal of Pediatric Otorhinolaryngology, 62,* 45–51.

Pulvermüller, F., Kujala, T., Shtyrov, Y., Simola, J., Tiitinen, H., Alku, P., Alho, K., Martinkauppi, S., Ilmoniemi, R., & Näätänen, R. (2001). Memory traces for words as revealed by the mismatch negativity. *NeuroImage, 14,* 607–616.

Purcell, D., John, M., Schneider, B., & Picton, T. (2004). Human temporal auditory acuity as assessed by envelope following responses. *Journal of the Acoustical Society of America, 116,* 3581–3593.

Purdie, J. A., & Cullen, P. M. (1993). Brainstem auditory evoked response during propofol anaesthesia in children. *Anaesthesia, 48,* 192–195.

Purdy, S. C., & Abbas, P. J. (1989). Auditory brainstem response audiometry using linearly and Blackman-gated tonebursts. *Asha, 31,* 115–116.

Purdy, S. C., & Abbas, P. J. (2002). ABR thresholds to tonebursts gated with Blackman and linear windows in adults with high-frequency sensorineural hearing loss. *Ear and Hearing, 23,* 358–368.

Purdy, S. C., Houghton, J. M., & Keith, W. J. (1989). Frequency-specific auditory brainstem responses. Effective masking levels and relationship to behavioral thresholds in normal hearing adults. *Audiology, 28,* 82–91.

Purdy, S. C., Kelly, A., & Davies, M. (2002). Auditory brainstem response, middle latency response, and late cortical evoked potentials in children with learning disabilities. *Journal of the American Academy of Audiology, 13,* 367–382.

Quick, C. A. (1980). Chemical and drug effects on the inner ear. In M. M. Paparella & D. A. Shumrick (Eds.), *Otolaryngology* (2nd ed., pp. 1804–1827). Philadelphia: WB Saunders.

Radionova, E. A. (1989). Off-responses in the auditory system in relation to the signal end phase and neuronal characteristic frequency. *Hearing Research, 35,* 229–236.

Raggazoni, A., Amantini, A., Rossi, L., & Bindi, A. (1982). Brain-stem auditory evoked potentials and vertebral-basilar reversible ischemic attacks. *Advances in Neurology, 32,* 187–194.

Raimondi, A. J., & Hirschauer, J. (1984). Head injury in the infant and toddler: Coma scoring and outcome scale. *Child's Brain, 11,* 12–35.

Rance, G., Beer, D., Cone-Wesson, B., Shepherd, R., Dowell, R., King, A., Rickards, F., & Clark, G. (1999). Clinical findings for a group of infants and young children with auditory neuropathy. *Ear and Hearing, 20,* 238–252.

Rance, G., & Briggs, R. (2002). Assessment of hearing in infants with moderate to profound impairment: The Melbourne experience with steady-state evoked potential testing. *Annals of Otology, Rhinology, and Laryngology, 111,* 22–28.

Rance, G., Dowell, R., Rickards, F., Beer, D., & Clark, G. (1998). Steady-state evoked potential and behavioral hearing thresholds in a group of children with absent click-evoked auditory brain stem response. *Ear and Hearing, 19,* 48–61.

Rance, G., & Rickards, F. (2002). Prediction of hearing threshold in infants using auditory steady-state evoked potentials. *Journal of the American Academy of Audiology, 13,* 236–245.

Rance, G., Rickards, F., Cohen, L., Burton, M., & Clark, G. (1993). Steady-state evoked potentials: A new tool for the accurate assessment of hearing in cochlear implant candidates. *Advances in Otorhinolaryngology, 48,* 44–48.

Rance, G., Rickards, F., Cohen, L., De Vidi, S., & Clark, G. (1995). The automated prediction of hearing thresholds in sleeping subjects using auditory steady-state evoked potentials. *Ear and Hearing, 16,* 499–507.

Rance, G., Roper, R., Symons, L., Moody, L., Poulis, C., Dourlay, M., & Kelly, T. (2005). Hearing threshold estimation in infants using Auditory Steady-State Responses. *Journal of the American Academy of Audiology. 16,* 291–300.

Rapin, I. (1964). Practical considerations in using the evoked potential technique for audiometry. *Acta Otolaryngologica Supp, 206,* 117–122.

Rapin, I., & Gravel, J. (2003). "Auditory neuropathy": Physiologic and pathologic evidence calls for more diagnostic specificity. *International Journal of Pediatric Otorhinolaryngology, 67,* 707–728.

Rapin, I., & Gravel, J. S. (2006) Auditory neuropathy: A biologically inappropriate label unless acoustic nerve involvement is documented. *Journal of the Academy of Audiology, 17,* 147–150.

Rapin, I., & Graziani, L. J. (1967). Auditory evoked responses in normal, brain-damaged and deaf infants. *Neurology, 17,* 881–894.

Rapin, I., Ruben, R. J., & Lyttle, M. (1970). Diagnosis of hearing loss in infants using auditory evoked responses. *Laryngoscope, 80,* 712–722.

Rapin, I., Schimmel, H., & Cohen, M. M. (1972). Reliability in detecting the auditory evoked response (AER) for audiometry in sleeping subjects. *Electroencephalography and Clinical Neurophysiology, 32,* 521–528.

Rapin, I., Schimmel, H., Tourk, L. M., Krasnegor, N. A., & Pollak, C. (1966). Evoked responses to clicks and tones of varying intensity in waking adults. *Electroencephalography and Clinical Neurophysiology, 21,* 335–344.

Rappaport, M., Hall, K., Hopkins, K., Belleza, T., Berrol, S., & Reynolds, G. (1977). Evoked brain potentials and disability in brain-damaged patients. *Archives of Physical Medicine and Rehabilitation, 58,* 333–338.

Rasco, L., Skinner, R. D., & Garcia-Rill, E. (2000). Effect of age on sensory gating of the sleep state-dependent P1/P50 midlatency auditory evoked potential. *Brain Research Online, 3,* 97–105.

Ratke, R. A., Erwin, A., & Erwin, C. W. (1986). Abnormal sensory evoked potentials in amyotrophic lateral sclerosis. *Neurology, 36,* 796–801.

Raudzens, P. A. (1982). Intraoperative monitoring of evoked potentials. *Annals of the New York Academy of Science, 388,* 308–326.

Raudzens, P. A., & Shetter, A. G. (1982). Intraoperative monitoring of brain-stem auditory evoked potentials. *Journal of Neurosurgery, 57,* 341–348.

Rawool, V. W., & Ballachanda, B. B. (1990). Homo- and anti-phasic stimulation in ABR. *Scandinavian Audiology, 19,* 9–15.

Rea, P. A., & Gibson, W. P. (2003). Evidence for surviving outer hair cell function in congenitally deaf ears. *Laryngoscope, 113,* 2030–2034.

Recart, A., Gasanova, I., White, P. F., Thomas, T., Ogunnaike, B., Hamza, M., & Wang, A. (2003). The effect of cerebral monitoring on recovery after general anaesthesia: A comparison of the auditory evoked potential and bispectral index devices with standard clinical practice. *Anaesthesia and Analgesia, 97,* 1667–1674.

Reddy, S. N., & Kirlin, R. L. (1979). Spectral analysis of auditory evoked potentials with pseudorandom noise excitation. *IEEE Transactions on Biomedical Engineering BME, 26,* 479–487.

Rees, A., Green, G. G. R., & Kay, R. H. (1986). Steady-state evoked responses to sinusoidally amplitude-modulated sounds recorded in man. *Hearing Research, 23,* 123–133.

Reese, N. B., Garcia-Rill, E., & Skinner, R. D. (1995). Auditory input to the pedunculopontine nucleus: I. Evoked potentials. *Brain Research Bulletin, 37,* 257–264.

Regan, D. (1966). Some characteristics of steady-state and transient responses evoked by modulated light. *Electroencephalography and Clinical Neurophysiology, 20,* 238–248.

Reich, D. S., & Wiatrak, B. J. (1996). Methods of sedation for auditory brainstem response testing. *International Journal of Pediatric Otorhinolaryngology, 38,* 131–141.

Reid, A., Birchall, J. P., & Moffat, D. A. (1984). Auditory brainstem responses: Masking related changes in wave VI. *British Journal of Audiology, 18,* 17–22.

Reid, A., & Thornton, A. R. D. (1983). The effects of contralateral masking upon brainstem electric responses. *British Journal of Audiology, 17,* 155–162.

Reilly, E. L., Kelley, J. T., Pena, Y. M., Overall, J. E., & Faillace, L. A. (1983). Short latency brainstem and somatosensory evoked potentials in alcoholics. *Clinical Electroencephalography, 14,* 8–16.

Reite, M., Teale, P., Zimmerman, J., Davis, K., Whalen, J., & Eldrich, J. (1988). Source origin of a 50-msec latency auditory evoked field component in young schizophrenic men. *Biological Psychiatry, 24,* 495–506.

Reneau, J. P., & Hnatiow, G. Z. (1975). *Evoked response audiometry: a topical and historical review.* University Park Press, Baltimore.

Renvall, H., & Hari, R. (2003). Diminished auditory mismatch fields in dyslexic adults. *Annals of Neurology, 53,* 551–557.

Reske-Nielsen, E., Lundbaek, K., & Rafaelson, O. (1968). Pathological changes in peripheral and central nervous system of young long-term diabetics. Diabetic encephalophaty. *Diabetologica, 1,* 233–241.

Reuter, B. M., & Linke, D. B. (1989). P300 and coma. In K. Maurer (Ed.), *Topographic brain mapping of EEG and evoked potentials* (pp. 192–196). Berlin: Springer.

Rhee, C., Park, H., & Jang, Y. (1999). Audiologic evaluation of neonates with severe hyperbilirubinemia using transiently evoked otoacoustic emissions and auditory brainstem responses. *Laryngoscope, 109,* 2005–2008.

Rhode, W. W., & Greenberg, S. (1994). Encoding of amplitude modulation in the cochlear nucleus of the cat. *Journal of Neurophysiology, 56,* 261–286.

Rickards, F. W., & Clark, G. M. (1984). Steady-state evoked potentials to amplitude-modulated tones. In R. H. Nodar & C. Barber (Eds.), *Evoked potentials II: The Second International Evoked Potentials Symposium* (pp. 163–168). Boston: Butterworth.

Rickards, F. W., Tan, L., Cohen, L., Wilson, O., Drew, J., & Clark, G. (1994). Auditory steady-state evoked potentials in newborns. *British Journal of Audiology, 28,* 327–337.

Riekkinen, P., Jr., Paakkonen, A., Karhu, J., Partanen, J., Soininen, H., Laakso, M., & Riekkinen, P., Sr. (1997). THA disrupts mismatch negativity in Alzheimer disease. *Psychopharmacology (Berlin), 133,* 203–206.

Rinne, T., Alho, K., Ilmoniemi, R. J., Virtanen, J., & Näätänen, R. (2000). Separate time behaviors of the temporal and frontal mismatch negativity sources. *Neuroimage, 12,* 14–19.

Rintelmann, W., Church, M., Simpson, T., & Root, L. (1995). Effects of maternal alcohol and/or cocaine on maternal ABRs. *American Auditory Society Bulletin, 20,* 14.

Ritter, W., Deacon, D., Gomes, H., Javitt, D.C., & Vaughan, H. G., Jr. (1995). The mismatch negativity of event-related potentials as a probe of transient auditory memory: A review. *Ear and Hearing, 16,* 52–67.

Ritter, W., Gomes, H., Cowan, N., Sussman, E., & Vaughan, H. G., Jr. (1998). Reactivation of a dormant representation of an auditory stimulus feature. *Journal of Cognitive Neuroscience, 10,* 605–614.

Ritter, W., Paavilainen, P., Lavikainen, J., Reinikainen, K., Alho, K., Sams, M., & Näätänen, R. (1992). Event-related potentials to repetition and change of auditory stimuli. *Electroencephalography and Clinical Neurophysiology, 83,* 306–321.

Ritter, W., Simson, R., Vaughan, H. G., Jr., & Friedman, D. (1979). A brain event related to the making of a sensory discrimination. *Science, 203,* 1358–61.

Ritter, W., Simson, R., Vaughan, H. G., Jr., & Macht, M. (1982). Manipulation of event-related potential manifestations of information processing stages. *Science, 218,* 909–911.

Ritter, W., Sussman, E., Deacon, D., Cowan, N., & Vaughan, H. G., Jr. (1999). Two cognitive systems simultaneously prepared for opposite events. *Psychophysiology, 36,* 835–838.

Ritter, W., Vaughan, H. G., Jr., & Costa, L. D. (1968). Orienting and habituation to auditory stimuli: A study of short term changes in average evoked responses. *Electroencephalography and Clinical Neurophysiology, 25,* 550–556.

Rizzo, P. A., Pierelli, F., Pozzessere, G., Floris, R., & Morocutti, C. (1983). Subjective posttraumatic syndrome: A comparison of visual and brain stem auditory evoked responses. *Neuropsychobiology, 9,* 78–82.

Rizzo, P. A., Pierelli, F., Pozzessere, G., Verardi, S., Casciani, C. U., & Morocutti, C. (1982). Pattern visual evoked potentials and brainstem auditory evoked responses in uremic patients. *Acta Neurologica Belgium, 82,* 72–79.

Roberson, J. J., Jackson, L., & McAuley, J. (1999). Acoustic neuroma surgery: Absent auditory brainstem response does not contraindicate attempted hearing preservation. *Laryngoscope, 109,* 904–910.

Roberson, J. J., O'Rourke, C., & Stidham, K. (2003). Auditory steady-state response testing in children: Evaluation of a new technology. *Archives of Otolaryngology—Head & Neck Surgery, 129,* 107–113.

Roberson, J., Senne, A., Brackmann, D., Hitselberger, W., & Saunders, J. (1996). Direct cochlear nreve action potentials as an aid to hearing preservation in middle fossa acoustic neuroma resection. *American Journal of Otology, 17,* 653–657.

Roberts, T. P., Ferrari, P., Stufflebeam, S. M., & Poeppel, D. (2000). Latency of the auditory evoked neuromagnetic field components: Stimulus dependence and insights toward perception. *Journal of Clinical Neurophysiology, 17,* 114–129.

Robertson, D. D., & Ireland, D. J. (1995). Vestibular evoked myogenic potentials. *The Journal of Otolaryngology, 24,* 3–8.

Robier, A., & Reynaud, J. (1984). Auditory-evoked brainstem potentials and stapedius muscle reflex: Intersubject variability. *Audiology, 23,* 490–497.

Robier, A., Saudeau, D., Autret, A., & Reynaud, J. (1981). Cerebrovascular accidents affecting the brain stem and evoked auditory potentials. *Revue de Oto-Neuro-Ophthalmologie, 53,* 301–310.

Robinette, M., Bauch, C., Olsen, W., & Cevette, M. (2000). Auditory brainstem response and magnetic resonance imaging for acoustic neuromas: Costs by prevalence. *Archives of Otolaryngology—Head & Neck Surgery, 126,* 963–966.

Robinson, G., Baumann, S., Kleinbaum, D., Barton, C., Schroeder, S., Mushak, P., & Otto, D. (1985). Effects of low-to-moderate lead exposure on brainstem auditory evoked potentials in children. In *Environmental health, 3: Neurobehavioral methods in occupational and enviromental health.* (pp 177–182). Copenhagen: World Health Organization.

Robinson, K., & Rudge, P. (1977). Abnormalities of the auditory evoked potentials in patients with multiple sclerosis. *Brain, 100,* 19–40.

Robinson, K., & Rudge, P. (1980). The use of the auditory evoked potential in the diagnosis of multiple sclerosis. *Journal of Neurology Sciences, 45,* 235–244.

Robinson, K., & Rudge, P. (1983). The differential diagnosis of cerebellopontine angle lesions: A multidisciplinary approach with special emphasis on the brainstem auditory evoked potential. *Journal of Neurological Science, 60,* 1–21.

Rodin, E., Khabbazeh, Z., Twitty, G., & Schmaltz, S. (1989). The cognitive evoked potential in epilepsy patients. *Clinical Electroencephalography, 20,* 176–182.

Rodriguez-Ballesteros, M., del Castillo, F. J., Martin, Y., Moreno-Pelayo, M. A., Morera, C., Prieto, F., Marco, J., Morant, A., Gallo-Teran, J., Morales-Angulo, C., Navas, C., Trinidad, G., Tapia, M. C., Moreno, F.,

& del, C., I (2003). Auditory neuropathy in patients carrying mutations in the otoferlin gene (OTOF). *Human Mutation, 22,* 451–456.

Rodriguez-Holguin, S., Corral, M., & Cadaveira, F. (2001). Middle-latency auditory evoked potentials in children at high risk for alcoholism. *Neurophysiology Clinics, 31,* 40–47.

Roland, P. S., Rosenbloom, J., Yellin, W., & Meyerhoff, W. L. (1993). Intrasubject test-retest variability in clinical electrocochleography. *Laryngoscope, 103,* 963–966.

Roland, P. S., Yellin, M. W., Meyerhoff, W. L., & Frank, T. (1995). Simultaneous comparison between transtympanic and extratympanic electrocochleography. *American Journal of Otology, 16,* 444–450.

Roman, S., Canevet, G., Marquis, P., Triglia, J., & Liegeois-Chauvel, C. (2005). Relationship between auditory perception skills and mismatch negativity recorded in free field in cochlear-implant users. *Hearing Research, 201,* 10–20.

Romero, R., & Polich, J. (1986). P3(00) habituation from auditory and visual stimuli. *Physiology and Behavior, 59,* 517–522.

Ropper, A., & Chiappa, K. (1986). Evoked potentials in Guillain-Barre syndrome. *Neurology, 36,* 587–590.

Rosburg, T. (2004). Effects of tone repetition on auditory evoked neuromagnetic fields. *Clinical Neurophysiology, 115,* 898–905.

Rosburg, T., Haueisen, J., & Kreitschmann-Andermahr, I. (2004). The dipole location shift within the auditory evoked neuromagnetic field components N100m and mismatch negativity (MMNm). *Clinical Neurophysiology, 115,* 906–913.

Rosburg, T., Haueisen, J., & Sauer, H. (2002). Stimulus duration influences the dipole location shift within the auditory evoked field component N100m. *Brain Topography, 15,* 37–41.

Rosburg, T., Kreitschmann-Andermahr, I., & Sauer, H. (2004). Mismatch negativity in schizophrenia research. An indicator of early processing disorders of acoustic information. *Nervenarzt, 75,* 633–641.

Rosburg, T., Marinou, V., Haueisen, J., Smesny, S., & Sauer, H. (2004). Effects of lorazepam on the neuromagnetic mismatch negativity (MMNm) and auditory evoked field component N100m. *Neuropsychopharmacology, 29,* 1723–1733.

Rosburg, T., Trautner, P., Korzyukov, O. A., Boutros, N. N., Schaller, C., Elger, C. E., & Kurthen, M. (2004). Short-term habituation of the intracranially recorded auditory evoked potentials P50 and N100. *Neuroscience Letters, 372,* 245–249.

Roschke, J., Wagner, P., Mann, K., Prentice-Cuntz, T., & Frank, C. (1998). Amplitude frequency characteristics of evoked potentials during sleep: An analysis of the brain's transfer properties in depression. *Biological Psychiatry, 40,* 736–743.

Rose, A. S., Ellison, G. W., Myers, L. W., & Tourtelotte, W. W. (1976). Criteria for the clinical diagnosis of multiple sclerosis. *Neurology, 26,* 20–22.

Rose, D. E., & Malone, J. C. (1965). Some aspects of the acoustically evoked response to the cessation of stimulus. *Journal of Auditory Research, 5,* 27–40.

Rosenberg, C., Wogensen, K., & Starr, A. (1984). Auditory brainstem and middle- and long-latency evoked potentials in coma. *Archives of Neurology, 41,* 835–838.

Rosenberg, S. (2000). Natural history of acoustic neuromas. *Laryngoscope, 110,* 497–508.

Rosenblatt, B., & Majnemer, A. (1984). Brainstem auditory evoked potentials in children with brainstem encephalitis. In R. H. Nodar & C. Barber (Eds.), *Evoked potentials II: The Second International Evoked Potentials Symposium* (pp. 216–223). Boston: Butterworth.

Rosenblum, S. M., Ruth, R. A., & Gal, T. J. (1985). Brainstem auditory evoked potential monitoring during profound hypothermia and circulatory arrest. *Annals of Otology, Rhinology, & Laryngology, 94,* 281–283.

Rosenhall, U. (1981a). Brain stem electrical responses in cerebello-pontine angle tumours. *Journal of Laryngology & Otology, 95,* 931–940.

Rosenhall, U. (1981b). ABR and cerebellopontine angle tumors. *Scandinavian Audiology, 13,* 115.

Rosenhall, U., & Axelsson, A. 1995. Auditory brainstem response latencies in patients with tinnitus. *Scandinavian Audiology, 24,* 97–100.

Rosenhall, U., Bjorkman, G., Pedersen, K., & Kall, A. (1985). Brain-stem auditory evoked potentials in different age groups. *Electroencephalography and Clinical Neurophysiology, 62,* 426–430.

Rosenhall, U., Edstrom, S., Hanner, P., Badr, G., & Vahlne, A. (1983). Auditory brain stem response and abnormalities in patients with Bell's palsy. *Archives of Otolaryngology—Head & Neck Surgery, 91,* 412–416.

Rosenhall, U., Hadner, M.-.L., & Bjorkman, G. (1981). ABR in brain stem lesions. *Scandinavian Audiology Supplement, 13,* 117–123.

Rosenhall, U., Nordin, V., Brantberg, K., & Gillberg, C. (2003). Autism and auditory brain responses. *Ear and Hearing, 24,* 206–214.

Rosenhall, U., Pedersen, K., Johansson, E., & Kall, A. (1984). Auditory brain stem responses in patients with vertigo. *Clinical Otolaryngology, 9,* 149–154.

Rosenhall, U., & Roupe, G. (1981). Auditory brain-stem responses in syphilis. *British Journal of Venereal Diseases, 57,* 241–245.

Rosenhamer, H. J. (1977). Observations on electric brain-stem responses in retrocochlear hearing loss: A preliminary report. *Scandinavian Audiology, 6,* 179–196.

Rosenhamer, H. J. (1981). The auditory evoked brainstem electric response (ABR) in cochlear hearing loss. *Scandinavian Audiology Supplement, 13,* 83–93.

Rosenhamer, H. J., & Holmkvist, C. (1982). Bilaterally recorded auditory brainstem responses to monaural stimulation. *Scandinavian Audiology, 11,* 197–202.

Rosenhamer, H. J., & Holmkvist, C. (1983a). Latencies of ABR (waves III and V) to binaural clicks: Effects of interaural time and intensity differences. *Scandinavian Audiology, 12,* 201–207.

Rosenhamer, H. J., & Holmkvist, C. (1983b). Will contralateral white noise interfere with the monaural click-evoked brainstem response? *Scandinavian Audiology, 12,* 11–14.

Rosenhamer, H. J., Lindstrom, B., & Lundborg, T. (1978). On the use of click evoked responses in audiological diagnosis. I. The variability of the normal response. *Scandinavian Audiology, 7,* 193–205.

Rosenhamer, H. J., Lindstrom, B., & Lundborg, T. (1980). On the use of click-evoked electric brainstem responses in audiological diagnosis. II. Influence of sex and age upon normal response. *Scandinavian Audiology, 9,* 93–100.

Rosenhamer, H. J., Lindstrom, B., & Lundborg, T. (1981a). On the use of click-evoked electric brainstem responses in audiological diagnosis: III. Latencies in cochlear hearing loss. *Scandinavian Audiology, 10,* 3–11.

Rosenhamer, H. J., Lindstrom, B., & Lundborg, T. (1981b). On the use of click-evoked electric brainstem responses in audiological diagnosis: IV. Interaural latency differences (wave V) in cochlear hearing loss. *Scandinavian Audiology, 10,* 67–73.

Rosenhamer, H. J., & Silverskiold, B. P. (1980). Slower tremor and delayed brainstem auditory evoked responses in alcoholics. *Archives of Neurology, 37,* 293–296.

Rosenthal, E., Kileny, P., Boerst, A., & Telian, S. (1999). Successful cochlear implantation in a patient with MELAS syndrome. *American Journal of Otology, 20,* 187–191.

Rossi, L., Bindi, A., DeScisciolo, G., Russo, G., Marini, P., & Zappoli, R. (1984). [Electrophysiologic studies (auditory and somatosensory evoked potentials) in Friedreich's ataxia]. *Riv Patol Nerv Ment., 105,* 173–185.

Rössig, C., Wässer, S., & Oppermann, P. (1994). Audiologic manifestations in fetal alcohol syndrome assessed by brainstem auditory-evoked potentials. *Neuropediatrics, 25,* 245–249.

Rossini, P. M., & Cracco, J. B. (1987). Somatosensory and brainstem auditory evoked potentials in neurodegenerative system disorders. *European Neurology, 26,* 176–188.

Rossini, P. M., Di Stefano, E., Febbo, A., Di Paolo, B., & Basciani, M. (1984). Brain-stem auditory evoked responses (BAERs) in patients with chronic renal failure. *Electroencephalography and Clinical Neurophysiology, 57,* 507–514.

Rossini, P. M., Gambi, D., Marchionno, L., David, P., & Sollazzo, D. (1980). Cephalic and noncephalic references in brain stem evoked potential recording. *Applied Neurophysiology, 43,* 313–323.

Rossman, R. N., & Cashman, M. Z. (1985). Interinterpreter agreement for ABR tracings. *Scandinavian Audiology, 14,* 9–11.

Roth, W. T., & Cannon, E. H. (1972). Some features of the auditory evoked response in schizophrenics. *Archives of General Psychiatry, 27,* 466.

Roth, W. T., Ford, J. M., & Kopell, B. S. (1978). Long-latency evoked potentials and reaction time. *Psychophysiology, 15,* 17–23.

Roth, W. T., Ford, J. M., Lewis, S. J., & Kopell, B. S. (1976). Effects of stimulus probability and task-relevance on event-related potentials. *Psychophysiology, 13,* 311–317.

Roth, W. T., Krainz, J. M., & Ford, J. R. (1976). Parameters of temporal recovery of the human auditory evoked potential. *Electroencephalography and Clinical Neurophysiology, 40,* 623–632.

Roth, W. T., Pfefferbaum, A., Kelly, A. P., Berger, P. A., & Kopell, B. S. (1981). Auditory event related potentials in schizophrenia and depression. *Psychiatric Research, 4,* 199–212.

Roth, W. T., Shaw, J., & Green, J. (1956). The form, voltage distribution and physiological significance of the K complex. *Electroencephalography and Clinical Neurophysiology, 8,* 385–402.

Rothenberg, S. J., Poblano, A., & Schnaas, L. (2000). Brainstem auditory evoked responses at five years and prenatal and postnatal blood lead. *Neurotoxicology and Teratology, 22,* 503–510.

Rothenberg, S., Poblano, A., & Garza-Morales, S. (1994). Prenatal and perinatal low level lead exposure alters brainstem auditory evoked responses in infants. *Neurotoxicology, 15,* 695–700.

Rothenberger, A., Banaschewski, T., Heinrich, H., Moll, G., Schmidt, M., & van't Klooster, B. (2000). Comorbidity in ADHD-children: Effects of coexisting conduct disorder or tic disorder on event-related brain potentials in an auditory selective-attention task. *European Archives of Psychiatry and Clinical Neuroscience, 250,* 101–110.

Rothenberger, A., Szirtes, J., & Jurgens, R. (1982). Auditory evoked potentials to verbal stimuli in healthy, aphasic, and right hemisphere damaged subjects. *Archives of Psychiatry and Neurological Sciences, 231,* 155–170.

Rothman, H. H. (1970). Effects of high frequencies and intersubject variability on the auditory-evoked cortical response. *Journal of Acoustical Society of America, 47,* 569–573.

Rothman, H. H., Davis, H., & Hay, I. S. (1970). Slow evoked cortical potentials and temporal features of stimulation. *Electroencephalography and Clinical Neurophysiology, 29,* 225–232.

Rotteveel, J. J., Colon, E. J., Hombergen, G., Stoelinga, G. B. A., & Lippens, R. (1985). The application of evoked potentials in the diagnosis and follow-up of children with intracranial tumors. *Child's Nervous System, 1,* 172–178.

Rowe, M. J., III. (1978). Normal variability of the brain-stem auditory evoked response in young and old adult subjects. *Electroencephalography and Clinical Neurophysiology, 44,* 459–470.

Rowe, M. J., & Carlson, C. (1980). Brainstem auditory evoked potentials in postconcussion dizziness. *Archives of Neurology, 37,* 679–683.

Rubel, E. W., & Ryals, B. M. (1983). Development of the place principle: Acoustic trauma. *Science, 219,* 512–514.

Ruben, R. J., Bordley, J. E., & Lieberman, A. T. (1961). Cochlear potentials in man. *The Laryngoscope, 71,* 1141–1164.

Ruben, R. J., Elberling, C., & Salomon, G. (1976). *Electrocochleography.* Baltimore: University Park Press.

Ruben, R., Hudson, W., & Chiong, A. (1963). Anatomical and physiological effects of chronic section of the eighth nerve in cat. *Acta Otolaryngologica, 55,* 473–484.

Ruben, R., Sekula, J., & Bordley, J. (1960). Human cochlear response to sound stimuli. *Annals of Otology, Rhinology and Laryngology, 69,* 459–476.

Rubenstein, J. (2004). An introduction to the biophysics of the electrically evoked compound action potential. *International Journal of Audiology, 43,* S3–S9.

Ruchkin, D. S., & Sutton, S. (1978). Emitted P300 potentials and temporal uncertainty. *Electroencephalography and Clinical Neurophysiology, 45,* 268–277.

Ruchkin, D. S., Sutton, S., Kietzman, M., & Silver, K. (1980). Slow wave and P300 in signal detection. *Electroencephalography and Clinical Neurophysiology, 50,* 35–47.

Ruckenstein, M., Cueva, R., Morrison, D., & Press, G. (1996). A prospective study of ABR and MRI in the screening for vestibular schwannomas. *American Journal of Otology, 17,* 317–320.

Ruckenstein, M. J., Cueva, R. A., & Prioleau, G. R. (1997). Advantages of a new, atraumatic, self-retaining electrode for direct cochlear nerve monitoring. *Skull Base Surgery, 7,* 69–75.

Rugg, M., Pickles, C., Potter, D., Doyle, M., Pentland, B., & Roberts, R. (1993). Cognitive brain potentials in a three-stimulus auditory "oddball" task after closed head injury. *Neuropsychologia, 31,* 373–393.

Ruhm, H. B. (1971). Directional sensitivity and laterality of electroencephalic responses evoked by acoustic sweep frequencies. *Journal of Auditory Research, 11,* 9–16.

Ruhm, H. B., & Jansen, J. W. (1969). Rate of stimulus change and the evoked response: Signal rise-time. *Journal of Auditory Research, 9,* 211–216.

Rumsey, J., Grimes, A., Pikus, A., Duara, R., & Ismond, D. (1984). Auditory brainstem responses in pervasive developmental disorders. *Biological Psychiatry, 19,* 1403–1418.

Rupa, V., & Dayal, A. (1993). Wave V latency shifts with age and sex in normals and patients with cochlear hearing loss: Development of a predictive model. *British Journal of Audiology, 27,* 273–279.

Russo, N., Nicol, T., Musacchia, G., & Kraus, N. (2004). Brainstem responses to speech syllables. *Clinical Neurophysiology, 115*(9), 2021–2030.

Russolo, M., & Poli, P. (1983). Lateralization, impedance, auditory brainstem response, and synthetic sentence audiometry in brainstem disorders. *Audiology, 22,* 50–62.

Rust, J. (1977). Habituation and the orienting response in the auditory cortical evoked potential. *Psychophysiology, 14,* 123–126.

Ruth, R. A., Gal, T. J., DiFazio, C. A., & Moscicki, J. C. (1985). Brainstem auditory-evoked potentials during lidocaine infusion in humans. *Archives of Otolaryngology, 111,* 799–802.

Ruth, R. A., Hildebrand, D. L., & Cantrell, R. W. (1982). A study of methods used to enhance wave I in the auditory brain stem response. *Archives of Otolaryngology—Head & Neck Surgery, 90,* 635–640.

Ruth, R. A., & Lambert, P. R. (1989). Comparison of tympanic membrane to promontory electrode recordings of electrocochleographic responses in Meniere's patients. *Archives of Otolaryngology—Head & Neck Surgery, 100,* 546–552.

Ruth, R. A., Mills, J., & Jane, J. (1986). Intraoperative monitoring of electrocochleographic and auditory brainstem responses. *Seminars in Hearing, 7,* 307–327.

Ryerson, S. G., & Beagley, H. A. (1981). Brainstem electric responses and electrocochleography: A comparison of threshold sensitivity in children. *British Journal of Audiology, 15,* 41–48.

Saarinen, J., Paavilainen, P., Schoger, E., Tervaniemi, M., & Näätänen, R. (1992). Representation of abstract attributes of auditory stimuli in the human brain. *Neuroreport, 3,* 1149–1151.

Sabin, H. I., Prasher, D., Bentivoglio, P., & Symon, L. (1987). Preservation of cochlear potentials in a deaf patient fifteen months after excision of an acoustic neuroma. *Scandinavian Audiology, 16,* 109–111.

Sabo, D. L., Nozza, R. J., & Finegold, D. N. (1987). *Latency changes in children with diabetes mellitus.* Paper presented at annual convention of the American Speech-Language-Hearing Association, New Orleans.

Sabri, M., Labelle, S., Gosselin, A., & Campbell, K. B. (2003). Effects of sleep onset on the mismatch negativity (MMN) to frequency deviants using a rapid rate of presentation. *Cognitive Brain Research, 17,* 164–176.

Saha, S. N., Bhargava, V. K., Johnson, R. C., & McKean, C. M. (1978). Latency changes in brain stem auditory evoked potentials with impaired brain myelination. *Experimental Neurology, 58,* 111–118.

Saigal, S., Hoult, L. A., Streiner, D. L., Stoskopf, B. L., & Rosenbaum, P. D. (2000). School difficulties at adolescence in a regional cohort of children who were extremely low birth weight. *Pediatrics, 105,* 325–331.

Saito, A., Handa, J., & Kitahara, M. (1993). [Eighth cranial neuritis difficult to differentiate from intracanalicular acoustic neurinoma on MRI: case report.] *No Shinkei Geka, 21,* 341–344.

Saito, Y., Nishio, T., Arakawa, K., Ogawa, M., & Sunohara, N. (1997). [A case of spastic tetraplegia with medullo-cervical atrophy.]. *Rinsho Shinkeigaku, 37,* 1030–1033.

Sakakura, K., Takahashi, K., Takayasu, Y., Chikamatsu, K., & Furuya, N. (2005). Novel method for recording vestibular evoked myogenic potential: Minimally invasive recording on neck extensor muscles. *Laryngoscope, 115,* 1768–1773.

Sakai, Y., Kaga, K., Kodama, K., Higuchi, A. & Miyamoto, J. (2004). Hearing evaluation in two sisters with a T8993G point mutation of mitochondrial DNA. *International Journal of Pediatric Otorhinolaryngology, 68,* 1115–1119.

Salamy, A., Eldredge, L., & Wakely, A. (1985). Maturation of contralateral brain-stem responses in preterm infants. *Electroencephalography and Clinical Neurophysiology, 62,* 117–123.

Salamy, A., & McKean, C. M. (1976). Postnatal development of human brain stem potentials during the first year of life. *Electroencephalography and Clinical Neurophysiology, 41,* 418–426.

Salamy, A., & McKean, C. M. (1977). Habituation and dishabituation of cortical and brainstem evoked potentials. *International Journal of Neuroscience, 7,* 175–182.

Salamy, A., McKean, C. M., & Buda, F. B. (1975). Maturational changes in auditory transmission as reflected in human brainstem potentials. *Brain Research, 96,* 361–366.

Salamy, A., McKean, C. M., Pettett, G., & Mendelson, T. (1978). Auditory brainstem recovery processes from birth to adulthood. *Psychophysiology, 15,* 214–220.

Salisbury, D., & Squires, N. K. (1993). Response properties of long-latency event-related potentials evoked during NREM sleep. *Journal of Sleep Research, 2,* 232–240.

Sallinen, M., & Lyytinen, H. (1997). Mismatch negativity during objective and subjective sleepiness. *Psychophysiology, 34,* 694–702.

Salt, A. N., & Thornton, A. R. D. (1984a). The choice of stimulus polarity for brainstem auditory evoked potentials in the clinic. In R. H. Nodar & C. Barber (Eds.), *Evoked potentials II: The Second International Evoked Potentials Symposium,* pp. 203–215. Boston: Butterworth.

Salt, A. N., & Thornton, A. R. D. (1984b). The effects of stimulus rise-time and polarity on the auditory brainstem responses. *Scandinavian Audiology, 13,* 119–127.

Samar, V. (1999). Wavelet analysis of neuroelectric waveforms: A conceptual tutorial. *Brain and Language, 66,* 1–6.

Samar, V. J., Bopardikar, A., Rao, R., & Swartz, K. (1999). Wavelet analysis of neuroelectric waveforms: a conceptual tutorial. *Brain and Language, 66,* 7–60.

Sammeth, C. A., & Barry, S. J. (1985). The 40-Hz event-related potential as a measure of auditory sensitivity in normals. *Scandinavian Audiology 14,* 51–55.

Sammeth, C., Burkard, R., & Hecox, K. (1986). Effects of relative starting phase and frequency separation on two-tone auditory brainstem responses. *Journal of the Acoustical Society of America (Supplement 1), 80,* S47.

Samra, S. K., Krutak-Krol, H., Pohorecki, R., & Domino, E. F. (1985). Scopolamine, morphine and brain-stem auditory evoked potentials in awake monkeys. *Anesthesiology, 62,* 437–441.

Samra, S. K., Lilly, D. J., Rush, N. L., & Kirsh, M. M. (1984). Fentanyl anesthesia and human brain-stem auditory evoked potentials. *Anesthesiology, 61,* 261–265.

Sams, M., Alho, K., & Näätänen, R. (1983). Sequential effects on the ERP in discriminating two stimuli. *Biological Psychiatry, 17,* 41–58.

Sams, M., Alho, K., & Näätänen, R. (1984). Short-term habituation and dishabitation of the mismatch negativity of the mismatch negativity of the ERP. *Psychophysiology, 21,* 434–441.

Sams, M., Aulanko, R., Aaltonen, O., & Näätänen, R. (1990). Event-related potentials to infrequent changes in synthesized phonetic stimuli. *Journal of Cognitive Neuroscience, 2,* 344–357.

Sams, M., Hamalainen, M., Hari, R., & McEvoy, L. (1993). Human auditory cortical mechanisms of sound lateralization: I. Interaural time differences within sound. *Hearing Research, 67,* 89–97.

Sanchez-Turet, M., & Serra-Grabulosa, J. M. (2002). Auditory revoked potentials and alcohol: Characteristics of the mismatch negativity component in alcoholism. *Revista de Neurologia, 35,* 1049–1055.

Sand, T. (1986). BAEP subcomponents and wave form—relation to click phase and stimulus rate. *Electroencephalography and Clinical Neurophysiology, 65,* 72–80.

Sand, T. (1991). BAEP amplitudes and amplitude ratios: Relation to click polarity, rate, age, and sex. *Electroencephalography and Clinical Neurophysiology, 78,* 291–296.

Sand, T., & Vingen, J. (2000). Visual, long-latency auditory and brainstem auditory evoked potentials in migraine: relation to pattern size, stimulus intensity, sound and light discomfort thresholds and pre-attack state. *Cephalalgia, 20,* 804–820.

Sanders, R. A., Duncan, P. G., & McCullough, D. W. (1979). Clinical experience with brain stem audiometry performed under general anesthesia. *Journal of Otolaryngology, 8,* 24–31.

Sanderson, J., & Blades, J. (1988). Multicentre study of propofol in the day case surgery. *Anaesthesia, 43,* 70–72.

Sangal, B., & Sangal, J. M. (1996). Topography of auditory and visual P300 in normal adults. *Clinical Electroencephalography, 27,* 145–150.

Sanna, M., Zini, C., Mazzoni, A., et al. (1987). Hearing preservation in acoustic neuroma surgery. *American Journal of Otology, 8,* 500–506.

Santarelli, R., & Arslan, E. (2002). Electrocochleography in auditory neuropathy. *Hearing Research, 170,* 32–47.

Santarelli, R., Maurizi, M., Conti, G., Ottaviani, F., Paludetti, G., & Pettorossi, V. E. (1995). Generation of human auditory steady-state responses (SSRs). II: Addition of responses to individual stimuli. *Hearing Research, 83,* 9–18.

Santos-Sacchi, J. (1986). The temperature dependence of electrical coupling in the organ of Corti. *Hearing Research, 21,* 205–211.

Sasaki, H. (1991). [Influence of anesthesia on auditory evoked response.] *Nippon Jibiinkoka Gakkai Kaiho, 94,* 1834–1843.

Sasaki, H., Kikuoka, H., Emoto, M., Nanjo, K., & Miyamura, K. (1987). [Auditory brainstem responses and electroencephalographic findings in patients with occupational vibration disease.] *Japanese Journal of Industrial Health, 29,* 136–144.

Sass, K. (1998). Sensitivity and specificity of transtympanic electrocochleography in Meniere's disease. *Acta Otolaryngology, 118,* 150–156.

Sass, K., Densert, B., & Arlinger, S. (1998). Recording techniques for transtympanic electrocochleography in clinical practice. *Acta Otolaryngol,. 118,* 17–25.

Sass, K., Densert, B., & Magnusson, M. (1997). Transtympanic electrocochleography in the assessment of perilymphatic fistulas. *Audiology & Neuro-Otology, 2,* 391–402.

Sass, K., Densert, B., Magnusson, M., & Whitaker, S. (1998). Electrocochleographic signal analysis: condensation and rarefaction click stimulation contributes to diagnosis in Meniere's disorder. *Audiology, 37,* 198–206.

Sator, M., Franz, P., Egarter, C., Gruber, D., Wolfl, G., & Nagele, F. (1999). Effects of tibolone on auditory brainstem responses in post-menopausal women—a randomized, double-blind, placebo-controlled trial. *Fertility and Sterility, 72,* 885–888.

Satterfield, J., Schell, A., & Backs, R. (1987). Longitudinal study of AERPs in hyperactive and normal children: Relationship to antisocial behavior. *Electroencephalography and Clinical Neurophysiology, 67,* 531–536.

Satya-Murti, S., & Cacace, A. T. (1982). Brainstem auditory evoked potentials in disorders of the primary sensory ganglion. *Advances in Neurololgy, 32,* 219–225.

Satya-Murti, S., Cacace, A. T., & Hanson, P. A. (1979). Abnormal auditory evoked potentials in hereditary motor-sensory neuropathology. *Annals of Neurology, 5,* 445–448.

Satya-Murti, S., Cacace, A., & Hanson, P. (1980). Auditory dysfunction in Friedreich ataxia: Result of spiral ganglion degeneration. *Neurology, 30,* 1047–1053.

Satya-Murti, S., Wolpaw, J. R., Cacace, A. T., & Schaffer, C. A. (1983). Late auditory evoked potentials can occur without brain stem potentials. *Electroencephalography and Clinical Neurophysiology, 56,* 304.

Saul, L. J., & Davis, H. (1932). Action currents in the central nervous system: I. Action currents of the auditory tracts. *Archives of Neurology and Psychiatry, 28,* 1104–1116.

Sawaishi, Y., Tomita, Y., & Mito, T. (1990). [Neurological and pathophysiological analyses of patients with absent auditory brainstem evoked response.] *No To Hattatsu, 22,* 223–229.

Sayers, B. McA., Beagley, H. A., & Henshall, W. R. (1974). Mechanism of auditory evoked responses. *Nature, 247,* 481–483.

Schaefer, S., Finitzo, T., Ross, E., Close, L., Reisch, J., Freeman, F., Cannito, M., & Maravilla, K. (1985). Magnetic resonance imaging findings and correlations in spasmodic dysphonia patients. *Annals of Otology, Rhinology, and Laryngology, 94,* 595–601.

Schaefer, S. C., Gerling, I. J., Finitzo-Hieber, T., & Freeman, F. J. (1983). Brainstem conduction abnormalities in spasmodic dysphonia. *Annals of Otology, Rhinology & Laryngology, 92,* 59–63.

Schall, U., Johnston, P., Todd, J., Ward, P. B., & Michie, P. T. (2003). Functional neuroanatomy of auditory mismatch processing: An event-related fMRI study of duration-deviant oddballs. *NeuroImage, 20,* 729–736.

Schellart, N., & Wubbels, R. (1998). The auditory and mechanosensory lateral line system. In D. Evans (Ed.), *The physiology of fishes* (pp. 283–312). Boca Raton, FL: CRC Press.

Scherg, M. (1982a). Simultaneous recording and separation of early and middle latency auditory evoked potentials. *Electroencephalography and Clinical Neurophysiology, 54,* 339–341.

Scherg, M. (1982b). Distortion of the middle latency auditory response produced by analog filtering. *Scandinavian Audiology, 11,* 57–60.

Scherg, M., & Speulda, E. W. (1982). Brainstem auditory evoked potentials in the neurologic clinic: improved stimulation and analysis methods. In

J. Courjon, F. Mauguiere & M. Revol (Eds.), *Clinical applications of evoked potentials in neurology* (pp. 211–218). New York: Raven Press.

Scherg, M., & Volk, S. A. (1983). Frequency specificity of simultaneously recorded early and middle latency auditory evoked potentials. *Electroencephalography and Clinical Neurophysiology, 56,* 443–452.

Scherg, M., & von Cramon, D. (1984). Topographical analysis of auditory evoked potentials: Derivation of components. In R. H. Nodar & C. Barber (Eds.), *Evoked potentials II: The Second International Evoked Potentials Symposium* (pp. 73–101). Boston: Butteworths.

Scherg, M., & von Cramon, D. (1985a). A new interpretation of the generators of BAEP waves I–V: Results of a spatio-temporal dipole model. *Electroencephalography and Clinical Neurophysiology, 62,* 290–299.

Scherg, M., & von Cramon, D. (1985b). Two bilateral sources of the late AEP as identified by a spatio-temporal dipole model. *Electroencephalography and Clinical Neurophysiology, 62,* 32–44.

Scherg, M., & von Cramon, D. (1986). Evoked dipole source potentials of the human auditory cortex. *Electroencephalography and Clinical Neurophysiology, 65,* 344–360.

Scherler, M., & Bohmer, A. (1995). [The value of clinical examination methods in diagnosis of acoustic neuroma.]. *HNO, 43,* 487–491.

Schiff, A., Cracco, R., & Cracco, J. (1985). Brainstem auditory form of Landry-Guillain-Barre syndrome. *Neurology, 35,* 771–773.

Schimmel, H., Rapin, I., & Cohen, M. M. (1975). Improving evoked response audiometry: Results of normative studies for machine scoring. *Audiology, 14,* 466–469.

Schlake, H. P., Milewski, C., Goldbrunner, R. H., Kindgen, A., Riemann, R., Helms, J., & Roosen, K. (2001). Combined intra-operative monitoring of hearing by means of auditory brainstem responses (ABR) and transtympanic electrocochleography (ECochG) during surgery of intra- and extrameatal acoustic neurinomas. *Acta Neurochirurgica (Wiene) 143,* 985–995.

Schmidt, P. H., Eggermont, J. J., & Odenthal, D. W. (1974). Study of Ménière's disesase by electrocochleography. *Acta Otolaryngologica, Supplement, 316,* 75–84.

Schmidt, R., Sataloff, R., Newman, J., Spiegel, J., & Myers, D. (2001). The sensitivity of auditory brainstem response testing for the diagnosis of acoustic neuromas. *Archives of Otolaryngology—Head & Neck Surgery, 127,* 19–22.

Schmidt, S., Traber, F., Block, W., Keller, E., Pohl, C., von Oertzen, J., et al. (2001). Phenotype assignment in symptomatic female carriers of X-linked adrenoleukodystrophy. *Journal of Neurology, 248,* 36–44.

Schmulian, D., Swanepoel, D., & Hugo, R. (2005). Predicting pure-tone thresholds with dichotic multiple frequency auditory steady state responses. *Journal of the American Academy of Audiology, 16,* 5–17.

Schoonhoven, R. (1992). Dependence of auditory brainstem response on click polarity and high-frequency sensorineural hearing loss. *Audiology, 31,* 72–86.

Schoonhoven, R., Fabius, M. A., & Grote, J. J. (1995). Input/output curves to tone bursts and clicks in extratympanic and transtympanic electrocochleography. *Ear and Hearing, 16,* 619–630.

Schoonhoven, R., Lamore, P. J., de Laat, J. A., & Grote, J. J. (1999). The prognostic value of electrocochleography in severely hearing-impaired infants. *Audiology, 38,* 141–154.

Schoonhoven, R., Prijs, V. F., & Grote, J. J. (1996). Response thresholds in electrocochleography and their relation to the pure tone audiogram. *Ear and Hearing, 17,* 266–275.

Schramm, J., Mokrusch, T., Fahlbusch, R., & Hochstetter, A. (1985). Intra- and perioperative acoustic evoked brain-stem responses in cerebellopontine angle surgery. *HNO, 33,* 495–498.

Schroeder, M. M., Ritter, W., & Vaughan, H. G., Jr. (1995). The mismatch negativity to novel stimuli reflects cognitive decline. *Annals of the New York Academy of Science, 769,* 399–401.

Schröger, E. (1994). Automatic detection of frequency change is invariant over a large intensity range. *Neuroreport, 5,* 825–828.

Schröger, E. (2005). Part III: Mental representations of music—combining behavioral and neuroscience tools. Introduction. *Annals of the New York Academy of Science, 1060,* 98–99.

Schröger, E., Näätänen, R., & Paavilainen, P. (1992). Event-related potentials reveal how non-attended complex sound patterns are represented by the human brain. *Neuroscience Letters, 146,* 183–186.

Schröger, E., Tervaniemi, M., Wolff, C., & Näätänen, R. N. (1996). Preattentive periodicity detection in auditory patterns as governed by time and intensity information. *Brain Research & Cognitive Brain Research, 4,* 145–148.

Schröger, E., & Wolff, C. (1998). Behavioral and electrophysiological effects of task-irrelevant sound change: A new distraction paradigm. *Brain and Cognitive Brain Research, 7,* 71–87.

Schrott, A., Stephan, K., & Spoendlin, H. (1989). Hearing with selective inner hair cell loss. *Hearing Research, 40,* 213–219.

Schuckit, M. (1980). Biological markers: Metabolism and acute reactions to alcohol in sons of alcoholics. *Pharmacology Biochemistry and Behavior, 13,* 9–16.

Schuckit, M., Gold, E., Croot, K., Finn, P., & Polich, J. (1988). P300 latency after ethanol ingestion in sons of alcoholics and in controls. *Biological Psychiatry, 24,* 310–315.

Schulman-Galambos, C., & Galambos, R. (1975). Brain stem auditory evoked responses in premature infants. *Journal of Speech and Hearing Research, 18,* 456–465.

Schulte-Körne, G., Deimel, W., Bartling, J., & Remschmidt, H. (1998). Auditory processing and dyslexia: evidence for a specific speech processing deficit. *Neuroreport, 9,* 337–340.

Schulte-Körne, G., Deimel, W., Bartling, J., & Remschmidt, H. (1999). Preattentive processing of auditory patterns in dyslexic human subjects. *Neuroscience Letters, 276,* 41–44.

Schwaber, M. K., & Hall, J. W., III. (1990). A simplified approach for transtympanic electrocochleography. *American Journal of Otology, 11,* 260–265.

Schwaber, M. K., & Hall, J. W., III. (1992). Cochleovestibular nerve compression syndrome. I. Clinical features and audiovestibular findings. *Laryngoscope, 102,* 1020–1029.

Schwartz, D. M., & Berry, G. A. (1985). Normative aspects of the ABR. In J. T. Jacobson (Ed.), *The auditory brainstem response* (pp. 65–97). San Diego: College-Hill Press.

Schwartz, D. M., Bloom, M. J., & Dennis, J. M. (1985). Perioperative monitoring of auditory brainstem responses. *The Hearing Journal, 38,* 9–13.

Schwartz, D. M., Bloom, M. J., Pratt, R. E., Jr., & Costello, J. A. (1988). Anesthetic effects on neuroelectric events. *Seminars in Hearing, 9,* 99–111.

Schwartz, D. M., Larson, V., & DeChicchis, A. R. (1985). Spectral characteristics of air and bone transducers used to record the auditory brainstem response. *Ear and Hearing, 6,* 274–277.

Schwartz, D. M., Morris, M. D., Spydell, J. D., Brink, C. T., Grim, M. A., & Schwartz, J. A. (1990). Influence of click polarity on the brain-stem auditory evoked response (BAER) revisited. *Electroencephalography and Clinical Neurophysiology, 77,* 445–457.

Schwartz, D. M., Pratt, R. E. Jr., & Schwartz, J. A. (1989). Auditory brainstem responses in preterm infants: Evidence of peripheral maturity. *Ear and Hearing, 10,* 14–22.

Schwartz, D. M., & Schwartz, R. H. (1978). Acoustic impedance and otoscopic findings in young children with Down's syndrome. *Archives of Otolaryngology, 104,* 652–656.

Schweitzer, V. G., & Shepard, N. (1989). Sudden hearing loss: An uncommon manifestation of multiple sclerosis. *Archives of Otolaryngology—Head & Neck Surgery, 100,* 327–332.

Schwender, D., Kaiser, A., Klasing, S., Peter, K., & Poppel, E. (1994). Mid-latency auditory evoked potentials and explicit and implicit memory in patients undergoing cardiac surgery. *Anesthesiology, 80,* 493–501.

Schwender, D., Weninger, E., Schnatmann, N., Mulzer, S., Klasing, S., & Peter, K. (1995). [Acoustic evoked potentials mid-latency following anaesthesia with sufentanil]. *Anaesthesist, 44,* 478–482.

Schwent, V. L., & Hillyard, S. A. (1975). Evoked potential correlates of selective attention with multi-channel auditory input. *Electroencephalography and Clinical Neurophysiology, 38,* 131–138.

Schwent, V. L., Snyder, E., & Hillyard, S. A. (1976). Auditory evoked potentials during multichannel selective listening: Role of pitch and localization cues. *Journal of Experimental Psychology: Human Perception and Performance, 2,* 313–325.

Seales, D. M., Rossiter, V. S., & Weinstein, M. E. (1979). Brainstem auditory evoked responses in patients comatose as a result of blunt head trauma. *Journal of Trauma, 19,* 347–353.

Seales, D. M., Torkelson, R. D., Shuman, R. M., Rossiter, V. S., & Spencer, J. D. (1981). Abnormal brainstem auditory evoked potentials and neuropathology in "locked-in" syndrome. *Neurology, 31,* 893–896.

Sebel, P., Flynn, P., & Ingram, D. (1984). Effects of nitrous oxide on visual, auditory and somatosensory evoked potentials. *British Journal of Anaesthesia, 56,* 1403–1407.

Segalowitz, S., & Barnes, K. (1993). The reliability of ERP components in the auditory oddball paradigm. *Psychophysiology, 30,* 451–459.

Sekiya, T., Iwabuchi, T., Kamata, S., & Ishida, T. (1985). Deterioration of auditory evoked potentials during cerebellopontine angle manipulations. *Journal of Neurosurgery, 63,* 598–607.

Sellick, P. M., & Russell, I. J. (1980). The responses of inner hair cells to basilar membrane velocity during low frequency auditory stimulation in the guinea pig cochlea. *Hearing Research, 2,* 439–445.

Sells, J., & Hurley, R. (1994). Acoustic neuroma in an adolescent without neurofibromatosis: Case study. *Journal of the American Academy of Audiology, 5,* 349–354.

Selmani, Z., Pyykko, I., Ishizaki, H., & Ashammakhi, N. (2002). Use of electrocochleography for assessing endolymphatic hydrops in patients with Lyme disease and Ménière's disease. *Acta Otolaryngology, 122,* 173–178.

Selters, W. A., & Brackmann, D. E. (1977). Acoustic tumor detection with brain stem electric response audiometry. *Archives of Otolaryngology, 103,* 181–187.

Seo, T., Node, M., Yukimasa, A., & Sakagami, M. (2003). Furosemide loading vestibular evoked myogenic potential for unilateral Ménière's disease. *Otology and Neuro-Otology, 24,* 283–288.

Seri, S., Cerquiglini, A., Pisani, F., & Curatolo, P. (1999). Autism in tuberous sclerosis: Evoked potential evidence for a deficit in auditory sensory processing. *Clinical Neurophysiology, 110,* 1825–1830.

Serpanos, Y., O'Malley, H., & Gravel, J. (1997). The relationship between loudness intensity functions and the click-ABR wave V latency. *Ear and Hearing, 18,* 409–419.

Serra, J. M., Escera, C., Sanchez-Turet, M., Sanchez-Sastre, J., & Grau, C. (1996). The H1-receptor antagonist chlorpheniramine decreases the ending phase of the mismatch negativity of the human auditory event-related potentials. *Neuroscience Letters, 203,* 77–80.

Setou, M., Kurauchi, T., Tsuzuku, T., & Kaga, K. (2001). Binaural interaction of bone-conducted auditory brainstem responses. *Acta Otolaryngologica, 121,* 486–489.

Setzen, G., Cacace, A., Eames, F., Riback, P., Lava, N., McFarland, D., Artino, L., & Kerwood, J. (1999). Central deafness in a young child with Moyamoya disease: Paternal linkage in a caucasian family. Two case reports and a review of the literature. *International Journal of Pediatric Otorhinolaryngology, 48,* 53–76.

Shafer, V. L., Morr, M. L., Datta, H., Kurtzberg, D., & Schwartz, R. G. (2005). Neurophysiological indexes of speech processing deficits in children with specific language impairment. *Journal of Cognitive Neuroscience, 17,* 1168–1880.

Shafer, V. L., Morr, M. L., Kreuzer, J. A., & Kurtzberg, D. (2000). Maturation of mismatch negativity in school-age children. *Ear and Hearing, 21,* 242–251.

Shagass, C., Straumanis, J. J., & Roemer, R. A. (1982). Psychotropic drugs and evoked potentials. *Electroencephalography and Clinical Neurophysiology, Supplement, 36,* 538–548.

Shallop, J. K., Beiter, A., Goin, D., & Mischke, R. (1990). Electrically evoked auditory brainstem responses and middle latency responses (EMLR) obtained from patients with the nucleus multichannel cochlear implant. *Ear and Hearing, 11,* 5–15.

Shallop, J. K., Facer, G., & Peterson, A. (1999). Neural response telemetry with the Nucleus CI24M cochlear implant. *Laryngoscope, 109,* 1755–1759.

Shallop, J. K., Jin, S., Driscoll, C., & Tibesar, R. (2004). Characteristics of electrically evoked potentials in patients with auditory neuropathy/auditory dys-synchrony. *International Journal of Audiology, 43,* S22–S27.

Shallop, J. K., & Osterhammel, P. A. (1983). A comparative study of measurements of SN-10 and the 40/sec middle latency responses in newborns. *Scandinavian Audiology, 12,* 91–95.

Shallop, J. K., Peterson, A., Facer, G., Fabry, L., & Driscoll, C. (2001). Cochlear implants in five cases of auditory neuropathy: Postoperative findings and progress. *Laryngoscope, 111,* 555–562.

Shallop, J. K., VanDyke, L., Goin, D. W., & Mischke, R. E. (1991). Prediction of behavioral threshold and comfort values for Nucleus 22-channel implant patients from electrical auditory brain stem response test results. *Annals of Otology, Rhinology & Laryngology, 100,* 896–898.

Shankar, N., Tandon, O., Bandhu, R., Madan, N., & Gomber, S. (2000). Brainstem auditory evoked potential responses in iron-deficient anemic children. *Indian Journal of Physiology and Pharmacology, 44,* 297–303.

Shanon, E., Gold, S., & Himelfarb, M. Z. (1981a). Auditory brain stem responses in cerebellopontine angle tumors. *Laryngoscope, 91*(2): 254–259.

Shanon, E., Gold, S., & Himmelfarb, M. Z. (1981b). Assessment of functional integrity of brain stem auditory pathways by stimulus stress. *Audiology, 20,* 65–71.

Shanon, E., Himelfarb, M. Z., & Zikk, D. (1985). Measurement of auditory brain stem potentials in Bell's palsy. *Laryngoscope, 95,* 206–209.

Shapiro, S. M., & Conlee, J. W. (1991). Brainstem auditory evoked potentials correlate with morphological changes in Gunn rat pups. *Hearing Research, 57,* 16–22.

Sharma, A., Dorman, M. F., & Kral, A. (2005). The influence of a sensitive period on central auditory development in children with unilateral and bilateral cochlear implants. *Hearing Research, 203,* 134–143.

Sharma, A., Dorman, M., & Spahr, T. (2002). A sensitive period for the development of the central auditory system in children with cochlear implants. *Ear and Hearing, 23,* 532–539.

Sharma, A., Kraus, N., McGee, T. J., & Nicol, T. G. (1997). Developmental changes in P1 and N1 central auditory responses elicited by consonant-vowel syllables. *Electroencephalography and Clinical Neurophysiology, 104,* 540–545.

Sharma, A., Marsh, C. M., & Dorman, M. D. (2000). Relationship between N1 evoked potential morphology and the perception of voicing. *Journal of the Acoustical Society of America, 108,* 3030–3035.

Sharma, A., Tobey, E., Dorman, M., Bharadwaj, S., Martin, K., Gilley, P., & Kunkel, F. (2004). Central auditory maturation and babbling development in infants with cochlear implants. *Archives of Otolaryngology—Head and Neck Surgery, 130,* 511–516.

Sharma, M., Purdy, S. C., Newall, P., Wheldall, K., Beaman, R., & Dillon, H. (2004). Effects of identification technique, extraction method, and stimulus type on mismatch negativity in adults and children. *Journal of the American Academy of Audiology, 15,* 616–632.

Shaw, N. A. (1991). A possible thalamic component of the auditory evoked potential in the rat. *Brain Research Bulletin, 27,* 133–136.

Shea, J. J., & Howell, M. (1978). Management of tinnitus aurium with lidocaine and carbamazepine. *Laryngoscope, 88,* 1477–1480.

Shehata-Dieler, W., Shimizu, H., Soliman, S. M., & Tusa, R. J. (1991). Middle latency auditory evoked potentials in temporal lobe disorders. *Ear and Hearing, 12,* 377–388.

Shelley, A. M., Silipo, G., & Javitt, D.C. (1999). Diminished responsiveness of ERPs in schizophrenic subjects to changes in auditory stimulation parameters: Implications for theories of cortical dysfunction. *Schizophrenia Research, 37,* 65–79.

Shelley, A. M., Ward, P. B., Catts, S. V., Michie, P. T., Andrews, S., & McConaghy, N. (1991). Mismatch negativity: an index of a preattentive processing deficit in schizophrenia. *Biological Psychiatry, 30,* 1059–1062.

Shelton, C., Hitselberger, W. E., House, W. F., & Brackmann, D. E. (1990). Hearing preservation after acoustic tumor removal: Long-term results. *Laryngoscope, 100,* 115–119.

Shelton, C., & House, W. F. (1990). Hearing improvement after acoustic tumor removal. *Archives of Otolaryngology—Head & Neck Surgery, 103,* 963–965.

Shera, C., & Guinan, J. (2000). Frequency dependence of stimulus-frequency-emission phase: Implications for cochlear mechanics. In H. Wada, T. Takasaka, K. Ikeda, K. Ohyama, & T. Koike (Eds.), *Recent developments in auditory mechanics* (pp. 381–387). Singapore: World Scientific.

Shestakova, A., Huotilainen, M., Čeponiene, R., & Cheour, M. (2003). Event-related potentials associated with second language learning in children. *Clinical Neurophysiology, 114,* 1507–1512.

Sheykholeslami, K., Habiby, K. M., & Kaga, K. (2001a). Bone-conducted vestibular evoked myogenic potentials in patients with congenital atresia of the external auditory canal. *International Journal of Pediatric Otorhinolaryngology, 57,* 25–29.

Sheykholeslami, K., Habiby, K. M., & Kaga, K. (2001b). Frequency sensitivity range of the saccule to bone-conducted stimuli measured by vestibular evoked myogenic potentials. *Hearing Research, 160,* 58–62.

Sheykholeslami, K., Kaga, K., & Kaga, M. (2001). An isolated and sporadic auditory neuropathy (auditory nerve disease): report of five patients. *Journal of Laryngology & Otology, 115,* 530–534.

Sheykholesami, K., Kaga, K., Megerian, C., & Arnold, J. (2005). Vestibular-evoked myogenic potentials in infancy and early childhood. *Laryngoscope, 115,* 1440–1444.

Sheykholesami, K., Kaga, K., Murofushi, T., & Hughes, D. W. (2000). Vestibular function in auditory neuropathy. *Acta Otolaryngological, 120,* 849–854.

Sheykholesami, K., Murofushi, T., Kermany, M., & Kaga, K. (2000). Bone conducted evoked myogenic potentials from the sternocleidmastoid muscle. *Acta Otolaryngologica, 120,* 731–734.

Sheykholesami, K., Schmerber, S., Kermany, M., & Kaga, K. (2004). Vestibular-evoked myogenic potentials in three patients with large vestibular aqueduct. *Hearing Research, 190,* 161–168.

Shigematsu, Y., Hori, C., Nakai, A., Kuriyama, M., Kikawa, Y., Konishi, Y., et al. (1991). Mucopolysaccharidosis VI (Maroteaux-Lamy syndrome) with hearing impairment and pupillary membrane remnants. *Acta Paediatrica, 33,* 476–481.

Shimizu, H. (1968). Evoked response in eighth nerve lesions. *Laryngoscope, 78,* 2140–2152.

Shimizu, K., Murofushi, T., Sakurai, M., & Halmagyi, G. (2000). Vestibular evoked myogenic potentials in multiple sclerosis. *Journal of Neurology Neurosurgery and Psychiatry, 69,* 276–277.

Shimotake, T., & Iwai, N. (1994). Auditory brainstem response in children with total intestinal aganglionosis. *Lancet, 343,* 1362.

Shinozaki, N., Yabe, H., Sato, Y., Hiruma, T., Sutoh, T., Nashida, T., Matsuoka, T., & Kaneko, S. (2002). The difference in mismatch negativity between the acute and post-acute phase of schizophrenia. *Biological Psychology, 59,* 105–119.

Shiraishi, K., Eura, Y., Kato, T., Shibata, K., Sakata, T., & Soda, T. (1997). [Negative potential auditory brainstem response with 3-msec latency in profoundly deaf patients: Characteristics and relationship to vestibular evoked response.] *Nippon Jibiinkoka Gakkai Kaiho, 100,* 1382–1393.

Shivashankar, N., Satishchandra, P., Shashikala, H., & Gore, M. (2003). Primary auditory neuropathy: An enigma. *Acta Neurologica Scandinavia, 108,* 130–135.

Shtyrov, Y., Kujala, T., Ahveninen, J., Tervaniemi, M., Alku, P., Ilmoniemi, R. J., & Näätänen, R. (1998). Background acoustic noise and the hemispheric lateralization of speech processing in the human brain: Magnetic mismatch negativity study. *Neuroscience Letters, 251,* 141–144.

Shtyrov, Y., & Pulvermüller, F. (2002a). Memory traces for inflectional affixes as shown by mismatch negativity. *European Journal of Neuroscience, 15,* 1085–1091.

Shtyrov, Y., & Pulvermüller, F. (2002b). Neurophysiological evidence of memory traces for words in the human brain. *Neuroreport, 13,* 521–525.

Shtyrov, Y., Pulvermüller, F., Näätänen, R., & Ilmoniemi, R. J. (2003). Grammar processing outside the focus of attention: An MEG study. *Journal of Cognitive Neuroscience, 15,* 1195–1206.

Shucard, J. L., Shucard, D. W., & Cummins, K. R. (1981). Auditory evoked potentials and sex-related differences in brain development. *Brain and Language, 13,* 91–102.

Shutara, Y., Koga, Y., Fujita, K., Takeuchi, H., Mochida, M., & Takemasa, K. (1996). An event-related potential study on the impairment of automatic processing of auditory input in schizophrenia. *Brain Topography, 8,* 285–289.

Siegel, C., Waldo, M., Mizner, G., Adler, L. E., & Freedman, R. (1984). Deficits in sensory gating in schizophrenic patients and their relatives. Evidence obtained with auditory evoked responses. *Archives of General Psychiatry, 41,* 607–612.

Sieger, A., White, N. H., Skinner, M. W., & Spector, G. J. (1983). Auditory function in children with diabetes mellitus. *Annals of Otology, Rhinology, and Laryngology, 92,* 237–241.

Sikorski, C., & Ruth, R. A. (1982). *The use of ABR in assessing hearing function of institutionalized mentally retarded.* Paper presented at the Second International Evoked Potentials Symposium, Cleveland.

Silverstein, H., McDaniel, A., Norrell, H., & Haberkamp, T. (1986). Hearing preservation after acoustic neuroma surgery with intraoperative direct eighth cranial nerve monitoring: Part II. A classification of results. *Archives of Otolaryngology—Head & Neck Surgery, 95,* 285–291.

Silverstein, H., McDaniel, A., Wazen, J., & Norrell, H. (1985). Retrolabyrinthine vestibular neurectomy with simultaneous monitoring of eighth nerve and brain stem auditory evoked potentials. *Archives of Otolaryngology—Head & Neck Surgery, 93,* 736–742.

Silverstein, H., Wazen, J., Norrell, H., & Hyman, S. M. (1984). Retrolabyrinthine vestibular neurectomy with simultaneous monitoring of VIIIth nerve action potentials and electrocochleography. *American Journal of Otology, 5,* 552–555.

Simmons, F. B., Lusted, H. S., Meyers, T., & Shelton, C. (1984). Electrically induced auditory brainstem response as a clinical tool in estimating nerve survival. *Annals of Otology, Rhinology, and Laryngology (Supp), 112,* 97–100.

Simmons, F. B., & Russ, F. N. (1974). Automated newborn hearing screening: The Crib-O-Gram. *Archives of Otolaryngology—Head & Neck Surgery, 100,* 1–7.

Simson, R., Vaughan, H. G., Jr., & Ritter, W. (1976). The scalp topography of potentials in auditory and visual discrimination tasks. *Electroencephalography and Clinical Neurophysiology, 40,* 33–42.

Sindou, M., Fobe, J., Ciriano, D., & Fischer, C. (1990). [Intraoperative brainstem auditory evoked potential in the microvascular decompression of the 5th and 7th cranial nerves.] *Revue Laryngologie Otologie et Rhinologie (Bord.) 111,* 427–431.

Singhal, A., Doerfling, P., & Fowler, B. (2002). Effects of a dual task on the N100-P200 complex and the early and late Nd attention waveforms. *Psychophysiology, 39,* 236–245.

Sininger, Y. S. (1995). Filtering and spectal characteristics of averaged auditory brainstem response and background noise in infants. *Journal of the Acoustic Society of America, 98,* 2048–2055.

Sininger, Y. S., Abdala, C., & Cone-Wesson, B. (1997). Auditory threshold sensitivity of the human neonate as measured by the auditory brainstem response. *Hearing Research, 104,* 27–38.

Sininger, Y. S., Cone-Wesson, B., & Abdala, C. (1998). Gender distinctions and lateral asymmetry in the low-level auditory brainstem response of the human neonate. *Hearing Research, 126,* 58–66.

Sininger, Y. S., Cone-Wesson, B., Folsom, R. C., Gorga, M. P., Vohr, B., Widen, J. E., Ekelid, M., & Norton, S. J. (2000). Identification of neonatal hearing impairment: Auditory brainstem responses in the perinatal period. *Ear and Hearing, 21,* 383–399.

Sininger, Y. S., & Don, M. (1989). Effects of click rate and electrode orientation on threshold of the auditory brainstem response. *Journal of Speech and Hearing Research, 32,* 880–886.

Sininger, Y. S., Hood, L. J., Starr, A., & Berlin, C. I. (1995). Hearing loss due to auditory neuropathy. *Audiology Today, 7,* 10–13.

Sininger, Y. S., & Masuda, A. (1990). Effect of click polarity on ABR threshold. *Ear and Hearing, 11,* 206–209.

Sininger, Y. S., & Oba, S. (2001). Patients with auditory neuropathy: Who are they and what can they hear. In Y. Sininger & A. Starr (Eds.), *Auditory neuropathy: New perspectives on hearing disorders* (pp. 15–36). San Diego CA: Singular-Thomson Learning.

Sinkkonen, J., & Tervaniemi, M. (2000). Towards optimal recording and analysis of the mismatch negativity. *Audiology & Neuro-Otology, 5,* 235–246.

Sjogren, B., Iregren, A., Frech, W., Hagman, M., Johansson, L., Tesarz, M., & Wennberg, A. (1996). Effects on the nervous system among welders exposed to aluminium and manganese. *Occupational & Environmental Medicine, 53,* 32–40.

Skinner, P. H., & Antinoro, F. (1971). The effects of signal rise time and duration on the early components of the auditory evoked cortical response. *Journal of Speech and Hearing Research, 14,* 552–558.

Skinner, P. H., & Jones, H. C. (1968). Effects of stimulus duration and rise time on the auditory evoked potential. *Journal of Speech and Hearing Research, 11,* 301–306.

Skinner, P. H., & Shimota, J. (1975). A comparison of the effects of sedatives on the auditory evoked cortical response. *Journal of the American Audiology Society, 1,* 71–78.

Sklar, F. H., Ehle, A. L., & Clark, W. K. (1979). Visual evoked potentials: A noninvasive technique to monitor patients with hydrocephalus. *Neurosurgery, 4,* 529–534.

Sklare, D. A., & Lynn, G. E. (1984). Latency of the P3 event-related potential: Normative aspects and within subject variability. *Electroencephalography and Clinical Neurophysiology, 59,* 420–424.

Skoff, B., Mirsky, A., & Turner, D. (1980). Prolonged brainstem transmission time in autism. *Psychiatric Research, 2,* 157–166.

Skrandies, W. (1990). Global field power and topographic similarity. *Brain Topography, 3,* 137–141.

Sloan, T. B. (1998). Anesthetic effects on electrophysiologic recordings. *Clinical Neurophysiology, 15,* 217–226.

Sloan, T. B. (2002). Anesthetics and the brain. *Anesthesiology Clinics of North America, 20,* 265–292.

Small, J. G., Milstein, V., Kellams, J. H., & Small, I. F. (1981). Auditory brain stem evoked responses in hospitalized patients undergoing drug treatment or ECT. *Biological Psychiatry, 16,* 287–290.

Small, S. A., Hatton, J., & Stapells, D. R. (2004). *Multiple auditory steady-state response thresholds to bone-conduction stimuli in premature infants.* Paper presented at the International Conference on Newborn Hearing Screening, Diagnosis, and Intervention, Como, Italy.

Small, S., & Stapells, D. (2004). Artifactual responses when recording auditory steady-state responses. *Ear and Hearing, 25,* 611–623.

Small, S., & Stapells, D. (2005). Multiple auditory steady-state response thresholds to bone-conduction stimuli in adults with normal hearing. *Journal of the American Academy of Audiology, 16,* 172–183.

Smith, D. A., Boutros, N. N., & Schwarzkopf, S. B. (1994). Reliability of P50 auditory event-related potential indices of sensory gating. *Psychophysiology, 31,* 495–502.

Smith, D. B. D., Michalewski, H. J., Brent, G. A., & Thompson, L. W. (1980). Auditory averaged evoked potentials and aging: Factors of stimulus, task and topography. *Biological Psychology, 11,* 135–151.

Smith, D. I., & Kraus, N. (1987). Effects of chloral hydrate, pentobarbital, ketamine, and curare on the auditory middle latency response. *American Journal of Otolaryngology, 8,* 241–248.

Smith, J., Marsh, J., & Brown, W. (1975). Far-field recorded frequency-following responses: Evidence for the locus of brainstem sources. *Electroencephalography and Clinical Neurophysiology, 39,* 465–472.

Smith, L. E., & Simmons, F. B. (1982). Accuracy of auditory brain stem-evoked response with hearing level unknown. *Annals of Otology, Rhinology, and Laryngology, 91,* 266–267.

Smith, L., & Simmons, F. B. (1983). Estimating eighth nerve survival by electrical stimulation. *Annals of Otology, Rhinology & Laryngology, 92,* 19–25.

Smoorenburg, G., Willeboer, C., & Van Dijk, J. (2002). Speech perception in Nucleus CI24M cochlear implant users with processing settings based on electrically evoked compound action potential thresholds. *Audiology and Neurootology, 7,* 335–347.

Smyth, V. (1985). On the effect of cross-hearing and clinical masking on the auditory brain-stem evoked response. *Electroencephalography and Clinical Neurophysiology, 61,* 26–29.

Snell, R. S. (1987). *Clinical neuroanatomy for medical students.* Boston: Little, Brown & Co.

Sobe, T., Vreugde, S., Shahin, H., Berlin, M., Davis, N., Kanaan, M., Yaron, Y., Orr-Urtreger, A., Frydman, M., Shohat, M., & Avraham, K. (2000). The prevalence and expression of inherited connexin 26 mutations associated with nonsyndromic hearing loss in the Israeli population. *Human Genetics, 106,* 50–57.

Sohmer, H., & Feinmesser, M. (1967). Cochlear action potentials recorded from the external ear in man. *Annals of Otology, Rhinology, and Laryngology, 76,* 427–435.

Sohmer, H., Feinmesser, M., & Szabo, G. (1974). Sources of electrocochleographic responses as studied in patients with brain damage. *Electroencephalography and Clinical Neurophysiology, 37,* 663–669.

Sohmer, H., Kinarti, R., & Gafni, M. (1980). The source along the basilar membrane of the cochlear microphonic potential recorded by surface electrodes in man. *Electroencephalography and Clinical Neurophysiology, 49,* 506–514.

Sohmer, H., Kinarti, R., & Gafni, M. (1981). The latency of auditory nerve-brainstem responses in sensorineural hearing loss. *Archives of Otorhinolaryngology, 230,* 189–199.

Sohmer, H., & Pratt, H. (1976). Recording of the cochlear microphonic potential with surface electrodes. *Electroencephalography and Clinical Neurophysiology, 40,* 253–260.

Sohmer, H., Pratt, H., & Kinarti, R. (1977). Sources of frequency following responses (FFRs) in man. *Electroencephalography and Clinical Neurophysiology, 42,* 656–664.

Sohmer, H., & Student, M. (1978). Auditory nerve and brain stem evoked responses in normal, autistic, minimal brain dysfunction and psychomotor retarded children. *Electroencephalography and Clinical Neurophysiology, 44,* 380–388.

Soininen, H. S., Karhu, J., Partanen, J., Paakkonen, A., Jousmaki, V., Hanninen, T., & Hallikainen, M. (1995). Habituation of auditory N100 correlates with amygdaloid volumes and frontal functions in age-associated memory impairment. *Physiology and Behavior, 57,* 927–935.

Sokolov, Y., Zhang, R., & Long, G. (2005). Wireless communications in otoacoustic emissions and auditory evoked potentials. *Abstracts of the 28th Annual Midwinter Research Meeting, Association for Research in Otolaryngology, 505,* 177–178.

Solbakk, A., Reinvang, I., Nielsen, C., & Sundet, K. (1999). ERP indicators of disturbed attention in mild closed head injury: A frontal lobe syndrome? *Psychophysiology, 36,* 802–817.

Soliman, S. M. (1987). Low-frequency sensorineural hearing loss: A syndrome. *Audiology, 26,* 332–338.

Solliway, B. M., Schaffer, A., Erez, A., Mittleman, N., Pratt, H., & Yannai, S. (1995). The effect of lead exposure on target detection and memory scanning differs. *Journal of Neurological Science, 134,* 171–177.

Sood, S., & Mahapatra, A. (1991). Effects of CSF shunt on brainstem auditory evoked potential in hydrocephalus secondary to brain tumor. *Acta Neurochirurgica, 111,* 92–95.

Soucek, S., & Mason, S. (1992). Effects of adaptation on electrocochleography and auditory brain-stem response in the elderly. *Scandinavian Audiology, 21,* 149–152.

Souliere, C. R., Kava, C. R., Barrs, D. M., & Bell, A. F. (1991). Sudden hearing loss as the sole manifestation of neurosarcoidosis. *Otolaryngology—Head & Neck Surgery, 105,* 376–381.

Soustiel, J. F., Hafner, H., Chistyakov, A. V., Barzilai, A., & Feinsod, M. (1995). Trigeminal and auditory evoked responses in minor head injuries and post-concussion syndrome. *Brain Injury, 9,* 805–813.

Sparacino, G., Milani, S., Magnavita, V., & Arslan, E. (2000). Electrocochleography potentials evoked by condensation and rarefaction clicks independently derived by a new numerical filtering approach. *Audiology & Neuro-Otology, 5,* 276–291.

Spinelli, E. M., Pallàs-Areny, R., & Mayosky, M. A. (2003). AC-coupled front-end for biopotential measurements, *IEEE Transactions on Biomedical Engineering, 50,* 1–2.

Spink, U., Johannsen, H. S., & Pirsig, W. (1979). Acoustically evoked potential: Dependence upon age. *Scandinavian Audiology, 8,* 11–14.

Spirduso, W. (1980). Physical fitness, aging, and psychomotor speed: A review. *Journal of Gerontology, 35,* 850–865.

Spitzer, J., & Newman, C. (1987). Brainstem auditory evoked potentials in detoxified alcoholics. *Journal of the Study of Alcohol, 48,* 9–13.

Spivak, L. G., & Seitz, M. R. (1988). Response asymmetry and binaural interaction in the auditory brain stem evoked response. *Ear and Hearing, 9,* 57–64.

Spoendlin, H. (1972). Innervation densities of the cochlea. *Acta Otolaryngologica, 73,* 235–248.

Spoor, A., & Eggermont, J. J. (1976). Electroencephalography as a method for objective audiogram determination. In S. K. Hirsh, D. H. Eldredge & I. J. Hirsh (Eds.), *Hearing and Davis: Essays honoring Hallowell Davis.* St. Louis: CID Press.

Spoor, A., Timmer, F., & Odenthal, D. W. (1969). The evoked auditory response (EAR) to intensity modulated and frequency modulated tones and tone bursts. *International Audiology, 8,* 410–415.

Spydell, J. D., Pattee, G., & Goldie, W. D. (1985). The 40 hertz auditory event-related potential: normal values and effects of lesions. *Electroencephalography and Clinical Neurophysiology, 62,* 193–202.

Squires, K. C., Chu, N.-S., & Starr, A. (1978). Acute effects of alcohol on auditory brainstem potentials in humans. *Science, 201,* 174–176.

Squires, K. C., & Donchin, E. (1976). Beyond averaging: The use of discriminant functions to recognize event related potentials elicited by single auditory stimuli. *Electroencephalography and Clinical Neurophysiology, 41,* 449–459.

Squires, K. C., Donchin, E., Herning, R., & McCarthy, G. (1977). On the influence of task relevance and stimulus probability on event-related potential components. *Electroencephalography and Clinical Neurophysiology, 42,* 1–14.

Squires, K. C., & Hecox, K. E. (1983). Electrophysiological evaluation of higher level auditory processing. *Seminars in Hearing, 4*(4), 415–433.

Squires, K. C., Squires, N., & Hillyard, S. (1975). Decision-related cortical potentials during an auditory signal detection task with cued observation intervals. *Journal of Experimental Psychology: Human Perception and Performance, 1,* 268–279.

Squires, N., Aine, C., Buchwald, J., Norman, R., & Galbraith, G. (1980). Auditory brainstem response abnormalities in severely profoundly retarded children. *Electroencephalography and Clinical Neurophysiology, 50,* 172–185.

Squires, N., Buchwald, J., Liley, F., & Strecher, J. (1982). Brainstem auditory evoked potential abnormalities in retarded adults. In J. Courjon, F. Mauquierre & M. Revol (Eds.), *Clinical applications of evoked potentials in neurology.* New York: Raven Press.

Squires, N., Ollo, C., & Jordan, R. (1986). Auditory brainstem responses in the mentally retarded: Audiometric correlates. *Ear and Hearing, 7,* 83–92.

Squires, N., Squires, K., & Hillyard, S. (1975). Two varieties of long-latency positive waves evoked by unpredictable auditory stimuli in man. *Electroencephalography and Clinical Neurophysiology, 38,* 387–401.

St. Clair, D., Blackwood, D., & Muir, W. (1989). P300 abnormality in schizophrenic subtypes. *Journal of Psychiatric Research, 23,* 49–55.

Stach, B. A. (1986). *Optimum stimulus rate for measurement of the auditory steady-state evoked potential.* Houston: Baylor College of Medicine.

Stach, B., Stoner, W., Smith, S., & Jerger, J. (1994). Auditory evoked potentials in Rett syndrome. *Journal of the American Academy of Audiology, 5,* 226–230.

Stach, B. A., Westerberg, B. D., & Roberson, J. B., Jr. (1998). Auditory disorder in central nervous system miliary tuberculosis: Case report. *Journal of the American Academy of Audiology, 9,* 305–310.

Staller, S. S. (1986). Electrocochleography in the diagnosis and management of Ménière's disease. *Seminars in Hearing, 7,* 267–278.

Stanton, S. G., Cashman, M. Z., Harrison, R. V., Nedzelski, J. M., & Rowed, D. W. (1989). Cochlear nerve action potentials during cerebellopontine angle surgery: Relationship of latency, amplitude, and threshold measurements in hearing. *Ear and Hearing, 10,* 23–28.

Stapells, D. R. (1989). Auditory brainstem response assessment of infants and children. *Seminars in Hearing, 10,* 229–251.

Stapells, D. R. (2000). Threshold estimation by the tone-evoked auditory brainstem response: A literature meta-analysis. *Journal of Speech-Language Pathology and Audiology, 24,* 74–83.

Stapells, D., R., Galambos, R., Costello, J., & Makeig, S. (1988). Inconsistency of auditory middle latency and steady-state responses in infants. *Electroencephalography and Clinical Neurophysiology, 71,* 289–295.

Stapells, D. R., Gravel, J. A., & Martin, B. A. (1995). Thresholds for auditory brain stem responses to tones in notched noise from infants and young children with normal hearing or sensorineural hearing loss. *Ear and Hearing, 16,* 361–371.

Stapells, D. R., Herdman, A., Small, S., Dimitrijevic, A., & Hatton, J. (2005). Current status of the auditory steady-state responses for estimating an infant's audiogram. In: A sound foundation through early amplification. Phonak, pp. 1–18.

Stapells, D. R., Linden, D., Suffield, J. B., Hamel, G., & Picton, T. W. (1984). Human auditory steady state potentials. *Ear and Hearing, 5,* 105–113.

Stapells, D. R., Makeig, S., & Galambos, R. (1987). Auditory steady-state responses: Threshold prediction using phase coherence. *Electroencephalography and Clinical Neurophysiology, 67,* 260–270.

Stapells, D. R., & Picton, T. W. (1981). Technical aspects of brainstem evoked potential audiometry using tones. *Ear and Hearing, 2,* 20–29.

Stapells, D. R., Picton, T. W., Abalo, M. P., Read, D., & Smith, A. (1985). Frequency specificity in evoked potential auditory. In J. Jacobsen (Ed.), *The auditory brainstem response* (pp. 147–177). San Diego: College Hill Press.

Stapells, D. R., Picton, T. W., & Durieux-Smith, A. (1994). Electrophysiologic measures of frequency-specific auditory function. In J. T. Jacobson (Ed.), *Principles and applications in auditory evoked potentials* (pp. 251–283). Boston: Allyn and Bacon.

Stapells, D. R., Picton, T. W., Durieux-Smith, A., Edwards, C. G., & Moran, L. M. (1990). Thresholds for short-latency auditory-evoked potentials to tones in notched noise in normal-hearing and hearing-impaired subjects. *Audiology, 29,* 262–274.

Stapells, D. R., Picton, T. W., & Smith, A. D. (1982). Normal hearing thresholds for clicks. *Journal of Acoustical Society of America, 72,* 74–79.

Stapells, D. R., & Oates, P. (1997). Estimation of the pure-tone audiogram by the auditory brainstem response: A review. *Audiology and Neurootology, 2,* 257–280.

Stapells, D. R., & Ruben, R. (1989). Auditory brainstem responses to bone-conducted tones in infants. *Annals of Otology Rhinology and Laryngology, 98,* 941–949.

Starr, A. (1976). Auditory brainstem response in brain death. *Brain, 99,* 543–554.

Starr, A., & Achor, L. J. (1975). Auditory brainstem responses in neurological disease. *Archives of Neurology, 32,* 761–768.

Starr, A., Amlie, R. N., Martin, W. H., & Sanders, S. (1977). Development of auditory function in newborn infants revealed by auditory brainstem potentials. *Pediatrics, 60,* 831–839.

Starr, A., & Brackmann, D. E. (1979). Brain stem potentials evoked by electrical stimulation of the cochlea in human subjects. *Annals of Otology, Laryngology & Rhinology, 88,* 59–67.

Starr, A., & Hamilton, A. E. (1976). Correlation between confirmed sites of neurological lesions and abnormalities of far-field auditory brainstem responses. Electroencephalography and clinical *Neurophysiology, 41,* 595–608.

Starr, A., Isaacson, B., Michalewski, H., Zeng, F., Kong, Y., Beale, P., Paulson, G., Keats, B., & Lesperance, M. (2004). A dominantly inherited progressive deafness affecting distal auditory nerve and hair cells. *Journal of the Association for Research in Otolaryngology, 5,* 411–426.

Starr, A., McPherson, D., Patterson, J., Don, M., Luxford, W., Shannon, R., Sininger, Y., Tonakawa, L., & Waring, M. (1991). Absence of both auditory evoked potentials and auditory percepts dependent on timing cues. *Brain, 114* (Pt 3), 1157–1180.

Starr, A., Michalewski, H., Zeng, F., Fujikawa-Brooks, S., Linthicum, F., Kim, C., Winnier, D., & Keats, B. (2003). Pathology and physiology of auditory neuropathy with a novel mutation in the MPZ gene (Tyr 145-Ser). *Brain, 126,* 1604–1619.

Starr, A., Picton, T. W., & Kim, R. (2001). Pathophysiology of auditory neuropathy. In Y. Sininger & A. Starr (Eds.), *Auditory neuropathy: New perspectives on hearing disorders* (pp. 67–82). San Diego, CA: Singular-Thomson Learning.

Starr, A., Picton, T., Sininger, Y., Hood, L., & Berlin, C. (1996). Auditory neuropathy. *Brain, 119,* 741–753.

Starr, A., Sininger, Y. S., & Pratt, H. (2000). The varieties of auditory neuropathy. *Journal of Basic Clinical Physiology & Pharmacology, 11,* 215–230.

Starr, A., Sininger, Y., Winter, M., Derebery, M., Oba, S., & Michalewski, H. (1998). Transient deafness due to temperature sensitive auditory neuropathy. *Ear and Hearing, 19,* 169–179.

Starr, A., & Squires, K. (1982). Distribution of auditory brainstem potentials over the scalp and nasopharynx in humans. *Annals of New York Academy of Sciences, 388,* 427–442.

Steel, K., & Bock, G. (1983). Hereditary inner ear abnormalities in animals. Relationships with human abnormalities. *Archives of Otolaryngology, 109,* 22–29.

Stein, H., Barth, H., Eichmann, T., & Mehdorn, H. M. (1996). [Primary traumatic midbrain syndrome—follow-up and prognosis of acute primary brain stem damage.] *Zentralblatt für Chirurgie, 121,* 985–989.

Stein, L. K., Clark, S., & Kraus, N. (1983). The hearing-impaired infant: patterns of identification and habilitation. *Ear and Hearing, 4,* 232–236.

Stein, L. K., & Kraus, N. (1988). Auditory evoked potentials with special populations. *Seminars in Hearing, 9,* 35–45.

Stein, L., Kraus, N., Özdamar, O., Cartee, C., Jabaley, T., Jeantet, C., & Reed, N. (1987). Hearing loss in an institutionalized mentally retarded population. *Archives of Otolaryngology, 113,* 32–35.

Stein, L. K., Özdamar, O., Kraus, N., & Paton, J. (1983). Follow-up of infants screened by auditory brainstem response in the neonatal intensive care unit. *Journal of Pediatrics, 103,* 447–453.

Stein, L. K., Özdamar, O., & Schnabel, M. (1981). Auditory brainstem responses (ABR) with suspected deaf-blind children. *Ear and Hearing, 2,* 30–40.

Steinschneider, M., Volkov, I. O., Noh, M. D., Garell, P. C., & Howard, M. A., III. (1999). Temporal encoding of the voice onset time phonetic parameter by field potentials recorded directly from human auditory cortex. *Journal of Neurophysiology, 82,* 2346–2357.

Stenklev, N., & Laukli, E. (2004). Cortical cognitive potentials in elderly persons. *Journal of the American Academy of Audiology, 15,* 401–413.

Stephenson, W. A., & Gibbs, F. A. (1951). A balanced non-cephalic reference electrode. *Electroencephalography and Clinical Neurophysiology, 3,* 237–240.

Sterkers, J., Morrison, G., Sterkers, O., et al. (1994). Preservation of facial, cochlear, and other nerve functions in acoustic neuroma treatment. *Archives of Otolaryngology—Head & Neck Surgery, 110,* 146–155.

Stevens, A. A., Skudlarski, P., Gatenby, J. C., & Gore, J. C. (2000). Event-related fMRI of auditory and visual oddball tasks. *Magnetic Resonance Imaging, 18,* 495–502.

Stevens, S. S. (1961). The psychophysics of sensory function. In W. A. Rosenblith (Ed.), *Sensory communication* (pp. 1–33). New York: Wiley.

Stewart, D., Mehl, A., Hall, J. W., III, Thompson, V., Carrol, M., & Hamlett, J. (2000). Universal newborn hearing screening with automated auditory brainstem response: A multisite investigation. *Journal of Perinatology, 20,* S128-S131.

Stewart, M. G., Jerger, J., & Lew, H. L. (1993). Effect of handedness on the middle latency auditory evoked potential. *American Journal of Otology, 14,* 595–600.

Stidham, K., & Roberson, J. J. (2001). Hearing improvement after middle fossa resection of vestibular schwannoma. *Otology and Neurotology, 22,* 917–921.

Stockard, J. E., & Stockard, J. J. (1983). Recording and analyzing. In E. J. Moore (Ed.), *Bases of auditory brain-stem evoked responses,* (pp. 255–286). New York: Grune and Stratton.

Stockard, J. E., Stockard, J. J., & Coen, R. (1983). Auditory brain stem response variability in infants. *Ear and Hearing, 4,* 11–23.

Stockard, J. E., & Westmoreland, B. F. (1981). Technical considerations in the recording and interpretation of the brainstem auditory evoked potential for neonatal neurologic diagnosis. *American Journal of EEG Technology, 21,* 31–54.

Stockard, J. E., Stockard, J. J., Westmoreland, B. F., & Corfits, J. L. (1979). Brainstem auditory-evoked responses: Normal variation as a function of stimulus and subject characteristics. *Archives of Neurology, 36,* 823–831.

Stockard, J. J. (1982). Brainstem auditory evoked potentials in adult and infant sleep apnea syndromes, including sudden infant death syndrome and near-miss for sudden infant death. *Annals of New York Academy of Science, 388,* 443–465.

Stockard, J. J. (1983). Prognostic value of brain-stem auditory evoked potentials in neonates. *Archives of Neurology, 40,* 360–365.

Stockard, J. J., & Hecox, K. (1981). Brainstem auditory evoked potentials in sudden infant death syndrome, "near-miss-for-SIDS," and infant apnea sydnromes. *Electroencephalography and Clinical Neurophysiology, 51,* 43–47.

Stockard, J. J., & Rossiter, V. S. (1977). Clinical and pathologic correlates of brain stem auditory response abnormalities. *Neurology, 27,* 316–325.

Stockard, J. J., Rossiter, V. S., Wiederholt, W. C., & Kobayashi, R. M. (1976). Brain stem auditory-evoked responses in suspected central pontine myelinolysis. *Archives of Neurology, 33,* 726–728.

Stockard, J. J., Sharbrough, F. W., Staats, B. A., & Westbrook, P. R. (1980). Brain stem auditory evoked potentials (BAEPs) in sleep apnea. *Electroencephalography and Clinical Neurophysiology, 50,* 167p.

Stockard, J. J., Sharbrough, F. W., & Stockard, F. E. (1977). Detection and localization of occult lesions with brainstem auditory responses. *Mayo Clinic Proceedings, 52,* 761–769.

Stockard, J. J., Stockard, J. E., & Sharbrough, F. W. (1978). Nonpathological factors influencing brainstem auditory evoked potentials. *American Journal of EEG Technology, 18,* 177–209.

Stockard, J. J., Stockard, J. E., & Sharbrough, F. W. (1980). Brainstem auditory evoked potentials in neurology: Methodology, interpretation, clinical application. In M J. Aminoff (Ed.). *Electrodiagnosis in clinical neurology* (pp. 370–413). New York: Churchill Livingstone.

Stockard, J. J., Stockard, J. E., & Sharbrough, F. W. (1986). Brainstem auditory evoked potentials in neurology: Methodology, interpretation, and clinical application. In M J. Aminoff (Ed.). *Electrodiagnosis in clinical neurology* (2nd ed.; pp. 467–503). New York: Churchill Livingston.

Stollman, M., Snik, A., Hombergen, G., Nieuwenhuys, R., & ten Koppel, P. (1996). Detection of the binaural interaction component in the auditory brainstem response. *British Journal of Audiology, 30,* 227–232.

Streletz, L. J., Katz, L., Hohenberger, M., & Cracco, R. Q. (1977). Scalp recorded auditory evoked potentials and sonomotor responses: An evaluation of components and recording techniques. *Electroencephalography and Clinical Neurophysiology, 43,* 192–206.

Struys, M. M., Jensen, E. W., Smith, W., Smith, N. T., Rampil, I., Dumortier, F. J., Mestach, C., & Mortier, E. P. (2002). Performance of the ARX-derived auditory evoked potential index as an indicator of anesthetic depth: A comparison with bispectral index and hemodynamic measures during propofol administration. *Anesthesiology, 96,* 803–816.

Stuart, A., & Yang, E. (1994). Effects of high-pass filtering on the neonatal auditory brainstem response to air- and bone-conducted clicks. *Journal of Speech and Hearing Research, 37,* 475–479.

Stuart, A., & Yang, E. (2001). Gender effects in auditory brainstem responses to air- and bone- conducted clicks in neonates. *Journal of Communicative Disorders, 34,* 229–239.

Stuart, A., Yang, E., & Botea, M. (1996). Neonatal auditory brainstem responses from four electrode montages. *Journal of Communicative Disorders, 29,* 125–139.

Stuart, A., Yang, E., & Green, W. (1994). Neonatal auditory brainstem response thresholds to air- and bone-conducted clicks: 0 to 96 hours postpartum. *Journal of the American Academy of Audiology, 5,* 163–172.

Stuart, A., Yang, E., & Stenstrom, R. (1990). Effect of temporal area bone vibrator placement on auditory brainstem response in newborn infants. *Ear and Hearing, 11,* 363–369.

Stuart, A., Yang, E., Stenstrom, R., & Reindorp, A. (1993). Auditory brainstem response thresholds to air and bone conducted clicks in neonates and adults. *American Journal of Otology, 14,* 176–182.

Studebaker, G. A. (1962). Placement of vibrator in bone-conduction testing. *Journal of Speech and Hearing Research, 5,* 321–331.

Stueve, M., & O'Rourke, C. (2003). Estimation of hearing loss in children: Comparison of auditory steady-state response, auditory brainstem response, and behavioral test methods. *American Journal of Audiology, 12,* 125–136.

Stürzebecher, E., & Cebulla, M. (1997). Objective detection of auditory evoked potentials: Comparison of several statistical tests in the frequency domain on the basis of near-threshold ABR data. *Scandinavian Audiology, 26,* 7–14.

Stürzebecher, E., Cebulla, M., & Pschirrer, U. (2001). Efficient stimuli for recording of the amplitude modulation following response. *Audiology, 40,* 63–68.

Stürzebecher, E., Kevanishvili, Z., Werbs, M., Meyer, E., & Schmidt, D. (1985). Interpeak intervals of auditory brainstem response, interaural differences in normal-hearing subjects and patients with sensorineural hearing loss. *Scandinavian Audiology, 14,* 83–87.

Stürzebecher, V. E., Werbs, M., & Kevanishvili, Z. (1985). BERA-Normal values for the early detection of acoustic neuromas. *HNO-Praxis, 10,* 243–250.

Stypulkowski, P. H., & Staller, S. (1987). Clinical evaluation of a new ECochG recording electrode. *Ear and Hearing, 8,* 304–310.

Stypulkowski, P. H., & van den Honert, C. (1984). Physiological properties of the electrically stimulated auditory nerve. I. Compound action potential recordings. *Hearing Research, 14,* 205–223.

Stypulkowski, P. H., van den Honert, C., & Kvistad, S. D. (1986). Electrophysiologic evaluation of the cochlear implant patient. *Otolaryngology Clinics of North America, 19,* 249–257.

Su, H., Huang, T., Young, Y., & Cheng, P. (2004). Aging effect on vestibular evoked myogenic potential. *Otology and Neurotology, 25,* 977–980.

Sugg, M. J., & Polich, J. (1995). P300 from auditory stimuli: Intensity and frequency effects. *Biological Psychology, 41,* 255–269.

Sugimoto, T., Yasuhara, A., Ohta, T., Nishida, N., Saitoh, S., Hamabe, J., et al. (1992). Angelman syndrome in three siblings: characteristic epileptic seizures and EEG abnormalities. *Epilepsia, 33,* 1078–1082.

Sundaramoorthy, V., Pont, M., Degg, C., & Cook, J. (2000). A computerized database of 'normal' auditory brainstem responses. *British Journal of Audiology, 34,* 197–201.

Sundel, R., Cleveland, S., Beiser, A., Newburger, J., McGill, T., Baker, A., Koren, G., Novak, R., Harris, J., & Burns, J. (1992). Audiologic profiles of children with Kawasaki disease. *American Journal of Otology, 13,* 512–515.

Suppeij, A., Montini, G., Casara, G., Polo, A., Zacchello, G., & Zacchello, F. (1992). Evoked potentials before and after anemia correction with recombinant human erythropoietin in end-stage renal disease. *Child Nephrology and Urology, 12,* 197–201.

Sutton, L. N., Frewen, T., Marsh, R. R., Jaffi, J., & Bruce, D. A. (1982). The effects of deep barbiturate coma on multimodality evoked potentials. *Journal of Neurosurgery, 57,* 178–185.

Sutton, S., Braren, M., Zubin, J., & John, E. R. (1965). Evoked potential correlates of stimulus uncertainty. *Science, 150,* 1187–1188.

Sutton, S., Tueting, P., Zubin, J., & John, E. R. (1967). Information delivery and the sensory evoked potential. *Science, 155,* 1436–1439.

Suwazono, S., Shibasaki, H., Nishida, S., Nakamura, M., Honda, M., Nagamine, T., Ikeda, A., & Ito, J. (1994). Automatic detection of P300 in single sweep records of auditory event-related potential. *Journal of Clinical Neurophysiology, 11*, 448–460.

Suzaki, F., Suzuki, R., & Sugiyama, M. (2002). [Relationship between location of stress erosive gastritis and brain damage in resuscitated patients]. *Nippon Shokakibyo Gakkai Zasshi, 99*, 264–269.

Suzuki, M., & Suzuki, J. I. (1977). Clinical application of the auditory evoked brain stem response in children. *ANL, 4*, 19–26.

Suzuki, T., & Asawa, I. (1957). Evoked potential of waking human brain to acoustic stimuli. *Acta Otolaryngologica, 48*, 508–515.

Suzuki, T., Hirabayashi, M., & Kobayashi, K. (1983). Auditory middle responses in young children. *British Journal of Audiology, 17*, 5–9.

Suzuki, T., Hirabayashi, M., & Kobayashi, K. (1984). Effects of analog and digital filterings on auditory middle latency responses in adults and young children. *Annals of Otology, Rhinology, and Laryngology, 93*.

Suzuki, T., Hirai, Y., & Horiuchi, K. (1977). Auditory brain stem responses to pure tone stimuli. *Scandinavian Audiology, 6*, 51–56.

Suzuki, T., Hirai, Y., & Horiuchi, K. (1981). Simultaneous recording of early and middle components of auditory electric response. *Ear and Hearing, 2*, 276–282.

Suzuki, T., & Horiuchi, K. (1977). Effect of high-pass filter on auditory brain stem responses to tone pips. *Scandinavian Audiology, 6*, 123–126.

Suzuki, T., & Horiuchi, K. (1981). Rise time pure-tone stimuli in brain stem response audiometry. *Audiology, 20*, 101–112.

Suzuki, T., & Kobayashi, K. (1984). An evaluation of 40-Hz event-related potentials in young children. *Audiology, 23*, 599–604.

Suzuki, T., Kobayashi, K., Aoki, K., & Umegaki, Y. (1992). Effect of sleep on binaural interaction in auditory brainstem response and middle latency response. *Audiology, 31*, 25–30.

Suzuki, T., Kobayashi, K., & Hirabayashi, M. (1983). Frequency composition of auditory middle responses. *Brititsh Journal of Audiology, 17*, 1–4.

Suzuki, T., Kobayashi, K., & Takagi, N. (1985). Effects of stimulus repetition rate on slow and fast components of auditory brain-stem responses. *Electroencephalography and Clinical Neurophysiology, 65*, 150–156.

Suzuki, T., Sakabe, N., & Miyashita, Y. (1982). Power spectral analysis of auditory brain stem responses to pure tone stimuli. *Scandinavian Audiology, 11*, 25–30.

Suzuki, T., & Taguchi, K. (1965). Cerebral evoked response to auditory stimuli in waking man. *Annals of Otology, Rhinology, Laryngology, 74*, 128–139.

Suzuki, T., & Taguchi, K. (1968). Cerebral evoked response to auditory stimuli in young children during sleep. *Annals of Otology, Rhinology, and Laryngology, 77*, 102–110.

Swanepoel, D. C. D., Delport, S. D., & Swart, J. G. (2004c). Universal newborn hearing screening in South Africa—a first-world dream? *South African Medical Journal, 94*, 634–635.

Swanepoel, D., & Hugo, R. (2004). Estimations of auditory sensitivity for young cochlear implant candidates using the ASSR: Preliminary results. *International Journal of Audiology, 43*, 377–382.

Swanepoel, D., Hugo, R., & Roode, R. (2004). Auditory steady-state responses for children with severe to profound hearing loss. *Archives of Otolaryngology—Head & Neck Surgery, 130*, 531–535.

Swanepoel, D., Schmulian, D., & Hugo, R. (2004). Establishing normal hearing with the dichotic multiple-frequency auditory steady-state response comapred to an auditory brainstem response protocol. *Acta Otolaryngologica, 124*, 62–68.

Symon, L., Sabin, H. I., Bentivoglio, P., Cheesman, A. D., Prasher, D., & Barratt, H. (1988). Intraoperative monitoring of the electrocochleogram and the preservation of hearing during acoustic neuroma excision. *Acta Neurochir Supplement (Wien), 42*, 27–30.

Syndulko, K., Hansch, M. A., Cohen, S. N., Pearce, J. W., Goldberg, Z., Montan, B., & Tourtelotte, B. (1982). Long-latency event-related potentials in normal aging and dementia. In F. Courjon, F. Mauguiere, & M. Revol (Eds.), *Clinical applications of evoked potentials in neurology* (pp. 279–285). New York: Raven Press.

Szyfter, W., Dauman, R., & Charlet de Savage, R. (1984). 40 Hz middle latency responses to low frequency tone pips in normally hearing adults. *Journal of Otolaryngology, 13*, 275–280.

Szymanski, M. D., Bain, D. E., Kiehl, K., Pennington, S., Wong, S., & Henry, K. R. (1999). Killer whale (*Orcinus orca*) hearing: Auditory brainstem response and behavioral audiograms. *Journal of the Acoustical Society of America, 106*, 1134–1141.

Tachibana, H., Aragane, K., Miyata, Y., & Sugita, M. (1997). Electrophysiological analysis of cognitive slowing in Parkinson's disease. *Journal of Neurological Sciences, 149*, 47–56.

Tachibana, H., Toda, K., & Sugita, M. (1992). Event-related potentials in patients with multiple lacunar infarcts. *Gerontology, 38*, 322–329.

Tackmann, W., Ettlin, T., & Strenge, H. (1982). Multimodality evoked potentials and electrically elicited blink reflex in optic neuritis. *Journal of Neurology, 227*, 157–163.

Tackmann, W., Ettlin, T., Wuthrich, R., & Strenge, H. (1984). Can multimodal evoked potentials and the electrically elicited blink reflex really increase the diagnostic probability of multiple sclerosis. In R. H. Nodar & C. Barber (Eds.), *Evoked potentials II: The second international evoked potentials symposium*, (pp. 632–636). Boston: Butterworth Publishers.

Taguchi, K., Picton, T. W., Orpin, J., & Gordman, J T. (1969). Evoked response audiometry in newborn infants. *Acta Oto-Laryngologica (Suppl) (Stockholm), 252*, 5–17.

Takagi, K. N., Suzuki, T., & Kobayashi, K. (1985). Effect of tone-burst frequency on fast and slow components of auditory brain-stem response. *Scandinavian Audiology, 14*, 75–79.

Takegata, R., Roggia, S. M., & Näätänen, R. (2003). A paradigm to measure mismatch negativity responses to phonetic and acoustic changes in parallel. *Audiology and Neuro-Otology, 8*, 234–241.

Takegoshi, H., & Murofushi, T. (2000). Vestibular evoked myogenic potentials in patients with spinocerebellar degeneration. *Acta Otolaryngologica, 120*, 821–824.

Takegoshi, H., & Murofushi, T. (2003). Effect of white noise on vestibular evoked myogenic potentials. *Hearing Research, 176*, 59–64.

Tanaka, F., Tsukasaki, N., Nakao, Y., Shigeno, K., & Kobayashi, T. (1999). Electrocochleographic evaluation of hearing loss in acoustic neuromas. *American Journal of Otology, 20*, 479–483.

Tanaka, M., Okubo, O., Fuchigami, T., & Harada, K. (2001). A study of mismatch negativity in newborns. *Pediatrics International, 43*, 281–286.

Tandon, O., Bhatia, R., & Goel, N. (1996). P3 event related evoked potentials in pregnancy. *Indian Journal of Physiology and Pharmacology, 40*, 345–349.

Tandon, O., Misra, R., & Tandon, I. (1990). Brainstem auditory evoked potentials (BAEPs) in pregnant women. *Indian Journal of Physiology and Pharmacology, 34*, 42–44.

Tang, T. P., McPherson, B., Yuen, K. C., Wong, L. L., & Lee, J. S. (2004). Auditory neuropathy/auditory dys-synchrony in school children with hearing loss: Frequency of occurrence. *International Journal of Pediatric Otorhinolaryngology, 68*, 175–183.

Tang, Y., Lopez, I., & Baloh, R. (2001). Age-related change of neuronal number in the human medial vestibular nucleus: A stereological investigation. *Journal of Vestibular Research, 11*, 357–363.

Tanguay, P., Edwards, R. M., Buchwald, J., Schwafel, J., & Allen, V. (1982). Auditory brain stem responses in autistic children. *Archives of General Psychiatry, 39*, 174–180.

Tarkka, I. M., Stokic, D. S., Basile, L. F., & Papanicolaou, A. C. (1995). Electric source localization of the auditory P300 agrees with magnetic source localization. *Electroencephalography and Clinical Neurophysiology, 96*, 538–545.

Tasaki, I. (1954). Nerve impulses in individual auditory nerve fibres of guinea pig. *Journal of Comparative Neurophysiology, 17*, 97–122.

Tasaki, I., Davis, H., & Eldredge, D. H. (1954). Exploration of cochlear potentials in guinea pig with a micro-electrode. *Journal of Acoustical Society of America, 26*, 765–773.

Tasman, A., Hahn, T., & Maiste, A. (1999). Menstrual cycle synchronized changes in brain stem auditory evoked potentials and visual evoked potentials. *Biological Psychiatry, 45*, 1516–1519.

Tator, C. H., & Nedzelski, J. M. (1985). Preservation of hearing in patients undergoing excision of acoustic neuromas and other cerebellopontine angle tumors. *Journal of Neurosurgery, 63*, 168–174.

Taylor, I., & Irwin, J. (1978). Some audiological aspects of DM. *Journal of Laryngology and Otology, 9*, 99–113.

Taylor, M. J., Houston, B. D., & Lowry, N. J. (1983). Recovery of auditory brain-stem responses after a severe hypoxic ischemic insult. *New England Journal of Medicine, 309*, 1169–1170.

Taylor, M. J., McMenamin, J. B., Andermann, E., & Watters, G. V. (1982). Electrophysiological investigation of the auditory system in Friedreich's ataxia. *Canadian Journal of Neurology, 9*, 131–135.

Taylor, M. J., Rosenblatt, B., & Linschoten, L. (1982). Auditory brainstem response abnormalities in autistic children. *Canadian Journal of Neurological Sciences, 9,* 429–433.

Taylor, M. J., Voros, J., Logan, W., & Malone, M. (1993). Changes in event-related potentials with stimulant medication in children with attention deficit hyperactivity disorder. *Biological Psychiatry, 36,* 139–156.

Teas, D.C. (1965). Analysis of evoked and ongoing electrical activity at the scalp of human subjects. *Journal of Speech and Hearing Research, 8,* 371–387.

Teas, D.C., Eldridge, D. H., & Davis, H. (1962). Cochlear responses to acoustic transients and interpretation of the whole nerve action potentials. *Journal of the Acoustical Society of America, 34,* 1438–1459

Telian, S. A., & Kileny, P. R. (1988). Pitfalls in neurotologic diagnosis. *Ear and Hearing, 9,* 86–91.

Telian, S. A., & Kileny, P. R. (1989). Usefulness of 1000 Hz tone-burst-evoked responses in the diagnosis of acoustic neuroma. *Otolaryngology Head and Neck Surgery, 101,* 466–471.

Telian, S. A., Kileny, P. R., Niparko, J. K., Kemink, J. L., & Graham, M. D. (1989). Normal auditory brainstem response in patients with acoustic neuroma. *Laryngoscope, 99,* 10–14.

Tempest, W., & Bryan, M. E. (1966). Objective audiometry. *Journal of the Acoustical Society of America, 40,* 914.

Teo, R. K., & Ferguson, D. A. (1986). The acute effects of ethanol on auditory event-related potentials. *Psychopharmacology (Berlin), 90,* 179–184.

Terkildsen, K., & Osterhammel, P. (1981). The influence of reference electrode position on recordings of the auditory brain stem response. *Ear and Hearing, 2,* 9–14.

Terkildsen, K., Huis in't Veld, F., & Osterhammel, P. (1977). Auditory brain stem responses in the diagnosis of cerebellopontine angle tumours. *Scandinavian Audiology, 6,* 43–45.

Terkildsen, K., Osterhammel, P., & Huis in't Veld, F. (1974). Far field electrocochleography: Electrode position. *Scandinavian Audiology, 3,* 123.

Terkildsen, K., Osterhammel, P., & Huis in't Velt, F. (1975). Far field electrocochleography. Frequency specificity of the response. *Scandinavian Audiology, 41,* 167–172.

Terkildsen, K., Osterhammel, P., & Thomsen, J. (1981). The ABR and the MLR in patients with acoustic neuromas. *Scandinavian Audiology (Suppl), 13,* 103–107.

Tervaniemi, M., & Brattico, E. (2004). From sounds to music—Towards understanding the neurocognition of musical sound perception. *Journal of Consciousness Studies, 11,* 9–27.

Tervaniemi, M., & Huotilainen, M. (2003). The promises of change-related brain potentials in cognitive neuroscience of music. *Neurosciences and Music, 999,* 29–39.

Tervaniemi, M., Maury, S., & Näätänen, R. (1994a). Neural representations of abstract stimulus features in the human brain as reflected by the mismatch negativity. *Neuroreport, 5,* 844–846.

Tervaniemi, M., Radil, T., Radilova, J., Kujala, T., & Näätänen, R. (1999). Pre-attentive discriminability of sound order as a function of tone duration and interstimulus interval: a mismatch negativity study. *Audiology & Neuro-Otology, 4,* 303–310.

Tervaniemi, M., Rytkonen, M., Schroger, E., Ilmoniemi, R. J., & Näätänen, R. (2001). Superior formation of cortical memory traces for melodic patterns in musicians. *Learning & Memory, 8,* 295–300.

Tervaniemi, M., Saarinen, J., Paavilainen, P., Danilova, N., & Näätänen, R. (1994b). Temporal integration of auditory information in sensory memory as reflected by the mismatch negativity. *Biological Psychology, 38,* 157–167.

Thai-Van, H., Chanal, J., Coudert, C., Veuillet, E., Truy, E., & Collet, L. (2001). Relationship between NRT measurements and behavioral levels in children with the Nucleus 24 cochlear implant may change over time: Preliminary report. *International Journal of Pediatric Otorhinolaryngology, 58,* 153–162.

Thelin, J. W., & Fussner, J. C. (2005). Factors related to the development of communication in CHARGE syndrome. *American Journal of Medical Genetics, 15,* 282–90.

Theodore, W. H., Comite, F., Sato, S., Loriaux, L., & Cutler, G. (1983). EEG and evoked potentials in precocious puberty. *Electroencephalography and Clinical Neurophysiology, 55,* 69–72.

Thivierge, J., Bedard, C., Cote, R., & Maziade, M. (1990). Brainstem auditory evoked response and subcortical abnormalities in autism. *American Journal of Psychiatry, 147,* 1609–1613.

Thoma, J., Gerull, G., & Mrowinski, D. (1986). A long-term study of hearing in children following neonatal hyperbilirubinemia. *Archives of Otorhinolaryngology, 243,* 133–137.

Thoman, E. B., Davis, D. H., & Denenberg, V. H. (1987). The sleeping and waking states of infants: Correlations across time and person. *Physiology & Behavior, 41,* 531–537.

Thomas, K. (2003). Assessing brain development using neurophysiologic and behavioral measures. *Journal of Pediatrics, 143,* S46-S53.

Thompson, D. C., McPhillips, H., Davis, R. L., Lieu, T. L., Homer, C. J., & Helfand, M. (2000). Universal newborn hearing screening: Summary of evidence. *Journal of the American Medical Association, 286,* 2000-2010.

Thompson, D. S., Woodward, J. B., Ringel, S. P., & Nelson, L. M. (1983). Evoked potential abormalities in myotonic dystrophy. *Electroencephalography and Clinical Neurophysiology, 56,* 453–456.

Thomsen, J., Nyboe, J., Borum, P., Tos, M., & Barfoed, C. (1981). Acoustic neuromas Diagnostic efficiency of various test combinations. *Archives of Otolaryngology, 107,* 601–607.

Thomsen, J., Terkildsen, K., & Osterhammel, P. (1978). Auditory brainstem responses in patients with acoustic neuromas. *Scandinavian Audiology, 7,* 179–183.

Thornton, A. R. D. (1975). Distortion of averaged post-auricular muscle responses due to system bandwidth limits. *Electroencephalography and Clinical Neurophysiology, 39,* 195–197.

Thornton, A. R. D., & Coleman, M. J. (1975). The adaptation of cochlear and brainstem auditory evoked potentials in humans. *Electroencephalography and Clinical Neurophysiology, 39,* 399–406.

Thornton, A. R. D., Farrell, G., & McSporran, E. L. (1989). Clinical methods for the objective estimation of loudness discomfort level (LDL) using auditory brainstem responses in patients. *Scandinavian Audiology, 18,* 225–230.

Thornton, A. R. D., Farrell, G., Reid, A., & Peters, J. (1991). Isochronic mapping: A preliminary report of a new technique. *British Journal of Audiology, 25,* 275–282.

Thornton, A. R. D., Mendel, M. I., & Anderson, C. (1977). Effect of stimulus frequency and intensity on the middle components of the averaged auditory electroencephalic response. *Journal of Speech and Hearing Research, 20,* 81–94.

Thornton, A. R., Shin, K., Gottesman, E., & Hine, J. (2001). Temporal nonlinearities of the cochlear amplifier revealed by maximum length sequence stimulation. *Clinical Neurophysiology, 112,* 768–777.

Thornton, A. R. D., & Slaven, A. (1993). Auditory brainstem responses recorded at fast stimulation using maximum length sequences. *British Journal of Audiology, 27,* 205–210.

Thornton, A. R. D., Yardley, L., & Farrell, G. (1987). The objective estimation of loudness discomfort level using auditory brainstem evoked responses. *Scandinavian Audiology, 16,* 219–225.

Thornton, C., Catley, D. M., Jordan, C., Royston, D., Lehange, J. R., & Jones, J. G. (1981). Enflurane increases the latency of early components of the auditory evoked response man. *British Journal of Anesthesia, 53,* 1102–1103.

Thornton, C., Creagh-Barry, P., Jordan, C., Luff, N. P., Dore, C. J., Henley, M., & Newton, D. E. (1992). Somatosensory and auditory evoked responses recorded simultaneously: Differential effects of nitrous oxide and isoflurane. *British Journal of Anesthesia, 68,* 508–514.

Thornton, C., Heneghan, C., James, M., & Jones, J. (1984a). Effects of halothane and enflurane with controlled ventilation an auditory evoked potentials. *British Journal of Anaesthesia, 56,* 315–323.

Thornton, C., Heneghan, C. P. H., James, M. F. M., & Jones, J. G. (1984b). The effects of halothane and enflurane anesthesia on the early auditory evoked potentials in humans. In R. H. Nodar & C. Barber (Eds.), *Evoked potentials II: The second international evoked potentials symposium* (pp. 483–489). Boston: Butterworth Publishers.

Thornton, C., Heyderman, R. S., Thorniley, M., Curtis, N., Mielke, J., Pasvol, G., & Newton, D. E. (2002). Auditory- and somatosensory-evoked potentials in cerebral malaria and anaesthesia: A comparison. *European Journal of Anesthesiology, 19,* 717–726.

Thornton, C., Konieczko, K. M., Knight, A. B., Kaul, B., Jones, J. G., Dore, C. J., & White, D.C. (1989). Effect of propofol on the auditory evoked response and oesophageal contractility. *British Journal of Anaesthesia, 63,* 411–417.

Tian, J., Juhola, M., & Gronfors, T. (1997). Latency estimation of auditory brainstem response by neural networks. *Artificial Intelligence in Medicine, 10,* 115–128.

Tietze, G. (1980). Stimulation methods for a simultaneous derivation of acoustically evoked brainstem and cortical responses. *Scandinavian Audiology, 11,* 97–104.

Tiitinen, H., Sinkkonen, J., May, P., & Näätänen, R. (1994). The auditory transient 40-Hz response is insensitive to changes in stimulus features. *Neuroreport, 6,* 190–192.

Tiitinen, H., Sivonen, P., Alku, P., Virtanen, J., & Näätänen, R. (1999). Electromagnetic recordings reveal latency differences in speech and tone processing in humans. *Brain Research & Cognitive Brain Research, 8,* 355–363.

Tobimatsu, S., Fukui, R., Kato, M., Kobayashi, T., & Kuroiwa, Y. (1985). Multimodality evoked potentials in patients and carriers with adrenoleukodystrophy and adrenomyeloneuropathy. *Electroencephalography and Clinical Neurophysiology, 62,* 18–24.

Todd, N. P., Cody, F. W. & Banks, J. R. (2000). A saccular origin of frequency tuning in myogenic vestibular evoked potentials? Implications for human responses to loud sounds. *Hearing Research, 41,* 180–188.

Tokimura, H., Asakura, T., Tokimura, Y., Atsuchi, M., Kimotsuki, K., Sato, E., et al (1990). [Intraoperative ABR monitoring during cerebello-pontine angle surgery.] *No Shinkei Geka, 18,* 1023–1027.

Tolosa, E. S., & Zeese, J. A. (1979). Brainstem auditory evoked responses in progressive supranuclear palsy. *Annals of Neurology, 6,* 369.

Tonn, J., Schlake, H., Goldbrunner, R., Milewski, C., Helms, J., & Roosen, K. (2000). Acoustic neuroma surgery as an interdisciplinary approach: A neurosurgical series of 508 patients. *Journal of Neurology Neurosurgery and Psychiatry, 69,* 161–166.

Tonndorf, J. (1966). Bone conduction—studies in experimental animals. *Acta Otolaryngologica (Supp), 213,* 132.

Tonnquist-Uhlen, I. (1996). Topography of auditory evoked long-latency potentials in children with severe language impairment: The P2 and N2 components. *Ear and Hearing, 17,* 314–326.

Tooley, M. A., Stapleton, C. L., Greenslade, G. L., & Prys-Roberts, C. (2004). Mid-latency auditory evoked response during propofol and alfentanil anaesthesia. *British Journal of Anaesthesia, 92,* 25–32.

Tooth, G. (1947). On the use of mental tests for the measurement of disability after head injury: With a comparison between the results of these tests in patients after head injury and psychoneurotics. *Journal of Neurology, Neurosurgery and Psychiatry, 10,* 467–471.

Tos, M., & Thomsen, J. (1982). The price of preservation of hearing in acoustic neuroma surgery. *Annals of Otology, Rhinology & Laryngology, 91,* 240–245.

Totsuka, G., Nakamura, K., & Kirikae, I. (1954). Studies of the acoustic reflex. I. Electromyographic studies of the acoustic-auricular reflex. *Annals of Otology, Rhinology & Laryngology, 63,* 939–949.

Townsend, G. I., & Cody, D. T. (1971). The averaged inion response evoked by acoustic stimulation: Its relation to the saccule. Anna. *Annals of Otology, Rhinology & Laryngology, 80,* 121–131.

Toyama, Y., Kobayashi, T., Nishiyama, Y., Satoh, K., Ohkawa, M., & Seki, K. (2005). CT for acute stage of closed head injury. *Radiation Medicine, 23,* 309–316.

Tramo, J. M., Schneck, M. J., & Lee, B. C. P. (1985). Evoked potentials and MRI in the diagnosis of multiple sclerosis. *Neurology, 35,* 105.

Trautwein, P., Sininger, Y., & Nelson, R. (2000). Cochlear implantation of auditory neuropathy. *Journal of the American Academy of Audiology, 11,* 309–315.

Tremblay, K. L., Billings, C., & Rohila, N. (2004). Speech evoked cortical potentials: effects of age and stimulus presentation rate. *Journal of the American Academy of Audiology, 15,* 226–237.

Tremblay, K. L., Friesen, L., Martin, B. A., & Wright, R. (2003). Test-retest reliability of cortical evoked potentials using naturally produced speech sounds. *Ear and Hearing, 24,* 225–232.

Tremblay, K. L., & Kraus, N. (2002). Auditory training induces asymmetrical changes in cortical neural activity. *Journal of Speech, Language & Hearing Research, 45,* 564–572.

Tremblay, K. L., Kraus, N., Carrell, T. D., & McGee, T. (1997). Central auditory system plasticity: Generalization to novel stimuli following listening training. *Journal of the Acoustical Society of America, 102,* 3762–3773.

Tremblay, K. L., Kraus, N., & McGee, T. (1998). The time course of auditory perceptual learning: Neurophysiological changes during speech-sound training. *Neuroreport, 9,* 3557–3560.

Tremblay, K. L., Kraus, N., McGee, T., Ponton, C., & Otis, B. (2001). Central auditory plasticity: Changes in the N1-P2 complex after speech-sound training. *Ear and Hearing, 22,* 79–90.

Tremblay, K. L., Piskosz, M., & Souza, P. (2003). Effects of age and age-related hearing loss on the neural representation of speech cues. *Clinical Neurophysiology, 114,* 1332–1343.

Triana, R., Suits, G., Garrison, S., Prazma, J., Brechtelsbauer, P., et al. (1991). Inner ear damage secondary to diabetes mellitus. *Archives of Otolaryngology—Head & Neck Surgery, 117,* 635–640.

Trillo-Urrutia, L., Fernandez-Galinski, S., & Castano-Santa, J. (2003). Awareness detected by auditory evoked potential monitoring. *British Journal of Anaesthesia, 91,* 290–292.

Truy, E., Gallego, S., Chanal, J., Collet, L., & Morgon, A. (1998). Correlation between electrical auditory brainstem response and perceptual thresholds in Digisonic Cochlear Implant users. *Laryngoscope, 108,* 554–559.

Tsubokawa, T., Nichimoto, H., Yamamoto, T., Kitamura, M., Katayama, Y., & Moriyasu, N. (1980). Assessment of brainstem damage by the auditory brainstem response in acute severe brain injury. *Journal of Neurology, Neurosurgery, and Psychiatry, 43,* 1005–1011.

Tsuchitani, C. (1983). Physiology of the auditory system. In E. J. Moore (Ed.). *Bases of auditory brain-stem evoked responses* (pp. 67–108). New York: Grune and Stratton.

Tsuji, S., Muracka, S., Kuroina, Y., Chen, K. M., & Gajdusek, C. (1981). Auditory brainstem evoked response of Parkinson-dementia complex and amyotrophic lateral sclerosis in Guam and Japan. *Rirsho Shinkeigaku (Clinical Neurology Tokyo), 21,* 37–41.

Tsutsumi, T., Nishida, H., Noguchi, Y., Komatsuzaki, A., & Kitamura, K. (2001). Audiological findings in patients with myoclonic epilepsy associated with ragged-red fibres. *Journal of Laryngology & Otology, 115,* 777–781.

Tucci, D., Telian, S., Kileny, P., Hoff, J., & Kemink, J. (1994). Stability of hearing preservation following acoustic neuroma surgery. *American Journal of Otology, 15,* 183–188.

Tucker, A., Slattery, W., III, Solcyk, L., & Brackmann, D. (2001). Intraoperative auditory assessments as predictors of hearing preservation after vestibular schwannoma surgery. *Journal of the American Academy of Audiology, 12,* 471–477.

Tucker, D. A., & Ruth, R. A. (1996). Effects of age, signal level, and signal rate on the auditory middle latency response. *Journal of the American Academy of Audiology, 7,* 83–91.

Tullio, P. (1929). *Some experiments and considerations on experimental otology and phonetics.* Bologna: Licinio Cappelli.

Turner, R. G., & Nielsen, D. (1984). Application of clinical decision analysis to audiological tests. *Ear and Hearing, 5,* 125–133.

Turner, R. G., Shepard, N. T., & Frazer, G. J. (1984). Clinical performance of audiological and related diagnostic tests. *Ear and Hearing, 5,* 187–194.

Uc, E. Y., Skinner, R. D., Rodnitzky, R. L., & Garcia-Rill, E. (2003). The midlatency auditory evoked potential P50 is abnormal in Huntington's disease. *Journal of Neurological Sciences, 212,* 1–5.

Umbricht, D., Javitt, D., Novak, G., Bates, J., Pollack, S., Lieberman, J., & Kane, J. (1998). Effects of clozapine on auditory event-related potentials in schizophrenia. *Biological Psychiatry, 44,* 716–725.

Umbricht, D., Koller, R., Vollenweider, F. X., & Schmid, L. (2002). Mismatch negativity predicts psychotic experiences induced by NMDA receptor antagonist in healthy volunteers. *Biological Psychiatry, 51,* 400–406.

Umbricht, D., Schmid, L., Koller, R., Vollenweider, F. X., Hel, D., & Javitt, D.C. (2000). Ketamine-induced deficits in auditory and visual context-dependent processing in healthy volunteers: Implications for models of cognitive deficits in schizophrenia. *Archives of General Psychiatry, 57,* 1139–1147.

Umbricht, D., Vollenweider, F. X., Schmid, L., Grubel, C., Skrabo, A., Huber, T., & Koller, R. (2003). Effects of the 5-HT2A agonist psilocybin on mismatch negativity generation and AX-continuous performance task: Implications for the neuropharmacology of cognitive deficits in schizophrenia. *Neuropsychopharmacology 28,* 170–181.

Umbricht, D., Vyssotky, D., Latanov, A., Nitsch, R., Brambilla, R., D'Adamo, P., & Lipp, H. P. (2004). Midlatency auditory event-related potentials in mice: Comparison to midlatency auditory ERPs in humans. *Brain Research, 1019,* 189–200.

Uno, A., Kaga, K., Tsuzuku, T., & Kuroki, M. (1993). Middle-latency responses of awake and anesthetized Japanese macaques. *Audiology, 32,* 302–307.

Urbani, L., & Lucertini, M. (1994). Effects of hypobaric hypoxia on the human auditory brainstem responses. *Hearing Research, 76,* 73–77.

Uri, N., Schuchman, G., & Pratt, H. (1984). Auditory brain-stem evoked potentials in Bell's palsy. *Archives of Otolaryngology, 110,* 301–304.

Ushio, M., Kaga, K., Sakata, H., Ogawa, Y., Makiyama, Y., & Nishimoto, H. (2001). Auditory brainstem repsonse and temporal bone pathology findings in a brain-dead infant. *International Journal of Pediatric Otorhinolaryngology, 58,* 249–253.

Ushio, M., Matsuzaki, M., Takegoshi, H., & Murofushi, T. (2001). Click and short tone burst evoked myogenic potentials in cerebellopontine angle tumors. *Acta Otolaryngologica, 545,* 133–135.

Valdes, J., Perez-Abalo, M., Martin, V., Savio, G., Sierra, C., Rodriguez, E., et al. (1997). Comparison of the statistical indicators for the automatic detection of 80 Hz auditory steady state responses. *Ear and Hearing, 18,* 420–429.

Valente, M., Peterein, J., Goebel, J., & Neely, J. (1995). Four cases of acoustic neuromas with normal hearing. *Journal of the American Academy of Audiology, 6,* 203–210.

Valkama, A., Laitakari, K., Tolonen, E., Vayrynen, M., Vainionpaa, L., & Koivisto, M. (2000). Prediction of permanent hearing loss in high-risk preterm infants at term age. *European Journal of Pediatrics, 159,* 459–464.

Valvassori, G. E. (1986). Applications of magnetic resonance imaging in otology. *American Journal of Otology, 7,* 262–266.

Van, H., Deguine, O., Esteve-Fraysse, M., Bonafe, A., & Fraysse, B. (1999). Relationship between cochleovestibular disorders in hemifacial spasm and neurovascular compression. *Laryngoscope, 109,* 741–747.

Vanagaite Vingen, J., Pareja, J., Storen, O., White, L., & Stovner, L. (1998). Phonophobia in migraine. *Cephalalgia, 18,* 243–249.

Vanasse, M., Fischer, C., Berthezene, F., Roux, Y., Volman, G., & Mornex, R. (1989). Normal brainstem auditory evoked potentials in adult hypothyroidism. *Laryngoscope, 99,* 302–306.

Van Campen, L. E., Hall, J. W., III, Grantham, D. W. (1997). Human offset auditory brainstem response: Effects of stimulus acoustic ringing and rise-fall time. *Hearing Research, 103,* 35–46.

Van Campen, L. E., Sammeth, C. A., Hall, J. W., III, & Peek, B. F. (1992). Comparison of Etymotic insert and TDH supra-aural earphones in auditory brainstem response measurement. *Journal of the American Academy of Audiology, 3,* 315–323.

van Deelen, G. W., Ruding, P. R., Smoorenburg, G. G., Veldman, J. E.,& Huizing, E. H. (1988). Electrocochleographic changes in relation to cochlear histopathology in experimental endolymphatic hydrops. *Acta Otolaryngologica, 105,* 193–201.

van den Honert, C., & Stypulkowski, P. H. (1986). Characterization of the electrically evoked auditory brainstem response (ABR) in cats and humans. *Hearing Research, 21,* 109–126.

Vanderbilt University Deafness and Heredity Study Group. (1968). Dominantly inherited low-frequency hearing loss. *Archives of Otolaryngology, 88,* 242.

van der Drift, J. F. C., Brocaar, M. P., & van Zanten, G. A. (1987). The relation between the pure-tone audiogram and the click auditory brainstem response threshold in cochlear hearing loss. *Audiology, 26,* 1–10.

van der Drift, J. F. C., Brocaar, M. P., & van Zanten, G. A. (1988a). Brainstem response audiometry. I. Its use in distinguishing between conductive and cochlear hearing loss. *Audiology, 27,* 260–270.

van der Drift, J. F. C., Brocaar, M. P., & van Zanten, G. A. (1988b). Brainstem response audiometry. II. Classification of hearing loss by discriminant analysis. *Audiology, 27,* 271–278.

van der Meyden, C., Bartel, P., Sommers, D., Blom, M., Becker, P., Erasmus, S., et al. (1992). Effect of acute doses of controlled-release carbamazepine on clinical, psychomotor, electrophysiological and cognitive parameters of brain function. *Epilepsia, 33,* 335–342.

Vander Werff, K. R., & Brown, C. J. (2005). Effect of audiometric configuration on threshold and suprathreshold auditory steady-state responses. *Ear and Hearing, 26,* 310–326.

Vander Werff, K., Brown, C., Gienapp, B., & Schmidt Clay, K. (2002). Comparison of auditory steady-state response and auditory brainstem

response thresholds in children. *Journal of the American Academy of Audiology, 13,* 227–235.

Van Nechel, C., Deltenre, P., Strul, S., & Capon, A. (1982). Value of simultaneous recording of brainstem auditory evoked potentials, blink reflex, and short-latency somatosensory evoked potentials for the assessment of brainstem function in clinical neurology. In J. Courjon, F. Mauguiere, & M. Revol (Eds.), *Clinical applications of evoked potentials in neurology* (pp. 203–210). New York: Raven Press.

Vannier, E., Adam, O., Karasinski, P., Ohresser, M., & Motsch, J. (2001). Computer-assisted ABR interpretation using the automatic construction of the latency-intensity curve. *Audiology, 40,* 191–201.

Vannier, E., Adam, O., & Motsch, J. (2002). Objective detection of brainstem auditory evoked potentials with a priori information from higher presentation levels. *Artificial Intelligence in Medicine, 25,* 283–301.

van Olphen, A. F., Rodenburg, M., & Vervey, C. (1978). Distribution of brain stem responses to acoustic stimuli over the human scalp. *Audiology, 17,* 511–518.

van Olphen, A. F., Rodenburg, M., & Vervey, C. (1979). Influence of the stimulus repetition rate on brain-stem evoked responses in man. *Audiology, 18,* 388–394.

Van Riper, L. A., & Kileny, P. R. (1999). ABR hearing screening for high-risk infants. *The American Journal of Otology, 20,* 516–521.

Van Riper, L. A., & Kileny, P. R. (2002). ABR hearing screening for high-risk infants. *Neonatal Intensive Care, 15,* 47–54.

van Strääten, H. (1999). Automated auditory brainstem response in neonatal hearing screening. *Acta Paediatrica, 432,* 76–79.

van Strääten, H. L., Groote, M. E., & Oudesluys-Murphy, A. M. (1996). Evaluation of an automated auditory brainstem response infant hearing screening method in at risk neonates. *European Journal of Pediatrics, 155,* 702–705.

van Strääten, H. L., Tibosch, C. H., Dorrepaal, C., Dekker, F. W., & Kok, J. H. (2001). Efficacy of automated auditory brainstem response hearing screening in very preterm newborns. *Journal of Pediatrics, 138,* 674–678.

van Weert, S., Stokroos, R., Rikers, M., & Van Dijk, P. (2005). Effect of peri-modiolar cochlear implant positioning on auditory nerve responses: A neural response telemetry study. *Acta Otolaryngologica, 125,* 725–731.

van Zanten, G. A., & Brocaar, M. P. (1984). Frequency-specific auditory brainstem responses to clicks masked by notched noise. *Audiology, 23,* 253–264.

van Zuijen, T. L., Sussman, E., Winkler, I., Näätänen, R., & Tervaniemi, M. (2004). Grouping of sequential sounds—an event-related potential study comparing musicians and nonmusicians. *Journal of Cognitive Neuroscience, 16,* 331–338.

Varga, R., Kelley, P., Keats, B., Starr, A., Leal, S., Cohn, E., & Kimberling, W. (2003). Non-syndromic recessive auditory neuropathy is the result of mutations in the otoferlin (OTOF) gene. *Journal of Medical Genetics, 40,* 45–50.

Vaughan, H. G., & Arezzo, J. C. (1988). The neural basis of event-related potentials. In T. W. Picton (Ed.), *Human event related potentials: EEG handbook.* Amsterdam: Elsevier Science Publishers.

Vaughan, H. G., Jr. (1982). The neural origins of human event-related potentials. *Annals of New York Academy of Sciences, 388,* 125–138.

Vaughan, H. G., Jr., & Ritter, W. (1970). The sources of auditory evoked responses recorded from the human scalp. *Electroencephalography and Clinical Neurophysiology, 28,* 360–367.

Vaz, C., & Thakor, N. (1989). Adaptive Fourier estimation of time-varying evoked potentials. *IEEE Transactions in Biomedical Engineering, 36,* 448–455.

Velasquez-Villasenor, L., Merchant, S., Tsuji, K., Glynn, R., Wal, C. I., & Rauch, S. (2001). Temporal bone studies of the human peripheral vestibular system. Normative Scarpa's ganglion cell data. *Annals of Otology Rhinology and Laryngology, 181,* 14–19.

Veniselli, E., Biancheri, R., DiRocco, M., & Tortorelli, S. (1998). Neurophysiological findings in a case of carbohydrate-deficient glycoprotein (CDG) syndrome type I with phosphomannomutase deficiency. *European Journal of Paediatrics and Neurology, 2,* 239–244.

Venkataramana, N. K., Satishchandra, P., Hegde, A. S., Reddy, G. N., & Das, B. S. (1988). Evaluation of brainstem auditory evoked responses in congenital hydrocephalus. *Child's Nervous System, 4,* 334–348.

Verbaten, M., Overtoom, C. C., Koelega, H. S., Swaab-Barneveld, H., & van der Gaag, R. J. (1994). Methylphenidate influences on both early and late ERP waves of ADHD children in a continuous performance test. *Journal of Abnormal Child Psychology, 22,* 561–578.

Vercruyssen, A., Martin, J. J., & Mercelis, R. (1982). Neurophysiological studies in adrenomyeloneuropathy. A report on five cases. *Journal of Neurological Science, 56,* 327–336.

Verleger, R. (1998). Event-related potentials ond cognition: A critique of the context updating hypothesis and an alternative interpretation of P3. *Behavior, Brain and Science, 11,* 343–356.

Verleger, R., Kompf, D., & Neukater, W. (1992). Event-related EEG potentials in mild dementia of the Alzheimer type. *Electroencephalography and Clinical Neurophysiology, 84,* 332–343.

Verleger, R., Lefebre, C., Wieschemeyer, R., & Kompf, D. (1997). Event-related potentials suggest slowing of brain processes in generalized epilepsy and alterations of visual processing in patients with partial seizures. *Brain Research & Cognitive Brain Research, 5,* 205–219.

Verma, A., Bisht, M. S., & Ahuja, G. K. (1984). Involvement of central nervous system in diabetes mellitus. *Journal of Neurology, Neurosurgery, and Psychiatry, 47,* 414–416.

Verma, N. P., Nigro, M. A., & Hart, Z. H. (1987). Rett syndrome—a gray matter disease? Electrophysiologic evidence. *Electroencephalography and Clinical Neurophysiology, 67,* 327–329.

Versino, M., Bergamaschi, R., Romani, A., Banfi, P., Callieco, R., Citterio, A., Gerosa, E., & Cosi, V. (1992). Middle latency auditory evoked potentials improve the detection of abnormalities along auditory pathways in multiple sclerosis patients. *Electroencephalography and Clinical Neurophysiology, 84,* 296–299.

Vesco, K. K., Bone, R. C., Ryan, J. C., & Polich, J. (1993). P300 in young and elderly subjects: auditory frequency and intensity effects. *Electroencephalography and Clinical Neurophysiology, 88,* 302–308.

Viemeister, N. F. (1979). Temporal modulation transfer functions based upon modulation thresholds. *Journal of the Acoustical Society of America, 66,* 164–180.

Virtaniemi, J., Kuusisto, J., Karjalainen, S., Karjalainen, L., & Laakso, M. (1995). Improvement of metabolic control does not normalize auditory brainstem latencies in subjects with insulin-dependent diabetes mellitus. *American Journal of Otolaryngology, 16,* 172–176.

Virtaniemi, J., Laakso, M., Karja, J., Nuutinen, J., & Karjalainen, S. (1993). Auditory brainstem latencies in Type 1 (insulin-dependent) diabetic patients. *American Journal of Otolaryngology, 14,* 413–418.

Vivion, M. C., Hirsch, J. E., Frye-Osier, J. L., & Goldstein, R. (1980). Effects of stimulus rise-fall time and equivalent duration on middle components of AER. *Scandinavian Audiology, 9,* 223–232.

Vivion, M. C., Wolf, K. E., Goldstein, R., Hirsch, J. C., & MacFarland, W. H. (1979). Toward objective analysis for electroencephalic audiometry. *Journal of Speech and Hearing Research, 22,* 88–102.

Vohr, B. R., Lester, B., Rapisardi, G., O'Dea, C., Brown, L., Peucker, M., Cashore, W., & Oh, W. (1989). Abnormal brain-stem function (brain-stem auditory evoked response) correlates with acoustic cry features in term infants with hyperbilirubinemia. *Journal of Pediatrics, 115,* 303–308.

Vohr, B., Carty, L. M., Moore, P. E., & Letourneau, K. (1998). The Rhode Island Hearing Assessment Program: Experience with statewide hearing screening. *Journal of Pediatrics, 13,* 353–357.

Vohr, B. R., Oh, W., Stewart, E. J., Bentkover, J. D., Gabbard, S., Lemons, J., Papile, L. A., & Pye, R. (2001). Comparison of costs and referral rates of 3 universal newborn hearing screening protocols. *Journal of Pediatrics, 139,* 238–244.

von Deuster, C., & Axmann, D. (1995). [Reliability of brain stem audiometry in specific learning disorders (disorders of sensory integration).] *Laryngorhinootologie, 74,* 539–542.

von Glass, W., Haid, C., Cidlinsky, K., Stenglein, C., & Christ, P. (1991). False-positive MR imaging in the diagnosis of acoustic neuromas. *Archives of Otolaryngology—Head & Neck Surgery, 104,* 863–867.

von Knorring, L., & Perris, C. (1981). Biochemistry of the augmenting-reducing response in visual evoked potentials. *Neuropsychobiology, 7,* 1–8.

Wackym, P., Firszt, J., Gaggl, W., Runge-Samuelson, C., Reeder, R., & Raulie, J. (2004). Electrophysiologic effects of placing cochlear implant electrodes in a perimodiolar position in young children. *Laryngoscope, 114,* 71–76.

Wade, P. J., & House, W. (1984). Hearing preservation in patients with acoustic neuromas via the middle fossa approach. *Archives of Otolaryngology—Head & Neck Surgery, 92,* 184–193.

Waldo, M. C., Cawthra, E., Adler, L. E., Dubester, S., Staunton, M., Nagamoto, H., Baker, N., Madion, A., Simon, J., & Scherzinger, A. (1995). Auditory sensory gating, hippocampal volume, and catecholamine metabolism in schizophrenics and their siblings. *Schizophrenia Research, 12,* 93–106.

Waldo, M. C., Gerhardt, G., Baker, N., Drebing, C., Adler, L., & Freedman, R. (1992). Auditory sensory gating and catecholamine metabolism in schizophrenic and normal subjects. *Psychiatry Research, 44,* 21–32.

Walker, J. E., Jacobson, J. L., & Cody, D. T. R. (1964). Comparison of cerebral and myogenic components of the averaged response to sound stimulation in man. *Electroencephalography and Clinical Neurophysiology, 17,* 456.

Walker, M. L., Mayer, T. A., Storrs, B. B., & Hylton, P. D. (1985). Pediatric head injury—factors which influence outcome. *Concepts in Pediatric Neurosurgery, 6,* 84–97.

Wall, L. G., Dalebout, S. D., Davidson, S. A., & Fox, R. A. (1991). Effect of hearing impairment on event-related potentials for tone and speech distinctions. *Folia Phoniatr (Basel), 43,* 265–274.

Wall, L., Davidson, S., & Dalebout, S. (1991). Determining latency and amplitude for multiple peaked P300 waveforms. *Journal of the American Academy of Audiology, 2,* 189–194.

Walser, H., Kriss, A., Cunningham, K., Halliday, A. M., Jones, S. J., & Taube, D. (1984). A multimodal evoked potential assessment of uremia. In R. H. Nodar & C. Barber (Eds.), *Evoked potentials II: The Second International Evoked Potentials Symposium* (pp. 643–649). Boston: Butterworth Publishers.

Walsh, S. M., & Leake-Jones, P. A. (1982). Chronic electrical stimulation of auditory nerve in cat: Physiological and histological results. *Hearing Research, 7,* 281–304.

Walter, B., & Blegvad, B. (1981). Identification of wave I by means of an atraumatic ear canal electrode. *Scandinavian Audiology (Suppl), 13,* 63–64.

Walter, D. O. (1969). A posteriori "Weiner filtering" of average evoked responses. *Electroencephalography and Clinical Neurophysiology (Suppl), 27,* 61–70.

Walton, J., Orlando, M., & Burkard, R. (1999). Auditory brainstem response forward-masking recovery functions in older humans with normal hearing. *Hearing Research, 127,* 86–94.

Wang, C., Hsu, W., & Young, Y. (2005). Vestibular evoked myogenic potentials in neurofibromatosis 2. *Annals of Otology, Rhinology & Laryngology, 114,* 69–73.

Wang, C., Tien, H., & Hsu, C. (2001). Diagnosis and treatment of lipomas of the internal auditory canal. *Ear Nose and Throat Journal, 80,* 340–342.

Wang, C., & Young, Y. (2004). Earlier and later components of tone burst evoked myogenic potentials. *Hearing Research, 191,* 59–66.

Wang, L., Jiang, W., Gong, J., & Zheng, X. (1994). Saturation diving with heliox to 350 meters. Observation of hearing threshold, brainstem evoked response and acoustic impedance. *Chinese Medical Journal, 107,* 934–938.

Wang, S. J., Hsu, W. C., & Young, Y. H. (2003). Reversible cochleo-vestibular deficits in two cases of jugular foramen tumor after surgery. *European Archives of Otorhinolaryngology.*

Wang, S. J., & Young, Y. (2003). Vestibular evoked myogenic potentials using simultaneous binaural acoustic stimulation. *Hearing Research, 185,* 43–48.

Wang, W., & Schoenen, J. (1998). Interictal potentiation of passive "oddball" auditory event-related potentials in migraine. *Cephalalgia, 18,* 261–265.

Wang, W., Wang, Y. H., Fu, X. M., Sun, Z. M., & Schoenen, J. (1999). Auditory evoked potentials and multiple personality measures in migraine and post-traumatic headaches. *Pain, 79,* 235–242.

Waring, M. D. (1992). Electrically evoked auditory brainstem response monitoring of auditory brainstem implant integrity during facial nerve tumor surgery. *Laryngoscope, 102,* 1293–1295.

Waring, M. D. (1995). Intraoperative electrophysiological monitoring to assist placement of auditory brainstem implant. *Annals of Otology, Rhinology & Laryngology, 104,* 33–36.

Waring, M. D. (1996). Properties of auditory brainstem responses evoked by intra-operative electrical stimulation of the cochlear nucleus in human subjects. *Electroencephalography and Clinical Neurophysiology, 100,* 538–548.

Warrier, C. M., Johnson, K. L., Hayes, E. A., Nicol, T., & Kraus, N. (2004). Learning impaired children exhibit timing deficits and training-related improvements in auditory cortical responses to speech in noise. *Experimental Brain Research, 157,* 431–441.

Wasch, H. H., Estrin, W. J., Yip, P., Bowler, R., & Cone, J. E. (1989). Prolongation of the P-300 latency associated with hydrogen sulfide exposure. *Archives of Neurology, 46,* 902–904.

Wastell, D. G. (1977). Statistical detection of individual evoked responses: An evaluation of Woody's adaptive filter. *Electroencephalography and Clinical Neurophysiology, 42,* 835–839.

Wasterstrom, S.-.A. (1985). Auditory brainstem-evoked response after single-dose injection of lidocaine and tocainide. *Scandinavian Audiology, 14,* 41–45.

Watanabe, K., Yamada, H., Hara, K., Miyazaki, S., & Nakamura, S. (1984). Neurophysiological evaluation of newborns with congenital hydrocephalus. *Clinical Electroencephalography, 15,* 22–31.

Watanabe, T., Miwa, H., Wada, K., Sugano, K., Hatori, K., Tanaka, S., et al. (1999). [Rhythmic involuntary movement of the neck in a patient with brainstem encephalitis.] *No To Shinkei, 51,* 1045–1048.

Waters, C., French, G., & Burt, M. (2004). Difficulty in brainstem death testing in the presence of high spinal cord injury. *British Journal of Anaesthesia, 92,* 760–764.

Watkin, P., & Baldwin, M. (1999). Confirmation of deafness in infancy. *Archives of Disease in Childhood, 81,* 380–389.

Watson, D. (1996). The effects of cochlear hearing loss, age and sex on the auditory brainstem response. *Audiology, 35,* 246–258.

Watson, S., & Colebatch, J. (1998). Vestibulocollic reflexes evoked by short-duration galvanic stimulation in man. *Journal of Physiology, 513,* 587–597.

Watson, S., Halmagyi, G., & Colebatch, J. (2000). Vestibular hypersensitivity to sound (Tullio phenomenon): Structural and functional assessment. *Neurology, 54,* 722–728.

Wazen, J. J. (1994). Intraoperative monitoring of auditory function: Experimental observations and new applications. *Laryngoscope, 104,* 446–455.

Webb, K. C., & Greenberg, H. J. (1984). Bone-conduction masking for threshold assessment in brainstem auditory evoked potential testing. In R. H. Nodar & C. Barber (Eds.), *Evoked potentials II: The Second International Evoked Potentials Symposium* (pp. 169–176). Boston: Butterworth Publishers.

Weber, B. A. (1982). Comparison of auditory brain stem response latency norms for premature infants. *Ear and Hearing, 3,* 257–262.

Weber, B. A. (1983a). Pitfalls in auditory brain stem response audiometry. *Ear and Hearing* 4(4): 179–184.

Weber, B. A. (1983b). Masking and bone conduction testing in brainstem response audiometry. *Seminars in Hearing, 4,* 343–352.

Weber, B. A., & Fujikawa, S. M. (1977). Brainstem evoked responses (BER) audiometry at various stimulus presentation rates. *Journal of American Auditory Society, 3,* 59–62.

Weber, B. A., & Roush, P. A. (1993). Application of maximum length sequence analysis to auditory brainstem response testing of premature newborns. *Journal of the American Academy of Audiology, 4,* 157–162.

Weber, C., Hahne, A., Friedrich, M., & Friederici, A. D. (2004). Discrimination of word stress in early infant perception: Electrophysiological evidence. *Cognitive Brain Research, 18,* 149–161.

Wegman, W. E. (1982). Annual summary of vital statistics—1981. *Pediatrics, 75,* 835–843.

Wegner, O., & Dau, T. (2002). Frequency specificity of chirp-evoked auditory brainstem responses. *Journal of the Acoustical Society of America, 111,* 1318–1329.

Weiner, R. D., Erwin, C. W., & Weber, B. A. (1981). Acute effects of electroconvulsive therapy on brain stem auditory evoked potentials. *Electroencephalography and Clinical Neurophysiology, 52,* 202–204.

Weir, N. (1977). Sensorineural deafness associated with recessive hypophosphatemic rickets. *Journal of Laryngology and Otology, 91,* 717–722.

Weisz, N., Voss, S., Berg, P., & Elbert, T. (2004). Abnormal auditory mismatch response in tinnitus sufferers with high-frequency hearing loss is associated with subjective distress level. *BMC Neuroscience, 5,* 8.

Weitzman, E., Fishbein, W., & Graziani, L. J. (1965). Auditory evoked responses obtained from the scalp electroencephalogram of the full-term neonate during sleep. *Pediatrics, 35,* 458–562.

Weitzman, E. D., & Kremen, H. (1965). Auditory evoked responses during different stages of sleep in man. *Electroencephalography and Clinical Neurophysiology, 18,* 65–70.

Welgampola, M., & Colebatch, J. (2001a). Characteristics of tone burst-evoked myogenic potentials in the sternocleidomastoid muscles. *Neurology and Neurootology, 22,* 796–802.

Welgampola, M., & Colebatch, J. (2001b). Vestibulocollic reflexes: Normal values and the effect of age. *Clinical Neurophysiology, 112,* 1971–1979.

Welgampola, M., & Colebatch, J. (2005). Characteristics and clinical applications of vestibular-evoked myogenic potentials. *Neurology, 64,* 1682–1688.

Welgampola, M., Rosengren, S., Halmagyi, G., & Colebatch, J. (2003). Vestibular activation by bone conducted sound. *Journal of Neurology Neurosurgery and Psychiatry, 74,* 771–778.

Wennberg, R. P., Ahlfors, C. E., Bickers, R., McMurtry, C. A., & Shetter, J. L. (1982). Abnormal auditory brainstem response in a newborn infant with hyperbilirubinemia: Improvement with exchange transfusion. *Journal of Pediatrics, 100,* 624–626.

Werner, L. A., Folsom, R. C., & Mancl, L. R. (1993). The relationship between auditory brainstem response and behavioral thresholds in normal hearing infants and adults. *Hearing Research, 68,* 131–141.

Werner, L. A., Folsom, R., & Mancl, L. (1994). The relationship between auditory brainstem response latencies and behavioral thresholds in normal hearing infants and children. *Hearing Research, 77,* 88–98.

Werner, L. A., Folsom, R., Mancl, L., & Syapin, C. (2001). Human auditory brainstem response to temporal gaps in noise. *Journal of Speech, Language, and Hearing Research, 44,* 737–750.

Werner, R. A., & Vanderzant, C. W. (1991). Multimodality evoked potential testing in acute mild closed head injury. *Archives of Physical Medicine and Rehabilitation, 72,* 31–34.

Westmoreland, B. F., Sharbrough, F. W., Stockard, J. J., & Dale, A. J. D. (1983). Brainstem auditory evoked potentials in 20 patients with palatal myoclonus. *Archives of Neurology, 40,* 155–158.

Weston, P. F., Manson, J. I., & Abbott, K. J. (1986). Auditory brainstem-evoked response in childhood brainstem glioma. *Child's Nervous System, 2,* 301–305.

Wetmore, R., Henry, W., & Konkle, D. (1993). Acoustical factors of noise created by suctioning middle ear fluid. *Archives of Otolaryngology—Head & Neck Surgery, 119,* 762–766.

Wever, E. G., & Bray, C. W. (1930). Auditory nerve impulses. *Science, 71,* 215.

Wharton, J., & Church, G. (1990). Influence of menopause on the auditory brainstem response. *Audiology, 29,* 196–201.

Wheeland, R., & Roundtree, J. (1985). Calcinosis cutis resulting from percutaneous penetration and depositing of calcium. *Journal of the American Academy of Dermatology, 12,* 172–175.

White, M., Merzenich, M., & Gardi, J. (1984). Multichannel cochlear implants. Channel interactions and processor design. *Archives of Otolaryngology, 110,* 501.

White, P. F., Ma, H., Tan, J., Wender, R. H., Sloninsky, A., & Kariger, R. (2004). Does the use of electroencephalographic bispectral index or auditory evoked potential index monitoring facilitate recovery after desflurane anaesthesia in the ambulatory setting? *Anesthesiology, 100,* 811–817.

Whitfield, I., & Ross, H. (1965). Cochlear microphonic and summating potentials and the outputs of individual hair cell generators. *Journal of Acoustical Society of America, 38,* 126–131.

Whiting, K. A., Martin, B. A., & Stapells, D. R. (1998). The effects of broadband noise masking on cortical event-related potentials to speech sounds /ba/ and /da/. *Ear and Hearing, 19,* 218–231.

Wible, B., Nicol, T. G., & Kraus, N. (2002). Abnormal neural encoding of repeated speech stimuli in noise in children with learning problems. *Clinical Neurophysiology, 113,* 485–494.

Wible, B., Nicol, T., & Kraus, N. (2005). Correlation between brainstem and cortical auditory processes in normal and language-impaired children. *Brain, 128* (Pt 2), 417–423.

Wiederholt, W. C., Kobayashi, M. K, Stockard, J. J., & Rossiter, V. S. (1977). Central pontine myelinolysis. A clinical reappraisal. *Archives of Neurology, 34,* 220–223.

Wieland, R., & Kemp, B. (1979). Auditory brainstem evoked responses in brainstem compression due to posterior fossa tumors. *Clinical Neurology and Neurosurgery, 81,* 185–193.

Wiley, H., & Eaglstein, W. (1979). Calcinosis cutis in children following electroencephalography. *Journal of the American Medical Association, 242*, 455–456.

Wilkinson, R. T., & Morlock, H. C. (1967). Auditory evoked response and reaction time. *Electroencephalography and Clinical Neurophysiology, 23*, 50–56.

Williams, H. L., Tepas, D. I., & Morlock, H. C. (1962). Evoked responses to clicks and electroencephalography stages of sleep in man. *Science, 138*, 685–686.

Wilson, D., Hodgson, R., Gustafson, M., Hogue, S., & Mills, L. (1992). The sensitivity of auditory brainstem response testing in small acoustic neuromas. *Laryngoscope, 102*, 961–964.

Wilson, K. S., Wilson, L. A., & Cant, W. (1984). The effect of halothane upon auditory evoked potentials. In R. H. Nodar & C. Barber (Eds.), *Evoked potentials II: The second international evoked potentials symposium* (pp. 490–496). Boston: Butterworth.

Wilson, M. J., Kelly-Ballweber, D., & Dobie, R. A. (1985). Binaural interaction in auditory brain stem responses: parametric studies. Ear and Hearing, 6, 80–88.

Wilson, W., & Aghdasi, F. (2001). The importance of pre-analysis windowing on auditory brainstem response fast Fourier transform analysis. *Scandinavian Audiology, 30*, 3–12.

Wilson, W. J., & Bowker, C. A. (2002). The effects of high stimulus rate on the electrocochleogram in normal-hearing subjects. *International Journal of Audiology, 41*, 509–517.

Winkler, I., & Näätänen, R. (1995). The effects of auditory backward masking on event-related brain potentials. *Electroencephalography and Clinical Neurophysiology, Supplement 44*, 185–189.

Winkler, I., Paavilainen, P., Alho, K., Reinikainen, K., Sams, M., & Näätänen, R. (1990). The effect of small variation of the frequent auditory stimulus on the event-related brain potential to the infrequent stimulus. *Psychophysiology, 27*, 228–235.

Winkler, I., Reinikainen, K., & Näätänen, R. (1993). Event-related brain potentials reflect traces of echoic memory in humans. *Perception & Psychophysics, 53*, 443–449.

Winsberg, B. G., Javitt, D.C., & Silipo, G. S. (1997). Electrophysiological indices of information processing in methylphenidate responders. *Biological Psychiatry, 42*, 434–445.

Winsberg, B. G., Javitt, D.C., Silipo, G. S., & Doneshka, P. (1993). Mismatch negativity in hyperactive children: Effects of methylphenidate. *Psychopharmacology Bulletin, 29*, 229–233.

Winter, O., Kok, A., Kenemans, J. L., & Elton, M. (1995). Auditory event-related potentials to deviant stimuli during drowsiness and stage 2 sleep. *Electroencephalography and Clinical Neurophysiology, 96*, 398–412.

Wioland, N., Rudolf, G., & Metz-Lutz, M. (2001). Electrophysiological evidence of persisting unilateral auditory cortex dysfunction in the late outcome of Landau and Klaffner syndrome. *Clinical Neurophysiology, 112*, 319–323.

Wisniewski, K. E., Segan, S. M., Miezejeski, C. M., Sersen, E. A., & Rudelli, R. D. (1991). The fragile X syndrome: Neurological, electrophysiological, and neuropathological abnormalities. *American Journal of Medical Genetics, 38*, 476–480.

Witelson, S. F. (1991). Neural sexual mosaicism: Sexual differentiation of the human temporo-parietal region for functional asymmetry. *Psychoneuroendocrinology, 16*, 131–53.

Witelson, S. F. (1992). Cognitive neuroanatomy: A new era. *Neurology, 42*, 709–713.

Wolf, K. E., & Goldstein, R. (1978). Middle component averaged electroencephalic responses to tonal stimuli from normal neonates. *Archives of Otolaryngology, 104*, 508–513.

Wolf, K. E., & Goldstein, R. (1980). Middle component AERs from neonates to low-level tonal stimuli. *Journal of Speech and Hearing Research, 23*, 185–201.

Wolfe, J. A., Skinner, P., & Burns, J. (1978). Relationship between sound intensity and the latency and amplitude of the brainstem auditory evoked response. *Journal of Speech and Hearing Research, 21*, 387–400.

Wolpaw, J. R., & Penry, J. K. (1975). A temporal component of the auditory evoked response. *Electroencephalography and Clinical Neurophysiology, 39*, 609–620.

Wolpaw, J. R., & Penry, J. K. (1978). Effects of ethanol, caffeine, and placebo on the auditory evoked response. *Electroencephalography and Clinical Neurophysiology, 44*, 568–574.

Wong, M. L., & Brackmann, D. E. (1981). Computed tomography in acoustic tumor diagnosis. *Journal of the American Medical Association, 245*, 2497–2500.

Wong, P. K. H., & Bickford, R. G. (1980). Brain stem auditory evoked potentials: The use of noise estimate. *Electroencephalography and Clinical Neurophysiology, 50*, 25–34.

Wong, S. H.-W., Gibson, W. P. R., & Sanli, H. (1997). Use of transtympanic round window electrocochleography for threshold estimations in children. *The American Journal of Otology, 18*, 632–636.

Wong, V. (1997). A neurophysiological study in children with Miller Fisher syndrome and Guillain-Barre syndrome. *Brain and Development, 19*, 197–204.

Wong, V., Ng, T., & Yeung, C. (1991). Electrophysiologic study in acute lead poisoning. *Pediatric Neurology, 7*, 133–136.

Wong, V., & Wong, S. (1991). Brainstem auditory evoked potential study in children with autistic disorder. *Journal of Autism and Developmental Disorders, 21*, 329–340.

Wood, C. C., & Allison, T. (1981). Interpretation of evoked potentials: A neurophysiologic perspective. *Canadian Journal of Psychology, 35*, 113–135.

Wood, C., Allison, T., Goff, W., Williamson, P., & Spencer, D. (1980). On the neural origin of P300 in man. *Progress in Brain Research, 54*, 51–56.

Wood, C. C., & Wolpaw, J. R. (1982). Scalp distribution of human evoked potentials. II. Evidence for overlapping sources and involvement of auditory cortex. *Electroencephalography and Clinical Neurophysiology, 54*, 25–38.

Wood, M., Siltz, M. R., & Jacobson, J. T. (1979). Brainstem electrical responses from selected tone pip stimuli. *Journal of American Auditory Society, 5*, 156–162.

Wood, S., Mason, S., Farnsworth, A., Davis, A., Curnock, D., & Lutman, M. (1998). Anomalous screening outcomes from click-evoked otoacoustic emissions and auditory brainstem response tests. *British Journal of Audiology, 32*, 399–410.

Woods, D. L., Alain, C., Covarrubias, D., and Zaidel, O. (1995). Middle latency auditory evoked potentials to tones of different frequency. *Hearing Research, 85*, 69–75.

Woods, D. L., & Clayworth, C. C. (1985). Click spatial position influences latency auditory evoked potentials (MAEPs) in humans. *Electroencephalography and Clinical Neurophysiology, 60*, 122–129.

Woods, D. L., & Clayworth, C. C. (1986). Age-related changes in human middle latency auditory evoked potentials. *Electroencephalography and Clinical Neurophysiology, 65*, 297–303.

Woods, D. L., Clayworth, C. C., Knight, R. T., Simpson, G. V., & Naeser, M. A. (1987). Generators of middle- and long-latency auditory evoked potentials: implications from studies of patients with bitemporal lesions. *Electroencephalography and Clinical Neurophysiology, 68*, 132–148.

Woodward, S., McManis, M., Kagan, J., Deldin, P., Snidman, N., Lewis, M., & Kahn, V. (2001). Infant temperament and the brainstem auditory evoked response in later childhood. *Developmental Psychology, 37*, 533–538.

Woodworth, W., Reisman, S., & Fontaine, A. (1983). The detection of auditory evoked responses using a matched filter. *IEEE Transactions in Biomedical Engineering, 30*, 369–376.

Woody, C. D. (1967). Characterization of an adaptive filter for the analysis of variable latency neuroelectric signals. *Medical Biological Engineering, 5*, 539–553.

Woolsey, C. N., & Walzl, E. M. (1942). Topical projection of nerve fibers from local regions of the cochlea to the cerebral cortex of the cat. *Bulletin of Johns Hopkins Hospital, 71*, 315–344.

Worden, F. G., & Marsh, J. T. (1968). Frequency following (microphonic-like) neural response evoked by sound. *Electroencephalography and Clinical Neurophysiology, 25*, 42–52.

Worthington, D. W., Brookhauser, P. E., Mohiuddin, S. M., & Gorga, M. P. (1985). The effects of tocainide on audiological and electrophysiological responses in humans. *Ear and Hearing, 6*, 179–183.

Worthington, D. W., & Peters, J. F. (1980). Quantifiable hearing and no ABR: Paradox or error? *Ear and Hearing, 1*, 281–285.

Wrege, K. S., & Starr, A. (1981). Binaural interaction in human auditory brainstem evoked potentials. *Archives of Neurology, 38*, 572–580.

Wright, D. R., Thornton, C., Hasan, K., Vaughan, D. J., Dore, C. J. & Brunner, M. D. (2004). The effect of remifentanil on the middle latency auditory evoked response and haemodynamic measurements with and without the stimulus of orotracheal intubation. *European Journal of Anaesthesiology, 21,* 509–516.

Wu, C., Qi, Y., Zhang, S., & Lu, J. (1993). Neonatal hearing impairment complicated by neonatal pneumonia. Application of auditory evoked potentials in neonatology. *Chinese Medical Journal, 106,* 292–297.

Wu, C., Young, Y., & Murofushi, T. (1999). Tone burst-evoked myogenic potentials in the human neck flexor and extensor. *Acta Otolaryngologica, 119,* 741–744.

Wu, X., Zhao, D., Ling, Q., Bu, D., & Zuo, C. (1988). Rett syndrome in China: Report of 9 patients. *Pediatric Neurology, 4,* 126–127.

Wunderlich, J. L., & Cone-Wesson, B. K. (2001). Effects of stimulus frequency and complexity on the mismatch negativity and other components of the cortical auditory-evoked potential. *Journal of the Acoustical Society of America, 109,* 1526–1537.

Wuyts, F. L., Van de Heyning, P. H., Van Spaendonck, M. P., Molenberghs, G. (1997). A review of electrocochleography: Instrumentation settings and meta-analysis of criteria for diagnosis of endolymphatic hydrops. *Acta Otolaryngolica (Supplement) 526,* 14–20.

Wuyts, F. L., Van de Heyning, P. H., Van Spaendonck, M., Van der Stappen, A., D'Haese, P., Erre, J., Charlet de Sauvage, R., & Aran, J. (2001). Rate influences on tone burst summating potential amplitude in electrocochleography: Clinical (a) and experimental (b) data. *Hearing Research, 152,* 1–9

Xu, S. H., Cai, Y. L., & Yang, R. M. (1997). [Contrast analysis of brainstem auditory evoked potential in untreated and treated hepatolenticular degeneration patients with treatment of combining traditional Chinese and Western medicine.] *Zhongguo Zhongxiyi. jiehe, zazhi, 17,* 17–19.

Yabe, H., Saito, F., & Fukushima, Y. (1983). Median method for detecting endogenous event-related brain potentials. *Electroencephalography and Clinical Neurophysiology, 89,* 403–407.

Yagi, T., & Baba, N. (1983). Evaluation of the brain-stem function by the brainstem response and the caloric vestibular reaction in comatose patients. *Archives of Otorhinolaryngology, 238,* 33–43.

Yagi, T., & Hughes, D. W. (1975). Effect of click repetition rate and intensity on the auditory brainstem response (BSR). *Audiology Japan, 18,* 336–341.

Yagi, T., & Kaga, K. (1979). The effect of the click repetition rate on the latency of the auditory evoked brainstem response and its clinical use for a neurological diagnosis. *Archives of Otorhinolaryngology, 222,* 91–97.

Yagi, T., Kaga, K., & Baba, S. (1980). A study of cases with partial disappearance of the waves in the auditory brain stem response. *Archives of Otorhinolaryngology, 226,* 251–258.

Yamada, O., Ashikawa, H., Kodera, K., & Yamane, H. (1983). Frequency-selective auditory brain-stem response in newborns and infants. *Archives of Otolaryngology, 109,* 79–82.

Yamada, O., Kodera, K., & Yagi, T. (1979). Cochlear processes affecting Wave V latency of the auditory evoked brainstem response: A study of patients with sensory hearing loss. *Scandinavian Audiology, 8,* 67–70.

Yamada, O., Marsh, R. R., & Handler, S. D. (1982). Contributing generator of frequency-following response in man. *Scandinavian Audiology, 11,* 53–56.

Yamada, T., Nakamura, A., Horibe, K., Washimi, Y., Bundo, M., Kato, T., Ito, K., Kachi, T., & Sobue, G. (2003). Asymmetrical enhancement of middle-latency auditory evoked fields with aging. *Neuroscience Letters, 337,* 21–4.

Yamaguchi, J., Yagi, T., Baba, S., Aoki, H., & Yamanobe, S. (1991). Relationship between auditory brainstem response waveform and head size. *ORL: Journal of Otorhinolaryngology and Related Specialties, 53,* 94–99.

Yamakami, I., Ushikubo, O., Uchino, Y., Kobayashi, E., Saeki, N., Yamaura, A., & Oka, N. (2002). [Intraoperative monitoring of hearing function in the removal of cerebellopontine angle tumor: Auditory brainstem response and cochlear nerve compound action potential.] *No Shinkei Geka, 30,* 275–282.

Yamamoto, K., Sakabe, N., & Kaiho, I. (1979). Power spectral analysis of auditory evoked response. *Journal of Acoustical Society of America, 5,* 107–111.

Yamamoto, K., Uno, A., Kawashima, T., Iwaki, T., Doi, K., & Kubo, T. (1998). [Clinical significance of electrically evoked auditory brainstem response.] *Nippon Jibiinkoka Gakkai Kaiho, 101,* 1328–1334.

Yamamoto, N., Watanabe, K., Sugiura, J., Okada, J., Nagae, H., & Fujimoto, Y. (1990). Marked latency change of auditory brainstem response in preterm infants in the early postnatal period. *Brain Development, 12,* 766–769.

Yang, E. Y., Rupert, A. L., & Moushegian, G. (1987). A developmental study of bone conduction auditory brain stem response in infants. *Ear and Hearing, 8,* 244–251.

Yang, E. Y., & Stuart, A. (2000). The contribution of the auditory brainstem responses to bone-conducted stimuli in newborn hearing screening. *Journal of Speech-Language Pathology and Audiology, 24,* 84–91.

Yang, E. Y., Stuart, A., Mencher, G., Mencher, L., & Vincer, M. (1993). Auditory brainstem responses to air- and bone-conducted clicks in the audiological assessment of at-risk infants. *Ear and Hearing, 14,* 175–182.

Yang, E. Y., Stuart, A., Stenstrom, R., & Green, W. (1993). Test-retest variability of the auditory brainstem response to bone-conducted clicks in newborn infants. *Audiology, 32,* 89–94.

Yang, E. Y., Stuart, A., Stenstrom, R., & Hollett, S. (1991). Effect of vibrator to head coupling force on the auditory brainstem response to bone-conducted clicks in newborn infants. *Ear and Hearing, 12,* 55–60.

Yang, T., & Young, Y. (2003). Comparison of tone burst and tapping evocation of myogenic potentials in patients with chronic otitis media. *Ear and Hearing, 24,* 191–194.

Yanz, J., & Dodd, H. (1985). An ear-canal electrode for the measurement of the human auditory brainstem response. *Ear and Hearing, 6,* 98–104.

Yasuhara, A., & Hori, A. (2002). A comparison of the three-dimensional auditory brainstem response and the conventional auditory brainstem response in children. *Brain and Development, 24,* 750–757.

Yee, C. M., & Miller, G. A. (1987). Affective valence and information processing. In R. Johnson, Jr., J. W. Rohrbaugh & R. Parasuraman (Eds.), *Current trends in event-related potential research* (EEG Supplement 40) (pp. 300–307). Amsterdam: Elsevier.

Yee, C. M., Nuechterlein, K. H., Morris, S. E., & White, P. M. (1998). P50 suppression in recent-onset schizophrenia: Clinical correlates and risperidone effects. *Journal of Abnormal Psychology, 107,* 691–698.

Yellin, A. M., Lodwig, A. K., & Jerison, H. J. (1980). Auditory evoked brain potentials as a function of interstimulus interval in adults with Down's syndrome. *Audiology, 19,* 255–262.

Yellin, M. W., & Chase K. K. (1991). A comparison of electrocochleography recording techniques. *Ear and Hearing, 12,* 434–436.

Yilmaz, Y., Degirmenci, S., Akdas, F., Kulekci, S., Ciprut, A., Yuksel, S., Yildiz, F., Karadeniz, L., & Say, A. (2001). Prognostic value of auditory brainstem response for neurologic outcome in patients with neonatal indirect hyperbilirubinemia. *Journal of Child Neurology, 16,* 772–775.

Yokoyama, J., Aoyagi, M., Suzuki, T., Kiren, T., & Koike, Y. (1994). Three frequency component waveforms of auditory evoked brainstem response in spinocerebellar degeneration. *Acta Otolaryngologica, 511,* 52–55.

Yokoyama, K., Araki, S., Yamashita, K., Murata, K., Nomiyama, K., Nomiyama, H., et al. (2002). Subclinical cerebellar anterior lobe, vestibulocerebellar and spinocerebellar afferent effects on young female lead workers in China: Computerized posturography with sway frequency analysis and brainstem auditory evoked potentials. *Industrial Health, 40,* 245–253.

Yokoyama, K., Nishida, H., Noguchi, Y., & Komatsuzaki, A. (1996). [Assessment of cochlear functions of patients with acoustic neuromas]. *Nippon Jibiinkoka Gakkai Kaiho, 99,* 586–593.

Yokoyama, T., Ryu, H., Uemura, K., Miyamoto, T., & Imamura, Y. (1987). Study of the constant wave form of ML-AEP in humans. *Electroencephalography and Clinical Neurophysiology, 67,* 372–378.

Yokoyama, Y., Nakashima, K., Shimoyama, R., Urakami, K., & Takahashi, K. (1995). Distribution of event-related potentials in patients with dementia. *Electromyography and Clinical Neurophysiology, 35,* 431–437.

Yoshida, Y., Ichikawa, G., Sakurai, A., Nakagawa, M., Uozaki, S., & Musha, T. (1991). [Dipole tracing method analysis for source of auditory brainstem response (wave V) in two normal hearing subjects.] *Nippon Jibiinkoka Gakkai Kaiho, 94,* 1880–1887.

Yoshie, N. (1968). Auditory nerve action potential responses to clicks in man. *Laryngoscope, 78,* 198–215.

Yoshie, N. (1971). Clinical cochlear response audiometry by means of an average response computer: Non-surgical technique and clinical use. *Revue de Laryngologie (Supplement), 92,* 646–672.

Yoshie, N. (1973). Diagnostic significance of the electrocochleogram in clinical audiometry. *Audiology, 12,* 504–539.

Yoshie, N. (1976). Electrocochleographic study of Ménière's disease: Pathological pattern of the cochlear nerve compound action potential in man. In R. J. Ruben, C. Elberling & G. Salomon (Eds.), *Electrocochleography*, (pp. 353–386). Baltimore: University Park Press.

Yoshie, N., & Ohashi, T. (1969). Clinical use of cochlear nerve action potential responses in man for differential diagnosis of hearing losses. *Acta Otolaryngologica (Supp)*, 252, 71–87.

Yoshie, N., Ohashi, T., & Suzuki, T. (1967). Non-surgical recording of auditory nerve action potentials in man. *Laryngoscope, 77*, 76.

Yoshie, N., & Okidura, T. (1969). Myogenic evoked click responses in man. *Acta Otolaryngologica, 252*, 89–103.

Yoshikawa, H., & Takamori, M. (2001). Benign segmental myoclonus: Electrophysiological evidence of transient dysfunction in the brainstem. *Journal of Clinical Neuroscience, 8*, 54–56.

Yoshinaga, H., Ogino, T., Ohtahara, S., Sakuta, R., Nonaka, I., & Horai, S. (1993). A T-to-G mutation at nucleotide pair 8993 in mitochondrial DNA in a patient with Leigh's syndrome. *Journal of Child Neurology, 8*, 129–133.

Yoshinaga-Itano, C., Sedley, A., Coulter, D., & Mehl, A. (1998). Language of early- and later-identified children with hearing loss. *Pediatrics, 102*, 1171.

Young, E., Fernandez, C., & Goldberg, J. (1977). Responses of squirrel monkey vestibular neurons to audio-frequency sound and head vibration. *Acta Otolaryngologica, 84*, 352–360.

Young, I. R., Bydder, G. M., & Hall, A. S. (1983). The role of NMR imaging in the diagnosis and management of acoustic neuroma. *American Journal of Neuroradiology, 4*, 223–224.

Young, N., & Grohne, K. (2001). Comparison of pediatric Clarion recipients with and without the electrode positioner. *Otology and Neurotology, 22*, 195–199.

Young, Y., & Kuo, S. (2004). Side-difference of vestibular evoked myogenic potentials in healthy subjects. *Hearing Research, 198*, 93–98.

Young, Y., Wu, C., & Wu, C. (2002). Augmentation of vestibular evoked myogenic potentials: An indication for distended saccular hydrops. *Laryngoscope, 112*, 509–512.

Yuksul, A., Sarslan, O., Devranoglu, K., Dirican, A., Hattat, N., Cenani, A., & Yalcin, E. (1995). Effects of valproate and carbamazepine on brainstem auditory evoked potentials in epileptic children. *Child's Nervous System, 11*, 474–477.

Zackeim, H., & Pinkus, H. (1957). Calcium chloride necrosis of the skin. Report of two cases. *Archives of Dermatology, 76*, 244–246.

Zani, A. (1989). Brain evoked responses reflect information processing changes with the menstrual cycle in young female athletes. *Journal of Sports Medicine and Physical Fitness, 29*, 113–121.

Zapala, D., & Brey, R. (2004). Clinical experience with vestibular evoked myogenic potentials. *Journal of the American Academy of Audiology, 15*, 198–215.

Zappalla, R. A., Greenblatt, E., & Karmel, V. C. (1982). The effects of acoustic neuromas on ipsilateral and contralateral brainstem auditory evoked responses during stimulation of the unaffected ear. *American Journal of Otology, 4*, 118–122.

Zappalla, R. A., Greenblatt, E., Kaye, S., & Malis, L. (1984). A quantitative assessment of the brain stem auditory evoked response during intraoperative monitoring. *Neurosurgery, 15*, 186–191.

Zappia, J. J., O'Connor, C. A., Wiet, R. J., & Dinces, E. A. (1997). Rethinking the use of auditory brainstem response in acoustic neuroma screening. *Laryngoscope, 107*, 1388–1392.

Zappia, J. J., Wiet, R. J., O'Connor, C. A., & Martone, L. (1996). Intraoperative auditory monitoring in acoustic neuroma surgery. *Archives of Otolaryngology—Head & Neck Surgery, 115*, 98–106.

Zattore, R. J., & Krumhansl, C. L. (2002). Neuroscience. Mental models and musical minds. *Science, 298*, 2138–2139.

Zealear, D. L., Herzon, G. D., & Korff, M. (1988). Evoked accelerometry: a sensitive and accurate method for evaluating facial nerve function using a portable device. *Laryngoscope, 98*, 568–572.

Zealear, D. L., & Kurago, Z. (1985). Facial nerve recording from the ear canal: A possible method for evaluating Bell's palsy. *Archives of Otolaryngology—Head & Neck Surgery, 93*, 474–481.

Zeng, F. G., Oba, S., Garde, S., Sininger, Y., & Starr, A. (1999). Temporal and speech processing deficits in auditory neuropathy. *Neuroreport, 10*, 3429–3435.

Zerlin, S. (1986). Electrophysiological evidence for the critical bands in humans. *Journal of the Acoustical Society of America, 79*, 1612–1616.

Zerlin, S., & Nauton, R. F. (1974). Auditory brainstem and middle latency evoked response sensitivity near threshold. *Annals of Otology, Rhinology & Laryngology, 90*, 236–240.

Zgorzalewicz, M., & Galas-Zgorzalewicz, B. (2000). Visual and auditory evoked potentials during long-term vigabatrin treatment in children and adolescents with epilepsy. *Clinical Neurophysiology, 111*, 2150–2154.

Zgorzalewicz, M., Galas-Zgorzalewicz, B., & Nowak, R. (2001). Analysis of the measurement methods of endogenous, cognitive P300 potential in school children and adolescents. *Folio Neuropathy, Supplement A*, 1–6.

Zgorzalewicz, M., Galas-Zgorzalewicz, B., & Steinborn, B. (1995). Effects of anti-epileptic drugs on visual and auditory evoked potentials in children and adolescents with epilepsy. *Developmental Medicine and Child Neurology, 37*, 137.

Zhang, Y., Ji, W., & Jiang, X. (1997). The value of the ratio of –SP/AP in diagnosing Ménière's disease. *Zhonghua Er. Bi Yan.Hou Ke. Za Zhi., 32*, 77–80.

Zheng, X. Y., Ding, D. L., McFadden, S. L., & Henderson, D. (1997). Evidence that inner hair cells are the major source of cochlear summating potentials. *Hearing Research, 113*, 76–88.

Zhou, J., & Durrant, J. D. (2003). Effects of interaural frequency difference on binaural fusion evidenced by electrophysiological versus psychoacoustical measures. *Journal of the Acoustical Society of America, 114*, 1508–1515.

Zoghbi, H., Percy, A., Glaze, D., Butler, I., & Riccardi, V. (1985). Reduction of biogenic amine levels in the Rett syndrome. *New England Journal of Medicine, 313*, 921–924.

Zöllner, C. H., & Eibach, H. (1981a). Criteria for the differential diagnosis of cochlear-retrocochlear disorders with brainstem audiometry. *Archives of Otorhinolaryngology, 230*, 135–147.

Zöllner, C. H., & Eibach, H. (1981b). Can the differential diagnosis of cochlear retrocochlear disorder be improved using the brain stem potentials with changing stimulus rates? *HNO, 29*, 240–245.

Zöllner, C., Karnahl, T., & Stange, G. (1976). Input-output function and adaptation behaviour of the five early potentials registered with the earlobe-vertex pick-up. *Archives of Otorhinolaryngology, 212*, 23–33.

Zouridakis, G., & Boutros, N. N. (1992). Stimulus parameter effects on the P50 evoked response. *Biological Psychiatry, 32*, 839–841.

Zubick, H. H., Fried, M. P., Thebeau, R., Feudo, P., Jr., & Strome, M. (1983). "How do I do it" - Otology and neurotology. A specific issue and its solution: A new head set for eliciting auditory evoked potentials in the neonate. *Laryngoscope 93*(5): 659–660.

Zurbuchen, P., LeCoultre, C., Calza, A., & Halperin, D. (1996). Cutaneous necrosis after contact with calcium chloride: A mistaken diagnosis of child abuse. *Pediatrics, 97*, 257–258.

Zwicker, E. (1955). Der ungewöhnliche Amplitudengang der nichtlinearen Verzerungen des Ohres. *Acustica, 5*, 67–74.

Zwirner, P., & Wilichowski, E. (2001). Progressive sensorineural hearing loss in children with mitochondrial encephalomyopathies. *Laryngoscope, 111*, 515–521.

Zwislocki, J. J. (1975). Phase opposition between inner and outer hair cells and auditory sound analysis. *Audiology, 14*, 443–455.

Aaltonen, O., 555, 556, 575
Abbas, P., 260, 263, 585, 586, 588, 589, 590, 595, 596, 597
Abbate, C., 414
Abdala, C., 225
Abe, M., 26, 499
Abrahamian, H.A., 240, 310, 471, 509
Abramovich, S.J., 234, 257, 417
Abramson, M., 429
Abubakr, A., 545
Acevedo, J.C., 427
Achor, L.J., 44
Ackley, R., 614
Adams, D., 238, 309
Adler, G., 494, 495
Adler, L.E., 23, 450, 476, 480, 482
Adour, K.K., 617
Agrawal, V., 341
Aguilar, E.A., 437
Aguirre, M., 542
Ahveninen, J., 472, 476, 578
Ainslie, P.J., 193, 194, 195, 196, 197, 198
Akaboshi, S., 347
Akin, F., 606, 610, 612
Akiyama, Y., 504
Alain, C., 490, 493, 502, 571, 575, 578
Alexander, J., 507, 528, 533, 535
Alexander, M., 415
Alho, K., 491, 502, 508, 521, 557, 571, 572
Allison, R.S., 399
Allison, T., 233, 235, 382
Almadori, G., 369
Alonso-Prieto, E., 545
Amadeo, M., 134
Amantini, A., 411, 481
Amatuzzi, M.G., 141
Ambrosini, A., 449, 450, 542
Amenedo, E., 452, 461, 462, 463, 506
American Academy of Pediatrics Task Force on Newborn and Infant Hearing, 315, 322
American National Standards Institute (ANSI), 75, 195
American Psychiatric Association, 358
Amin, S.B., 145, 230, 231, 232
Anand, N., 340
Anderer, P., 535
Anderson, D.C., 439, 483, 486
Anderson, D.J., 121
Anderson, H., 429

Anft, D., 155
Annett, M., 464
Anteby, I., 334
Antinoro, F., 490, 494, 495
Antonelli, A.R., 174, 379, 380, 381, 389, 392, 393, 399
Anyanwu, E., 414
Aoyagi, M., 235, 264, 298, 300, 427
Arakawa, K., 155
Aran, J.M., 7, 10, 38, 109, 110, 113, 129, 133, 136, 157, 256
Arehole, S., 479, 512, 544
Arenberg, I.K., 161, 166
Arezzo, J., 46, 50, 52
Arikan, M., 527
Arinami, T., 346
Arlinger, S.D., 8, 74, 75, 175, 210
Arriaga, M., 426
Arsenault, M.D., 111
Arslan, E., 196, 197, 198, 227
Asai, H., 160
Aso, S., 110, 116, 136, 155, 158, 160, 161
Atienza, M., 538, 572
Ayerbe, I., 407
Azumi, T., 461
Azzena, C.B., 449
Babkoff, H., 182
Bacon, S.P., 285
Baiocco, F., 354, 411
Baldeweg, T., 555, 569, 576, 577
Baldwin, R.L., 373
Baldy-Moulinier, M., 406
Balfour, P., 172, 176, 251, 258, 264
Balkany, T.J., 359
Bancaud, J., 26
Bank, J., 421
Bao, X., 341, 351
Bar-Haim, Y., 579
Barajas, J.J., 227, 253
Baran, J.A., 397, 478, 510
Baranak, C.C., 308, 312
Barkovich, A.J., 390
Barnet, A., 7, 26, 504, 514
Barnett, S.B., 236
Barratt, H., 193, 202, 204, 205
Barrett, G., 506
Barrs, D., 376, 389, 390
Barry, R.J., 575
Bartel, D.R., 399, 401
Barth, P., 347

Bartnik, E.A., 486
Basar, E., 24
Basta, D., 606, 607, 612, 635
Bastuji, H., 492, 508, 526, 538, 539
Bath, A., 114, 115, 125, 612
Batra, R., 48
Battista, R., 427, 433, 434
Battmer, R., 588, 589, 593
Bauch, C.D., 63, 137, 172, 209, 253, 257, 264, 377, 378, 380, 381, 383, 392
Beagley, H.A., 225, 233, 234, 382, 494, 495
Beattie, R.C., 173, 185, 208, 264
Beauchaine, K.A., 73
Beckerman, R., 363
Begleiter, H., 241, 412, 539, 543
Beiser, M., 234
Beiter, R.C., 441, 446
Békèsy, G.v., 40, 74, 77, 603
Bell, S.L., 93, 107, 448, 485
Bellman, S., 136
Benita, M., 236
Benna, P., 398
Bennett, M.J., 314
Beresford, H.R., 439
Bergenius, J., 385
Bergsmark, J., 345
Berlad, I., 526
Berlin, C.I., 7, 10, 138, 139, 142, 146, 147, 149, 151, 152, 153
Bernal, J., 512
Bernard, P., 237
Bess, F.J., 313, 365
Beynon, A., 601
Beynon, G.J., 114, 134
Bhargava, V.K., 241
Bickford, R.G., 6, 21, 26, 465, 466, 603, 605, 608
Black, F., 593
Black, J.A., 344, 402
Blegvad, B., 193, 198, 253
Bobbin, R.P., 240, 310
Bock, G.R., 365
Bockenheimer, S.T., 388
Bodis-Wollner, I., 31
Boezeman, E.H., 74, 78, 189
Bojrab, D.I., 166
Bolz, J., 420
Bomba, M., 541
Bonafe, A., 388, 389

Madden, C., 140, 144, 145, 146, 149, 152
Maddox III, H.E., 429
Madhavan, G., 227
Maeshima, S., 542, 546
Magdziarz, D., 375
Magliulo, G., 615, 616
Mair, I.W.S., 259, 270
Maiste, A.C., 557
Majkowski, J., 53
Makashima, K., 415
Mäkelä, A.M., 53, 491
Mäkelä, J.P., 17, 442, 463
Makhdoum, M.J., 597, 600, 601
Malinoff, R., 226
Mancuso, G., 82
Mangham, C., 375
Manley, J.A., 134, 236
Manninen, P., 239, 310, 424
Mantzaridis, H., 486
Marangos, N., 116, 118, 121, 131, 156,
157, 158, 159, 391, 392
Markand, O.N., 343, 344, 348, 402
Marsh, J.T., 47
Marsh, R.R., 225, 240, 310
Marshall, L.F., 435
Marshall, N.K., 236
Martin, B.A., 56, 491, 512, 573, 575
Martin, L.J., 533, 535
Martin, M.E., 201
Martini, A., 415, 476
Marvel, J.B., 479
Maslan, M.J., 389
Mason, J.A., 153, 242, 323, 324, 590
Mason, S., 324, 361, 479, 590, 591, 594,
595, 596
Mast, T.E., 6, 466
Mathalon, D.H., 546
Matheson, J.K., 409
Mathiak, K., 557
Matsuura, K., 111, 155
Matsuyama, Z., 414
Matsuzaki, M., 614
Matsuzawa, T., 413
Matthews, W.B., 399, 401, 402
Matthies, C., 165, 434
Mauldin, L., 74, 189
Maurer, J., 600
Maurer, K., 185, 186, 187, 379, 386,
388, 389
Maurer, U., 573, 577
Maurizi, M., 181, 185, 209, 231, 233,
360, 421
May, P., 559
Maybeck, P.S., 96
Mazzini, L., 515
McAlpine, D., 399
McArthur, G.M., 567
McCall, S., 182
McCallum, W.C., 497, 503, 527
McCandless, G.A., 26, 495
McCarley, R.W., 546
McCarthy, G., 525

McClelland, R.J., 234, 357
McCue, M., 603, 604, 606
McDonald, J.M., 259, 264, 270
McDonald, W.I., 184, 399
McDonnell, D.E., 429
McFadden, D., 463
McFarland, W.H., 95, 441, 446, 447, 448,
474
McFarlane, A.C., 482
McGee, T.J., 49, 256, 333, 337, 341, 366,
367, 442, 456, 458, 468, 567
McIssac, H., 505, 507, 520, 533, 633
McLeod, B., 239
McPherson, D.L., 193, 196, 201, 204,
207, 217, 218, 364, 536
McRandle, C.C., 459, 509
McSherry, J.W., 364
Meador, K., 545
Megala, A.L., 498
Meister, M., 348, 349
Menard, M., 597, 598
Mendel, M.I., 459, 467, 468, 469, 507,
509, 540
Mendelson, T., 333, 334, 459
Mens, L., 592
Merchart, S., 612
Messick, J.M., 435
Messner, A., 322, 323
Metrick, S.A., 241, 413
Metting Van Rijn, A.C., 108
Metzger, L.J., 482
Meurer, J., 322
Meyer, C., 323
Meyerhoff, W.L., 161
Micco, A., 600, 601
Michael, R., 543
Michalewski, H.J., 235
Michie, P.T., 508, 578
Middleton, M., 396, 421
Miezejeski, C., 346
Mikulec, A., 616
Milford, C.A., 176
Milhorat, T.H., 364
Miller, A.L., 585
Minami, T., 353, 406
Minoda, R., 353
Minoli, I., 364
Mitchell, C., 177
Miyamoto, R.T., 429
Miyao, M., 355
Mizrahi, E.M., 205
Mizukoshi, K., 154, 155
Mochizuki, Y., 230, 234
Moffatt, D.A., 116, 155
Mogensen, F., 399, 400
Mohamed, A.S., 476
Mokotoff, B., 169, 238, 309, 469
Mokrusch, R., 425
Møller, A.R., 8, 39, 40, 41, 43, 44, 45, 46,
107, 121, 164, 165, 168, 172, 175, 176,
181, 202, 204, 210, 249, 250, 254, 263,
378, 379, 380, 386, 422, 425, 433, 618

Møller, M.B., 379, 404, 422
Mongey, A.B., 418
Monobe, H., 615
Mononen, L.J., 53
Montandon, P.B., 110, 230, 256
Moore, E.J., 14, 15, 175
Moore, J.K., 41, 45, 46, 231
Moore, R.D., 365
Mora, J.A., 448, 455
Morawski, K., 167
Morgan, D.E., 230, 231
Mori, K., 356
Mori, N., 155, 156, 158, 160
Morita, Y., 535, 539
Morlet, T., 325
Morr, M.L., 572
Morrison, A.W., 129, 160, 161
Mosko, S.S., 422
Mouney, D.F., 120
Moushegian, G., 7, 47
Muchnik, C., 188, 420
Mulert, C., 517
Müller, V., 56
Müller-Gass, A., 559, 575
Munte, T.F., 560
Murakami, T., 574
Murata, K., 350, 414, 422, 510, 540
Murofushi, T., 603, 606, 607, 608, 611,
613, 614, 615, 616, 617
Murphy, M., 390
Murray, G., 323
Musiek, F.E., 23, 37, 111, 137, 233, 339,
349, 361, 376, 377, 378, 379, 380, 381,
385, 386, 388, 389, 392, 397, 398, 399,
400, 401, 404, 406, 407, 411, 414, 454,
459, 474, 475, 476, 478, 479, 483
Mustillo, P., 399
Muthane, U., 410

Näätänen, R., 30, 31, 32, 53, 490, 491,
496, 497, 499, 502, 503, 508, 537, 548,
549, 550, 551, 553, 554, 556, 558, 561,
566, 567, 570, 571, 572, 574, 579
Nadol, J., 426
Naessens, B., 391
Naganuma, Y., 534
Nagata, K., 408
Nager, W., 560
Nagy, E., 573
Naito, R., 396
Nakano, S., 396
Nakagawa, M., 49
Narayan, R.K., 423, 439, 483, 486
Nash, C.L., 164
National Institutes of Health, 325, 371
National Instruments, 295
Naunton, R.F., 109, 133
Navaratnarajah, M., 471, 509
Negishi, H., 341
Negri, M., 116, 117
Nelson, C., 545
Nelson, D.A., 496